MILLER'S REVIEW OF
ORTHOPAEDICS

MILLER'S REVIEW OF
ORTHOPAEDICS

SEVENTH EDITION

MARK D. MILLER, MD

S. Ward Casscells Professor
Head, Division of Sports Medicine
Department of Orthopaedic Surgery
University of Virginia
Charlottesville, Virginia
Team Physician
James Madison University
Founder and Director
Miller Review Course
Denver, Colorado

STEPHEN R. THOMPSON, MD, MEd, FRCSC

Cooperating Associate Professor of Sports Medicine
The University of Maine
Medical Director
EMMC Sports Health
Deputy Editor
The Journal of Bone and Joint Surgery
Eastern Maine Medical Center
Bangor, Maine
Cofounder and Codirector
Miller Review Course Part II
Denver, Colorado

ELSEVIER

CONTRIBUTORS

Ermias S. Abebe, MD
Resident
Department of Orthopaedic Surgery
University of Pittsburgh Medical Center
Pittsburgh, Pennsylvania

James A. Browne, MD
Assistant Professor
Department of Orthopaedic Surgery
University of Virginia
Charlottesville, Virginia

Lance M. Brunton, MD
Clinical Assistant Professor
Department of Orthopaedic Surgery
University of Pittsburgh Medical Center
Pittsburgh, Pennsylvania
Attending Staff
Excela Health Orthopaedics and Sports Medicine
Latrobe, Pennsylvania

M. Tyrrell Burrus, MD
Resident Physician
Department of Orthopaedic Surgery
University of Virginia Health System
Charlottesville, Virginia

Bobby Chhabra, MD
Professor and Chair
Department of Orthopaedic Surgery
University of Virginia Health System
Charlottesville, Virginia

Marc McCord DeHart, MD
Clinical Assistant Professor
Orthopaedic Surgery and Rehabilitation
University of Texas Medical Branch
Galveston, Texas
Clinical Assistant Professor
Department of Surgery
Texas A&M Health Science Center
College of Medicine
Round Rock, Texas

F. Winston Gwathmey, Jr., MD
Assistant Professor
Department of Orthopaedic Surgery
University of Virginia
Charlottesville, Virginia

David J. Hak, MD, MBA, FACS
Professor
Department of Orthopaedic Surgery
Denver Health/University of Colorado
Denver, Colorado

Joseph M. Hart, PhD, ATC
Associate Professor
Kinesiology
University of Virginia
Director, Clinical Research
Department of Orthopaedic Surgery
University of Virginia
Charlottesville, Virginia

MaCalus Vinson Hogan, MD
Assistant Professor
Department of Orthopaedic Surgery
University of Pittsburgh Medical Center
Associate Residency Program Director
Department of Orthopaedic Surgery
University of Pittsburgh Medical Center
Pittsburgh, Pennsylvania

Ginger E. Holt, MD
Associate Professor
Orthopaedic Surgery and Rehabilitation
Orthopaedic Oncologist
Vanderbilt Medical Center
Nashville, Tennessee

Anish Kadakia, MD
Staff Orthopedic Surgeon
Department of Orthopedic Surgery
Illinois Bone and Joint Institute
Glenview, Illinois
Clinical Educator
Department of Orthopedic Surgery
University Of Chicago
Chicago, Illinois

Cyril Mauffrey, MD
Associate Professor
Department of Orthopaedic Surgery
Denver Health/University of Colorado
Denver, Colorado

Edward J. McPherson, MD
Director and Founder
LA Orthopedic Institute
Los Angeles, California

Todd A. Milbrandt, MD, MS
Pediatric Orthopaedic Surgeon
Orthopaedic Surgery
Mayo Clinic
Rochester, Minnesota

Mark D. Miller, MD
S. Ward Casscells Professor
Head, Division of Sports Medicine
Department of Orthopaedic Surgery
University of Virginia
Charlottesville, Virginia
Team Physician
James Madison University
Founder and Director
Miller Review Course
Denver, Colorado

Zain N. Qazi, MD
Surgery Resident
University of Washington Medical Center
Seattle, Washington
Former Research Fellow
Department of Orthopaedic Surgery
Joan C. Edwards School of Medicine
Marshall University
Huntington, West Virginia

Jeremy Rush, MD
Pediatric Orthopaedic Surgeon
San Antonio Military Medical Center
Fort Sam Houston
San Antonio, Texas
Assistant Professor
Department of Surgery
Herbert School of Medicine
Uniformed Services University of the Health Sciences
Bethesda, Maryland

Matthew R. Schmitz, MD
Chief, Pediatric Orthopaedics and Young Adult Hip
   Preservation
Department of Orthopaedics and Rehabilitation
San Antonio Military Medical Center
San Antonio, Texas
Assistant Professor
Department of Surgery
Herbert School of Medicine
Uniformed Services University of the Health Sciences
Bethesda, Maryland

Jeffrey D. Seybold, MD
Orthopaedic Surgeon
Twin Cities Orthopedics
Edina, Minnesota

Francis H. Shen, MD
Warren G. Stamp Endowed Professor
Division Head, Spine Division
Co-Director, Spine Center
Department of Orthopaedic Surgery
University of Virginia Health Systems
Charlottesville, Virginia

Franklin D. Shuler, MD, PhD
Professor of Orthopedic Traumatology
Orthopedics
Marshall University Joan C. Edwards School of Medicine
Vice Chairman of Research
Orthopedics
Cabell Huntington Hospital
Huntington, West Virginia

Stephen R. Thompson, MD, MEd, FRCSC
Cooperating Associate Professor of Sports Medicine
The University of Maine
Medical Director
EMMC Sports Health
Deputy Editor
The Journal of Bone and Joint Surgery
Eastern Maine Medical Center
Bangor, Maine
Cofounder and Codirector
Miller Review Course Part II
Denver, Colorado

PREFACE

Congratulations! You have in your hands one of the most popular books in the history of orthopaedic surgery. The odyssey from the first edition—which began as little more than compiled notes with a working title of *Basic Orthopaedic Notes Edited (BONE)* and "scrapbook art" picked up from other Saunders/Mosby (now Elsevier) textbooks—to the seventh edition has been quite an adventure. What has made that adventure especially rewarding is the crew that we have assembled along the way. The seventh edition of this book personifies, in all ways, a team effort. We invited many new but seasoned authors, mostly from our popular Miller Review Course (MRC), to participate in the creation in this edition. Most were assigned new coauthors and/or sections that they had not worked on before.

All chapters in the seventh edition have undergone major revisions:

- Chapter 1, "Basic Science": We assembled the team that covers this exhaustive topic for MRC and asked them to completely revise the text.
- Chapter 2, "Anatomy": We asked Dr. Gwathmey, who has taken over the orthopaedic anatomy course at the University of Virginia, to reorganize and update this material.
- Chapter 3, "Pediatric Orthopaedics": Dr. Schmitz, a young and energetic pediatric orthopaedic surgeon, took the lead in doing a major overhaul of this chapter.
- Chapter 4, "Sports Medicine": Drs. Thompson and Miller spent a lot of time and much of the art budget in replacing the scrapbook images with new artwork, including composite images.
- Chapter 5, "Adult Reconstruction": Because we have recently broken up the topics of hip and knee arthroplasty for MRC, we took a similar approach for this chapter, and it is new and improved as a result. Advances in shoulder arthroplasty are also incorporated.
- Chapter 6, "Disorders of the Foot and Ankle": Dr. Kadaka took the lead on expanding and revitalizing this part of the book. It is more organized and includes great new images.
- Chapter 7, "Hand, Upper Extremity, and Microvascular Surgery": Drs. Chhabra and Brunton took one of the best chapters from the last edition and made it even better.
- Chapter 8, "Spine": We invited Dr. Shen, new MRC lecturer (and veteran AAOS lecturer), to work on this chapter, and he made major changes, including tripling the number of images. We would be remiss if we did not recognize the former spine chapter author, the late Dr. William

Lauerman. Please note the tribute to him in Dr. Shen's chapter.
- Chapter 9, "Orthopaedic Pathology": Dr. Holt made updating this important area of practice her personal mission, and it is a masterpiece (just like her lectures at MRC).
- Chapter 10, "Rehabilitation": Dr. Hogan, new to both MRC and this book, did a great job with a very thorough revision.
- Chapter 11, "Trauma": Dr. Hak took on the challenge of reorganizing and revising this important chapter, and it is much improved.
- Chapter 12, "Principles of Practice": Dr. DeHart, one of the few remaining original MRC faculty members, has done his usual excellent job in updating this difficult chapter.
- Chapter 13, "Biostatistics and Research Design": Dr. Hart has a knack for making statistics and research understandable, if not fun (OK, we won't go that far).

A lot of thought went into the reorganization of this popular text. We tried to put things where they belong, based on what subspecialty would most likely be used to treat a given condition. We began by cleaning up the sports medicine chapter by removing much of the overlap with other subspecialties. Sports foot and ankle was transferred to the foot and ankle chapter; sports elbow and hand was transferred to become part of the hand chapter; and spine injuries were moved to the spine chapter. Next we tackled the trauma chapter, shifting spine trauma to the spine chapter. Foot and ankle injuries distal to the tibial pilon were transferred to the foot and ankle chapter. Hand injuries were consolidated in the already great hand chapter. And, appropriately, some things were left the same. We continued the popular highlighting of key points and use of highlighter icons for important figures. We also kept the end of chapter Testable Concepts summaries, which residents have told us are invaluable for last minute test preparation.

Finally, above all else, we have made every attempt to maintain C.C. Colton's mantra from the preface of the first edition of *Miller's Review of Orthopaedics*: "The writer does the most who gives the reader the most knowledge and takes from him the least time."

Mark D. Miller, MD
Stephen R. Thompson, MD, MEd, FRCSC

CONTENTS

5 ADULT RECONSTRUCTION, 403

*Edward J. McPherson, James A. Browne,
and Stephen R. Thompson*

CHAPTER 1

BASIC SCIENCES

Matthew R. Schmitz, Marc McCord DeHart, Zain Qazi, and Franklin D. Shuler

CONTENTS

SECTION 1 ORTHOPAEDIC TISSUES

BONE

- **Histologic features of bone**
- Types (Figure 1-1, Table 1-1)
  - Normal bone: lamellar or mature; either cortical or cancellous
  - Immature and pathologic bone: woven; more random, more osteocytes, increased turnover, weaker
    - Lamellar bone is stress oriented; woven bone is not.
  - Cortical (compact) bone
    - Constitutes 80% of the skeleton
    - Consists of tightly packed osteons or haversian systems
      - Connected by haversian (or Volkmann) canals
      - Contains arterioles, venules, capillaries, nerves, possibly lymphatic channels
    - Interstitial lamellae: between osteons
      - Fibrils connect lamellae but do not cross cement lines.
      - Cement lines define the outer border of an osteon.
    - Bone resorption has stopped and new bone formation has begun.
    - Nutrition provided by intraosseous circulation through canals and canaliculi (cell processes of osteocytes)
    - Characterized by slow turnover rate, higher Young's modulus of elasticity, more stiffness
  - Cancellous bone (spongy or trabecular bone)
    - Less dense, more remodeling according to lines of stress (Wolff's law)
    - Characterized by high turnover rate, smaller Young's modulus, more elasticity
- Cellular biology (Figure 1-2)
  - Osteoblasts
    - **Appear as cuboid cells aligned in layers along immature osteoid**
    - Derived from undifferentiated mesenchymal stem cells

- Have more endoplasmic reticulum, Golgi apparatus, and mitochondria than do other cells (for synthesis and secretion of matrix)
- RUNX2 is a multifunctional transcription factor that directs mesenchymal cells to the osteoblast lineage.
- Bone surfaces lined by more differentiated, metabolically active cells
- "Entrapped cells": less active cells in "resting regions"; maintain the ionic milieu of bone
- Disruption of the active lining cell layer activates entrapped cells.
- Two main functions:
  - **Form bone**
  - **Regulate osteoclastic activity**
- Osteoblast differentiation:
  - Bone morphogenetic protein (BMP) stimulates mesenchymal cells to become osteoprogenitor cells.
  - Core-binding factor α-1 stimulates differentiation.
  - β-Catenin stimulates differentiation into osteoblasts, with resulting intramembranous bone formation.
  - Platelet-derived growth factor (PDGF)
  - Insulinlike growth factor (IGF)
- Receptor-effector interactions in osteoblasts (Table 1-2)
- Osteoblasts produce the following:
  - Alkaline phosphatase
  - Osteocalcin (stimulated by 1,25 dihydroxyvitamin D)
  - Type I collagen
  - Bone sialoprotein
  - **Receptor activator of nuclear factor (NF)-κB ligand (RANKL)**
  - **Osteoprotegrin—binds RANKL to limit its activity**
- **Osteoblast activity stimulated by intermittent (pulsatile) exposure to parathyroid hormone (PTH)**

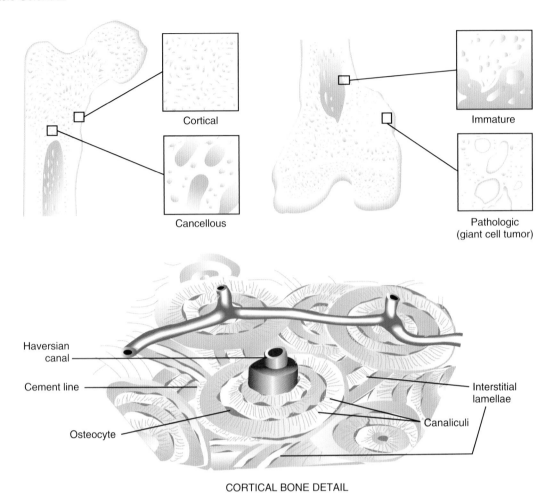

CORTICAL BONE DETAIL

FIGURE 1-1 Types of bone. *Cortical* bone consists of tightly packed osteons. *Cancellous* bone consists of a meshwork of trabeculae. In *immature* bone, unmineralized osteoid lines the immature trabeculae. *Pathologic* bone is characterized by atypical osteoblasts and architectural disorganization. (Colorized from Brinker MR, Miller MD: *Fundamentals of orthopaedics,* Philadelphia, 1999, WB Saunders, p 2.)

Table 1-1	Types of Bone		
MICROSCOPIC APPEARANCE	**SUBTYPES**	**CHARACTERISTICS**	**EXAMPLES**
Lamellar	Cortical	Structure is oriented along lines of stress Strong	Femoral shaft
Woven	Cancellous Immature	More elastic than cortical bone Not stress oriented	Distal femoral metaphysis Embryonic skeleton Fracture callus
	Pathologic	Random organization Increased turnover Weak Flexible	Osteogenic sarcoma Fibrous dysplasia

Modified from Brinker MR, Miller MD: *Fundamentals of orthopaedics,* Philadelphia, 1999, WB Saunders, p 1.

- **Osteoblast activity inhibited by tumor necrosis factor (TNF)-α**
- Wnts are proteins that promote osteoblast survival and proliferation.
  - Deficient wnt causes osteopenia; excessive wnt expression causes high bone mass.
  - **Wnts can be sequestered by other secreted molecules such as sclerostin (Scl) and dickkopf-related protein 1 (dkk1).**
- Certain antiseptics toxic to cultured osteoblasts:
  - Hydrogen peroxide
  - Povidone-iodine (Betadine)
  - Bacitracin (believed to be less toxic)
- Osteocytes (see Figure 1-1)
  - Maintain bone
  - Constitute 90% of the cells in the mature skeleton
  - Former osteoblasts surrounded by newly formed matrix

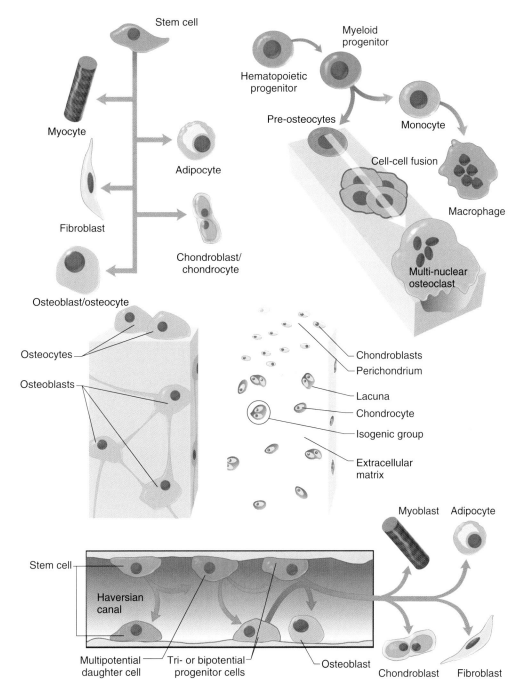

FIGURE 1-2 Cellular origins of bone and cartilage cells.

Table 1-2	Bone Cell Types, Receptor Types, and Effects	
CELL TYPE	**RECEPTOR**	**EFFECT**
Osteoblast	PTH	Releases a secondary messenger (exact mechanism unknown) to stimulate osteoclastic activity Activates adenylyl cyclase
	1,25(OH)$_2$ vitamin D$_3$	Stimulates matrix and alkaline phosphatase synthesis and production of bone-specific proteins (e.g., osteocalcin)
	Glucocorticoids	Inhibits DNA synthesis, collagen production, and osteoblast protein synthesis
	Prostaglandins	Activates adenylyl cyclase and stimulates bone resorption
	Estrogen	Has anabolic (bone production) and anticatabolic (prevents bone resorption) properties Increases mRNA levels for alkaline phosphatase Inhibits activation of adenylyl cyclase
Osteoclast	Calcitonin	Inhibits osteoclast function (inhibits bone resorption)

mRNA, Messenger RNA; *PTH,* parathyroid hormone.

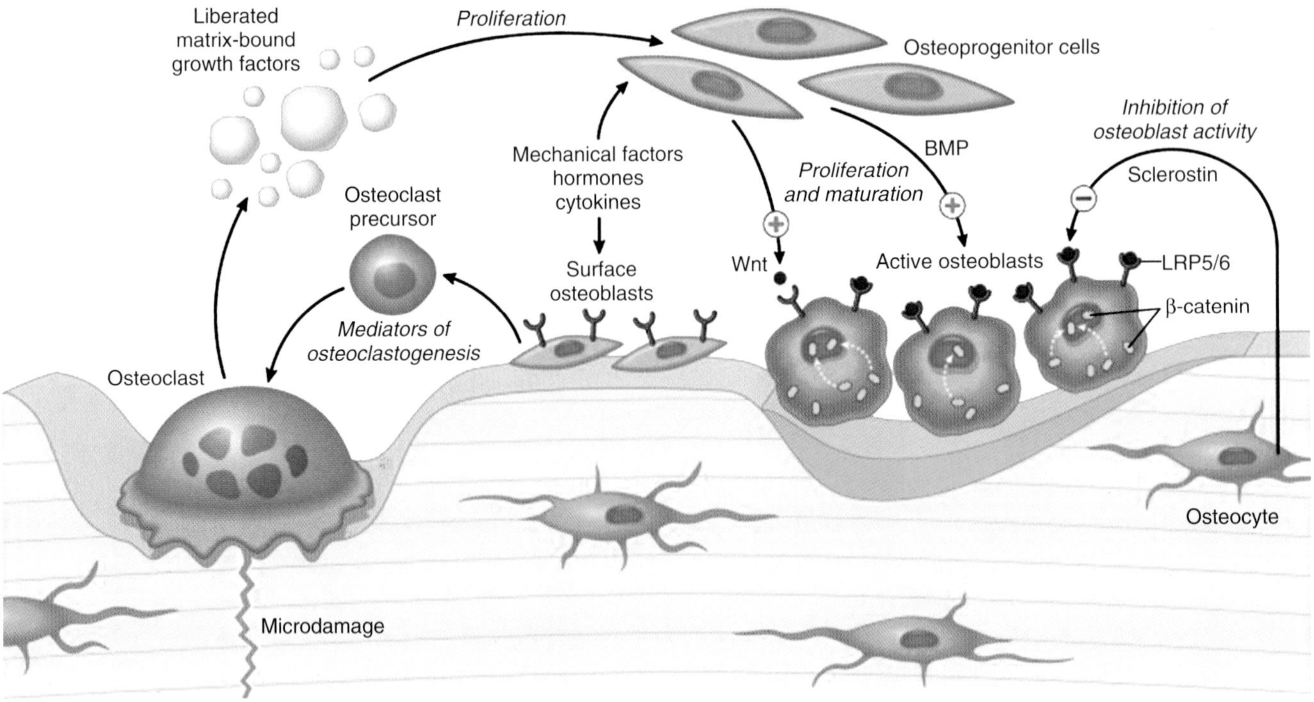

FIGURE 1-3 Paracrine crosstalk between osteoblasts and osteoclasts. *BMP,* Bone morphogenic protein; *LRP5/6,* LDL receptor related proteins 5 and 6. (From Kumar V et al, editors: Bones, joints, and soft tissue tumors. In *Robbins and Cotran pathologic basis of disease,* ed 9, Philadelphia, 2014, Saunders, Figure 26-5.)

- High nucleus/cytoplasm ratio
- Long interconnecting cytoplasmic processes projecting through the canaliculi
- Less active in matrix production than are osteoblasts
- Important for control of extracellular calcium and phosphorus concentration
- Directly stimulated by calcitonin, inhibited by PTH
- Sclerostin secreted by osteocytes helps negative feedback on osteoblasts' bone deposition (Figure 1-3).
  - Differentially regulated based on mechanical loading, with decreased sclerostin in areas of concentrated strain
  - Downregulation is associated with increased bone formation (via sclerostin antibody).
  - Potential for use in fracture healing, bone loss, implant osseous integration, and genetic bone diseases via upregulating sclerostin
- Osteoclasts
  - Formation
    - Multinucleated irregular giant cells
  - Derived from hematopoietic cells in macrophage lineage
  - Monocyte progenitors form giant cells by fusion
  - Function
    - Resorb bone
      - Occurs both normally and in certain conditions including multiple myeloma and metastatic bone disease
      - Possess a ruffled ("brush") border and surrounding clear zone
      - Border consists of plasma membrane enfoldings that increase surface area for resorption.

- Bone resorption occurs in depressions: Howship lacunae.
- Formation and resorption are linked ("coupled").
- Resorption occurs more rapidly.
- Synthesize tartrate-resistant acid phosphate
- Bind to bone surfaces through cell attachment (anchoring) proteins
- Integrin, specifically $\alpha_v\beta_3$ or vitronectin receptor
- Effectively seal the space below the osteoclast
- Produce hydrogen ions through carbonic anhydrase
- Lower PH
- Increase solubility of hydroxyapatite crystals
- Organic matrix then removed by proteolytic digestion through activity of the lysosomal enzyme cathepsin K
  - Osteoblasts (and tumor cells) express RANKL (Figure 1-4), which acts as follows:
    - Binds to receptors on osteoclasts
    - Stimulates differentiation into mature osteoclasts
    - Increases bone resorption
    - **Inhibited by osteoprotegerin binding to RANKL**
- Signaling
  - Have specific receptors for calcitonin, which inhibits osteoclastic resorption
  - Interleukin (IL)-1: potent stimulator of osteoclast differentiation and bone resorption
    - Found in membranes surrounding loose total joint implants
- In contrast, IL-10 suppresses osteoclasts.
- Bisphosphonates
  - Inhibit osteoclastic bone resorption—direct anabolic effect on bone
  - **Categorized into two classes on the basis of presence or absence of a nitrogen side group:**

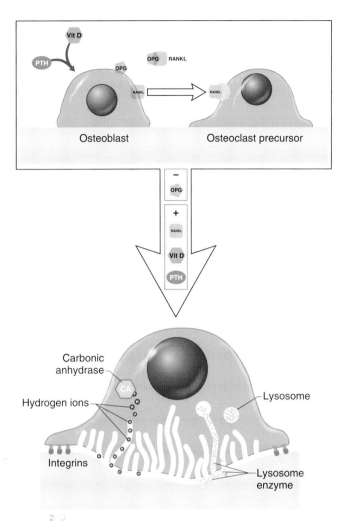

FIGURE 1-4 Control and function of the osteoclast. *OPG,* Osteoprotegerin; *PTH,* parathyroid hormone; *RANKL,* receptor activator of nuclear factor κB ligand; *Vit,* vitamin.

- **Nitrogen-containing bisphosphonates**—up to 1000-fold more potent in their antiresorptive activity:
  - Zoledronic acid (Zometa) and alendronate (Fosamax)
  - **Inhibit protein prenylation within the mevalonate pathway, blocking farnesyl pyrophosphate synthase**
  - **Results in a loss of guanosine triphosphatase (GTPase) formation, which is needed for ruffled border formation and cell survival**
- Non–nitrogen-containing bisphosphonates:
  - Metabolized into a nonfunctional adenosine triphosphate (ATP) analogue, inducing apoptosis
  - Decreases skeletal events in multiple myeloma
  - Associated with osteonecrosis of the jaw
- Orthopaedic implications of bisphosphonate use:
  - Spine—reduced rate of spinal fusion in animal model; withholding bisphosphonate is recommended after surgery
  - Hip and knee—safe for use in cementless hip arthroplasty and cemented knee arthroplasty; may decrease rate of acetabular component subsidence

- Fracture healing—no good data to recommend for or against use
- Osteoprogenitor cells
  - Originate from mesenchymal stem cells
  - Become osteoblasts under conditions of low strain and increased oxygen tension
  - Become cartilage under conditions of intermediate strain and low oxygen tension
  - Become fibrous tissue under conditions of high strain
  - Line haversian canals, endosteum, and periosteum
    - Awaiting the stimulus to differentiate
- Matrix (Table 1-3)
  - Organic components: 40% of dry weight of bone
  - Collagen (90% of organic component)
    - **Primarily type I (mnemonic: *bone* contains the word *one*)**
      - **Type I collagen provides tensile strength of bone**
    - Hole zones (gaps) exist within the collagen fibril between the ends of molecules.
    - Pores exist between the sides of parallel molecules.
    - Mineral deposition (calcification) occurs within the hole zones and pores (Figure 1-5).
    - Cross-linking decreases collagen solubility and increases its tensile strength.
  - Proteoglycans
  - Matrix proteins (noncollagenous)
    - Osteocalcin: most abundant noncollagenous protein in bone
    - Inhibited by PTH and stimulated by 1,25-dihydroxyvitamin D_3
    - Can be measured in serum or urine as a marker of bone turnover
    - Growth factors and cytokines
  - Inorganic (mineral) components: 60% of dry weight of bone
    - Calcium hydroxyapatite $[Ca_{10}(PO_4)_6(OH)_2]$
    - Calcium phosphate (brushite)
- Bone remodeling
  - General
    - Cortical and cancellous bone is continuously remodeled throughout life by osteoclastic and osteoblastic activity (Figure 1-6).
    - **Wolff's law: remodeling occurs in response to mechanical stress.**
      - Increasing mechanical stress increases bone gain.
      - Removing external mechanical stress increases bone loss, which is reversible (to varying degrees) on remobilization.
      - Piezoelectric remodeling occurs in response to electric charge.
    - The compression side of bone is electronegative, stimulating osteoblasts (formation).
    - The tension side of bone is electropositive, stimulating osteoclasts (resorption).
    - **Hueter-Volkmann law**: remodeling occurs in small packets of cells known as *basic multicellular units (BMUs)*.
      - Such remodeling is modulated by hormones and cytokines.
      - **Compressive forces inhibit growth; tension stimulates it.**

Table 1-3	Components of Bone Matrix			
TYPE OF MATRIX	**FUNCTION**	**COMPOSITION**	**TYPES**	**NOTES**
ORGANIC MATRIX				
Collagen	Provides tensile strength	Primarily type I collagen		Constitutes 90% of organic matrix Structure: triple helix of one α_2 and two α_1 chains, quarter-staggered to produce a fibril
Proteoglycans	Partly responsible for compressive strength	Glycosaminoglycan-protein complexes		Inhibit mineralization
Matrix proteins (noncollagenous)	Promote mineralization and bone formation		Osteocalcin (bone γ-carboxyglutamic acid–containing protein)	Attracts osteoclasts; direct regulation of bone density; most abundant noncollagenous matrix protein (10%-20% of total)
			Osteonectin (SPARC)	Secreted by platelets and osteoblasts; postulated to have a role in regulating calcium or organizing mineral in matrix
			Osteopontin	Cell-binding protein, similar to an integrin
Growth factors and cytokines	Aid in bone cell differentiation, activation, growth, and turnover		TGF-β IGF IL-1, IL-6 BMPs	Present in small amounts in bone matrix
INORGANIC MATRIX				
Calcium hydroxyapatite [$Ca_{10}(PO_4)_6(OH)_2$]	Provides compressive strength			Most of the inorganic matrix; primary mineralization in collagen gaps (holes and pores), secondary mineralization on periphery
Osteocalcium phosphate (brushite)				Makes up the remaining inorganic matrix

BMP, Bone morphogenetic proteins; *IGF,* insulinlike growth factor; *IL,* interleukin; *SPARC,* secreted protein, acidic, rich in cysteine; *TGF-β,* transforming growth factor-β.

Progressively increasing mineral mass due to:
1. Increased number of new mineral phase particles (nucleation)
   a. Heterogeneous nucleation by matrix in collagen holes (and pores)
   b. Secondary crystal–induced nucleation in holes and pores
2. Initial growth of particles to ~400 Å × 15-30 Å × 50-75 Å

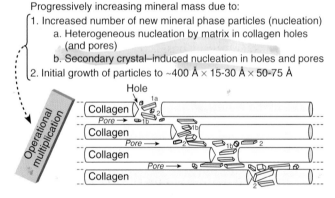

FIGURE 1-5 Biological considerations of mineral accretion: heterogeneity within a collagen fibril. (From Simon SR, editor: *Orthopaedic basic science,* Rosemont, Ill, 1994, American Academy of Orthopaedic Surgeons, p 139.)

- Suggests that mechanical factors influence longitudinal growth, bone remodeling, and fracture repair
- May play a role in scoliosis and Blount disease
- Cortical bone remodeling
  - Osteoclastic tunneling (cutting cones; Figure 1-7)
    - Followed by layering of osteoblasts and successive deposition of layers of lamellae
    - The head of the cutting cone is made up of osteoclasts.
      - Behind the osteoclast front are capillaries.
      - Followed by the laying down of osteoid by osteoblasts

- Cancellous bone remodeling
  - Osteoclastic resorption occurs, and then osteoblasts lay down new bone.
- Bone circulation
  - Anatomy
    - Bone receives 5% to 10% of the cardiac output.
      - Bones with a tenuous blood supply include the scaphoid, talus, femoral head, and odontoid.
    - Long bones receive blood from three sources (systems):
      - Nutrient artery system
        - Branch from systemic arteries, enter the diaphyseal cortex through the nutrient foramen, enter the medullary canal, and branch into ascending and descending arteries (Figure 1-8)
        - Further branch into arterioles in the endosteal cortex; enables blood supply to at least **the inner two thirds** of the mature diaphyseal cortex via the haversian system (Figure 1-9)
        - Blood pressure (BP) in the nutrient artery system is high.
        - **60% of cortical bone vascularized by nutrient arteries**
      - Metaphyseal-epiphyseal system
        - Arises from the periarticular vascular plexus (e.g., geniculate arteries)
      - Periosteal system
        - Consists mostly of capillaries that supply the outer third (at most) of the mature diaphyseal cortex
        - **BP in the periosteal system is low.**

BONE REMODELING

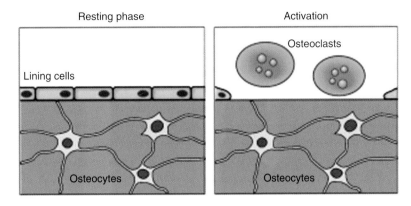

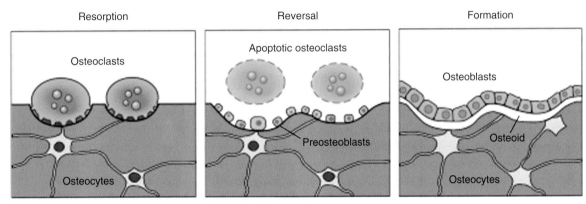

FIGURE 1-6 Bone remodeling. Osteoclasts dissolve the mineral from the bone matrix. Osteoblasts produce new bone (osteoid) that fills in the resorption pit. Some osteoblasts are left within the bone matrix as osteocytes. (From Firestein GS et al, editors: *Kelley's textbook of rheumatology,* ed 8, Philadelphia, 2008, Saunders.)

- Physiologic features
  - Direction of flow (Figure 1-10)
    - Arterial flow in mature bone is centrifugal (inside to outside), which is the net effect of the high-pressure nutrient artery system and the low-pressure periosteal system.
    - When fracture disrupts the nutrient artery system, the periosteal system pressure predominates and blood flow is centripetal (outside to inside).
    - Flow in immature developing bone is centripetal because the highly vascularized periosteal system is the predominant component.
    - Venous flow in mature bone is centripetal.
      - Cortical capillaries drain to venous sinusoids, which drain to the emissary venous system.
  - Fluid compartments of bone:
    - Extravascular: 65%
    - Haversian: 6%
    - Lacunar: 6%
    - Red blood cells (RBCs): 3%
    - Other: 20%
  - Physiologic states
    - Hypoxia, hypercapnia, and sympathectomy increase flow.
- Fracture healing
  - **Bone blood flow is the major determinant of how well a fracture heals.**
  - Delivers nutrients to the injury site
    - Initial response is a decrease in bone blood flow after vascular disruption at the fracture site.

  - Within hours to days, bone blood flow increases (as part of the regional acceleratory phenomenon), **peaks at approximately 2 weeks,** and returns to normal in 3 to 5 months.
    - Unreamed intramedullary nails preserve endosteal blood supply.
  - Reaming devascularizes the inner 50% to 80% of the cortex and delays revascularization of endosteal blood supply.
  - Loose-fitting nails spare cortical perfusion and allow more rapid reperfusion than do canal-filling nails.
- Regulation of bone blood flow
  - Influenced by metabolic, humoral, and autonomic inputs
    - Arterial system: great potential for vasoconstriction (from the resting state), less potential for vasodilation
    - Vessels within bone: have several vasoactive receptors (β-adrenergic, muscarinic, thromboxane/ prostaglandin)
- Tissues surrounding bone
  - Periosteum
    - Connective tissue membrane covers bone.
    - More highly developed in children
    - Inner periosteum, or cambium, is loose and vascular and contains cells capable of becoming osteoblasts.
      - Cells enlarge the diameter of bone during growth and form periosteal callus during fracture healing.
    - Outer (fibrous) periosteum is less cellular and is contiguous with joint capsules.

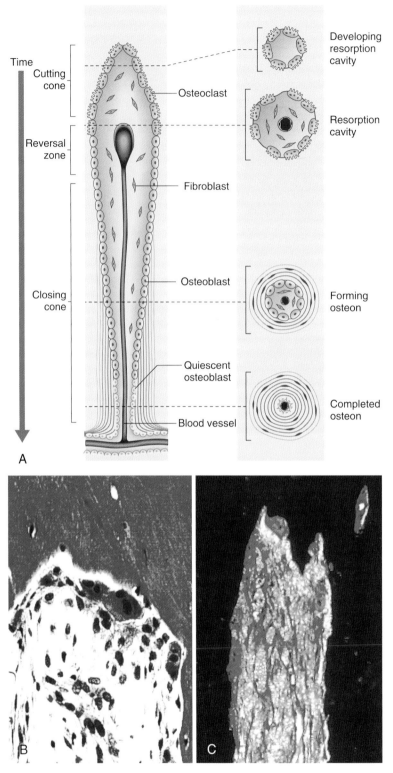

FIGURE 1-7 Cortical bone remodeling. **A,** Longitudinal and cross sections of a time line illustrating formation of an osteon. Osteoclasts cut a cylindrical channel through bone. Osteoblasts follow, laying down bone on the surface of the channel until matrix surrounds the central blood vessel of the newly formed osteon (closing cone of a new osteon). **B,** Photomicrograph of a cutting cone. **C,** Higher-magnification photomicrograph; osteoclastic resorption can be more clearly appreciated. (**A** from Standring S et al, editors: Functional anatomy of the musculoskeletal system. In *Gray's anatomy,* ed 40, London, 2008, Elsevier, Figure 5-19.)

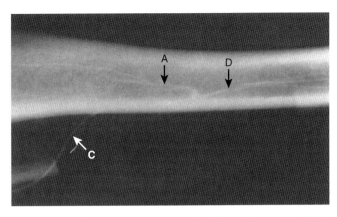

FIGURE 1-8 Intraoperative arteriogram (canine tibia) demonstrating ascending (A) and descending (D) branches of the nutrient artery. *C,* Cannula. (From Brinker MR et al: Pharmacological regulation of the circulation of bone, *J Bone Joint Surg Am* 72:964–975, 1990.)

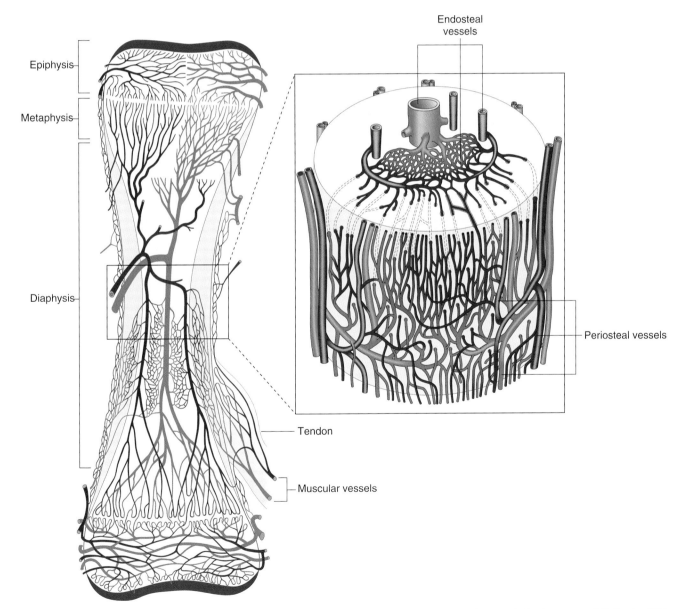

FIGURE 1-9 Blood supply to bone. (From Standring S et al, editors: Functional anatomy of the musculoskeletal system. In *Gray's anatomy,* ed 40, London, 2008, Elsevier, Figure 5-20.)

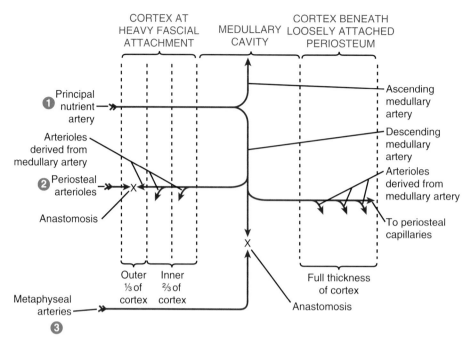

FIGURE 1-10 Major components of the afferent vascular system of long bone. Components 1, 2, and 3 constitute the total nutrient supply to the diaphysis. Arrows indicate the direction of blood flow. (From Rhinelander FW: Circulation in bone. In Bourne G, editor: *The biochemistry and physiology of bone,* ed 2, vol 2, Orlando, Fla, 1972, Academic Press, pp 1-77.)

Table 1-4	Types of Bone Formation		
TYPE OF OSSIFICATION	**MECHANISM**	**EXAMPLES OF NORMAL MECHANISMS**	**EXAMPLES OF DISEASES WITH ABNORMAL OSSIFICATION**
Enchondral	Bone replaces a cartilage model	Embryonic formation of long bones Longitudinal growth (physis) Fracture callus Bone formed with the use of demineralized bone matrix	Achondroplasia
Intramembranous	Aggregates of undifferentiated mesenchymal cells differentiate into osteoblasts, which form bone	Embryonic flat bone formation Bone formation during distraction osteogenesis Blastema bone	Cleidocranial dysostosis
Appositional	Osteoblasts lay down new bone on existing bone	Periosteal bone enlargement (width) The bone formation phase of bone remodeling	Paget disease of bone Infantile hyperostosis (Caffey disease) Melorheostosis

- Bone marrow—source of progenitor cells; controls inner diameter of bone
  - Red marrow
    - Hematopoietic (40% water, 40% fat, 20% protein)
    - Slowly changes to yellow marrow with age, first in appendicular skeleton and later in axial skeleton
  - Yellow marrow
    - Inactive (15% water, 80% fat, 5% protein)
- Types of bone formation (Table 1-4)
  - Enchondral bone formation and mineralization
    - General
      - Undifferentiated cells secrete cartilaginous matrix and differentiate into chondrocytes.
      - Matrix mineralizes and is invaded by vascular buds that bring osteoprogenitor cells.
      - Osteoclasts resorb calcified cartilage; osteoblasts form bone.
      - **Bone replaces the cartilage model; cartilage is not converted to bone.**
    - Examples of enchondral bone formation:
      - Embryonic formation of long bones
      - Longitudinal growth (physis)
      - Fracture callus
      - Bone formed with demineralized bone matrix
  - Embryonic formation of long bones (Figures 1-11 and 1-12)
    - These bones are formed from the mesenchymal anlage at 6 weeks' gestation.
    - Vascular buds invade the mesenchymal model, bringing osteoprogenitor cells that differentiate into osteoblasts and form the primary ossification centers at 8 weeks.
    - Differentiation stimulated in part **by binding of WNT protein to the LRP5 or LRP6 receptor**
    - Cartilage model increases in size through appositional (width) and interstitial (length) growth
    - Marrow forms by resorption of the central cartilage anlage by invasion of myeloid precursor cells that are brought in by capillary buds.

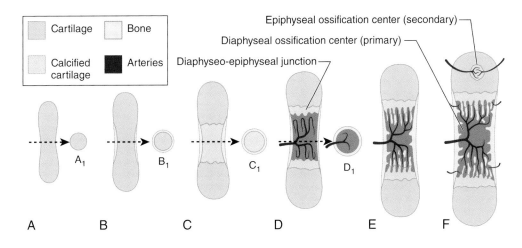

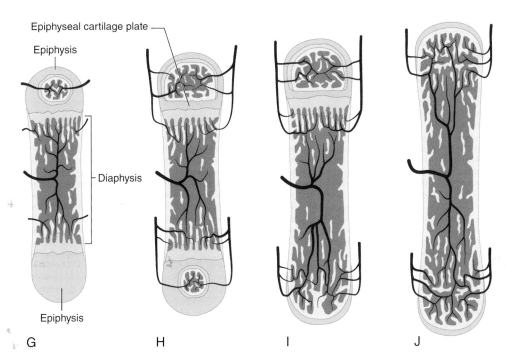

FIGURE 1-11 Enchondral ossification of long bones. Note that phases F through J often occur after birth. (From Moore KL: *The developing human*, Philadelphia, 1982, WB Saunders, p 346.)

- Secondary ossification centers develop at bone ends, forming the epiphyseal centers (growth plates) responsible for longitudinal growth.
- Arterial supply is rich during development, with an epiphyseal artery (terminates in the proliferative zone), metaphyseal arteries, nutrient arteries, and perichondrial arteries. (Figure 1-13)
- Physis
  - Two growth plates exist in immature long bones: (1) horizontal (the physis) and (2) spherical (growth of the epiphysis)
    - The spherical plate is less organized than the horizontal plate.
  - Perichondrial artery—major source of nutrition of growth plate
  - Acromegaly and spondyloepiphyseal dysplasia affect the physis; multiple epiphyseal dysplasia affects the epiphysis.

- Delineation of physeal cartilage zones is based on growth (see Figure 1-13) and function (Figures 1-14 and 1-15; also see Figure 1-17).
  - **Reserve zone:** cells store lipids, glycogen, and proteoglycan aggregates; decreased oxygen tension occurs in this zone.
    - Lysosomal storage diseases (e.g., Gaucher disease) can affect this zone.
  - **Proliferative zone:** growth is longitudinal, with stacking of chondrocytes (the top cell is the dividing "mother" cell), cellular proliferation, and matrix production; increased oxygen tension and increased proteoglycans inhibit calcification.
    - Achondroplasia causes defects in this zone (see Figure 1-14).
    - Growth hormone exerts its effect in the proliferative zone.

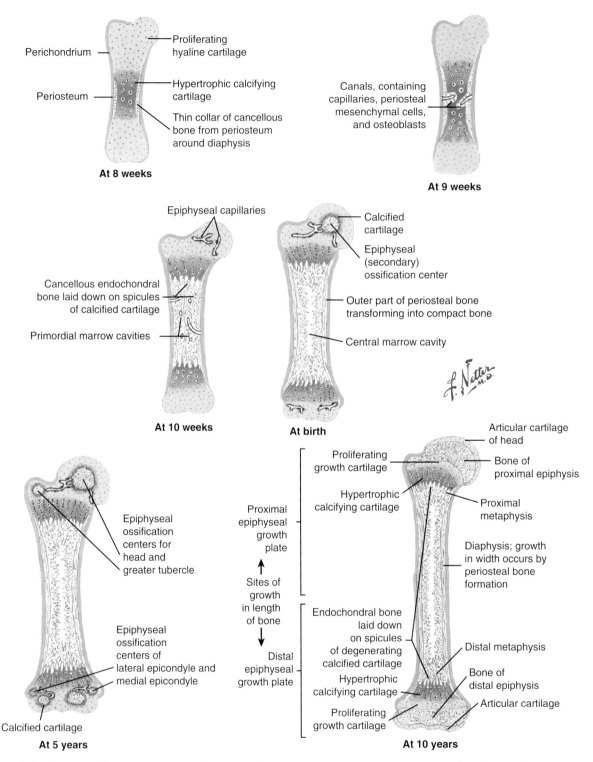

FIGURE 1-12 Development of a typical long bone: formation of the growth plate and secondary centers of ossification. (From Netter FH: *CIBA collection of medical illustrations,* vol 8: *Musculoskeletal system,* part I: *Anatomy, physiology and developmental disorders,* Basel, Switzerland, 1987, CIBA, p 136.)

CLOSE-UP VIEW OF DEVELOPING EPIPHYSIS AND EPIPHYSEAL GROWTH PLATE

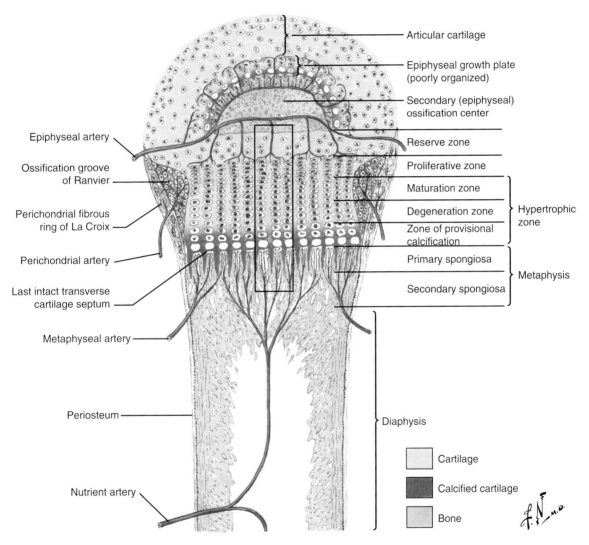

FIGURE 1-13 Structure and blood supply of a typical growth plate. (From Netter FH: *CIBA collection of medical illustrations,* vol 8: *Musculoskeletal system,* part I: *Anatomy, physiology and developmental disorders,* Basel, Switzerland, 1987, CIBA, p 166.)

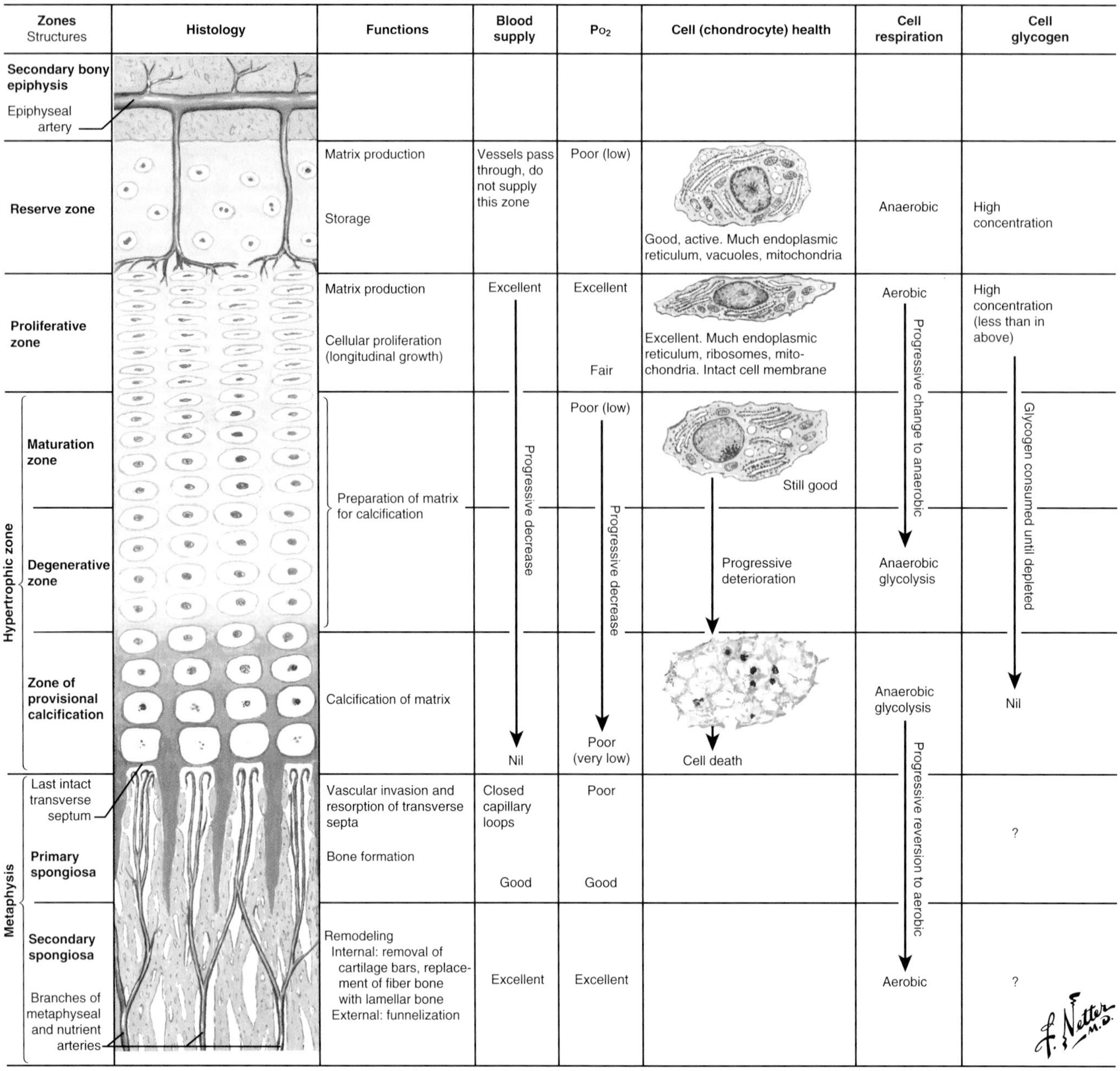

Zones / Structures	Histology	Functions	Blood supply	Po2	Cell (chondrocyte) health	Cell respiration	Cell glycogen
Secondary bony epiphysis — Epiphyseal artery							
Reserve zone		Matrix production; Storage	Vessels pass through, do not supply this zone	Poor (low)	Good, active. Much endoplasmic reticulum, vacuoles, mitochondria	Anaerobic	High concentration
Proliferative zone		Matrix production; Cellular proliferation (longitudinal growth)	Excellent	Excellent / Fair	Excellent. Much endoplasmic reticulum, ribosomes, mitochondria. Intact cell membrane	Aerobic	High concentration (less than in above)
Hypertrophic zone — Maturation zone / Degenerative zone		Preparation of matrix for calcification	*(Progressive decrease)*	Poor (low) *(Progressive decrease)*	Still good → Progressive deterioration	*(Progressive change to anaerobic)* Anaerobic glycolysis	*(Glycogen consumed until depleted)*
Zone of provisional calcification		Calcification of matrix	Nil	Poor (very low)	Cell death	Anaerobic glycolysis	Nil
Metaphysis — Last intact transverse septum / Primary spongiosa		Vascular invasion and resorption of transverse septa; Bone formation	Closed capillary loops / Good	Poor / Good		*(Progressive reversion to aerobic)*	?
Secondary spongiosa — Branches of metaphyseal and nutrient arteries		Remodeling Internal: removal of cartilage bars, replacement of fiber bone with lamellar bone; External: funnelization	Excellent	Excellent		Aerobic	?

FIGURE 1-14 Zone structure, function, and physiologic features of the growth plate. (From Netter FH: *CIBA collection of medical illustrations,* vol 8: *Musculoskeletal system,* part I: *Anatomy, physiology and developmental disorders,* Basel, Switzerland, 1987, CIBA, p 164.)

- **Hypertrophic zone**—sometimes divided into three zones: maturation, degeneration, and provisional calcification
  - Normal matrix mineralization occurs in the lower hypertrophic zone: chondrocytes increase five times in size, accumulate calcium in their mitochondria, die, and release calcium from matrix vesicles.
  - Chondrocyte maturation is regulated by systemic hormones and local growth factors (PTH-related peptide inhibits chondrocyte maturation; Indian hedgehog is produced by chondrocytes and regulates the expression of PTH-related peptide).
  - Osteoblasts migrate from sinusoidal vessels and use cartilage as a scaffolding for bone formation.
  - Low oxygen tension and decreased proteoglycan aggregates aid in this process.
  - This zone widens in rickets (see Figure 1-15), with little or no provisional calcification.
  - Enchondromas originate here.
  - Mucopolysaccharide diseases (see Figure 1-15) affect this zone, leading to chondrocyte degeneration.
  - Physeal fractures probably traverse several zones, depending on the type of loading (Figure 1-16).
  - **Slipped capital femoral epiphysis (SCFE) believed to occur here** (through metaphyseal spongiosa with renal failure)
- Metaphysis
  - Adjacent to the physis and expands with skeletal growth

Zones Structures	Histology	Functions	Exemplary diseases	Defect (if known)
Secondary bony epiphysis Epiphyseal artery				
Reserve zone		Matrix production Storage	Diastrophic dwarfism.................. (also, defects in other zones)	Defective type II collagen synthesis
			Pseudoachondroplasia................. (also, defects in other zones)	Defective processing and transport of proteoglycans
			Kneist syndrome......................... (also, defects in other zones)	Defective processing of proteoglycans
Proliferative zone		Matrix production Cellular proliferation (longitudinal growth)	Gigantism.................................... Achondroplasia........................... Hypochondroplasia..................... Malnutrition, irradiation.............. injury, glucocorticoid excess	Increased cell proliferation (growth hormone increased) Deficiency of cell proliferation Less severe deficiency of cell proliferation Decreased cell proliferation and/or matrix synthesis
Hypertrophic zone · **Maturation zone**		Preparation of matrix for calcification	Mucopolysaccharidosis............... (Morquio syndrome, Hurler syndrome)	Deficiencies of specific lysosomal acid hydrolases, with lysosomal storage of mucopolysaccharides
Hypertrophic zone · **Degenerative zone**				
Hypertrophic zone · **Zone of provisional calcification**		Calcification of matrix	Rickets, osteomalacia.................. (also, defects in metaphysis)	Insufficiency of Ca^{2+} and/or for normal calcification of matrix
Metaphysis · Last intact transverse septum **Primary spongiosa**		Vascular invasion and resorption of transverse septa Bone formation	Metaphyseal chondro-................. dysplasia (Jansen and Schmid types) Acute hematogenous................... osteomyelitis	Extension of hypertrophic cells into metaphysis Flourishing of bacteria due to sluggish circulation, low PO_2, reticuloendothelial deficiency
Metaphysis · **Secondary spongiosa** Branches of metaphyseal and nutrient arteries		Remodeling Internal: removal of cartilage bars, replacement of fiber bone with lamellar bone External: funnelization	Osteopetrosis............................. Osteogenesis imperfecta............ Scurvy....................................... Metaphyseal dysplasia................ (Pyle disease)	Abnormality of osteoclasts (internal remodeling) Abnormality of osteoblasts and collagen synthesis Inadequate collagen formation Abnormality of funnelization (external remodeling)

 FIGURE 1-15 Zone structure and pathologic defects of cellular metabolism. (From Netter FH: *CIBA collection of medical illustrations*, vol 8: *Musculoskeletal system*, part I: *Anatomy, physiology and developmental disorders*, Basel, Switzerland, 1987, CIBA, p 165.)

- Osteoblasts from osteoprogenitor cells align on cartilage bars produced by physeal expansion.
- Primary spongiosa (calcified cartilage bars) mineralizes to form woven bone and remodels to form secondary spongiosa and a "cutback zone" at the metaphysis.
- Cortical bone forms as physeal (enchondral), and intramembranous bone remodels in response to stress along the periphery of the growing long bone.
- Periphery of the physis
  - Groove of Ranvier: supplies chondrocytes to the periphery for lateral growth (width)
  - Perichondrial ring of La Croix: dense fibrous tissue, primary membrane anchoring the periphery of the physis

- Mineralization
  - Collagen hole zones are seeded with calcium hydroxyapatite crystals through branching and accretion (crystal growth)
  - Hormones and growth factors (Figure 1-17, Table 1-5)
- Intramembranous ossification
  - Occurs without a cartilage model
  - Undifferentiated mesenchymal cells aggregate into layers (or membranes), differentiate into osteoblasts, and deposit an organic matrix that mineralizes.
  - Examples:
    - Embryonic flat bone formation
    - Bone formation during distraction osteogenesis
    - Blastema bone (in young children with amputations)

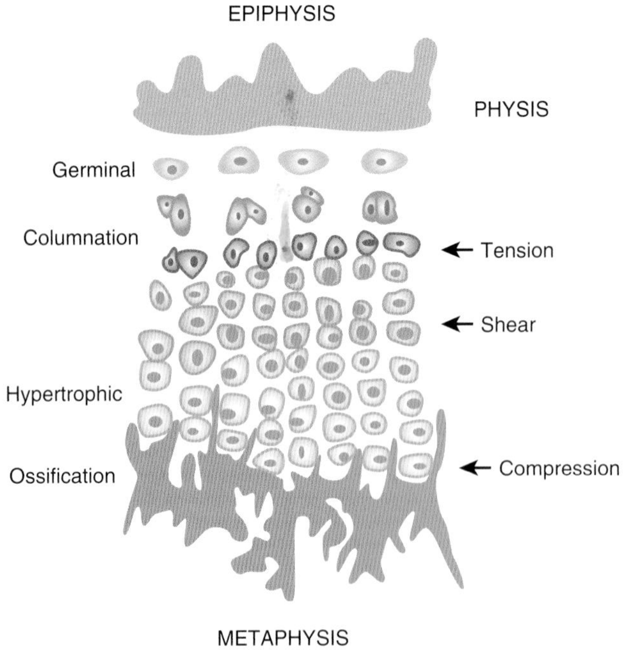

EPIPHYSIS

PHYSIS

Germinal

Columnation

← Tension

← Shear

Hypertrophic

Ossification

← Compression

METAPHYSIS

FIGURE 1-16 Histologic zone of failure varies with the type of loading applied to a specimen. (From Moen CT, Pelker RR: Biomechanical and histological correlations in growth plate failure, *J Pediatr Orthop* 4:180–184, 1984.)

- Appositional ossification
  - Osteoblasts align on the existing bone surface and lay down new bone
  - Examples:
    - Periosteal bone enlargement (width)
    - Bone formation phase of bone remodeling
- ■ **Bone injury and repair**
- ▨ Fracture repair (Table 1-6)
  - Continuum: inflammation to repair (soft callus followed by hard callus), ending in remodeling
  - **Blood supply (bone blood flow): the most important factor**
  - Stages of fracture repair
    - Inflammation
      - Bleeding creates a hematoma, which provides hematopoietic cells capable of secreting growth factors.
      - Subsequently, fibroblasts, mesenchymal cells, and osteoprogenitor cells form granulation tissue around the fracture ends.
      - Osteoblasts (from surrounding osteogenic precursor cells) and fibroblasts proliferate.
    - Repair
      - Primary callus response within 2 weeks
      - For bone ends not in continuity, bridging (soft) callus occurs.
        - Soft callus is later replaced through enchondral ossification by woven bone (hard callus).

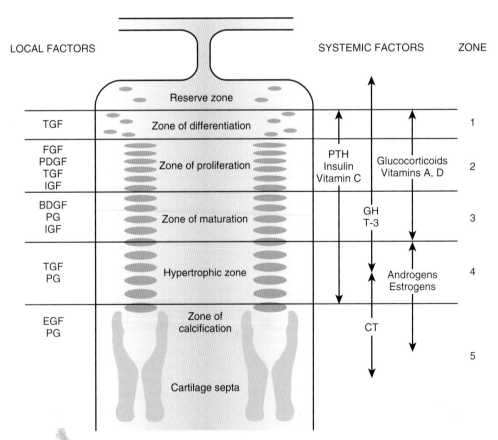

FIGURE 1-17 Growth plate demonstrating proposed sites of action of hormones, growth factors, and vitamins. *BDGF,* bone-derived growth factor; *CT,* calcitonin; *EGF,* epidermal growth factor; *FGF,* fibroblast growth factor; *GH,* growth hormone; *IGF,* insulinlike growth factor; *PDGF,* platelet-derived growth factor; *PG,* proteoglycan; *PTH,* parathyroid hormone; *T-3,* triiodothyronine; *TGF,* transforming growth factor. (From Simon SR, editor: *Orthopaedic basic science,* Rosemont, Ill, 1994, American Academy of Orthopaedic Surgeons, p 197.)

Table 1-5   Effects of Hormones and Growth Factors on the Growth Plate

BIOLOGICAL EFFECT OF HORMONE/FACTOR	SYSTEMIC/LOCAL DERIVATION	PROLIFERATION	MACROMOLECULE BIOSYNTHESIS	MATURATION DEGRADATION	MATRIX CALCIFICATION	ZONE PRIMARILY AFFECTED
Thyroid hormone	Systemic (thyroid)	+ (T_3 with IGF-1)	0	+ (T_3 alone)	0	Proliferative zone and upper hypertrophic zone
Parathyroid	Systemic (parathyroid)	+	++ (Proteoglycan)	0	0	Entire growth plate
Calcitonin	Systemic (thyroid)	0	0	+	+	Hypertrophic zone and metaphysis
Excess corticosteroids	Systemic (adrenal glands)	–	–	–	0	Entire growth plate
Growth hormone	Systemic (pituitary)	+ (Through IGF-1 locally)	+ (Slight)	0	0	Proliferative zone
Somatomedins	Systemic local paracrine (liver, chondrocytes)	+	+ (Slight)	0	0	Proliferative zone
Insulin	Systemic (pancreas)	+ (Through IGF-1 receptor)	0	0	0	Proliferative zone
1,25(OH)$_2$-vitamin D$_3$	Systemic (liver, kidney)	0	0	+ Indirect effect serum Ca and PO	0	Hypertrophic zone
24,25(OH)2D$_3$	Systemic (liver, kidney)	+	+ (Collagen II)	0	0	Proliferative zone and hypertrophic zone
Vitamin A	Systemic (diet)	0	0	–	0	Hypertrophic zone
Vitamin C	Systemic (diet)	0	+ (Collagen)	0	+ (Matrix vesicles)	Proliferative zone and hypertrophic zone
EGF	Local paracrine (endothelial cells)	+	– (Collagen)	0	0	Metaphysis
FGF	Local paracrine (endothelial cells)	+	0	0	0	Proliferative zone
PDGF	Local paracrine (platelets)	+	+ (Noncollagenous proteins)	0	0	Proliferative zone
TGF-β	Local paracrine (platelets, chondrocytes)	±	±	0	0	Proliferative zone and hypertrophic zone
BDGF	Local paracrine (bone matrix)	0	+ (Collagen)	0	0	Upper hypertrophic zone
IL-1	Local paracrine (inflammatory cells, synoviocytes)	0	–	++ (Activates tissue metalloproteinases)	0	Entire growth plate
Prostaglandin	Local autocrine	±	+ (Proteoglycan) – (Collagen and alkaline phosphatase)	0	Bone resorption with osteoclasts	Hypertrophic zone and metaphysis

From Simon SR, editor: *Orthopaedic basic science*, ed 2, Rosemont, Ill, 1994, American Academy of Orthopaedic Surgeons, p 196.

+, Increase stimulation; 0, no known effect; –, inhibitory; ±, depending on the local hormonal milieu.
BDGF, Bone-derived growth factor; *EGF,* epidermal growth factor; *FGF,* fibroblast growth factor; *IGF-1,* insulinlike growth factor; *IL-1,* interleukin-1; *PDGF,* platelet-derived growth factor; T_3, triiodothyronine; *TGF-β,* transforming growth factor-β.

Table 1-6	Biological and Mechanical Factors Influencing Fracture Healing	
BIOLOGICAL FACTORS	**MECHANICAL FACTORS**	
Patient age	Soft tissue attachments to bone	
Comorbid medical conditions		
Functional level	Stability (extent of immobilization)	
Nutritional status		
Nerve function	Anatomic location	
Vascular injury	Level of energy imparted	
Hormones	Extent of bone loss	
Growth factors		
Health of the soft tissue envelope		
Sterility (in open fractures)		
Cigarette smoke		
Local pathologic conditions		
Level of energy imparted		
Type of bone affected		
Extent of bone loss		

Table 1-7	Type of Fracture Healing Based on Type of Stabilization
TYPE OF STABILIZATION	**PREDOMINANT TYPE OF HEALING**
Cast (closed treatment)	**Periosteal bridging callus and interfragmentary enchondral ossification**
Compression plate	Primary cortical healing (cutting-cone type or haversian remodeling)
Intramedullary nail	Early: periosteal bridging callus; enchondral ossification Late: medullary callus and intramembranous ossification
External fixator	Dependent on extent of rigidity: Less rigid: periosteal bridging callus; enchondral ossification More rigid: primary cortical healing; intramembranous ossification
Inadequate immobilization with adequate blood supply	Hypertrophic nonunion (failed enchondral ossification); type II collagen predominates
Inadequate immobilization without adequate blood supply	**Atrophic nonunion**
Inadequate reduction with displacement at the fracture site	Oligotrophic nonunion

- Medullary callus supplements the bridging callus, forming more slowly and later.
- Fracture healing varies with treatment method (Table 1-7).
  - In unstable fracture, type II collagen is expressed early, followed by type I collagen.
  - Amount of callus is inversely proportional to extent of immobilization
- Progenitor cell differentiation:
  - High strain promotes development of fibrous tissue.
  - Low strain and high oxygen tension promote development of woven bone.
  - Intermediate strain and low oxygen tension promote development of cartilage.
- Remodeling
  - Remodeling begins in middle of repair phase and continues long after clinically healing (up to 7 years).
  - Allows bone to assume its normal configuration and shape according to stress exposure (Wolff's law)
  - Throughout, woven bone is replaced with lamellar bone.
  - Fracture healing is complete when the marrow space is repopulated.
- Biochemistry of fracture healing (Table 1-8)
- Growth factors of bone (Table 1-9)
  - BMP-2: acute open tibial fractures
  - **BMP-3: no osteogenic activity**
  - **BMP-4: associated with fibrodysplasia ossificans progressiva**
  - BMP-7: tibial nonunions
- Endocrine effects on fracture healing (Table 1-10)
- Head injury
  - Can increase the osteogenic response to fracture

Table 1-8	Biochemical Steps of Fracture Healing
STEP	**COLLAGEN TYPE**
Mesenchymal	I, II, III, V
Chondroid	II, IX
Chondroid-osteoid	I, II, X
Osteogenic	I

Table 1-9	Growth Factors of Bone		
GROWTH FACTOR	**ACTION**		**NOTES**
Bone morphogenetic protein (BMP)	Osteoinductive; stimulates bone formation Induces metaplasia of mesenchymal cells into osteoblasts		Target cells of BMP are the undifferentiated perivascular mesenchymal cells; signal through serine-threonine kinase receptors Intracellular molecules called SMADs serve as signaling mediators for BMPs
Transforming growth factor (TGF)-β	Induces mesenchymal cells to produce type II collagen and proteoglycans Induces osteoblasts to synthesize collagen		Found in fracture hematomas; believed to regulate cartilage and bone formation in fracture callus; signal through serine/threonine kinase receptors Coating porous implants with TGF-β enhances bone ingrowth
Insulinlike growth factor (IGF)-2	Stimulates type I collagen, cellular proliferation, cartilage matrix synthesis, and bone formation		Signal through tyrosine kinase receptors
Platelet-derived growth factor (PDGF)	Attracts inflammatory cells to the fracture site (chemotactic)		Released from platelets; signal through tyrosine kinase receptors

- Nicotine (smoking)
  - Increases time to fracture healing
  - Increases nonunion risk (particularly in the tibia)
  - Decreases fracture callus strength
  - Increases pseudarthrosis risk after lumbar fusion up to 500%
- Nonsteroidal antiinflammatory drugs (NSAIDs)
  - Have adverse effects on fracture healing and healing of lumbar spinal fusions
  - Cyclooxygenase (COX)-2 activity is required for normal enchondral ossification during fracture healing.
- Quinolone antibiotics
  - Toxic to chondrocytes and inhibit fracture healing
- Ultrasonography and fracture healing
  - Low-intensity pulsed ultrasonography accelerates fracture healing and increases the mechanical strength of callus (30 mw/cm^2)
  - A cellular response to the mechanical energy of ultrasonography has been postulated.
- Effect of radiation on bone
  - High-dose irradiation causes long-term changes within the haversian system and decreases cellularity.
- Diet and fracture healing
  - Protein malnutrition results in negative effects in fracture healing:
    - Decreased periosteal and external callus
    - Decreased callus strength and stiffness
    - Increased fibrous tissue within callus
  - In experimental models, oral supplementation with essential amino acids improves bone mineral density in fracture callus.
- Electricity and fracture healing
  - Definitions
    - Stress-generated potentials
      - Piezoelectric effect: tissue charges are displaced secondary to mechanical forces.
      - Streaming potentials: occur when electrically charged fluid is forced over a cell membrane that has a fixed charge
    - Transmembrane potentials: generated by cellular metabolism
  - Types of electrical stimulation
    - **Direct current (DC): stimulates an inflammatory-like response, resulting in decreased oxygen concentrations and increase in tissue pH (similar to an implantable bone stimulator).**
    - Alternating current (AC): "capacity coupled generators"; affects cyclic adenosine monophosphate (cAMP) synthesis, collagen synthesis, and calcification during repair stage
    - Pulsed electromagnetic fields (PEMFs): initiate calcification of fibrocartilage (but not fibrous tissue)
- Pathologic fracture
  - In bone weakened by tumor, infection, or metabolic bone disease
  - Risk factors: pain, anatomic location, and pattern of bony destruction (scoring system of Mirels)
  - Risk for such fractures: highest in subtrochanteric femur
- Bone grafting (Table 1-11)
  - Graft properties
    - Osteoconductive matrix: acts as a scaffold or framework for bone growth
    - Osteoinductive factors: growth factors (BMP) that stimulate bone formation
    - Osteogenic cells: primitive mesenchymal cells, osteoblasts, and osteocytes
    - Structural integrity
  - Overview
    - Autografts (from same person) or allografts (from another person)

Table 1-10	Endocrine Effects on Fracture Healing	
HORMONE	**EFFECT**	**MECHANISM**
Cortisone	−	Decreased callus proliferation
Calcitonin	+?	Unknown
TH, PTH	+	Bone remodeling
Growth hormone	+	Increased callus volume

PTH, Parathyroid hormone; *TH*, thyroid hormone.

Table 1-11	Types of Bone Grafts and Bone Graft Properties				
	PROPERTIES				
GRAFT	**OSTEOCONDUCTION**	**OSTEOINDUCTION**	**OSTEOGENIC CELLS**	**STRUCTURAL INTEGRITY**	**OTHER PROPERTIES**
Autograft					
Cancellous	Excellent	Good	Excellent	Poor	Rapid incorporation
Cortical	Fair	Fair	Fair	Excellent	Slow incorporation
Allograft	Fair	Fair	None	Good	Fresh has the highest immunogenicity
					Freeze dried is the least immunogenic but has the least structural integrity (weakest)
					Fresh frozen preserves BMP
Ceramics	Fair	None	None	Fair	
Demineralized bone matrix	Good	Fair	None	Poor	
Bone marrow	Poor	Poor	Good	Poor	

Modified from Brinker MR, Miller MD: *Fundamentals of orthopaedics*, Philadelphia, 1999, WB Saunders, p 7.
BMP, Bone morphogenetic protein.

- Cancellous bone: for grafting nonunions or cavitary defects; remodels quickly and incorporates through the laying down of new bone on old trabeculae ("creeping substitution")
- Cortical bone: slower to turn over; used for structural defects
- Osteoarticular (osteochondral) allograft used for tumor surgery
  - Immunogenic (cartilage is vulnerable to inflammatory mediators of immune response)
  - Articular cartilage preserved with glycerol or dimethyl sulfoxide (DMSO)
  - Cryogenically preserved grafts (leave few viable chondrocytes)
  - Tissue-matched (syngeneic) osteochondral grafts (produce minimal immunogenic effects and incorporate well)
- Osteoarticular autograft used for cartilage defects
  - Cortical bone becomes incorporated
  - Overlying cartilage remains viable
- Vascularized bone grafts
  - Although technically difficult to implant, allow more rapid union and cell preservation; best for irradiated tissues or large tissue defects (morbidity may occur at donor site [e.g., fibula])
  - Nonvascular bone grafts are more common
- Allograft bone
  - **Fresh: increased immunogenicity**
  - Fresh frozen: less immunogenic than fresh; BMP preserved
  - Freeze dried (lyophilized "croutons"): loses structural integrity and depletes BMP, is least immunogenic, is purely osteoconductive, has lowest risk of viral transmission
  - Bone matrix gelatin (a digested source of BMP): demineralized bone matrix is osteoconductive and osteoinductive.

- Antigenicity
  - Allograft bone possesses a spectrum of potential antigens, primarily from cell surface glycoproteins.
  - Classes I and II cellular antigens in allograft are recognized by T lymphocytes in the host.
  - Primary mechanism of rejection is cellular rather than humoral.
    - Incorporation related to cellularity and major histocompatibility complex (MHC) incompatibility
  - Cellular components that contribute to antigenicity are marrow origin, endothelium, and retinacular activating cells.
    - Marrow cells incite the greatest immunogenic response.
  - Extracellular matrix components that contribute to antigenicity are as follows:
    - Type I collagen (organic matrix): stimulates cell-mediated and humoral responses
    - Noncollagenous matrix (proteoglycans, osteopontin, osteocalcin, other glycoproteins)
  - Hydroxyapatite does not elicit immune response.
- Five stages of graft healing (Urist) (Table 1-12)
  - Factors influencing incorporation (Figure 1-18)

Table 1-12	Stages of Graft Healing
STAGE	**ACTIVITY**
1: Inflammation	Chemotaxis stimulated by necrotic debris
2: Osteoblast differentiation	From precursors
3: Osteoinduction	Osteoblast and osteoclast function
4: Osteoconduction	New bone forming over scaffold
5: Remodeling	Process continues for years

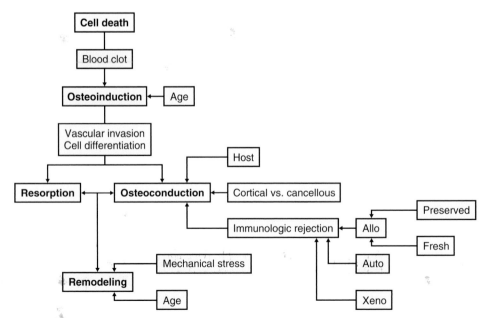

FIGURE 1-18 Major factors influencing bone graft incorporation. *Allo,* Allograft; *Auto,* autograft; *Xeno,* xenograft. (From Simon SR, editor: *Orthopaedic basic science,* Rosemont, Ill, 1994, American Academy of Orthopaedic Surgeons, p 284.)

- Specific bone graft types
  - Cortical bone grafts
    - Slower incorporation: remodels existing haversian systems through resorption (weakens the graft) and then deposits new bone (restores strength)
    - Resorption confined to osteon borders; interstitial lamellae are preserved
    - Used for structural defects
    - Insufficiency fracture eventually occurs in 25% of massive grafts.
  - Cancellous grafts
    - Revascularize and incorporate quickly
    - Osteoblasts lay down new bone on old trabeculae, which are later remodeled ("**creeping substitution**").
  - Demineralized bone matrix
    - Acidic extraction of bone matrix from allograft
    - Osteoconductive without structural support
    - **Minimally osteoinductive despite preservation of osteoinductive molecules**
  - Synthetic bone grafts: calcium, silicon, or aluminum
    - Calcium phosphate–based grafts: capable of osseoconduction and osseointegration
      - Biodegrade very slowly
      - **Highest compressive strength of any graft material**
      - Many prepared as ceramics (heated apatite crystals fuse into crystals [sintered])
        - Tricalcium phosphate
        - Hydroxyapatite; purified bovine dermal fibrillar collagen plus ceramic hydroxyapatite granules and tricalcium phosphate granules
    - Calcium sulfate: osteoconductive
      - Rapidly resorbed
    - Calcium carbonate (chemically unaltered marine coral): resorbed and replaced by bone (osteoconductive)
    - Coralline hydroxyapatite: calcium carbonate skeleton is converted to calcium phosphate through a thermoexchange process.
    - Silicate-based incorporate silicon as silicate (silicon dioxide); bioactive glasses and glass-ionomer cement
    - Aluminum oxide: alumina ceramic bonds to bone in response to stress and strain between implant and bone
- Distraction osteogenesis
  - Definition: distraction-stimulated formation of bone
  - Clinical applications:
    - Limb lengthening
    - Hypertrophic nonunions
    - Deformity correction (via differential lengthening)
    - Segmental bone loss (via bone transport)
  - Biological features:
    - Under optimal stability, intramembranous ossification occurs.
    - Under instability, bone forms through enchondral ossification.
      - Pseudarthrosis may occur under extreme instability.
    - Three histologic phases:
      - Latency phase (5-7 days)
      - **Distraction phase (1 mm/day [≈1 inch/mo])**
      - Consolidation phase (typically twice as long as distraction phase)
  - Optimal conditions during distraction osteogenesis:
    - Low-energy corticotomy/osteotomy
    - Minimal soft tissue stripping at corticotomy site (preserves blood supply)
    - Stable external fixation and elimination of torsion, shear, and bending moments
    - Latency period (no lengthening) 5 to 7 days
    - Distraction: 0.25 mm three or four times per day (0.75-1.0 mm/day)
    - Neutral fixation interval (no distraction) during consolidation
    - Normal physiologic use of the extremity, including weight bearing
- Heterotopic ossification
  - Ectopic bone forms in soft tissues.
    - Most commonly in response to injury or surgical dissection
    - Myositis ossificans: heterotopic ossification in muscle
  - Increased risk with traumatic brain injury
    - Recurrence after resection is likely if neurologic compromise is severe.
    - Timing of surgery for heterotopic ossification after traumatic brain injury is important:
      - Time since injury (3-6 months)
      - Evidence of bone maturation on radiographs (sharp demarcation, trabecular pattern)
  - Heterotopic ossification may be resected after total hip arthroplasty (THA).
    - Resection should be delayed for 6 months or longer after THA.
    - Adjuvant radiation therapy may prevent recurrence of heterotopic ossification.
    - Optimal therapy: single postoperative dose of 600 to 700 rad
    - Prevents proliferation and differentiation of primordial mesenchymal cells into osteoprogenitor cells
  - Preoperative radiation (600-800 rad) may be used in treatment.
    - Helps prevent heterotopic ossification after THA in patients at high risk for this development
    - Incidence of heterotopic ossification after THA among patients with Paget disease is approximately 50%.
  - When oral bisphosphonate therapy is discontinued, heterotopic ossification may occur.
    - Oral bisphosphonate inhibits mineralization.
      - However, it does not prevent formation of osteoid matrix.

- **Normal bone metabolism**
- Calcium
  - Important in muscle and nerve function, clotting, and many other areas
  - More than 99% of the body's calcium is stored in bones.
    - Plasma calcium is about equally free and bound (usually to albumin).
    - Approximately 400 mg of calcium is released from bone daily.
  - Absorbed in the duodenum by active transport
    - Requires ATP and calcium-binding protein
    - Regulated by $1,25(OH)_2$-vitamin D_3

- Absorbed in the jejunum by passive diffusion
- Kidney reabsorbs 98% of calcium (60% in proximal tubule)
  - Calcium may be excreted in stool.
- Primary homeostatic regulators of serum calcium are PTH and $1,25(OH)_2$-vitamin D_3
- Dietary requirement of elemental calcium:
  - Approximately 600 mg/day for children
  - **Approximately 1300 mg/day for adolescents and young adults (ages 10-25 years)**
  - 750 mg/day for adults (ages 25-50 years)
  - **1200-1500 over the age of 50**
  - 1500 mg/day for pregnant women
  - 2000 mg/day for lactating women
  - **1500 mg/day for postmenopausal women and for patients with a healing fracture in a long bone**
- Calcium balance is usually positive in the first three decades of life and negative after the fourth decade.
- Phosphate
  - A key component of bone mineral
    - Approximately 85% of the body's phosphate stores are in bone.
    - Plasma phosphate is mostly unbound.
  - Also important in enzyme systems and molecular interactions as a metabolite and buffer
  - Dietary intake of phosphate is usually adequate.
    - Daily requirement is 1000 to 1500 mg.
  - Reabsorbed by the kidney (proximal tubule)
    - Phosphate may be excreted in urine.
- Parathyroid hormone
  - PTH is an 84–amino acid peptide
    - Synthesized in and secreted from **chief cells** of the (four) parathyroid glands
    - N-terminal fragment 1-34 is the active portion.

- **Teriparatide, the synthetic form of recombinant human PTH, contains this active sequence.**
  - Used to treat some forms of osteoporosis
  - Increased risk of osteosarcoma
- Effect of PTH mediated by the cAMP second-messenger mechanism downstream in osteocytes
- PTH helps regulate plasma calcium.
  - Decreased calcium levels in extracellular fluid stimulate β_2 receptors to release PTH, which acts at the intestines, kidneys, and bones (Table 1-13).
- PTH directly activates osteoblasts.
- PTH modulates renal phosphate filtration.
- PTH may accentuate bone loss in elderly persons.
- PTH-related protein and its receptor have been implicated in metaphyseal dysplasia.
- Vitamin D
  - Naturally occurring steroid
    - Activated by ultraviolet radiation from sunlight or utilized from dietary intake (Figure 1-19)
  - Hydroxylated to $25(OH)$-vitamin D_3 in the liver and hydroxylated a second time in the kidney to one of the following:
    - $1,25(OH)_2$-vitamin D_3, the active hormone
    - $24,25(OH)_2$-vitamin D_3, the inactive form (Figure 1-20)
  - $1,25(OH)_2$-vitamin D_3 works at the intestines, kidneys, and bones (see Table 1-13).
  - Phenytoin (Dilantin) impairs metabolism of vitamin D.
- Calcitonin
  - A 32–amino acid peptide hormone produced by **clear cells** in the parafollicles of the thyroid gland
  - Limited role in calcium regulation (see Table 1-13)
  - Increased extracellular calcium levels cause secretion of calcitonin.

Table 1-13 Regulation of Calcium and Phosphate Metabolism

PARAMETER	PTH (PEPTIDE)	1,25(OH)2D (STEROID)	CALCITONIN (PEPTIDE)
Origin	Chief cells of parathyroid glands	Proximal tubule of kidney	Parafollicular cells of thyroid gland
Factors stimulating production	Decreased serum Ca^{2+}	Elevated PTH level Decreased serum Ca^{2+} level Decreased serum P_i	Elevated serum Ca^{2+} level
Factors inhibiting production	Elevated serum Ca^{2+} Elevated $1,25(OH)_2D$	Decreased PTH Elevated serum Ca^{2+} Elevated serum P_i	Decreased serum Ca^{2+}
Effect on end-organs for hormone action			
Intestine	No direct effect Acts indirectly on bowel by stimulating production of $1,25(OH)_2D$ in kidney	Strongly stimulates intestinal absorption of Ca^{2+} and P_i	?
Kidney	Stimulates $25(OH)D$ 1α-hydroxylase in mitochondria of proximal tubular cells to convert $25(OH)D$ to $1,25(OH)_2D$ Increases fractional resorption of filtered Ca^{2+} Promotes urinary excretion of P_i	?	?
Bone	Stimulates osteoclastic resorption of bone Stimulates recruitment of preosteoclasts	Strongly stimulates osteoclastic resorption of bone	Inhibits osteoclastic resorption of bone ? Role in normal human physiology
Net effect on Ca^{2+} and P_i concentrations in extracellular fluid and serum	Increased serum Ca^{2+} level Decreased serum P_i level	Increased serum Ca^{2+} level Increased serum P_i level	Decreased serum Ca^{2+} level (transient)

Adapted from Netter FH: *CIBA collection of medical illustrations*, vol 8: *Musculoskeletal system*, part I: *Anatomy, physiology and developmental disorders*, Basel, Switzerland, 1987, CIBA, p 179.
1,25(OH)₂D, 1,25-dihydroxyvitamin D; *25(OH)D*, 25-hydroxyvitamin D; *Pᵢ*, inorganic phosphate; *PTH*, parathyroid hormone.

- Controlled by a β_2 receptor
- Inhibits osteoclastic bone resorption
  - Osteoclasts have calcitonin receptors.
  - Calcitonin decreases osteoclast number and activity.
- Decreases serum calcium level
- May also have a role in fracture healing and in reducing vertebral compression fractures in high-turnover osteoporosis
- Other hormones affecting bone metabolism
  - Estrogen
    - Prevents bone loss by inhibiting bone resorption
      - Decrease in urinary pyridinoline cross-links
    - Because bone formation and resorption are coupled, estrogen therapy also decreases bone formation.
    - Supplementation is helpful in postmenopausal women only if started within 5 to 10 years after onset of menopause.
      - Risk of endometrial cancer is reduced when estrogen therapy is combined with cyclic progestin therapy.
    - Certain regimens of hormone replacement therapy may increase risk of heart disease and breast cancer.
    - Other postmenopausal pharmacologic interventions (alendronate, raloxifene) should be strongly considered.
  - Corticosteroids
    - Increase bone loss
      - Decrease gut absorption of calcium by decreasing binding proteins

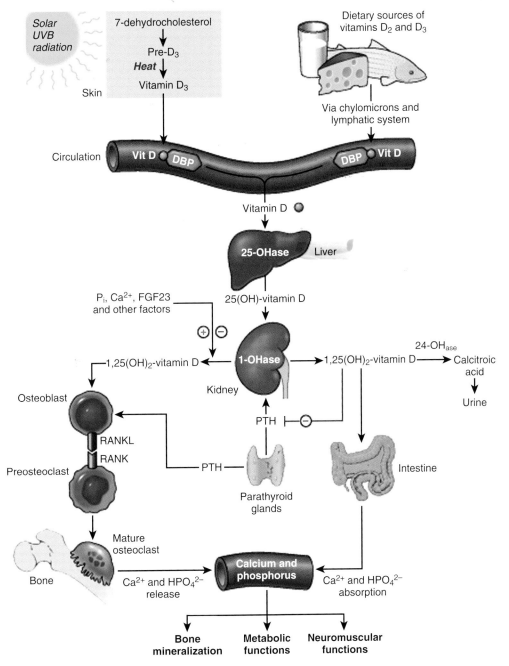

FIGURE 1-19 Vitamin D metabolism. *1,25(OH)₂D*, 1,25-dihydroxyvitamin D; *25(OH)D*, 25-hydroxyvitamin D; *DBP*, vitamin D–binding protein; *FGF23*, fibroblast growth factor 23; *OHₐₛₑ*, 1α-hydroxylase; *Pᵢ*, inorganic phosphate; *PTH*, parathyroid hormone; *UVB*, ultraviolet B. (From Kumar V et al, editors: *Robbins and Cotran pathologic basis of disease*, Philadelphia, 2010, Saunders.)

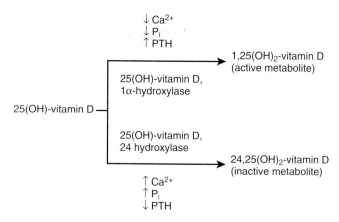

FIGURE 1-20 Vitamin D metabolism in the renal tubular cell. *P$_i$,* Inorganic phosphate; *PTH,* parathyroid hormone. (From Simon SR, editor: *Orthopaedic basic science,* Rosemont, Ill, 1994, American Academy of Orthopaedic Surgeons, p 165.)

- Decrease bone formation (cancellous more than cortical) by inhibiting collagen synthesis and osteoblast productivity
    - Do not affect mineralization
  - Alternate-day therapy may reduce the effects.
- Thyroid hormones
  - Affect bone resorption more than bone formation
    - Large (thyroid-suppressive) doses of thyroxine can lead to osteoporosis.
  - Regulates skeletal growth at the physis
    - Stimulates chondrocyte growth, type X collagen synthesis, and alkaline phosphatase activity
- Growth hormone
  - Causes positive calcium balance by increasing gut absorption of calcium more than it increases urinary excretion
  - Insulin and somatomedins participate in this effect.
- Growth factors
  - Transforming growth factor (TGF)-β, PDGF, monokines, and lymphokines have roles in bone and cartilage repair.
- Interactions
  - Calcium and phosphate metabolism
    - Affected by an elaborate interplay of hormones and the levels of the metabolites themselves
  - Feedback mechanisms: important in the regulation of plasma levels of calcium and phosphate
- Bone aging
  - Peak bone mass
    - Believed to occur between 16 and 25 years of age
    - Higher in men and in African Americans
  - After peak, bone loss occurs at a rate of 0.3% to 0.5% per year
    - Rate of bone loss is 2% to 3% per year in untreated women during the sixth through tenth years after menopause.
    - Affects trabecular more than cortical bone
      - Increase in trabecular rods results in increased anisotropy.
      - Cortical bone becomes thinner and intracortical porosities increase.
      - Cortical bone becomes more brittle, less strong, and less stiff.
  - Long bones have increased inner and outer diameter.

- Bone loss
  - Occurs at the onset of menopause when both bone formation and resorption are accelerated
    - A net negative change in calcium balance: menopause decreases intestinal absorption and increases urinary excretion of calcium
  - Both urinary hydroxyproline and pyridinoline cross-links are elevated when bone resorption occurs.
  - Serum alkaline phosphatase level is elevated when bone formation is increased.
  - Estrogen therapy is recommended for patients at high risk for osteoporosis.
    - Decreases urinary pyridinoline (decreased bone resorption)
    - Decreases serum alkaline phosphatase (decreased bone formation)
    - Increases bone density of the femoral neck, reducing the rate of hip fracture

- **Conditions of bone mineralization (Tables 1-14 through 1-18)**
- Hypercalcemia
  - Can manifest in a number of ways:
    - Polyuria
    - Polydipsia
    - Kidney stones
    - Excessive bony resorption with or without fibrotic tissue replacement (osteitis fibrosa cystica)
    - Central nervous system (CNS) effects (confusion, stupor, weakness)
    - Gastrointestinal (GI) effects (constipation)
  - Can also cause anorexia, nausea, vomiting, dehydration, and muscle weakness
  - Primary hyperparathyroidism
    - Overproduction of PTH usually a result of a parathyroid adenoma (surgical parathyroidectomy is curative)
      - Generally affects only one parathyroid gland
    - Reflected in a net increase in plasma calcium and a decrease in plasma phosphate (as a result of enhanced urinary excretion)
    - Increased osteoclastic resorption and failure of repair attempts (poor mineralization as a result of low phosphate level)
    - Diagnosis
      - Signs and symptoms of hypercalcemia
      - Characteristic laboratory results
        - Increased serum calcium, PTH, urinary phosphate
        - Decreased serum phosphate
    - Bony changes
      - Osteopenia
      - Osteitis fibrosa cystica (fibrous replacement of marrow)
        - "Brown tumors" (Figure 1-21): increased giant cells, extravasation of RBCs, hemosiderin staining, fibrous tissue hemosiderin
      - Chondrocalcinosis
    - Radiographs
      - Deformed, osteopenic bones
      - Fractures
      - "Shaggy" trabeculae
      - Radiolucent areas (phalanges, distal clavicle, skull)
      - Destructive metaphyseal lesions
      - Calcification of soft tissues
    - Histologic changes

Table 1-14	Overview of Clinical and Radiographic Aspects of Metabolic Bone Diseases		
DISEASE	**CAUSE**	**CLINICAL FINDINGS**	**RADIOGRAPHIC FINDINGS**
Hypercalcemia			
Hyperparathyroidism	PTH overproduction: adenoma	Kidney stone, hyperreflexia	Osteopenia, osteitis fibrosa cystica
Familial syndromes	PTH overproduction: MEN/renal	Endocrine and renal abnormalities	Osteopenia
Hypocalcemia			
Hypoparathyroidism	PTH underproduction: idiopathic	Neuromuscular irritability, cataracts	Calcified basal ganglia
PHP/Albright syndrome	PTH receptor abnormality	Short MC/MT, obesity	Brachydactyly, exostosis
Renal osteodystrophy	CRF: ↓ phosphate excretion	Renal abnormalities	"Rugger jersey" spine
Rickets (osteomalacia)			
Vitamin D–deficiency rickets	↓ Vitamin D diet; malabsorption	Bone deformities, hypotonia	"Rachitic rosary," wide growth plates, fractures
Vitamin D–dependent (types I and II) rickets	See Table 1-15	Total baldness	Poor mineralization
Vitamin D–resistant (hypophosphatemic) rickets	↓ Renal tubular phosphate resorption	Bone deformities, hypotonia	Poor mineralization
Hypophosphatasia	↓ Alkaline phosphatase	Bone deformities, hypotonia	Poor mineralization
Osteopenia			
Osteoporosis	↓ Estrogen: ↓ bone mass	Kyphosis, fractures	Compression vertebral fractures, hip fractures
Scurvy	Vitamin C deficiency: defective collagen	Fatigue, bleeding, effusions	Thin cortices, corner sign
Osteodensity			
Paget disease of bone	Osteoclastic abnormality: ↑ bone turnover	Deformities, pain, CHF, fractures	Coarse trabeculae, "picture-frame" vertebrae
Osteopetrosis	Osteoclastic abnormality: unclear	Hepatosplenomegaly, anemia	Bone within bone

↓, Decreased; ↑, increased; *CHF,* congestive heart failure; *CRF,* chronic renal failure; *MC,* metacarpal; *MEN,* multiple endocrine neoplasia; *MT,* metatarsal; *PHP,* pseudohypoparathyroidism; *PTH,* parathyroid hormone.

- Osteoblasts and osteoclasts active on both sides of the trabeculae (as in Paget disease)
- Areas of destruction
- Wide osteoid seams
- Other causes of hypercalcemia
  - Familial syndromes
    - Pituitary adenomas associated with multiple endocrine neoplasia (MEN) types I and II
    - Familial hypocalciuric hypercalcemia
      - Poor renal clearance of calcium
  - Other disorders
    - Malignancy (most common)
      - Can be life threatening; commonly associated with muscle weakness
      - Initial treatment should include hydration with normal saline (reverses dehydration).
      - Can occur in the absence of extensive bone metastasis
      - **Most commonly results from release of systemic growth factors and cytokines that stimulate osteoclastic bone resorption at bony sites not involved in the tumor process (RANKL pathway)**
    - PTH-related protein secretion (lung carcinoma)
    - Lytic bone metastases and lesions (e.g., multiple myeloma)
    - Hyperthyroidism
    - Vitamin D intoxication
    - Prolonged immobilization
    - Addison disease
    - Steroid administration
    - Peptic ulcer disease (milk-alkali syndrome)
    - Kidney disease
    - Sarcoidosis
    - Hypophosphatasia
  - Treatment of hypercalcemia
    - Hydration (saline diuresis)
    - Loop diuretics
    - Dialysis (for severe cases)
    - Mobilization (prevents further bone resorption)
    - Specific drugs (bisphosphonates, mithramycin, calcitonin, and gallium nitrate)
- Hypocalcemia (Figure 1-22)
  - Findings
    - Low plasma calcium
    - Results from low levels of PTH or vitamin D_3
    - Neuromuscular irritability (tetany, seizures, Chvostek sign), cataracts, fungal nail infections, electrocardiographic (ECG) changes (prolonged QT interval), and other signs and symptoms
  - Hypoparathyroidism
    - Decreased PTH level causes decrease in plasma calcium level and increase in plasma phosphate level
      - Urinary excretion not enhanced because of the lack of PTH
    - Common findings:
      - Fungal nail infections
      - Hair loss
      - Blotchy skin (pigment loss, vitiligo)
    - Skull radiographs may show basal ganglia calcification.
    - Iatrogenic hypoparathyroidism most commonly follows thyroidectomy.

Text continued on p. 30

Table 1-15 Laboratory Findings and Clinical Data Regarding Patients with Metabolic Bone Diseases Causing Hypercalcemia

DISORDER	CHANGES IN LEVEL OR CONCENTRATION						OTHER FINDINGS OR POSSIBLE FINDINGS	TREATMENT	COMMENTS
	SERUM CALCIUM	SERUM PHOS	ALK PHOS	PTH	25(OH)-VITAMIN D	1,25(OH)₂-VITAMIN D	URINARY CALCIUM			
Primary hyperparathyroidism	↑	None or ↓	None or ↑	↑	None	None or ↑	↑	Active turnover observed on bone biopsy with peritrabecular fibrosis Brown tumors	Surgical excision of parathyroid edema Treat hypercalcemia (see text)	Most commonly caused by parathyroid adenoma Because PTH stimulates conversion of the inactive form to the active form [1,25(OH)₂-vitamin D] in the kidney, ↑ production of PTH leads to ↑ levels of 1,25(OH)₂-vitamin D
Malignancy with bony metastases	↑	None or ↑	None or ↑	None or ↓	None	None or ↓	↑	Destructive lesions in bone	Treat cancer and hypercalcemia (see text)	↑ Calcium levels may lead to ↓ PTH production through feedback mechanism ↓ 1,25(OH)₂-vitamin D levels result from ↓ PTH (responsible for conversion of inactive to active form of vitamin D in the kidney) Patients with multiple myeloma display abnormal urinary and serum protein electrophoresis
Hyperthyroidism	↑	None	None	None or ↓	None	None	↑	↑ Free thyroxin index ↓ Thyroid-stimulating hormone Tachycardia, tremors	Treat hyperthyroidism	↑ Calcium levels caused by ↑ bone turnover (hypermetabolic state)
Vitamin D intoxication	↑	None or ↑	None or ↑	None or ↓	↑↑↑	None	↑		Normalize vitamin D intake and levels	History of excessive vitamin D intake Dietary vitamin D is converted to 25(OH)-vitamin D in the liver; very high concentrations of 25(OH)-vitamin D cross-react with intestinal vitamin D receptors to ↑ resorption of calcium and cause hypercalcemia

↓, Decreased; ↑, increased; *Alk,* alkaline; *BUN,* blood urea nitrogen; *Phos,* phosphatase; *PTH,* parathyroid hormone.

Table 1-16 Laboratory Findings and Clinical Data Regarding Patients with Metabolic Bone Diseases Causing Hypocalcemia

DISORDER	CHANGES IN LEVEL OR CONCENTRATION							OTHER FINDINGS OR POSSIBLE FINDINGS	TREATMENT	COMMENTS
	SERUM CALCIUM	SERUM PHOS	ALK PHOS	PTH	25(OH)-VITAMIN D	1,25(OH)$_2$-VITAMIN D	URINARY CALCIUM			
Hypoparathyroidism	↓	↑	None	↓	None	↓	↓	Basal ganglia calcification; Hypocalcemic findings	Calcium and vitamin D supplementation	↓ PTH production most commonly follows surgical ablation of the thyroid (with the parathyroid) gland. ↓ PTH leads to ↓ serum calcium and ↑ serum phosphate (as result of ↓ urinary excretion of phosphate). Because PTH stimulates conversion from the inactive to the active form of vitamin D (in the kidney), 1,25(OH)$_2$-vitamin D is also ↓
Pseudohypoparathyroidism	↓	↑	None or ↑	None or ↑	None	↓	↓	Hypocalcemic findings	Calcium and vitamin D supplementation	PTH has no effect on the target cells (in the kidney, bone, and intestine) because of a PTH receptor abnormality. Leads to a ↓ in the active form of vitamin D. Therefore, serum calcium levels are ↓ as result of (1) lack of effect of PTH on bone and (2) ↓ levels of 1,25(OH)$_2$-vitamin D
Renal osteodystrophy (high-turnover bone disease resulting from renal disease [secondary hyperparathyroidism])	↓ or none	↑↑↑	↑	↑↑↑	None	↓	—	Findings of secondary hyperparathyroidism: "rugger jersey" spine; Osteitis fibrosa; Amyloidosis	1. Correct underlying renal abnormality 2. Maintain normal serum phosphorous and calcium 3. Dietary phosphate restriction 4. Phosphate-binding antacid (calcium carbonate) 5. Administration of the active form of vitamin D: 1,25(OH)$_2$-vitamin D (calcitriol)	↓ Renal phosphorus excretion leads to hyperphosphatemia. Phosphorus retention leads to ↓ serum calcium and ↑↑ PTH (which can lead to secondary hyperparathyroidism). Elevated BUN and creatinine levels. Associated with long-term hemodialysis
Renal osteodystrophy (low-turnover bone disease due to renal disease [aluminum toxicity])	↑ or none	None or ↑	↑	None or mildly elevated	None	↓	—	"Rugger jersey" spine; Osteitis fibrosa; Amyloidosis; Osteomalacia may be observed	Treat the urinary obstruction or kidney disease	PTH levels may be suppressed because of (1) frequent episodes of hypercalcemia and (2) direct inhibitory effect of aluminum on PTH. No secondary hyperparathyroidism is present. Elevated BUN and creatinine levels. Associated with long-term hemodialysis

↓, Decreased; ↑, increased; *Alk*, alkaline; *BUN*, blood urea nitrogen; *Phos*, phosphatase; *PTH*, parathyroid hormone.

Table 1-17 Laboratory Findings and Clinical Data Regarding Patients with Rickets and Related Diseases

DISORDER	CHANGES IN LEVEL OR CONCENTRATION							OTHER FINDINGS OR POSSIBLE FINDINGS	TREATMENT	COMMENTS
	SERUM CALCIUM	SERUM PHOS	ALK PHOS	PTH	25(OH)-VITAMIN D	1,25(OH)$_2$-VITAMIN D	URINARY CALCIUM			
Nutritional rickets: vitamin D deficiency	↓ or none	↓	↑	↑	↓	↓	↓	Osteomalacia, hypotonia, Muscle weakness, tetany, Bowing deformities of the long bones, Rachitic rosary	Oral vitamin D (1500–5000 IU/day)	With ↓ vitamin D intake, intestinal calcium and phosphate absorption is reduced, leading to hypocalcemia. ↓ Serum calcium stimulates ↑ PTH (secondary hyperparathyroidism), which leads to bone resorption and ↑ serum calcium (toward or to normal levels). Sources of vitamin D include sunlight, fish-liver foods, and fortified milk
Nutritional rickets: calcium deficiency	↓ or none	↓	↑	↑	None	↑ or none	↓	Clinical findings similar to those for vitamin D deficiency	Oral calcium (700 mg/day)	Hypocalcemia leads to secondary hyperparathyroidism. ↑ PTH leads to enhanced renal conversion of 25(OH)-vitamin D to 1,25(OH)$_2$-vitamin D
Nutritional rickets: phosphate deficiency	None	↓	↑	None	None	↑↑↑	None	No changes of secondary hyperparathyroidism are observed	Oral supplementation of phosphate	Neither secondary hyperparathyroidism nor vitamin D deficiency is present. ↓ Serum phosphate leads to ↑ renal production of 1,25(OH)$_2$-vitamin D
Hereditary vitamin D–dependent rickets type I ("pseudo–vitamin D deficiency")	↓	↓	↑	↑	None or ↑	↓↓↓	↓	Osteomalacia, Clinical findings similar to (but more severe than) those of nutritional rickets caused by vitamin D deficiency	Oral physiologic doses (1–2 µg/day) of 1,25(OH)$_2$-vitamin D	There is a defect in renal 25(OH)-vitamin D 1α-hydroxylase. This enzymatic defect inhibits conversion from the inactive form [25(OH)-vitamin D] to the active form [1,25(OH)$_2$-vitamin D] of vitamin D in the kidney
Hereditary vitamin D–dependent rickets type II ["hereditary resistance to 1,25(OH)$_2$-vitamin D"]	↓	↓	↑	↑	None or ↑	↑↑↑	↓	Osteomalacia, Alopecia, Clinical findings similar to (but more severe than) nutritional rickets caused by vitamin D deficiency	Long-term (3–6 months) daily administration of high-dose vitamin D analogue [1,25(OH)$_2$-vitamin D or (OH)-vitamin D 1α-hydroxylase] plus 3 g/day of elemental calcium	There is an intracellular receptor defect for 1,25(OH)$_2$-vitamin D. Patients with this disorder have the highest 1,25(OH)$_2$-vitamin D levels observed in humans; this ↑↑↑ level of 1,25(OH)$_2$-vitamin D distinguishes hereditary vitamin D–dependent rickets type II from type I, in which the level of 1,25(OH)$_2$-vitamin D is ↓↓↓
Hypophosphatemic rickets (also known as vitamin D-resistant rickets and "phosphate diabetes"; Albright syndrome is an example of a hypophosphatemic syndrome)	None	↓↓↓	↑	None	None	None	None or ↑	Osteomalacia, No changes of secondary hyperparathyroidism, Classic triad: 1. Hypophosphatemia 2. Lower limb deformities 3. Stunted growth rate	Oral administration of elemental phosphate (1–3 g/day) plus high-dose vitamin D (20,000–70,000 IU/day). Vitamin D administration is needed to counterbalance the hypocalcemic effect of phosphate administration, which otherwise could lead to severe secondary hyperparathyroidism	There is an inborn error in phosphate transport (probably located in the proximal nephron); this leads to failure of reabsorption of phosphate in the kidney and "spilling" of phosphate (phosphate diabetes) in the urine. Although the absolute levels of 1,25(OH)$_2$-vitamin D are normal, they are inappropriately low with regard to the degree of phosphaturia; production of 1,25(OH)$_2$-vitamin D is normally stimulated by ↓ serum phosphorous (see Table 1-13). This is the most commonly encountered form of rickets
Hypophosphatasia	↑	↑	↓↓↓	None	None	None		Osteomalacia, Early loss of teeth	There is no established medical therapy	There is an inborn error in the tissue-nonspecific (kidney, bone, liver) isoenzyme of alkaline phosphatase. Elevated urinary phosphoethanolamine is diagnostic

Table 1-18   Differential Diagnosis of Metabolic Bone Diseases, Based on Blood Chemistry Findings

CALCIUM LEVEL			PHOSPHORUS LEVEL		
INCREASED	**DECREASED**	**NORMAL**	**INCREASED**	**DECREASED**	**NORMAL**

CALCIUM LEVEL

INCREASED
- Primary hyperparathyroidism
- Hyperthyroidism
- Vitamin D intoxication
- Malignancy without bony metastasis
- Malignancy with bony metastasis
- Multiple myeloma
- Lymphoma
- Sarcoidosis
- Milk-alkali syndrome
- Severe generalized immobilization
- Multiple endocrine neoplasias
- Addison disease
- Steroid administration
- Peptic ulcer disease
- Hypophosphatasia
- Primary hyperparathyroidism
- Pseudohypoparathyroidism
- Renal osteodystrophy
- Nutritional rickets: vitamin D deficiency
- Nutritional rickets: calcium deficiency
- Hereditary vitamin D–dependent rickets (types I and II)

DECREASED
- Hypoparathyroidism
- Pseudohypoparathyroidism
- Renal osteodystrophy (high-turnover bone disease)
- Nutritional rickets: vitamin D deficiency
- Nutritional rickets: calcium deficiency
- Nutritional rickets: phosphate deficiency
- Hereditary vitamin D–dependent rickets (types I and II)
- Malignancy with bony metastasis
- Malignancy without bony metastasis
- Multiple myeloma
- Lymphoma
- Hyperthyroidism
- Vitamin D intoxication
- Hypoparathyroidism
- Sarcoidosis
- Milk-alkali syndrome
- Severe generalized immobilization

NORMAL
- Osteoporosis
- Pseudohypoparathyroidism
- Nutritional rickets: vitamin D deficiency
- Nutritional rickets: calcium deficiency
- Nutritional rickets: phosphate deficiency
- Hypophosphatemic rickets
- Osteoporosis
- Malignancy with bony metastasis
- Multiple myeloma
- Lymphoma
- Vitamin D intoxication
- Pseudohypoparathyroidism
- Renal osteodystrophy (only low-turnover bone disease)
- Nutritional rickets: phosphate deficiency
- Hypophosphatemic rickets
- Hypophosphatasia
- Sarcoidosis
- Hyperthyroidism
- Milk-alkali syndrome
- Severe generalized immobilization

PHOSPHORUS LEVEL

INCREASED
- Malignancy with bony metastasis
- Multiple myeloma
- Lymphoma
- Vitamin D intoxication
- Hypoparathyroidism
- Pseudohypoparathyroidism
- Renal osteodystrophy
- Hypophosphatasia
- Sarcoidosis
- Milk-alkali syndrome
- Severe generalized immobilization
- Primary hyperparathyroidism
- Nutritional rickets: calcium deficiency
- Nutritional rickets: phosphate deficiency
- Hereditary vitamin D–dependent rickets type II
- Sarcoidosis

DECREASED
- Primary hyperparathyroidism
- Malignancy without bony metastasis
- Nutritional rickets: vitamin D deficiency
- Nutritional rickets: calcium deficiency
- Nutritional rickets: phosphate deficiency
- Hereditary vitamin D–dependent rickets (types I and II)
- Hypophosphatemic rickets
- Malignancy with bony metastasis
- Malignancy without bony metastasis
- Multiple myeloma
- Lymphoma
- Hypoparathyroidism
- Pseudohypoparathyroidism
- Renal osteodystrophy
- Nutritional rickets: vitamin D deficiency
- Hereditary vitamin D–dependent rickets type I

NORMAL
- Osteoporosis
- Primary hyperparathyroidism
- Malignancy with bony metastasis
- Multiple myeloma
- Lymphoma
- Hyperthyroidism
- Vitamin D intoxication
- Renal osteodystrophy (only low-turnover bone disease)
- Sarcoidosis
- Milk-alkali syndrome
- Severe generalized immobilization
- Osteoporosis
- Primary hyperparathyroidism
- Malignancy with bony metastasis
- Multiple myeloma
- Lymphoma
- Hyperthyroidism
- Vitamin D intoxication
- Nutritional rickets: calcium deficiency
- Hypophosphatemic rickets
- Hypophosphatasia

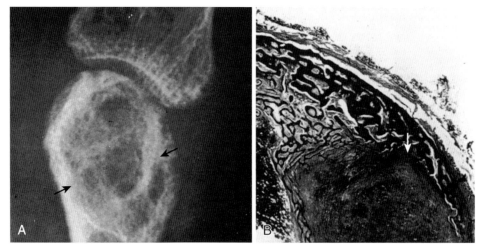

FIGURE 1-21 Radiograph **(A)** and photomicrograph **(B)** showing delineation of brown tumor *(arrows)* of hyperparathyroidism. (From Resnick D, Kransdorf MJ, editors: *Bone and joint imaging,* ed 3, Philadelphia, 2005, Saunders, p 608.)

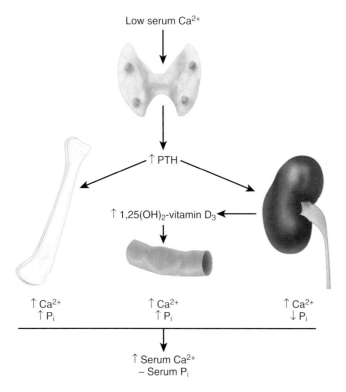

FIGURE 1-22 Body's reaction to hypocalcemia, with consequent resorption of bone. When calcium level falls, parathyroid hormone (PTH) is secreted, which releases calcium and inorganic phosphate (P_i) from bone. PTH increases renal reabsorption of calcium while inhibiting phosphate reabsorption. These actions in combination restore calcium concentration. If hypocalcemia persists, PTH stimulates renal production of 1,25(OH)$_2$-vitamin D$_3$, which increases intestinal calcium absorption. (From Goldman L, Ausiello D, editors: *Cecil medicine,* ed 23, Philadelphia, 2008, Saunders Elsevier.)

- Pseudohypoparathyroidism (PHP)
  - A rare genetic disorder caused by lack of effect of PTH on the target cells
  - PTH is normal or high.
  - PTH action is blocked by an abnormality at the receptor, by the cAMP system, or by a lack of required cofactors (e.g., Mg^{2+})
  - Defect in *GNAS* gene from mother

- Albright hereditary osteodystrophy, a form of PHP
  - Short first, fourth, and fifth metacarpals and metatarsals
  - Brachydactyly
  - Exostoses
  - Obesity
  - Diminished intelligence
- Pseudo-pseudohypoparathyroidism (pseudo-PHP)
  - Normocalcemic disorder that is phenotypically similar to PHP
  - However, response to PTH is normal
- Renal osteodystrophy (Figure 1-23)
  - A spectrum of bone mineral metabolism disorders in chronic renal disease.
  - Due to impaired excretion, which compromises mineral homeostasis
  - Leads to abnormalities in bone mineral metabolism
  - High-turnover renal bone disease
    - Chronically elevated serum PTH level leads to secondary hyperparathyroidism (hyperplasia of parathyroid gland chief cells).
    - Factors contributing to sustained increased PTH and secondary hyperparathyroidism include:
      - Diminished renal phosphorus excretion; phosphorus retention promotes PTH secretion by three mechanisms:
        - Hyperphosphatemia lowers serum calcium, stimulating PTH.
        - Phosphorus impairs renal 1α-hydroxylase activity, impairing production of 1,25(OH)$_2$-vitamin D$_3$.
        - Phosphorus retention may directly increase the synthesis of PTH.
          - Hypocalcemia
          - Impaired renal calcitriol [1,25(OH)$_2$-vitamin D$_3$]
          - Alterations in the control of *PTH* gene transcription secretion
          - Skeletal resistance to the actions of PTH
  - Low-turnover renal bone disease (adynamic lesion of bone and osteomalacia)
    - Secondary hyperparathyroidism is not characteristic with this condition.
      - Serum PTH level is normal or mildly elevated.

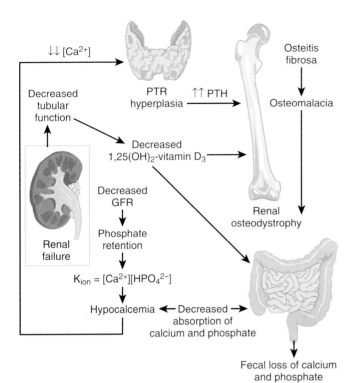

FIGURE 1-23 Pathogenesis of bony changes in renal osteodystrophy. *GFR,* Glomerular filtration rate; *PTR,* proximal tubule reabsorption. (From McPherson RA, Pincus MR, editors: *Henry's clinical diagnosis and management by laboratory methods,* ed 21, Philadelphia, 2007, Saunders Elsevier.)

- Bone formation and turnover are reduced.
- Excess deposition of aluminum into bone (aluminum toxicity) negatively affects bone mineral metabolism.
  - Impairs differentiation of precursor cells to osteoblasts
  - Impairs proliferation of osteoblasts
  - Impairs PTH release from the parathyroid gland
  - Disrupts the mineralization process
  - Adynamic lesion: accounts for the majority of cases of low-turnover bone disease in patients with chronic renal failure
  - Osteomalacia: defects in mineralization of newly formed bone
- Radiographs may demonstrate a "rugger jersey" spine (vertebral bodies appear to have increased density in the upper and lower zones in a striated appearance, like that in childhood osteopetrosis) and soft tissue calcification.
- β_2-Microglobulin may accumulate with chronic dialysis, leading to amyloidosis.
  - Amyloidosis may be associated with carpal tunnel syndrome, arthropathy, and pathologic fractures.
  - In amyloidosis, Congo red stain causes material to turn pink.
- Laboratory test results:
  - Abnormal glomerular filtration rate (GFR)
  - Increased alkaline phosphatase, blood urea nitrogen (BUN), and creatinine levels
  - Decreased venous bicarbonate level
- Treatment directed at relieving the urologic obstruction or kidney disease

---

Box 1-1 | **Causes of Rickets and Osteomalacia**

NUTRITIONAL DEFICIENCY
Vitamin D deficiency
Dietary chelators (rare) of calcium
Phytates
Oxalates (spinach)
PHOSPHORUS DEFICIENCY (UNUSUAL)
Abuse of antacids (which contain aluminum), leading to severe dietary phosphate binding
GASTROINTESTINAL ABSORPTION DEFECTS
Postgastrectomy (rare today)
Biliary disease (interference with absorption of fat-soluble vitamin D)
Enteric absorption defects
Short bowel syndrome
Rapid transit (gluten-sensitive enteropathy) syndromes
Inflammatory bowel disease
- Crohn disease
- Celiac disease
RENAL TUBULAR DEFECTS (RENAL PHOSPHATE LEAK)
X-linked dominant hypophosphatemic vitamin D–resistant rickets or osteomalacia
Classic Albright syndrome or Fanconi syndrome type I
Fanconi syndrome type II
Phosphaturia and glycosuria
Fanconi syndrome type III
Phosphaturia, glycosuria, aminoaciduria
Vitamin D–dependent rickets (or osteomalacia) type I (a genetic or acquired deficiency of renal tubular 25-hydroxyvitamin D 1α hydroxylase enzyme that prevents conversion of 25-hydroxyvitamin D to the active polar metabolite 1,25-dihydroxyvitamin D)
Vitamin D–dependent rickets (or osteomalacia) type II (which represents enteric end-organ insensitivity to 1,25-dihydroxyvitamin D and is probably caused by an abnormality in the 1,25-dihydroxyvitamin D nuclear receptor)
Renal tubular acidosis
Acquired: associated with many systemic diseases
Genetic
- Debré–De Toni–Fanconi syndrome
- Lignac-Fanconi syndrome (cystinosis)
- Lowe syndrome
RENAL OSTEODYSTROPHY: MISCELLANEOUS CAUSES
Soft tissue tumors secreting putative factors
Fibrous dysplasia
Neurofibromatosis
Other soft tissue and vascular mesenchymal tumors
Anticonvulsant medication (induction of the hepatic P450 microsomal enzyme system by some anticonvulsants—e.g., phenytoin, phenobarbital, and primidone [Mysoline]—causes increased degradation of vitamin D metabolites)
Heavy metal intoxication
Hypophosphatasia
High-dose diphosphonates
Sodium fluoride

Adapted from Simon SR, editor: *Orthopaedic basic science,* ed 2, Rosemont, Ill, 1994, American Academy of Orthopaedic Surgeons, p 169.

- Rickets (osteomalacia in adults; Box 1-1)
  - Failure of mineralization, leading to changes in the physis in the **zone of provisional calcification** (increased width and disorientation) and bone (cortical thinning, bowing)
  - Nutritional rickets (see Table 1-17)
    - Vitamin D–deficiency rickets
      - Rare after addition of vitamin D to milk, except in the following populations:
        - Asian immigrants
        - Patients with dietary peculiarities
        - Premature infants

- Patients with malabsorption (celiac sprue)
- Patients receiving chronic parenteral nutrition
- Decreased intestinal absorption of calcium and phosphate leads to secondary hyperparathyroidism.
- Laboratory studies
  - Low-normal calcium level (maintained by high PTH level)
  - Low phosphate level (excreted because of the effect of PTH)
  - Increased alkaline phosphatase level
  - Low vitamin D level
  - Increased PTH level leads to increased bone absorption
- Examination
  - Enlargement of the costochondral junction ("rachitic rosary")
  - Bowing of the knees
  - Muscle hypotonia
  - Dental disease
  - Pathologic fractures (Looser zones: pseudofracture on the compression side of bone)
  - Milkman's fracture (Figure 1-24)
  - Waddling gait
- Radiographic findings
  - Physeal widening and cupping
  - Coxa vara
  - "Codfish" vertebrae
  - Retarded bone growth (defect in the hypertrophic zone, widened osteoid seams)
- In affected children, height is commonly below the fifth percentile for age.
- Treatment with vitamin D (5000 IU daily) resolves most deformities.
- Calcium-deficiency rickets (Figure 1-25)
- Phosphate-deficiency rickets

- Hereditary vitamin D–dependent rickets
  - Rare disorders with features similar to vitamin D deficiency (nutritional) rickets, except that symptoms may be worse and patients may have total baldness
    - Type I: defect in renal 25(OH)-vitamin D 1α-hydroxylase, inhibiting conversion of inactive vitamin D to its active form
      - Autosomal recessive inheritance
      - Gene on chromosome 12q14
    - Type II: defect in an intracellular receptor for 1,25(OH)$_2$-vitamin D$_3$
- Familial hypophosphatemic rickets (vitamin D–resistant rickets or "phosphate diabetes")
  - Most commonly encountered form of rickets
  - X-linked dominant inheritance
    - Impaired renal tubular reabsorption of phosphate
  - Normal GFR with an impaired vitamin D$_3$ response
  - **Normal levels of serum calcium, low serum phosphorus and 1,25 vitamin D, elevated alkaline phosphatase**
    - Treatment:
      - Phosphate replacement (1-3 g daily)
      - High-dose vitamin D$_3$
- Hypophosphatasia (Figure 1-26)
  - Autosomal recessive
  - **Error in the tissue-nonspecific isoenzyme of alkaline phosphatase**
    - Leads to low levels of alkaline phosphatase, required for synthesis of inorganic phosphate and important in bone matrix formation
  - Features are similar to those of rickets.
  - Increased urinary phosphoethanolamine is diagnostic.
  - Treatment may include phosphate therapy.

■ **Conditions of bone mineral density**

▨ Bone mass is regulated by rates of deposition and withdrawal (Figure 1-27).

▨ Osteoporosis
- Age-related decrease in bone mass
  - Usually associated with estrogen loss in postmenopausal women (Figure 1-28)
- A quantitative defect, not qualitative
  - Mineralization remains normal
- World Health Organization's definition
  - Lumbar (L2-L4) density is 2.5 or more standard deviations less than mean peak bone mass of a healthy 25-year-old (T-score).
  - Osteopenia: bone density is 1.0 to 2.5 standard deviations less than the mean peak bone mass of a healthy 25-year-old.
- Responsible for more than 1 million fractures per year
  - Fractures of the vertebral body are most common.
  - History of osteoporotic vertebral compression fractures are strongly predictive of subsequent vertebral fracture.
    - After initial vertebral fracture, the risk for a second vertebral fracture is 20%.
  - Vertebral compression fracture is associated with increased mortality rate.
    - Incidence of vertebral compression fractures is higher among men than women.

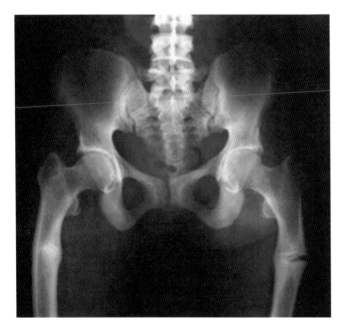

FIGURE 1-24 Pseudofracture in both femurs in an adult patient with X-linked hypophosphatemic osteomalacia. (From Adam A, Dixon AK: *Grainger & Allison's diagnostic radiology: a textbook of medical imaging*, ed 5, Philadelphia, 2008, Elsevier Churchill Livingstone.)

Nutritional Calcium Deficiency

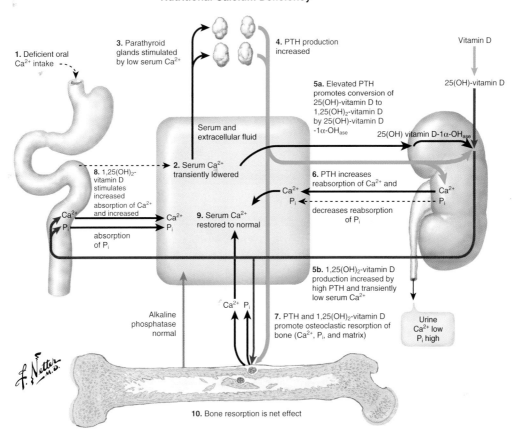

1. Deficient oral Ca²⁺ intake

3. Parathyroid glands stimulated by low serum Ca²⁺

4. PTH production increased

Vitamin D

25(OH)-vitamin D

5a. Elevated PTH promotes conversion of 25(OH)-vitamin D to 1,25(OH)₂-vitamin D by 25(OH)-vitamin D -1α-OH$_{ase}$

25(OH) vitamin D-1α-OH$_{ase}$

Serum and extracellular fluid

8. 1,25(OH)₂-vitamin D stimulates increased absorption of Ca²⁺ and increased absorption of P$_i$

2. Serum Ca²⁺ transiently lowered

6. PTH increases reabsorption of Ca²⁺ and decreases reabsorption of P$_i$

Ca²⁺
P$_i$

Ca²⁺
P$_i$

Ca²⁺
P$_i$

Ca²⁺
P$_i$

9. Serum Ca²⁺ restored to normal

5b. 1,25(OH)₂-vitamin D production increased by high PTH and transiently low serum Ca²⁺

Alkaline phosphatase normal

Ca²⁺ P$_i$

Urine
Ca²⁺ low
P$_i$ high

7. PTH and 1,25(OH)₂-vitamin D promote osteoclastic resorption of bone (Ca²⁺, P$_i$, and matrix)

10. Bone resorption is net effect

FIGURE 1-25 Nutritional calcium deficiency. *1,25(OH)₂D,* 1,25(OH)₂-vitamin D; *25(H)D,* 25(OH)-vitamin D; *OH$_{ase}$,* hydroxylase; *P$_i$,* inorganic phosphate; *PTH,* parathyroid hormone. (From Netter FH: *CIBA collection of medical illustrations,* vol 8: *Musculoskeletal system,* part I: *Anatomy, physiology and developmental disorders,* Basel, Switzerland, 1987, CIBA, p 184.)

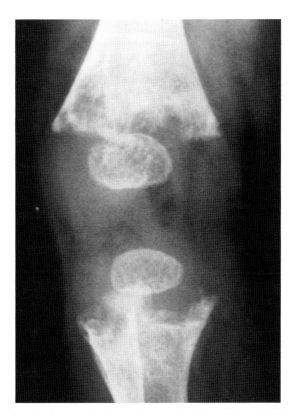

FIGURE 1-26 Hypophosphatasia. Deossification is present adjacent to growth plates. Characteristic radiolucent areas extend from the growth plates into the metaphysis. (From Resnick D, Kransdorf MJ, editors: *Bone and joint imaging,* ed 3, Philadelphia, 2005, Saunders, p 574.)

Four Mechanisms of Bone Mass Regulation

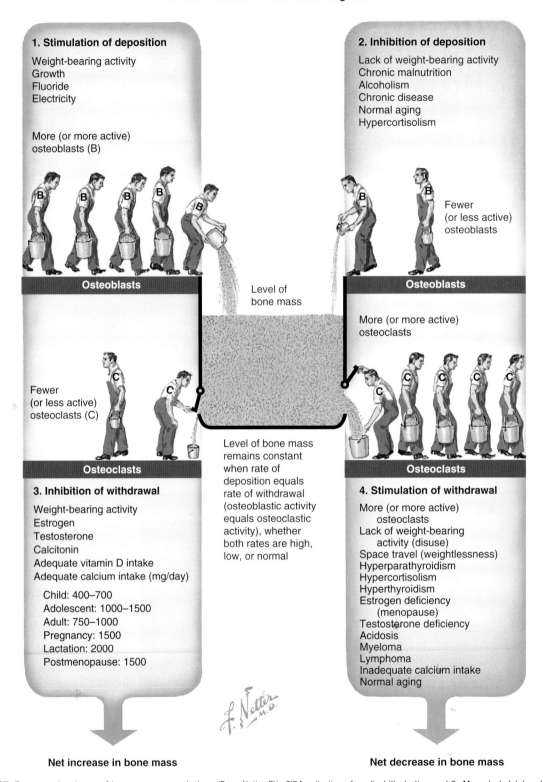

1. Stimulation of deposition

Weight-bearing activity
Growth
Fluoride
Electricity

More (or more active)
osteoblasts (B)

Osteoblasts

Fewer
(or less active)
osteoclasts (C)

Osteoclasts

3. Inhibition of withdrawal

Weight-bearing activity
Estrogen
Testosterone
Calcitonin
Adequate vitamin D intake
Adequate calcium intake (mg/day)

Child: 400–700
Adolescent: 1000–1500
Adult: 750–1000
Pregnancy: 1500
Lactation: 2000
Postmenopause: 1500

2. Inhibition of deposition

Lack of weight-bearing activity
Chronic malnutrition
Alcoholism
Chronic disease
Normal aging
Hypercortisolism

Fewer
(or less active)
osteoblasts

Osteoblasts

Level of
bone mass

More (or more active)
osteoclasts

Level of bone mass
remains constant
when rate of
deposition equals
rate of withdrawal
(osteoblastic activity
equals osteoclastic
activity), whether
both rates are high,
low, or normal

Osteoclasts

4. Stimulation of withdrawal

More (or more active)
   osteoclasts
Lack of weight-bearing
   activity (disuse)
Space travel (weightlessness)
Hyperparathyroidism
Hypercortisolism
Hyperthyroidism
Estrogen deficiency
   (menopause)
Testosterone deficiency
Acidosis
Myeloma
Lymphoma
Inadequate calcium intake
Normal aging

Net increase in bone mass

Net decrease in bone mass

FIGURE 1-27 Four mechanisms of bone mass regulation. (From Netter FH: *CIBA collection of medical illustrations*, vol 8: *Musculoskeletal system*, part I: *Anatomy, physiology and developmental disorders,* Basel, Switzerland, 1987, CIBA, p 181.)

- Lifetime risk of fracture in white women after 50 years of age: 75%
   - The risk for hip fracture is 15% to 20%.
- Risk factors (Box 1-2)
- Cancellous bone is most affected.

- Clinical features:
   - Kyphosis and vertebral fractures
      - Compression fractures of T11-L1 that create an anterior wedge-shaped defect or a centrally depressed "codfish" vertebra

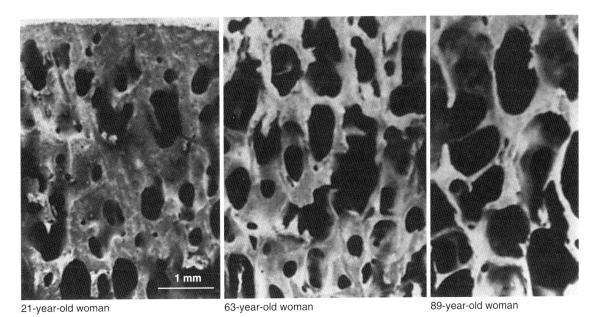

21-year-old woman   63-year-old woman   89-year-old woman

FIGURE 1-28 Age-related changes in density and architecture of human trabecular bone from the lumbar spine. With progressive age, there is a quantitative decrease in bone, but the mineralization (qualitative) remains the same.

Box 1-2	Risk Factors for the Development of Osteoporosis

- White race, female gender, northern European descent (fair skin and hair)
- Sedentary lifestyle
- Thinness
- Smoking
- Heavy drinking
- Phenytoin (impairs vitamin D metabolism)
- Diet low in calcium and vitamin D
- History of breastfeeding
- Positive family history of osteoporosis
- Premature menopause

From Keaveney TM, Hayes WC: Mechanical properties of cortical and trabecular bone, Bone, 7:285-344, 1993.

- Hip fractures
- Distal radius fractures
- Type I osteoporosis (postmenopausal)
  - Primarily affects trabecular bone
  - Vertebral and distal radius fractures common
- Type II osteoporosis (age-related)
  - Patients older than 75 years
  - Affects both trabecular and cortical bone
  - Related to poor calcium absorption
  - Hip and pelvic fractures are common
- Laboratory studies
  - Obtained to rule out secondary causes of low bone mass
    - Vitamin D deficiency, hyperthyroidism, hyperparathyroidism, Cushing syndrome, hematologic disorders, malignancy
  - Complete blood cell count (CBC); measurements of serum calcium, phosphorus, 25(OH)-vitamin D, alkaline phosphatase, liver enzymes, creatinine, and total protein and albumin levels; and measurement of 24-hour urinary calcium excretion
  - Results of these studies are usually unremarkable in osteoporosis.
- Plain radiographs not helpful unless bone loss exceeds 30%

- Special studies
  - Single-photon (appendicular) absorptiometry
  - Double-photon (axial) absorptiometry
  - Quantitative computed tomography (CT)
  - Dual-energy x-ray absorptiometry (DEXA)
    - Most accurate with less radiation
- Biopsy
  - After tetracycline labeling
  - To evaluate the severity of osteoporosis and identify osteomalacia
- Histologic changes:
  - Thinning trabeculae
  - Decreased osteon size
  - Enlarged haversian and marrow spaces
- Treatment (Figure 1-29):
  - Physical activity
  - Calcium supplements
    - 1000 to 1500 mg plus 400 to 800 IU of vitamin D per day
    - More effective in type II (age-related) osteoporosis
  - Fluoride
    - Inhibits bone resorption
    - However, bone is more brittle.
  - Bisphosphonates: bind to bone resorption surfaces and inhibit osteoclastic membrane ruffling without destroying the cells
  - Other drugs (e.g., intramuscular calcitonin) may be helpful.
    - Expensive
    - May cause hypersensitivity reactions
  - Efficacy of bone augmentation with PTH, growth factors, prostaglandin inhibitors, and other therapies remains to be determined.
- Prophylaxis for patients at risk for osteoporosis:
  - Diet with adequate calcium intake
  - Weight-bearing exercise program
  - Estrogen therapy evaluation at menopause
- Other causes for decreased mineral density
  - Idiopathic transient osteoporosis of the hip
    - Uncommon; diagnosis of exclusion

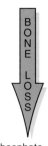
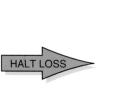

- Phosphate
- Bisphosphonates

- Calcium
- Vitamin D
- Alendronate (Fosamax)
- Calcitonin (+Ca)
- Mild exercise (biomechanical-electrical coupling)
- Pamidronate (Aredia)
- Raloxifene (Evista)
- Etidronate (Didronel)
- Tamoxifen

- Fluoride
  plus
  -Calcium
  -Vitamin D
  -Calcitonin
- Extensive exercise (biomechanical-electrical coupling)

FIGURE 1-29 Treatment options for osteoporosis. (Adapted from Simon SR, editor: *Orthopaedic basic science,* Rosemont, Ill, 1994, American Academy of Orthopaedic Surgeons, p 174.)

- Most common during third trimester of pregnancy in women but can occur in men
- Groin pain, limited range of motion (ROM), and localized osteopenia without a history of trauma
  - Treatment: analgesics and limited weight bearing
  - Generally self-limiting and tends to resolve spontaneously after 6 to 8 months
    - This feature distinguishes idiopathic transient osteoporosis from osteonecrosis, which has progressive symptoms and does not resolve spontaneously.
  - Stress fractures may occur.
  - Joint space remains preserved on radiographs.
- Bone loss related to spinal cord injury
  - Bone mineral loss occurs throughout the skeleton (except the skull) for approximately 16 months.
    - Levels off when bone mass reaches two thirds of the original value
  - High risk of fracture
  - Bone loss greatest in the lower extremities
- Osteomalacia
  - Femoral neck fractures are common.
  - Qualitative defect
  - Defect of mineralization results in a large amount of unmineralized osteoid.
  - Causes:
    - Vitamin D–deficient diet
    - GI disorders
    - Renal osteodystrophy
    - Certain drugs
      - Aluminum-containing phosphate-binding antacids; aluminum deposition in bone prevents mineralization
      - Phenytoin (Dilantin)
    - Alcoholism
  - Radiographic findings:
    - Looser zones (microscopic stress fractures)

- Other fractures
- Biconcave vertebral bodies
- Trefoil pelvis
- Biopsy (transiliac) required for diagnosis
  - Widened osteoid seams are histologic findings.
- Treatment: usually includes large doses of vitamin D
- Osteoporosis and osteomalacia are compared in Figure 1-30.
- Scurvy
  - Vitamin C (ascorbic acid) deficiency
  - Produces a decrease in chondroitin sulfate synthesis
    - Leads to defective collagen growth and repair
    - Also leads to impaired intracellular hydroxylation of collagen peptides
  - Clinical features:
    - Fatigue
    - Gum bleeding
    - Ecchymosis
    - Joint effusions
    - Iron deficiency
  - Radiographic findings:
    - May include thin cortices and trabeculae and metaphyseal clefts (corner sign)
  - Laboratory studies: normal results
  - Histologic features:
    - Primary trabeculae replaced with granulation tissue
    - Areas of hemorrhage
    - Widening of the zone of provisional calcification in the physis
      - Greatest effect on bone formation in the metaphysis
- Marrow packing disorders
  - Myeloma, leukemia, and other such disorders can cause osteopenia.
- Osteogenesis imperfecta
  - Caused by abnormal collagen synthesis
    - Failure of normal collagen cross-linking as a result of glycine substitutions in procollagen
      - Caused primarily by a mutation in genes responsible for metabolism and synthesis of type I collagen
  - Increased bone turnover
- Lead poisoning
  - Results in short stature and reduced bone density
  - Lead alters the chondrocyte response to PTH-related protein and TGF-β.
- Increased osteodensity
  - Osteopetrosis (marble bone disease)
    - *Osteopetrosis* is the term for a group of bone disorders characterized by increased sclerosis and obliteration of the medullary canal.
    - Result of decreased osteoclast (and chondroclast) function: failure of bone resorption
    - **Associated with loss of function mutation in carbonic anhydrase II gene**
      - Osteoclast numbers may be increased, decreased, or normal.
      - May result from an abnormality of the immune system (thymic defect)
      - Osteoclasts lack the normal ruffled border and clear zone.
      - Marrow spaces fill with necrotic calcified cartilage.
      - Cartilage may be trapped within the osteoid.

Comparison of Osteoporosis and Osteomalacia

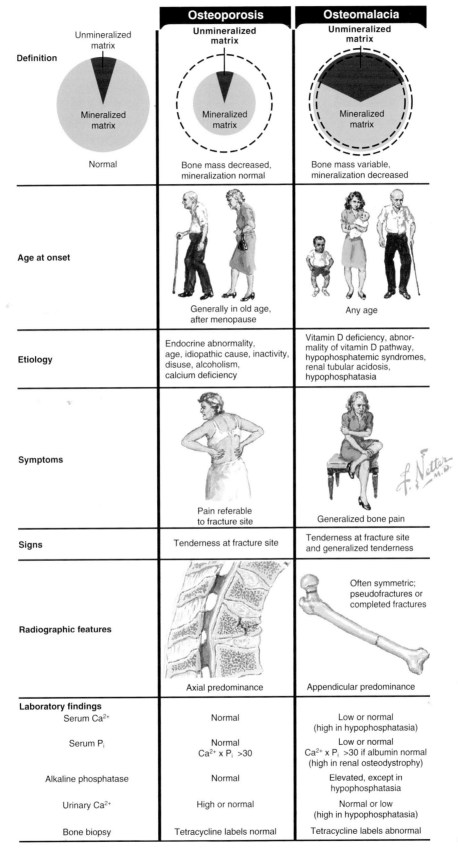

	Osteoporosis	**Osteomalacia**
Definition	Unmineralized matrix Mineralized matrix Bone mass decreased, mineralization normal	Unmineralized matrix Mineralized matrix Bone mass variable, mineralization decreased
Age at onset	Generally in old age, after menopause	Any age
Etiology	Endocrine abnormality, age, idiopathic cause, inactivity, disuse, alcoholism, calcium deficiency	Vitamin D deficiency, abnormality of vitamin D pathway, hypophosphatemic syndromes, renal tubular acidosis, hypophosphatasia
Symptoms	Pain referable to fracture site	Generalized bone pain
Signs	Tenderness at fracture site	Tenderness at fracture site and generalized tenderness
Radiographic features	Axial predominance	Often symmetric; pseudofractures or completed fractures Appendicular predominance
Laboratory findings		
Serum Ca^{2+}	Normal	Low or normal (high in hypophosphatasia)
Serum P_i	Normal $Ca^{2+} \times P_i > 30$	Low or normal $Ca^{2+} \times P_i > 30$ if albumin normal (high in renal osteodystrophy)
Alkaline phosphatase	Normal	Elevated, except in hypophosphatasia
Urinary Ca^{2+}	High or normal	Normal or low (high in hypophosphatasia)
Bone biopsy	Tetracycline labels normal	Tetracycline labels abnormal

FIGURE 1-30 Comparison of osteoporosis and osteomalacia. P_i, Inorganic phosphate. (From Netter FH: *CIBA collection of medical illustrations,* vol 8: *Musculoskeletal system,* part I: *Anatomy, physiology and developmental disorders,* Basel, Switzerland, 1987, CIBA, p 228.)

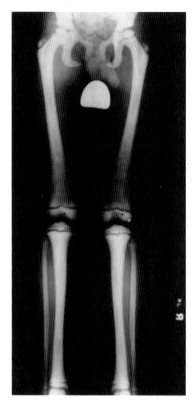

FIGURE 1-31 Typical "marble bone" appearance of osteopetrosis. (From Herring JA, editor: *Tachdjian's pediatric orthopaedics,* ed 5, Philadelphia, 2014, Saunders Elsevier.)

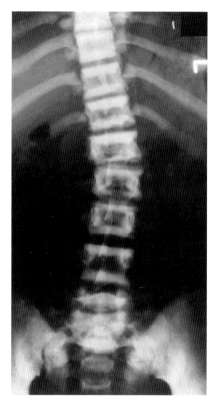

FIGURE 1-32 Typical "rugger jersey" spine observed in osteopetrosis. (From Herring JA, editor: *Tachdjian's pediatric orthopaedics,* ed 5, Philadelphia, 2014, Saunders Elsevier.)

- Empty lacunae and plugging of haversian canals are also observed.
- One of these disorders is infantile autosomal recessive ("malignant") osteopetrosis.
  - Most severe form
  - "Bone within a bone" appearance on radiographs
  - Hepatosplenomegaly
  - Aplastic anemia
  - Can lead to death during infancy
  - Bone marrow transplantation (e.g., osteoclast precursors) can be lifesaving during childhood.
  - High doses of calcitriol with or without steroids may also be helpful.
- Another disorder is autosomal dominant "tarda" (benign) osteopetrosis (Albers-Schönberg disease).
  - Generalized osteosclerosis, including **the typical "rugger jersey" spine**
  - Usually without other anomalies (Figures 1-31 and 1-32)
  - Pathologic fractures are common (brittle bone).
- Osteopoikilosis ("spotted bone disease")
  - Islands of deep cortical bone appear within the medullary cavity and the cancellous bone of the long bones
    - Especially in the hands and feet
  - These areas are usually asymptomatic
  - This disease is accompanied by no known incidence of malignant degeneration.
- Paget disease of bone (osteitis deformans)
  - Elevated serum alkaline phosphatase and urinary hydroxyproline levels
  - **Virus-like inclusion bodies in osteoclasts— abnormal function of osteoclasts**

- Both decreased and increased osteodensity may be present.
  - Depends on phase of disease
    - Active phase
      - Lytic phase: intense osteoclastic bone resorption
      - Mixed phase
      - Sclerotic phase: osteoblastic bone formation
    - Inactive phase

■ **Conditions of bone viability**

▧ Osteonecrosis
- Death of bony tissue from causes other than infection
  - Usually adjacent to a joint surface
- Caused by loss of blood supply as a result of trauma or another event (e.g., slipped capital femoral epiphysis)
- Idiopathic osteonecrosis of the femoral head and Legg-Calvé-Perthes disease may occur in patients with coagulation abnormalities.
  - Deficiency of antithrombin factors protein C and protein S
  - Increased levels of lipoprotein (a)
- Commonly affects the hip joint
- Leads to collapse and flattening of the femoral head, most frequently the anterolateral region
- **Associated with the following conditions:**
  - Steroid and heavy alcohol use
  - Blood dyscrasias (e.g., sickle cell disease)
  - Dysbarism (caisson disease)
  - Excessive radiation therapy
  - Gaucher disease
- Cause
  - Theories vary (Figure 1-33)

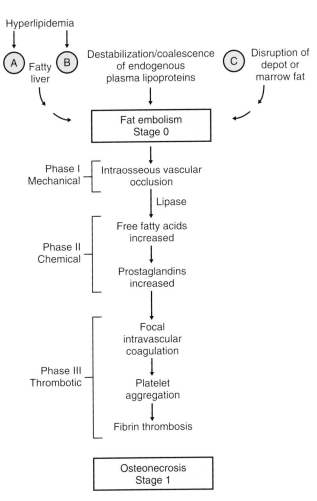

FIGURE 1-33 Possible mechanisms by which intraosseous fat embolism leads to focal intravascular coagulation and osteonecrosis. (From Jones JP Jr: Fat embolism and osteonecrosis, *Orthop Clin North Am* 16:595–633, 1985.)

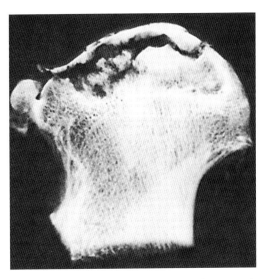

FIGURE 1-34 Fine-grain micrograph demonstrating space between articular surface and subchondral bone: "crescent sign" of osteonecrosis. (From Steinberg ME: *The hip and its disorders*, Philadelphia, 1991, WB Saunders, p 630.)

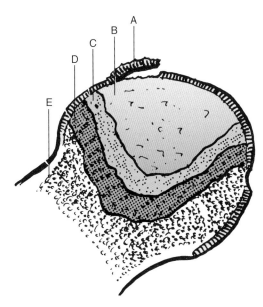

FIGURE 1-35 Pathologic features of avascular necrosis. Illustration of articular cartilage (A), necrotic bone (B), reactive fibrous tissue (C), hypertrophic bone (D), and normal trabeculae (E). (From Steinberg ME: *The hip and its disorders*, Philadelphia, 1991, WB Saunders, p 630.)

- Osteonecrosis may be related to enlargement of space-occupying marrow fat cells, which lead to ischemia of adjacent tissues.
- Vascular insults and other factors may also be significant.
- Idiopathic (or spontaneous) osteonecrosis is diagnosed when no other cause can be identified.
- Chandler disease: osteonecrosis of the femoral head in adults
- Medial femoral condyle osteonecrosis: most common in women older than 60 years
  - Idiopathic, alcohol, and dysbaric forms of osteonecrosis are associated with multiple insults.
  - These may be secondary to a hemoglobinopathy (e.g., sickle cell disease) or marrow disorder (e.g., hemochromatosis).
  - Cyclosporine has reduced the incidence of osteonecrosis of the femoral head among renal transplant recipients.
- Pathologic changes
  - Grossly necrotic bone, fibrous tissue, and subchondral collapse (Figures 1-34 and 1-35)
- Histologic findings:
  - Early changes (14-21 days) involve autolysis of osteocytes and necrotic marrow.
- Followed by inflammation with invasion of buds of primitive mesenchymal tissue and capillaries
- Newly woven bone is laid down on top of dead trabecular bone.
- Followed by resorption of dead trabeculae and remodeling through "creeping substitution"
  - The bone is weakest during resorption and remodeling.
  - Collapse (crescent sign on radiographs) and fragmentation can occur.
- Evaluation
  - A careful history (to discern risk factors) and physical examination (e.g., to discern decreased ROM, limp) should precede additional studies.
  - Other joints (especially the contralateral hip) should be evaluated to identify the disease process early.

- The process is bilateral in the hip in 50% of cases of idiopathic osteonecrosis and up to 80% of cases of steroid-induced osteonecrosis.
- Magnetic resonance imaging (MRI) and bone scanning are helpful for early diagnosis.
  - MRI: earliest study to yield positive results; highest sensitivity and specificity
- Femoral head pressure measurement is possible but invasive.
  - Pressure higher than 30 mm Hg or increased more than 10 mm Hg with injection of 5 mL saline (stress test) is considered abnormal.
  - Values vary widely from one investigation to another.
- Treatment
  - Arthroplasty of the hip is associated with increased loosening.
  - Nontraumatic osteonecrosis of the distal femoral condyle and proximal humerus may improve spontaneously without surgery.
  - Precise role of core decompression remains unresolved
  - Results are best when core decompression is performed in early hip disease (Ficat stage I).
- Osteochondrosis (Table 1-19)
  - Can occur at traction apophyses in children
  - May or may not be associated with trauma, joint capsule inflammation, vascular insult, or secondary thrombosis
  - Pathologic process is similar to that of osteonecrosis in the adult.

JOINTS

- **Hyaline cartilage structure and function**
- Hyaline cartilage: articular bearing surface
  - Slick bearing surface: decreases friction and distributes loads
    - Coefficient of friction less than ice on ice
  - Shock-absorbing cushion resists shear/compression.
    - Withstands impact loads up to 25 N/mm^2
  - Avascular, aneural, and alymphatic
    - Receives nutrients and oxygen from synovial fluid via diffusion

Table 1-19	Common Types of Osteochondrosis	
DISORDER	**SITE**	**AGE (YR)**
Van Neck disease	Ischiopubic synchondrosis	4-11
Legg-Calvé-Perthes disease	Femoral head	4-8
Osgood-Schlatter disease	Tibial tuberosity	11-15
Sinding-Larsen-Johansson syndrome	Inferior patella	10-14
Blount disease (in infants)	Proximal tibial epiphysis	1-3
Blount disease (in adolescents)	Proximal tibial epiphysis	8-15
Sever disease	Calcaneus	9-11
Köhler disease	Tarsal navicular	3-7
Freiberg infarction	Metatarsal head	13-18
Scheuermann disease	Discovertebral junction	13-17
Panner disease	Capitellum of humerus	5-10
Thiemann disease	Phalanges of hand	11-19
Kienböck disease	Carpal lunate	20-40

- Cartilage is hypoxic; ATP from glycolysis
  - Heals poorly
- Anisotropic—properties of material vary with direction of force
- Biphasic—property of liquid and solid
- Viscoelastic—strain (change in L/L) varies by rate of loading
- Cartilage homeostasis disrupted by:
  - Direct trauma/excess or inadequate forces
  - Loss of underlying bone structure
  - Genetic defects in normal structure/function
  - Chemical/enzymatic threats
- **Composition of hyaline cartilage**
- Water makes up approximately 75% of wet weight
  - Highest at surface layers
  - Recurrent low-level forces shifts synovial fluid in and out of cartilage.
  - Responsible for nutrition and lubrication
  - More at the surface
  - H_2O decreases with aging
  - H_2O increases in osteoarthritis (Figure 1-36)
    - Increased permeability
    - Decreased strength
    - Decreased Young's modulus of elasticity
- Collagen makes up approximately 15% of wet weight (≈60% of dry weight) (Figure 1-37, Table 1-20)
  - Chains of hydroxyproline
  - Vitamin C (deficiency leads to scurvy) puts hydroxyl group (-OH) on proline
  - -OH allows sharp molecular twists of "triple helix" of three α-procollagen chains
  - Stable molecule (long half-life [>20 years])
  - Forms tough flexible meshwork
  - Provides tensile strength and stiffness
  - Many types: **cartilage has approximately 95% type II collagen.**
    - Genetic defects of type II cause:
      - Achondrogenesis (lethal at birth)
      - Spondyloepiphyseal dysplasia congenita
      - Precocious arthritis
    - IX and XI are "linking collagen"
    - **X collagen only found near calcified cartilage**
      - Calcified zone of articular cartilage's tidemark
      - Hypertrophic zone of the physis (genetic defect of type X leads to Schmid metaphyseal chondrodysplasia)
      - Fracture callus and calcifying cartilaginous tumors
- Proteoglycans make up approximately 10% of wet weight (≈30% of dry weight) (Figure 1-38).
  - Protein polysaccharides (glycosaminoglycans, specifically aggrecan)
    - Chondroitin sulfate—most prevalent glycosaminoglycan of cartilage
      - Chondroitin 4-sulfate decreases with age.
      - Chondroitin 6-sulfate remains constant.
    - Keratin sulfate increases with age.
      - Provides compressive strength
  - Proteoglycans have half-life of 3 months
  - Large macromolecules shaped like "bristle brushes" (see Figure 1-38)
    - HA backbone
    - Link protein
    - Keratan sulfate

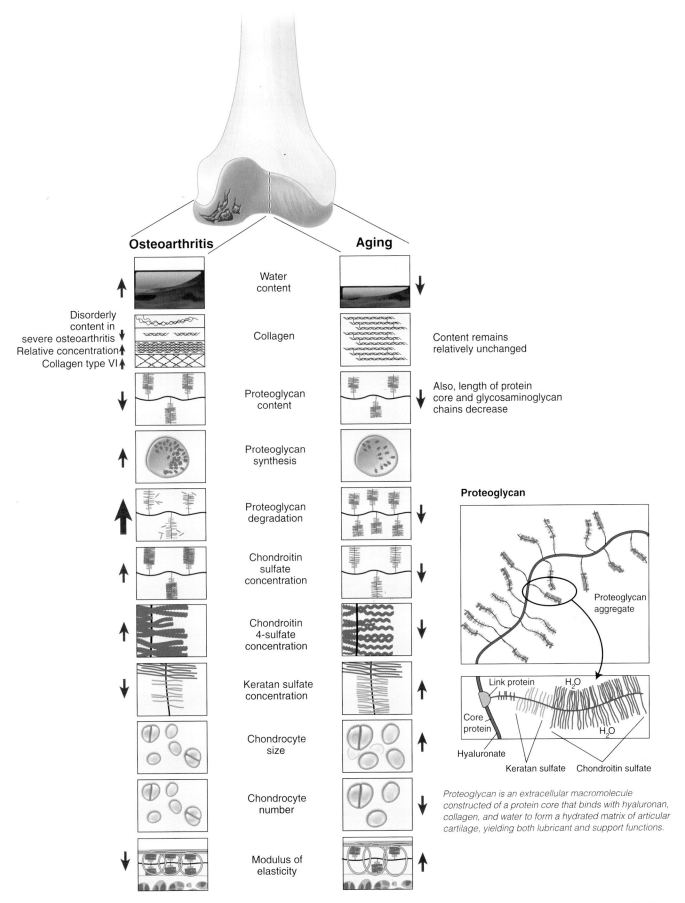

FIGURE 1-36 Articular cartilage changes in osteoarthritis and aging. Proteoglycan aggregate and aggrecan molecule. (From Brinker MR, Miller MD: *Fundamentals of orthopaedics,* Philadelphia, 1999, WB Saunders, p 9.)

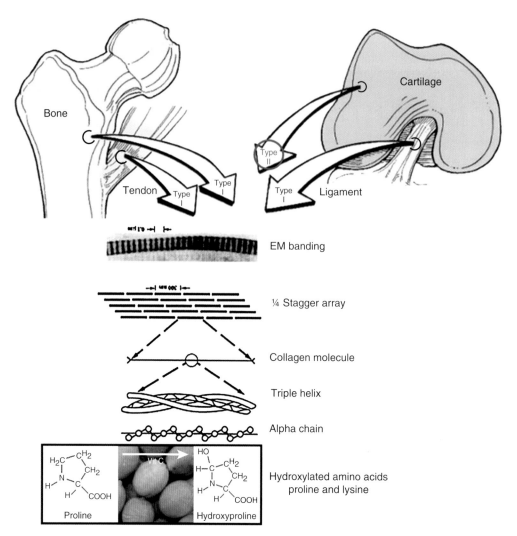

FIGURE 1-37 Macrostructure to microstructure of collagen. Although the majority of the collagen in bone, tendon, and ligament is type I, most of the collagen in cartilage is type II. Collagen is composed of microfibrils that are quarter-staggered arrangements of tropocollagen. Note hole and pore regions for mineral deposition (for calcification). Vitamin C (ascorbic acid) is an enzymatic cofactor needed to form the hydroxylated version of the amino acids proline and lysine, which allow the twists to form the triple helix from the polypeptide α chains. (Modified from Brinker MR, Miller MD: *Fundamentals of orthopaedics,* Philadelphia, 1999, WB Saunders.)

Table 1-20	Collagen Types, Locations, and Related Genetic Disorders*	
TYPE	**LOCATION**	**GENETIC DISEASE**
I	Bone, tendon, meniscus	**Osteogenesis imperfecta**
	Disc annulus, eye (sclera), skin	**Ehlers-Danlos**
II	Articular cartilage	**Achondrogenesis (lethal)**
	Disc nucleus pulposus, eye (vitreous humor)	Hypochondrogenesis
		Spondyloepiphyseal dysplasia congenita
		Kniest dysplasia
		Stickler syndrome
		Precocious arthritis
III	Skin, blood vessels	**Ehlers-Danlos**
IV	Basement membrane: kidney, ear, eye (basal lamina)	Alport syndrome
V	Articular cartilage (in small amounts)	**Ehlers-Danlos**
VI	Articular cartilage (in small amounts); tethers chondrocyte to pericellular matrix	Bethlem myopathy
		Ullrich congenital muscular dystrophy
VII	Basement membrane (epithelial)	Epidermolysis bullosa
VIII	Basement membrane (epithelial)	Corneal endothelial dystrophy
IX	Articular cartilage (in small amounts)	**Multiple epiphyseal dysplasia** (one type)
X	Hypertrophic zone or tidemark of cartilage (associated with calcified cartilage)	Metaphyseal chondroplasia, Schmid type
XI	Articular cartilage (in small amounts); acts as an adhesive	Otospondylomegaepiphyseal dysplasia
XII	Tendon	
XIII	Endothelial cells	

*More common orthopaedic diseases are in **bold.**

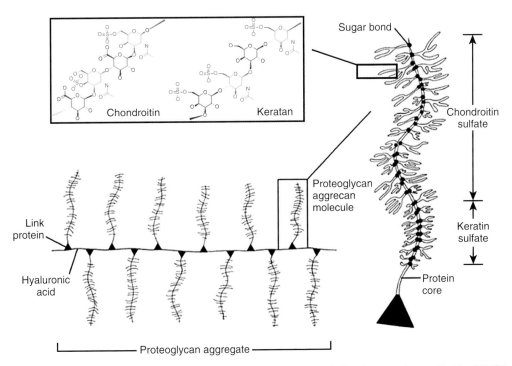

FIGURE 1-38 Proteoglycan aggregate and bristle brush–shaped aggrecan molecule. Sulfate ions are transmitted by DTDST protein; when genetically defective, this causes diastrophic dysplasia (short stature with "hitchhiker's thumbs" and cauliflower ears). (Modified from Brinker MR, Miller MD: *Fundamentals of orthopaedics,* Philadelphia, 1999, WB Saunders, p 9.)

- Chondroitin sulfate
- C-terminal
- Sulfate ions on ends of molecules with negative charges
  - Repel each other but attract positive cations
  - Increase osmotic pressure that traps and holds water
  - Provides turgor of matrix
  - Cell SO_4^- transporter (protein DTDST)
    - Genetic defect causes diastrophic dysplasia
    - Dwarfism with short extremities, hitchhiker's thumbs, and cauliflower ears
- Provide structural properties, chiefly compressive and elastic strength
- Produce cartilage's porous structure
- Produced by chondrocytes, secreted into the extracellular matrix
- Chondrocytes (1%-5% of wet weight)—the only cell of cartilage
  - Mechanotransduction—metabolism modulated via mechanical stimulation
    - Cyclical loads of walking stimulate chondrocytes to form matrix.
      - Low loads (1-5 MPa) at moderate frequency (≈1 Hz)
    - Primary cilia are the mechanosensory organ "antennae" for cells.
      - (Bardet-Biedl syndrome [genetic ciliopathy])
  - Integrins—transmembrane proteins that help transmit signals
  - Chondrocytes are derived from undifferentiated mesenchymal precursors.
    - SOX9—transcriptional factor to stimulate chondrocyte formation
  - Produce the extracellular matrix of collagen and proteoglycans (Figure 1-39)

- Intracellular synthesis of procollagen, link peptide, hyaluronic acid, proteoglycans
- Extracellular assembly of component parts
- Produce proteins and enzymes and maintain matrix
  - IL-1β (also from synovium and white blood cells [WBCs]): main cartilage destroyer
  - Metalloproteinases—break down cartilage matrix
    - Collagenase—dissolves collagen (MMP-13)
    - Aggrecanase—degrades proteoglycans (ADAMT)
  - Enzyme inhibitors—protect cartilage
    - Tissue inhibitors of metalloproteinases (TIMPs)
    - Plasminogen activator inhibitor-1 (PAI-1)
- Chondrocytes are most dense and most active in the superficial zone.
- Deeper cartilage zone chondrocytes less metabolically active:
  - Decreased rough endoplasmic reticulum
  - Increased intraplasmic filaments (degenerative products)
- Other matrix components:
  - Adhesives—noncollagenous proteins:
    - Fibronectin—binds to integrins (transmembrane receptors)
      - Increased in osteoarthritis
    - Chondronectin—mediates attachment of chondrocytes to collagen type II
    - Anchorin CII—binds collagen type II to chondrocytes
  - Lipids—unknown function
- **Articular cartilage layers (Figure 1-40)**
- Tangential-superficial zone
  - Thin lamina splendens
  - **Flat chondrocytes**
  - **Highest [superficial zone protein] (same as lubricin or PRG4)**

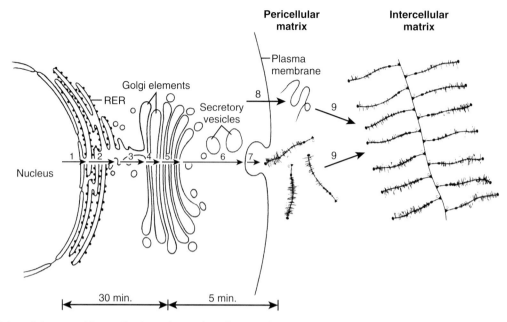

FIGURE 1-39 Extracellular assembly, synthesis, and secretion of proteoglycan aggrecan molecules and link protein by a chondrocyte. *1,* Transcription of aggrecan and link protein genes to messenger RNA. *2,* Translation of messenger RNA to form protein core. *3,* Transportation. *4* and *5, cis*-Golgi and medial *trans*-Golgi compartments, respectively, where glycosaminoglycan chains are added to the protein core. *6,* Transportation to the secretory vesicles. *7,* Release into the extracellular matrix. *8* and *9,* Hyaluronate from the plasma membrane binds with the aggrecan and link proteins to form aggregates in the extracellular matrix. *RER,* Rough endoplasmic reticulum. (From Simon SR, editor: *Orthopaedic basic science,* Rosemont, Ill, 1994, American Academy of Orthopaedic Surgeons, p 13.)

- Collagen fibers:
  - Highest concentration
  - Parallel to joint surface strength against shear
  - Greatest tensile stiffness
- Least concentration of proteoglycans
- **Highest concentration of water**
- Deeper middle zones—transitional/radial
  - Have increased chondrocyte volume
  - **Highest concentration of proteoglycans**
  - Collagen fibers become perpendicular to joint surface/bone surface.
  - Lower H_2O
- Calcified cartilage zone—begins at "tidemark"
  - Transitions stiffness from flexible cartilage to rigid subchondral bone
  - **Type X collagen found here**
  - **Injuries superficial to this level do not heal.**
- **Lubrication and wear mechanisms of articular cartilage (Figure 1-41)**
- Coefficient of friction in healthy human joint is less than ice on ice (0.002-0.04)
- Mechanisms enhancing the coefficient of friction of healthy cartilage:
  - Elastohydrodynamic lubrication—wet deformable surface
    - Predominant mechanism as the joint moves under load
    - Elastic deformation of surfaces separated by lubricants
  - Boundary lubrication—specialized molecules permit surface-surface contact
    - Lubricant only partially separates surfaces
    - Lubricin—superficial zone protein (proteoglycan 4)
    - "Slippery surfaces"
  - Boosted lubrication—fluid entrapment

- Lubricant trapped between regions of bearing surfaces that make contact
- Friction coefficient generally worse than with elastohydrodynamic lubrication
- Hydrodynamic lubrication
  - Fluid separates surfaces when joint slides on the other.
- Weeping lubrication
  - Fluid squeezed out in response to load, separating the surfaces by hydrostatic pressure

- **Hyaline cartilage damage and healing**
- Avascular tissue with very limited healing response
- Chondrocyte viability disrupted by:
  - High-impact loads—trauma or lacerations
  - Prolonged excessive stress—obesity, dysplasia, varus/valgus
  - Prolonged lack of stress—inactivity/disuse
  - Chemical issues:
    - PH changes: (normally at 7.4)
    - Enzymes—metalloproteases
  - Laceration depth is key factor
    - Tidemark: the landmark between vascular bone and avascular cartilage
    - Lacerations above tidemark demonstrate "chondrocyte cloning"
      - Limited increases in numbers of chondrocytes
    - Lacerations extending below the tidemark:
      - Penetrate to vascular subchondral bone
      - Cause an inflammatory response and stem cells
      - Marrow mesenchymal stem cells respond.
      - May heal with less durable fibrocartilage (collagen type I)
  - Forms the basis of the ICRS (International Cartilage Repair Society) grading system
    - Grade 0: normal cartilage

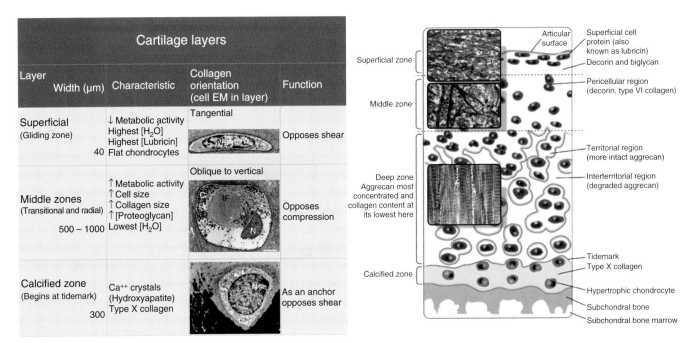

Cartilage layers				
Layer Width (μm)	Characteristic	Collagen orientation (cell EM in layer)		Function
Superficial (Gliding zone) 40	↓ Metabolic activity Highest [H₂O] Highest [Lubricin] Flat chondrocytes	Tangential		Opposes shear
Middle zones (Transitional and radial) 500 – 1000	↑ Metabolic activity ↑ Cell size ↑ Collagen size ↑ [Proteoglycan] Lowest [H₂O]	Oblique to vertical		Opposes compression
Calcified zone (Begins at tidemark) 300	Ca⁺⁺ crystals (Hydroxyapatite) Type X collagen			As an anchor opposes shear

FIGURE 1-40 Cartilage layers, characteristics, and function. *C,* Cytoplasm; *EM,* electron micrograph; *IF,* intermediate filaments; *N,* nucleus. (Composite from Mark R. Brinker MR, Daniel P, O'Connor DP: Basic science. In Miller MD et al, editors: *Miller orthopaedic review,* Philadelphia, 2012, Saunders, Fig 1-40; Buckwalter JA, Mankin HJ: Articular cartilage. Part I: tissue design and chondrocyte-matrix interactions, *J Bone Joint Surg Am* 79:600–611, 1997.)

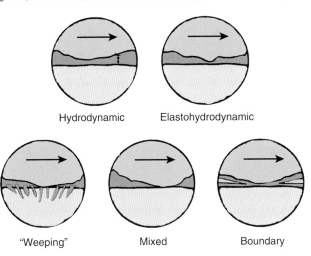

FIGURE 1-41 Types of lubrication of articular cartilage. (From Simon SR, editor: *Orthopaedic basic science,* Rosemont, Ill, 1994, American Academy of Orthopaedic Surgeons, p 465.)

- Grade 1: nearly normal (superficial lesions)
- Grade 2: abnormal (lesions extend < 50% of cartilage depth)
- Grade 3: severely abnormal (>50% of cartilage depth)
- Grade 4: severely abnormal (through the subchondral bone)
- Blunt trauma and strenuous loading causes cell apoptosis.
  - Effects look similar to osteoarthritis.
  - Cartilage thinning and proteoglycan loss
- Joint immobilization leads to atrophy or cartilage degeneration.
  - Continuous passive motion is believed to benefit cartilage healing.
  - Four weeks of immobilization decreases proteoglycan/collagen ratio.

- Ratio returns to normal after 8 weeks of joint mobilization.
- Joint instability allows abnormal shearing loads.
  - Early (≈4 weeks), decreases proteoglycan/collagen ratio
  - Later (≈12 weeks), proteoglycan/collagen is elevated and hydration is increased.
  - Instability markedly decreases hyaluronan (disuse does not).

■ **Aging cartilage—lack of anabolic response (see Figure 1-36)**
▨ Characteristics
- Decreased number of chondrocytes (but larger in size)
- Increased lysosomal enzymes
- Senescence markers of chondrocytes
  - Telomere erosion and β-galactosidase
- Decreased response to growth factors (TGF-β)
  - Decreased matrix production and matrix maintenance
  - Decreased chondroitin SO₄⁻ (but increased keratan SO₄⁻)
- Proteoglycan molecules smaller, so less able to hold water
  - **Decreased water content**—"dried up old cartilage"
- Increased advanced glycosylation end products
  - Yellows and stiffens cartilage
- Increased decorin—"decorates collagen for cross-links"—stiffens cartilage
- Collagen—increased cross-links and diameter—stiffens cartilage
- Increased protein
- Decreased tensile strength
- Increased modulus of elasticity (more stiff)
- **"DRIED UP OLD CARTILAGE IS YELLOW, WEAK, BRITTLE, & STIFF"**

■ **Cartilage of osteoarthritis degraded by matrix metalloproteinases (MMPs)**
▨ Characteristics
- Increase in cells early ("cloning")

- Loss of smooth lamina leads to fibrillation/fissures.
  - Increases coefficient of friction
- Chondrocytes react to IL-1β and tumor necrosis factor.
- Chondrocytes produce nitric oxide (NO).
- MMPs degrade matrix.
  - Collagenases (MMP-13)—first irreversible step
  - Aggrecanase—proteoglycans (ADAMTs)
  - Stromelysin
- Proteoglycans are degraded by enzymes.
  - Decreased size and content of proteoglycan molecules
- Decreased keratan SO_4^-
- Increase in percentage of nonaggregated glycosaminoglycans
- Increase in permeability of matrix
- Increased water content—**OA IS WET**
- Collagen becomes disorganized.
- Mechanical properties suffer.
- **Decreased modulus of elasticity (less stiff)**
- Decreased tensile strength

■ **Other joint tissues**

▨ Synovium
- Loose connective tissue rich in capillaries
- Lacks a basement membrane
- No tight junctions
- No epithelial cells
- Type A synovial cells—macrophage-like
  - Phagocytosis
  - From bone marrow
- **Type B** synovial cells—fibroblast-like
  - **Make golden synovial fluid with lubricin**
  - Mesenchymal derived

▨ Synovial fluid
- **Ultrafiltrate of plasma**
- Hyaluronic acid, lubricin, proteinase, collagenases, and prostaglandins
- Nourishes and lubricates cartilage
- **Non-newtonian fluid: "shear thinning" (thixotropic)**
  - Viscosity decreases with increased shear rate.
- Normal knee has approximately 2 mL.
- Normally contains no RBCs, WBCs, clotting factors, or hemoglobin (Hb).
- Joint fluid analysis: evaluate effusions
  - Cell count with differential, crystals, cultures
    - Noninflammatory arthritis
      - WBCs: fewer than 200/mL, with 25% polymorphonuclear leukocytes (PMNs)
      - Straw color
      - Clear
      - Normal high viscosity
    - Inflammatory arthritis
      - WBCs: 2000 to 75,000/mL, up to 50% PMNs
      - Yellow-green tinged
      - Low viscosity
      - Translucent
      - RA has decreased complement (normal in ankylosing spondylitis).
      - Crystals seen in gout and calcium pyrophosphate (dihydrate crystal) deposition disease (CPPD)
    - Septic arthritis
      - WBCs above 50,000 to 80,000/mL
      - Cloudy to opaque
      - Gram stain and cultures often positive
      - May have low glucose
      - May have high lactate

- Traumatic
  - Often as mild inflammatory
  - Often with blood
  - If fat globules—intraarticular fracture
  - MRI "neapolitan effusion"—fat above plasma above RBCs

▨ Meniscus (labrum in hip/shoulder)
- Curved wedge-shaped "shock absorber"
- Increases contact area and distributes load
- Deepens the articular surface of various synovial joints
- 90% type I collagen (as is bone)
- **Fibroelastic cartilage** (Figure 1-42)
- Fibrochondrocyte is responsible for meniscal healing
- More elastic and less permeable than articular cartilage
- Blood supplies only the peripheral 25%.
- Nerve fibers found in peripheral two thirds.
- Three years after meniscectomy, 70% show radiographic changes.

■ **Noninflammatory arthritides**

▨ Affect 21% of U.S. population (70 million)

▨ Osteoarthritis—degenerative joint disease
- Defined: progressive loss of cartilage structure and function
- Most common form of arthritis—multifactorial
  - Leading cause of disability
  - May be idiopathic
  - May be secondary to:
    - Genetics (*Col2* defect), women affected more than men
    - Overload: obesity, labor, dysplasia/femoral acetabular impingement, varus/valgus
    - Trauma: fractures, ligament injuries, impact
- Tissue changes:
  - Cartilage: as noted earlier—enzymatic degradation and loss (Figure 1-43)
  - Synovium: inflammation, vascular hypertrophy
  - Ligaments: tighten on concave side of deformity
  - Bone: sclerosis, osteophytes, and subchondral cysts
  - Muscles: atrophy from inactivity
- Radiographic findings (Figures 1-44 and 1-45):
  - Joint space narrowing—asymmetric
    - One side of body/one side of joint
  - Osteophytes
  - Eburnation of bone
  - Subchondral cysts "geodes"
- Advanced imaging—rarely needed
  - MRI—"bone bruises" predict cartilage lesions and OA progression

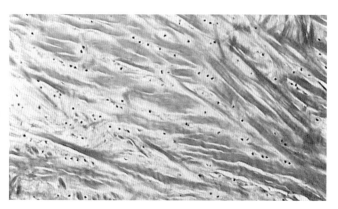

FIGURE 1-42 Histologic appearance of menisci.

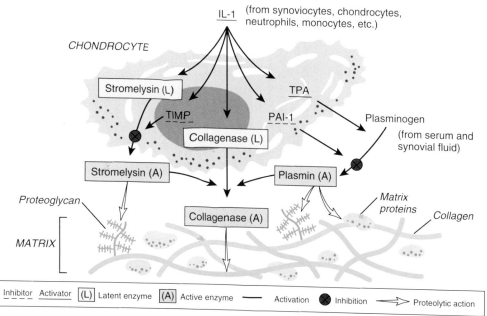

FIGURE 1-43 Enzyme cascade of interleukin-1–stimulated degradation of articular cartilage. (From Simon SR, editor: *Orthopaedic basic science,* Rosemont, Ill, 1994, American Academy of Orthopaedic Surgeons, p 40.)

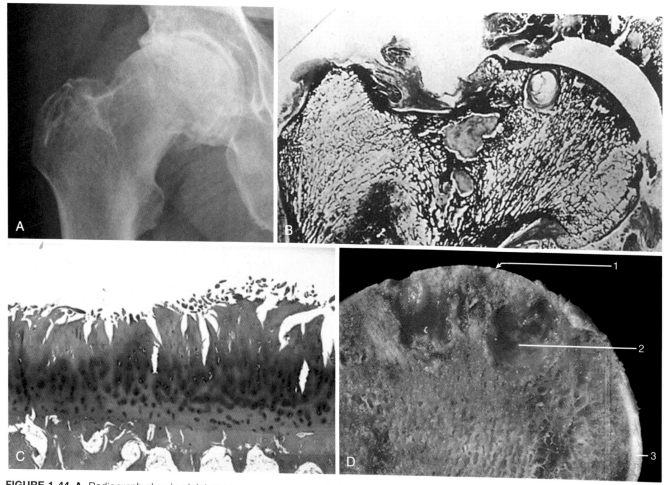

FIGURE 1-44 A, Radiograph showing joint space narrowing, osteophytes, and bony sclerosis. **B,** Macrosection of an osteoarthritic human femoral head demonstrating subarticular cysts, sclerotic bone formation, and a superior femoral head osteophyte. **C,** Low-power micrograph of osteoarthritis demonstrating fibrillation, fissures, and cartilage loss. **D,** Gross pathology of femoral head demonstrating cartilage thinning *(1),* subarticular cyst (*2* ["geode"]), and normal hyaline cartilage remaining *(3).* (**A,** Courtesy of Marc DeHart, MD, and Texas Orthopedics; **B,** Simon SR, editor: *Orthopaedic basic science,* Rosemont, Ill, 1994, American Academy of Orthopaedic Surgeons; **C** and **D** from Horvai A: Bones, joints, and soft tissue tumors. In Kumar V et al, editors: *Robbins and Cotran pathologic basis of disease,* ed 9, Philadelphia, 2015, Elsevier, Fig. 26-93.)

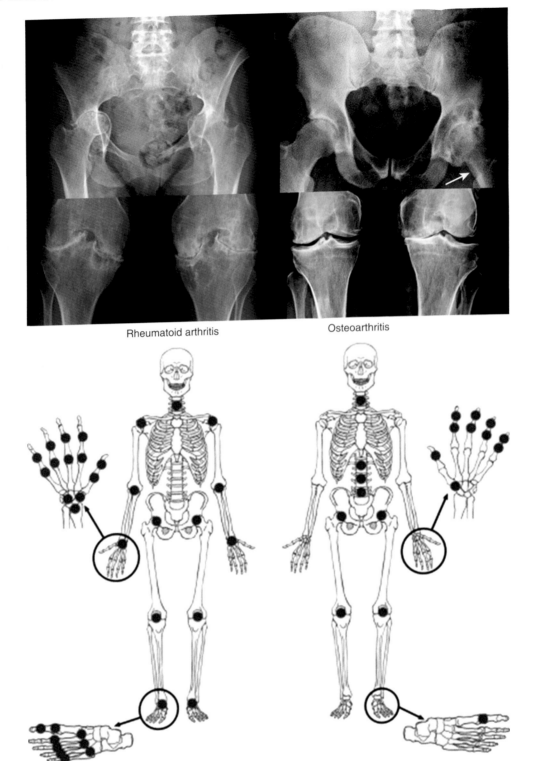

Rheumatoid arthritis   Osteoarthritis

FIGURE 1-45 Differences between rheumatoid arthritis (RA) and osteoarthritis. Left side of illustration demonstrates the main historical characteristics of RA, including symmetric involvement (both right and left joints as well as both medial and lateral compartments of the knees). Bilateral hand involvement is characteristic and usually involves wrist joints and proximal metacarpal joints. Right side of figure demonstrates osteoarthritis, which often is much more severe in one joint or one compartment of the knee. Hand involvement more commonly involves the distal interphalangeal joints (Heberden nodes) and proximal interphalangeal joints (Bouchard nodes) joints as well as the base of the thumb.

ARTHRITIS TYPES DEMONSTRATED IN HANDS

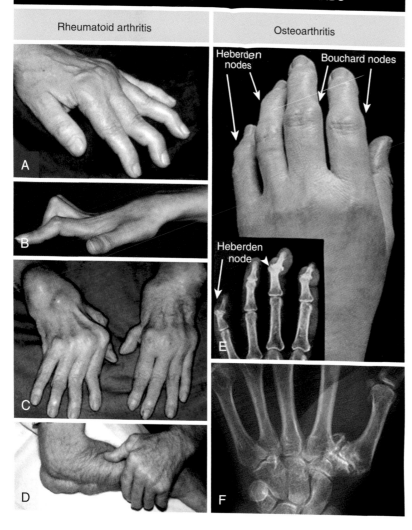

Rheumatoid arthritis | Osteoarthritis

Heberden nodes — Bouchard nodes

Heberden node

FIGURE 1-46 Upper extremity changes in common arthritis types. Left side of figure shows rheumatoid changes. **A,** "Swan neck deformity" of index, middle, and ring fingers, with proximal interphalangeal (PIP) joints extended and distal interphalangeal (DIP) joints flexed. **B,** "Boutonnière deformity": PIP joints flexed, DIP joints extended. **C,** Bilateral wrist swelling with both ulnar metacarpal phalangeal joint deformities and Swan neck deformities of fingers and left thumb. **D,** Rheumatoid nodes noted on posterior olecranon region. Right side of figure shows osteoarthritic changes. **E,** DIP changes (Heberden nodes) and PIP changes (Bouchard nodes). **F,** Radiograph showing osteoarthritic changes at the base of the thumb. (From O'Dell JD: Rheumatoid arthritis. In Goldman L, Schafer AI, editors: *Goldman-Cecil medicine*, Philadelphia, 2016, Elsevier, Fig 264-3; Sweeney SE et al: Clinical features of rheumatoid arthritis. In Firestein GS et al: *Kelley's textbook of rheumatology*, Philadelphia, 2013, Elsevier, Fig 70-4; and http://medsci.indiana.edu/c602web/602/c602web/jtcs/docs/heber1.html)

- dGEMRIC—delayed gadolinium-enhanced MRI of cartilage
  - Research for early diagnosis
- Microscopic changes (see Figure 1-44)
  - Fissuring and loss of superficial chondrocytes
  - Chondrocyte "cloning" (>1 chondrocyte per lacuna)
- Physical examination
  - Decreased ROM and crepitus
  - Knee: asymmetric involvement
  - Hand: distal interphalangeal (DIP), proximal interphalangeal (PIP), and thumb carpometacarpal joints (Figure 1-46)
  - Hip: superolateral versus central-medial involvement
- Treatment
  - Activity modification and low-level exercise
  - Weight loss, use of a cane
  - NSAIDs and COX-2 inhibitors
  - Corticosteroid injections for short-term release
  - Hyaluronic acid injections: controversial and expensive
  - Surgical procedures: arthroplasty and osteotomy
- Neuropathic arthropathy (Charcot joint disease)
  - Extreme form of arthritis caused by **disturbed sensory** innervation
  - Less pain than would be expected, considering radiographs
  - Etiology: two theories
    - Neuropathic loss of proprioception
      - Repetitive trauma causes microfractures.
    - Sympathetic-loss hyperemia
      - Stimulates osteoclasts, weakens bones
  - Diagnosis—clinical:
    - **Unstable, painless, swollen, red joint**
    - Effusion may show hemarthrosis.
    - Histology: osteochondral fragments imbedded in synovium
  - Radiographic findings (Figure 1-47):
    - Severe destructive changes on both sides of the joint
    - Scattered "chunks" of bone embedded in fibrous tissue
    - Joint distension by fluid
    - Heterotopic ossification

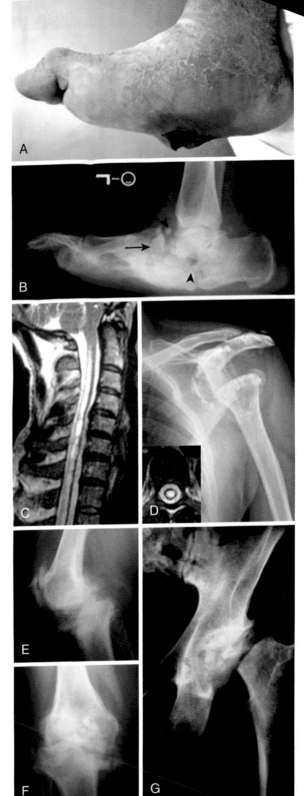

FIGURE 1-47 Neuropathic arthritis. Arthritic degeneration due to lack of sensation can be caused by many diseases. All share radiographic findings that are more severe than the symptoms (often painless) and the fragments from bony destruction. Often findings take many years to develop. **A** and **B,** Diabetic Charcot arthropathy of the foot is easily recognized by most of the industrialized world. **C** and **D,** The most common cause of upper extremity neuropathic joint is syringomyelia (syrinx = fluid-filled sac in central cord that causes insidious loss of pain and temperature early). **E** through **G,** Tabetic arthropathy (tertiary syphilis) is the most common neuropathic arthritis of the knee and can often involve the hip. (From Yablon CM et al: A review of Charcot neuroarthropathy of the midfoot and hindfoot: what every radiologist needs to know, *Curr Probl Diagn Radiol* 39:187–199, 2010; Atalar AC et al: Neuropathic arthropathy of the shoulder associated with syringomyelia: a report of six cases, *Acta Orthop Traumatol Turc* 44:328–336, 2010; and Allali F et al: Tabetic arthropathy. A report of 43 cases, *Clin Rheumatol* 25:858–860, 2006.)

- Charcot arthropathy versus osteomyelitis:
  - May be difficult with physical examination and radiograph
  - Both:
    - Swelling, warmth, erythema, variable pain
    - Variable WBCs and erythrocyte sedimentation rate (ESR)
  - Both entities common in diabetic patients
  - Technetium bone scan: may be "hot" (positive) for both
- Indium WBC scan:
  - "Hot" (positive) for osteomyelitis
  - "Cold" (negative) for Charcot arthropathy

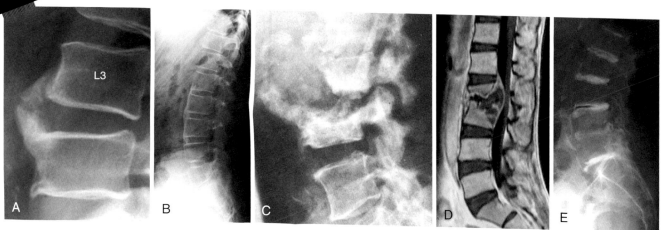

FIGURE 1-48 Arthritis in the spine. **A,** Diffuse idiopathic skeletal hyperostosis (Forestier disease), characterized by ossification of the entheses and flowing nonmarginal osteophytes with normal disc height (no sacroiliac [SI] or facet joint fusions). **B,** Ankylosing spondylitis, squaring lumbar and thoracic vertebrae with bridging marginal osteophytes ("bamboo spine"); SI fusion common (not shown). **C,** Neuropathic arthritis of the spine, characterized by more impressive radiograph findings than pain with scattered bony fragments in surrounding soft tissue. **D,** Tuberculous involvement of the spine (Pott disease); kyphotic collapse of lumbar or thoracic spine centered at the disc, involving both disc above and disc below. **E,** Ochronosis, showing thin, calcified discs in alkaptanuric patients with defect of homogentisic acid oxidase (black urine, cartilage and ears; see Fig. 1-49) (From Mazières B: Diffuse idiopathic skeletal hyperostosis (Forestier-Rotes-Querol disease): what's new? *Joint Bone Spine* 80:466–470, 2013; Jang JH et al: Ankylosing spondylitis: patterns of radiographic involvement—a re-examination of accepted principles in a cohort of 769 patients, *Radiology* 258:192–198, 2011; Crim JR et al: Spinal neuroarthropathy after traumatic paraplegia, *AJNR Am J Neuroradiol* 9:359–362, 1988; Ansari S: Pott's spine: diagnostic imaging modalities and technology advancements, *N Am J Med Sci* 5:404–411, 2013; and Miller MD et al: *Review of orthopaedics,* ed 6, Philadelphia, 2012, Saunders.)

- Treatment: limitation of activity
  - Bracing or casting (total contact cast)
  - May discontinue when skin temperature normal
  - Fusion after inflammatory phase in feet
  - Usually a contraindication for total joint arthroplasty (TJA)
- Causes and common sites:
  - Diabetes—most common cause (1% of those with neuropathy)
    - Charcot joint disease
    - Foot and ankle most commonly involved (see Figure 1-47, *A* and *B*)
  - Tabes dorsalis (syphilitic myelopathy)
    - Increasing rates seen in United States
    - Knee most common (see Figure 1-47, *E* and *F*)
  - Syringomyelia—syrinx by MRI of neck (see Figure 1-47, *C*)
    - Most common cause of upper extremity neuroarthropathy
    - 80% shoulder and elbow (see Figure 1-47, *D*)
    - Joint disease develops in 25% of patients with syringomyelia.
  - Leprosy—Hansen disease
    - Second most common cause in upper extremity
  - Other neurologic problems
    - Myelomeningocele: ankle and foot
    - Spina bifida and spinal trauma: (Figure 1-48, *C*; also see Figure 1-47, *G*)
      - Hip, knee, ankle, and spine
    - Congenital insensitivity to pain: ankle and foot
- Ochronosis arthritis from alkaptonuria (Figure 1-49; also see Figure 1-48, *D*)
  - Rare inborn metabolic
    - Autosomal recessive defect of homogentisic acid oxidase
    - Tyrosine and phenylalanine catabolism
  - Excess homogentisic acid deposited in the joints

- Accumulation of homogentisic acid causes cartilage destruction.
  - Spine, hips, knees, and shoulders
- Polymerizes with O_2
  - Tints matrix black
  - Stiffens cartilage
  - Leads to early arthritis, thin spinal discs
- Deposited in other tissues: heart valves, ears
- Patients may also present with black urine.
- Ochronotic spondylitis
  - Usually fourth decade of life
  - Progressive degenerative changes, disc space narrowing, and calcification
- Hemochromatosis arthritis (Figure 1-50)
  - Common inborn metabolic (frequently undiagnosed)
    - Abnormal excessive iron absorption
    - Genetic—*HFE* gene, *C282Y* mutation
      - 1 in 10 Caucasians are carriers
    - More common in Northern Europeans
      - So-called Celtic curse or Viking disease (Dupuytren contracture)
  - Classic triad—late findings:
    - Skin tints, diabetes, cirrhosis
      - "Bronze diabetes"—iron deposits in pancreas
      - "Pigmented cirrhosis"—iron deposits in liver
    - Presents in late middle age as iron accumulates
    - Males earlier than females (menses protects)
  - 50% to 80% of hereditary hemochromatosis patients have arthritis (most frequent presentation).
    - Hemosiderin deposition in synovium and chondrocytes
    - Chondrocalcinosis (CPPD)/pseudogout in 20% to 50%
    - Hook-like osteophytes on second and third metacarpal heads
    - Severe metacarpophalangeal (MCP) osteoarthritis
    - Hip, knee, ankle, wrist arthritis

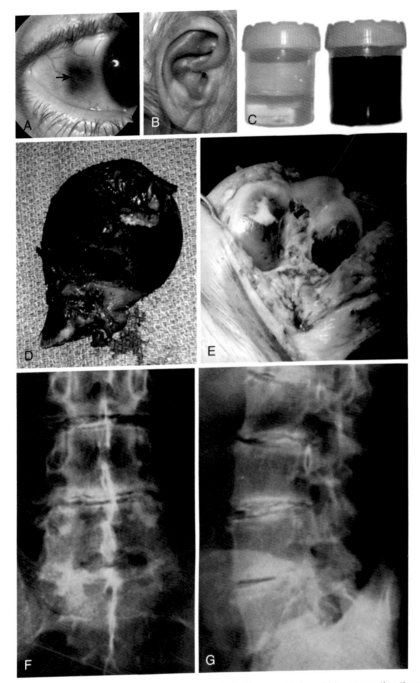

FIGURE 1-49 Ochronosis: so-called black arthritis of alkaptonuria. **A** and **B,** Homogentisic acid in connective tissues is noted most often in the eyes and ears. **C,** Urine left standing turns dark. **D** and **E,** When deposited into cartilage, arthritis develops, revealing dark/black cartilage. **F** and **G,** Characteristic irregular calcification and narrowing of intervertebral discs. Radiolucent streaks, evident anteriorly between the vertebral bodies, are not uncommon. (From Miller MD et al: *Review of orthopaedics*, ed 6, Philadelphia, 2012, Saunders; Ryan A, O'Toole L: Images in clinical medicine. Ochronosis, *N Engl J Med* 367:e26, 2012; Fisher AA, Davis MW: Alkaptonuric ochronosis with aortic valve and joint replacements and femoral fracture: a case report and literature review, *Clin Med Res* 2:209–215, 2004; and Harun M et al: A rare cause of arthropathy: an ochronotic patient with black joints, *Int J Surg Case Rep* 5:554–557, 2014.)

- High liver enzyme tests, cirrhosis
- Hypogonadism, diabetes
- Diagnosis depends on high degree of suspicion
  - Suspect if arthritis with high liver enzyme tests, especially if CPPD
    - Screen:
      - High ferritin (>200 µg/L)
      - High transferrin saturation (>45%)
    - Prove:
      - Genetic test
      - Liver biopsy of cirrhosis

- Treatment: phlebotomy, low-iron diet
  - Liver-friendly life
- Hypertrophic osteoarthropathy (Figure 1-51)
  - Clinical diagnosis; cause unknown
    - May be related to increased:
      - PDGF
      - Vascular endothelial growth factor (VEGF)
  - Primary hypertrophic osteoarthropathy—rare
    - Children (<20)
    - Autosomal dominant, male/female 9:1
    - Pachydermoperiostosis—skin hypertrophy

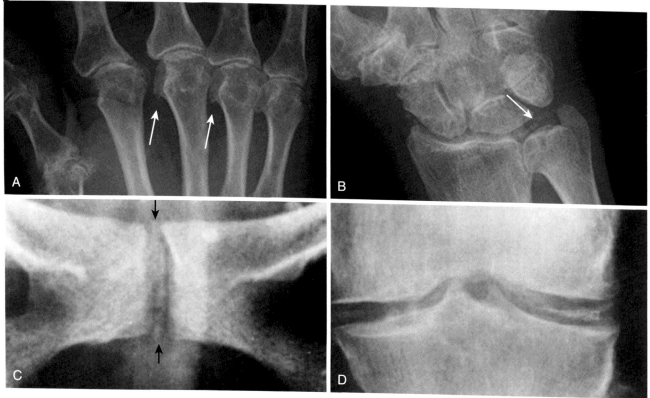

FIGURE 1-50 Hemochromatosis. Hemochromatosis arthropathy is often the first clinical hint of this preventable cause of cirrhosis. **A,** Hand radiographs show characteristic "hook-like" osteophytes on radial metacarpal heads *(arrows)* and joint space narrowing and subchondral sclerosis of metacarpophalangeal joints. **B,** Chondrocalcinosis present in the wrist *(arrow)*. **C,** Pubic symphyseal calcifications *(arrow)*. **D,** Knee chondrocalcinosis. (From Husar-Memmer et al: HFE-related hemochromatosis: an update for the rheumatologist, *Curr Rheumatol Rep* 16:393, 2014; Jensen PS: Hemochromatosis: a disease often silent but not invisible, *AJR Am J Roentgenol* 126:343–351, 1976.)

- Classic secondary pulmonary hypertrophic osteoarthropathy
  - **Clubbing of fingers/toes**—acropachy (see Figure 1-51, *B*)
  - Bilateral leg swelling
  - **Bilateral symmetric periostitis of long bone–diaphyseal pain**
  - Large joint effusions (<500 WBCs)
  - **Lung tumor,** chronic lung infection, or cyanotic heart disease
- Diagnosis: radiographs show periosteal new bone in diaphysis
  - Bone scan—symmetrical distal tubular bones uptake
    - "Double stripe" "parallel track" (see Figure 1-51, *A*)
- Treatment: symptomatic with NSAIDs, bisphosphonates
  - Resect lung tumor—symptoms resolve

■ **Inflammatory arthritides**
■ Collection of varied diseases that cause joint inflammation
■ Clinical factors often help distinguish specific diagnosis:
  - Joint locations involved
  - Chronology of presentation
  - Associated disorders
  - Prudent use of laboratory studies
■ Diagnosis and best treatment often involves rheumatology consultation.
■ Rheumatoid arthritis (Table 1-21)
  - Most common inflammatory arthritis
  - Chronic systemic autoimmune disease

- Mononuclear cells—primary mediator of RA tissue damage
- 0.5% to 1% of population, women three times the rate of men
- 15% concordance rate in monozygotic twins
- 50% have to stop working in 10 years
- Articular erosions present within 1 to 2 years
- Early diagnosis prevents deformity and maintains function.
- Clinical presentation (see Figure 1-45)
  - Insidious subacute onset over 6 weeks
  - Fatigue, malaise, anemia
  - Morning stiffness and polyarthritis with swelling
- Hands/wrists have early involvement: MCP and PIP
  - Later develop characteristic changes (see Figure 1-46):
    - Ulnar deviation and MCP subluxation
    - "Piano-key" ulna—hypermobile distal radioulnar joint (DRUJ)
    - "Swan-neck deformity"—PIP extended/DIP flexed
    - "Boutonnière deformity"—PIP flexed/DIP extended
    - "Z-line deformity"—thumb IP extended/MP flexed
- Feet affected early—30% present with foot pain
  - Metatarsophalangeal (MTP) joints, claw toes, and hallux valgus

Table 1-21 Comparison of Common Arthritides

ARTHRITIS	AGE GROUP AFFECTED	INCIDENCE BY SEX	SYMMETRY	JOINTS	PHYSICAL EXAMINATION	LABORATORY TESTS	RADIOGRAPHIC FINDINGS	SYSTEMIC MANIFESTATIONS	TREATMENT
NONINFLAMMATORY									
Osteoarthritis	Elderly	M > F	Asymmetric	Hip, knee, CMC	↓ ROM, crepitus	Nonspecific	Asymmetric narrowing, eburnation, cysts, osteophytes	None	NSAIDs, arthrodesis, osteotomy, TJA
Neuropathic	Elderly	M > F	Asymmetric	Foot, ankle, lower extremity	Effusion, unstable	For underlying disease	Destruction/ heterotopic bone	None	Brace; TJA contraindicated
Acute rheumatic fever	Children	M = F	Asymmetric	Migratory; large joints	Red, tender joint; rash	ASO titer	Usually normal	Erythema marginatum nodules, carditis	Symptomatic
Ochronosis	Adults	M = F	Asymmetric	Large joints/ spine	↓ ROM, locking	Urine homogentisic acid	Destruction, disc calcification	Spondylosis	Supportive
INFLAMMATORY									
Rheumatoid	Young adults	F > M	Symmetric	Hands, feet	Ulnar deviation, claw toes	ESR, CRP, RF	Symmetric narrow, periarticular resorption	Pericardial and pulmonary disease	Pyramid treatment for synovitis, reconstructive surgery
Systemic lupus erythematosus	Young adults	F > M	Symmetric	PIP joint, MCP joint, knee	Red, swollen joint; rash	ANA	Less destruction	Cardiac, renal, pancytopenia	Drug therapy as for rheumatoid arthritis
Juvenile rheumatoid arthritis	Children	F > M	Symmetric	Knee, multiple	Swollen joint, normal color	RF/ANA	Juxta-articular late, osteopenia	Iridocyclitis, rash	ASA; 75% remission
Relapsing polychondritis	Elderly	M = F	Symmetric	All joints	Eye, ear involved	ESR	Normal	Otic, cardiac	Supportive, dapsone?
SPONDYLOARTHROPATHIES									
Ankylosing spondylitis	Young adults	M > F	Symmetric	Sacroiliac, spine, hip	Rigid spine, "chin on chest"	ESR, alkaline phosphatase, CPK, HLA-B27	Sacroiliac arthritis, bamboo spine	Uveitis	Physical therapy, NSAID, osteotomy
Reactive Arthritis (Reiter syndrome)	Young adults	M > F	Asymmetric	Weight-bearing	Urethral discharge, conjunctivitis	ESR, WBC count, HLA-B27	MT head erosion, periostitis	Urethritis, conjunctivitis, ulcer	Physical therapy, NSAID, sulfa?
Psoriatic	Young adults	M = F	Asymmetric	DIP joint, small joints	Rash, sausage digit, pitting	ESR, HLA-B27	DIP joint: pencil-in-cup deformity	Rash, conjunctivitis	Drug therapy as for rheumatoid arthr˙
Enteropathic	Young adults	M > F	Asymmetric	Weight-bearing	Synovitis, gastrointestinal manifestations	ESR, HLA-B27	Normal	Erythema nodosum, pyoderma	Treatment for bo˙ disease, symptomatic therapy

	Age	Sex	Pattern	Location	Clinical	Diagnosis	Radiographic	Associated	Treatment
CRYSTAL DEPOSITION DISEASE									
Gout	Young	M > F	Asymmetric	Great toe, lower extremity	Tophi, red, swollen	Uric acid: Birefringent crystals	Soft tissue swelling, erosions	Tophi, renal stones	Colchicine, indomethacin
Chondrocalcinosis	Elderly	M = F	Asymmetric	Knee, lower extremity	Acute swelling	Birefringent rhombus-shaped crystals	Articular fibrocartilage calcified	Ochronosis, hyperparathyroidism, hypothyroidism	Symptomatic therapy: avoid surgery
INFECTIOUS									
Pyogenic	All	M = F	Asymmetric	Any joint	Red, hot, swollen	WBC count, ESR, bacterial cultures	Joint narrowing (late)	Fever, chills, infection	I&D, intravenous antibiotics
Tuberculous	Elderly	M > F	Asymmetric	Spine, lower extremity	Indolent, swelling	PPD, AFB, cultures	Both sides, cysts	Lung, multiorgan	Antibiotics ± I&D
Lyme disease	Young	M = F	Asymmetric	Any joint	Acute effusion	Culture, ELISA	Usually normal	ECM rash, neurologic, cardiac	Penicillin, tetracycline
Fungal	All	M > F	Asymmetric	Any joint	Indolent	Special studies/cultures	Minimal changes	Immunocompromised	5-flucytosine, amphotericin
HEMORRHAGIC									
Hemophilia	Young	M	Asymmetric	Knee, upper extremity (elbow, shoulder)	↓ ROM, swelling	PTT, factor VIII	Squared-off patella	Soft tissue bleeding	Support, synovectomy, TJA
Sickle cell disease	Young	M = F	Asymmetric	Hip, any bone	Pain, ↓ ROM	Sickle preparation	Osteonecrosis	Infarcts, osteonecrosis	Supportive and symptomatic therapy
Pigmented villonodular synovitis	Young	M = F	Asymmetric	Knee, lower extremity	Pain, synovitis	Aspirate, biopsy	Juxtacortical erosion	None	Surgical excision

AFB, Acid-fast bacilli; *ANA,* antinuclear antibody; *ASA,* acetylsalicylic acid; *ASO,* antistreptolysin O; *CMC,* carpometacarpal; *CPK,* creatine phosphokinase; *CRP,* C-reactive protein; *DIP,* distal interphalangeal; *ECM,* erythema chronicum migrans; *ELISA,* enzyme-linked immunosorbent assay; *ESR,* erythrocyte sedimentation rate; *HLA,* human leukocyte antigen; *I&D,* incision and drainage; *MCP,* metacarpophalangeal; *MT,* metatarsal; *NSAID,* nonsteroidal antiinflammatory drug; *PIP,* proximal interphalangeal; *PPD,* purified protein derivative; *PTT,* partial thromboplastin time; *RF,* rheumatoid factor; ↓ *ROM,* decreased range of motion; *TJA,* total joint arthroplasty; *WBC,* white blood cell.

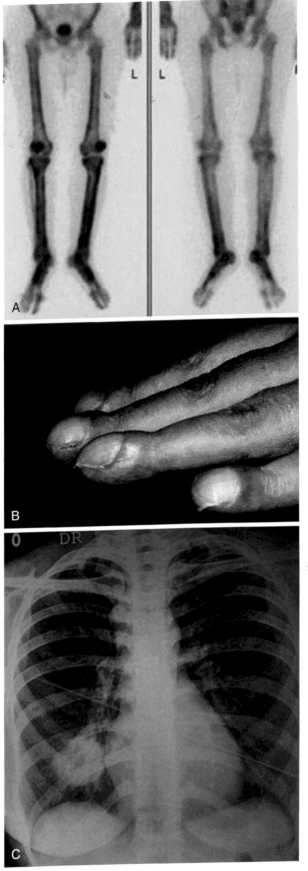

FIGURE 1-51 Hypertrophic osteoarthropathy (secondary pulmonary). Bilateral lower extremity swelling with diaphyseal symmetric periostitis of long bones associated with pulmonary tumors, chronic lung infections, and cyanotic heart disease. May be associated with joint effusions. A clinical diagnosis with unknown cause that may be related to platelet-derived growth factor (PDGF) or vascular endothelial growth factor (VEGF). **A,** Bone scan demonstrates "double track" sign (or "parallel track" sign), which represents the painful periosteal new bone that forms in the diaphysis of long bones in hypertrophic osteoarthropathy. **B,** Clubbing of fingers/toes (acropachy). **C,** Lung tumor, a cause of secondary pulmonary hypertrophic osteoarthropathy. (From Yao Q et al: Periostitis and hypertrophic pulmonary osteoarthropathy: report of 2 cases and review of the literature, *Semin Arthritis Rheum* 38:458–466, 2009; and Firestein GS et al: *Kelley's textbook of rheumatology,* ed 9, Philadelphia, Saunders, 2012.)

- Also common in the knees, elbows, shoulders, ankles, and cervical spine
- Subcutaneous "rheumatoid nodules" (see Figure 1-46)
- Diagnostic criteria of American Rheumatism Association:
  - **Morning stiffness lasting longer than 60 minutes**
  - **Swelling—symmetric, both hands/feet**
  - Nodules—20% of RA patients over life
  - **Positive laboratory test results** often found:
    - ESR, C-reactive protein (CRP)
    - Rheumatoid factor (RF) titer:
      - Autoantibodies (immunoglobulin [Ig]M or IgG) to Fc portion of IgG
      - Positive in about 80%
      - Positive years before symptoms develop
    - Anticyclic citrullinated protein (anti-CCP)
      - Also known as *anticitrullinated protein antibodies* (ACPAs)
      - Most sensitive and specific test (≈90% specific)
      - Positive years before symptoms develop
      - Linked to more aggressive disease
    - Aspiration:
      - WBCs: typically 5000 to 50,000
      - Often increased RF
      - Decreased complement
  - Radiographic findings are symmetric (see Figure 1-45)
    - Juxta-articular erosions and periarticular osteopenia
- Pathogenesis: probably related to a T cell–mediated immune response from an infectious or environmental antigen (smoking is one known trigger) that stimulates a genetically susceptible individual (HLA-DR4 and HLA-Dw4)
  - Incites a delayed inflammatory response
  - Initial response on soft tissues—neovascularization and synovitis
    - Intimal lining hyperplasia with **mononuclear** WBC cells:
      - CD4$^+$ **T lymphocytes**: "helper cells"
        - Activate both synovial cell types though **direct cell-cell contact**
    - Both synoviocytes produce cytokines:
      - Macrophages (type-A): main source for TNF-α, IL-1
      - Fibroblast (type-B): main source for MMPs, proteases, and RANKL
    - B lymphocytes (plasma cells): make RF, anti-CCP antibodies
  - Cytokines upregulated: TNF-α, IL-1, IL-6, IL-7
    - IL-1:
      - Regulator of inflammation and matrix destruction
    - TNF-α:
      - Upregulates endothelial adhesion molecules
      - Promotes influx of leukocytes
      - Activates synovial fibroblasts
      - Stimulates angiogenesis
      - Promotes pain receptor pathways
      - **Drives osteoclastogenesis**
    - IL-6:
      - From fibroblast-like T cells and monocytes
      - Stimulates immunoglobulin from plasma cells
  - Later response destroys:
    - Cartilage: chondrolysis from externally and from within

- Synovial cells invade cartilage "pannus" and release MMPs.
- PMNs in synovial fluid release MMPs.
- Chondrocytes under stress release MMPs.
- Bone: periarticular erosions
  - Cytokines stimulate osteoblasts and synovial B cells to make RANKL.
  - RANKL joins RANK receptor to activate osteoclasts.
  - Osteoclasts secrete:
    - Cathepsin K dissolves collagen.
    - Carbonic anhydrase dissolves crystals.
- Systemic manifestations
  - Rheumatoid vasculitis:
    - Distal splinter hemorrhage to gangrene
    - Cutaneous ulcers (pyoderma gangrenosum) (see Figure 1-56, C)
    - Visceral arteritis
  - Pericarditis:
    - Pericardial effusion
  - Pulmonary disease:
    - Pleurisy, nodules, fibrosis
- Named syndromes of RA:
  - Felty syndrome:
    - Severe erosive RA
    - Splenomegaly and leukopenia
  - Still disease:
    - Acute-onset juvenile RA (JRA)
    - Fever, rash, and splenomegaly
  - Sjögren syndrome:
    - Autoimmune exocrinopathy (IgA)
    - Lymphoid proliferation of exocrine glands
    - Decreased saliva and tears (sicca complex)
    - Often associated with RA
- Treatment and their perioperative considerations:
  - Treatment goals:
    - Remission
    - Control synovitis and pain.
    - Maintain joint function.
    - Prevent deformities.
    - Limit adverse drug reactions (ADRs).
  - Treatment regimen:
    - Variable, dependent on patient response
    - Usually multiple agents
  - NSAIDs: help symptoms early—antiinflammatory effects
    - COX inhibitors
    - ADRs: GI, hypertension (HTN), renal, cardiac
    - Hold for 7 to 10 days preoperatively.
  - Low-dose steroids help with inflammation.
    - Decrease prostaglandins and leukotrienes.
    - Used initially as "bridge therapy" to disease-modifying antirheumatic drugs (DMARDs)
    - ADRs: osteoporosis, HTN, diabetes, cataracts
    - Doses higher than 7.5 mg/day and longer than 3 weeks:
      - "Stress dose" (50-100 mg) prednisone for day of surgery
  - DMARDs
    - Intended to address underlying autoimmune response
    - Markedly successful
    - Decrease symptoms and need for surgery
    - Conventional DMARDs: take 2 to 6 months to work

- Methotrexate: folate analogue
  - Inhibits purine metabolism and T-cell activation
  - Inhibits neovascularization
  - ADRs: toxic to bone marrow, liver, and lung
    - Need CBC and liver enzyme tests
  - Usually can continue through surgery
  - Hold preoperatively for renal insufficiency, severe diabetes, alcohol abuse
- Azathioprine: immunosuppressive agent
  - ADR: neutropenia
- Cyclosporine: immunosuppressive agent
  - Inhibits activation of CD4$^+$ T cells
  - ADRs: nephrotoxic, neurotoxic, gingival hyperplasia
- Leflunomide: inhibits pyrimidine in rapidly dividing cells
  - ADR: diarrhea
  - Stop for major procedures
- Hydroxychloroquine (Plaquenil)
  - Inhibits toll-like receptor (TLR9)
  - ADR: retinal toxicity—ophthalmology visits
  - Can continue for all procedures
- Sulfasalazine
  - Decrease synthesis of inflammatory mediators
  - ADRs: granulocytopenia, hemolytic anemia (G6PD)
  - Can continue for all procedures
- Minocycline—a tetracycline
  - Inhibits MMP collagenase
  - ADR: cutaneous hyperpigmentation
- Biologic DMARDs:
  - Target TNF-α—etanercept, infliximab, adalimumab
  - Target IL-1—anakinra
  - Usually hold for 2 weeks before and after major surgery
  - Risks of atypical infections/reactivate tuberculosis (TB)/lymphoma
  - Azathioprine
- Surgical treatment:
  - Joint surgery
    - Synovectomy—less commonly used
      - May decrease pain and swelling
      - Does not prevent radiographic progression
      - Does not prevent need for arthroplasty
      - Does not improve ROM
        - Total joint replacement (not osteotomy or partial)
  - RA patients have increased risks for surgery
  - Perioperative considerations:
    - Clear C-spine:
      - Atlantoaxial subluxation
      - Basilar invagination
      - Subaxial subluxation
    - Increased infection risk:
      - Nearly twice normal controls
      - Autoimmune disease: altered immunity
      - Prednisone
      - Biologic DMARDs
      - Anemia—increases transfusion risk
- Juvenile idiopathic arthritis (JIA) (also JRA; see Table 1-21)
  - Autoimmune arthritis in children
  - Most common chronic rheumatic disease of childhood

- More than 6 weeks of persistent joint swelling . someone younger than age 16
- No specific lab
- Classified by age, number of joints, extraarticular symptoms
- Prompt treatment can avoid complications:
  - Macrophage activation syndrome (MAS)
  - Contractures
  - Growth retardation
  - Loss of vision
- Oligoarticular (pauciarticular) JIA: approximately 40%
  - Most common and best prognosis
    - Child younger than age 8 (girls > boys)
    - Fewer than five joints involved
  - Asymmetric
    - Knees most common
    - Not involving hips/spine
  - Painless iridocyclitis/uveitis :
    - Can prevent blindness with slit lamp exams
    - Kids with chronic arthritis get eye exams!
  - Laboratory findings: nondiagnostic; positive ANA can be present
- Seronegative polyarticular JIA: approximately 20%
  - Affects 8- to 12-year-olds; girls and boys equally
  - Many joints (>4)
  - Large joints: knees (not hips/spine)
  - Poor weight gain/growth
  - Negative RF
- Seropositive polyarticular JIA: approximately 15%
  - Teenage girls affected more than boys—resembles adult RA
    - Positive HLA-DR4, 10% with nodules
  - Many joints: hands/wrists
  - Symmetric (not hips/spine)
  - Aggressive (+RF) erosive disease
    - May have vasculitis, rheumatoid lung
    - May have Felty syndrome:
      - RA, splenomegaly, neutropenia
- Systemic onset JIA (Still disease): approximately 10% to 20%
  - Any age
  - Number of joints involved vary, sometimes hip
  - Myalgic back pain
  - Systemic involvement: **CAN BE FATAL**
    - **Diurnal fevers** ("rabbit-ear" graph)
    - Nonpruritic **salmon macular evanescent rash**
    - **Lymphadenopathy, hepatosplenomegaly**
    - Serositis
    - **Macrophage activation syndrome (MAS)**
      - "Cytokine storm" by T-cell activation
      - Disseminated intravascular coagulation (DIC) causes bruising and mucosal bleeding
      - Causes elevated ferritin but decrease in ESR
  - Laboratory findings: elevated ESR, CRP, liver enzymes, WBCs, platelets
  - Anemia
- Psoriatic JIA: less than 10%
  - Any age, varied, frequently peripheral small joints
  - Asymmetric, sometimes hip, **OFTEN SPINE**
    - **DIP joints, nail pitting, dactylitis**
    - 20% painful uveitis and painless iridocyclitis
      - **Need eye screen**
  - Laboratory findings: nondiagnostic

- ...sitis-related JIA (juvenile ankylosing spondylitis): less than 10%
  - Children 8 to 12 years of age; **affects more boys than girls**
  - Number of joints involved vary; lower extremity
  - **HIPS AND SPINE**
  - Enthesitis/sacroiliac joint
  - Dactylitis, heel pain, oral ulcers
  - May have inflammatory bowel disease
  - Positive Schober lumbar flexion test:
    - A line 10 cm above L5 above while erect
    - Should grow to 15 cm when spine flexed
  - Laboratory findings: positive HLA-B27; may have elevated ESR, CRP
- Relapsing polychondritis (RPC) (Figure 1-52; see Table 1-21)
  - Migratory nonerosive arthritis with ear, nose, and throat (ENT) issues
  - Rare disorder; episodic inflammation of cartilage
  - **70% self-limiting nonerosive joint arthritis**
    - Costochondral, sternoclavicular, and manubriosternal
    - Ankles, wrists, hands, and feet
  - Progressive cartilage destruction of **ear, nose, and trachea**
    - **Thickening of the auricle, floppy ear**
    - **"Saddle nose" deformity**
    - Also may involve eye and heart valves
  - Ocular: scleritis, episcleritis, and conjunctivitis
  - Unknown cause: genetic predisposition to external trigger
    - **Often antibodies to type II collagen**
    - **Matrilin-1** (fetal epiphyseal protein) in adults; unique to certain cartilage:
      - Auricular, nasal, tracheal, and costochondral
    - **HLA-DR4 more often positive**
  - One third occur with other disorders
    - Vasculitis
    - Connective tissue disorders, RA, SLE
    - Myelodysplastic disorders
  - Treatment: NSAIDs, dapsone, prednisone
- Systemic lupus erythematosus (SLE) (Figure 1-53; see Table 1-21)
  - Chronic inflammatory disease of unknown origin
  - **90% women** (black > white)
  - Initially mediated by **tissue-binding autoantibodies and immune complexes**
    - **Type III hypersensitivity**
  - Pathophysiology:
    - Susceptible genetics stimulated by environment
    - Damage to self-cells
      - Ultraviolet light damages skin
      - Epstein-Barr virus (EBV) infection
      - Smoking, exposure to silica
    - Dendritic cells sample nuclear DNA/proteins
    - Immune system autoregulatory failure
    - Sustained production of antibody to self-antigens
      - **Antinuclear antibodies (ANA)**—best screen; positive in 95%
      - **Anti-dsDNA**—double-stranded DNA SLE specific
      - **Anti-Sm**—nuclear RNA SLE specific
      - **Antihistone antibodies**—drug-induced lupus
      - Anti-Ro (SS-A)—SICCA (not SLE specific)
      - Anti-La (SS-B)—anti RNA
    - **Immune complexes** accumulate in various tissues.
      - Chronic inflammation causes pathology:
        - Skin/joints—rash, arthritis are most common
        - Heart/kidney—pericarditis/**nephritis**
        - Blood vessels—vasculitis
  - Clinical findings:
    - Joint involvement—most common feature
      - Nonerosive polyarthritis affects over 75%
      - PIP, MCP, carpus, knees, and others
    - **Butterfly malar rash—classic feature**
    - Fever, pancytopenia
    - **Osteonecrosis (especially with steroids)**
  - Laboratory findings:
    - Positive ANA
    - HLA-DR3 titers and may have positive RF titers
  - Treatment: same medications as for RA
- Polymyalgia rheumatica
  - Common among elderly persons (>50 years)
  - Women twice the rate of men
  - Caucasians of Northern European descent
  - Symmetric aching and longer than 30 minutes of morning stiffness
    - Bilateral shoulders and pelvic girdle
  - Associated with malaise, anorexia, fever, and headaches
    - Associated with giant cell arteritis/systemic vasculitis
    - **If temporal arteritis, then prevent blindness**
      - Need temporal artery biopsy
      - High-dose steroids
  - Physical examination findings: usually unremarkable
  - Laboratory findings: **markedly elevated ESR,** elevated CRP
    - Anemia
  - Treatment:
    - Usually symptomatic
    - Steroids for refractory cases
- Seronegative spondyloarthritis: SpA
  - Overlapping inflammatory disorders
    - Unified by similar clinical manifestation
  - Characterized by **negative RF titer**
  - Other laboratory findings nonspecific:
    - ESR and CRP often elevated
  - Common genetic predisposition:
    - Positive HLA-B27 (if negative, SpA is unlikely)
      - Higher percentage positive when axial involvement
      - Lower percentage positive when peripheral arthritis
    - Frequent first- or second-generation family history of SpA
  - Symptoms: musculoskeletal—peripheral versus axial
    - Inflammatory back pain
    - Peripheral arthritis
    - Enthesitis—heel pain
    - Dactylitis—"sausage digit"
    - Eye—uveitis (iritis), conjunctivitis
    - Skin, mucosal, GI, urethral
  - Most with very similar treatment routines
    - NSAIDs and/or DMARDs early
    - Biologics later: anti-TNF-α
- Ankylosing spondylitis: AS (Figure 1-54, Table 1-22; also see Table 1-21)
  - **Male/female ratio 3:1;** aged 20 to 40
  - Most common in Northern European whites
  - **90% HLA-B27 positive** (Table 1-23)

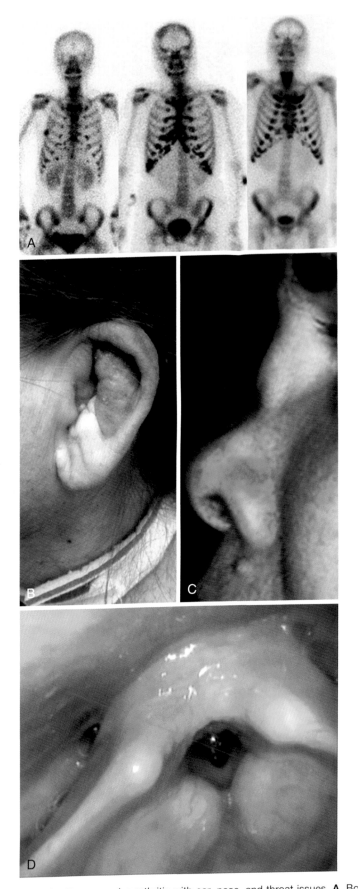

FIGURE 1-52 Relapsing polychondritis. Episodic nonerosive arthritis with ear, nose, and throat issues. **A,** Bone scans on three patients demonstrate "beaded string" uptake pattern at costochondral and sternoclavicular joints and nasopharyngeal cartilage. **B,** Lobe-sparing auricular chondral inflammation. **C,** "Saddle-nose" from nasal chondritis. **D,** Tracheal stenosis resulting from tracheobronchial chondritis. (From Shi XH et al: The value of 99mTc methylene diphosphonate bone scintigraphy in diagnosing relapsing polychondritis, *Chin Med J (Engl)* 119:1129–1132, 2006; and Iowa Head and Neck Protocols: Case example subglottic stenosis and relapsing polychondritis. Available at: https://wiki.uiowa.edu/display/protocols/Case+Example++Subglottic+Stenosis+and+Relapsing+Polychondritis.)

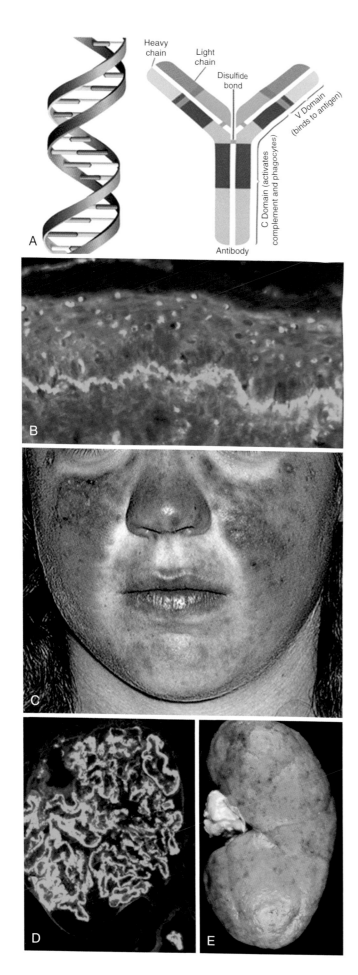

FIGURE 1-53 Systemic lupus erythematosus (SLE). **A,** Autoantibodies to DNA and DNA binding proteins form immune complexes that stimulate immune system–directed inflammation throughout the body (type III hypersensitivity reaction). **B,** Direct immunofluorescence with anti-immunoglobulin (Ig)G antibodies shows immune complex deposits at two different places: a bandlike deposit along the epidermal basement membrane—"lupus band test"—and within the nuclei of the epidermal cells (antinuclear antibodies [ANA]). **C,** Most patients have skin and joint involvement. The classic butterfly rash of SLE occurs in 10% to 50% of patients with acute SLE. **D,** The same immune complexes are seen in the basement membrane of the renal glomerulus. **E,** "Flea-bitten" appearance of kidney specimen, with lupus nephritis causing various degrees of proteinuria, hematuria, and cellular casts. (From Habif TP: *Clinical dermatology,* ed 5, St Louis, Mosby/Elsevier, 2009; Wikimedia Commons: Diffuse proliferative lupus nephritis. Available at: http://en.wikipedia.org/wiki/Lupus_nephritis#mediaviewer/File:Diffuse_proliferative_lupus_nephritis.jpg ; and Wikimedia Commons: Lupus band test. Available at: http://en.wikipedia.org/wiki/Systemic_lupus_erythematosus#mediaviewer/File:Lupus_band_test.jpg.)

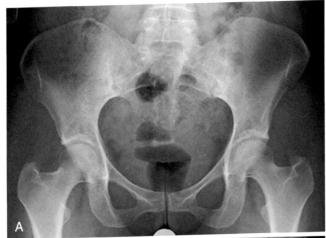

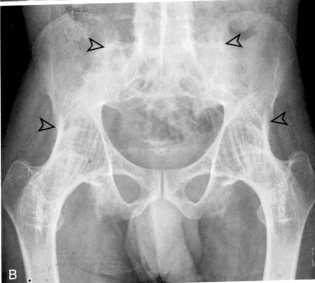

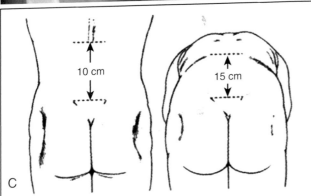

FIGURE 1-54 Ankylosing spondylitis (AS) is an axial seronegative spondyloarthropathy that causes progressive cervical and thoracic kyphosis and "bamboo spine" (also see Figure 1-48, *B*) but has earliest involvement in the sacroiliac joints. **A,** Early sacroiliitis demonstrated by loss of clarity and sclerosis in the lower third of the sacroiliac joints, particularly affecting the iliac side of the right sacroiliac joint (hip joints are normal). **B,** Advanced AS with ankylosis or fusion of both the sacroiliac and hip joints. **C,** Schober test; the difference between 2 marks 10 cm apart when erect versus flexed forward should be less than 4 to 5 cm. (From Raychaudhuri S: The classification and diagnostic criteria of ankylosing spondylitis, *J Autoimmun* 48-49:128–133, 2014.)

Table 1-22	Commonly Confused Laboratory Findings Inflammatory Arthritic Conditions	
FINDING	**CONDITIONS IN WHICH FINDING MAY BE POSITIVE**	**CONDITIONS IN WHICH FINDING IS USUALLY NEGATIVE**
Rheumatoid factor	Rheumatoid arthritis	Ankylosing spondylitis
	Sjögren syndrome	Gout
	Sarcoid	Psoriatic arthritis
	Systemic lupus erythematosus	Reactive arthritis (Reiter syndrome)
Positivity for HLA-B27*	Ankylosing spondylitis	
	Reactive arthritis (Reiter syndrome)	
	Psoriatic arthritis	
	Enteropathic arthritis	
Antinuclear antibody (ANA)	Systemic lupus erythematosus	
	Sjögren syndrome	
	Scleroderma	

Modified from Brinker MR, Miller MD: *Fundamentals of orthopaedics,* Philadelphia, 1999, WB Saunders, p 27.
*Approximately 6% of all white people are HLA-B27 positive.

- Insidious onset of **back pain (spondylitis) in a patient younger than 40**
  - Improves with exercise, no better with rest, night pain
- Pathophysiology: granulation tissue at enthesis
  - Spine enthesis—annulus fibrosis and vertebral bone
  - Tissue has CD4$^+$, CD8$^+$ T cells and macrophages
- Axial skeleton:
  - Bilateral sacroiliitis—earliest symptom
  - Associated morning stiffness
  - Progressive spinal flexion deformities over life
    - Ascending ankyloses from thoracic to entire
    - "Chin-on-chest" deformity
  - Hip involvement at young age—poor prognosis
  - Enthesitis: inflammation of tendon insertion
- Examination:
  - Modified Schober test (lumbar flexion loss) (see Figure 1-54, *C*)
    - Mark lumbar spine 10 cm
    - Maximum spinal flexion: less than 4 cm increase is positive.
  - Chest expansion loss:
    - Circumference at fourth rib space
    - Max inspiration versus max expiration
    - Normally over 5 cm
- Diagnostic criteria:
  - More than 3 months of low back pain in someone younger than age 45
  - Definite x-ray or MRI sacroiliitis
- Radiographic changes (see Figure 1-48, *B*)
  - Squaring of the vertebrae
  - Vertical syndesmophytes
  - **"Bamboo spine"**
  - **Autofusion of sacroiliac joints (see Figure 1-54, *B*)**
  - "Whiskering" of the enthesis
- Extraskeletal issues:
  - Uveitis—red, painful eye in 40%
  - Colitis—5% to 10%; aortic insufficiency
  - Pulmonary function tests: pulmonary restriction, chest excursion

Table 1-23	Associations between HLA Alleles and Susceptibility to Some Rheumatic Diseases			
DISEASE	HLA MARKER	FREQUENCY (%) IN PATIENTS (WHITES)	FREQUENCY (%) IN CONTROLS (WHITES)	RELATIVE RISK
Ankylosing spondylitis	B27	90	9	87
Reactive arthritis (Reiter syndrome)	B27	79	9	37
Psoriatic arthritis	B27	48	9	10
Inflammatory bowel disease with spondylitis	B27	52	9	10
Adult rheumatoid arthritis	DR4	70	30	6
Polyarticular juvenile rheumatoid arthritis	DR4	75	30	7
Pauciarticular juvenile rheumatoid arthritis	DR8	30	5	5
	DR5	50	20	4.5
	DR2.1	55	20	4
Systemic lupus erythematosus	DR2	46	22	3.5
	DR3	50	25	3
Sjögren syndrome	DR3	70	25	6

Adapted from Nepom BS, Nepom GT: Immunogenetics and the rheumatic diseases. In McCarty DJ, Koopman WJ, editors: *Arthritis and allied conditions: a textbook of rheumatology,* ed 12, Philadelphia, 1993, Lea & Febiger.
HLA, Human leukocyte antigen.

- Surgery:
  - Frequent THA
  - May require corrective cervical osteotomy ("chin-on-chest")
  - Severe kyphosis may need closing wedge.
  - Difficult cervical spine fractures (high mortality rate)
    - Associated with epidural hemorrhage
- Reactive arthritis (ReA; Reiter syndrome) (Figure 1-55; see Table 1-21)
  - Classical triad presentation: *"Can't see, pee, or bend the knee"*
    - Young white male (18-40 years) knee effusion
  - **Conjunctivitis, urethritis, and oligoarticular arthritis**
  - Sudden asymmetric swelling and pain in knee, ankle, hip
    - May persist 3 to 5 months
  - Feet more often than hands (heel pain)
    - Calcaneal periostitis and metatarsal head erosion
    - Dactylitis "sausage digit" of one finger/toe (see Figure 1-55, *E*)
  - History of infection 1 to 4 weeks before presentation
    - Often history of new sex partner
  - 60% with chronic disease have sacroiliitis.
  - Other common findings:
    - Painless mucocutaneous ulcers
      - Penis—circinate balanitis blisters to erosions (see Figure 1-55, *B*)
      - Oral stomatitis
    - Urethritis (dysuria), prostatitis, or cervicitis
    - **Pustular lesions on the extremities, palms, and soles** (keratoderma blennorrhagicum) (Figure 1-56, *B*)
    - Plantar heel pain—may have fluffy periosteal calcifications (see Figure 1-55, *D*)
  - Recurrence is common.
  - Pathophysiology: possible bacterial trigger
    - *Chlamydia*—most common in United States after urethritis
    - *Shigella*—most common after diarrhea
      - *Yersinia, Salmonella* also after diarrhea
    - Bacterial triggers share common traits:
      - Produce lipopolysaccharide
      - Attack mucosal surfaces
      - **Survive intracellularly**

- Treatment: NSAIDs (indomethacin 25 to 50 mg three times daily), physical therapy
  - Treat uveitis
  - Ensure no gonococcal/chlamydial arthritis: culture or polymerase chain reaction (PCR)
- Psoriatic arthropathy: PsA (see Table 1-21)
  - Affects 5% to 30% of patients with psoriasis
  - **Usually skin disease precedes arthritis** (see Figure 1-56, *A*)
  - Men and women (aged 30-40) equally affected
  - A version associated with human immunodeficiency virus (HIV)-positive patients is severe.
  - Characteristic changes:
    - **DIP involvement**
    - **Elsewhere in inflammatory arthritis, DIP is rare.**
    - **Nail changes in 90%**
      - Pitting, fragmentation, and discoloration
    - 30% "sausage" digits
    - Prominent enthesitis and tenosynovitis
  - Broad spectrum of arthritis:
    - Can be confined to DIP joints
    - Can be axial without peripheral involvement
    - Rare:
      - **Arthritis mutilans**—most destructive form
      - **"Telescoping" shortening of digits**
  - Pathophysiology:
    - Clonally expanded CD8+ cells common
    - Upregulated RANKL in synovium (B-type cells)
    - Marked increase in osteoclast precursors
  - Diagnostic criteria:
    - Current psoriasis, history or family history of psoriasis
    - Nail dystrophy
    - Negative RF
    - Dactylitis or history of dactylitis by rheumatologist
    - Juxtaarticular new bone in hand or foot
  - Radiography:
    - "Pencil-in-cup" deformity, DIP (Figure 1-57, *C*)
    - Small joint ankylosis
    - Osteolysis of MC and phalangeal bone
    - Periostitis
    - Bony enthesitis
- Enteropathic arthritis (see Tables 1-21 and 1-23)
  - Arthritis in face of inflammatory bowel disease
    - Crohn disease and ulcerative colitis

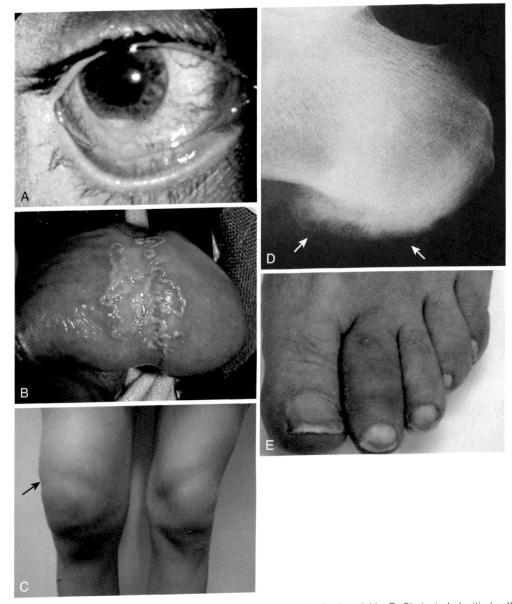

FIGURE 1-55 Reactive arthritis (ReA): "Can't see, can't pee, or bend the knee," **A,** Conjunctivitis. **B,** Circinate balanitis (urethritis not shown). **C,** Oligoarthritis (single knee effusion). **D,** "Fluffy" calcaneal periostitis. **E,** Dactylitis (sausage digit). (From Miller MD et al: *Review of orthopaedics*, ed 6, Philadelphia, 2012, Saunders; Wu IB, Schwartz RA: Reiter's syndrome: the classic triad and more, *J Am Acad Dermatol* 59:113–121, 2008.)

- Varied clinical picture, but joint erosions uncommon
- 10% to 50% experience peripheral joint arthritis.
  - Acute monoarticular synovitis precedes bowel symptoms.
  - Nondeforming arthritis
  - More common in large weight-bearing joints
  - 10% to 15% associated with ankylosing spondylitis
  - Nonarticular/non-GI involvement (see Figure 1-56):
  - Pyoderma gangrenosum
  - Erythema nodosum
  - Finger clubbing
- Pathophysiology: poorly understood
  - Mucosal leukocytes bind synovial vessels
- Crystal deposition arthropathy
  - Pathology from accumulation of crystal formation or deposition in or around joints
    - Gout—monosodium urate
    - CPPD "pseudogout"—calcium pyrophosphate

- Calcium apatite—tumoral calcinosis
- Calcium oxalate
- Gout (see Table 1-21)
  - Disorder of purine nucleic acid metabolism, causing hyperuricemia
  - **Deposition of monosodium urate crystals in joints**
  - Crystals activate inflammatory mediators:
    - Inflammatory mediators are inhibited by colchicine.
    - Activate platelets, IL-1 production, and the complement system
  - Attacks precipitated by:
    - Dehydration
    - Excess alcohol
    - Excess dietary purine
    - Chemotherapy for myeloproliferative disorders
  - Diagnosis
    - Recurrent acute joint pain
    - Men aged 40 to 60, postmenopausal women

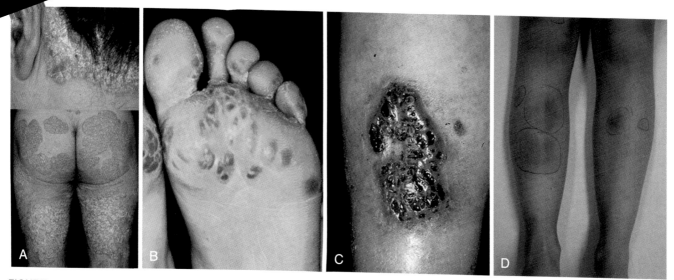

FIGURE 1-56 Skin lesions associated with various arthritides. **A,** Psoriasis: dry, silver, scaly patches on erythematous base associated with seronegative arthritis, which affects distal interphalangeal joints and pitting nails. **B,** Keratoderma blennorrhagica: vesicopustular waxy lesion with a yellow-brown color found in approximately 15% of patients with reactive arthritis (ReA). **C,** Pyoderma gangrenosum: neutrophilic dermatosis characterized by tissue necrosis causing deep ulcers that usually occur on the legs. Found in seronegative enteropathic arthritis associated with Crohn disease, ulcerative colitis, rheumatoid arthritis (RA), leukemias, and multiple myeloma. **D,** Erythema nodosum: sudden eruption of erythematous tender nodules and plaques, often over the extensor aspects of the lower extremities, most commonly in women aged 20 to 30. The lesions spontaneously resolve without ulceration, scarring, or atrophy, but recurrence is not uncommon. Associated with infections, lupus, enteropathic arthritis, reactive arthritis, RA, and sarcoidosis. (**A** and **C** from Habif TP: *Clinical dermatology,* ed 5, St Louis, Mosby/Elsevier, 2009; **B** from Rein MF: Centers for Disease Control and Prevention's Public Health Image Library; **D** from Wikimedia Commons: Erythema nodosum. Available at: http://commons.wikimedia.org/wiki/Category:Erythema_nodosum#/media/File:ENlegs.JPG.)

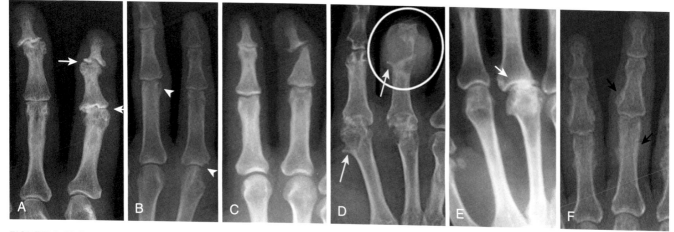

FIGURE 1-57 Radiographs of finger arthritis. Erosive osteoarthritis: distal interphalangeal (DIP) joint "gull wing" *(top arrow)* as well as proximal interphalangeal (PIP) joint "zig-zag" finger deformity. **B,** Rheumatoid arthritis (early): metacarpal and PIP periarticular marginal erosions of the bony "bare areas" due to synovial pannus. **C,** Psoriatic arthritis: mostly involves DIP joints of hands more than feet; classic deformity is "cup-in-pencil" deformity (frequent nail changes not shown). **D,** Gout: soft tissue swelling *(tophi circled),* "punched out" "rat bite" periarticular erosions, and sclerotic overhangings bordering the joint *(yellow arrows).* **E,** Hemochromatosis: characteristic metacarpophalangeal joint arthritis with radial "hook-like" osteophytes. **F,** Hypertrophic osteoarthropathy (secondary pulmonary): bilateral symmetric periostitis of long bones and phalanx with diaphyseal pain; up to 90% of cases are associated with primary or metastatic pulmonary neoplasms in adults. (From Gupta KB et al: Radiographic evaluation of osteoarthritis, *Radiol Clin North Am* 42:11–41, 2004; McQueen FM et al: Imaging in the crystal arthropathies, *Rheum Dis Clin North Am* 40:231–249; and Rana RS et al: Periosteal reaction, *AJR Am J Roentgenol* 193:W259–272, 2009.)

- Usually lower extremity, great toe (podagra)
- Crystal deposition as tophi when chronic
  - Ear helix, eyelid, olecranon, Achilles tendon
- Renal disease or stones—second most common site
- Radiographic findings (see Figure 1-57, *D*):
  - Soft tissue swelling early: edema, tophi
  - "Punched-out" "rat bite" periarticular erosions
  - Sclerotic overhanging borders

- Serum:
  - Elevated serum uric acid; 6.8 mg/dL common
  - Level is not diagnostic
- Synovial fluid:
  - Cloudy and must rule out infection
  - WBCs: wide range (5000-80,000; average, 15,000-20,000), mostly PMNs
  - Crystals often seen in WBCs, fluid, or tophi

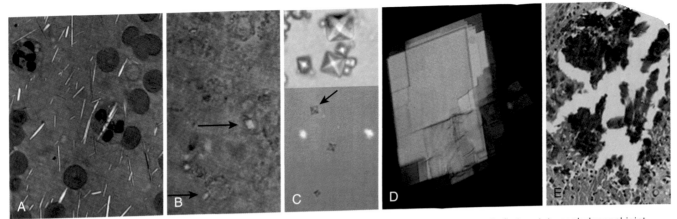

FIGURE 1-58 Synovial fluid crystals. **A,** Gout: yellow uric acid parallel to compensator, most common in first metatarsophalangeal joint. **B,** Calcium pyrophosphate (dihydrate crystal) deposition disease (CPPD—"pseudogout" crystals): blue rhomboid crystals most common in knees and wrists. **C,** Calcium oxalate crystals are pyramidal and almost exclusively seen in patients with renal damage and oxalosis. **D,** Platelike cholesterol crystals are rare and can be found in inflammatory synovial fluid and in fluids drained from bursas of patients with rheumatoid arthritis, systemic lupus erythematosus, and seronegative spondyloarthropathy. **E,** Calcium apatite crystals from tumoral calcinosis in histology slide from tissue. (From McPherson RA, Pincus MR, editors: *Henry's clinical diagnosis and management by laboratory methods*, ed 21, Philadelphia, 2007, Saunders Elsevier; Firestein GS et al, editors: *Kelley's textbook of rheumatology*, ed 8, Philadelphia, 2008, Saunders; Courtney P, Doherty M: Joint aspiration and injection and synovial fluid analysis, *Best Pract Res Clin Rheumatol* 23:161–192, 2013; Martínez-Castillo A et al: Synovial fluid analysis, *Rheumatol Clin* 6:316–321, 2010; and Topaz O et al: A deleterious mutation in *SAMD9* causes normophosphatemic familial tumoral calcinosis, *Am J Hum Genet* 79:759–764.)

- Yellow, needle-shaped when parallel to compensator
- Strongly "negatively birefringent" (Figure 1-58, *A*)
- Acute treatment:
  - NSAIDs: indomethacin 50 mg three times daily or ibuprofen 800 three times daily
  - Colchicine (microtubule inhibitor that inhibits mitosis)
  - ADR: diarrhea (*"patients run before they can walk"*)
- Chronic/maintenance:
  - Weight loss, low-purine diet, limit alcohol
  - Uricosuric agents: Probenecid
  - Allopurinol—xanthine oxidase inhibitor
  - Febaxostat for renally impaired
- Chondrocalcinosis (see Table 1-21)
- Caused by several disorders, including:
- CPPD or "pseudogout"
- Disorder of pyrophosphate metabolism
- Etiology:
  - Elderly patients
  - Genetic version: *ANKH* gene mutation
    - Increases extracellular pyrophosphate
  - Associated with several disease processes:
    - Ochronosis, hemochromatosis
    - Hyperparathyroidism, hypothyroidism
  - Meniscal calcifications, often after prior knee injury
- Occasionally causes acute attacks after trauma
  - Knee—most common, resembles gout/septic arthritis
  - Wrist most common in upper extremity (see Figure 1-50, *B* and *D*)
- Diagnosis: synovial fluid WBC counts from 5000 to 100,000 (average, 24,000)
  - Rhomboid-shaped crystals in WBCs
  - Weakly positively (blue) birefringent when parallel (see Figure 1-58, *B*)
- Radiographs: fine linear calcification in hyaline cartilage and more diffuse calcification of menisci (see Figure 1-50, *D*) and other fibrocartilage (triangular fibrocartilage complex, acetabular labrum)

- Treatment:
  - NSAIDs often helpful
  - Cortisone injections
  - Recurrent attacks: colchicine
- Calcium hydroxyapatite crystal deposition disease
- Apatite is primary crystal of normal bone
- Accumulates abnormally in:
  - Areas of tissue damage
  - Hypercalcemic or hyperparathyroid states (chronic kidney disease [CKD])
  - Genetic response
- Associated with:
  - Acute attacks of bursitis/synovitis
  - Severe degenerative joint disease
  - Calcific tendonitis of rotator cuff and hip abductors
- Destructive arthropathy can occur in the knee and shoulder.
  - "Milwaukee shoulder": calcium phosphate deposition, with cuff tear arthropathy
- Tumoral calcinosis—large subcutaneous masses (extracapsular)
  - Black patients
  - Caused by **hyperphosphatemia**
  - Primary—rare genetic renal tubular disorder
    - GalNAc transferase 3 (*GALNT3*)
    - *KLOTHO* or fibroblast growth factor 23 (*FGF23*)
    - *SAMD9* gene (normal phosphatemic)
  - Secondary—hyperparathyroidism
    - Renal failure—long-term dialysis
- Diagnosis: usually less than 2000 WBCs in synovial fluid; may be "bloody effusion"
  - Apatite crystals are too small to see with light microscopy.
  - Non-birefringent globules
  - Wright stain—purple aggregates (see Figure 1-58, *E*)
- Treatment is generally supportive
- Calcium oxalate deposition
  - Primary oxalosis—rare genetic defect of liver enzymes

- Alanine glyoxylate aminotransferase (AGT)
- Glyoxylate reductase (GR)
- Nephrocalcinosis, renal failure, and death by 20
- Treatment: liver/kidney transplant
- Secondary oxalosis—more common
  - Metabolic abnormalities of chronic renal insufficiency
  - Vitamin C makes worse
  - Associated with:
    - Calcium oxalate arthritis/periarthritis
    - Nephrolithiasis, kidney stones
- Diagnosis: synovial fluid usually contains fewer than 2000 WBCs.
  - Birefringent bipyramidal crystals (see Figure 1-58, C)
- Hemarthrosis
  - Posttraumatic:
    - Bony or osteochondral fracture:
      - Fat droplets or "neapolitan effusion"
    - Ligament, meniscus tear, dislocation
  - Spontaneous
    - Chronic trauma to tumor tissue:
      - Pigmented villonodular synovitis, synovial hemangioma (children>adults)
      - Malignant tumors in or near joint
    - Chronic trauma to insensate bone:
      - Neuropathic joints: Charcot, syrinx, tabes dorsalis
    - Vascular disorders: rare
      - Scurvy—vitamin C deficiency, vascular fragility, arterial aneurysms
    - Coagulopathy:
      - Iatrogenic
      - Severe illness:
        - Thrombocytopenia
        - Hemophilia
  - Hemophilic arthropathy (Figure 1-59):
    - X-linked recessive defect of factor VIII (A) or IX (B)
      - Intrinsic pathway severely impaired
    - Knee, elbow, ankle effusion in a 3- to 15-year-old
    - Joints become large and "knobby."
    - Decreased ROM to ankylosis
    - Pathophysiology:
      - Recurrent bleeds
      - Chronic synovitis
      - Synovial hypertrophy/hyperplasia
      - Iron-laden phagocytic type A synovial cells
      - No giant cells or PMNs, few lymphocytes
      - Synovium destroys cartilage
    - Radiographs:
      - Bulbous, flat condylar surface
      - Widened notch
      - Inferior patellar squaring
      - Talar flattening
    - Treatment:
      - Early: prevent bleeds/factor replacement
      - Radiation ablation of synovium
        - Yttrium-90 and phosphorus-32
      - Late: arthroplasty-knee/fusion-ankle
- Infectious arthritis (see Infection and Microbiology section of Section 2 in this chapter for details)
- Bacterial: gram-positive bacteria most common
- Fungal: *Candida* most common
- TB: spine is most common (see Figure 1-48, D), then hip and knee
- Unusual arthritis related to unusual infections or their immune response

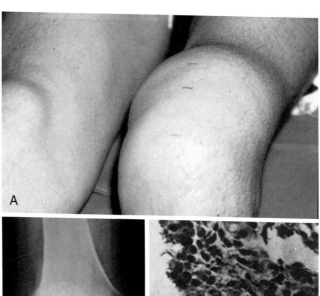
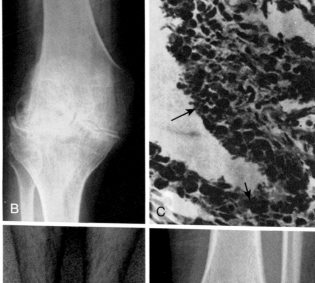
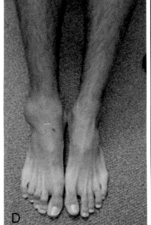
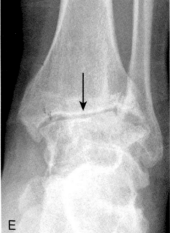

FIGURE 1-59 Hemophilic arthropathy. **A,** Recurrent knee effusions and synovitis. **B,** Radiograph of end-stage arthropathy. **C,** Synovial proliferation of hemophilic arthropathy demonstrates phagocytic (type A) synovial cells laden with iron pigment but no giant cells, polymorphonuclear leukocytes, and rare lymphocytes. **D,** Bloody ankle effusion presentation of teen with grandfather with history of bleeding disorder. **E,** End-stage hemophilic arthropathy of ankle demonstrates flattening of the talus. (From Rodriguez-Merchan EC: Musculoskeletal complications of hemophilia, *HSS J* 6:37–42, 2010; Mainardi CL et al: Proliferative synovitis in hemophilia: biochemical and morphologic observations, *Arthritis Rheum* 21:137–144, 1978; photo courtesy Texas Orthopedics Sports Medicine and Rehabilitation; and Rodriguez-Merchan EC: Prevention of the musculoskeletal complications of hemophilia, *Adv Prev Med* 2012:201271, 2012.)

- All have negative Gram stains/cultures of the effusion
- All require high index of clinical suspicion to diagnose
- Uncommon or hard to diagnose
- Acute rheumatic fever (see Table 1-21)
  - Once the most common cause of childhood arthritis
    - Acute painful arthralgias with effusions
      - Most common symptom of rheumatic fever
      - Migratory: multiple joints in rapid sequence
      - Knees, ankles, elbows, wrists
      - No joint lasts longer than a week.
    - Aged 5 to 15 years, 2 to 4 weeks after untreated strep throat
    - Group A β-hemolytic streptococcal infections
      - Antibodies to M protein of GAS
      - "Molecular mimicry" against joint and heart
      - Now rare because of antibiotics
      - Systemic manifestations (Jones criteria) (Figure 1-60):
    - Carditis
      - Prolonged PR interval on ECG
      - Thickened valves lead to regurgitation
  - Erythema marginatum
    - Painless macules with red margins
    - On trunk but not on face
  - Subcutaneous nodules
    - Extensor surfaces of the joints: olecranon
    - Skin moves over/not painful
  - Chorea—involuntary movements that stop in sleep
    - Sydenham chorea (St. Vitus dance)
    - "Milkmaid's grip": hand grip tightens and loosens
    - Tongue fasciculations
  - Diagnosis:
    - Jones criteria
      - Elevated ESR, CRP
      - Antistreptolysin O titers are elevated in 80%.
  - Treatment includes penicillin and salicylates
- Lyme arthritis: late manifestation of Lyme disease
  - Chronic episodic oligoarthritis/synovitis
    - Knee effusions with synovitis
    - U.S. Northeast or Pacific Northwest
    - *Ixodes* tick carrying *Borrelia burgdorferi* spirochete
    - Early: erythema migrans—"target lesion"
    - Later: arthritis and neurologic symptoms

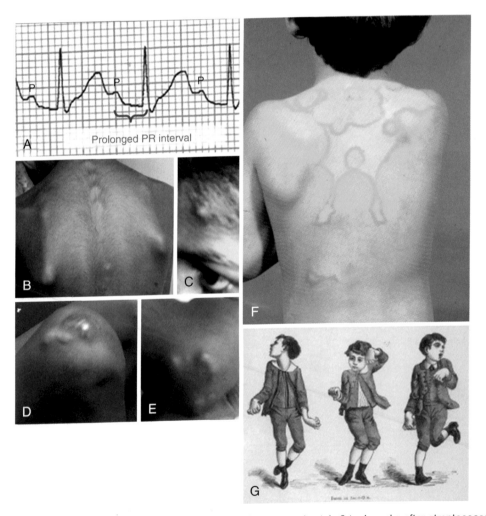

FIGURE 1-60 Acute rheumatic fever: acute migratory arthritis with effusions approximately 2 to 4 weeks after streptococcal infection ("A sore throat can lead to a broken heart."). Historically, *the most common cause of arthritis in children*. Pathology results from molecular mimicry between streptococcal organism and normal tissue. Diagnostic Jones criteria includes: **A,** carditis—characterized by prolonged PR interval and thickened valves; **B** through **E,** subcutaneous nodules on extensor surface of joints; **F,** erythema marginatum—painless macular rash on trunk (but not face); and **G,** chorea—(Sydenham chorea/St. Vitus dance), involuntary movements that stop in sleep. (From Singhi AK et al: Acute rheumatic fever: subcutaneous nodules and carditis, *Circulation* 121:946–947, 2010; and BMJ Best Practice: Rheumatic fever. Available at: http://bestpractice.bmj.com/best-practice/monograph/404/resources/image/bp/8.html.)

...er neurologic and arthritic manifestations develop:
- Neurologic:
  - Meningitis
  - Facial nerve (Bell) palsy
  - Peripheral radiculoneuropathy: motor and sensory
    - Distal paresthesias or spinal radicular pain
  - Cerebellar ataxia—more common in Europe
- Diagnosis:
  - Cerebrospinal fluid pleocytosis—increased WBCs
  - PCR serum IgG to *B. burgdorferi*
- Treatment: doxycycline or amoxicillin
- Whipple disease—intestinal lipodystrophy
  - Very rare chronic bacterial infection
  - Presents first as arthritis, often knees
  - **Untreated is fatal**—antibiotics cure
  - *Tropheryma whipplei*—ubiquitous actinomycete
  - Middle-aged white men
  - Farmer exposed to soil/animals/sewage
  - Most common symptoms:
    - 90% intermittent nondeforming migratory arthritis
    - Knees and large joints most common
    - Attacks last hours to days.
    - Complete remission between bouts
    - Precedes other symptoms by about 5 years
  - **Prolonged diarrhea**, abdominal pain, weight loss
  - Lymphadenopathy (50%): mesenteric and peripheral
  - Skin lesions:
    - Hyperpigmentation (≈50%) late—melanoderma
    - Subcutaneous nodules—erythema nodosum
    - Inflammatory rashes
  - 30% of the untreated get CNS symptoms
    - Dementia, memory loss, ataxia
    - **Pathognomonic:** (BUT IRREVERSIBLE)
      - Oculomasticatory
        - Involuntary blinking when talking/eating
      - Oculofacial-skeletal myorhythmia
        - Rapid, repetitive movements
      - Supranuclear vertical gaze palsy
        - Difficulty looking up
  - Pathophysiology:
    - Poor host immune response
    - Unable to degrade intracellular pathogens
    - Weak macrophage activation (CD11b cells few)
    - Defective T-lymphocyte function
  - Laboratory studies: CRP, ESR, RF
  - Diagnosis:
    - Duodenal or lymph node biopsy
      - PAS-positive foamy macrophages
      - Gram-positive bacilli
      - PCR available; is sensitive and specific
  - Treatment:
    - Two weeks of penicillin or ceftriaxone and streptomycin
    - Doxycycline for 2 years
- Viral arthritis:
  - Joint symptoms can be produced by:
  - **Virus in synovium or joint fluid**
  - Immune complexes deposition
  - Fever and rashes are common.
  - Joint aspirates usually reveal less than 3000 WBCs
  - HIV-associated arthritis: severe knee, ankle pain
    - Negative HLA-B27, negative RF
  - Hepatitis B—25% get arthritis, often of knees and hands

- Maculopapular or urticarial rash of lower extremity, elevated liver enzymes
- Rubella ("German measles")—classic rash; arthritis of hands, wrists, knees
- Acute maculopapular rash ("little red"): face to trunk to extremities
  - Not palms or soles
- Significant lymphadenopathy:
  - Behind ears, neck, and suboccipital
- Proximal interphalangeal and metacarpophalangeal joint arthritis in 60% of infected adults
- Alphaviruses: mosquito-borne RNA viruses live in synovial macrophages.
  - Arthritis, fever, and rash
  - Examples:
    - Ross River—Australia
    - Mayaro—South America
    - Chikungunya—Southeast Asia, Africa, Caribbean
- Dengue: "breakbone fever"
  - Severe muscle and joint pain, leukopenia, and thrombocytopenia

NEUROMUSCULAR AND CONNECTIVE TISSUES

- **Skeletal muscle**
- Noncontractile elements (Figure 1-61)
  - Fascial coverings of skeletal muscle
    - **Epimysium** surrounds the bundles of fascicles.
    - **Perimysium** surrounds individual muscle fascicles.
    - **Endomysium** surrounds individual fibers (myofibers).
  - Myotendinous junction
    - Skeletal muscle has myotendinous and bone-tendon junctions.
    - The **myotendinous junction** is often the site of tears, with eccentric contraction (forced lengthening of the myotendinous junction during contraction) placing maximum stress across this area.
    - Myofilament bundles are linked directly onto collagen fibrils, with sarcolemma filaments interdigitating with the basement membrane (type IV collagen) and tendon tissue (type I collagen).
  - Bone-tendon junction—**enthesis**
    - Two types of insertions: (1) direct or (2) indirect
    - **Direct insertion** (e.g., rotator cuff)—fibrocartilagenous transition zone composed of four elements: tendon, fibrocartilage, mineralized fibrocartilage, and bone
    - **Indirect insertion**—tendon fibers (Sharpey fibers) inserting directly onto periosteum
    - Inflammation of entheses is seen in HLA-B27–positive processes (e.g., **ankylosing spondylitis**), and subsequent ossification results in joint ankylosis. Commonly affected joints include:
      - Sacroiliac joints
      - Spinal apophyseal joints
      - Symphysis pubis
  - Sarcolemma and sarcoplasmic reticulum
    - **Sarcolemma** is the plasma membrane surrounding a skeletal muscle cell.
      - It surrounds the contractile elements, forming the **transverse tubules** (Figure 1-62).
    - **Sarcoplasmic reticulum** is a smooth endoplasmic reticulum that surrounds the individual myofibrils,

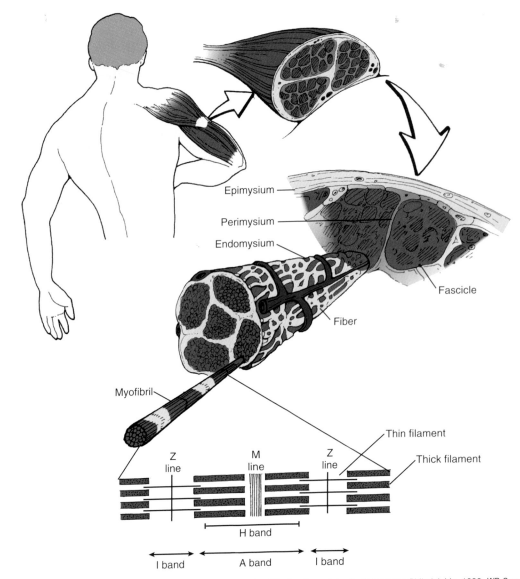

FIGURE 1-61 Skeletal muscle architecture. (From Brinker MR, Miller MD: *Fundamentals of orthopaedics*, Philadelphia, 1999, WB Saunders, p 10.)

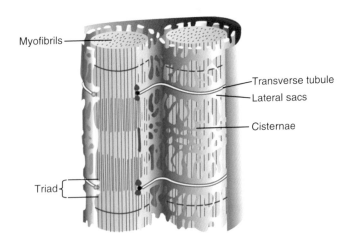

FIGURE 1-62 Sarcoplasmic reticulum. Action potentials travel down the transverse tubules, causing calcium release from the outer vesicles. (From DeLee JC et al, editors: *DeLee and Drez's orthopaedic sports medicine: principles and practice*, ed 3, Philadelphia, 2009, Saunders.)

storing calcium in intracellular membrane–bound channels.
- **Ryanodine receptors (RYR1)** regulate the release of calcium from the sarcoplasmic reticulum and serve as a connection between the sarcoplasmic reticulum and sarcolemma-derived transverse tubule.
- An abnormal ryanodine receptor in skeletal muscle is implicated in persons susceptible to **malignant hyperthermia**.
- Dantrolene decreases loss of calcium from the sarcoplasmic reticulum.
■ Contractile elements (see Figure 1-61)
- **Myoblasts** derived from precursor satellite stem cells
- Myofibrils (1-3 μm in diameter and 1-2 cm long) are highly organized, with individual contractile units called *sarcomeres*.
- Sarcomere organization causes the banding pattern (striations) seen in skeletal muscle (Table 1-24; see Figure 1-61).

- **Sarcomeres (Z line to Z line)** are arranged into bands and lines.
- Sarcomeres at the myotendinous junction are affected (decreased) by immobilization.
  - A **costamere** connects the sarcomere to the cell membrane at the Z disc.

Table 1-24	Sarcomere
BAND	**DESCRIPTION**
A band	Contains actin and myosin
I band	Contains actin only
H band	Contains myosin only
M line	Interconnecting site of the thick filaments
Z line	Anchors the thin filaments

From Brinker MR, Miller MD: *Fundamentals of orthopaedics,* Philadelphia, 1999, WB Saunders, p 11.

- **Thin filaments (actin [I band]**, troponin, and tropomyosin) attach to Z lines.
- I band thought to be involved in delayed-onset muscle soreness (DOMS)
- **Thick filaments (myosin [H band]**, M protein, C protein, titin, creatine kinase) have the globular domains that hydrolyze ATP, causing muscle contraction as a result of conformational changes in protein structure, with sequential cross-bridging to the actin molecules of the thin filaments.
- Muscle contraction and the motor unit
  - Contraction is in response to mechanical or electrochemical stimuli generated at the motor end plate (neuromuscular junction) where the axon contacts an individual myofiber (Figure 1-63).
    - An axon can contact multiple myofibers—**motor unit.**

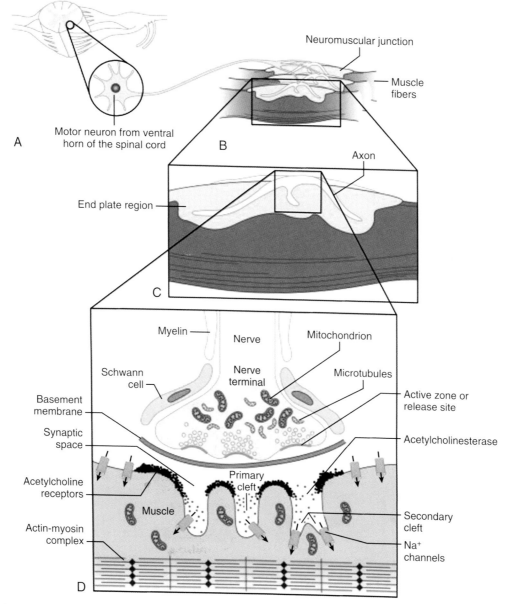

FIGURE 1-63 Structure of the adult motor end plate (neuromuscular junction). **A,** Motor nerve. **B,** Nerve branches that innervate many individual muscle fibers. **C,** Presynaptic boutons, which terminate on the muscle fiber. **D,** Nerve terminal. (From Miller RD et al: *Miller's anesthesia,* ed 7, Philadelphia, 2010, Churchill Livingstone.)

Table 1-25	Agents That Affect Neuromuscular Impulse Transmission		
AGENT	**SITE OF ACTION**	**MECHANISM**	**EFFECT**
Nondepolarizing drugs (curare, pancuronium, vecuronium)	Neuromuscular junction	Competitively binds to acetylcholine receptor to block impulse transmission	Paralytic agent (long-term)
Depolarizing drugs (succinylcholine)	Neuromuscular junction	Binds to acetylcholine receptor to cause temporary depolarization of muscle membrane	Paralytic agent (short-term)
Anticholinesterases (neostigmine, edrophonium)	Autonomic ganglia	Prevents breakdown of acetylcholine to enhance its effect	Reverses effect of nondepolarizing drugs; muscarinic effects (bronchospasm, bronchorrhea, bradycardia)

Table 1-26	Types of Muscle Contractions		
TYPE OF MUSCLE CONTRACTION	**DEFINITION**	**EXAMPLE**	**PHASES**
Isotonic	**Muscle tension is constant** throughout ROM. Muscle length changes throughout ROM. This is a measure of dynamic strength.	Biceps curls with free weights	Concentric contraction: muscle shortens during contraction. Tension within muscle is proportional to externally applied load. Example of an isotonic concentric contraction is the "curl" (elbow moving toward increasing flexion) portion of a biceps curl. Eccentric contraction: muscle lengthens during contraction (internal force < external force). Eccentric contractions are the most efficient way to strengthen muscle but have the greatest potential for high muscle tension and muscle injury. Example of an isotonic eccentric contraction is the "negative" (elbow moving toward increasing extension) portion of a biceps curl.
Isometric	Muscle tension is generated, but **muscle length remains unchanged.** This is a measure of static strength.	Pushing against an immovable object (e.g., wall)	
Isokinetic	Muscle tension is generated as muscle maximally contracts at a **constant velocity** over a full ROM. Isokinetic exercises are best for maximizing strength and are a measure of dynamic strength.	Isokinetic exercises require special equipment (e.g., Cybex machine).	Concentric contraction Eccentric contraction

ROM, Range of motion.

- Motor units can have ten to thousands of individual myofibers, with fine-control muscles having fewer myofibers in a motor unit.
- The conversion of electrical impulse to muscle contraction at the end plate region is facilitated by the neurotransmitter **acetylcholine** where it diffuses across the synaptic cleft (50 nm).
- Acetylcholine binds to its receptor on the muscle membrane, depolarizing the sarcoplasmic reticulum, releasing calcium, which exposes the actin on the thin filament owing to binding of calcium to tropomyosin, allowing for the formation of myosin cross-bridges, causing contraction/motion.
  - **Myasthenia gravis** has a shortage of **acetylcholine receptors.** Presents initially as ptosis and diplopia; worse with use owing to antibodies to receptors.
  - **Botulinum A** injections reduce spasticity by **blocking presynaptic acetylcholine release.** Commonly used for spastic muscles in cerebral palsy.
- Agents affecting impulse transmission can be found in Table 1-25.

- Types of muscle contractions (Table 1-26)
  - Skeletal muscle **cross-sectional area** is a reliable predictor of the potential for contractile force.
  - Muscle **tension** is determined by contractile force generated.
  - Muscle **contraction velocity** is determined by **fiber length.**
    - A well-conditioned muscle may be able to fire over 90% of its fibers simultaneously.
    - At any velocity, fast-twitch (type II) fibers produce more force.
  - **Isokinetic** exercises produce more strength gains than do isometric exercises (see Table 1-26).
  - **Isotonic** exercises produce a uniform strength increase throughout joint ROM.
  - **Plyometric** ("jumping") exercises, the most efficient method of improving power, consist of a muscle stretch followed immediately by a rapid contraction.
  - Closed-chain exercise involves loading an extremity with the most distal segment stabilized or not moving, allowing for muscular co-contraction around a joint, minimizing joint shear (e.g., less stress on the anterior cruciate ligament [ACL]).

Table 1-27	Characteristics of Types of Human Skeletal Muscle Fibers		
	TYPES		
CHARACTERISTIC	**TYPE I**	**TYPE IIA**	**TYPE IIB**
Other names	Red, slow-twitch Slow oxidative	White, fast-twitch Fast oxidative glycolytic	Fast glycolytic
Speed of contraction	Slow	Fast	Fast
Strength of contraction	Low	High	High
Fatigability	Fatigue-resistant	Fatigable	Most fatigable
Aerobic capacity	High	Medium	Low
Anaerobic capacity	Low	Medium	High
Motor unit size	Small	Larger	Largest
Capillary density	High	High	Low

From Simon SR, editor: *Orthopaedic basic science,* Rosemont, Ill, 1994, American Academy of Orthopaedic Surgeons, p 100.

- Open-chain exercise involves loading an extremity with the distal segment of the limb moving freely (e.g., biceps curls).
- Types of muscle fibers (Table 1-27)
  - Slow-twitch (**type I,** oxidative, "red") fibers— mnemonic "**slow red ox**"
    - **Aerobic**
    - Have more mitochondria, enzymes, and triglycerides (energy source) than do type II fibers
    - **Low concentrations** of glycogen and glycolytic enzymes (adenosine triphosphatase [ATPase])
    - Enable performing endurance activities, posture, balance
    - Are the first lost without rehabilitation
  - Fast-twitch (**type II,** glycolytic, "white") fibers
    - **Anaerobic**
    - Contract more quickly and have larger, stronger motor units (increased ATPase) than do type I fibers
    - Less efficient than type I but with large amount of force per cross-sectional area, with high contraction speeds and quick relaxation times
    - Well suited for **high-intensity, short-duration activities** (e.g., sprinting)
    - Rapid fatigue
    - Low intramuscular triglyceride stores
    - Types IIA and IIB fibers are associated with sprinting.
    - ATP–creatine phosphate system
      - Subtypes are based on myosin heavy chains.
- Energetics (Figure 1-64)
  - ATP–creatine phosphate system (phosphagen system) converts stored carbohydrates to energy without the use of oxygen and no lactate production.
    - For intense muscle activities lasting **up to 20 seconds**
    - Example: sprinting in a 100- or 200-m dash
  - **Lactic anaerobic system** (lactic acid metabolism)
    - For intense muscle activities lasting **20 to 120 seconds**
    - Example: a 400-m sprint
    - Involves hydrolysis of one glucose molecule to ultimately produce lactic acid plus energy
  - Aerobic system
  - The body depends on this system for muscle activities of **longer duration** and lower intensity with **replenishment of ATP** through oxidative phosphorylation and the Krebs (or citric acid or tricarboxylic acid) cycle.
  - Glucose or fatty acids are used to produce ATP.

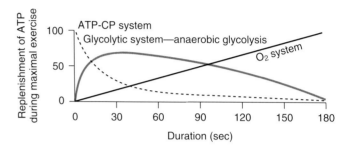

FIGURE 1-64 Energy sources for muscle activity. *ATP,* Adenosine triphosphate; *CP,* creatine phosphate. (From Simon SR, editor: *Orthopaedic basic science,* Rosemont, Ill, 1994, American Academy of Orthopaedic Surgeons, p 102.)

- Athletes and training
  - Genetics determines the distribution of fast-twitch versus slow-twitch fibers.
  - Specific training can selectively alter fiber composition.
  - Endurance athletes—higher percentage of slow-twitch fibers
  - Sprinters and athletes in "strength" sports—higher percentage of fast-twitch fibers
  - **Endurance training**—decreased tension and increased repetitions
    - Induces hypertrophy of slow-twitch fibers
    - Increases capillary density, mitochondria, and oxidative capacity
    - Increases resistance to fatigue
    - Improves blood lipid profiles
  - **Strength training**—increased tension and decreased repetitions
    - Increases myofibrils and fiber size
    - Induces **hypertrophy** (increased cross-sectional area) of fast-twitch (type II) fibers
  - Both endurance and strength training delay the lactate response to exercise.
  - Aerobic conditioning promotes cardiorespiratory fitness.
  - In contrast to resistance exercise, aerobic exercise increases stroke volume, which increases cardiac output, decreases the incidence of back injury in workers, and helps the elderly remain ambulatory.
  - A significant decline in aerobic fitness ("detraining") occurs after only 2 weeks of no training. Muscles that cross a single joint atrophy faster and atrophy occurs in a nonlinear fashion.

■ Anabolic (androgenic) steroids and growth hormone are widely used.
- Anabolic (androgenic) steroids do not increase aerobic power or capacity for muscular exercise; are more effective than corticosteroids for long-term contusion muscle recovery, with use detected by urine drug screening.
  - Anabolic (androgenic) steroids effects:
    - Increase muscle strength and mass
    - Increase messenger RNA and protein synthesis
    - Increase aggressive behavior that promotes increased weight training
    - Increase body weight
    - Increase erythropoiesis
  - Side effects
    - Testicular atrophy
    - Irreversible deepening of the female voice
    - Reduction in testosterone and gonadotropic hormones
    - Growth retardation
    - Oligospermia, azoospermia
    - Gynecomastia
    - HTN
    - Striae
    - Cystic acne
    - **Alopecia (irreversible)**
    - Liver tumors
    - Raised low-density lipoprotein (LDL) levels and **lower high-density lipoprotein (HDL)** levels
    - Abnormal amounts of the liver isoenzyme lactate dehydrogenase
- Abuse of the growth hormone somatotropin has adverse effects:
  - Selective hypertrophy of type I muscle fibers
  - Atrophy of type II fibers
  - Muscle hypertrophy with weakness and fatigue

■ Nutrition
- Weight reduction with fluid and food restriction (wrestlers, boxers, and jockeys trying to "make weight") may result in several pathologic developments:
  - Reduced cardiac output
  - Increased heart rate
  - Smaller stroke volume
  - Lower oxygen consumption
  - Decreased renal blood flow
  - Electrolyte loss
- Carbohydrate loading is often practiced by athletes:
  - Increasing carbohydrates and decreasing physical activity 3 days before an event (e.g., marathon)
- Fluid replacement regimen is recommended for competitive athletes:
  - Consuming enough water to maintain prepractice weight and maintaining a normal diet
  - Replacement of fluids, carbohydrates, and electrolytes is **most effective when the fluid's osmolality is less than 10%.**
  - Low-osmolality solutions enhance fluid absorption by the gut.
  - Glucose polymers minimize osmolality.
- Creatine supplements are used by some athletes to enhance performance.
  - Creatine is converted to phosphocreatine, which acts as an energy reservoir for ATP in muscle.

- Creatine supplementation can increase work produced in the first few maximum-effort anaerobic trials but does not increase peak force production.
- Creatine shifts fluid intracellularly; may present a risk for dehydration, though cramps are the more common side effect.

■ Muscle injury
- Muscle **strains**
  - Most common sports injury
  - Most occur at the **myotendinous junction.**
  - Occur primarily in muscles crossing two joints (hamstring, gastrocnemius) that have increased type II fibers
  - Initially there is inflammation and later fibrosis mediated by TGF-β.
- Muscle tears
  - Most occur at the **myotendinous junction** (e.g., rectus femoris tear at anterior inferior iliac spine).
  - Often occur during a rapid (high-velocity) eccentric contraction
  - Eccentric contractions develop the highest forces.
    - **Satellite cells** act as stem cells and are **most responsible for muscle healing.**
    - Alternatively, the defect can heal with bridging scar tissue. **TGF-β** stimulates **proliferation of myofibroblasts** and **increases fibrosis.**
  - Surgical repair of clean lacerations in the muscle midbelly usually results in minimal regeneration of muscle fibers distally, scar formation at the laceration, and recovery of about half the muscle strength.
  - Prevention of tears—muscle activation (through stretching) allows twice the energy absorption before failure.

■ Delayed-onset muscle soreness (DOMS)
- This phenomenon occurs 24 to 72 hours after intense exercise.
- May result from eccentric muscle contractions
- Caused by **edema and inflammation** in the **connective tissue,** with a **neutrophilic** response present after acute muscle injury.
- May be associated with changes in the I band of the sarcomere
- NSAIDs relieve DOMS in a dose-dependent manner.
- Massage has varying effects.
- Other modalities (ice, stretching, ultrasonography, electrical stimulation) have not been shown to affect DOMS.

■ Denervation
- Causes muscle atrophy and increased sensitivity to acetylcholine
- Leads to spontaneous fibrillations at 2 to 4 weeks after injury

■ Immobilization
- Accelerates granulation tissue response
- Immobilization in lengthened positions decreases contractures and maintains strength.
- Atrophy results from disuse or altered recruitment.
- Electrical stimulation can help offset these effects.

■ **Nervous system**
■ The spine and spinal trauma are covered in Chapter 8.
■ Organization of the nervous system and spinal cord anatomy

CNS—consists of over 100 billion neurons. Inputs and outputs to the CNS are through the spinal cord through afferent and efferent nerve fibers.

- **Afferent fibers**—transmission from sensory receptors in the peripheral nervous system (PNS) to the CNS and are composed of two types
  - *Somatic afferent fibers* originate in receptors in muscle, skin, and sense organs of the head (vision, hearing, taste, smell).
  - *Visceral afferent fibers* originate in viscera.
- **Efferent fibers**—transmission from the CNS to the PNS
  - *Motor efferent fibers* innervate skeletal muscle fibers.
  - *Somatic efferent fibers* innervate skin, skeletal muscle, and joints.
  - *Autonomic efferent fibers* (splanchnic fibers) innervate viscera.
- Key glial cells in the CNS include **oligodendrocytes** (form myelin) and **astrocytes** (most common).
- Injuries to CNS can have functional improvements up to 6 months after a stroke and up to 18 months after traumatic brain injury
- Spinal cord anatomy (Figure 1-65)
  - Spinal cord injury is most common through motor vehicle accident in adults, with organization of the columns covered in Chapter 8.
- Motor system
  - Organized into four areas:
    - Spinal cord
    - Brainstem
    - Motor cortex
    - Premotor cortical areas (basal ganglia and cerebellum)
- Spinal cord (Figure 1-66)
  - White matter (peripheral)
  - Ascending and descending fiber tracts
  - Myelinated and unmyelinated axons
  - Gray matter (central)
  - Contains neuronal cell bodies, glial cells, dendrites, and axons (myelinated and unmyelinated)
  - Contains three types of neurons
    - Motoneurons (α and γ): axons exit via ventral roots.
    - Interneurons: axons remain in the spinal cord.
    - Tract cells: axons ascend to supraspinal centers.
- Spinal cord reflexes (Table 1-28)
  - These reflexes are "stereotyped responses" to a specific sensory stimulus.
  - A reflex pathway involves a sensory organ (receptor), an interneuron, and a motoneuron.
  - Monosynaptic reflex: only one synapse is involved between receptor and effector.
  - Polysynaptic reflex: one or more interneurons are involved. Most human reflexes are polysynaptic.
- Motor unit
  - An α-motoneuron and the muscle fibers it innervates
  - Four types, based on physiologic demands (Table 1-29):
    - Type S (slow, fatigue resistant)
    - Type FR (fast, fatigue resistant)
    - Type FI (fast, fatigue intermediate)
    - Type FF (fast, fatigable)
- Upper and lower motoneurons
  - Upper motoneurons: located in the descending pathways of the cortex, brainstem, and spinal cord. Upper motor neuron pathology presents as spasticity with increased reflexive response (e.g., cerebral palsy, stroke)
  - Lower motoneurons: located in the ventral gray matter of the spinal cord. Lower motor neuron and distal axonal injury presents as fasciculations, fibrillations, and weakness.
  - ALS affects both upper and lower motor neurons, with complete sparing of afferent sensation.
- Motoneuron lesions (Table 1-30)
  - **Spasticity** is common in patients with an **upper motoneuron lesion.**
- Spinal (neurogenic) shock
  - A state of vasodilation: paradoxical hypotension and bradycardia; **absence of bulbocavernosus reflex**
  - Occurs after cervical or upper thoracic spinal cord injury
  - Occurs because the descending sympathetic pathways are disrupted
  - Treated by positioning, pressor agents, and atropine
- Patients with spinal cord injury may be given **methylprednisolone**:
  - If injury occurred less than 3 hours earlier: an initial bolus of 30 mg/kg over 15 minutes, followed by an infusion of 5.4 mg/kg/h for 23 hours
  - If injury occurred between 3 and 8 hours earlier: an initial bolus of 30 mg/kg over 15 minutes, followed by an infusion of 5.4 mg/kg/h for 47 hours
  - Decreases extent of cord hemorrhage
  - Does not affect cord edema
  - May improve root function at the level of the injury
  - Spinal cord function may or may not improve.
  - Not indicated for nerve root deficits, brachial plexus deficits, or gunshot wounds

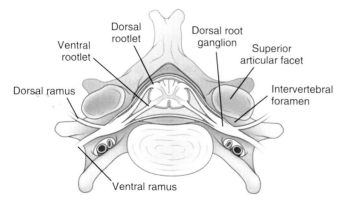

FIGURE 1-65 Spinal cord anatomy. Each spinal nerve has a dorsal (sensory) and a ventral (motor) root. Dorsal roots are branches from dorsal root ganglia cells; ventral roots are motor axons from cells in the ventral horn. (From Bradley WG et al, editors: *Neurology in clinical practice*, ed 5, Philadelphia, 2008, Butterworth-Heinemann.)

Table 1-31	Types and Characteristics of Nerve Fibers			
TYPE	**DIAMETER (μm)**	**MYELINATION**	**SPEED**	**EXAMPLES**
A	10-20	Heavy	Fast	Touch
B	<3	Intermediate	Medium	Autonomic nervous system
C	<1.3	None	Slow	Pain

- Somatosensory system has the following characteristics:
  - Conveys three types of modalities: mechanical, pain, and thermal
  - Each mediated by a specific type of sensory receptor (Table 1-32)
  - Input transmitted to spinal cord (or brainstem) via the dorsal root ganglion (see Figure 1-65)
- ■ Injury to the nervous system (Table 1-33)
  - Types of injuries
  - Preganglionic injuries
    - Imply CNS injury which do not heal appreciably
    - Proximal to the dorsal root ganglia
    - Presents with Horner syndrome
    - Medially winged scapula due to serratus anterior palsy (innervated by preganglionic long thoracic nerve)
    - EMG showing **loss of innervation** of cervical paraspinal muscle innervation
    - **Normal** or positive **histamine response test—** wheal and **flare** (see Immunology section).
  - Postganglionic injuries
    - Abnormal histamine response test (no flare)
    - EMG showing maintained innervation to the cervical paraspinal muscles
  - Peripheral nerve injury leads to death of the distal axons and **wallerian degeneration** (of myelin).
    - Extends distally from transection to the somatosensory receptor
    - Mechanical deformation of a compressed peripheral nerve is greatest in superficial regions and in zones between compressed and uncompressed segments.
    - Prolonged compression leads to **vascular obstruction** of **intraneural vessels**, which may cause **altered sensation** (e.g., cubital tunnel elbow flexion test).
    - Nerve stretching can affect function:
      - Microcirculation diminished at 8% elongation
      - Axons disrupted at 15% elongation
    - The nucleus pulposus induces an inflammatory response when in contact with the nerve roots.
      - Leukotaxis
      - Increased vascular permeability
      - Decreased nerve conduction velocities
      - Nerve regeneration
    - **Proximal axonal budding** occurs after a 1-month delay, and axon migration proceeds **antegrade.**
      - Leads to regeneration at the rate of approximately 1 mm/day
      - Possibly 3 to 5 mm/day in children
    - Nerve regeneration is influenced by three processes:
      - Contact guidance (attraction toward the basal lamina of Schwann cells)
      - Neurotrophism (factors enhancing growth)

Table 1-32	Receptor Types	
RECEPTOR TYPE	**FIBER TYPE**	**QUALITY**
NOCICEPTORS		
Mechanical	Aδ	Sharp, pricking pain
Thermal and mechanothermal	Aγ	Sharp, pricking pain
Thermal and mechanothermal	C	Slow, burning pain
Polymodal	C	Slow, burning pain
CUTANEOUS AND SUBCUTANEOUS MECHANORECEPTORS		
Meissner corpuscle	Aβ	Touch
Pacini corpuscle	Aβ	Flutter
Ruffini corpuscle	Aβ	Vibration
Merkel receptor	Aβ	Steady skin indentation
Hair-guard, tylotrich hair	Aβ	Steady skin indentation
Hair down	Aβ	Flutter
MUSCLE AND SKELETAL MECHANORECEPTORS		
Muscle spindle, primary	Aα	Limb proprioception
Muscle spindle, secondary	Aβ	Limb proprioception
Golgi tendon organ	Aα	Limb proprioception
Joint capsule mechanoreceptor	Aβ	Limb proprioception

Adapted from Kandel ER et al, editors: *Principles of neural science,* ed 3, Norwalk, Conn, 1991, Appleton & Lange, p 342.

Table 1-33	Types and Characteristics of Nerve Injuries	
INJURY	**PATHOPHYSIOLOGIC FEATURES**	**PROGNOSIS**
Neurapraxia	Reversible conduction block characterized by local ischemia and selective demyelination of axon sheath	Good
Axonotmesis	More severe injury; disruption of axon and myelin sheath but leaving epineurium intact	Fair
Neurotmesis	Complete nerve division, disruption of endoneurium	Poor

- Neurotropism (preferential attraction toward nerves rather than other tissues)
- **Pain is the first sensation to return.**
- ■ Testing and spinal cord monitoring
  - Neurologic studies:
    - Histamine testing
      - In a brachial plexus injury, a positive histamine response implies that the reflex arc is intact.
      - A positive response also indicates that the lesion is proximal to the ganglion (preganglionic).
    - Electromyography (EMG)/nerve conduction study (NCS)
      - May be useful for documenting the extent of injury
      - Insertional activity helps determine chronology.
      - Contraction activity

- Spontaneous activity
  - Normal displays end plate potentials and end plate spikes.
  - Abnormality of an individual muscle fiber demonstrates fibrillation. Abnormality of a group of fibers demonstrates fasciculations.
- Cortical evoked potential testing or **somatosensory evoked potential (SSEP)**
  - Most sensitive method of predicting neural compression
  - SSEPs are **not** reliable in monitoring **anterior** spinal cord **pathways.**
  - SSEPs monitor the integrity of the **dorsal column sensory pathways** of the spinal cord.
  - A **50% decrease in amplitude** and **a 10% increase in latency** typically indicate need for corrective action.
  - SSEPs are **less sensitive to anesthesia** than MEPs.
- Motor evoked potential (MEP) testing
  - Monitors integrity of the lateral and ventral **(anterior)** corticospinal **tracts** of the spinal cord directly
- Nerve repair
  - **Factors influencing nerve healing** after repair:
    - **Age** is the most important factor. Younger patients: better chance of recovery after operative repair of nerve transection.
    - **Level of injury**—the more **distal** an injury is the **better** chance at **recovery**
    - **Sharp transections** are more **easily healed** than crush injuries
    - **Repair delay**—the longer you wait until repair, the worse the recovery
    - **Proper alignment of nerve ends** during surgical repair: crucial for maximizing potential for functional recovery
    - **Direct muscular neurotization:**
      - Insertion of the proximal nerve stump into the affected muscle belly
      - Results in less than normal function but is indicated in selected cases
  - Epineural repair
    - Primary repair of the outer connective tissue layer at the site of injury
    - After resection of the proximal neuroma and distal glioma
    - Ensures proper rotation and lack of tension on the repair
  - Grouped fascicular repair
    - Identical to epineural repair but reapproximates individual fascicles under microscopic guidance
    - Used for large nerves (e.g., the **median** and **ulnar nerves** at the **distal third** of the **forearm,** the **sciatic nerve** at the thigh)
    - Improved results over epineural repair have not been demonstrated.
- Connective tissues
- **Tendons** (Figure 1-67)
  - Dense, regularly arranged groups of collagen bundles that attach muscle to bone at the enthesis, with either a rounded or flat shape (e.g., rotator cuff) and covered with synovium or paratenon (vascular)
  - Collagen bundles are arranged in parallel rows.

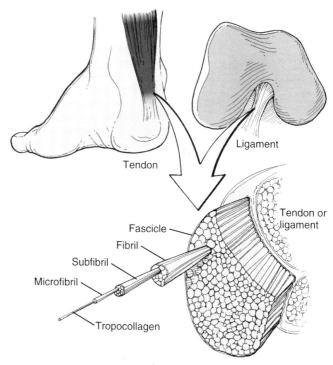

FIGURE 1-67 Tendon and ligament architecture. (From Brinker MR, Miller MD: *Fundamentals of orthopaedics,* Philadelphia, 1999, Saunders, p 15.)

- Composition
  - Collagen (75% dry weight; 95% type I collagen, 5% type III collagen)
  - Proteoglycans (decorin and biglycan—5% dry weight)
    - **Decorin**—most predominant proteoglycan in tendons. Regulates tendon diameter and provides cross-links between collagen fibers. Also shown to have **antifibrotic** properties via inhibition of TGF-β1.
    - **Aggrecan**—present at points of tendon compression
- **Tenocytes**—fibroblast-like differentiated cells; during embryogenesis, migrate from the mesoderm with myoblasts
  - Function to **synthesize extracellular matrix (ECM),** assemble early collagen fibrils, and produce matrix degrading enzymes (MMP)
  - Tenocyte production of collagen increases tendon healing and reduces repair ruptures.
  - Maintain extracellular environment; proposed role in tendinopathy (due to inflammatory mediator production)
    - Tenocytes **produce type III collagen in response to rupture.**
    - Greater proportion of type III collagen, naturally seen in Achilles tendon, predisposes tendons to rupture
- Structure
  - Fibers (individual fascicles) and bundles are surrounded by endotenon and epitenon. In tendons that endure less friction and are without synovial fluid and tendon sheath, paratenon functions as a sleeve.
  - Endotenon and epitenon are composed of type III collagen and carry the nerves, arteries, veins and lymphatics of tendons.

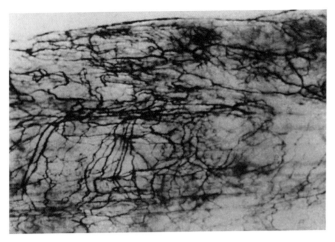

FIGURE 1-68 India ink injection of rabbit calcaneal tendon (Spalteholtz technique) demonstrates the vasculature of the paratenon. (From Simon SR, editor: *Orthopaedic basic science,* Rosemont, Ill, 1994, American Academy of Orthopaedic Surgeons, p 50.)

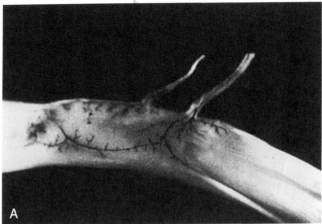

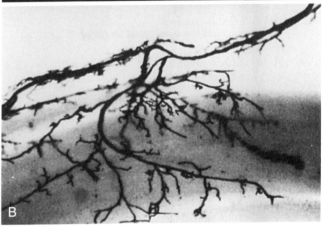

FIGURE 1-69 A and **B,** India ink specimens demonstrating the vascular supply of the flexor tendons via vincula. **B,** Close-up of the specimen. (From Simon SR, editor: *Orthopaedic basic science,* ed 2, Rosemont, Ill, 1994, American Academy of Orthopaedic Surgeons, p 51.)

- With age, more type I collagen interdigitates between type III.
- **Paratenon-covered tendons** (Achilles tendon): **high vascularity** of paratenon, with **better healing** results (Figure 1-68)
- Sheathed
  - Tendons in parts of the body that undergo significant friction require lubrication.
  - **Synovium-covered tendons** (flexor tendons): allow for gliding motion, with **vincula** that carry the blood supply to one tendon segment (Figure 1-69)
  - Areas not contacted by vincula receive nutrition via diffusion through paratenon.
  - Synovial fluid is found between the two layers of the synovial sheath.
- Insertion
  - Tendon inserts into bone by means of four transitional tissues (force dissipation) with direct insertions on bone and indirect insertions onto periosteum:
    - Tendon
    - Fibrocartilage
    - Mineralized fibrocartilage (Sharpey fibers interdigitate with periosteum)
    - Bone
- Injury and healing
  - Three stages of tendon healing: inflammation, proliferation (maximal type III collagen production) and remodeling phases (type I collagen)
  - In the **inflammatory phase, type III collagen** is produced at the injury site by tenocytes with maximal production in the proliferation phase.
  - Achilles, patellar, and supraspinatus tendons are prone to rupture at hypovascular areas.
    - **Achilles tendon is hypovascular 4 to 6 cm proximal to calcaneal insertion.**
  - Tenocytes are involved in tendon healing and scar formation.
  - Responsive to different cytokines and growth factors:
    - In vitro, PDGF genes transfected into tenocytes show collagen formation.

- In vitro, VEGF genes transfected into tenocytes show upregulation of TGF-β and adhesion formation.
- In vitro, when exposed to PMNs (as with inflammation), tenocytes upregulate genes for inflammatory cytokines, TGF-β, and MMP while suppressing type I collagen expression.
- The repair process is affected by treatment.
- **Surgical tendon repairs: weakest at 7 to 10 days**
  - Most of original strength regained at 21 to 28 days
  - Maximum strength achieved at 6 months, reaching two thirds of original strength
  - No evidence in favor of a trough (exposing tendon to cancellous bone) over direct repair to cortical bone
  - Early mobilization increases ROM and decreases repair strength.
  - Immobilization decreases strength at tendon-bone interface.
  - Bony avulsion: heals more rapidly than midsubstance tears
- **Ligaments** (see Figure 1-67)
  - Ligaments consist of dense connective tissue, similar to tendons.
  - Characteristics:
    - Originate and insert on bone
    - Stabilize joints and prevent displacement of bones

- Contain **mechanoreceptors** and nerve endings that facilitate **joint proprioception**
- Surrounding epiligamentous coat—analogous to the epitenon of tendons and carries neurovascular structures
- Composition:
  - Primarily **type I collagen** (80% of dry weight)
  - Water
  - **Elastin** (1% dry weight)
  - Lipids
  - **Proteoglycans** (1% dry weight)—function in water retention
- Compositional differences—compared to tendons, ligaments have:
  - Less collagen
  - More proteoglycans and therefore more water
  - Higher elastin content
  - Less organized collagen fibers that are more highly cross-linked
  - "Uniform microvascularity"—receive supply at insertion sites by the epiligamentous plexus
- Insertion
  - Collagen sliding plays an important role in changes in ligament length (**during growth and contracture**).
  - Ligament insertion into bone can be classified into two types:
    - **Indirect (fibrous) insertion**: superficial fibers insert into the periosteum and deep fibers insert into bone via Sharpey fibers (perforating calcified collagen fibers).
      - Insert at acute angles into the periosteum
    - **Direct (fibrocartilagenous) insertion (more common)**: superficial and deep fibers
      - Deep fibers attach at 90-degree angles.
  - Ligament-to-bone transition in **four phases (zones)**: ligament, fibrocartilage, mineralized fibrocartilage, bone
    - More **collagen type I** is seen at the **bony origin and insertion**, with collagen types II and III seen midsubstance.
- Injury
  - Most common ligaments injured—in the knee and ankle
  - Most common ligament injury—rupture of sequential series of collagen fiber bundles
    - Throughout the body of the ligament
    - Not localized to one specific area
  - Ligaments do not plastically deform.
    - They "break, not bend."
  - Midsubstance ligament tears are common in adults.
  - Avulsion injuries are more common in children.
  - Injury is more common in females.
  - Exercise increases strength and stiffness, preventing injury.
  - Typically occurs between unmineralized and mineralized fibrocartilage layers
- Healing
  - Three phases, as in bone:
    - **Inflammatory**—early acute mediators (PMNs and then macrophages), with production of **type III collagen** and growth factors
    - **Proliferative**—around 1 to 3 weeks, with replacement by **type I collagen** (Think of

macrophages as weakening the structure—weakest point.)
- **Remodeling** and maturation
- Factors that impair ligament healing:
  - Intraarticular ligamentous injury
  - Old age
  - Smokers
  - NSAID use
  - Diabetes mellitus
  - Alcohol use
  - Decrease in growth factors
  - Limited gene expression
  - Local injection of corticosteroids
- Factors that improve ligament healing experimentally:
  - Extraarticular ligamentous injury
  - Compromised immunity
  - IL-10 (antiinflammatory)
  - IL-1 receptor antagonists
  - Mesenchymal stem cells
  - Scaffolds
    - Example: collagen-platelet-rich-plasma hydrogels
  - Neuropeptides
  - Calcitonin gene–related peptide
- Immobilization
  - Adversely affects ligament strength: elastic modulus decreases
  - In rabbits, breaking strength reduced dramatically (66%) after 9 weeks of immobilization
  - Effects reverse slowly upon remobilization.
  - Prolonged immobilization
    - Disrupts collagen structure, which may not return to normal within insertion sites
- Exercise
  - Exercise increases mechanical and structural properties.
  - Increases strength, stiffness, and failure load
- Intervertebral discs (IVDs)
  - Allow spinal motion and stability
  - Also function as cushioning for axial loads on the spine
  - Two components:
    - Central nucleus pulposus
      - A hydrated gel with compressibility
      - **Low collagen (type II)/high proteoglycan** (and GAG) content
      - **Proteoglycans** make up **higher percentage** of dry weight
      - With time, the nucleus pulposus undergoes **loss of proteoglycans** and water (**desiccation**).
    - Surrounding annulus fibrosis
      - Extensibility and increased tensile strength
      - **High collagen (type I)/low proteoglycan** content
      - **Proteoglycans** make up **lower percentage** of dry weight
      - Superficial layer contains nerve fibers
  - Composition:
    - Water (85%)
    - Proteoglycans
    - **Type II collagen** (20% of dry weight) in the **nucleus pulposus**
    - **Type I collagen** (60% of dry weight) in the **annulus fibrosis**

- Neurovascularity:
  - Dorsal root ganglion gives rise to the **sinuvertebral nerve,** which then innervates the **superficial fibers of the annulus.**
  - **Avascular**—nutrients and fluid diffuse from the periphery inwards through pores in hyaline cartilage end plates. This is impaired by calcification with aging.
- Curvature and IVD load
  - Sagittal curvature (e.g., lordosis, kyphosis) influences compressive loading.
  - Adolescents stand with greater posterior sagittal balance.
  - Seniors have forward sagittal balance and increased thoracic kyphosis.
  - Altered curvature is implicated in lower back pain.
  - Increased kyphosis leads to increased IVD compression.
  - Less lumbar lordosis leads to greater lumbar shear load.
  - Shear stress greatest at L5-S1
  - Compressive stress greatest at midthoracic spine
- **Aging disc**
  - Early degenerative disc disease is an **irreversible process,** with **IL-1β** stimulating the release of MMPs, NO, IL-6, and prostaglandin-E$_2$ (PGE$_2$).
  - **Decreased water** content and conversion to **fibrocartilage**
    - A result of a lack of large proteoglycans and aggrecans
    - Also, **decrease and fragmentation of proteoglycans (loss of hydrostatic pressure)**
    - **Increase in keratan sulfate** concentration and **decreased chondroitin sulfate**
    - Increase in relative collagen concentration, with **no change in absolute quantity**
  - **Cigarette smoking: risk factor for degenerative disc disease**
- Neuropeptides
  - Involved in sensory transmission, nociceptive transmission, neurogenic inflammation, and skeletal metabolism
  - Several types:
    - Substance P
    - Calcitonin gene–related peptide
    - Vasoactive intestinal peptide
    - C-flanking peptide of neuropeptide Y
- Soft tissue healing
  - Four phases:
    - Hemostasis
      - A primary platelet plug is formed within 5 minutes of injury.
      - Secondary clotting occurs through the coagulation cascade and fibrin within 10 to 15 minutes.
      - Fibronectin, a large glycoprotein, binds fibrin to cells and acts as a chemotactic factor.
      - Platelets release factors that activate the next phase of healing.
    - Inflammation
      - Macrophages cause débridement of injured/necrotic tissue within 1 week.
      - Three stages:
        - Activation (immediate)
        - Amplification (in 48-72 hours)

- Débridement (bacteria, phagocytosis, and matrix [biochemical])
  - Prostaglandins mediate the response.
- Organogenesis
  - Tissue modeling (in 7-21 days)
  - Differentiation of mesenchymal precursors into myofibroblasts
  - Angiogenesis
  - Further differentiation, which leads to the final stage of healing
- **Remodeling** (of individual tissue lines)
  - Continues for up to 18 months
  - Collagen realignment and cross-linking: increase tensile strength
- Growth factors
  - Require activation, are redundant, have feedback loop mechanisms
  - Chemotactic factors (attract cells)
  - Prostaglandins: PMNs
  - Prostanoids: PMNs
  - Complement: PMNs and macrophages
  - PDGF: macrophages and fibroblasts
  - Angiokines: endothelial cells
  - Competence factors: activate dormant (G$_0$) cells
  - PDGF
  - Prostaglandins
  - Progression factors: allow cell growth
    - Induce epidermal growth factor, IL-1, somatomedins
  - Inductive factors: stimulate differentiation
    - Angiokines
    - BMP
    - Specific tissue growth factors
    - Transforming factors: cause differentiation and proliferation
  - Permissive factors: enhancing factors
    - Fibronectin
    - Osteonectin
- Soft tissue implants
  - Allografts
    - No donor-site morbidity
    - Incite an immune response
    - May transmit infection
    - Risk of HIV exposure from a ligament allograft is 1 : 1,600,000
    - Histologic recovery: slower and less predictable than that for autografts
  - Freeze drying
    - Reduces the immunogenic response
    - Decreases strength
    - Deep freezing without drying does not affect strength.
  - Cryopreservation
    - Controlled rate freezing in a protective medium
    - Prevents ice crystal formation
    - Preserves some cell viability and protein structure
    - Strength at 6 months comparable to that for autograft
    - If not harvested under sterile conditions, cold ethylene oxide gas may have adverse affects (graft failure).
  - Particularly in conjunction with irradiation with more than 4 megarad
    - Irradiation with 2 megarad with ethylene oxide: apparently has no significant effect on mechanical properties

- Fresh osteochondral allograft (lesion > 2 cm)
  - Osteoarticular allografts preserved with cryopreservation have no viable chondrocytes after clinical transplantation.
  - Fresh allografts are stored in culture medium at 4°C for 14 days to allow for microbiologic and serologic testing.
  - Chondrocyte viability is maintained for up to 45 days, but there is a significant decrease after 28 days.
- Osteochondral grafts
  - Fresh osteochondral **allograft**
    - Reserved for osteochondral **lesions larger than 2 cm**

- Osteochondral **autograft** (mosaicplasty)
  - Reserved for osteochondral **lesions smaller than 2 cm**
- Synthetic ligaments
  - No initial period of weakness, in contrast to autografts or allografts
  - Subject to wear (debris)
  - Associated with sterile joint effusions
  - Increase in neutral proteinases (collagenase and gelatinase)
  - Chondrocyte activation factor (IL-1)

SECTION 2 ORTHOPAEDIC BIOLOGY

CELLULAR AND MOLECULAR BIOLOGY

■ Chromosomes

- In the nucleus of every eukaryotic cell
  - Antibodies to nuclear contents—**ANA antibodies**—are seen in many systemic autoimmune disorders and used for screening.
  - Orthopaedic-relevant examples:
    - **Anti-Scl-70**—linked to scleroderma
    - **Anti-Jo-1**—linked to polymyositis and dermatomyositis
    - **Anti-dsDNA**—linked to SLE
    - **Anti-histone antibodies**—most commonly seen in drug-induced lupus and also in SLE, RA, and scleroderma
- In humans, **46 chromosomes** in 23 pairs
  - Of these: 22 pairs of autosomes, 1 pair of sex chromosomes
  - Each chromosome contains more than 150,000 genes.
- **DNA (deoxyribonucleic acid)**
  - All nuclear DNA resides in the 23 chromosome pairs.
  - DNA regulates cellular functions through protein synthesis that is determined by the arrangement of nitrogenous bases (adenine, guanine, cytosine, and thymine).
  - DNA has a double helix (double-stranded) structure with adenine linked to thymine and guanine linked to cytosine on a sugar-phosphate backbone.
    - **Anti–double-stranded DNA antibodies (anti-dsDNA) are specific for SLE.**
  - Histones are proteins that package DNA within the nuclei. They are the spools around which DNA is wound.
    - Antihistone antibodies are seen in drug-induced lupus.
- Nucleotide
  - A nucleotide consists of a DNA sugar molecule and phosphate group plus one nitrogenous base.
  - The nucleotide sequence in one strand of DNA determines the complementary nucleotide sequence in the other strand.
  - **Codons** are sequences of **three nucleotides**.
  - The genetic code is described in codons, or three-letter "words" that are templates for messenger (m)RNA generation then translation into proteins.

- Each codon specifies **one** of the 20 **amino acids** that are the basic units of all proteins.

■ Gene

- Portion of DNA that codes for a specific protein
- **Transcription—DNA to mRNA** (Figure 1-70)
  - Unwinding of DNA for transcription occurs by DNA topoisomerase.
    - Topoisomerase-1 (scl-70) antibodies are seen in scleroderma and CREST syndrome.
  - **Exons** are regions of DNA that code for mRNA. (**EX**ons are **EX**pressed)
  - DNA reverse transcribed from mRNA is called **cDNA.**
  - **Introns** are regions of DNA that are between exons; 97% of the human genome consists of noncoding DNA.

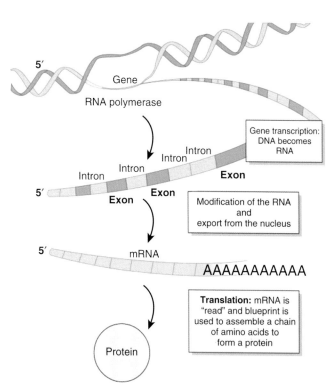

FIGURE 1-70 DNA information is transcribed into RNA in the nucleus. Messenger RNA (mRNA) is then transported to the cytoplasm where ribosomes complete translation into proteins. (From Jorde LB et al, editors: *Medical genetics*, ed 2, St. Louis, 1999, Mosby.)

- **Splicing** is the processing and removal of introns along with the combining of exons.
  - Small nuclear ribonucleoproteins (**sn-rnp**) are RNA-protein complexes that mediate this posttranscriptional modification.
  - Examples of these proteins are the U1 and Smith proteins.
    - **Anti-Smith** antibodies are specific to **SLE**.
    - **Anti-U1-rnp** antibodies are seen in **mixed connective tissue disease**.
- Gene enhancers
  - Binding sites for proteins (transcription factors)
  - Involved in the regulation of transcription
- Consensus sequences
  - Binding sites for specific proteins involved in gene regulation
  - Named for a specific nucleotide sequence

■ **RNA**
- Important differences from DNA: RNA is a single-stranded ribose sugar
- A hydroxyl group is attached to the pentose ring in the $2'$ position, making RNA less stable.
- Found in both nucleus and cytoplasm
- Nitrogenous bases: **adenine, guanine, cytosine, and uracil**
- **No thymine**
- Adenine is linked to uracil.
- mRNA is the strand of RNA transcribed by exons.
  - Micro- **(mi)RNA**—small, single-stranded noncoding RNA molecules that regulate gene expression by RNA silencing and modification
  - Small interfering **(si)RNA**—region of double-stranded RNA that loops back on itself to silence expression of genes by breaking down mRNA after transcription

■ **Translation** (see Figure 1-70)
- Building of a **protein** from **mRNA** through amino acids
  - Transfer **(t)RNA** carries a specific amino acid to the site of protein synthesis, based on the mRNA codon.
    - Antibodies to tRNA synthetase (**Anti-Jo-1 antibodies**) are seen in **dermatomyositis**.

■ **Cell cycle and ploidy**
- The cell cycle entails the events within a cell that result in DNA duplication, with production of two daughter cells. It is broken up into phases of interphase (G1, S, G2) and mitosis.
- **Ploidy** is the amount of DNA in a cell, and **haploid** is the amount of DNA in an individual sex cell (N = 23 chromosomes).
  - Growth 0 (G0)—stable phase of cells with **diploid (2N)** DNA content
  - Growth 1 (G1)—upon stimulus, cells begin growth but remain **diploid (2N)**.
  - Synthesis (S)—period of **DNA replication** that is **tetraploid (4N)** by the end
  - Growth 2 (G2)—phase of cell growth and protein synthesis that is **tetraploid (4N)** throughout
  - Mitosis (M)—sequence of events that result in two identical daughter cells
    - Separation of chromosomal material for daughter cells occurs by spindle fibers' attachment to centromeres that link sister chromatids

- **Anticentromere antibodies are seen in CREST syndrome.**
- Certain **proteins regulate progression** through the **cell cycle.** Genetic defects and alterations of these tumor suppressor proteins can predispose a cell to dysregulated growth.
- E2F, through its interaction with pRb-1, has a central role in cell cycle regulation.
  - **pRb-1 (retinoblastoma protein)** undergoes progressive cell cycle–regulated phosphorylation.
    - It is hypophosphorylated in G1 and is progressively phosphorylated as the cell cycle progresses.
    - Is phosphorylated by cyclin/CDK to facilitate progression from G1 to S
    - The phosphorylation is removed during mitosis by PP1.
    - The target for pRb-1 is **E2F,** a transcription factor that regulates genes important for cell cycle control.
      - Hypophosphorylated pRb (early G1) binds E2F.
      - Phosphorylated pRb (starting late G1) releases E2F, allowing the transcription of E2F target genes.
    - Implicated in retinoblastoma and osteosarcoma
  - p53—prevents entry to S phase
    - Implicated in osteosarcoma, rhabdomyosarcoma, and chondrosarcoma

■ **Techniques used to study genetic (inherited) disorders**
- Restriction enzymes
  - Used to cut DNA at precise reproducible cleavage locations
  - Produce restriction fragments
  - Identify polymorphisms (alternative gene expressions)
  - Linkage analysis
    - Estimates the probability that a genetic trait or disease is associated with polymorphisms
- **Agarose gel electrophoresis**
  - DNA (negatively charged) is suspended in agarose gel.
  - The gel is exposed to an electric field.
  - DNA moves through the gel toward the positive pole of the field.
  - The gel acts as a "sieve":
    - Small DNA fragments move farther than large fragments in a given time.
  - This technique is commonly used after and in conjunction with restriction enzymes.
- **DNA ligation**
  - Method of attaching genes from human DNA to pieces of nonhuman DNA known as *plasmids*
  - Facilitates the study of specific genes
  - DNA fragments linked by ligation form recombinant DNA
- Plasmid vectors
  - A plasmid is a **small, extrachromosomal, circular piece of DNA** that replicates independently of the host DNA. Plasmids can confer antibiotic resistance between bacteria.
  - Plasmid vectors are used to produce large quantities of a gene.
  - The gene is ligated to a plasmid (forming a recombinant plasmid).

- The recombinant plasmid is inserted into a bacterium (the vector) by a process called *transformation.*
- The recombinant plasmid replicates in the bacterium.
- Increases the recombinant DNA and its gene
- Cytogenetic analysis
  - Gross examination of chromosomes under microscope with the use of techniques of banding and fluorescent in situ hybridization
  - Used to detect **chromosomal translocations**
    - **t(X:18)**—in synovial sarcoma
    - **t(11:22)**—in Ewing sarcoma
    - **t(2:13)**—in rhabdomyosarcoma
    - **t(12:16)**—in myxoid liposarcoma
    - **t(12:22)**—in clear cell sarcoma
- Transgenic animals
  - Such animals are bred to investigate the function of cloned genes.
  - A foreign gene (transgene) is inserted into a single-cell embryo.
  - The cell replicates.
  - The transgene is carried by every cell in the body.
- **Southern blotting detects DNA by hybridization.**
  - Restriction enzymes and agarose gel electrophoresis
  - Identifies a particular **DNA sequence** in an extract of mixed DNA
- **Northern blotting detects RNA by hybridization.**
  - Restriction enzymes and agarose gel electrophoresis
  - Identifies a particular **RNA sequence** in an extract of mixed RNA
- **Western blotting detects protein.**
  - Sodium dodecyl sulfate–polyacrylamide gel electrophoresis (SDS-PAGE)
  - Identifies a particular **protein** in an extract of mixed proteins
- **PCR amplification**
  - Repetitive synthesis (amplification) of a specific DNA sequence in vitro
  - The number of copies of DNA doubles each cycle.
  - Has gained widespread use
  - Prenatal diagnosis of sickle cell disease
  - Screening DNA for gene mutations
- **Reverse transcription (RT)-PCR)**
  - Reverse transcriptase used to "reverse transcribe" **RNA to complementary DNA**
  - Typically used to study RNA viruses
- Cloning
  - The production of genetically identical biological entities
  - Therapeutic cloning
  - DNA removed from a patient is inserted into an embryo.
  - Stem cells are removed from the growing embryo (which dies).
  - These cells are stimulated to differentiate into a specific tissue.
  - The specific tissue (or organ) is transplanted back into the patient.
  - Avoids the need for transplantation of an organ from another person
  - Avoids organ rejection

- Avoids complications of immunosuppressive agents
- **Reproductive cloning**
  - DNA is removed from a host and inserted into an embryo.
  - The embryo is then implanted into a healthy womb and allowed to develop.
  - The goal is to produce an animal that is genetically identical to the host.
- Embryo cloning
  - One or more cells are removed from a fertilized embryo and stimulated to develop in utero.
  - The goal is to produce several genetically identical animals (e.g., twins or triplets).

Immunology

- The immune system is broadly categorized into two branches: the **innate** and **adaptive,** with interaction and overlap between the two (Figure 1-71).
  - The **innate system** is primitive, nonspecific, and the first line of defense; think of as hand-to-hand combat using complement and and leukocytes including NK cells, mast cells, basophils, eosinophils, macrophages, neutrophils, and dendritic cells.
  - The **adaptive system** is more complex; think of as advanced laser-targeted projectile weaponry using antigen presentation with B and T lymphocytes and antibodies.
    - Response to a pathogen generates an immunologic memory in the adaptive system.
  - Excessive immune responses can lead to host tissue damage. These are known as **hypersensitivity reactions.**
- Innate (nonspecific) response—first line of defense
  - Is **antigen independent** and involves the cells mentioned earlier
  - Barriers—physical and chemical components (e.g., enzymes, pH)
    - Skin—sebum, sweat (lysozyme, RNases and DNases, defensins, cathelicidins)
      - **α-Defensin**—example of an antimicrobial peptide secreted into synovial fluid
      - Highly sensitive and specific for periprosthetic joint infection
      - **Cathelicidins**—antimicrobial peptide that is regulated by sufficient stores of vitamin D
    - Mucous membranes (**IgA** most common immunoglobulin)
    - Respiratory epithelium
    - Urinary tract
  - Inflammation occurs in response to fracture, soft tissue injury, necrosis, infection or foreign body generating an environment that attracts neutrophils.
    - Signs of inflammation
      - Rubor (erythema)—pyrogens (e.g., LPS, PGE_2)
      - Calor (warmth)—increased blood flow from vasodilation
      - Dolor (pain)—sensitized nerve endings
      - Tumor (edema)—exudate from tissue injury
    - Cellular response in inflammation:
      - **Neutrophil** response—**first cells recruited** to sites of tissue injury
        - Margination, rolling, adhesion, chemotaxis, and phagocytosis
        - Destruction of phagocytosed material

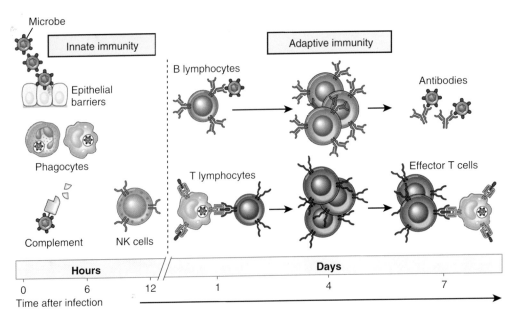

FIGURE 1-71 Innate and adaptive immunity. The mechanisms of innate immunity provide the initial defense against infections. Adaptive immune responses develop later and consist of activation of lymphocytes. *NK,* Natural killer. (From Abbas AK et al: *Cellular and molecular immunology,* ed 6, Philadelphia, 2009, Saunders.)

- **Macrophage** response—comes after neutrophils
  - **Initiate** inflammatory response in osteolysis or **aseptic loosening** (occurs in response to **particles < 1 μm** in diameter)
- **Mast cells**—activated by trauma, complement, or IgE cross-linking, releasing histamine granules
  - Histamine mediates the peripheral nerve axon reflex that results in flare—redness and warmth due to histamine granule release causing vascular smooth muscle relaxation.
    - Disruption of the postganglionic axon results in loss of flare.
  - Contracts endothelial cells to allow leakage of fluid from venules to cause edema (wheal).
  - Excessive endothelial vasodilation with respiratory smooth muscle constriction is an **emergency mediated by IgE–type I hypersensitivity reaction** and can lead to shock and death.
- Recognition of pathogens by innate system
  - Once physical barriers are breached, the innate immune response is activated through Toll-like receptors (TLRs).
  - **Pathogen-associated molecular patterns (PAMPs)** on microbes are recognized by TLRs on innate immune system cells (e.g., macrophages and dendritic cells).
    - Example of a PAMP is bacterial lipopolysaccharide (LPS), which is recognized by a **TLR** (TLR 4).
  - There is an upregulation of **NF-κB** transcription factor, resulting in immune mediator release (e.g., IL-1, IL-6, TNF-α).
    - IL-6 causes the liver to release inflammatory mediators such as **CRP.**
  - Arachidonic acid released from cell membranes is acted on by COX and 5-lipoxygenase to make:
    - Prostaglandins and leukotrienes that mediate exudation, chemotaxis, and bronchospasm.

- **Ibuprofen** inhibits COX and reduces prostaglandin production, preventing renal efferent arteriolar relaxation and increasing GFR.
- Factor (XII)—inflammatory protein made in the liver
  - When exposed to collagen under damaged endothelium, activates coagulation
  - Acute production of coagulation factors elevates ESR.
- Complement
  - Activated by IgM or IgG antigen (Ag) complexes, microbial products, or mannose on microorganisms
  - Mediate chemotaxis of PMNs, opsonization (tagging of evasive bacteria for elimination in the spleen), and MAC lysis of microbes, among other functions
- **Acquired** (specific or **adaptive**) response
  - Is **antigen dependent** and composed of the **cell mediated** and **humoral** responses. Cells involved include T and B lymphocytes.
  - Antigens are ligands recognized by the immune system. The smallest part of an antigen "seen" by a T- or B-cell receptor is an **epitope.**
  - Lymphocytes can mount specific reactions to millions of potential antigens.
    - They rearrange their genes (unique to lymphocytes).
    - They achieve antigenic diversity.
    - They produce millions of antibodies.
  - Adaptive response occurs in response to:
    - Persistent infection
    - Pathogens—viruses, mycobacteria, parasites, fungi
    - In autoimmune diseases
    - Foreign body
    - Cancer
  - **Cell mediated**—T lymphocytes (helper, CD4+; cytotoxic, CD8+), macrophages, natural killer cells
    - Targets intracellular bacteria, virus, fungi, parasites, tumors, and transplanted organs/orthopaedic hardware

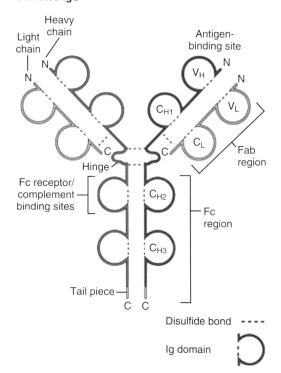

Secreted IgC

- Light chain
- Heavy chain
- Antigen-binding site
- N N N N N N
- V_H
- C_H1
- V_L
- C_L
- C C
- Fab region
- Hinge
- Fc receptor/complement binding sites
- C_H2
- Fc region
- C_H3
- Tail piece
- C C
- Disulfide bond ----
- Ig domain

FIGURE 1-72 Basic subunit structure of the immunoglobulin molecule. *C_H* and *C_L,* Constant regions; *Fab,* antigen-binding fragment; *Fc,* crystallizable fragment; *IgC,* immunoglobulin C; *V_H* and *V_L,* variable regions. (From Katz VL et al: *Comprehensive gynecology,* ed 5, Philadelphia, 2007, Mosby.)

- An example of excessive cell-mediated immunity is the **type IV hypersensitivity reaction**. This often occurs in response to **orthopaedic hardware.**
- Antigen-presenting cells (APCs—macrophages, dendritic cells, certain B cells, and Langerhans cells) process antigens.
  - The antigen specificity of receptors on APCs are genetically inherited and established before they are ever exposed to a PAMP.
- T cells that recognize these protein receptors, activate effector cells, and clone themselves
- **Humoral**—B lymphocytes and their matured counterpart, plasma cells. Both produce antibodies.
- Targets exotoxin-mediated disease, encapsulated bacterial infection, other viral infections
- Each B cell makes antibodies specific to one single epitope (antigen). B cells use immunoglobulins (IgM and IgD) as cell membrane receptors.
- Terminally differentiated B cells are called *plasma cells.* The difference is that they secrete immunoglobulins into fluid.
- Immunoglobulins (Figure 1-72)—mnemonic: MADGE
  - IgM: heaviest, first in the adaptive response
    - **RF is an IgM against** the Fc portion of **IgG.**
  - IgA: in mucosal surfaces (e.g., MALT [mucosa-associated lymphoid tissue]) and secretions
  - IgD: only on B-cell surfaces
  - IgG: also on B-cell surface but also secreted.
    - Mediates opsonization; later in the adaptive response

- IgE: on the surface of mast cells (allergic reactions), basophils, and eosinophils (response to parasite).
- Once secreted, antibodies can defend by a variety of mechanisms.
  - Neutralize viruses and toxins
  - Opsonization
  - Complement activation (IgG and IgM)
  - Antibody cellular cytotoxicity
  - Prevention of adherence and colonization (IgA)
- Excessive immune response
  - The innate immune system has evolved to efficiently recognize "self" epitopes
  - The adaptive immune response has mechanisms in place to help recognize "self"
    - Immunogenetics—HLA gene on chromosome 6 can be rearranged (VDJ recombination) to make an antigen-specific receptor on APCs for up to 10^{15} different epitopes.
      - **HLA-B27 is** associated with a variety of **rheumatologic diseases.** Mnemonic: **PAIR**
        - **Psoriatic arthritis**
        - **Ankylosing spondylitis**
        - Inflammatory bowel disease
        - **Reactive arthritis** (Reiter syndrome)
        - Also JRA
      - HLA-DR3: myasthenia gravis and SLE
      - HLA-DR4: RA
  - This leaves room for error and accidental "self" recognition.
  - Excessive self-recognition with subsequent tissue damage is known as *hypersensitivity.*
  - Hypersensitivity reactions
    - **Type I:** mediated by **IgE**
      - **Anaphylaxis** or allergic response, immediate response, mast cell degranulation
      - **Food allergy (milk, egg, peanut, seafood, etc.)**
      - **Penicillin allergy**
    - **Type II:** mediated by IgM or IgG, cytotoxic, antibody-mediated response
      - Heparin-induced thrombocytopenia
      - Rheumatic fever
      - Myasthenia gravis
    - **Type III:** immune complex mediated (antigen-antibody [e.g., IgG-Ag])
      - SLE
      - RA
    - **Type IV: cell-mediated** (no antibodies); helper T cells activate cytotoxic cells and macrophages to attack tissue; delayed response.
      - 2 to 3 days to develop—NOT antibody mediated
      - TB screening with **PPD/**Mantoux test
      - Type 1 diabetes mellitus
      - Multiple sclerosis
      - **Type IV response** to **metallic orthopaedic implants**
      - **Pseudotumor hypersensitivity response** can occur years after THA.
  - Autoimmunity
    - Recognition of epitopes from the "self" nuclear content of cells produces **antinuclear antibodies (ANAs),** which are seen in many disease processes.
      - **Anti-Sm**—SLE (specific but not sensitive—i.e., only one fifth with SLE present)

- Anti-RNP—mixed connective tissue disease
- Anti-scl-70—scleroderma
- Anti-ds-DNA—SLE and implicated in SLE nephritis
- Anti-histone—drug-induced lupus
- Anti-Ro and Anti-La—Sjögren syndrome

■ Origins of immune cells (B and T lymphocytes)
- Arise from primitive hematopoietic mesenchymal stem cells in the bone marrow
- B lymphocytes mature in lymph nodes.
  - Plasma cells are fully differentiated antibody-secreting B cells.
- T-lymphocytes
  - Originate in the bone marrow
  - Pass through the thymus during fetal development to mature
  - Finally, move into the lymph nodes and circulate through blood
  - Include: helper T cells, suppressor T cells, killer T cells, and regulatory T cells

■ Cytokines
- Low-molecular-weight proteins that bind to receptors and elicit cellular responses. Each cytokine can serve a variety of functions:
  - IL-1—initiates acute phase response
    - IL-1 induces **bone loss** through activation of osteoclasts via RANK/RANKL pathway.
  - IL-2—promotes growth and activation of lymphocytes
  - IL-6—induces synthesis of acute phase proteins from liver (e.g., CRP)
    - IL-6 is key for growth and survival of **multiple myeloma** (MM) cells.
      - Generated in autocrine (MM cells) and paracrine (bone marrow stromal cells and osteoblasts) fashion
    - IL-6 shifts dephosphorylated pRb-1 to its inactive phosphorylated form, promoting E2F gene transcription, releasing growth arrest of MM cells.
  - IL-10—antiinflammatory
  - TNF-α—helps mediate inflammatory response to intracellular infections
    - **Anti-TNF** antibody medications predispose individuals to **opportunistic infections**.
  - TGF-β—limits inflammation and **promotes fibrosis**

■ Additional considerations—response to stress
- Long-standing stress on an organ results in reprogramming of stem cells to produce a cell type more suitable to the new environment (metaplasia). If left unregulated, further dedifferentiation (neoplasia) can occur.
  - **Marjolin ulcer**—chronic inflammation over burns or draining sinus tract from **chronic osteomyelitis**, leading to ulceration.
    - Conversion to ulcerated squamous cell carcinoma can occur about **20 years later.**

■ Genetics
■ Mendelian inheritance
- Mendelian traits follow specific patterns of inheritance with an incidence of approximately 1%.
- Mendelian inheritance is due to transmission of alleles among offspring.
  - An individual is **homozygous** if the alleles on each of the paired chromosomes are identical.
  - An individual is **heterozygous** if the alleles differ.

- **Phenotype** refers to the features (traits) exhibited because of genetic makeup (genotype).
- Mendelian traits may be inherited by one of four modes (Tables 1-34 and 1-35):
  - **Autosomal dominant (AD)**
    - **Syndactyly/polydactyly, Marfan syndrome, hereditary multiple exostoses (HME), malignant hyperthermia, Ehlers-Danlos syndrome, achondroplasia, osteogenesis imperfecta (types I and IV)**
      - **Malignant hyperthermia—first sign is increased end-tidal CO_2** in patients with inhalational anesthetic agents and succinylcholine.
        - Other signs are acidosis, increased oxygen consumption, heat production, activation of SNS, DIC, and hyperkalemia.
        - There are over 30 mutations in malignant hyperthermia.
        - Treat with dantrolene—decreases loss of calcium from sarcoplasmic reticulum.
      - **Achondroplasia—constitutively active** mutation in the FGF-R3, affecting the proliferative growth plate zone.
        - 80% of cases are new mutations.
        - Most common cause of disproportionate short stature dwarfism.
  - **Autosomal recessive (AR)** (most enzyme/biochemical deficiencies)
    - Diastrophic dysplasia
      - Mutation in the DTDST (*SLC26A2*) gene on chromosome 5 that encodes for a sulfate transport protein—undersulfation of cartilage proteoglycans
      - Features include hitchhiker thumb, cauliflower ear, scoliosis, hip dysplasia, cleft palate (50%), foot deformities/club foot.
  - **X-linked dominant**
    - **Hypophosphatemic rickets**, Léri-Weil dyschondrosteosis
      - *PHEX* gene mutation (Xp.22) associated with hypophosphatemic rickets
        - *PHEX* regulates FGF-23, which normally prevents the kidney's reabsorption of phosphate.
        - The *PHEX* gene mutation therefore reduces phosphate reabsorption, leading to hypophosphatemia.
  - **X-linked recessive**
    - **Duchenne and Becker muscular dystrophy, Hunter syndrome, hemophilia, SED tarda**
    - **Duchenne muscular dystrophy—complete lack of dystrophin**
- Nonmendelian traits may be inherited through "polygenic" transmission.
  - Caused by the action of several genes:
    - Charcot-Marie-Tooth (AD, AR, and X-linked forms)
    - Osteopetrosis (AD and AR)
    - Osteogenesis Imperfecta (AD and AR)
    - Neurofibromatosis (AD and AR)
    - Spondyloepiphyseal dysplasia (SED) (AD and X-linked)

Text continued on p. 93

Table 1-34 Mendelian Inheritance

INHERITANCE PATTERN	DESCRIPTION	PUNNETT SQUARE(S)
Autosomal dominant*	Autosomal dominant disorders typically represent **structural defects.** Disorder is manifested in the heterozygous state (Aa). Affects 50% of offspring (assuming only one parent is affected) Normal offspring do not transmit the condition. There is no gender preference.	<table><tr><td></td><td>A</td><td>a</td></tr><tr><td>a</td><td>Aa</td><td>aa</td></tr><tr><td>a</td><td>Aa</td><td>aa</td></tr></table>
Autosomal recessive†	Autosomal recessive disorders typically represent **biochemical or enzymatic defects.** Disorder is manifested in the homozygous state (aa). Parents are unaffected (they are most commonly heterozygotes). Affects 25% of offspring (assuming each parent is a heterozygote). There is no gender preference.	<table><tr><td></td><td>A</td><td>a</td></tr><tr><td>A</td><td>AA</td><td>Aa</td></tr><tr><td>a</td><td>Aa</td><td>aa</td></tr></table>
X-linked dominant‡	X-linked dominant disorders are manifested in the heterozygous state (X′X or X′Y). Affected female (mating with unaffected male) transmits the X-linked gene to 50% of daughters and 50% of sons. Affected male (mating with unaffected female) transmits the X-linked gene to all daughters and no sons.	<table><tr><td></td><td>X</td><td>Y</td></tr><tr><td>X′</td><td>X′X</td><td>X′Y</td></tr><tr><td>X</td><td>XX</td><td>XY</td></tr></table> <table><tr><td></td><td>X′</td><td>Y</td></tr><tr><td>X</td><td>X′X</td><td>XY</td></tr><tr><td>X</td><td>X′X</td><td>XY</td></tr></table>
X-linked recessive§	Heterozygote (X′Y) male manifests the condition. Heterozygote (X′X) female is unaffected. Affected male (mating with unaffected female) transmits the X-linked gene to all daughters (who are carriers) and no sons. Carrier female (mating with unaffected male) transmits the X-linked gene to 50% of daughters (who are carriers) and 50% of sons (who are affected).	<table><tr><td></td><td>X′</td><td>Y</td></tr><tr><td>X</td><td>X′X</td><td>XY</td></tr><tr><td>X</td><td>X′X</td><td>XY</td></tr></table> <table><tr><td></td><td>X</td><td>Y</td></tr><tr><td>X′</td><td>X′X</td><td>X′Y</td></tr><tr><td>X</td><td>XX</td><td>XY</td></tr></table>

*"A" is the mutant dominant allele.
†"a" is the mutant recessive allele.
‡"X′" is the mutant dominant X allele.
§"X" is the mutant recessive X allele.

Table 1-35 Comprehensive Compilation of Inheritance Pattern, Defect, and Associated Gene in Musculoskeletal Disorders

DISORDER	INHERITANCE PATTERN	DEFECT	ASSOCIATED GENE
DYSPLASIAS			
Achondroplasia	Autosomal dominant	Defect in the fibroblast growth factor (FGF) receptor 3	**FGF3R**
Diastrophic dysplasia	Autosomal recessive	Mutation of a gene coding for a sulfate transport protein	DTDST
Kniest dysplasia	Autosomal dominant	Defect in type II collagen	COL 2A1
Laron dysplasia (pituitary dwarfism)	Autosomal recessive	Defect in the growth hormone receptor	
McCune-Albright syndrome (polyostotic fibrous dysplasia, café-au-lait spots, precocious puberty)	Sporadic mutation	Germline defect in the Gsα protein	**Mutation of Gsα subunit of the receptor/adenylyl cyclase–coupling G proteins**
Metaphyseal chondrodysplasia (Jansen form)	Autosomal dominant		PTH; PTH-related protein
Metaphyseal chondrodysplasia (McKusick form)	Autosomal recessive		RMRP
Metaphyseal chondrodysplasia (Schmid-tarda form)	Autosomal dominant	Defect in type X collagen	COL 10A1
Multiple epiphyseal dysplasia	Autosomal dominant (most commonly)	Cartilage oligomeric matrix protein	COMP
Spondyloepiphyseal dysplasia	Autosomal dominant (congenita form) X-linked recessive (tarda form)	Defect in type II collagen	Linked to Xp22.12-p22.31, SEDL (tarda), and COL 2A1 (congenita)
Achondrogenesis	Autosomal recessive	Fetal cartilage fails to mature	
Apert syndrome	Sporadic mutation/autosomal dominant		FGF2R
Chondrodysplasia punctata (Conradi-Hünerman)	Autosomal dominant		

Continued

Table 1-35 Comprehensive Compilation of Inheritance Pattern, Defect, and Associated Gene in Musculoskeletal Disorders—cont'd

DISORDER	INHERITANCE PATTERN	DEFECT	ASSOCIATED GENE
Chondrodysplasia punctata (rhizomelic form)	Autosomal recessive	Defect in subcellular organelles (peroxisomes)	
Cleidocranial dysplasia (dysostosis)	Autosomal dominant	Mutation of a gene coding for a protein related to osteoblast function	**CBFA1**
Dysplasia epiphysealis hemimelica (Trevor disease)	Unknown		
Ellis–van Creveld syndrome (chondroectodermal dysplasia)	Autosomal recessive		EVC
Fibrodysplasia ossificans progressiva	Sporadic mutation/autosomal dominant		
Geroderma osteodysplastica (Walt Disney dwarfism)	Autosomal recessive		
Grebe chondrodysplasia	Autosomal recessive		
Hypochondroplasia	Sporadic mutation/autosomal dominant		FGF3R
Kabuki makeup syndrome	Sporadic mutation		
Mesomelic dysplasia (Langer type)	Autosomal recessive		
Mesomelic dysplasia (Nievergelt type)	Autosomal dominant		
Mesomelic dysplasia (Reinhardt-Pfeiffer type)	Autosomal dominant		
Mesomelic dysplasia (Werner type)	Autosomal dominant		
Metatrophic dysplasia	Autosomal recessive		
Progressive diaphyseal dysplasia (Camurati-Engelmann disease)	Autosomal dominant		
Pseudoachondroplastic dysplasia	Autosomal dominant		COMP
Pyknodysostosis	Autosomal recessive		
Spondylometaphyseal chondrodysplasia	Autosomal dominant		
Spondylothoracic dysplasia (Jarcho-Levin syndrome)	Autosomal recessive		
Thanatophoric dwarfism	Autosomal dominant		FGF3R
Tooth-and-nail syndrome	Autosomal dominant		
Treacher Collins syndrome (mandibulofacial dysostosis)	Autosomal dominant		
METABOLIC BONE DISEASES			
Hereditary vitamin D–dependent rickets	Autosomal recessive	See Table 1-17	
Hypophosphatasia	Autosomal recessive	See Table 1-17	PHEX
Hypophosphatemic rickets (vitamin D–resistant rickets)	X-linked dominant	See Table 1-17	PHEX
Osteogenesis imperfecta	Autosomal dominant (types I and IV)	Defect in type I collagen (abnormal cross-linking)	COL IA1, COL IA2
	Autosomal recessive (types II and III)		COL IA1, COL IA2
Albright hereditary osteodystrophy (pseudohypoparathyroidism)	Uncertain	PTH has no effect at the target cells (in the kidney, bone, and intestine)	
Infantile cortical hyperostosis (Caffey disease)	Unknown		
Ochronosis (alkaptonuria)	Autosomal recessive	Defect in the homogentisic acid oxidase system	
Osteopetrosis	Autosomal dominant (mild, tarda form)		CLCN7, TC1RG1
	Autosomal recessive (infantile, malignant form)		
CONNECTIVE TISSUE DISORDERS			
Marfan syndrome	Autosomal dominant	Fibrillin abnormalities (some patients also have type I collagen abnormalities)	FBN1 or TGF-βR2
Ehlers-Danlos syndrome (there are at least 13 varieties)	Autosomal dominant (most common)	Defects in types I and III collagen have been described for some varieties; lysyl oxidase abnormalities	**COL 3A1 (for type III; most common)** **COL 1A2 (for type VII)**
Homocystinuria	Autosomal recessive	Deficiency of the enzyme cystathionine β-synthase	

Table 1-35 Comprehensive Compilation of Inheritance Pattern, Defect, and Associated Gene in Musculoskeletal Disorders—cont'd

DISORDER	INHERITANCE PATTERN	DEFECT	ASSOCIATED GENE
MUCOPOLYSACCHARIDOSIS			
Hunter syndrome ("gargoylism")	X-linked recessive		
Hurler syndrome	Autosomal recessive	Deficiency of the enzyme α-L-iduronidase	
Maroteaux-Lamy syndrome	Autosomal recessive		
Morquio syndrome	Autosomal recessive		
Sanfilippo syndrome	Autosomal recessive		
Scheie syndrome	Autosomal recessive	Deficiency of the enzyme α-L-iduronidase	
MUSCULAR DYSTROPHIES			
Duchenne muscular dystrophy	X-linked recessive	Defect on the short arm of the X chromosome	Dystrophin gene
Becker dystrophy	X-linked recessive		
Fascioscapulohumeral dystrophy	Autosomal dominant		
Limb-girdle dystrophy	Autosomal recessive		
Steinert disease (myotonic dystrophy)	Autosomal dominant		
HEMATOLOGIC DISORDERS			
Hemophilia (A and B)	X-linked recessive	Hemophilia A: factor VIII deficiency Hemophilia B: factor IX deficiency	
Sickle cell anemia	Autosomal recessive	Hemoglobin abnormality (presence of hemoglobin S)	
Gaucher disease	Autosomal recessive	*Deficient activity of the enzyme β-glucosidase (glucocerebrosidase)*	
Hemochromatosis	Autosomal recessive		
Niemann-Pick disease	Autosomal recessive	Accumulation of sphingomyelin in cellular lysosomes	
Smith-Lemli-Opitz syndrome	Uncertain		
Thalassemia	Autosomal recessive	Abnormal production of hemoglobin A	
von Willebrand disease	Autosomal dominant		
CHROMOSOMAL DISORDERS WITH MUSCULOSKELETAL ABNORMALITIES			
Down syndrome		Trisomy of chromosome 21	
Angelman syndrome		Chromosome 15 abnormality	
Clinodactyly		Associated with many genetic anomalies, including trisomy of chromosomes 8 and 21	
Edward syndrome		Trisomy of chromosome 18	
Fragile X syndrome	X-linked trait (does not follow the typical pattern of an X-linked trait)		Xq27-28
Klinefelter syndrome (XXY)		An extra X chromosome in affected boys and men	
Langer-Giedion syndrome	Sporadic mutation	Chromosome 8 abnormality	
Nail-patella syndrome	Autosomal dominant		LMX1B
Patau syndrome		Trisomy of chromosome 13	
Turner syndrome (XO)		One of the two X chromosomes missing in affected girls and women	SHOX
NEUROLOGIC DISORDERS			
Charcot-Marie-Tooth disease	Autosomal dominant (most common)	*Chromosome 17 defect for encoding peripheral myelin protein-22*	PMP22
Congenital insensitivity to pain	Autosomal recessive		
Dejerine-Sottas disease	Autosomal recessive		
Friedreich ataxia	Autosomal recessive		
Huntington disease	Autosomal dominant		
Menkes syndrome	X-linked recessive	Inability to absorb and use copper	
Pelizaeus-Merzbacher disease	X-linked recessive	Defect in the gene for proteolipid (a component of myelin)	
Riley-Day syndrome	Autosomal recessive		
Spinal muscular atrophy (Werdnig-Hoffman disease and Kugelberg-Welander disease)	Autosomal recessive		

Continued

Table 1-35	Comprehensive Compilation of Inheritance Pattern, Defect, and Associated Gene in Musculoskeletal Disorders—cont'd		
DISORDER	**INHERITANCE PATTERN**	**DEFECT**	**ASSOCIATED GENE**
Sturge-Weber syndrome	Sporadic mutation		
Tay-Sachs disease	Autosomal recessive	Deficiency in the enzyme hexosaminidase A	
DISEASES ASSOCIATED WITH NEOPLASIAS			
Ewing sarcoma			11;22 chromosomal translocation (EWS/FL11 fusion gene)
Multiple endocrine neoplasia (MEN) type I	Autosomal dominant		RET
MEN type II	Autosomal dominant		
MEN type III	Autosomal dominant	Chromosome 10 abnormality	
Neurofibromatosis (von Recklinghausen disease) type 1 (NF1) and type 2 (NF2)	Autosomal dominant	***NF1: chromosome 17 defect; codes for neurofibromin*** NF2: chromosome 22 defect	NF1, NF2
Synovial sarcoma			(X;18) (p11;q11) chromosomal translocations (STT/SSX fusion gene)
MISCELLANEOUS DISORDERS			
Malignant hyperthermia	Autosomal dominant		
Osteochondromatosis	Autosomal dominant		
Postaxial polydactyly	Autosomal dominant		GLI3 (types A, A/B) GJA1 (type IV)
Camptodactyly	Autosomal dominant		
Cerebro-oculofacioskeletal syndrome	Autosomal recessive		
Congenital contractural arachnodactyly			Fibrillin gene (chromosome 5)
Distal arthrogryposis syndrome	Autosomal dominant		
Dupuytren contracture	Autosomal dominant (with partial sex limitation)		
Fabry disease	X-linked recessive	Deficiency of α-galactosidase A	
Fanconi pancytopenia	Autosomal recessive		
Freeman-Sheldon syndrome (craniocarpotarsal dysplasia; whistling face syndrome)	Autosomal dominant Autosomal recessive		
GM1 gangliosidosis	Autosomal recessive		
Hereditary anonychia	Autosomal dominant		
Holt-Oram syndrome	Autosomal dominant		
Humeroradial synostosis	Autosomal dominant Autosomal recessive		
Klippel-Feil syndrome		Faulty development of spinal segments along the embryonic neural tube	
Klippel-Trénaunay-Weber syndrome	Sporadic mutation		
Krabbe disease	Autosomal recessive	Deficiency of galactocerebroside β-galactosidase	
Larsen syndrome	Autosomal dominant Autosomal recessive		
Lesch-Nyhan disease	X-linked trait	Absence of the enzyme hypoxanthine guanine phosphoribosyl transferase	
Madelung deformity	Autosomal dominant		
Mannosidosis	Autosomal recessive	Deficiency of the enzyme α-mannosidase	
Maple syrup urine disease	Autosomal recessive	Defective metabolism of the amino acids leucine, isoleucine, and valine	
Meckel syndrome (Gruber syndrome)	Autosomal recessive		
Möbius syndrome	Autosomal dominant		
Mucolipidosis (oligosaccharidosis)	Autosomal recessive	A family of enzyme deficiency diseases	
Multiple exostoses	Autosomal dominant		***EXT1: greater burden of disease and risk of malignancy*** EXT2/EXT3
Multiple pterygium syndrome	Autosomal recessive		
Noonan syndrome	Sporadic mutation		

Table 1-35	**Comprehensive Compilation of Inheritance Pattern, Defect, and Associated Gene in Musculoskeletal Disorders—cont'd**		
DISORDER	**INHERITANCE PATTERN**	**DEFECT**	**ASSOCIATED GENE**
Oral-facial-digital (OFD) syndrome			OFD I: X-linked dominant OFD II (Mohr syndrome): autosomal recessive
Osler-Weber-Rendu syndrome (hereditary hemorrhagic telangiectasia)	Autosomal dominant		
Pfeiffer syndrome (acrocephalosyndactyly)	Sporadic mutation/autosomal dominant		FGF2R
Phenylketonuria	Autosomal recessive	Enzyme deficiency characterized by the inability to convert phenylalanine to tyrosine because of a chromosome 12 abnormality	
Phytanic acid storage disease	Autosomal recessive		
Progeria (Hutchinson-Gilford progeria syndrome)	Autosomal dominant		
Proteus syndrome	Autosomal dominant		
Prune-belly syndrome	Uncertain	Localized mesodermal defect	
Radioulnar synostosis	Autosomal dominant		
Rett syndrome	Sporadic mutation/X-linked dominant		
Roberts syndrome (pseudothalidomide syndrome)	Sporadic mutation/autosomal recessive		
Russell-Silver syndrome	Sporadic mutation (possibly X-linked)		
Saethre-Chotzen syndrome	Autosomal dominant		
Sandhoff disease	Autosomal recessive	Enzyme deficiency of hexosaminidases A and B	
Schwartz-Jampel syndrome	Autosomal recessive		
Seckel syndrome (so-called bird-headed dwarfism)	Autosomal recessive		
Stickler syndrome (hereditary progressive arthro-ophthalmopathy)	Autosomal dominant	Collagen abnormality	
Thrombocytopenia-aplasia of radius (TAR) syndrome	Autosomal recessive		
Tarsal coalition	Autosomal dominant		
Trichorhinophalangeal syndrome	Autosomal dominant		
Urea cycle defects		A group of enzyme disorders characterized by high levels of ammonia in the blood and tissues	
Argininemia	Autosomal recessive		
Argininosuccinic aciduria	Autosomal recessive		
Carbamyl phosphate synthetase deficiency	Autosomal recessive		
Citrullinemia	Autosomal recessive		
Ornithine transcarbamylase deficiency	X-linked		
VATER association	Sporadic mutation		
Werner syndrome	Autosomal recessive		
Zygodactyly	Autosomal dominant		

PTH, Parathyroid hormone; *TGF-βR2,* transforming growth factor-β receptor 2; *VATER,* vertebral defects, imperforate anus, tracheoesophageal fistula, and radial and renal dysplasia.

■ Mutations
- Genetic disorders arise from alterations (mutations) in the genetic material.
- Inherited mutations are passed from generation to generation.
- A sporadic mutation may occur in the sperm or egg of the parents or in the embryo.
- Single gene mutation examples:
  - Most skeletal dysplasias are single gene mutations.
    - Collagen type I (bone) defects:
      - Osteogenesis imperfecta (types I-IV)—**COL1A1** and **COL1A2**
      - Ehlers-Danlos—**COL5A1** and **COL5A2**
  - Collagen type II (cartilage) defects:
    - Spondyloepiphyseal dysplasia (SED)—**COL2A1**, usually **random mutations**
  - Others:
    - Multiple epiphyseal dysplasia—**COMP** (cartilage oligomeric matrix protein gene also associated with pseudoachondroplasia)
    - Marfan syndrome—**FBN1** with superior lens dislocation
    - Achondroplasia—**FGFR3** (fibroblast growth factor receptor)
    - Spinal muscular atrophy—**SMN1** (**survival motor neuron-1**)

- Multiple concomitant anomalous phenotypes consistently seen with a disease process define a syndrome. The relevant osseous defects are:
  - VATER/VACTERL—spinal deformity, radius defects
  - Neurofibromatosis (NF)1 (AD)—scoliosis and congenital tibial pseudarthrosis
  - **McCune-Albright**—mutation in *GNAS* gene; fibrous dysplasia of bone with shepherd's crook deformity of hips, **café au lait** spots (**irregular/coast of Maine**), and endocrinopathy (e.g., early puberty)
  - Trisomy 21—ligamentous laxity, **atlanto-axial instability**, patellar and hip dislocations, severe flatfoot and bunions
- Epigenetics
  - Genetic alterations that are not caused by mutations in DNA sequence:
    - DNA methylation
    - Histone posttranslational modifications
  - **Genomic imprinting** is an epigenetic phenomenon that is independent of mendelian inheritance.
    - Genes are expressed in a parent-of-origin manner.
    - An example of genomic imprinting is the loss of a region in chromosome 15 with **Prader-Willi** (paternal; obesity, hypogonadism, hypotonia) and **Angleman syndromes** (maternal; epilepsy, tremors, smiling).
- Chromosomal abnormalities
  - Disruptions in the normal arrangement or number of chromosomes
  - Aneuploidy: an abnormal number of chromosomes
  - Triploidy: three copies of chromosomes (69 chromosomes)
  - Tetraploidy: four copies of chromosomes (92 chromosomes)
  - Monosomy: one chromosome of one pair is absent (total: 45 chromosomes)
  - **Trisomy**: one chromosome pair has an extra chromosome (total: 47 chromosomes)
    - **Trisomy 21 (Down syndrome)**—management of cervical spine instability, hip instability/hip dislocation
  - **Deletion**: a section of one chromosome (in a chromosome pair) is absent.
  - **Duplication**: an extra section of one chromosome (in a chromosome pair) is present.
  - **Translocation**: a portion of one chromosome is exchanged with a portion of another chromosome (see earlier in Section 2, Orthopaedic Biology, Cellular and Molecular Biology, and in Testable Concepts).
  - **Inversion**: a broken portion of a chromosome reattaches to the same chromosome in the same location but in a reverse direction.
- Genetics of musculoskeletal conditions and abnormalities (see Table 1-35)

INFECTIONS AND MICROBIOLOGY

- **Musculoskeletal infections overview**
- Treatment overview:
  - Empirical treatment: based on the presumed type of infection as determined from clinical findings and symptoms. *Staphylococcus* and *Streptococcus* are the most common organisms infecting skin, soft tissue,

and bone. The history of microbiology, infection diagnosis, and treatment of bacterial infection has been closely intertwined with *Staphylococcus aureus*, which is also the most common cause of surgical site infections.
- Definitive treatment: best based on final culture and sensitivity results when available
- Surgical treatment: drain contained infections, remove dead tissue, restore vascularity
- *Staphylococcus*: roughly 80% of orthopaedic infections
  - Antibiotic resistance
    - The bacteria Fleming's 1928 discovery of *Penicillium* mold killed were *S. aureus*.
    - **Penicillin (β-lactam antibiotics)—inhibits peptidoglycan bonds of bacterial cell walls**
    - Staphylococci that produce the enzyme **β-lactamase break penicillin found on *bla* gene**
    - **Often found on plasmids** selected and are penicillin resistant
    - Chemists altered penicillin in 1950s to defeat β-lactamase (methicillin, nafcillin, dicloxacillin) and, if susceptible, **methicillin-sensitive *S. aureus* (MSSA)**
    - *Staphylococcus* with the **staphylococcal chromosome cassette mobile element–carrying IV (SCCmecIV)**, which carries the ***mecA* gene, which codes for the penicillin-binding protein 2A, which binds poorly to penicillin** and selects these bacteria for survival. Known as *methicillin resistant*.
    - Growing percentage of staphylococci now resistant to penicillinase-resistant penicillin
    - Methicillin-resistant *Staphylococcus aureus* (MRSA)
    - **MRSA results from PBP2A coded by *mecA* gene that is carried on SCCmecIV.**
    - Consider vancomycin or linezolid for MRSA.
  - Community versus hospital
    - Hospital-acquired MRSA (HA-MRSA) or healthcare acquired (HC-MRSA)
      - Patients from nursing homes, recent hospitalization/surgery, prolonged catheters
      - Have larger SCCmec:
        - Multiple antibiotic resistance genes
        - **More drug resistance known as "super bugs"**
    - Community-acquired MRSA (CA-MRSA)
      - Have smaller SCCmec:
        - Less drug resistance
        - Almost all have **Panton-Valentine leukocidin (PVL) cytotoxin**
        - γ-Hemolysin: a pore-forming toxin that can lyse PMNs
        - Young adults with recurrent boils and severe hemorrhagic pneumonia
    - At-risk groups: athletes, intravenous (IV) drug abusers, homeless, military recruits, prisoners
    - Risk factors:
      - Previous antibiotic use within 1 year
      - Frequent skin-to-skin contact with others
      - Frequent sharing of personal items
      - Compromised skin integrity
- **Infection by tissue type**
- Soft tissue infections: superficial to deep (Table 1-36)
  - Erysipelas: infection of dermis and lymphatics—group A streptococcal

Table 1-36   Soft Tissue Infections

TYPE	AFFECTED TISSUES	CLINICAL FINDINGS	ORGANISMS	TREATMENT
Cellulitis, erysipelas	Superficial, subcutaneous	Erythema; tenderness; warmth; lymphangitis; lymphadenopathy	Group A streptococci (most common) *Staphylococcus aureus* (less common)	Initial antibiotic treatment: penicillin G or penicillinase-resistant synthetic penicillins (nafcillin or oxacillin) Alternative therapies: erythromycin, first-generation cephalosporins, amoxicillin/clavulanate, azithromycin, clarithromycin, tigecycline, or daptomycin
Necrotizing fasciitis	Muscle fascia	Aggressive, life-threatening; may be associated with an underlying vascular disease (particularly diabetes) Commonly occurs after surgery, trauma, or streptococcal skin infection	Four types: 1. Groups A, C, and G streptococci 2. Clostridia 3. Polymicrobial (aerobic plus anaerobic) 4. Methicillin-resistant *S. aureus* (MRSA)	Necessitates extensive emergency surgical débridement (involving the entire length of the overlying cellulitis) and intravenous antibiotics Initial antibiotic treatments: penicillin G for streptococcal or clostridial infection; imipenem, doripenem, or meropenem for polymicrobial infections Add vancomycin or daptomycin if MRSA suspected
Gas gangrene	Muscle; commonly in grossly contaminated, traumatic wounds, particularly those that are closed primarily	Progressive, severe pain; edema (distant from the wound); foul-smelling, serosanguineous discharge; high fever; chills; tachycardia; confusion Clinical findings consistent with toxemia Radiographs typically show widespread gas in the soft tissues (facilitates rapid spread of the infection)	Classically caused by *Clostridium perfringens, Clostridium septicum,* or other histotoxic *Clostridium* spp. These gram-positive, anaerobic, spore-forming rods produce exotoxins that cause necrosis of fat and muscle and thrombosis of local vessels	Primary treatment: surgical (radical) débridement with fasciotomies Hyperbaric oxygen may be a useful adjuvant therapy, although its effectiveness remains inconclusive Initial antibiotic treatment: clindamycin plus penicillin G Alternative therapies include ceftriaxone or erythromycin
Toxic shock syndrome (TSS): staphylococcal	Toxemia, not septicemia In orthopaedics, TSS is secondary to colonization of surgical or traumatic wounds (even after minor trauma) TSS can be associated with tampon use through colonization of the vagina with toxin-producing *S. aureus*	Fever, hypotension, an erythematous macular rash with a serous exudate (gram-positive cocci are present) The infected wound may look benign, which may belie the seriousness of the underlying condition	Caused by toxins produced by *S. aureus*	Irrigation and débridement and intravenous antibiotics with intravenous immune globulin plus antibiotics Initial antibiotic treatment: penicillinase-resistant penicillins (nafcillin or oxacillin), vancomycin if MRSA Alternative therapies include first-generation cephalosporins Patients may also require emergency fluid resuscitation
Toxic shock syndrome (TSS): streptococcal	Toxemia, not a septicemia Commonly associated with erysipelas or necrotizing fasciitis	Similar to staphylococcal TSS	Toxins from group A, B, C, or G *Streptococcus pyogenes*	Initial antibiotic treatment: clindamycin plus penicillin G Alternative therapies include ceftriaxone or clindamycin Intravenous immune globulin may be used; associated with decrease in organ failure, but no effect on all-cause mortality in children
Surgical wound infection	Varies		*S. aureus*; groups A, B, C, and G streptococci Other organism may be involved	Initial antibiotic treatment: trimethoprim-sulfamethoxazole or clindamycin MRSA species are best treated with vancomycin (alternatives for MRSA include daptomycin or ceftobiprole).
Marine injuries	Varies	History of fishing (or other marine activity) injury, with signs of infection Culture specimens at 30°C (60°F); organisms may take several weeks to grow on culture media	Marine injuries involve organisms that can cause indolent infections *Vibrio vulnificus* is the most likely organism in infected wounds that were exposed to brackish water or shellfish; can cause a devastating infection Consider atypical mycobacteria (e.g., *Mycobacterium marinum*) for injuries with indolent, low-grade infection	*V. vulnificus* is best treated with ceftazidime plus doxycycline; cefotaxime and ciprofloxacin are alternatives *M. marinum* is best treated with clarithromycin, minocycline, doxycycline, trimethoprim/sulfamethoxazole, or rifampin plus ethambutol

- Painful raised lesion with a red, edematous, indurated (peau d'orange) appearance and an advancing raised border
  - Treatment: penicillins or erythromycin
- Cellulitis: subcutaneous infection most commonly group A streptococci or *S. aureus*
  - Acute spreading infection with pain, erythema, and warmth, with or without lymphadenopathy; may develop into abscess (may surround abscess or ulcer)
  - Treatment: routine for cellulitis—penicillin, dicloxacillin (but IV cefazolin or nafcillin if systemic systems prominent or high risk [asplenia, neutropenia, immunocompromise, cirrhosis, cardiac or renal failure, local trauma, or preexisting edema])
- Abscess: pus-filled inflammatory subcutaneous nodule (furuncle = "boil") that may be multiple and coalesce (carbuncle): almost always *S. aureus*. Small lesions sometimes mistaken as spider bite.
  - Painful pus under pressure
  - **Treatment: incision and drainage (I&D), leave open,** with culture and sensitivities to select antibiotics.
  - For simple abscesses, systemic antibiotics **have not** been shown to improve cure rate or decrease recurrence above I&D alone.
  - Systemic antibiotics only for (Infectious Disease Society of America Guidelines):
    - Severe or extensive disease
    - Rapid progression in the presence of associated cellulitis
    - Signs and symptoms of systemic illness
    - Associated comorbidities or immunosuppression, extremes of age
    - Abscess in an area difficult to drain
    - Associated septic phlebitis
    - Lack of response to incision and drainage
  - Empirical antibiotics selected should aim at MRSA.
    - Dicloxacillin, clindamycin, macrolides versus vancomycin, linezolid or daptomycin
- Necrotizing fasciitis: rare, rapidly progressive, life-threatening infection of the fascia and subcutaneous tissue; causes liquefactive necrosis with thrombosis of the cutaneous microcirculation. Most commonly polymicrobial, but group A β-hemolytic streptococci ("flesh eating") most often monomicrobial cause (i.e., *Streptococcus pyogenes*).
  - Risk factors: diabetes, peripheral vascular disease, liver failure
  - **Mortality most related to delay in treatment for more than 24 hours**
  - Fascial infection spreads faster than the observed skin changes.
  - Skin microcirculation thrombosis and later necrosis:
    - Early—pain out of proportion, swelling and edema
    - Late:
      - Blisters/bullae
      - Skin that does not blanch (skin is dying)
      - Skin becomes numb (nerves are dying)
  - Difficult diagnosis—paucity of cutaneous findings need high clinical suspicion
    - Less than one fifth made at admission; preadmission antibiotics mask severity
    - Repeated examinations noting margins that migrate quickly despite antibiotic treatment

- Surgical findings:
- Grayish necrotic fascia
  - Lack of normal muscular fascial resistance to blunt dissection
  - Lack of bleeding of the fascia during dissection
  - **Foul-smelling "dishwater" pus**
- Treatment: broad-spectrum antibiotics
  - Early operative débridement of all necrotic tissue—select level ahead of infection
  - Consider amputation/disarticulation.
  - Second look 24 hours later to reevaluate
- Gas gangrene: *Clostridium perfringens* (obligate anaerobes) most common organism that produces gas and toxins in subcutaneous tissues and muscle
  - Dirty wound managed with primary closure: war wounds, tornado, lawn mower
  - Inadequate débridement of more severe devitalizing injuries
  - Clostridial dermonecrotizing exotoxin lecithinase
  - Crepitance of soft tissue, **soft tissue air on x-rays, foul "sweet"-smelling discharge**
  - Treatment:
    - Early, adequate, and thorough surgical débridement
    - Delayed closure and second look 24 hours later to reevaluate
    - High-dose IV penicillin and hyperbaric oxygen can help if available.
- Surgical site infection:
  - Infections are the product of **bacteria** that take hold in a favorable **wound** environment in a **host** with a susceptible immune system.
  - Bacterial issues:
    - Load:
      - Need more than 10^5 in normal host to cause infection
      - Need only about 100 if foreign object present
    - Bacterial source:
      - Skin: both patient and surgical team
        - Preoperative bathing (with or without chlorhexidine)
        - Low operating room personnel numbers
        - Space suites, pressurized rooms with HEPA filters, ultraviolet lights
    - Sterile technique:
      - Wash your hands.
      - Prep—chlorhexidine
      - Care with draping
      - Equipment processing issues
      - Dilution—solution to pollution
    - Virulence:
      - Antibiotic resistance—plasmid
        - β-Lactamase (bla)—makes staphylococci resistant to penicillin
        - Penicillin-binding protein 2a (*mecA* gene)—makes *S. aureus* MRSA
      - Increased surface adhesion
        - Fnb gene—fibronectin in *S. aureus*
          - Increases adhesion to titanium
        - Glycocalyx-biofilm-slime-polysaccharide capsule
          - Improves attachment to inert surfaces
          - Protects bacteria from desiccation

- ..ll protection from phagocytosis
  - Glycocalyx-biofilm-slime-polysaccharide capsule—inhibits phagocytosis
    - Hides PAMPs
    - Protects bacteria from toxic enzymes/chemicals
  - Protein A: *S. aureus*—inhibits phagocytosis
  - Binds immunoglobulins (Fc region of IgG)
  - M protein: group A *S. pyogenes*—inhibits phagocytosis
    - Inhibits activation of alt complement pathway on cell surface
- Toxins:
  - Endotoxin: gram-negative lipopolysaccharide capsules
  - Exotoxin:
    - *Clostridium perfringens*: lecithinase—tissue-destroying alpha toxin
      - Myonecrosis and hemolysis of gangrene
    - *Clostridium tetani*: tetanospasm—blocks inhibitory nerves
      - "Lockjaw" or muscle spasms
    - *Clostridium botulinum*: botulism—blocks acetylcholine release
      - "Floppy" baby (also wrinkle relaxers and antispasmodic for cerebral palsy)
    - CA-MRSA: Panton-Valentine leukocidin (PVL) cytotoxin
      - Pore-forming toxin specific to neutrophils
- Superantigens:
  - Activate approximately 20% of T cells
  - Trigger cytokine release
  - Systemic inflammation; appears as septic shock
    - *S. pyogenes* (GAS): M protein
    - *S. aureus*: TSS toxin-1 causes toxic shock syndrome
      - Acute febrile illness with a generalized scarlatiniform rash
      - Hypotension (shock) with organ system failure
      - Desquamation of palmar/plantar skin lesions (if the patient lives)
    - Treatment:
      - Remove foreign object (retained sponge or tampon).
      - Supportive care with fluids and anti-*Staphylococcus* antibiotics
- Wound issues:
  - Surgical technique:
    - Remove foreign objects
    - Débride devitalized necrotic tissue
    - Prevent/drain hematomas
    - Shorter procedures better
  - Local environment:
    - Shaving doubles infection rate; clip
    - Prophylactic antibiotics:
      - Less than 1 hour before until 24 hours after
      - Repeat if more than 4 hours (longer than half-life of antibiotic selected)
      - Repeat if blood loss more than 1000 mL
      - Double if patient weighs over 80 kg (>176 lb)
    - Warm patient
    - Adequate O_2, tight glucose control

- Host issues:
  - Avoid hematogenous seeding
    - No active infections in elective cases—check legs, feet, toes
    - If urologic symptoms: urinalysis and culture
      - Postpone surgery if:
        - Over 10^3 organisms and dysuria/frequency
        - Obstructive symptoms:
          - ↓ Force, hesitancy, straining
      - D/C Foleys as soon as possible after surgery.
  - MRSA: carrier screening and eradication, "active detection and isolation (ADI)"
    - Nasal carriage—important risk factor, some controversy; if high-risk population:
      - Screen:
        - Swab culture versus PCR
      - If positive screen: postoperative infection rates are two to nine times higher
    - If positive MRSA screen:
      - Use vancomycin 1 g every 12 hours
      - 2% intranasal mupirocin ointment twice daily × 5 days
      - 2% chlorhexidine showers daily × 5 days
  - Nutrition: malnutrition associated with wound dehiscence and infection
    - Clinical evaluation:
      - History of weight loss (10% over 6 months or 5% over 1 month)
      - Albumin less than 3.5, total lymphocyte count less than 1500, transferrin less than 200
    - Obesity—body mass index (BMI) above 30 kg/m^2; higher numbers, more wound problems
      - ↑ Duration of surgery, dissection, hematoma/seroma
      - Subcutaneous fat has little vascularity and less oxygen tension.
      - ↑ Diabetes/hyperglycemia
      - Consider **bariatric consultation:**
        - If BMI above 35 kg/m^2
        - Early in course of patients likely to progress to need large elective cases
        - No severe diets acutely preoperatively
      - Remember weight-adjusted antibiotics (>80 kg, get 2 g cefazolin)
  - Smoking: two to four times more infections/osteomyelitis
    - Hypoxia—CO binds to Hb = carboxyhemoglobin (HbCO)
    - Nicotine—microvascular vasoconstriction
    - ↓ Bone, skin, soft tissue healing
    - Stopping: ↓ postoperative complications
      - 4 to 6 weeks preoperatively (+6 weeks postoperatively!)
  - Alcohol: heavy alcohol use (blood alcohol > 200 mg/dL) increases rate of infections 2.6 times
    - ↓ Fibroblast production of collagen type I
    - Inhibits osteoblasts: ↓ osteocalcin, inhibits Wnt/β-catenin pathway
    - Impairs fracture healing
    - Associated with "bad behaviors," cirrhosis, and liver failure
  - Diabetes:
    - Chronic issues well known: cardiac, renal, peripheral vascular, neuropathy

- Best measured with HbA_{1c}—goal is less than 6.9
- Acute hyperglycemia is also a threat:
  - Collagen synthesis suppressed at 200 mg/dL—impaired wound healing
  - WBC phagocytosis impaired at 250 mg/dL—decreased ability to fight infection
- Post-splenectomy:
  - Decrease in IgM memory B cells
  - Decreased effectiveness against bacterial polysaccharide capsules
  - Susceptible to streptococcal pneumonia "pneumococcal" infections
- Special soft tissue infections
  - Bite infections (Table 1-37):
    - Initial treatment: exploring wound, removing foreign objects and irrigation with saline
    - Closure controversial: cosmesis/soft tissue coverage versus recurrence
    - Consider delayed primary closure at 48 to 72 hours
    - Antibiotic prophylaxis controversial:
      - Consider for bites to hands, feet, face
      - Wounds hard to clean—deep punctures, edema/crush injury
      - Bites involving tendon, cartilage, or bone
      - Bites in immunocompromised or asplenic host
    - Bite prophylaxis antibiotics: amoxicillin-clavulanate
      - If penicillin-allergic, trimethoprim-sulfamethoxazole plus clindamycin

- Antibiotic treatment: oral unless febrile, spreading, or high risk; then IV
- Bite organisms: Organisms causing infections from bites usually derive from the mouth of the biter, not the skin of the victim. Most oral flora are polymicrobial in nature. Some bacteria are more specific to source of "bite":
  - Human bites: *Streptococcus viridans* common, **Eikenella corrodens**
    - "Fight bite" x-rays for cartilage divots and broken teeth and formal identification
  - Cat bites: *Pasteurella multocida*
    - 50% require surgery—puncture wounds to tendons/joints
    - Cat scratch disease: *Bartonella henselae*
  - Dog bites: **Pasteurella multocida**, *Pasteurella canis*
  - "Fish bite" and marine injuries: *Mycobacterium marinum*
    - Atypical mycobacteria, acid fast bacilli
    - Slow culture **at low temperature** (30°C)
    - Aquarium, fresh or salt water
    - Noncaseating granulomas
    - Treatment: 3 months of minocycline or clarithromycin
  - Fish and marine: *Erysipelothrix rhusiopathiae*
    - Erysipeloid—"fish handler's disease" (also swine handler)
    - Gram-positive bacillus

Table 1-37	**Bite Injuries**	
SOURCE OF BITE	**ORGANISM**	**PRIMARY ANTIMICROBIAL (OR DRUG) REGIMEN**
Human	*Streptococcus viridans* (100%) *Bacteroides* spp. (82%) *Staphylococcus epidermidis* (53%) *Corynebacterium* spp. (41%) *Staphylococcus aureus* (29%) *Peptostreptococcus* spp. *Eikenella* spp.	Early treatment (not yet infected): amoxicillin/clavulanate (Augmentin) With signs of infection: ampicillin/sulbactam (Unasyn), cefoxitin, ticarcillin/clavulanate (Timentin), or piperacillin-tazobactam Patients with penicillin allergy: clindamycin plus either ciprofloxacin or trimethoprim/sulfamethoxazole *Eikenella* organisms are resistant to clindamycin, nafcillin/oxacillin, metronidazole, and possibly to first-generation cephalosporins and erythromycin; susceptible to fluoroquinolones and trimethoprim/sulfamethoxazole; treat with cefoxitin or ampicillin
Dog	*Pasteurella canis* *S. aureus* *Bacteroides* spp. *Fusobacterium* spp. *Capnocytophaga* spp.	Amoxicillin/clavulanate (Augmentin) or clindamycin (adults); clindamycin plus trimethoprim/sulfamethoxazole (children) *P. canis* is resistant to doxycycline, cephalexin, clindamycin, and erythromycin Consider antirabies treatment Only 5% of dog bite wounds become infected
Cat	*Pasteurella multocida* *S. aureus* Possibly tularemia	Amoxicillin/clavulanate, cefuroxime axetil, or doxycycline Do not use cephalexin *P. multocida* is resistant to doxycycline, cephalexin, and clindamycin; many strains are resistant to erythromycin Of cat bite wounds, 80% become infected; culture
Rat	*Streptobacillus moniliformis* *Spirillum minus*	Amoxicillin/clavulanate or doxycycline Antirabies treatment is not indicated
Pig	Polymicrobial (aerobes and anaerobes)	Amoxicillin/clavulanate, third-generation cephalosporin, ticarcillin/clavulanate (Timentin), ampicillin/sulbactam, or imipenem-cilastatin
Skunk, raccoon, bat	Varies	Amoxicillin/clavulanate or doxycycline Antirabies treatment is indicated
Pit viper (snake)	*Pseudomonas* spp. *Enterobacteriaceae* *S. epidermidis* *Clostridium* spp.	Antivenin therapy Ceftriaxone Tetanus prophylaxis
Brown recluse spider	Toxin	Dapsone
Catfish sting	Toxins (may become secondarily infected)	Amoxicillin/clavulanate prophylaxis

Adapted from Gilbert DN et al: *The Sanford guide to antimicrobial therapy*, Hyde Park, Vt, 2010, Antimicrobial Therapy, p 48.

- Painful, **itchy, spreading, purple ring**-shaped lesion
- Treatment: oral penicillin
- "Oyster bite": *Vibrio vulnificus*
- Bullae and necrotizing fasciitis from gram-negative motile rod
- Gastroenteritis from eating bad oyster
- Treatment: I&D and broad-spectrum antibiotics (ceftazidime)
- Tick bite (*Ixodes*): *Borrelia burgdorferi* (a **spirochete**)
  - **Erythema migrans, "bull's-eye" lesion**
  - White-footed deer mouse in northeast and Pacific north
  - Knee effusions
  - Neurologic disease: Bell palsy common
  - Lyme disease—treatment: amoxicillin versus doxycycline
- "Plant bite" sporotrichosis: *Sporothrix schenckii* (fungus)
  - Thorns and splinter: rose, mesquite, cactus
  - Nodule then ulcer: "rose grower's granuloma"
  - Lymphatic spread
  - Treatment: débridement and antifungals (itraconazole)
- Raccoon/skunk/bat: rabies—a neurotropic virus
  - CNS irritation, "hydrophobia," paralysis, and death
  - Death if not treated before symptoms
  - Treatment: **human rabies immune globulin**
- Paronychias
  - Acute paronychia—single finger
    - Red, hot, swollen, pus
    - Traumatic: nail biting, hangnails, poor manicures
    - Infection of the eponychium ("run-around infection")
    - *S. aureus* most common (also streptococci plus anaerobes)
    - Treatment:
      - Warm soaks
      - Spontaneous drainage versus I&D
  - Chronic paronychia—multiple fingers
    - Boggy, tender, red, rare fluctuance
    - Dishwashers, laundry, bartenders
    - Fungal infection after prolonged water exposure
    - *Candida albicans* most common
    - Treatment:
      - Keep dry
      - Antifungals: miconazole
      - Topical steroids
      - Eponychial marsupialization and nail removal
  - Herpetic whitlow: "viral paronychia"
    - Grouped vesicles on erythematous base
    - Dentists, anesthesia, toddlers
    - Exposure to oral secretions
    - Clear fluid with negative Gram stain
    - Tzanck test may be positive.
    - Herpes simplex virus types 1 and 2
    - Treatment:
      - Self-limited; no need for I&D
      - Antivirals may decrease duration.
- Septic bursitis:
  - Similar pathology of olecranon, prepatellar or pretibial

- Redness, swelling, pain, and subcutaneous fluctuance
- About 80% caused by *S. aureus*, others streptococci
- Chronic recurrent cases can be fungal, mycobacterial
- Gout, rheumatic, and traumatic causes common
- Aspiration with Gram stain and culture if redness
- Treatment:
  - Serial aspirations and oral antibiotics
  - IV antibiotics for systemic symptoms and immunocompromised
  - Bursectomy for persistent or recurrent cases
  - Can be done endoscopically
- Marjolin ulcer: cancer that looks like infection
  - Chronic draining wounds that fail to heal even with antibiotics
  - Squamous cell carcinoma in sites of inflammation
  - Chronic draining wounds, pressure ulcers, burns, osteomyelitis
  - Wide local resection and skin graft
- Tetanus:
  - **Potentially lethal neuroparalytic disease leading to trismus ("lockjaw")**
  - Exotoxin from anaerobe *Clostridium tetani*
    - Tetanospasm blocks inhibitory nerves.
  - Deep wounds and devitalized tissues are high risk.
    - More than 6 hours old, more than 1 cm deep, ischemic, crush, grade III
    - Contaminated with soil, feces, and animal bites
  - DTaP × 5 routine for children younger than age 7
  - Tetanus toxoid (Td) 0.5 mL diphtheria-tetanus toxoid for adult/ER
  - Tetanus immune globulin for unknown status in ER
  - Vaccination:
    - **Every 10 years with Td**
    - **Status unknown or history of fewer than three: give both Td and TIG**
- Tinea corporis: "ringworm of the body"
  - *Trichophyton rubrum*—dermatophytosis
  - **Most common superficial fungal infection**
  - Warm humid climates, close contact—wrestling, rugby
  - "Athlete's foot," tinea pedis; "jock rot," tinea cruris
  - Fungal folliculitis: tinea capitis (scalp), tinea barbae (beard)
  - Onychomycosis—fingernail infection
  - **Topical antifungals: clotrimazole, ketoconazole, tolnaftate**
- Bone infections—osteomyelitis
  - Exogenous: most common osteomyelitis in adults
    - Acute osteomyelitis from open fracture or bone exposed at surgery
    - Chronic osteomyelitis from neglected wounds: diabetic feet, decubitus ulcers
  - Hematogenous: most common osteomyelitis in children
    - Bloodborne organisms of sepsis (often positive blood cultures *before antibiotics given*)
    - Pediatric—immature immune system
      - Metaphysis or epiphysis of long bones
      - Lower extremity more often than upper
      - Boys more often than girls
    - Adults—immunocompromised—vertebrae most common adult hematogenous site
      - Dialysis patient—rib and spine osteomyelitis

- IV drug abuser—medial or lateral clavicle osteomyelitis
- Elderly, IV drug abuser, transplant patients
- Acute osteomyelitis:
  - Short duration, usually less than 2 weeks, gradual onset
  - Pain to palpation, with weight bearing, decreased use, limp
  - Fever and systemic symptoms variable
  - Laboratory findings:
    - **CRP—most sensitive test (increased in ≈ 97%)**
      - Most rapid rise and fall—good measure of treatment success
    - ESR—increased in approximately 90%
    - CBC—WBC increased in only a third
    - **Aspiration and biopsy cultures—most specific test**
  - **Histopathology: bony spicules with live osteocytes surrounded by inflammatory cells**
  - Treatment:
    - 6 weeks of antibiotics directed at specific cultures
    - Surgery is reserved for draining abscesses or failure to improve on antibiotics
    - No Esmarch exsanguination for infections or tumors
- Subacute osteomyelitis: Brodie abscess
  - Residual of acute osteomyelitis versus hematogenous seeding of growth plate trauma
  - Painful limp with no systemic signs
  - Adolescent to early adult (<25 years)—stronger immune system
  - Localized radiolucency with sclerotic rim at metaphysis of long bones
  - Almost exclusively S. aureus (may be lower virulence)
  - Treatment: surgical débridement and 6 weeks of IV antibiotics
  - Rule out tumors (chondroblastoma): *"biopsy all infections, culture all tumors"*
- Chronic osteomyelitis:
  - History:
    - Prior trauma/surgery or soft tissue wound
    - Previous acute osteomyelitis or septic arthritis
    - Consider in all nonunions
  - Often chronic wound or draining sinus
    - Chronic osteomyelitis is present if you can probe the bone or if the wound is > 2 × 2 cm
  - Laboratory findings:
    - Less helpful
    - **Open bone biopsy/culture best test (sinus tract cultures not helpful)**
  - Histopathology:
    - **Dead bone (avascular) (no nuclei of osteocytes)**
    - **Fibrosis of marrow space**
    - **Chronic inflammatory cells**
  - Treatment:
    - **Surgery needed to cure chronic osteomyelitis**
    - Basic principles:
      - Surgery must be individualized.
      - Multiple procedures frequently required
      - Remove infected hardware.
      - Remove dead bone that serves as a "foreign object."

Table 1-38	**Chronic Osteomyelitis: Infected Host Type**	
TYPE	**DESCRIPTION**	**RISK**
A	Normal immune response; nonsmoker	Minimal
B	Local or mild systemic deficiency; smoker	Moderate
C	Major nutritional or systemic disorder	High

- Débride bone until punctate bleeding is restored ("paprika sign")
- Débride compromised or necrotic soft tissue.
- Consider preoperative sinus tract injection with methylene blue.
- Consider antibiotic spacers: PMMA cement versus biologics.
- Restore vascularity or soft tissue muscle coverage.
- Six weeks of antibiotics directed at specific cultures
- Adequate minimal inhibitory concentration (MIC) of antibiotics at site of infection
- Classify host (Cierny-Mader [Table 1-38])
  - A: healthy patients
  - B: wound healing comorbidities
  - BL (local): compromised vascularity
    - Arterial disease, venous stasis, irradiation, scarring, or smoking
  - BS (systemic): compromised immune system
    - Diabetes mellitus, malnutrition, end-stage renal disease, malignancy, alcoholism, rheumatologic diseases, or immunocompromised status
      - HIV, immunosuppressive therapy, DMARDs
  - BL/S (combined)
  - C: compromised patient (palliative care or amputation)
    - No quality-of-life improvement if cured
    - Morbidity of procedure exceeds that of the disease.
    - Poor prognosis, poor cooperation in care
- Anatomic lesion classification with examples and treatment (Figure 1-73)
  - I: medullary—nidus endosteal
    - Residual hematogenous or intramuscular infected nonunion
    - Treatment: unroofing
  - II: superficial—infection on surface defect of coverage
    - Full-thickness soft tissue wounds: venous stasis/pressure ulcer
    - Treatment: decortication and soft tissue coverage
  - III: localized—cortical infection without loss of stability
    - Infected fracture union with butterfly fragment or prior plate
    - Treatment: sequestrectomy, soft tissue coverage, with or without bone graft
  - IV: diffuse—permeative throughout bone, unstable before or after débridement
    - Periprosthetic infection, septic arthritis or infected nonunions
    - Treatment: stabilization, soft tissue coverage, and bone graft

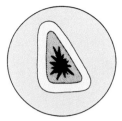
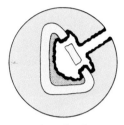
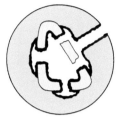

Medullary   Superficial

Localized   Diffuse

FIGURE 1-73 Cierny's anatomic classification of adult chronic osteomyelitis.

- Techniques:
  - Open bone grafting (Papineau):
    - Cancellous autograft bone in vascular bed of débrided defect
    - Consider negative pressure wound therapy: builds granulation tissue, drains region
    - If transfer or free flaps unavailable
    - If host inappropriate (smoker, adherence)
  - Antibiotic spacers/beads
    - Provide very high antibiotic levels at local area
    - 2 to 4 g per bag (40 g) of cement (**>2 g reduces compressive strength**)
    - Can form pouch and cover with adherent film
    - Antibiotics must be heat stable:
      - Cephalosporins, aminoglycosides, vancomycin, clindamycin
    - Avoid antibiotics inactivated by heat:
      - Tetracycline, fluoroquinolones, polymyxin B, chloramphenicol
    - Antibiotics elute out over 2 to 6 weeks.
    - Elution increased with:
      - Surface area—beads
      - Higher porosity—no vacuum mixing
      - Larger antibiotic crystals—mix cement until doughy, then add antibiotic
- Imaging of osteomyelitis
  - Radiographs
    - Acute osteomyelitis:
      - Soft tissue swelling (early)
      - Bone demineralization or regional osteopenia (≈2 weeks after infection)
    - Chronic osteomyelitis
      - Periosteal reaction, cortical erosions, bony lucency and sclerotic changes
      - Bony lysis around hardware and prosthetic joints
      - **Sequestra—dead bone nidus** with surrounding granulation tissue
      - **Involucrum—periosteal new bone** forming later

- Nuclear medicine
  - Technetium three-phase bone scan—shows bone turnover (osteoblast activity)
    - Most helpful in cases of normal x-rays
    - **If negative rules out osteomyelitis**
    - Sensitive but not specific
    - Useful if MRI not an option
  - Gallium scan: shows acute phase reactants
    - **If negative, rules out osteomyelitis**
    - Cellulitis may cause false positive
    - Useful in diabetic foot: chronic osteomyelitis versus neuropathic foot
  - Indium WBC: shows areas of inflammation
    - Shows where leukocytes go
    - Usually negative in neoplasia
    - **Low sensitivity for axial skeleton**
    - Best for appendicular chronic osteomyelitis
- MRI best test to show early osteomyelitis
  - **Best test to show anatomic localization**
  - **Penumbra sign:**
    - Bright signal in surrounding bone
    - Darker abscess and sclerotic bone
  - If negative, rules out osteomyelitis
  - When positive may over estimate extent of disease
- Fluorodeoxyglucose positron emission tomography (FDG-PET)
  - Shows malignancies and infections: ↑ glycolysis
  - **Most sensitive test for chronic osteomyelitis**
  - More specific than MRI or bone scan
- Empirical treatment for osteomyelitis prior to definitive culture findings:
  - Newborn (up to 4 months of age):
    - *S. aureus,* gram-negative bacilli, and group B streptococci
    - Nafcillin or oxacillin plus a third-generation cephalosporin
    - If MRSA: vancomycin plus a third-generation cephalosporin
  - Children 4 months of age or older:
    - *S. aureus* and group A streptococci
    - Nafcillin or oxacillin versus vancomycin (MRSA)
    - Immunization has almost eliminated *Haemophilus influenzae* bone infections.
  - Adults 21 years of age or older:
    - *S. aureus*
    - Nafcillin or oxacillin versus vancomycin (MRSA)
- Situations of unusual organisms and unusual osteomyelitis:
  - *Salmonella* **osteomyelitis—sickle cell**
    - Microinfarcts of bone and bowel
    - Spleen dysfunction
    - Bone crisis versus diaphyseal osteomyelitis
  - *Pseudomonas* osteomyelitis
    - IV drug abuse and osteomyelitis of medial/lateral clavicle
    - Puncture wounds through rubber/synthetic shoes
  - *Bartonella henselae:* cats (same as "cat scratch fever")
    - Long-bone lytic lesions in **late-stage AIDS and cats**
    - Hard to culture; if Gram stain negative, must use a silver stain

- TB osteomyelitis:
  - One third of the world is infected with TB.
  - One third of TB in pediatric and HIV-positive patients is extrapulmonary.
  - Spine most common: Pott disease ("spinal gibbus") (see Figure 1-48, D)
  - One fourth of extrapulmonary TB is in hips and knees.
  - Often involves bones on both side of joint
- Syphilitic osteomyelitis (*Treponema pallidum*, a spirochete):
  - Neuropathic (Charcot) joints from neurosyphilis
  - Granulation tissue radiolucency in bilateral tibial metaphysis: "Wimberger sign"
  - Periosteal reaction: metaphysitis, periostitis, dactylitis
  - "Saber shin tibia": cortical thickening and bowing
- Fungal osteomyelitis
  - Long-term IV meds or parental nutrition
  - Immunosuppression by disease or drugs (RA, transplant)
  - *Candida*—**most common** is a normal flora
  - *Aspergillus*—rare in bone
  - Regional varieties—via inhalation or direct inoculation
    - *Coccidioides*—**southwest United States** to South America
    - *Histoplasma*—soil and bird/bat guano, **Ohio and Mississippi river valleys**
    - *Blastomyces*—rotting wood, **central southeastern United States**
    - *Cryptococcus*—**pigeon droppings, northwest United States/Canada**
  - Treatment:
    - Débride osteonecrosis, resect sinuses and/or synovitis
    - Antifungals: amphotericin
- Chronic sclerosing osteomyelitis of Garré
  - Rare; insidious onset of pain in diaphyseal bones of adolescents
  - Proliferation of the periosteum, which leads to bony deposition
  - Dense, progressive sclerosis on radiographs
  - May be caused by anaerobic organisms (*Propionibacterium acnes*)
  - Temporary improvement with antibiotics
  - Surgical resection—cultures usually negative
  - Rule out malignancy: osteoid osteoma, Ewing sarcoma, eosinophilic granuloma
- Chronic regional multifocal osteomyelitis (CRMO) (also chronic nonbacterial osteomyelitis [CNO])
  - Children/adolescents with multifocal bone pain without systemic symptoms
  - Exacerbations and remissions, more than 6 months of pain
  - Autoinflammatory disease; a diagnosis of exclusion
  - No abscess, fistula, or sequestra
  - Laboratory findings: WBC count normal; ESR, CRP may be elevated
  - X-rays demonstrate multiple metaphyseal lytic or sclerotic lesions.

- Whole-body spin tau inversion recovery MRI more sensitive
- Cultures negative—antibiotics do not help
- Histology:
  - Early: PMNs and osteoclasts
  - Later: lymphocytes, fibrosis, and reactive bone
  - Especially in the medial clavicle, distal tibia, and distal femur
- Treatment: symptomatic, resolves spontaneously, NSAIDs help
- SAPHO (synovitis, acne, pustulosis, hyperostosis, osteitis) syndrome
  - Also acquired hyperostosis syndrome
  - Young to middle-aged adults with bone pain and skin involvement
  - Suspect *P. acnes* serving as antigenic trigger
  - Humoral induction of sclerosis and erosions
  - Sternoclavicular region most commonly involved
  - Axial skeleton and unilateral sacroiliitis common
  - Palmopustular psoriasis, acne, or hidradenitis suppurativa
  - Laboratory findings: ESR, CRP moderately elevated
  - Bone scan (gold standard): "bull's head sign," sacroiliac joint uptake
  - MRI: erosion of vertebral body corner
  - Pathology: sterile neutrophilic pseudoabscesses
  - Cultures: occasional *P. acnes*
  - Treatment: NSAIDs, rheumatology consult, methotrexate, and biologics
- Joint infections: septic arthritis
  - Sources:
    - Hematogenous spread
    - Extension of metaphyseal osteomyelitis at intraarticular physis
      - Proximal femur—most common
      - Proximal humerus, radial neck, distal fibula
    - Direct inoculation—penetrating trauma, iatrogenic complication
  - Diagnosis of septic arthritis:
    - Progressive development of joint pain, swelling (effusion), warmth, redness
    - Progressive loss of function
    - Loading or moving joint hurts
  - Differential diagnosis of acute monoarthritis:
    - Gout/pseudogout—may have history of prior episodes
    - Reactive arthritis—uveitis, urethritis, heel/back pain, colitis, psoriasis
    - Viral arthritis
    - Fever and systemic symptoms more common in younger patients
  - Laboratory:
    - ↑ CRP, ↑ ESR, ↑ WBC
    - Aspiration—best test
    - Cell count: greater than 50,000 WBCs, left shift
    - Gram stain—helpful if positive
    - Cultures: aerobic and anaerobic
    - Crystals
  - Treating septic arthritis
    - I&D of fluid collection
    - IV antibiotics best based on cultures
    - Empirical antibiotics based on Gram stain:
      - Gram-positive cocci: vancomycin
      - Gram-negative cocci: ceftriaxone

- Gram-negative: ceftazidime, carbapenem or floxacin
- Negative Gram stain: vancomycin and ceftazidime or floxacin
- Monitor progress with CBC, ESR, **CRP (best measure of success)**
- Most common organisms by age:
  - Neonates: **S. aureus**
  - Children younger than 2 years: **S. aureus** (*Haemophilus influenzae*; less with vaccine)
  - Children 1 to 4 years: *Kingella kingae*: diagnose by PCR
  - Children older than 2 years: **S. aureus**
  - Healthy young adults (sexually active): *Neisseria gonorrhoeae*
  - Adults: **S. aureus**, streptococci, gram-negatives
- Periprosthetic septic arthritis: see Chapter 5, Adult Reconstruction, for details.
  - Pain and effusion
  - Laboratory:
    - ↑ CRP, ↑ ESR, blood WBCs rarely elevated early
  - Aspiration—best test, but for periprosthetic infection:
    - **Synovial fluid WBCs only need be above 2000.**
    - Percentage of PMNs only need be above 60% to 70% for concern.
  - PCR: limited by false-positive rate
  - Biomarkers have demonstrated high accuracy
    - Synovial fluid IL-1β and IL-6 had sensitivity, specificity, PPV, NPV, and high diagnostic accuracy
    - Markers do not identify the organism or antibiotic sensitivities.
- Septic arthritis clinical situations by organism:
  - *S. aureus*—most common cause of septic joints
    - Baby with "irritable hip" or child stops walking
    - Ultrasound to look for fluid and aspirate
  - *Kingella kingae*
    - Toddler (aged 1-4) with painful joint
    - After upper respiratory infection in fall/winter
    - Gram-negative coccobacilli—hard to culture; use blood bottles
    - Consider PCR
  - Group A streptococci—septic arthritis after chickenpox
    - **Most common infecting organisms after varicella infection**
    - Gram-positive cocci in chains
  - *Staphylococcus epidermidis*
    - Most common organism in implant infections (then *S. aureus*)
    - Total joint infection that "smolders"
    - Tissue culture most accurate test
    - Prevention with prophylaxis: cefazolin 1 g less than 1 hour preoperatively and Q8 for 24 hours postoperatively
  - Gonorrhea
    - **Migratory septic joint with** pustular palmar/plantar skin lesions
    - Gram-negative intracellular diplococci
    - More common in women near menses
  - *P. acnes*
    - Most common cause after mini–open repair of rotator cuff

- Shoulder replacement (second only to *S. aureus*)
- Indolent low-grade common contaminant
- Need more than 1 culture; grows very slowly (7-10 days)
- Gram-positive anaerobic rod that fluoresces under ultraviolet light
- **Less sensitive to cefazolin** (penicillin, vancomycin, clindamycin)
- *Mycobacterium tuberculosis*
  - Elderly, world traveler, HIV positive, history of RA and immune drugs
  - Knee and hip second only to spine
  - Usually hematogenous spread
  - Then osteolytic lesions on both sides of joint
  - "Rice bodies" and acid-fast bacilli
  - Acid-fast bacilli cultures: approximately 6 weeks
- Fungal infections: all are rare causes of musculoskeletal infections
  - Chronic effusions, synovitis
  - Immunocompromised: especially cellular immunity
  - Disease or drugs (rheumatologic agents, chemotherapy)
  - **Cultures and Gram stain negative off antibiotics**
  - Aspiration: 10,000 to 40,000, 70% PMNs
  - Diagnosis: potassium hydroxide (KOH) versus 6 weeks' culture
- *Candida*
  - Severe diabetic, chronic renal failure, liver failure
  - Prolonged IV catheter and broad-spectrum antibiotics
  - After multiple knee injections versus joint surgery
  - IV drug abuse: sacral, spinal, or clavicular
  - **Most common *fungal* infection following TJA**
- Aspergillosis
  - Neutropenia and heavy glucocorticoid use
  - Recurrent leukemia or HIV patient
- Coccidiomycosis
  - **Immigrant from southwestern United States to Central America**
  - History of **"valley fever"** (nonspecific upper respiratory infection)
  - Single joint with chronic synovitis, arthritis
- Histoplasmosis
  - **Ohio and Mississippi river valleys**
  - Soil exposed to **bird/bat guano**
  - Spelunker, excavators, cleaning chicken coops
  - Compromised cellular immunity: AIDS
  - Drugs: methotrexate, prednisone, anti–TNF-α agents
- *Blastomyces:*
  - Africa and southeast/central United States
  - Exposure to soil/rotting wood
  - Common skin lesions: wartlike or ulcer
- *Cryptococcus:*
  - Pacific Northwest, British Columbia, and subtropics
  - Soil and eucalyptus trees
  - AIDS, steroids, transplants, cancer, sarcoidosis

■ **Infectious risks of practice**
■ HIV infection
  • Obligate intracellular retrovirus
  • Primarily affects lymphocyte and macrophage cell lines
  • Decreases T-helper cells (CD4 cells)
  • Approximately 50,000 new cases/year reported by CDC
  • Increased in: homosexual men, hemophilia, and IV drug abusers
  • One fifth know they are HIV positive.
  • AIDS (acquired immunodeficiency syndrome)
    • Diagnosis requires an HIV-positive test plus one of the following:
      • One of the opportunistic infections (e.g., pneumocystis)
      • CD4 count of less than 200 (normal, 700 to 1200)
  • Transmission rate:
    • Increases with amount of blood exposed and viral load
    • Decreases with postexposure antiviral prophylaxis
    • From a contaminated needlestick: 0.3%
    • From mucous membrane exposure: 0.09%
    • From a blood transfusion: approximately 1 per 500,000 per unit transfused
    • From frozen bone allograft: less than 1 per 1 million
      • Donor screening—most important factor in preventing viral transmission
      • No cases from fresh frozen bone allograft have been reported since 2001.
      • Most sensitive screen—nucleic acid amplification testing (NAAT)
  • HIV positivity is not a contraindication to performing required surgical procedures.
    • HIV-positive patients more likely to have THA
    • Increased association with liver disease, drug abuse, coagulopathy
    • More likely to develop acute renal failure and postoperative infection
    • Asymptomatic HIV-positive individuals have no significant difference in short-term infection risks.
  • Orthopaedic manifestations more common in later stages
    • Increased infections:
      • Polymyositis: viral muscle infection
      • Pyomyositis: *S. aureus*
      • TB
      • Bacillary angiomatosis (*B. henselae*) from cats
    • Reactive arthritis (Reiter syndrome)
    • Non-Hodgkin lymphoma and Kaposi sarcoma
    • Osteonecrosis
■ Hepatitis
  • Hepatitis A—no surgical transmission risks (fecal-oral)
    • Common in areas with poor sanitation and public health concerns
  • Hepatitis B
    • Blood transmission: bites/sexual/occupational
    • Single stick transmission in the unvaccinated: approximately 30%
    • Causes cirrhosis, liver failure, and hepatocellular carcinoma
    • Screening and vaccination have reduced the risk of transmission for healthcare workers.
    • Immune globulin is administered after exposure in unvaccinated persons.

Table 1-39 Mechanism of Action of Antibiotics

CLASS OF ANTIBIOTIC	EXAMPLES	MECHANISM OF ACTION
β-Lactam antibiotics	Penicillin Cephalosporins	Inhibit cross-linking of polysaccharides in the cell wall by blocking transpeptidase enzyme
Aminoglycosides	Gentamicin Tobramycin	Inhibit protein synthesis (the mechanism is through binding to cytoplasmic 30S-ribosomal subunit)
Clindamycin and macrolides	Clindamycin Erythromycin Clarithromycin Azithromycin	Inhibit the dissociation of peptidyl-transfer RNA from ribosomes during translocation (the mechanism is through binding to 50S-ribosomal subunit)
Tetracyclines		Inhibit protein synthesis (binds to 50S-ribosomal subunit)
Glycopeptides	Vancomycin Teicoplanin	Interfere with the insertion of glycan subunits into the cell wall
Rifampin		Inhibits RNA polymerase F
Quinolones	Ciprofloxacin Levofloxacin Ofloxacin	Inhibit DNA gyrase
Oxazolidinones	Linezolid	Inhibits protein synthesis (binds to 50S-ribosomal subunits)

  • Allografts are screened for HBsAg and HB core antibody.
  • Hepatitis C (non-A, non-B)
    • Blood transmission: two thirds of U.S. HCV-positive individuals have IV drug abuse history, 2% occupational
    • Single-stick transmission (≈3%)
    • Recent advances in screening have decreased the risk of transfusion-associated infection.
    • Most sensitive method to screen and early test:
      • PCR = NAAT
■ **Antibiotics**
■ Prophylactic treatment
  • Bone exposed
  • Hardware placed
  • Large hematomas
  • Open fractures
■ Gustilo classification of open fractures:
  • I and II: first-generation cephalosporins the treatment of choice
  • Type IIIA: first-generation cephalosporin plus an aminoglycoside
  • IIIB (grossly contaminated): first-generation cephalosporin plus aminoglycoside plus penicillin
■ Mechanism of action of antibiotics (Table 1-39)
■ Antibiotic indications and side effects (Table 1-40)

Table 1-40	Antibiotic Indications and Side Effects	
ANTIBIOTICS	**SENSITIVE ORGANISMS**	**COMPLICATIONS/OTHER INFORMATION**
Aminoglycosides	G–, PM	Auditory (most common) and vestibular damage is caused by destruction of the cochlear and vestibular sensory cells from drug accumulation in the perilymph and endolymph Renal toxicity Neuromuscular blockade
Amphotericin	Fungi	Nephrotoxic
Aztreonam	G–	Ineffective against anaerobes
Carbenicillin/ticarcillin/ piperacillin	Better against G– than for G+	Platelet dysfunction, increased bleeding times
Cephalosporins		
First generation	Prophylaxis (surgical)	Nausea, vomiting, diarrhea
Second generation	Some G+, some G–	Cefazolin is the drug of choice
Third generation	G–, fewer G+	
Chloramphenicol	*Haemophilus influenzae,* anaerobes	Hemolytic anemia (bleeding diathesis [moxalactam]) Bone marrow aplasia
Ciprofloxacin	G–, MRSA	Tendon ruptures; cartilage erosion in children; antacids reduce absorption of ciprofloxacin; theophylline increases serum concentrations of ciprofloxacin
Clindamycin	G+, anaerobes	Pseudomembranous enterocolitis
Daptomycin	G+, MRSA	Muscle toxicity
Erythromycin	G+	In cases of PCN allergy
Imipenem	G+, some G–	Ototoxic Resistance, seizure
Methicillin/oxacillin/nafcillin	Penicillinase resistant	Same as penicillin; nephritis (methicillin); subcutaneous skin slough (nafcillin)
Penicillin	Streptococcal, G+	Hypersensitivity/resistance; hemolytic
Polymyxin/nystatin	GU	Nephrotoxic
Sulfonamides	GU	Hemolytic anemia
Tetracycline	G+	In cases of PCN allergy Stains teeth/bone (contraindicated up to age 8)
Vancomycin	MRSA, *Clostridium difficile*	Ototoxic; erythema with rapid IV delivery

G–, Gram-negative; *G+,* gram-positive; *GU,* genitourinary; *IV,* intravenous; *MRSA,* methicillin-resistant *Staphylococcus aureus; PM,* polymicrobial; *PCN,* penicillin.

SECTION 3 PERIOPERATIVE AND ORTHOPAEDIC MEDICINE

PERIOPERATIVE PROBLEMS

- Orthopaedic surgeons who evaluate their patients with care *preoperatively* can be rewarded with fewer perioperative problems. Goals include finding correctable issues and identifying risks to provide accurate risk/benefit assessment for proper consent.
- Cardiac issues
- Heart disease—leading cause of death in United States
- Coronary artery disease (CAD): leading cause in those older than 35 years
  - Risk factors: hypercholesterolemia, HTN, obesity, smoking, diabetes
- Leading cause of cardiac death in young sports population: hypertrophic cardiomyopathy
- Myocardial infarction (MI) can present with nausea and back pain with exertion
- American College of Cardiology/American Heart Association (ACC/AHA) three elements for assessing risk:
  - Clinical risk factors of perioperative cardiac risk:
    - Major predictors:
      - Unstable/severe angina, recent MI (<6 weeks)
      - Worsening or new-onset congestive heart failure (CHF)
      - Arrhythmias:
        - Atrioventricular (AV) block
        - Symptomatic ventricular dysrhythmia: bradycardia (<30 beats/min), tachycardia (>100 beats/min)
      - Severe aortic stenosis or symptomatic mitral stenosis
    - Other:
      - Prior ischemic heart disease
      - Prior CHF
      - Prior stroke/transient ischemic attack (TIA)
      - Diabetes
      - Renal insufficiency (creatine > 2)
  - Functional exercise capacity—measured in metabolic equivalents (METs)
    - METs: 3.5 mL O_2 uptake/kg/min
    - Perioperative risk elevated if unable to meet 4-MET demand
      - Walk up flight of steps or hill (= 4 METs)
      - Heavy work around house (>4 METs)
      - Can you walk four blocks or climb two flights of stairs?
  - Surgery-specific risk:
    - High risk (>5% death/MI)
      - Aortic, major or peripheral vascular
    - Intermediate risk (1%-5% death/MI)
      - **Orthopaedic surgery**, ENT, abdominal/thoracic
    - Low risk (<1% death/MI)—usually do not need further clearance
      - Ambulatory surgery, endoscopic, superficial
- Twelve-lead ECG if:
  - CAD and intermediate-risk procedure
  - One clinical risk factor and intermediate-risk procedure

- Noninvasive evaluation of left ventricular function if:
  - Three or more clinical risk factors and intermediate-risk procedure
  - Dyspnea of unknown origin
  - CHF with worsening dyspnea without testing in 12 months
- β-Blockers and statins should be continued around the time of surgery.
- Aspirin:
  - Monotherapy—when used alone
    - Stop using 7 days prior to surgery—avoid bleeding
  - Dual antiplatelet therapy—clopidogrel, prasugrel
    - Balance risk of stent thrombosis with surgical bleed
    - Consult cardiologist

- **Shock**
  - Cardiovascular collapse with hypotension, followed by impaired tissue perfusion and cellular hypoxia. May be a result of orthopaedic pathology or complication of surgery.
  - Metabolic consequence:
    - O_2 is unavailable—no oxidative phosphorylation
    - Cells shift to anaerobic metabolism and glycolysis
    - Pyruvate is converted to lactate—metabolic acidosis
    - **Lactate—indirect marker of tissue hypoperfusion**
    - Best measures of adequate resuscitation:
      - **Clinical measure of organ function: urine output over 30 mL/h**
      - **Laboratory measure: lactate less than 2.5**
  - Immunologic consequence:
    - Damaged cells release intracellular products
      - Damage-associated molecular patterns (DAMPs)
    - Cell surface receptors (TLRs)
      - Pattern recognition receptors (PRRs)
      - Recognize PAMPs
        - Example: bacterial products—lipopolysaccharide
      - Signal immune system to destroy bacteria
        - Cytokine cascade—TNF-α and IL-1
        - Complement activation
        - Endothelial damage—acute respiratory distress syndrome (ARDS)
    - DAMPs stimulate similar response from PRRs
      - Source for systemic inflammatory response syndrome (SIRS)
      - Common end of all: uncompensated shock
  - Types of shock
    - Neurogenic shock:
      - High spinal cord injury (also anesthetic accidents)
      - Motor/sensory deficits of spinal damage
      - Loss of sympathetic tone
      - Loss of vasomotor tone to peripheral arterial bed
      - Diagnosis:
        - **Bradycardia**, hypotension
        - Extremities warm
      - Treatment: vasoconstrictors and volume
    - Septic shock: (vasogenic)
      - **Number one cause of intensive care unit (ICU) death**
      - Mortality 50%
      - Bacterial toxins stimulate cytokine storm.
        - Examples: gram-negative lipopolysaccharides
        - Toxic shock superantigen
      - Inflammatory mediators cause endothelial dysfunction.
      - Peripheral vasodilation

- Diagnosis:
  - Multiple causes
  - Most common in orthopaedics: necrotizing fasciitis
- Treatment:
  - Identify and treat infections.
  - Prompt resection of dead tissue
  - Appropriate antibiotics
- Cardiogenic
  - Bad pump
    - Extensive MI, arrhythmias
  - Blocked pump (obstructive shock)
    - Massive "saddle" pulmonary embolism
    - Diagnosis: spiral CT angiography
    - Treatment: anticoagulation
  - Tension pneumothorax
    - Diagnosis:
      - **Decreased lung sounds**
      - **Hypertympany**, tracheal deviation
    - Treatment:
      - Needle in second intercostal space
      - Tube thoracostomy
- Cardiac tamponade
- Diagnosis:
  - Beck triad:
    - Hypotension
    - **Muffled heart sounds**
    - Neck vein distension
  - Pulsus paradoxus
  - Decreased systolic BP with inspiration
  - Echocardiography
- Treatment:
  - Pericardiocentesis
  - 16-gauge IV catheter
- Hypovolemic:
  - **Most common shock of trauma**
  - Volume loss from bleeds or burns
    - "Third spacing" also a cause
    - Translocation of intravascular fluid to site of injury/surgery
  - Neuroendocrine response: save heart and brain
    - Peripheral vasoconstriction
      - BP may be normal
      - Pale, cold, clammy extremities
  - Percentage of blood loss key to symptoms/signs
    - I: up to 15% blood volume loss
      - Vital signs can be maintained.
      - Pulse below 100 beats/min
    - II: 15% to 30% blood volume loss
      - Tachycardia (>100 beats/min), orthostatic
      - Anxious
      - Increased diastolic BP
    - III: 30% to 40% blood volume loss
      - Decreased systolic BP
      - **Oliguria**
      - Confusion, mental status changes
    - IV: more than 40% blood volume loss
      - Life threatening, obtunded
      - Narrowed pulse pressure
      - Immeasurable diastolic BP
- Treatment:
  - Start with ABCs: stop the bleeding
  - Two large-bore IV
  - 1 to 2 L lactated Ringers or normal saline
  - Some centers use packed RBCs (PRBCs)

Perioperative pulmonary complications

- Higher in cases that involve thorax
  - Orthopaedic cases: scoliosis
- Highest in patients with prior disease
  - Favor spinal/epidural anesthesia over general
  - Maximize medical treatment around surgery
- Chronic obstructive pulmonary disease (COPD)
  - Symptomatic COPD: anticholinergic inhalers (ipratropium)
  - May require corticosteroids
  - If sputum or lung fluid: delay surgery and give antibiotics
- Asthma
  - If wheezes or shortness of breath: β-agonist inhalers (albuterol)
  - Perioperative oral steroids safe
    - Consider systemic glucocorticoids if:
      - FEV_1 or peak expiratory flow rate (PEFR) below 80% predicted values/personal best
- Postoperative atelectasis
  - Like the cough associated, the workup is usually nonproductive.
  - Deep breathing/incentive spirometry—equally effective
- Postoperative pneumonia takes up to 5 days to present.
  - Productive cough, fever/chills, increased WBCs
  - Radiograph: pulmonary infiltrates
- Postoperative physical examination
  - **X-rays: normal early versus "oligemia"**
- Smoking cessation: improves outcomes
  - Stop 6 to 8 weeks preoperatively
  - Nicotine supplements no harm to wound
  - Less pulmonary complications
    - Smokers have six times more pulmonary complications.
  - Less wound healing issues (breakdowns, hematomas)
  - Less nonunions, wound infections
  - Less lung cancer:
    - Shoulder, neck, and thoracic pain in smokers
      - Prompts careful evaluation of lung fields

- Superior sulcus tumor ("Pancoast tumor")
  - Shoulder pain, weight loss
  - Intrinsic atrophy of hand—C8-T1
  - Horner syndrome—destroyed preganglionic fibers
    - Ptosis—eyelid droop
    - Miosis—pupil small (anisocoria)
    - Anhidrosis—decreases facial sweating
- **Acute respiratory distress syndrome (ARDS)**
- Pulmonary failure by edema (Figure 1-74, *A*)
- Pathophysiology:
  - Complement pathway activated:
    - Recruits leukocytes, oxygen free radicals
    - TNF, IL-1, IL-8, proteases
  - Increased pulmonary capillary permeability
  - Intravascular fluid floods alveoli
  - Results:
    - Hypoxia, pulmonary HTN
    - Right heart failure
  - 50% mortality
- Etiology:
  - Blunt chest trauma, aspiration, pneumonia
    - Shock, burns, smoke inhalation, near drowning
    - Orthopaedic:
  - **Long-bone trauma**
  - **Sepsis**
- Clinical symptoms:
  - Tachypnea, dyspnea, hypoxia, decreased lung compliance
  - $PaO_2:FIO_2$ below 200 mm Hg
- Imaging
  - **Radiographs: diffuse bilateral infiltrates, "snowstorm"**
  - CT: "ground glass"
- Treatment:
  - Prompt diagnosis and treatment of musculoskeletal infections
  - Prompt treatment of long-bone fractures
  - Ventilation with **positive end-expiratory pressure (PEEP)**
  - 100% O_2

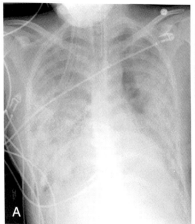 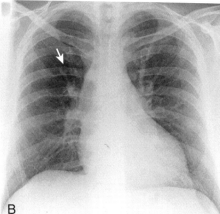 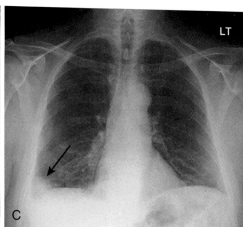

FIGURE 1-74 A, Chest x-ray (CXR) shows diffuse bilateral fluffy patchy infiltrates, worse at bases, consistent with ARDS (acute respiratory distress syndrome). **B,** CXR with a focal area of oligemia in the right middle zone (Westermark sign *[white arrow]*) and cutoff of the pulmonary artery in the upper lobe of the right lung. Seen with acute pulmonary embolism. **C,** CXR with a peripheral wedge-shaped density without air bronchograms at lateral right lung base (Hampton hump *[black arrow]*) that develops over time after a pulmonary embolism. (**B** from Krishnan AS, Barrett T: Images in clinical medicine: Westermark sign in pulmonary embolism, *N Engl J Med* 366:e16, 2012; **C** from Patel UB et al: Radiographic features of pulmonary embolism: Hampton hump, *Postgrad Med J* 90:420–421, 2014.)

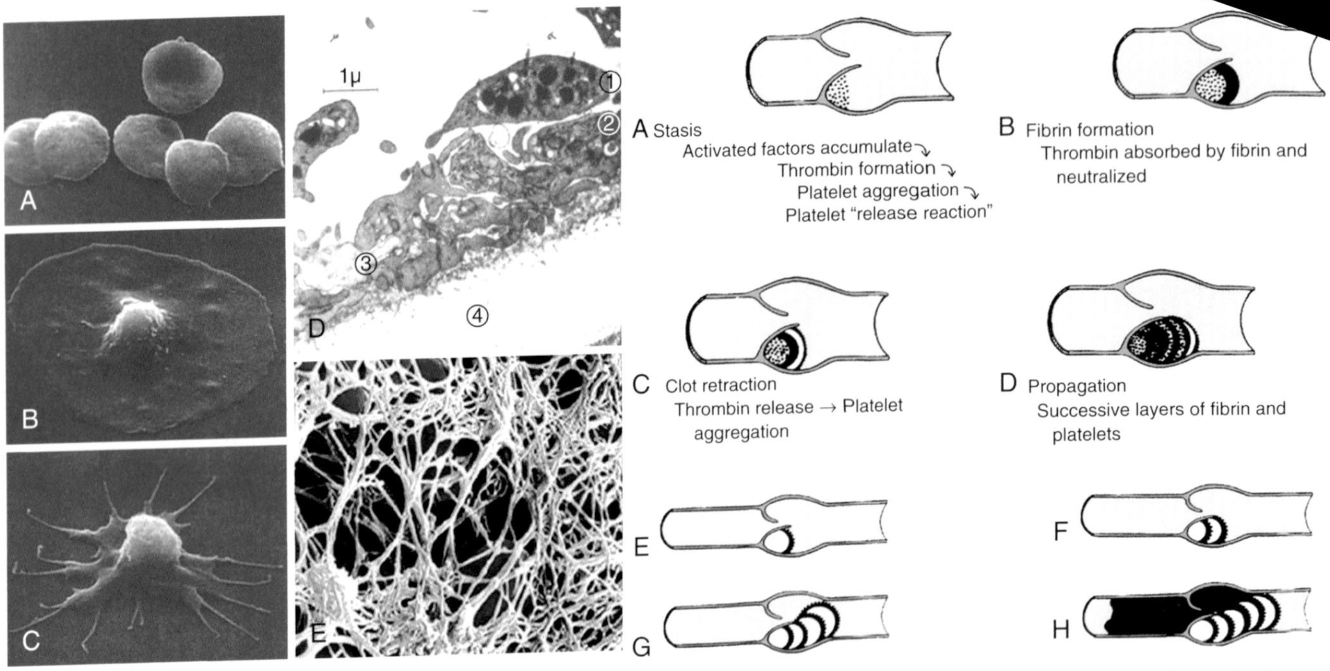

FIGURE 1-75 Electromicrograph panel (**A** through **E** on left). **A,** Scanning electron micrograph (SEM) of free platelets. **B,** SEM of platelet adhesion. **C,** SEM of platelet activation. **D,** Transmission electron micrograph of aggregating platelets. *1,* Platelet before secretion; *2* and *3,* platelets secreting contents of granules; *4,* collagen of endothelium. **E,** SEM of fibrin mesh encasing colorized red blood cells. Cartoon panel: (**A** through **H** on right) venous thromboembolus formation. **A,** Stasis. **B,** Fibrin formation. **C,** Clot retraction. **D,** Propagation. **E** through **H,** Continuation of this process until the vessel is effectively occluded. (From Miller MD, Thompson SR, editors: *DeLee and Drez's orthopaedic sports medicine: principles and practice,* ed 4, Philadelphia, 2014, Saunders; platelet electron micrographs courtesy James G. White, MD, Department of Laboratory Medicine and Pathology, University of Minnesota School of Medicine; Miller MD et al: *Review of orthopaedics,* ed 6, Philadelphia, 2012, Saunders; and Simon SR, editor: *Orthopaedic basic science,* Rosemont, Ill, 1994, American Academy of Orthopaedic Surgeons, p 492.)

■ **Fat emboli syndrome—classic clinical triad**
■ Long-bone fractures cause tiny fat emboli.
  • **Petechial rash**—pathognomonic: fat to skin
    • Upper anterior aspect of body—fat floats
      • Chest, neck, upper arm/axilla, shoulder
      • Neck, conjunctivae
  • Neurologic symptoms: fat to brain
    • **Mental status changes:** confusion, stupor
    • Rigidity, convulsions, coma
  • Pulmonary collapse: fat showers lung
  • **ARDS:** hypoxia, tachypnea, dyspnea
■ After asymptomatic interval with long-bone fractures
  • Immediate:
    • Long bones cause fat emboli in 90%
    • Fat emboli spread throughout body
    • Emboli block vessels in end organs
  • Late:
    • After 24 to 72 hours "asymptomatic interval"
    • Fat globules converted to toxic fatty acids
    • Fatty acids irritate endothelium of end organs
■ **Thromboembolic disease**
■ Common orthopaedic complication
  • Thrombosis: clotting at improper site
  • Embolism: clot that migrates
■ Most clinically silent but can be fatal
■ Complications of thromboembolic disease:
  • Postthrombotic syndrome: chronic venous insufficiency
    • Venous HTN
    • Chronic skin issue with swelling, pain
    • Pigmentation, induration, ulceration
    • Larger clots have worse symptoms
    • Delayed symptoms

  • Recurrent deep venous thrombosis (DVT): four to eight times increased after first DVT
  • Pulmonary embolism (PE):
    • Cause of readmission
    • Potentially fatal
■ Pathophysiology: (Virchow triad) (Figure 1-75)
  • **Endothelial damage:** trauma or surgery
    • Exposes collagen—triggers platelets
    • Platelets—three roles:
      • Adhesion and activation
      • Secretion of prothrombotic mediators
      • Aggregation of many platelets
  • **Stasis:** allows bonds of clotting proteins and cells
    • Immobility: pain, stroke, paralysis
    • Blood viscosity: polycythemia, cancer, estrogen
    • Decreased inflow: tourniquet, vascular disease
    • Decreased outflow: venous scarring, CHF
  • **Hypercoagulability**
    • Clotting cascades final product is **thrombin**
    • Converts soluble fibrinogen to **insoluble fibrin**
■ Risk factors and epidemiology:
  • Reported risks of thromboembolic disease vary by:
    • Definitions: asymptomatic versus symptomatic
    • Distal: below popliteal have very low PE risk
    • Proximal: above popliteal have greater PE risk
    • Total DVT: distal + proximal
    • Fatal PE: worth preventing
  • Patient specific risks factors (Figure 1-76)
    • **Prior thromboembolic disease strong risk factor**
    • **Risk is exponential with age (>40 years)** (Figure 1-77)

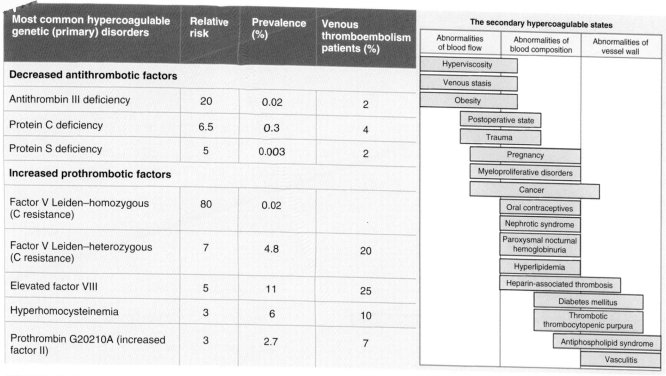

Most common hypercoagulable genetic (primary) disorders	Relative risk	Prevalence (%)	Venous thromboembolism patients (%)
Decreased antithrombotic factors			
Antithrombin III deficiency	20	0.02	2
Protein C deficiency	6.5	0.3	4
Protein S deficiency	5	0.003	2
Increased prothrombotic factors			
Factor V Leiden–homozygous (C resistance)	80	0.02	
Factor V Leiden–heterozygous (C resistance)	7	4.8	20
Elevated factor VIII	5	11	25
Hyperhomocysteinemia	3	6	10
Prothrombin G20210A (increased factor II)	3	2.7	7

FIGURE 1-76 Genetic (primary) disorders *(table on left)* and secondary hypercoagulable states *(figure on right)*. (Data from Ginsberg MA: Venous thromboembolism. In Hoffman R et al, editors: *Hematology: basic principles and practice,* ed 4, Philadelphia, 2005, Churchill Livingstone, pp 2225–2236; Perry SL, Ortel TL: Clinical and laboratory evaluation of thrombophilia, *Clin Chest Med* 24:153–170, 2003; and Schafer AI: Thrombotic disorders: hypercoagulable states. In Goldman L, Ausiello D, editors: *Cecil textbook of medicine,* ed 22, Philadelphia, 2004, Saunders, pp 1082–1087.)

- Genetic factors—thrombophilias
  - Decreased anticlotting factors
    - Antithrombin III deficiency
    - Protein C deficiency
    - Protein S deficiency
  - Increased clotting factors
    - Factor V Leiden (homozygous≫hetero)
    - Elevated factor VIII
    - Hyperhomocysteinemia
    - Prothrombin II G20210A
- Procedure-specific factors (Figure 1-78)
  - PE risk lower with distal cases versus hip
  - Risk higher with longer cases
  - TKA has higher total DVT risk but lower PE risk
  - Hip fracture risk is higher than THA risk.
  - Arthroscopy risk too low for prophylaxis
- Diagnosis:
  - Clinical diagnosis favors assessment of risk factors.
  - **Physical exam is unreliable: most are asymptomatic.**
    - DVTs can cause calf pain, palpable cords, swelling.
      - 50% with classic signs have no DVT by studies
      - 50% with venogram positive for clot have normal exam
    - PEs: most asymptomatic
      - Healthy lungs need over 60% occlusion prior to symptoms.
      - Signs/symptoms found in over 50% of patients with PEs:
        - Chest pain (often pleuritic)
        - Shortness of breath (dyspnea)
        - Tachypnea (>20/min)

- Saddle emboli can present with death.
  - PE is a common cause of rare death after arthroplasty.
  - PE is a common cause of readmission.
- Lab studies:
  - D-Dimer studies not helpful post injury/surgery
  - If negative, rules out significant clot
- ECG: rule out MI
  - Nonspecific findings; most common: sinus tachycardia
- Radiologic studies (Figure 1-79):
  - Venogram—best for distal below popliteal (clinical relevance?)
  - Duplex compression ultrasound—most practical
    - Noninvasive, easily repeatable bedside test
    - "Noncompressible vein" about 95% sensitive/specific
    - Helpful between popliteal space and inguinal ligament
    - **Guidelines strongly against routine duplex screening**
  - Chest x-ray—early: usually normal, "oligemia," or prominent hilum (see Figure 1-74, *B*)
    - Late findings: wedge or platelike atelectasis (see Figure 1-74, *C*)
  - Spiral CT angiography– best for suspected PE
    - Use linked to increase in diagnosis and treatment of PE
    - **No evidence of decreased mortality**
  - Ventilation-perfusion (V̇/Q̇) scan—most helpful for **dye-sensitive patients**
- Thromboembolic prophylaxis
  - Preventing DVTs has been shown possible.
  - **Preventing mortality unproven**

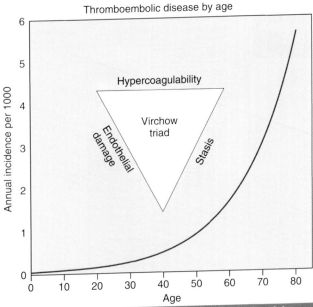

FIGURE 1-77 The three primary influences of thromboembolic disease (Virchow triad) and the relative risks of various patient conditions; note that age has an exponentially increasing risk. (Composite from Miller MD, Thompson SR, editors: *DeLee and Drez's orthopaedic sports medicine: principles and practice*, ed 3, Philadelphia, 2014, Saunders; and data from Anderson FA Jr et al: A population-based perspective of the hospital incidence and case-fatality rates of deep vein thrombosis and pulmonary embolism. The Worcester DVT Study, *Arch Intern Med* 151:933–938, 1991.)

Condition	Relative risk
Age > 70 yr	10–15×
Cancer	6×
Pregnancy	5×
Lupus antiphospholipid antibodies	4×
Oral contraceptive pills	3–4×
Obesity (body mass index ≥ 29)	3×
Smoking	3×
Diabetes	2×
Hypertension	2×

- Guidelines vary in their recommendations (Figure 1-80).
- Prophylaxis recommended for all arthroplasty patients
  - THA may benefit for extended treatment (≈30 days).
- For standard patients, not recommended for:
  - Upper extremity, arthroscopic, isolated fractures at knee and below
- Mechanical measures:
  - Early mobilization
  - Graduated elastic hose—not sufficient alone
  - Intermittent pneumatic compression devices (IPCDs)
    - Stimulates fibrinolytic system
    - Low bleeding risks
    - Grade IC by 2012 American College of Chest Physicians (ACCP) guidelines
  - CPM of no benefit
- Drug prophylaxis:
  - Surgical Care Improvement Project (SCIP) quality measures require DVT prophylaxis.
    - Highest compliance with DVT medicines
    - Linked to highest infection risks (suspect to bleeds/reoperations)
      - Encouraged for patients with high clot risk
      - Discouraged for patients with high bleed risks
    - Drug efficacy related to bleeding risks
    - Earlier a drug used postoperatively, the more bleeding seen
    - Longer the drug used, the more bleeding seen
  - Aspirin:
    - Irreversibly binds COX in platelets
    - Weakest; use of IPCD encouraged
    - Low bleeding risk
    - Long effect—stop 1 week prior to surgery
    - Consider for patients at higher risk for bleeding.
  - Warfarin (Coumadin):
    - Prevents vitamin K γ-carboxylation in liver
    - Inhibits factors II, VII, IX, X, and proteins C and S
    - Vitamin K and fresh frozen plasma can reverse
    - Multiple reactions with drugs and diet
    - Must monitor with international normalized ratio (INR; goal, 2 to 3)
    - Can cause fetal warfarin syndrome, skin necrosis
  - Heparin:
    - Reversibly Xa through ATIII and II, IX, XI, XII
    - Protamine sulfate can reverse
    - Short half-life: 2 hours
    - High bleeding rate in arthroplasty
    - Binds platelets—heparin-induced thrombocytopenia
  - Low-molecular-weight heparin (LMWH):
    - Reversibly Xa through ATIII and II
    - Protamine sulfate can reverse
    - Better pharmacokinetics: twice-daily dose
    - No monitoring needed
    - Less heparin-induced thrombocytopenia
    - Higher risk for bleeding than warfarin
  - Fondaparinux:
    - Irreversibly binds X through ATIII
    - Synthetic pentasaccharide
    - Good pharmacokinetics
    - No monitoring
    - No antidote
    - Higher risk for bleeding than LMWH
  - Rivaroxaban:
    - Direct Xa inhibitor
    - Oral drug
    - Higher risk for bleeding than LMWH
  - Hirudin:
    - Direct thrombin (IIa) inhibitor
    - Intramuscular and oral (dabigatran) versions
    - No antidote
  - Inferior vena cava filter use: controversial
    - May be used:
      - If contraindication to prophylaxis
      - Cerebral bleed/trauma
      - Spine surgery
      - If complication of prophylaxis
- Treatment of thromboembolic disease:
  - Blood-thinning medicines:
    - Early: strong medicines given for 1 week
    - Prolonged therapy often recommended
      - DVT approximately 3 months, PE approximately 12 months
  - Early mobilization—**NO BED REST**
    - Risk of dislodgment less than risk of more clots in these high-risk patients

Procedure	sDVT (%)	PE (%)
All hospital admission	0.048–0.07	0.023–0.03
Major orthopaedic procedures: THA, TKA, HFS		
In 2 weeks no prophylaxis	1.8	1
In 35 days no prophylaxis	2.8	1.5
In hospital with prophylaxis	0.26–0.8	0.14–0.35
In 35 days with prophylaxis	0.45	0.20
Knee arthroscopy	0.25–9.9	0.028–0.17
ACL reconstruction	0.3	0.8
Hip arthroscopy	0–3.7	0
Shoulder arthroscopy	0.01–0.26	0.01–0.21
Shoulder fracture	0	0.2
Shoulder arthroplasty	0.19–0.2	0.1–0.4
Elbow arthroplasty		0.25
Foot and ankle surgery	0–0.22	0.02–0.15
Ankle fracture	0.05–2.5	0.17–0.47
Ankle arthroscopy	0	0

ACL, Anterior cruciate ligament; *HFS*, hip fracture surgery; *PE*, pulmonary embolism; *sDVT*, symptomatic deep vein thrombosis; *THA*, total hip arthroplasty; *TKA*, total knee arthroplasty.

FIGURE 1-78 Rates of symptomatic thromboembolism in orthopaedic sports medicine. (From DeHart M: Deep venous thrombosis and pulmonary embolism. In Miller MD, Thompson SR, editors: *DeLee and Drez's orthopaedic sports medicine: principles and practice,* ed 4, Philadelphia, 2014, Saunders, p 207.)

- No decrease in PE with bed rest
- Pain and swelling improve with early mobilization.
- Graduated elastic compression hose for 2 years.
  - May prevent postthrombotic syndrome
- Thrombolytics, thrombectomy, embolectomy controversial
- Special clot situations:
- Isolated calf thrombosis smaller than 5 cm rarely needs treatment
  - Follow with serial ultrasound.
- Upper extremity blood clot in athlete
  - "Effort thrombosis" (Paget-Schroetter syndrome)
  - Axillary-subclavian vein thrombosis
  - Complaints:
    - Pain, swelling
    - Dilated veins
    - Feeling of heaviness
  - Diagnosis: duplex ultrasound
  - Treatment: consider thoracic outlet decompression
- Thromboembolic risks of flying
  - Flights longer than 8 hours—increased risks
  - Eight times the risks of non-flyers
  - Consider elastic compression hose—no drugs.
- **Bleeding and blood products**
- Avoid bleeding complications by identifying risk preoperatively.
- Historical clues:
  - "Easy bleeder"
    - Abnormal bruising, petechiae
    - Menorrhagia, epistaxis, gum bleed

- History of poor wound healing
- Liver/renal disease
- Previous bleeding complications
- Family history of bleeding complications
- Medicines or supplements
- Common inherited bleeding disorders
  - Von Willebrand disease: autosomal dominant
    - Most common genetic coagulation disorder
    - Von Willebrand factor dysfunction
      - Binds platelets to endothelium
      - Carrier for factor VIII
    - Treatment: desmopressin
  - Hemophilia A (VIII): X-linked recessive
  - Hemophilia B (IX) Christmas disease: X-linked recessive
- Medicines/supplements to stop prior to surgery
  - Platelet-inhibitor drugs
    - Aspirin, clopidogrel, prasugrel, NSAIDs
  - Drugs that cause thrombocytopenia:
    - Penicillin, quinine, heparin, LMWH
  - Anticoagulants (see earlier DVT section)
  - Supplements:
    - Fish oil, omega-3 fatty acids, vitamin E
    - Garlic, ginger, *Ginkgo biloba*
    - Dong quai, feverfew
- Diseases associated with increased bleeding
  - Chronic renal disease—uremia causes platelet dysfunction
  - Chronic liver failure—decreased liver proteins of clotting cascade

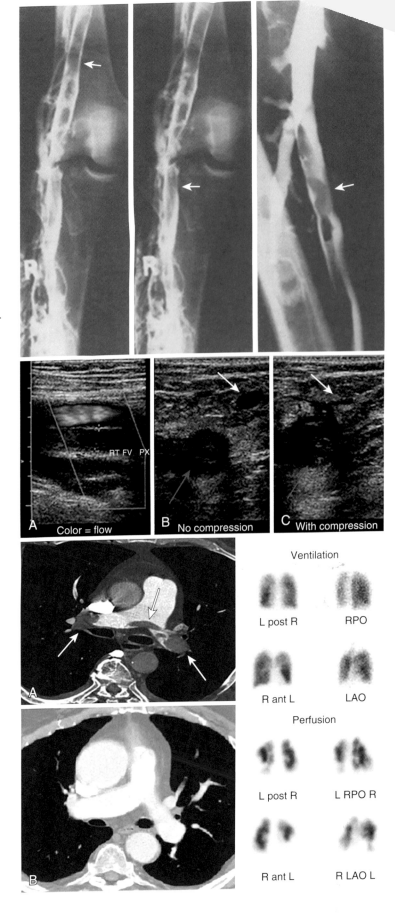

FIGURE 1-79 *Top series,* Venogram showing deep vein thrombosis (DVT). Intraluminal filling defects seen on two or more views of a venogram. The left two images are at the knee, and the right image is at the hip. *Middle series,* Doppler ultrasound for proximal DVT in femoral vein thrombosis. **A,** Longitudinal view shows presence of flow *(light blue)* in the more superficial vein over an occlusive thrombus *(dark gray).* **B,** A transverse view without compression shows an open superficial vein seen as a black oval *(white arrow)* and a thrombosed deeper vein as a dark gray circle with an echogenic center *(red arrow).* **C,** A transverse view with compression shows the flattened compressible superficial vein *(white arrow)* and the unchanged noncompressible thrombosed deeper vein *(red arrow). Bottom series (left images),* Spiral computed tomography (CT) pulmonary angiography. **A,** Large pulmonary embolism (PE) *(arrows).* **B,** Normal CT. *Right images,* high probability V/Q scan showing full lung fields on ventilation scan above and multiple areas lacking tracer on the perfusion scan below. (DVT panel from Jackson JE, Hemingway AP: Principles, techniques and complications of angiography. In Grainger RG, editor: *Grainger & Allison's diagnostic radiology: a textbook of medical imaging,* ed 4, Philadelphia, 2011, Churchill Livingstone. Original images courtesy Austin Radiological Association and Seton Family of Hospitals.)

Recommendations on prevention of VTE in hip and knee arthroplasty

Grade of recommendation: ! Strong + Moderate ~ Weak * Consensus ? Inconclusive	Notes from other guidelines: 1 ACCP, 2 NICE, 3 AHRQ
!	No "screening" duplex US	
+	History of normal risks of VTE and bleeding, use drugs **and/or** IPC	
+	D/C platelet inhibitors preop (aspirin, clopidogrel, prasugrel)	Discuss with medical team, stop 1 week prior[2]
+	Neuraxial anesthesia to decrease bleeding (no effect on VTE)	Caution with drugs and neuraxial[1]; wait 12 hours after drugs[2]
~	Ask history of previous VTE	
*	Hx of VTE, get IPC **and** drugs	DRUGS: LMWH, fondaparinux, dabigatran, rivaroxaban, VKA, aspirin[1]
*	Ask Hx of bleeding disorder (hemophilia) and active liver disease	
*	Hx of bleeding disorder (hemophilia or active liver disease) **only** IPC	If bleeding risk, IPC or nothing[1]; if bleeding risk > clotting risk, IPC[2]
*	Discuss duration with patient	≥10 days, consider 35 days[1]
*	Early mobilization	
?	Assess other clotting risk factors	
?	Assess other bleeding risk factors	
?	No one technique optimal	Drugs and IPC[1,2] ; D/C drugs when TKA mobile[2]
?	IVC filter	If VTE risks high and contraindication to prophylaxis[2]

Guideline title	Source:
2011 AAOS Preventing Venous Thromboembolic Disease	http://www.aaos.org/research/guidelines
2012 ACCP Prevention of VTE in Orthopedic Surgery Patient	http://journal.publications.chestnet.org/
2012 AHRQVTE Prophylaxis in Orthopedic Surgery, CER 49	http://effectivehealthcare.ahrq.gov/
2010 NICE Reducing the Risk of VTE in patients admitted to hospital	http://guidance.nice.org.uk/CG92/

FIGURE 1-80 Rates by procedure: symptomatic thromboembolism in orthopaedic sports medicine. *AAOS,* American Academy of Orthopaedic Surgeons; *ACCP,* American College of Chest Physicians; *AHRQVTE,* Agency for Healthcare Research and Quality Venous Thromboembolism Prophylaxis; *CER,* comparative effectiveness research; *D/C,* discontinue; *Hx.,* history; *IPC,* intermittent pneumatic compression devices; *IVC,* inferior vena cava; *LMWH,* low-molecular-weight heparin; *NICE,* National Institute for Health and Care Excellence; *TKA,* total knee arthroplasty; *US,* ultrasound; *VKA,* vitamin K antagonist; *VTE,* venous thromboembolism. (From DeHart M: Deep venous thrombosis and pulmonary embolism. In Miller MD, Thompson SR, editors: *DeLee and Drez's orthopaedic sports medicine: principles and practice,* ed 4, Philadelphia, 2014, Saunders, p 207.)

- Techniques to avoid blood loss at surgery
  - Tourniquets: tissue effect relates to time and pressure
    - Use no longer than 2 hours
      - Time to restore equilibrium:
        - 5 minutes after 90 minutes of use
        - 15 minutes after 3 hours
    - Prolonged use can cause tissue damage.
      - Nerve damage compressive (not ischemic)
      - Electromyography: subclinical abnormalities in 70% routine use
      - Slight increase in pain
    - Wider tourniquets distribute forces
      - Peak pressure at center of cuff (less at edges)
    - Pad under to prevent skin blisters in TKA
    - Lowest pressure needed for effect
      - 100 to 150 mm Hg above systolic BP
        - 200 mm Hg upper extremity
        - 250 mm Hg lower extremity
    - Esmarch elastic band to exsanguinate (not for infections or tumors)
  - Tranexamic acid:
    - Multiple trials show clinical and statistical improvements.
    - Reduces blood loss enough to show fewer transfusions
    - Cost-effective and safe
    - **Synthetic lysine analogue,** acts on fibrinolytic system
    - **Competitive inhibitor of plasminogen activation**
    - Plasmin dissolves fibrin clots
    - **No increase in DVT has been noted.**
  - Temperature:
    - Mild hypothermia increases bleeding time and blood loss.
  - Intraoperative "cell saver" may be cost-effective if:
    - Expecting about 1000 mL blood loss
    - Anticipate recovering 1 or more unit of blood
  - Techniques not yet found to be effective or cost-effective:
    - Bipolar sealant, topical sealants, autologous donation
    - Reinfusion systems, **routine transfusions over 8 g/dL Hb**
- Bleeding classifications:
  - Major bleeding:
    - Fatal or into critical organ:
    - Retroperitoneal, intracranial, intraspinal
    - Requiring reoperation
    - Bleeding index: 2 or greater
      - PRBCs transfused plus preoperative/postoperative Hb
  - Minor bleeding:
    - Any other clinically overt bleeding
- Preoperative techniques to address anemia
  - Anemia-associated vitamins:
    - Iron 256 mg, vitamin C 1 g, folate 5 mg/day
    - For 30 to 45 days preoperatively, decreased transfusion rate
    - Erythropoietin if preoperative Hb below 13

- Transfusions
  - Risks of needing transfusion after surgery:
  - Preoperative Hb
    - Most significant risk factor
    - Below 13 g/dL, more likely
  - Patient size, age, lateral release
  - Longer surgery, women
  - PRBCs: Hct 60% to 70%
  - 1 unit increases Hb approximately 1 g/dL
  - Trigger—no absolute; clinical judgment
    - Various guidelines:
      - Below 6 g/dL: transfuse
      - 7-8 g/dL: transfuse postoperative patients
      - 8-10 g/dL: transfuse symptomatic patients
        - Orthostatic hypotension
        - Tachycardia unresponsive to fluids
      - Above 10 g/dL: transfusion not routinely indicated
  - Restrictive transfusion strategies:
    - Lower 30-day mortality trend (relative risk [RR], .85)
    - Lower infection risk trend (RR .81)
      - Greatest benefits to orthopaedic patients
    - No difference in functional recovery
  - Prevent transfusion by anticipating lowest Hb by procedure
    - If preoperative Hb is less than 7 (2.1% transfused), consider erythropoietin preoperatively.
- Platelets
  - Can help prevent bleeding
  - **Blood component most likely contaminated**
    - Stored at room temperature
    - Infected cases: 10 cases/million units transfused
    - Gram-positive organisms more common
  - Thrombocytopenia
    - Platelet count below 5000/mm^3—give to avoid spontaneous bleed
    - Platelet count below 50,000/mm^3—give before surgery
    - Platelet count above 100,000/mm^3—no need to give
- Transfusions risks:
  - Leading risk: transfusing wrong blood to patient
    - Occurs in 1 in 10 to 20,000 RBC units transfused
    - Autologous donations decrease preoperative Hb
      - Increase likelihood of needing transfusion
      - Risks and cost exceed benefits
- Transfusion reactions:
  - Febrile nonhemolytic transfusion reaction
    - Most common
    - Fever/chills with or without mild dyspnea
    - One to 6 hours post transfusion
    - From leukocyte cytokines released from stored cells
      - Luekoreduction decreases incidence
      - Related to length of storage
  - Acute hemolytic transfusion reaction
    - Medical emergency
    - ABO incompatibility
      - **Clinical errors lead to highest risk of transfusion reactions**
      - IgM anti-A and anti-B, which fix complement
      - Rapid intravascular hemolysis

- Classic triad: fever, flank pain, rec/u.. urine (rare)
  - Can cause DIC, shock, and acute renal failure (ARF) due to acute tubular necrosis (ATN)
  - Fever/chills, "pink plasma"
  - Positive direct antiglobulin test (Coombs)
- Delayed hemolytic transfusion reactions
  - Reexposure to previous antigen (i.e., Rh or Kidd)
  - History of pregnancy, prior transfusion, transplantation
  - 3 to 30 days post transfusion
  - Anemia, mild elevation of unconjugated bilirubin, spherocytosis
- Anaphylactic reactions: about 1 in 20,000
  - Rapid hypotension, angioedema
    - Shock, respiratory distress
  - **Frequently involve anti-IgA and IgE antibodies**
  - **Stop transfusions, ABCs, epinephrine**
- Urticarial reactions: about 1% to 3%
  - Mast cell/basophils release of histamine—hives
  - Only reaction that may allow continued transfusion
  - Stop, give diphenhydramine
    - If urticaria resolves and there is no hypotension, shortness of breath, or anaphylaxis, then may resume transfusion
- Infectious risks:
  - Bacterial: 0.2/million PRBC units transfused
    - Gram positive
    - **Cryophilic organisms: *Yersinia, Pseudomonas***
  - HTLV—approximately 1 in 2 million
  - HIV—approximately 1 in 2 million
  - Hepatitis C—approximately 1 in 2 million
  - Hepatitis B—approximately 1 in 250,000

- ■ **Renal and urologic issues:**
- ■ ARF (acute kidney injury [AKI])
  - Edema, HTN, urinary output less than 30 mL/hour (<0.5 mL/kg/h)
  - Laboratory findings: increased creatinine over 1.5 times baseline
    - Hyperkalemia can be fatal.
      - Above 5.5, consider dialysis
    - Urinalysis: protein, sediment
  - Prerenal renal failure (most common ARF): decreased kidney perfusion
    - Hypovolemia/hypotension from blood loss
  - Intrinsic renal failure:
    - ATN: most frequent intrinsic ARF
      - Does not respond to fluid
  - Ischemia, sepsis
  - Myoglobin from rhabdomyolysis
  - Nephrotoxic dyes/drugs:
    - Radiocontrast
    - Aminoglycosides
    - Amphotericin
  - Acute interstitial nephritis (AIN): fever, eosinophils in blood/urine
    - Allergy
    - Infections
    - Medications—**most common cause of AIN**
      - NSAIDs, penicillin, cephalosporins, sulfonamides
      - Furosemide, hydrochlorothiazide

- Glomerular disease: hematuria, proteinuria, HTN, edema
  - SLE, poststreptococcal, IgA nephropathy, hepatorenal
- Postrenal ARF: obstruction
  - Bladder catheter to empty bladder
- Chronic kidney disease (CKD):
  - Definition
    - More than 3 months
    - GFR below 60 or
    - Urine albumin loss greater than 30 mg/day
  - Retained phosphate and secondary to hyperparathyroidism
  - Causes increased extraskeletal calcification
    - Vascular calcification—**increased cardiovascular risk**
    - Increased chondrocalcinosis, tumoral calcinosis
    - Decreased calcitriol (active form of vitamin D is 1,25 dihydroxycholecalciferol)
      - *Two kidneys* put the *second OH* on vitamin D in the **ONE** spot to make it active.)
  - High perioperative complications
    - Increased cardiovascular risk
    - **Hyperkalemia** and fluid adjustments
    - Increased bleeding complications
    - Poor BP control
    - Higher infection rates
    - Higher complications/revisions
    - Higher morbidity
- Nephrogenic systemic fibrosis (NSF) (also nephrogenic fibrosing dermopathy)
  - Occurs in patients with CKD or ARF who get IV gadolinium for MRI
  - Skin thickening and fibrosis (appears similar to scleroderma)
    - Skin plaques, cobblestone appearance, peau d'orange
  - Rapid joint contractures and disability
  - Systemic changes of cardiomyopathy and pulmonary fibrosis
- Perioperative urinary retention:
  - Outflow obstructions: benign prostatic hypertrophy (BPH) in men (common)
  - Bladder muscle (detrusor) compromise
  - Overdistention:
    - Excess fluid/long cases
      - Leads to atonic bladder
    - Neurogenic:
      - Spinal trauma, tumor, stroke, diabetes
      - "Neurogenic" atonic bladder
    - Medications:
      - Anticholinergic and sympathomimetic drugs
      - Opioids, antidepressants, pseudoephedrine, diphenhydramine
  - Can cause postrenal ARF (AKI)
  - Associated with higher rates of urinary tract infections
  - Increased 2-year mortality after hip fracture
  - Risk factors: men>women
    - BPH
      - Screen: International Prostate Symptom Score (I-PSS)
        - Incomplete emptying, weak stream
        - Frequency, urgency, straining
        - Nocturia, intermittency

- Age, symptoms, prostate volume, urine flow rate
- Epidural > spinal > PCA > peripheral blocks
- HTN
- Treatment:
  - α-Blockers—tamsulosin 0.4 mg/day
  - Bladder ultrasound if no voiding by 3 to 4 hours
  - If ultrasound shows more than 400 to 600 mL, then in-and-out (IO) urinary catheter
  - Continuous Foley if more than 2 IOs
  - Transurethral retrograde prostatectomy (TURP) prior to elective arthroplasty preferred
- **Trauma patients—no catheter if:**
  - Bloody meatus or scrotal hematoma
- Perioperative urinary tract infection (UTI)
  - "Irritative symptoms": dysuria, urgency, frequency
  - 30% to 40% of hospital-acquired infections
    - Upper UTI: pyelonephritis, perinephric abscess
      - Need urgent treatment; defer elective surgery
    - Lower UTI: urethritis, cystitis, prostatitis
  - Most common organisms: *Escherichia coli* and *Enterococcus*
  - Risk factors: women more at risk than men
    - Duration of Foley catheter: increase of 10%/day
    - SCIP measure—discontinue by 24 hours postoperatively
  - Diagnosis:
    - If symptoms, urinalysis and culture/sensitivities
    - WBCs (leukocyte esterase positive)
    - Bacterial count over 10^3 CFU/mL, treat preoperatively
  - Treatment:
    - Antibiotics for gram-negative organisms
    - Trimethoprim-sulfamethoxazole or fluoroquinolone
- **GI motility disorders (Figure 1-81):**
- 1.5% of hip/knee arthroplasty
- Common presentation:
  - Abdominal pain
  - Distension
  - Nausea with or without vomiting
- Prevention:
  - Chew gum: vagal (parasympathetic stimulation)
  - Early mobility
  - Spinal (sympathetic block)
  - Limit dose and length of IV opioids
- Postoperative adynamic ileus
  - Gut autonomic nerve imbalance:
    - Excess sympathetics
    - Deficient parasympathetics
  - Large and small bowel involved
  - More common in spine (≈7%) and joint arthroplasty (≈1%)
  - Risk factors:
    - Older, male, history of alcohol abuse
    - Anemia, fluid/electrolyte disorder—low potassium
    - Prior abdominal surgery
    - Spine (anterior > posterior), increased with greater than two levels
    - THA > TKA
  - X-ray: dilated small and large bowel (see Figure 1-81, *A*)
  - Treatment: nothing by mouth, nasogastric tube
    - Electrolyte control
    - Stop narcotics

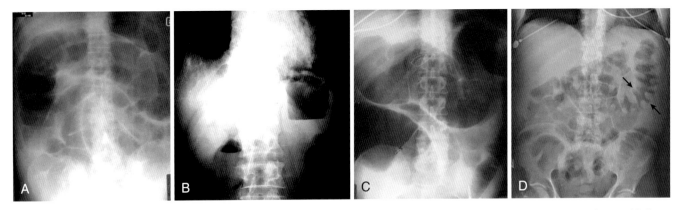

FIGURE 1-81 Perioperative gastrointestinal mobility radiographs. **A,** Dilated loops of both small bowel and large bowel consistent with ileus. **B,** Characteristic dilation with fluid air levels of stomach and right-sided upper duodenum seen in mesenteric artery syndrome ("cast syndrome"). **C,** Isolated dilation of the large bowel seen in acute colonic pseudo-obstruction ("Ogilvie syndrome"). **D,** Dilated loops of both small and large bowel in a patient with watery diarrhea after antibiotic use. Wide, thickened, transverse bands of nodular colon wall replace normal haustral folds ("thumb printing") as seen in pseudomembranous colitis. (A and C from Nelson JD et al: Acute colonic pseudo-obstruction (Ogilvie syndrome) after arthroplasty in the lower extremity, *J Bone Joint Surg Am* 88:604–610, 2006; B from Tidjane A et al: [Superior mesenteric artery syndrome: rare but think about it], [Article in French] *Pan Afr Med J* 17:47, 2014; and D from Thomas A et al: "Thumbprinting," *Intern Med J* 40:666, 2010.)

- Superior mesenteric artery (SMA) syndrome ("cast syndrome")
  - Occlusion of duodenum by SMA
  - Gastric dilatation with duodenal obstruction
  - Epigastric pain
  - Nausea plus **intermittent bilious vomiting**
  - Risk factors: often **tall patient with low BMI**
  - Orthopaedic causes:
    - Hip spica cast
    - Following scoliosis surgery
    - Following THA with severe hip flexion contracture
    - Following traumatic quadriplegia
  - Also found in patients with **rapid, large weight loss**
    - Anorexia nervosa, drug abuse, and bariatrics
  - X-ray: distended stomach and upper duodenum (see Figure 1-81, *B*)
  - CT:
    - Aortomesenteric artery angle less than 25 degrees
    - Aortomesenteric distance is less than 8 mm
  - Treatment: nothing by mouth, nasogastric tube
    - General surgery:
      - Divide ligament of Treitz
      - Duodenojejunal bypass
- Acute colonic pseudo-obstruction (Ogilvie syndrome)
  - Large bowel dilation
  - Abdominal distension prominent symptom
  - AVOID COLONIC PERFORATION
  - Risk factors:
    - Elderly, male
    - Previous bowel surgery
    - Diabetes, hypothyroidism
    - Electrolyte disorders
  - X-ray:
    - **Distended transverse, descending, and cecum** (see Figure 1-81, *C*)
    - **Colonic diameters over 10 cm risk perforation.**
  - Treatment:
    - Nothing by mouth
    - **Neostigmine**
    - **Colonic decompression**

- Pseudomembranous colitis: *potentially fatal diarrhea*
  - Most common antibiotic-associated colitis
  - Change in colon flora favors *Clostridium difficile*
    - Makes enterotoxin-A and cytotoxin-B
  - Many antibiotics:
    - Clindamycin, fluoroquinolones
    - Penicillins and cephalosporins
  - Can become severe fulminant colitis
    - Toxic megacolon and perforations
  - Risk factors:
    - Elderly hospitalized
    - Severe illness
    - Antibiotic use
    - Proton pump inhibitor use
  - Diagnosis:
    - **Watery diarrhea with fever**
    - Leukocytosis, lower abdominal pain
  - Laboratory findings:
    - WBC count above 15,000
    - Send stool for *C. difficile* toxin
    - PCR or enzyme-linked immunosorbent assay (ELISA)
  - KUB (kidney, ureter, bladder [plain abdominal radiograph]):
    - "Toxic megacolon": greater than 7 cm
    - "Thumbprinting" (see Figure 1-81, *D*)
  - Treatment:
    - Oral metronidazole
    - Oral vancomycin (IV will not work)
    - Fidaxomicin
    - Colectomy if unresponsive and severe
      - Megacolon, WBCs over 20,000
- **Perioperative hepatic issues**
- Liver failure: critical for producing proteins and metabolizing toxins
  - Mental status changes: encephalopathy
  - Bleeding, jaundice, ascites
  - Asterixis—flapping wrists
  - Late: spider telangiectasias, gynecomastia, splenomegaly
    - Palmar erythema, clubbing of fingers (biliary cirrhosis)

aspartate aminotransferase (AST), alanine aminotransferase (ALT), and bilirubin
  - INR above 1.5, low platelets (<150,000)
- Acute—most commonly viral and drug induced
  - Acetaminophen—number one cause in United States
    - Guidelines recommend using less than 3 to 4 g/day
  - Other toxins: alcohol, occupational, mushrooms
  - Viral hepatitis
- Chronic—cirrhosis is end-stage fibrosis of liver
  - Common: hepatitis (B, C), alcoholic, hemochromatosis
- Classifications can be helpful to estimate risks:
  - Child classification—most widely used
    - Based on laboratory results and physical examination
    - Difficulty assessing encephalopathy/ascites
    - Child class A: some elective surgery tolerated
      - Bilirubin below 1.5, albumin over 3.5, partial thromboplastin time (PTT) less than 4 seconds prolonged
      - No encephalopathy and no ascites
    - Child class B: may be permissible
      - Bilirubin 1.5 to 3.0, albumin 2.8 to 3.5, PTT 4 to 6 seconds prolonged
      - Moderate encephalopathy and slight ascites
    - Child class C: surgery contraindicated
      - Bilirubin above 3.0, albumin less than 2.8, PTT more than 6 seconds prolonged
      - **Severe encephalopathy and moderate ascites**
  - Model for End-Stage Liver Disease (MELD) score
    - Formula based on bilirubin, INR, creatinine
    - http://www.mayoclinic.org/medical-professionals/model-end-stage-liver-disease/meld-model
    - Studies highlight mortality at 90 days relative to MELD score:
      - Less than 9: about 2% mortality
      - 10 to 19: about 6% mortality
      - 20 to 29: about 20% mortality
      - 30 to 39: about 53% mortality
      - Above 40: about 71% mortality
- Orthopaedic importance:
  - Surgery is frequently to be avoided in liver failure.
  - Complication rates from surgery are extremely high.
    - In arthroplasty patients, MELD score above 10 predicted:
      - Three times the complication rate
      - Four times the rate death
    - Arthroplasty infections:
      - From 6% to 10% if any cirrhosis
      - Approximately 20% if hepatic decompensation or variceal bleeding
      - Two-stage failure after infection in cirrhosis: 30%
      - Hip arthroplasty for trauma:
        - 80% complication
        - 60% death

■ **Perioperative CNS**

▨ Stroke
  - Rare (0.2% of joint arthroplasty)
  - Mortality roughly 25% at 1 year
  - Ischemic more common than hemorrhagic
  - Risk factors:
    - Advanced age, cerebrovascular accident (CVA), TIA
    - MI, coronary artery bypass graft, atrial fibrillation, or ECG rhythm abnormality
    - Left ventricular dysfunction
    - Cardiac valvular disease
  - General greater than regional
  - Higher anesthesia ASA risk score, rhythm problems during surgery
  - Blood transfusion (and number of units transfused)
  - Diagnosis: head CT or MRI
  - Treatment: ABCs, hospitalist/neurology consult

▨ Delirium: approximately 40% in hip fractures
  - Fluctuating levels of consciousness
  - Impairment of memory and attention
  - Disorientation, hallucinations, agitation
  - Associated with increased length of stay
    - Decubitus ulcers, failure to regain function
    - Feeding issues, urinary incontinence
    - Mortality and nursing home placement
  - Risk factors: elderly
    - History of prior postoperative confusion
    - History of alcohol abuse
    - Acute surgery more than elective
    - Night-time surgery
    - Long duration of anesthesia
    - Intraoperative pressures below 80 mm Hg
    - Use of meperidine (Demerol)
  - Diagnosis: rule out anemia, infection, electrolyte issues
    - Urinalysis, urine culture and sensitivity, chest x-ray
    - CT if trauma or stroke signs
    - Spinal tap if fever or nuchal rigidity
    - Serum ammonia if hepatic history
  - Treatment: O_2 saturation above 95%, systolic BP above 90 mm Hg
    - Correct medical issues
    - Family/friends
  - Treatment: haloperidol (beware torsades de pointes)
    - Lorazepam
    - Restraints as last resort

■ **Special anesthesia issues:**

▨ Obstructive sleep apnea (OSA)
  - Intermittent hypercapnia and hypoxia
    - "Obesity hypoventilation syndrome"
    - Daytime hypercapnia while awake
    - Decreased CO_2-induced respiratory drive
    - Extreme sensitivity to opioids
    - Leads to:
      - Pulmonary HTN
      - Cardiac arrhythmias
  - GERD (reflux) directly related to BMI
    - Delayed gastric emptying
    - Higher intragastric pressure
    - Increased risks for aspiration/intubation
    - Obese anatomy makes mask/intubation difficult
  - Higher risk for complications (2-4 times greater)
    - Respiratory failure, ICU transfers, length of stay increased
    - Increased postoperative O_2 desaturation
    - Increased intubation, aspiration pneumonia, ARDS
    - Increased MI, arrhythmias (atrial fibrillation)
  - Screening tools: STOP-BANG (Figure 1-82)
    - Snoring, Tired, Observed apnea, Pressure (HTN)
    - BMI over 35, Age older than 50, Neck circumference larger than 40 cm, Gender male
    - Five or more—high risk of severe OSA
  - Best practices:
    - Initiate or continue continuous positive airway pressure (CPAP) use

```
┌─────────────────────────────────────────────┐
│           STOP-BANG scoring method          │
│ Every Yes answer = 1 point                  │
│                                             │
│ Snoring: Do you snore loudly (loud enough to be   ☐ Yes  ☐ No │
│   heard through closed doors)?              │
│ Tired: Do you often feel tired, fatigued, or sleepy ☐ Yes  ☐ No │
│   during daytime?                           │
│ Observed: Has anyone observed you stop breathing ☐ Yes ☐ No │
│   during your sleep?                        │
│ Blood Pressure: Do you have or are you being   ☐ Yes  ☐ No │
│   treated for high blood pressure?          │
│ BMI more than 35?                           ☐ Yes  ☐ No │
│ Age older than 50 years?                    ☐ Yes  ☐ No │
│ Neck circumference greater than 40 cm?      ☐ Yes  ☐ No │
│ Gender male?                                ☐ Yes  ☐ No │
│                                             │
│    5 or more = high risk for Obstructive Sleep Apnea │
│       Initiate or continue CPAP machine     │
│    Avoid/minimize narcotics – maximize local blocks │
└─────────────────────────────────────────────┘
```

FIGURE 1-82 STOP-BANG screening questionnaire to identify obstructive sleep apnea. *CPAP,* Continuous positive airway pressure. (From Shilling AM et al: Anesthesia and perioperative medicine. In Miller MD, Thompson SR, editors: *DeLee and Drez's orthopaedic sports medicine: principles and practice,* ed 4, Philadelphia, 2014, Saunders, p 365.)

- More than 2 weeks' preoperative CPAP improved HTN, O_2 saturation, apneic events
- Pulmonary HTN: in 20% to 40% of OSA
- Preoperative serum bicarbonate predicts hypoxia in OSA
  - Chronic respiratory acidosis
- Site of service: (American Society of Anesthesiology consensus statement)
  - Ambulatory surgery under local/regional—lower risk
  - Avoid procedures requiring opioids—greater risk
  - Comorbid conditions must be optimized for outpatient surgery:
    - HTN, arrhythmias, CHF, cardiovascular disease, and metabolic syndrome
- Anesthesia techniques:
  - Prolonged preoxygenation with 100% O_2
  - Avoid preoperative sedatives and excess opioids
  - Rapid intubation after H_2 blockers
  - Avoid long-acting opioids: morphine, hydromorphone
  - Better :
    - NSAIDs, COX-2 inhibitors, acetaminophen
    - Dexamethasone
    - Fentanyl (shorter acting)
  - Avoid flat supine position; sitting position opens airway
- Cervical stability:
  - Adult trauma: C-spine clearance
    - Needed for:
      - Cervical pain
      - Altered mental status
      - Neurologic deficits
      - Distracting injuries
    - Can "clear" with:
      - C-spine with flexion/extension
      - CT of head and neck
  - Children—injury usually higher (occiput, C1-C2)
    - Spinal cord injury without radiographic abnormality (SCIWORA)
      - Ligamentously lax

- Head relatively large
- More likely associated with
- MRI best test
- Anterior ADI over 5 mm is abnormal
  - RA—C spine involved in up to 90%
    - Atlanto-axial synovitis associated with instability
    - Basilar invagination
      - Occipital headaches, neck pain
    - If symptoms, need flexion/extension views
      - Anterior atlanto-dens interval greater than 3.5 abnormal
      - Posterior posterior atlanto-dens interval (space available for the cord) less than 14 mm needs fusion
    - If abnormalities: fiberoptic bronchoscope
- Malignant hyperthermia
  - Genetic defect of T-tubule of sarcoplasmic reticulum
    - Ryanodine receptor defect *(RYR1)*
    - Dihydropyridine receptors *(DHP)*
  - Triggered by volatile anesthetics and succinylcholine
  - Creates an uncontrolled release of Ca^{2+}
    - Sustained muscular contraction—masseter rigidity
      - CO_2—increasing end-tidal CO_2
        - Earliest and most sensitive/specific sign
        - Mixed respiratory and metabolic acidosis
      - Heat: "hyperthermia" is classic but later finding
    - Muscle cell damage (type I slow aerobic marathon)
      - Myoglobin—rhabdomyolysis, ARF
        - Elevated creatine kinase
      - Hyperkalemia—ventricular arrhythmias
  - Risks increased:
    - Male/female, 2 : 1
    - Central core disease (myopathy)
    - Muscular dystrophy:
    - Duchenne and Becker
  - Treatment: dantrolene
    - Decreases intracellular Ca^{2+}
    - Stabilizes sarcoplasmic reticulum
  - Support:
    - 100% O_2,
    - Treat high K^+
    - Hydrate to protect kidneys
    - Cool

■ Wound healing

- A complex response to tissue injury that initially involves cells of the immune system and then progresses to collagen deposition and remodeling by fibroblasts. Also see section on neuromuscular and soft tissue earlier in this chapter.
- Granulation tissue:
  - Mesenchymal cells and capillaries
  - Fibroplasia:
    - Fibroblasts proliferate
    - Synthesize and secrete collagen
    - Continues for 6 weeks
  - Angiogenesis:
    - Endothelial buds (pseudopodia)
    - Form from capillaries
    - Grow new capillaries
  - Maturation:
    - Increased collagen cross-linking
    - 80% strength by 6 weeks
  - Peripheral arterial disease (PAD):
    - Compromises delivery of oxygen and nutrients
    - Absence of pedal pulses
    - Ankle-brachial pressure index by Doppler

- Below 0.9 predicts angiogram will be positive for PAD
- Below 0.5 predicts poor wound healing
- Transcutaneous O_2 below 20 mm Hg
- Diabetes:
  - Chronic issues: DM ($HbA_{1c} < 6.9$)
  - Macrovascular disease: ischemia/hypoxia
    - PAD, coronary artery disease, cardiovascular disease, chronic renal failure
  - Peripheral neuropathy—sensory and motor nerves
    - Loss of protective sensation: increased plantar ulcer risk
      - **5.07 (10 g) monofilament**
      - **Loss of pain and vibration**
  - Acute hyperglycemia:
    - Collagen synthesis suppressed at 200 mg/dL
      - Impaired wound healing
    - WBC phagocytosis impaired at 250 mg/dL
      - Decreased ability to fight infection
- Smoking:
  - Hypoxia
    - **Nicotine—microvascular vasoconstriction**
    - **CO binds to Hb = HbCO**
- Glucocorticoids:
  - Reduce collagen synthesis and wound strength
  - Inhibits:
    - Inflammatory phase
    - Epithelialization
- Nutrition—healing requires:
  - Energy: calories
    - Metabolic increase related to multitrauma: 50%
  - Building blocks: amino acids
    - Collagen—hydroxyproline/lysine
  - Enzymes and cofactors to catalyze reactions:
    - Vitamin C:
      - Converts proline to hydroxyproline
      - Converts lysine to hydroxylysine

- Vitamin A:
  - Increases inflammatory response
  - Effect on lysosomal enzymes
  - Reverses inhibitory effects of prednisone
- Zinc:
  - 150 enzymes use as cofactor
  - When deficient:
    - Decreased fibroblast proliferation
    - Decreased collagen synthesis
    - Impaired wound strength
    - Delayed epithelialization
- Malnutrition: five to seven times greater wound complication rates
  - Screen at-risk patients:
    - Cachexia, morbid obesity, malignancy,
    - History of wound healing issues or alcoholism
  - Diagnosis with history and physical:
    - Weight loss over 6 months—5%, mild; over 10%, severe
    - Arm circumference
      - 60% to 90% of sex matched—moderate
      - Less than 60% of sex matched—severe malnutrition
    - Triceps skinfold and infection in arthroplasty
      - 30 mm ≈ 5% infection
      - 20 mm ≈ 10% infection
    - BMI below 20
  - Diagnosis of malnutrition with laboratory studies:
    - Serum albumin less than 3.5 g/dL
      - Half-life 20 days
    - Serum transferrin less than 200 mg/dL
      - Half-life 8 to 9 days
    - Serum prealbumin less than 22.5 mg/dL
      - Half-life 2 to 3 days
    - Total lymphocyte count less than 1500 cells/mm^3
- Plan:
  - Nutrition consult
  - When gut works, use enteral feeding.

SECTION 4   OTHER BASIC PRINCIPLES

IMAGING AND SPECIAL STUDIES

■ Radiation safety
- Should be considered for every fluoroscopic case
- Increased radiation exposure associated with:
  - Imaging larger body parts
  - Positioning the extremity closer to the x-source
  - Use of large c-arm rather than mini c-arm
- Factors to decrease the amount of radiation exposure
  - **Minimizing exposure time**
  - **Using collimation to manipulate the x-ray beam**
  - **Use of protective shielding**
  - **Maximizing the distance between the surgeon and the radiation beam**
  - **Utilizing mini c-arm whenever feasible (associated with minimal radiation exposure)**
  - **Surgeon control of the c-arm**

■ Nuclear medicine
- Bone scan (Table 1-41)
  - Technetium-99m phosphate complexes
    - Reflect increased blood flow and metabolism

- Absorbed onto hydroxyapatite crystals in bone
  - Areas of infection, trauma, and neoplasia
- Whole-body views and more detailed (pinhole) views possible

Table 1-41	Nuclear Medicine Studies	
STUDY	**USES**	**COMMENTS**
Bone scan	Subtle fractures Avascular necrosis Osteomyelitis Total joint loosening Osteochondritis	Three-phase scan useful for osteomyelitis, reflex sympathetic dystrophy, acute scaphoid fractures
Gallium	Inflammation Neoplasms	Localizes in sites of inflammation Requires prolonged uptake
Indium-111	Acute infections Possible arthroplasty infections	Labeled WBC uptake in areas of infection

- Evaluative uses:
  - Subtle fractures
  - Avascular necrosis
    - Hypoperfused early
    - Increased uptake in reparative phase
  - Osteomyelitis
    - Especially triple-phase study
    - Also in conjunction with gallium or indium scan
  - THA and TKA loosening
    - Especially femoral components
    - In conjunction with gallium scan to rule out infection
  - Patellofemoral overload
  - Osteochondritis dissecans of the talus
- Phase studies
  - Three-phase (or even four-phase) studies
    - Helpful for reflex sympathetic dystrophy and osteomyelitis
    - Most reliable test for nondisplaced scaphoid fracture
  - First phase (blood flow, immediate)
    - Blood flow through the arterial system
  - Second phase (blood pool, 30 minutes)
    - Equilibrium of tracer throughout the intravascular volume
  - Third phase (delayed, 4 hours)
    - Displays sites of tracer accumulation
  - May be negative in pediatric septic arthritis
- Gallium (Gallium-67 citrate) scan
  - Localizes in sites of inflammation and neoplasia
    - Exudation of labeled serum proteins
  - Delayed imaging required (24-48 hours or more)
  - Less dependent on vascular flow than is technetium
    - May identify foci otherwise missed
  - Difficulty differentiating cellulitis from osteomyelitis
- Indium-111 scan
  - Labeled WBCs (leukocytes)
    - Collect in areas of inflammation
    - Do not collect in areas of neoplasia
  - Uses:
    - Acute infections (e.g., osteomyelitis)
    - Possibly TJA infections
- Technetium-labeled WBC scan: similar to indium scan
- Radiolabeled monoclonal antibodies
  - May identify primary malignancies and metastatic disease
- DVT/PE scan
  - Radioactive iodine
    - Labels fibrinogen in clot on scanning
    - Inaccurate near surgical wounds
  - Lung scans: may help evaluate pulmonary blood flow
    - Limited at present
- Single-photon emission computed tomography (SPECT)
  - Scintigraphy with CT to evaluate overlapping structures
    - Femoral head osteonecrosis
    - Patellofemoral syndrome
    - Spondylolysis
- **Arthrography (Table 1-42)**
- **MRI**
- Introduction
  - Excellent for evaluating soft tissues and bone marrow
  - Ineffective in evaluating trabecular bone and cortical bone
    - These tissues have virtually no hydrogen nuclei

- Used to evaluate osteonecrosis, neoplasms, infection, and trauma
- Allows both axial and sagittal representations
- Contraindications:
  - Pacemakers
  - Cerebral aneurysm clips
  - Shrapnel or hardware, in certain locations
- Basic principles of MRI (Tables 1-43 through 1-46)
  - Radiofrequency pulses on tissues in a magnetic field
  - Images in any desired plan
  - Nuclei with odd numbers of protons/neutrons (with a normally random spin) aligned parallel to a magnetic field
    - Field strength: 0.5 to 15 T (1 T = 10,000 G)
      - **3.0 T has 9 times greater proton energy**
    - No ionizing radiation
  - Nuclear magnetic moments of these particles deflected by radiofrequency pulses; results in an image
  - The use of surface coils decreases the signal-to-noise ratio.
    - Body coils are used for large joints
    - Smaller coils are available
  - Sequences developed to demonstrate the differences in T1 and T2 relaxation between tissues
  - T1 images weighted toward fat with TR (time to repetition) values lower than 1000 ms
  - T2 images weighted toward water with TR values higher than 1000 ms
  - Dark on T1- and bright on T2-weighted images
    - Water
    - Cerebrospinal fluid
    - Acute hemorrhage
    - Soft tissue tumors
  - Tissues showing similar intensity on both T1- and T2-weighted images:
    - Dark: cortical bone, rapid flowing blood, fibrous tissue
    - Gray: muscle and hyaline cartilage
    - Bright: fatty tissue, nerves, slow flowing (venous) blood, bone marrow
  - T1-weighted images best for demonstrating anatomic structure
  - T2-weighted images best for contrasting normal and abnormal tissues
  - "Magic angle phenomena":
    - Tendon or ligament tissue oriented near 55 degrees to the field produces bright T1-weighted images
    - False appearance of pathologic process
    - Most common in shoulder, ankle, knee
  - Techniques for identifying contrast between fluid and nonfluid elements (e.g., bone, fat)
    - Spin tau inversion recovery (STIR)
    - Fat-suppressed T2-weighted images
- Specific applications
  - Osteonecrosis
    - Highest sensitivity and specificity for early detection
      - Detects early marrow necrosis
      - Detects ingrowth of vascularized mesenchymal tissue
    - Specificity of 98% and high reliability for estimating age and extent of disease
    - Diseased marrow dark on T1-weighted images
      - Allows direct assessment of overlying cartilage
  - Infection and trauma
    - Excellent sensitivity to increased free water
    - Shows areas of infection and fresh hemorrhage

Table 1-42	Arthrographic Findings	
ANATOMIC LOCATION	**CONDITIONS**	**DESCRIPTION**
Shoulder		Technique can entail single or double contrast agents (better detail)
	Rotator cuff tear	Extravasation of contrast through the tear into the subacromial bursa
	Adhesive capsulitis	Demonstrates diminished joint capsule size and loss of the normal axillary fold
		May be therapeutic (distends the capsule)
	Recurrent dislocations	May demonstrate a distended capsule or disruption of the glenoid labrum
		Use with tomography or computed tomography to better demonstrate capsular or labral disease
	Other	Bicipital tendon abnormalities
		Articular disease
		Impingement syndrome
Elbow	Articular cartilage defects/loose bodies	Especially helpful when used with tomography
	Osteochondral fractures	
Wrist	Posttraumatic ligament disruption	Communication between compartments is used to determine pathologic process, but communication is common in asymptomatic patients older than 40 years
		Communication at the radiocarpal and midcarpal joints: suspect scapholunate or lunoquitetral ligament tear
		Communication at the radiocarpal and distal radioulnar joints: suspect a triangular fibrocartilage complex (TFCC) tear
Hip		
Infants and children	"Septic" hip	Obtain aspirate and assess joint damage
	Developmental dysplasia of the hip	Degree of joint incongruity: interposed limbus
	Legg-Calvé-Perthes disease	Severity of deformity
Adolescents and adults	Arthritis	Cartilage destruction and loose bodies
	Osteochondral fractures, chondrolysis, and THA loosening	Digital subtraction arthrography can be useful for suspected loose THAs
Knee	Meniscal tears (except posterior horn of the lateral meniscus) and discoid lateral menisci	Can be useful for screening patients with equivocal history or findings
		Evaluation of cruciate ligaments yields less accurate findings than does evaluation of the menisci
	Articular cartilage evaluation	
	Loose bodies	Only air contrast is recommended for evaluation of loose bodies
	Pathologic synovial tissue	PVNS, popliteal cysts, synovial chondromatosis, plicae
Ankle	Acutely torn ligaments	
	Chronic osseous and osteocartilaginous abnormalities	
Spine	Facet joints	May be useful combined with therapeutic injections (anesthetics and steroids)

PVNS, Pigmented villonodular synovitis; *THA*, total hip arthroplasty.

- Dark on T1-weighted images, bright on T2-weighted images
- Excellent (accurate and sensitive) for occult fractures
  - Particularly in hip in elderly patients
- Neoplasms
  - MRI has many applications in the study of primary and metastatic bone tumors
  - Primary tumors are well demonstrated
    - Particularly tumors in soft tissue (extraosseous and marrow)
  - Used in evaluating skip lesions and spinal metastases
    - Nuclear medicine studies remain the procedure of choice for seeking metastatic foci in bone
  - Demonstrates benign bony tumors
    - Typically bright on T1-weighted images and dark on T2-weighted images
  - Demonstrates malignant bony lesions
    - Often bright on T2-weighted images
  - Differential diagnosis is best made on the basis of plain radiographs.
- Spine
  - Disc disease is well demonstrated on T2-weighted images.

Table 1-43	Magnetic Resonance Imaging Terminology
TERM	**EXPLANATION**
T1	Time constant of exponential growth of magnetism; T1 signal measures how rapidly a tissue gains magnetism
T2	Time constant of exponential decay of signal after an excitation pulse; a tissue with a long T2 signal (such as that with a high water content) maintains its signal (is bright on T2-weighted image)
T2*	Similar to T2 but includes the effects of magnetic field homogeneity
TR	Time to repetition; the time between successive excitation pulses; short TR is less than 80 ms, long TR is greater than 80
TE	Time to echo; the time that an echo is formed by the refocusing pulse; short TE is less than 1000 ms, long TE is greater than 1000
NEX	Number of excitations; higher NEX results in decreased noise with better images
FOV	Field of view
Spin-echo	A commonly used pulse sequence
FSE	Fast spin-echo; a type of pulse sequence
GRE	Gradient-recalled echo; a type of pulse sequence

Table 1-44	Signal Intensities on Magnetic Resonance Imaging	
TISSUE	**APPEARANCE ON T1-WEIGHTED IMAGE**	**APPEARANCE ON T2-WEIGHTED IMAGE**
Cortical bone	Dark	Dark
Osteomyelitis	Dark	Bright
Ligaments	Dark	Dark
Fibrocartilage	Dark	Dark
Hyaline cartilage	Gray	Gray
Meniscus	Dark	Dark
Meniscal tear	Bright	Gray
Yellow bone marrow (fatty-appendicular)	Bright	Gray
Red bone marrow (hematopoietic-axial)	Gray	Gray
Marrow edema	Dark	Bright
Fat	Bright	Gray
Normal fluid	Dark	Bright
Abnormal fluid (pus)	Gray	Bright
Acute blood collection	Gray	Dark
Chronic blood collection	Bright	Bright
Muscle	Gray	Gray
Tendon	Dark	Dark
Intervertebral disc (central)	Gray	Bright
Intervertebral disc (peripheral)	Dark	Gray

Modified from Brinker MR, Miller MD: *Fundamentals of orthopaedics*, Philadelphia, 1999, WB Saunders, p 24.

Table 1-45	Magnetic Resonance Imaging of Bone Marrow Disorders		
DISORDER	**PATHOLOGIC FEATURES**	**EXAMPLES**	**MRI CHANGES**
Reconversion	Yellow→red	Anemia, metastasis	↓ T1-weighted intensity
Marrow infiltration		Tumor, infection	↓ T1-weighted intensity
Myeloid depletion		Anemia, chemotherapy	↓ T1-weighted intensity
Marrow edema		Trauma, CRPS	↓ T1-weighted intensity, ↑ T2-weighted intensity
Marrow ischemia		Osteonecrosis	↓ T1-weighted intensity

↑, Increased; ↓, decreased; *CRPS*, complex regional pain syndrome.

Table 1-46	Magnetic Resonance Imaging Changes of Meniscal Disease
DISEASE GROUP	**CHARACTERISTICS**
I	Globular areas of hyperintense signal
II	Linear hyperintense signal
III	Linear hyperintense signal that communicates with the meniscal surface (tears)
IV	Vertical longitudinal tear/truncation

- Degenerated discs lose water.
- Appear dark on T2-weighted studies
- Extent of herniation of discs is also well shown.
- Recurrent disc herniation is best diagnosed with gadolinium MRI scan.
  - Differentiation from scar:
    - On T1-weighted image:
      - Scar: decreased signal
      - Free fragment: increased signal
      - Extruded disc: decreased signal
    - On T2-weighted image:
      - Scar: increased signal
      - Free fragment: increased signal
      - Extruded disc: decreased signal
  - MRI is most sensitive for diagnosing early discitis.
    - Decreased signal on T1-weighted images, increased signal on T2-weighted images

- MRI can help evaluate the spine in asymptomatic persons:
  - Cervical spine abnormality is seen in 28% of those older than age 40.
  - Lumbar disc herniation is seen in 20% to 30% of those younger than age 40.
  - Evidence of degeneration or bulging of lumbar discs is seen in 93% of those older than age 60.
  - Biochemical studies show degenerative disc changes as early as the second decade of life.
- Bone marrow changes
  - Best demonstrated by MRI (poor specificity) (see Table 1-45)
- Knee MRI
  - Arthrography with MRI
    - Accomplished with instillation of saline, which creates iatrogenic effusion
    - Improves joint definition
  - Knee derangements well demonstrated on MRI
    - ACL rupture correctly diagnosed in 95% of cases
    - Meniscal changes also demonstrated (see Table 1-46)
    - Best radiologic test for posterior cruciate ligament (PCL) rupture
- Shoulder MRI
  - Rotator cuff tears
    - Sensitivity and specificity: about 90%
    - Grade 0 tears: normal signal intensity
    - Grades 1, 2, and 3 tears: increased signal intensity

- Morphologic features:
  - Grades 0 and 1 tears: normal
  - Grade 2 tears: abnormal
  - Grade 3 tears: discontinuity
  - Capsular/labral tears
- Efficacy of MRI equals that of CT arthrography in presence of effusion.
- MRI spectroscopy may help measure metabolic changes (ischemia)

■ **Other imaging studies**

▨ CT
- Demonstrates details of bony anatomy better than any other study
- Hounsfield units used to identify tissue types
  - −100 = air
  - −100 to 0 = fat
  - 0 = water
  - 100 = soft tissue
  - 1000 = bone
- Multiple-detector row arrays
  - Improved resolution in the longitudinal axis
  - Decreased data acquisition times
  - Improved spatial resolution
  - Improved quality of reconstructing algorithms
  - Reduced artifact caused by hardware
- Shows herniated nucleus pulposus better than myelography alone
  - CT may be helpful differentiating disc herniation from scar
  - IV contrast material is taken up in scar tissue but not in disc tissue.
- Frequently used with contrast material
  - Arthrographic CT, myelographic CT
- CT digital radiography (CT scanography)
  - Accurate demonstration of leg length discrepancy with minimal radiation exposure
    - Particularly when joint contractures exist (lateral scanography)
- Best demonstrates joint incongruity after closed reduction of hip dislocation
- Useful for measuring the cross-sectional dural area in the workup of cervical spinal stenosis
  - Spinal stenosis is diagnosed if this area is less than 100 mm^2.
- Important for evaluating subtalar joint injuries and diagnosing tarsal coalitions
  - Talocalcaneal tarsal coalitions also well visualized on axial (Harris) radiographs
- Dynamic CT scanning: test of choice for atlantoaxial rotatory subluxation
  - Grisel syndrome: spontaneous atlantoaxial subluxation in conjunction with soft tissue inflammation in the neck, such as pharyngitis
- Images distorted by metal implants

▨ Ultrasonography
- Shoulder—diagnosing rotator cuff tears
- Hip
  - Diagnosis and follow-up of developmental hip dysplasia
  - Identification of iliopsoas bursitis in adults
- Knee
  - Determination of articular cartilage thickness
  - Identification of intraarticular fluid

- Soft tissue masses
- Hematoma
- Tendon rupture
- Abscesses
- Foreign body location
- Intraspinal disorders in infants
- Aorta
  - In patients at increased risk for aortic dilation or rupture
  - In patients with Marfan syndrome
- Fractures—to evaluate progression of fracture healing

▨ Guided biopsy
- Workup of musculoskeletal lesions
- Commonly in conjunction with CT

▨ Myelography
- Procedure of choice for extramedullary intradural pathologic processes
- Cervical radiculopathy
- Subarachnoid cysts
- Failed back syndrome
- Can be used with other studies such as CT

▨ Discography
- Use controversial
- Helpful for evaluating symptomatic disc degeneration
- Pathologic discs: reproduction of pain with injection and characteristic changes on discograms
- Commonly used with CT

▨ Measurement of bone density (noninvasive)
- Single-photon absorptiometry
  - Cortical bone density is inversely proportional to quantity of photons passing through it
  - Radioisotope ^{125}I emits a single energy beam of photons.
    - ^{125}I passes through bone.
    - A sodium iodide scintillation counter detects the transmitted photons.
  - Denser bone attenuates the photon beam.
    - Fewer photons reach the scintillation counter.
  - Best used in the appendicular skeleton
    - Radius: diaphysis or distal metaphysis
  - Findings are unreliable in the axial skeleton
    - Soft tissue depth alters the beam.
- Dual-photon absorptiometry
  - Also an isotope-based method
  - Allows for measurement of the axial skeleton and the femoral neck
    - Accounts for soft tissue attenuation
- Quantitative CT
  - Preferred for measurement of trabecular bone density
    - Trabecular bone is at greatest risk for early metabolic changes
  - Simultaneous scanning of phantoms of known density
    - Creating a standard calibration curve
  - Accuracy within 5% to 10%
  - Radiation dose higher than that for dual-energy x-ray absorptiometry (DEXA)
- DEXA
  - Most accurate and reliable for predicting fracture risk
  - Radiation dose lower than that for quantitative CT
  - Measures bone mineral content and soft tissue components

Table 1-47	Nerve Conduction Study Results		
CONDITION	**LATENCY**	**CONDUCTION VELOCITY**	**EVOKED RESPONSE**
Normal study	Normal	Upper extremities: >45 m/sec; lower extremities: >40 m/sec	Biphasic
Axonal neuropathy	Increased	Normal or slightly decreased	Prolonged, decreased amplitude
Demyelinating neuropathy	Normal	Decreased (10%-50%)	Normal or prolonged, with decreased amplitude
Anterior horn cell disease	Normal	Normal (rarely decreased)	Normal or polyphasic, with prolonged duration and decreased amplitude
Myopathy	Normal	Normal	Decreased amplitude; may be normal
Neurapraxia			
Proximal to lesion	Absent	Absent	Absent
Distal to lesion	Normal	Normal	Normal
Axonotmesis			
Proximal to lesion	Absent	Absent	Absent
Distal to lesion	Absent	Absent	Normal
Neurotmesis			
Proximal to lesion	Absent	Absent	Absent
Distal to lesion	Absent	Absent	Absent

Modified from Jahss MH: *Disorders of the foot,* Philadelphia, 1982, WB Saunders.

■ Electrodiagnostic studies
- Nerve conduction studies
  - Evaluation of peripheral nerves
    - Sensory and motor responses along their courses
  - Nerve impulses stimulated and recorded by surface electrodes
    - Allows calculation of conduction velocity
  - Measures latency (time from stimulus onset to response) and response amplitude
  - Late responses (F wave, H reflex) allow evaluation of proximal lesions.
    - Impulse travels to the spinal cord and returns
  - Somatosensory evoked potentials
    - Used to evaluate brachial plexus injuries
    - Used for spinal cord monitoring
- Electromyography
  - Intramuscular needle electrodes to evaluate muscle units
  - Used to evaluate denervation
    - Fibrillations; earliest sign usually at 4 weeks
    - Sharp waves
    - Abnormal recruitment pattern
- Interpretation
  - Peripheral nerve entrapment syndromes
    - **Distal motor and sensory latencies longer than 35 m/sec**
    - **Nerve conduction velocities shorter than 50 m/sec**
    - Changes over a distinct interval (Table 1-47)

BIOMATERIALS AND BIOMECHANICS

■ Basic concepts
- Definitions
  - Biomechanics—science of forces, internal or external, on the living body
  - Statics—action of forces on rigid bodies in a system in equilibrium
    - At rest
    - Moving at a constant velocity
  - Dynamics—bodies that are accelerating and the related forces
    - Kinematics—study of motion (displacement, velocity, and acceleration) without reference to forces
    - Kinetics—relates the effects of forces to motion

- Kinesiology—study of human movements and motions
  - Kinematics
  - Kinetics
  - Anatomy
  - Physiology
  - Motor control
- Principal quantities
  - Basic quantities—described by International System of Units (SI); metric system
    - Length: meters (m)
    - Mass (quantity of matter): kilograms (kg)
    - Time: seconds (sec)
  - Derived quantities: derived from basic quantities
    - Velocity
      - Time rate of change of displacement (meters/second)
      - Rate of translational displacement: *linear velocity*
      - Rate of rotational displacement: *angular velocity*
    - Acceleration
      - Time rate of change of velocity (m/sec^2)
      - Can also be linear or angular
    - Force
      - Action causing acceleration of a mass (body) in a certain direction
      - Unit of measure: newton (N) = kg • m/sec^2
- Newton's laws
  - First law: inertia
    - If the net external force (F) acting on a body is zero, the body will remain at rest or move with a constant velocity.
    - This law allows static analysis: $\Sigma F = 0$ (sum of external forces = zero)
  - Second law: acceleration
    - Acceleration (*a*) of an object of mass (*m*) is directly proportional to the force (*F*) applied to the object:

$$F = ma$$

  - This law is used in dynamic analysis.
  - Third law: reactions
    - For every action (force), there is an equal and opposite reaction (force).
    - This law leads to free-body analysis.
    - This law also assists in the study of interacting bodies.

- Scalar and vector quantities
  - Scalar quantities
    - Have magnitude but no direction
    - Examples: volume, time, mass, and speed (not velocity)
  - Vector quantities
    - Have magnitude and direction
    - Examples: force and velocity
    - Vectors have four characteristics:
      - Magnitude (length of the vector)
      - Direction (head of the vector)
      - Point of application (tail of the vector)
      - Line of action (orientation of the vector)
    - Vectors can be added, subtracted, and split into components (resolved)
      - Resultant of two vectors: principle of "parallelogram of forces"
  - Tensors
    - Tensors are arrays of numbers or functions that represent the physical properties of a system.
      - Scalars (e.g., mass) are tensors of rank 0.
      - Vectors (e.g., force) are tensors of rank 1.
      - Stress (force per unit area) is an example of a tensor of rank 2.
        - Stress has magnitude and direction and is determined over a plane (surface) rather than a line.
    - Higher order tensors represent properties more complex than can be represented by vectors.
- Free-body analysis
  - Forces, moments, and free-body diagrams to analyze the action of forces on bodies
  - Know how to solve these problems!
  - Force
    - A mechanical push or pull (load) that causes external (acceleration) and internal (strain) effects
    - Unit of measure: the newton (N)
    - Force vectors (F): can be split into independent components for analysis
      - Usually in the x and y directions (F_x, F_y).
      - With angle (θ) between F_x and F_y.
    - Some elementary knowledge of trigonometry is helpful.
      - $F_x = F \cos \theta$
      - $F_y = F \sin \theta$
    - Also remember the following approximations:

$$\sin 30 = \cos 60 \cong 0.5$$

$$\sin 45 = \cos 45 \cong 0.7$$

$$\sin 60 = \cos 30 \cong 0.9$$

  - A *normal* force is perpendicular to the surface on which it acts.
  - A *tangential* force is parallel to the surface.
  - A *compressive* force shrinks a body in the direction of the force.
  - A *tensile* force elongates a body.
  - Moment (M)
    - Rotational effect of a force
    - Moment = force (F) multiplied by the perpendicular distance (the moment arm or lever arm = d) from point of rotation:

$$M = F \times d$$

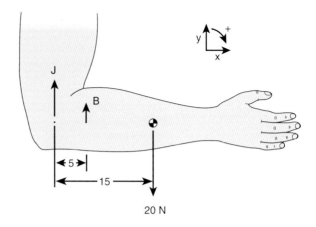

$$\sum M_J = 0 \qquad \sum F_j = 0$$
$$-B(.05\text{ m}) + 20\text{ N}(.15\text{ m}) = 0 \qquad J + B - 20\text{ N} = 0$$
$$B(.05\text{ m}) = 3\text{ Nm} \qquad J = 20\text{ N} - B$$
$$B = 60\text{ N} \qquad J = 20\text{ N} - 60\text{ N} = -40\text{ N}$$

FIGURE 1-83 Free-body diagram (see text for explanation). *B,* Biceps force; *J,* joint compressive force; *M,* moment; *N,* newton (mass).

  - *Torque* is a moment from a force perpendicular to the long axis of a body, causing rotation.
  - A *bending moment* is from a force parallel to the long axis.
  - The *mass moment of inertia* is the resistance to rotation.
    - Product of mass times the square of the moment arm:

$$I = m \times d^2$$

    - Affects angular acceleration
- Free-body diagram
  - A free-body diagram is a sketch of a body (or segments) isolated from other bodies, showing all forces acting on it.
  - The weight of each object acts through its center of gravity.
  - **Center of gravity in the human body is just anterior to S2**
- Free-body analysis
  - The following steps are used in the analysis:
    - Identify the system (objective, known quantities, assumptions).
    - Select a coordinate system.
    - Isolate free bodies (free-body diagram).
    - Apply Newton's laws; establish equilibrium ($\Sigma F = 0$ and $\Sigma M = 0$).
    - Solve for unknown quantities.
  - Assumptions
    - No change in motion
    - No deformation
    - No friction
  - Example (Figure 1-83)
    - Calculate biceps force (B) needed to hold the 20-N weight of the forearm:
      - Elbow flexed 90 degrees
      - Biceps insertion: 5 cm distal to the elbow

- Center of gravity of the forearm: 15 cm distal to the elbow
  - *Answer:* 60 N
- Also solve for the joint (compressive) force (J):
  - Answer: −40 N
- Finite element analysis
  - Complex geometric forms and material properties are modeled.
  - A structure is modeled as a finite number of simple geometric forms.
    - Typically triangular or trapezoidal elements
  - A computer matches forces and moments between neighboring elements.
  - Finite element analysis is often used to estimate internal stresses and strains.
    - Example: stress/strain at bone-implant interface
- Other important basic concepts are as follows:
  - Work
    - The product of a force and the displacement it causes
    - Work (W) = force (F; vector components parallel to displacement) × distance (displacement produced by F)
    - Unit of measure: joule (J) = N • *m*
  - Energy
    - Ability to perform work (unit of measure is also joule)
    - Laws of conservation of energy:
      - Energy is neither created nor destroyed.
      - It is transferred from one state to another.
    - Potential energy
      - Stored energy
      - Potential of a body to do work as a result of its position or configuration (e.g., strain energy)
    - Kinetic energy—energy caused by motion ($\frac{1}{2}mv^2$)

  - Friction (*f*)
    - Resistance to motion when one body slides over another
      - Produced at points of contact
    - Oriented opposite to the applied force
    - When applied force exceeds *f*, motion begins.
    - Proportional to coefficient of friction and applied normal (perpendicular) load
      - Independent of contact area and surface shape
  - Piezoelectricity
    - Electrical charge when a force deforms a crystalline structure (e.g., bone)
    - Concave (compression) side: charge is electronegative
    - Convex (tension) side: charge is electropositive
- **Biomaterials**
- Strength of materials
  - Branch of mechanics—study of relations between externally applied loads and resulting internal effects
  - Loads
    - Forces acting on a body
    - Compression, tension, shear, and torsion
  - Deformations
    - Temporary (elastic) or permanent (plastic) change in shape
    - Load changes produce deformational changes
  - Elasticity—ability to return to resting length after undergoing lengthening or shortening
  - Extensibility—ability to be lengthened

- Stress
  - Intensity of internal force
    - Stress = force/area
    - *Internal* resistance of a body to a load
  - Unit of measure: pascal (Pa) = N/m^2
  - Helps in selection of materials
  - Normal stresses
    - Compressive or tensile
    - Perpendicular to the surfaces on which they act
  - Shear stresses
    - Parallel to the surfaces on which they act
    - Cause a part of a body to be displaced in relation to another part
  - Stress differs from *pressure:*
    - Pressure is the distribution of an *external* force to a solid body.
    - However, they share the same definition (force/area) and unit of measure (Pa).
- Strain
  - Relative measure of deformation (six components) resulting from loading
  - Strain = change in length/original length
  - Can also be normal or shear
  - Strain is a proportion; it has no units.
  - Strain rate
    - Strain divided by time load is applied (units = sec^{-1}).
- Hooke's law: stress is proportional to strain up to a limit.
  - The proportional limit
  - Within the elastic zone
- Young's modulus of elasticity (E)
  - Measure of material stiffness
    - Also a measure of the material's ability to resist deformation in tension
    - E = stress/strain
    - E is the slope in the elastic range of the stress-strain curve.
  - The critical factor in load-sharing capacity
  - Linearly perfect elastic material
    - A straight stress-strain curve to the point of failure
    - Modulus = stress at failure (ultimate stress) divided by strain at failure (ultimate strain)
  - E is unique for every type of material
    - A material with a higher E can withstand greater forces than can material with a lower E
- Shear modulus
  - Ratio of shear stress to shear strain
  - A measure of stiffness
  - Unit of measure: pascal (Pa)
- Stress-strain curve (Figure 1-84)
  - Derived by loading a body and plotting stress versus strain
    - The curve's shape varies by material.
  - Proportional limit—transition point at which stress and strain are no longer proportional
    - The material returns to its original length when stress removed: elastic behavior
  - Elastic limit (yield point)
    - This is the transition point from elastic to plastic behavior.
    - Beyond this point, the material's structure is irreversibly changed.
    - The elastic limit equals 0.2% strain in most metals.

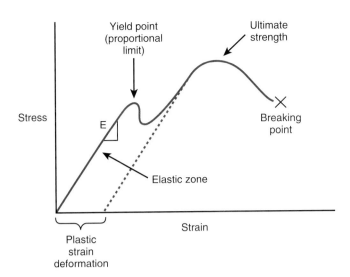

FIGURE 1-84 Stress-strain curve. *E,* Young's modulus of elasticity.

- Plastic deformation—irreversible change after load is removed
  - Occurs in the plastic range of the curve
  - After the elastic limit, before the breaking point
- Ultimate strength—maximum strength obtained by the material
- Breaking point—point at which the material fractures
  - If deformation between elastic limit and breaking point is large, material is **ductile.**
  - If deformation between elastic limit and breaking point is small, material is **brittle.**
- Strain energy (toughness)
  - Capacity of material (e.g., bone) to absorb energy
  - Area under the stress-strain curve
  - Total strain energy = recoverable strain energy (resilience) + dissipated strain energy
  - **A measure of the toughness of material**
    - Ability to absorb energy before failure
▥ Materials and structures
- Material
  - Related to a substance or element
    - Mechanical properties:
      - Force
      - Stress
      - Strain
    - Rheologic properties:
      - Elasticity
      - Plasticity
      - Viscosity: resistance to flow or shear stress
      - Strength
  - Brittle materials (e.g., PMMA)
    - Stress-strain curve is linear up to failure.
    - These materials undergo only recoverable (elastic) deformation before failure.
    - They have little or no capacity for plastic deformation.
  - Ductile materials (e.g., metal)
    - These materials undergo large plastic deformation before failure.
    - Ductility is a measure of postyield deformation.
  - Viscoelastic materials (e.g., bone and ligaments)
    - Stress-strain behavior is time-rate dependent.
      - Depend on load magnitude and rate at which the load is applied

- A function of internal friction
- Exhibit both fluid (viscosity) and solid (elasticity) properties
- Modulus increases as strain rate increases.
- Exhibit hysteresis
  - Loading and unloading curves differ.
  - Energy is dissipated during loading.
- Most biological tissues exhibit viscoelasticity.
- Isotropic materials
  - Mechanical properties are the same for all directions of applied load (e.g., as with a golf ball)
- Anisotropic materials
  - Mechanical properties vary with the direction of the applied load.
  - Example: bone is stronger with axial load than with radial load
- Homogeneous materials
  - Have a uniform structure or composition throughout
- Structure
  - Material, shape, and loading characteristics
  - Load deformation curve:
    - Constructed similarly to stress-strain curve
    - Slope in the elastic range is the rigidity of the structure.
  - Bending rigidity of a rectangular structure:
    - Proportional to the base multiplied by the height cubed:

$$bh^3/12$$

- Bending rigidity of a cylinder
  - Related to the fourth power of the radius
  - Intramedullary nails, half-pins
  - Closely related to area moment of inertia (I)
    - Resistance to bending
    - Function of width, thickness, and the polar moment of inertia (J)
    - J: resistance to torsion (twisting)
    - I and J: functions of the distribution of material in cross section
      - Distance squared of mass distribution from the center of mass
  - Deflection associated with bending
    - Proportional to applied force (F) divided by elastic modulus (E) and then multiplied by area moment of inertia (I):

$$\text{Deflection} = (F/E) \times (I)$$

- Metals
  - Fatigue failure
    - Occurs with cyclic loading at stress below ultimate tensile strength
    - Depends on magnitude of stress and number of cycles
    - Endurance limit
      - Maximum stress under which the material will not fail regardless of number of loading cycles
      - If the stress is below this limit, the material may be loaded cyclically an infinite number of times ($>10^6$ cycles) without breaking.
      - Above this limit, fatigue life is expressed by the *S-n* curve:
        - Stress (S) versus the number of cycles (n)

Table 1-48	Types of Corrosion
CORROSION	**DESCRIPTION**
Galvanic	Dissimilar metals*; electrochemical destruction
Crevice	Occurs in fatigue cracks with low O_2 tension
Stress	Occurs in areas with high stress gradients
Fretting	From small movements abrading outside layer
Other	For example, inclusion, intergranular

*Metals such as 316 L stainless steel and cobalt-chromium-molybdenum (Co-Cr-Mo) alloy produce galvanic corrosion.

- Creep (cold flow)
  - Progressive deformation response to constant force over an extended period of time
  - Sudden stress followed by constant loading causes continued deformation.
  - Can produce permanent deformity
  - May affect mechanical function (e.g., in TJA)
- Corrosion (Table 1-48)
  - Chemical dissolving of metals
    - May occur in the body's high-saline environment
  - Stainless steel (316 L)
    - The metal most susceptible to both crevice corrosion and galvanic corrosion
    - **Risk of galvanic corrosion highest between 316 L stainless steel and cobalt-chromium (Co-Cr) alloy**
  - Modular components of THA
    - Direct contact between similar or dissimilar metals at the modular junctions
    - Results in corrosion products
      - Examples: metal oxides, metal chlorides
  - Corrosion can be decreased in the following ways:
    - Using similar metals
    - Proper implant design
    - Passivation by an adherent oxide layer
      - Effectively separates metal from solution
      - Example: stainless steel coated with chromium oxide
- Types of metals
  - Orthopaedic implants
    - Three types of alloys: steel (iron-based), cobalt-based, titanium-based
    - 316 L stainless steel
      - Iron-carbon, chromium, nickel, molybdenum, manganese
      - Nickel: increases corrosion resistance and stabilizes molecular structure
      - Chromium: forms a passive surface oxide, improving corrosion resistance
      - Molybdenum: prevents pitting and crevice corrosion
      - Manganese: improves crystalline stability
      - "L"—low carbon: greater corrosion resistance
    - Cobalt alloys
      - Cobalt-chromium-molybdenum (Co-Cr-Mo)
        - 65% cobalt, 35% chromium, 5% molybdenum
        - Special forging process
        - Nickel may be added to improve ease of forging.
        - Increased ultimate strength compared to titanium

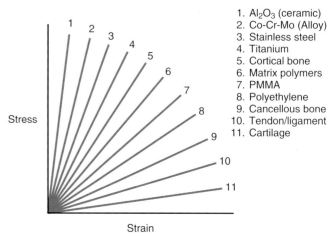

1. Al_2O_3 (ceramic)
2. Co-Cr-Mo (Alloy)
3. Stainless steel
4. Titanium
5. Cortical bone
6. Matrix polymers
7. PMMA
8. Polyethylene
9. Cancellous bone
10. Tendon/ligament
11. Cartilage

Stress / Strain

FIGURE 1-85 Comparison of Young's modulus (relative values, not to scale) for various orthopaedic materials. *Al2O3,* Alumina; *Co-Cr-Mo,* cobalt-chromium-molybdenum; *PMMA,* polymethylmethacrylate.

- Titanium alloy (Ti-6Al-4 V)
  - Stiffness (*E*) differences (Figure 1-85)
- Problems with certain metals:
  - Wear
  - Stress shielding
    - Increased in metals with a higher *E*
  - Ion release
    - Co-Cr: macrophage proliferation and synovial degeneration
    - Ions excreted through the kidneys
- Titanium: poor resistance to wear (notch sensitivity)
  - Particulate may incite a histiocytic response.
  - The relationship between titanium and neoplasms is uncertain.
  - Polishing, passivation, and ion implantation improve its fatigue properties.
  - Titanium is extremely biocompatible:
    - Rapidly forms an adherent oxide coating (self-passivation); decreases corrosion
    - A nonreactive ceramic coating
  - Other advantages of titanium:
    - Relatively low *E*
    - Most closely emulates axial and torsional stiffness of bone
    - High yield strength
- Co-Cr alloy
  - Generates less metal debris (in THA) than does titanium alloy
  - Better resistance to corrosion than stainless steel
  - Problems with orthosis fabrication
- Tantalum—passive material designed to elicit a response (bone ingrowth)
  - Surface oxide layer as barrier to corrosion
  - Used as augmentation of cancellous defects
- Nonmetal materials
  - Polyethylene
    - Ultra-high-molecular-weight polyethylene (UHMWPE)
      - Polymer of long carbon chains
      - **Direct molding resin into finished part leads to the net shape**

- Used in weight-bearing components of TJAs
  - Acetabular cups, tibial trays
- Wear characteristics superior to those of high-density polyethylene
  - Tough, ductile, resilient, resistant to wear, low friction
- Polyethylene: viscoelastic and highly susceptible to abrasion
  - Wear damage to a UHMWPE articulating surface is most often caused by third-body inclusions
- UHMWPE: also thermoplastic
  - May be altered by temperature or high-dose radiation
- Oxidative polyethylene degradation after γ-irradiation in air
  - This degradation is related to free radical formation.
    - Increases susceptibility to oxidation
  - γ-Irradiation increases polymer chain cross-links.
    - **Greatly improves wear characteristics**
    - However, reduces resistance to fatigue and fracture
    - Decreases elastic modulus, tensile strength, ductility, and yield stress
- Annealing
  - Heating to below melting point
  - **Decreases free radicals**
  - Good mechanical properties; does not disrupt crystalline areas
- Polyethylene is weaker than bone in tension and has a low E.
- **Wear debris associated with a histiocytic osteolytic response**
  - Particles with a size range of 0.1 to 1.0 μm are most reactive
  - This response is increased with thinner (<6 mm), flatter, carbon fiber–reinforced polyethylene.
- Metal backing may help minimize plastic deformation of high-density polyethylene and loosening.
  - But decreases effective thickness of polyethylene
- Catastrophic wear of polyethylene tibial inserts associated with:
  - Varus knee alignment
  - Thin inserts (<6 mm)
  - Flat, nonconforming inserts
  - Heat treatments of the insert
- Polyethylene wear debris: main factor affecting THA longevity
  - Fatigue wear more prevalent in TKA than in THA
  - Volumetric wear most affected by relative motion between the two surfaces in contact
- PMMA (bone cement)
  - Used for fixation and load distribution for implants
    - Act as a grout, not an adhesive
    - Mechanically interlocks with bone
  - Reaches ultimate strength within 24 hours
  - Can be used as an internal splint for patients with poor bone stock
    - PMMA can be used as a temporary internal splint until the bone heals
    - If bone fails to heal, PMMA will ultimately fail

- Poor tensile and shear strength
- Is strongest in compression and has a low E
  - Not as strong as bone in compression
- Reducing voids (porosity) increases cement strength and decreases cracking.
  - Vacuum mixing, centrifugation, good technique
  - Cement failure often caused by microfracture and fragmentation
- Insertion can lead to a precipitous drop in BP.
- Wear particles can incite a macrophage response
  - Leads to prosthesis loosening
- Silicones
  - Polymers for replacement in non–weight-bearing joints
  - Poor strength and wear capabilities
    - Frequent synovitis with extended use
- Ceramics
  - Metallic and nonmetallic elements bonded ionically in a highly oxidized state
    - Good insulators (poor conductors)
    - Biostable (inert) crystalline materials such as Al_2O_3 (alumina) and ZrO_2 (zirconium dioxide)
    - Bioactive (degradable) noncrystalline substances such as bioglass
  - **Typically brittle (no elastic deformation)**
  - High modulus (E)
  - High compressive strength
  - Low tensile strength
  - Low yield strain
  - Poor crack resistance characteristics
    - Low resistance to fracture
  - **Best wear characteristics, with polyethylene and a low oxidation rate**
  - High surface wettability and high surface tension
    - Highly conducive to tissue bonding
    - Less friction and diminished wear ("smooth surface")
  - Small grain size allows an ultrasmooth finish.
    - Less friction
  - Calcium phosphates (e.g., hydroxyapatite) may be useful as a coating (plasma sprayed) to increase attachment strength and promote bone healing.
- Other materials
  - Investigational
    - Polylactic acid–coated carbon and new polymer composites with carbon fiber reinforcement
      - "Piles" of carbon fibers impregnated with matrix polymer (polysulfone or polyetherketone)
      - **Material undergoes hydrolysis, resulting in lactic acid, which is excreted from the lungs as carbon dioxide.**
  - Bioabsorbable polymers induce foreign body reactions in many patients.
- Biomaterials
  - Possess certain unique characteristics
    - Viscoelasticity
    - Creep
    - Stress relaxation
      - Internal stress decreases with time.
      - Deformation remains constant.
  - Capable of self-adaptation and repair
    - Characteristics change with aging and sampling.
      - Comparison of common orthopaedic materials (see Figure 1-85)

■ Orthopaedic structures
- Bone
  - Mechanical properties
    - Composite of collagen and hydroxyapatite
      - Collagen: low E, good tensile strength, poor compressive strength
      - Calcium apatite: stiff, brittle, good compressive strength
    - Anisotropic
      - Strongest in compression
      - Weakest in shear
      - Intermediate in tension
      - Resists rapidly applied loads better than slowly applied loads
    - Mineral content is the main determinant of the elastic modulus of cortical bone.
    - Cancellous bone is 25% as dense, 10% as stiff, and 500% as ductile as cortical bone.
      - Cortical bone excellent at resisting torque.
      - Cancellous bone good at resisting compression and shear.
    - Bone is dynamic.
      - Able to self-repair
      - Changes with aging: stiffer and less ductile
      - Changes with immobilization: weaker
    - Bone aging
      - To offset loss in material properties, bone remodels to increase inner and outer cortical diameters.
      - Area moment of inertia increases.
        - Bending stresses decrease.
    - Stress concentration effects
      - Occur at defect points within bone or implant-bone interface (stress risers)
      - Reduce overall loading strength
    - Stress shielding by load-sharing implants
      - Induces osteoporosis in adjacent bone
        - Decreases normal physiologic bone stresses
      - Common under plates and at the femoral calcar in high-riding THAs
    - A hole 20% to 30% of bone diameter reduces strength up to 50%.
      - Regardless of whether it is filled with a screw
      - Area returns to normal 9 to 12 months after screw removal
    - Cortical defects can reduce strength 70% or more.
      - Oval defects less than rectangular defects
        - Smaller stress riser (concentration)
  - Fracture
    - Type is based on mechanism of injury.
    - Tension
      - Muscle pull, typically transverse
      - Perpendicular to load and bone axis
    - Compression
      - Axial loading of cancellous bone
      - Crush fracture
    - Shear
      - Commonly around joints
      - Load parallel to the bone surface
      - Fracture parallel to the load
    - Bending
      - Eccentric loading or direct blows
      - Begins on the tension side of the bone
      - Continues transversely/obliquely
      - Eventually bifurcates to produce a butterfly fragment
      - High-velocity bending: produces comminuted butterfly fracture
      - Four-point bending: produces segmental fracture
    - Torsion
      - Shear and tensile stresses around the longitudinal axis
      - Most likely to result in a spiral fracture
      - Torsional stresses proportional to the distance from the neutral axis to the periphery of a cylinder
        - Greatest stresses in a long bone under torsion are on the outer (periosteal) surface
    - Comminution
      - A function of the amount of energy transmitted to bone
- Ligaments and tendons
  - These structures can sustain 5% to 10% tensile strain before failure.
    - In contrast, bone can sustain only 1% to 4% tensile strain.
    - Failure commonly results from tension rupture of fibers and shear failure among fibers
  - Most ligaments can undergo plastic strain to the point that function is lost but structure remains in continuity.
  - Soft tissue implants have the following characteristics:
    - Tendons
      - Strong in tension only
      - E is 10% that of bone; increases with slower loading
      - Parallel fiber orientation
      - Demonstrate stress relaxation and creep
    - Ligament fibers
      - Oriented parallel if they resist major joint stress
        - More randomly if they resist forces from different directions
      - Stiffness = force/strain
        - As depicted on a force deformation graph
        - Similar to E but does not account for cross-sectional area
        - Bone-ligament complex is softer; less stiff implies decreased E
      - Prolonged immobilization lowers yield point and tensile strength.
- Stents
  - Internal splint devices:
    - Proplast Tendon Transfer Stabilizer
    - Gore-Tex prosthetic ligaments
    - Xenotech (bovine tendon)
    - Polyester implants
  - Stents do not allow adequate collagen ingrowth.
    - All eventually fail.
  - Synthetic ligaments produce wear particles.
    - Increase proteinases, collagenase, gelatinase, and chondrocyte activation factor
- Ligament augmentation devices (LADs)
  - Kennedy LAD (polypropylene yarn) and Dacron LADs.
    - LADs do allow some fibrous ingrowth.
    - However, their use is limited.

- Biodegradable tissue scaffolding
  - Immediate stability
  - Long-term replacement with host tissue
  - Carbon fiber and polylactic acid–coated carbon fiber devices
    - Limited success
    - Slow ingrowth is improved with polylactic acid coating
- Articular cartilage
  - Ultimate tensile strength is only 5% that of bone.
    - E is only 0.1% that of bone.
    - However, because of its viscoelastic properties, it is well-suited for compressive loading.
  - Articular cartilage is biphasic.
    - Solid phase depends on structural matrix
    - Fluid phase depends on deformation and shift of water within solid matrix
  - Relatively soft and impermeable solid matrix requires high hydrodynamic pressure to maintain fluid flow
    - Significant support provided by the fluid component
    - Stress-shielding effect on the matrix
- Metal implants
  - Screws
    - Have the following characteristics:
      - Pitch: distance between threads
      - Lead: distance advanced in one revolution
      - Root diameter: minimal/inner diameter is proportional to tensile strength
      - Outer diameter: determines holding power (pullout strength)
    - To maximize pullout strength
      - Large outer diameter
      - Small root diameter
      - Fine pitch
    - Pedicle screw pullout strength most affected by degree of osteoporosis
  - Plates
    - Strength varies with material and moment of inertia.
    - **Bending stiffness is proportional to the third power of the thickness (t^3).**
      - Doubling thickness increases bending stiffness eightfold.
    - Plates are load-bearing devices.
      - Most effective on a fracture's tension side
    - Types include:
      - Static compression
        - Best in upper extremity
        - Can be stressed for compression
      - Dynamic compression
        - Example: tension band plate
      - Neutralization
      - Resists torsion
      - Buttress
        - Protects bone graft
    - Stress concentration at open screw holes can lead to implant failure.
      - Screw holes that remain after removal of plate and screw represent a stress riser.
        - At risk for refracture
    - Blade plates
      - Increased resistance to torsional deformation
- Locking plates
  - Absorb axial forces transmitted from screws
  - Do not require compression to bone; preserve periosteal blood supply
  - Biomechanical advantages for osteoporotic fractures without cortical contact
- Hybrid locking plates
  - Both nonlocked and locked screws are used.
  - Nonlocked screws assist in reduction.
  - Locked screws create a fixed-angle device or can be used in patients with osteoporosis.
  - **Bicortical locked screws provide strength difference compared to unicortical locked screws in torsion.**
- Intramedullary nails
  - Load-sharing devices
    - Require high polar moment of inertia to maximize torsional rigidity and strength
  - Mechanical characteristics
    - Torsional rigidity
      - Amount of torque needed to produce a unit angle of torsional deformation
      - Depends on both material properties (shear modulus) and structural properties (polar moment of inertia)
    - Bending rigidity
      - Amount of force required to produce a unit amount of deflection
      - Depends on both material properties (elastic modulus) and structural properties (area moment of inertia, length)
      - **Related to the fourth power of the nail's radius**
        - Increasing nail diameter by 10% increases bending rigidity by 50%.
      - Better at resisting bending forces than rotational forces
  - Reaming
    - Allows increased torsional resistance
      - Increased contact area
      - A larger nail; increased rigidity and strength
  - Unslotted nails
    - Smaller diameter
    - Stronger fixation
    - At the expense of flexibility
    - Increased torsional stiffness: greatest advantage of closed-section nails over slotted nails
  - Intramedullary nail insertion for femoral shaft fracture
    - Hoop stresses are lowest for a slotted titanium alloy nail with a thin wall
    - Posterior starting points decrease hoop stresses and iatrogenic comminution of fractures
    - Implant failure is more frequent with smaller-diameter unreamed nails
- External fixators
  - Conventional external fixators
    - Allowing fracture ends to come into contact is the most important factor for stability of fixation with external fixation.
    - Other factors to enhance stability (rigidity) include:
      - Larger-diameter pins (second most important factor)

- Additional pins
- Decreased bone-rod distance
- Pins in different planes
- Pins separated by more than 45 degrees
- Increased mass of the rods or stacked rods
- A second rod in the same plane increases resistance to bending.
- Rods in different planes
- Increased spacing between pins
- Place central pins closer to the fracture site
- Place peripheral pins farther from the fracture site (near-near, far-far).
  - Tibial shaft fractures
    - Additional lag screws with external fixation are associated with a higher refracture rate than is external fixation alone.
- Circular (Ilizarov) external fixators
  - Thin wires (usually 1.8 mm in diameter)
    - Fixed under tension (usually between 90 and 130 kg)
    - Circular rings
  - Half-pins may also be used.
    - Offer better purchase in diaphyseal (not metaphyseal) bone
  - Optimum orientation of implants on the ring
    - At a 90-degree angle to each other
    - Maximizes stability
    - A 90-degree angle not always possible
      - Anatomic constraints such as neurovascular structures
  - Bending stiffness of frame
    - Independent of the loading direction
    - Because the frame is circular
  - Each ring should have at least two implants.
    - Wires or half-pins may be used.
    - The construct is most stable when an olive wire and a half-pin are at a 90-degree angle to each other on a ring.
    - Two wires are used on a ring.
      - One wire should be superior to the ring and one inferior.
      - Tensioned wires on the same side can cause the ring to deform.
  - Factors that enhance stability of circular external fixators:
    - Larger-diameter wires (and half-pins)
    - Decreased ring diameter
    - Use of olive wires
    - Additional wires or half-pins (or both)
    - Wires (or half-pins or both) crossing at a 90-degree angle
    - Increased wire tension (up to 130 kg)
    - Placement of the two central rings close to the fracture site
    - Decreased spacing between adjacent rings
    - Increased number of rings
- Total hip arthroplasty
  - Evolving design has led to reduction in biomechanical constraints
  - Cemented versus cementless
    - Femoral components designed for use with or without cement
    - Cementless

- Proximal porous coating: should be circumferential
- Seals the diaphysis from wear debris
- Cemented
  - Mantle less than 2 mm thick increases incidence of crack formation
- Stem length
  - Directly related to rigidity
  - Metal heads: more neck-length options than ceramic heads
  - Compressive and tensile stresses in adjacent structures can be minimized:
    - Broad medial surface
    - Broader lateral surface
    - Large moment of inertia
- Moment arms
  - Femoral component design must account for rotational forces.
    - Rotational torque in retroversion
      - Most responsible for initiating loosening in cemented femoral stems
      - Increased in femoral stems with a higher offset
- Femoral component
  - This can be used in cases of neutral or slight valgus angulation.
  - It decreases moment arm, cement stress, and abductor length.
  - Increasing offset moves the abductor attachment away from the joint center.
    - **Increases the abductor moment arm**
    - **Reduces abductor force required in normal gait**
    - Reduces resulting hip joint reaction force
    - Increases the bending moment (strain) on the implant
    - Increases strain on the medial cement mantle
- Femoral head size
  - Small (22-mm) components
    - Decrease ROM and stability
    - Decrease friction and torque and polyethylene volumetric wear
  - Large (36-mm) components
    - **Increase ROM and stability**
    - Increase friction and torque and polyethylene volumetric wear
    - Wear: less of an issue with modern bearings
- Durability
  - Survival of surface replacement hip arthroplasty is poor as a result of volumetric wear of polyethylene.
    - This wear is 4 to 10 times that of a THA when a 28-mm head is used.
  - Metal-backing acetabular components are used.
    - Decrease stress in cement and cancellous bone
  - Polyethylene on titanium makes a poor bearing surface.
    - Excessive volumetric wear
  - Titanium on weight-bearing surfaces is not recommended.
    - May lead to fretting, wear debris, and blackening of soft tissues
  - Wear synovitis can occur in TJA.
    - Associated with histiocyte injection of submicron polyethylene debris

- UHMWPE serves as a "shock absorber."
  - Should be at least 6 mm thick to prevent creep
- Ceramic femoral head on a ceramic acetabulum has the lowest coefficient of friction
- Wear rates:
  - UHMWPE in the acetabulum: 0.1 mm (100 μm) per year
  - Metal-on-metal bearings for THA: 0.002 to 0.005 mm (2-5 μm) per year
    - Smaller particles than UHMWPE, but more numerous
  - Ceramic bearing surfaces: 0.0005 to 0.0025 mm (0.5-25 μm) per year
- Newer concepts
  - Computer design of THA stems
  - Modularity
    - Increased corrosion at modular metallic junction sites
    - Such as junction of the head and stem
  - Custom designs
  - More flexible stems
  - Forging of components appears to be superior to casting.
- Total knee arthroplasty
  - Design has evolved significantly.
    - Original designs did not account for human knee kinematics.
    - Appropriate compromise is sought between the following designs:
      - Total-contact designs
        - Excess stability (less motion)
        - Less wear
      - Low-contact designs
        - Less stability (better motion)
        - Increased wear
  - Metal alloys are typically used.
  - Cemented cruciate ligament–substituting TKA designs are available.
    - Associated with low polyethylene wear rates
    - Minimal osteolysis
      - High tibiofemoral conformity
- Compression hip screws
  - Loading characteristics superior to those of blade plates
    - Higher angled plates subjected to lower bending loads
      - However, may be more difficult to insert
  - Sliding of the screw proportional to two aspects:
    - Angle of screw to side plate
    - Length of the screw in the barrel
- Implant fixation
  - Interference fit
    - Mechanical or press-fit components
      - Rely on formation of fibrous tissue interface
    - Loosening
      - Can occur if stability is not maintained and high-E substances are used
        - Increases bone resorption and remodeling
  - Interlocking fit
    - PMMA allows gradual transfer of stress to bone.
      - Microinterlocking of cement within cancellous bone
        - May not be achievable with cemented revision of previously cemented TKA

- Aseptic loosening can occur over time
  - **Macrophages initiate the inflammatory cascade, which leads to aseptic loosening.**
  - Careful technique yields the best results:
    - Limiting porosities and gaps
    - Use of a 3- to 5-mm cement thickness
  - Other improvements are as follows:
    - Low-viscosity cement
    - Better bone bed preparation
    - Plugging and pressurization
    - Better (vacuum) cement mixing
- Biological fit
  - Tissue ingrowth
    - Fiber-metal composites
    - Void metal composites
    - Microbeads
    - Key: to create pore sizes of 100 to 400 μm (ideally 100-250 μm)
  - Mechanical stability required
  - Ingrowth typically limited to 10% to 30% of the surface area
  - Problems:
    - Fiber or bead loosening
    - Increased cost
    - Proximal bone resorption
      - Monocyte/macrophage mediated
    - Corrosion
    - Decreased implant fatigue strength
  - Uncemented TJA
    - Bone ingrowth in the tibial component of TKA occurs adjacent to fixation pegs and screws.
    - Bone ingrowth depends on the avoidance of micromotion at the bone-implant interface.
      - Observed on radiographs as radiodense reactive lines about the prosthesis
    - Canal filling (maximal endosteal contact) of more fully coated femoral stems: important for bone ingrowth
- Bone-implant unit
  - The composite structure of this unit has shared properties.
  - More accurate bone cross-section reconstruction with metallic support improves loading characteristics.
  - Plates should act as tension bands.
  - Materials with increased E may result in bone resorption.
  - Materials with decreased E may result in implant failure.
  - Placement of the implant initiates a race between bone healing and implant failure.

▣ Biomechanics

- Joint biomechanics: general
  - Degrees of freedom
    - Rotations and translations each occur in the x, y, and z planes
      - Thus six parameters, or degrees of freedom, describe motion.
    - Translations may be relatively insignificant for many joints.
      - Are often ignored in biomechanical analyses
  - Joint reaction force (R)
    - R is the force within a joint in response to forces acting on the joint.

- Both intrinsic and extrinsic
  - Muscle contraction about a joint: the major contributing factor
- R is correlated with predisposition to degenerative changes.
  - Joint contact pressure (stress) can be minimized:
    - Decrease R
    - Increase contact area
- Coupled forces—rotation about one axis causes obligatory rotation about another axis (occurs in some joints).
  - Such movements (and associated forces) are *coupled*.
  - Example: lateral bending of the spine accompanied by axial rotation
- Joint congruence
  - Related to the fit of two articular surfaces
    - A necessary condition for joint motion
  - Can be evaluated radiographically
  - High congruence increases joint contact area
  - Low congruence decreases joint contact area
  - Movement out of a position of congruence increases stress in cartilage
    - Allows less contact area for distribution of joint reaction force
    - Predisposes the joint to degeneration
- Instant center of rotation
  - Point about which a joint rotates
  - In some joints (knee), the instant center changes during the arc of motion, following a curved path.
    - Effect of joint translation and morphologic features
  - It normally lies on a line perpendicular to the tangent of the joint surface at all points of contact.
- Rolling and sliding (Figure 1-86)
  - During motion, almost all joints roll and slide to remain in congruence.
  - Pure rolling:
    - Instant center of rotation is at the rolling surfaces.
    - Contacting points have zero relative velocity.
      - No "slipping" of one surface on the other
  - Pure sliding:
    - Occurs with pure translation or rotation about a stationary axis
    - No angular change in position
    - No instant center of rotation
      - "Slipping" of one surface on the other
- Friction and lubrication
  - Friction: resistance between two objects as one slides over the other
    - Not a function of contact area
    - Coefficient of friction: 0 = no friction
  - Lubrication: decreases resistance between surfaces
    - Articular surfaces, lubricated with synovial fluid, have a coefficient of friction 10 times better than the best synthetic systems.
  - Coefficient of friction for human joints: 0.002 to 0.04
  - Coefficient of friction for metal-on-UHMWPE joint arthroplasty: 0.05 to 0.15
    - Not as good as human joints
  - Elastohydrodynamic lubrication
    - Primary lubrication mechanism for articular cartilage during dynamic function

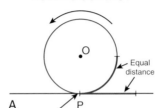
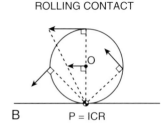
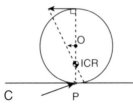
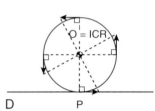

FIGURE 1-86 A, Rolling contact occurs when the circumferential distance of the rolling object equals the distance traced along the plane. This can occur only when there is no sliding—that is, when the relative velocity at the point of contact (P) is zero. **B,** For rolling contact, the point P of the wheel has zero velocity because it is in contact with the ground. Therefore P is the instant center of rotation (ICR) of the wheel. This diagram shows the actual velocity of points along the wheel as it rolls along the ground. **C,** Rolling and sliding contact occurs when the relative velocity at the contact point is not zero. **D,** Pure sliding occurs when the wheel rotates about a stationary axis (O). In this case, the wheel would have no forward motion. (From Buckwalter JA et al: *Orthopaedic basic science: biology and biomechanics of the musculoskeletal system,* ed 2, Rosemont, Ill, 2000, American Academy of Orthopaedic Surgeons, p 145.)

Table 1-49	Hip Biomechanics: Range of Motion	
MOTION	**AVERAGE RANGE (DEGREES)**	**FUNCTIONAL RANGE (DEGREES)**
Flexion	115	90 (120 to squat)
Extension	30	
Abduction	50	20
Adduction	30	
Internal rotation	45	0
External rotation	45	20

- Hip biomechanics
  - Kinematics
    - ROM (Table 1-49)
    - Instant center
      - Simultaneous triplanar motion for this ball-and-socket joint makes analysis impossible.
  - Kinetics
    - Joint reaction force (R) in the hip can reach three to six times body weight (W).
      - Primarily as a result of contraction of the muscles crossing the hip
    - Hip kinetics demonstrated in Figure 1-87
      - If $A = 5$ and $B = 12.5$, then according to standard free-body diagram analysis:

$$\Sigma M = 0 \text{ (sum of moments} = 0)$$

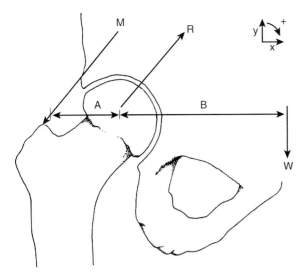

FIGURE 1-87 Free-body diagram of the hip (see text for explanation). *M,* Moment; *R,* joint reaction force; *W,* work.

$$-5\,M_y + 12.5W = 0$$

$$M_y = 2.5W$$

$$\Sigma F_y = 0 \text{ (sum of forces} = 0)$$

$$-M_y - W + R_y = 0$$

$$R_y = 3.5W$$

$$R = R_y / (\cos 30 \text{ degrees})$$

$$R \cong 4W$$

- An increase in the ratio of *A/B* decreases *R*.
  - For example, medialization of the acetabulum, long-neck prosthesis, or lateralization of the greater trochanter
  - If *A* = 7.5 and *B* = 10, *R* ≅ 2.3 *W*.
- Both *R* and abductor moment are reduced by shifting body weight over the hip.
  - Trendelenburg gait
- A cane in the contralateral hand produces an additional moment.
  - This can reduce *R* up to 60%.
  - Carrying a load in the ipsilateral hand also decreases *R* at the hip.
- Energy expenditure is 264% of normal with a resection arthroplasty of the hip.
- The hip and trunk generate 50% of the force during a tennis serve.
- Other considerations
  - Stability
    - Deep-seated "ball-and-socket" joint is intrinsically stable.
  - Sourcil
    - Condensation of subchondral bone under superomedial acetabulum
    - *R* is maximal at this point
  - Gothic arch
    - Remodeled bone supporting the acetabular roof
    - Sourcil at its base

- Neck-shaft angle
  - Varus angulation
    - Decreases *R*
    - Increases shear across the neck
    - Leads to shortening of the lower extremity
    - Alters muscle tension resting length of the abductors
      - May cause a persistent limp
  - Valgus angulation
    - Increases *R*
    - Decreases shear
    - Neutral or valgus angulation better for THA
    - PMMA resists shear poorly
- Arthrodesis
  - Position: 25 to 30 degrees of flexion, 0 degrees of abduction and rotation
    - External rotation is better than internal rotation.
  - If the implant is fused in abduction, the patient will lurch over the affected lower extremity with an excessive trunk shift.
    - This will later result in low back pain.
  - Effects:
    - Increases oxygen consumption
    - Decreases gait efficiency to approximately 50% of normal
    - Increases transpelvic rotation of the contralateral hip
- Knee biomechanics
  - Kinematics
    - ROM
      - Ten degrees of extension (recurvatum) to 130 degrees of flexion
      - Functional ROM is nearly full extension to about 90 degrees of flexion.
      - 117 degrees: required for squatting and lifting
      - 110 degrees: required for rising from a chair after TKA
    - Rotation varies with flexion
      - At full extension, rotation is minimal.
      - At 90 degrees of flexion, ROM is 45 degrees of external rotation and 30 degrees of internal rotation.
    - Amount of abduction or adduction is essentially 0 degrees.
      - A few degrees of passive motion is possible at 30 degrees of flexion.
    - Knee motion is complex about a changing instant center of rotation.
      - Polycentric rotation
    - Excursions of 0.5 cm for the medial meniscus and 1.1 cm for the lateral meniscus are possible during 120-degree arc of motion.
  - Joint motion
    - Instant center traces a J-shaped curve about the femoral condyle.
      - Moves posteriorly with flexion
    - Flexion and extension involve both rolling and sliding.
    - Femur internally rotates (external tibial rotation) during the last 15 degrees of extension
      - "Screw home" mechanism
      - Related to different in radii of curvature for the medial and lateral femoral condyles and the musculature

- Posterior rollback increases maximum knee flexion.
  - Tibiofemoral contact point moves posteriorly.
  - Normal rollback is compromised by PCL sacrifice, as in some TKAs
- Axis of rotation of the intact knee is in the medial femoral condyle.
- Patellofemoral joint has sliding articulation:
  - Patella slides 7 cm caudally with full flexion.
  - Instant center is near the posterior cortex above the condyles.
- Kinetics
  - Knee stabilizers
    - Ligaments and muscles play the major stabilizing role (Table 1-50).
      - ACL:
        - Typically subjected to peak loads of 170 N during walking
        - Up to 500 N with running
        - Ultimate strength in young patients: about 1750 N
        - Failures by serial tearing at 10% to 15% elongation
      - PCL: Sectioning increases contact pressures in the medial compartment and the patellofemoral joint.
- Joint forces
  - Tibiofemoral joint
    - Knee joint surface loads
      - Three times body weight during level walking
      - Up to four times body weight with stair walking
    - Menisci
      - Help with load transmission
      - Bear one third to half body weight
      - Removal increases contact stresses
        - Up to four times the load transfer to bone
      - Quadriceps produces maximum anterior force on the tibia at 0 to 60 degrees of knee flexion
  - Patellofemoral joint
    - Patella aids in knee extension.
      - Increases the lever arm
      - Stress distribution
    - Has the thickest cartilage in the entire body
      - Bears the greatest load
      - Bears half the body weight with normal walking

- Bears seven times the body weight with squatting and jogging
- Loads proportional to ratio of quadriceps force to knee flexion
- In descending stairs, compressive force reaches two to three times body weight.
- Patellectomy
  - Length of the moment arm is decreased by width of patella: 30% reduction
  - Power of extension is decreased by 30%.
- During TKA, the following enhance patella tracking:
  - External rotation of the femoral component
  - Lateral placement of the femoral and tibial components
  - Medial placement of the patellar component
  - Avoidance of malrotation of the tibial component
    - These actions avoid internal rotation.
- Axes of the lower extremity (Figure 1-88)
  - Mechanical axis of the lower extremity
    - Center of femoral head to center of ankle
    - Normally passes just medial to the medial tibial spine

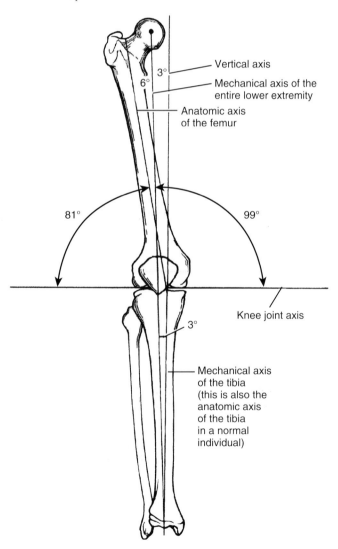

FIGURE 1-88 Axes of the lower extremity. (Modified from Helfet DL: Fractures of the distal femur. In Browner BD et al, editors: *Skeletal trauma*, Philadelphia, 1992, WB Saunders, p 1645.)

Table 1-50	Knee Stabilizers
DIRECTION	**STRUCTURES**
Medial	Superficial MCL (primary), joint capsule, medial meniscus, ACL/PCL
Lateral	Joint capsule, IT band, LCL (middle), lateral meniscus, ACL/PCL (90 degrees)
Anterior	ACL (primary), joint capsule
Posterior	PCL (primary), joint capsule; PCL tightens with internal rotation
Rotatory	Combinations: MCL checks external rotation; ACL checks internal rotation

ACL, Anterior cruciate ligament; *IT*, iliotibial; *LCL*, lateral collateral ligament complex; *MCL*, medial collateral ligament complex; *PCL*, posterior cruciate ligament.

- Vertical axis
  - From the center of gravity to the ground
- Anatomic axes
  - Along the shafts of the femur and tibia
  - Where these axes intersect at the knee, valgus angle is normal.
- Mechanical axis of the femur
  - From center of the femoral head to center of the knee
- Mechanical axis of the tibia
  - From center of the tibial plateau to center of the ankle
- Relationships
  - Mechanical axis of the lower extremity is in 3 degrees of valgus angulation from the vertical axis.
  - Anatomic axis of the femur is in 6 degrees of valgus angulation from the mechanical axis.
    - Nine degrees versus the vertical axis
  - Anatomic axis of the tibia is in 2 to 3 degrees of varus angulation from the mechanical axis.
- Arthrodesis
  - Position: 0 to 7 degrees of valgus angulation, 10 to 15 degrees of flexion
- Ankle and foot biomechanics
  - Ankle
    - Kinematics
      - Instant center of rotation within the talus
        - Lateral and posterior points at the tips of the malleoli
        - Change slightly with movement
      - Talus described as a cone
        - Body and trochlea wider anteriorly and laterally
        - Therefore talus and fibula externally rotate slightly with dorsiflexion
      - Dorsiflexion and abduction are coupled.
      - ROM:
        - Dorsiflexion: 25 degrees
        - Plantar flexion: 35 degrees
        - Rotation: 5 degrees
    - Kinetics
      - Tibiotalar articulation
        - Major weight-bearing surface of the ankle
        - Supports compressive forces up to five times body weight (W)
        - Shear (backward to forward) forces up to Wt
      - Large weight-bearing surface area decreases joint stress
      - Fibular/talar joint transmits about one sixth of the force
      - Highest net muscle moment occurs during terminal-stance phase of gait.

- Other considerations
  - Stability based on articulation shape (mortise maintained by talar shape) and ligament support
    - Stability is greatest in dorsiflexion.
    - During weight bearing, tibial and talar articular surfaces contribute most to stability.
  - Windlass action
    - Full dorsiflexion is limited by the plantar aponeurosis.
    - Further tension on the aponeurosis (toe dorsiflexion) raises the arch.
  - A syndesmosis screw limits external rotation.
  - Arthrodesis: neutral dorsiflexion, 5 to 10 degrees of external rotation, 5 degrees of hindfoot valgus angulation
    - Anticipate 70% loss of sagittal plane motion of the foot.
- Subtalar joint (talus-calcaneus-navicular)
  - Axis of rotation:
    - In the sagittal plane: 42 degrees
    - In the transverse plane: 16 degrees
  - Functions like an oblique hinge
    - Pronation coupled with dorsiflexion, abduction, and eversion
    - Supination coupled with plantar flexion, adduction, and inversion
  - ROM
    - Pronation: 5 degrees
    - Supination: 20 degrees
    - Functional ROM: approximately 6 degrees
- Transverse tarsal joint (talus-navicular, calcaneal-cuboid)
  - Motion based on foot position
    - Two axes of rotation: talonavicular and calcaneocuboid
  - Eversion (early stance)
    - The joint axes are parallel.
    - ROM is allowed.
  - Inversion (late stance)
    - External rotation of the lower extremity causes the joint axes to intersect.
    - Motion is limited.
- Foot
  - Transmits 1.2 times body weight with walking
    - Three times body weight with running
  - Has three arches (Table 1-51)
  - Second metatarsal (Lisfranc) joint is "keylike"
    - Stabilizes second metatarsal
    - Allows it to carry the most load with gait
    - First metatarsal bears the most load during standing

Table 1-51	Arches of the Foot			
ARCH	**SKELETAL COMPONENTS**	**KEYSTONE**	**LIGAMENT SUPPORT**	**MUSCLE SUPPORT**
Medial longitudinal	Calcaneus, talus, navicular, three cuneiform bones, first to third metatarsals	Talus head	Spring (calcaneonavicular)	Tibialis posterior, flexor digitorum longus, flexor hallucis longus, adductor hallucis
Lateral longitudinal	Calcaneus, cuboid, fourth and fifth metatarsals		Plantar aponeurosis	Abductor digiti minimi, flexor digitorum brevis
Transverse	Three cuneiform bones, cuboid, metatarsal bases			Peroneus longus, tibialis posterior, adductor hallucis (oblique)

Table 1-52	Range of Motion of Spinal Segments			
LEVEL	**FLEXION/ EXTENSION (DEGREES)**	**LATERAL BENDING (DEGREES)**	**ROTATION (DEGREES)**	**INSTANT CENTER**
Occiput-C1	13	8	0	Skull, 2-3 cm above dens
C1-C2	10	0	45	Waist of odontoid
C2-C7	10-15	8-10	10	Vertebral body below
T-spine	5	6	8	Vertebra below/disc centrum
L-spine	15-20	2-5	3-6	Disc annulus

C, Cervical; L, lumbar; T, thoracic.

- Expected life of Plastazote shoe insert in active adults is less than 1 month
  - Fatigues rapidly in compression and shear
  - Should be replaced frequently or supported with other materials such as Spenco or PPT foam
- Spine biomechanics
  - Kinematics
    - ROM by anatomic segment (Table 1-52)
    - Analysis based on the functional unit
      - Motion segment: two vertebrae and the intervening soft tissues
    - Six degrees of freedom exist about all three axes.
    - Coupled motion
      - Simultaneous rotation, lateral bending, and flexion or extension
      - Especially axial rotation with lateral bending
    - Instant center of rotation within the disc
    - Normal sagittal alignment of the lumbar spine: 55 to 60 degrees of lordosis
      - The lordosis exists because of the disc spaces (not the vertebrae).
      - Most lordosis occurs between L4 and S1.
      - Loss of disc space height can cause loss of normal lumbar lordosis.
    - Iatrogenic flat back syndrome of the lumbar spine
      - Result of a distraction force
  - Supporting structures
    - Anterior supporting structures
      - Anterior longitudinal ligament
      - Posterior longitudinal ligament
      - Vertebral disc
    - Posterior supporting structures
      - Intertransverse ligaments
      - Capsular ligaments and facets
      - Ligamentum flavum (yellow ligament)
    - Halo vest—most effective device for controlling cervical motion
      - Because of pin purchase in the skull
    - Apophyseal joints
      - Resist torsion during axial loading
        - Attached capsular ligaments resist flexion.
      - Guide the motion segment
      - Direction of motion determined by orientation of the facets of the apophyseal joint
        - Varies with each level
      - Cervical spine facet
        - Orientation: 45 degrees to the transverse plane
        - Parallel to the frontal plane
      - Thoracic spine facet
        - Orientation: 60 degrees to the transverse plane
        - Also 20 degrees to the frontal plane
    - Lumbar spine facet
      - Orientation: 90 degrees to the transverse plane
      - Also 45 degrees to the frontal plane
      - They progressively tilt up (transverse) and inward (frontal).
    - Cervical facetectomy of more than 50% causes loss of stability in flexion and torsion.
    - Torsional load resistance in the lumbar spine:
      - Facets contribute 40%
      - Disc contributes 40%
      - Ligamentous structures contribute 20%
  - Kinetics
    - Disc
      - Behaves viscoelastically
      - Demonstrates creep
        - Deforms with time
      - Demonstrates hysteresis
        - Absorbs energy with repeated axial loads
        - Later decreases in function
      - Compressive stresses highest in the nucleus pulposus
      - Tensile stresses highest in the annulus fibrosus
      - Stiffness increases with compressive load.
      - Higher loads increase deformation and creep rate.
      - Repeated torsional loading (shear forces)
        - Such repeated loading may separate the nucleus pulposus from the annulus and end plate.
        - This in turn may force nuclear material through an annular tear.
      - Loads increase with bending and torsional stresses.
      - After subtotal discectomy, extension is the most stable loading mode.
      - Disc pressures are lowest with lying supine, higher with standing, and highest with sitting.
      - Carrying loads
        - Disc pressures are lowest when the load is close to the body.
    - Vertebrae
      - Strength is related to bone mineral content and vertebrae size.
        - Increased in lumbar spine
      - Fatigue loading may lead to pars fractures.
      - Compression fractures occur at the end plate.
      - Vertebral body stiffness is decreased in osteoporosis.
        - Caused by loss of horizontal trabeculae
      - Spinal arthrodesis is helpful:
        - Increasing implant stiffness
          - Increases probability of successful fusion
          - Increases likelihood of decreased bone mineral content of the bridged vertebrae

Table 1-53	Shoulder Biomechanics: Muscle Forces	
MOTION	**MUSCLE FORCES**	**COMMENTS**
GLENOHUMERAL		
Abduction	Deltoid, supraspinatus	Cuff depresses head
Adduction	Latissimus dorsi, pectoralis major, teres major	
Forward flexion	Pectoralis major, deltoid (anterior), biceps	
Extension	Latissimus dorsi	
Internal rotation	Subscapularis, teres major	
External rotation	Infraspinatus, teres minor, deltoid (posterior)	
SCAPULAR		
Rotation	Upper trapezius, levator scapulae (anterior), serratus anterior, lower trapezius	Works through a force couple
Adduction	Trapezius, rhomboid, latissimus dorsi	
Abduction	Serratus anterior, pectoralis minor	

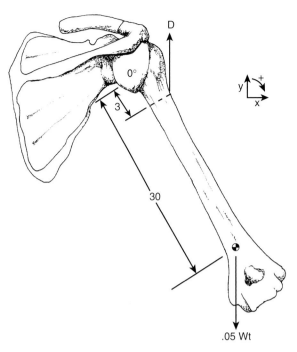

FIGURE 1-89 Free-body diagram of the deltoid force (D) (see text for explanation). *Wt,* Weight of arm (N).

- Shoulder biomechanics (Table 1-53)
  - Kinematics
    - Scapular plane
      - Positioned 30 degrees anterior to the coronal plane
      - The preferred reference plane for ROM
    - Abduction requires external rotation of the humerus.
      - To prevent greater tuberosity impingement
      - With internal rotation contractures, abduction limited to 120 degrees
    - Abduction
      - Glenohumeral motion: 120 degrees
      - Scapulothoracic motion: 60 degrees
      - In ratio of 2 : 1
        - Varies over the first 30 degrees of motion
    - Scapulothoracic motion
      - Acromioclavicular joint movement during the early part
      - Sternoclavicular movement during the later portion
        - With clavicular rotation along the long axis
    - Surface joint motion in the glenohumeral joint is a combination of rotation, rolling, and translation.
  - Kinetics
    - Zero position
      - Abduction of 165 degrees in the scapular plane
      - Minimal deforming forces about the shoulder
      - Ideal position for reducing shoulder dislocations
        - Also for reducing "fractures with traction"
    - Free-body analysis of deltoid force (*D*) (Figure 1-89):

$$\Sigma M_0 = 0$$

$$3D - 0.05W(30) = 0$$

$$D = 0.5W$$

  - Stability
    - Limited about the glenohumeral joint
    - Humeral head surface area larger than glenoid area:
      - 48 × 45 mm versus 35 × 25 mm
    - Bony stability is limited
      - Relies on humeral head inclination (125 degrees) and retroversion (25 degrees)
      - Also relies on slight glenoid retrotilt
    - Inferior glenohumeral ligament (anterior band)
      - The most important static stabilizer
      - Superior and middle glenohumeral ligaments: secondary stabilizers to anterior humeral translation
    - Inferior subluxation prevented by negative intraarticular pressure
    - Rotator cuff muscles
      - Dynamic contribution to stability
    - Arthrodesis: 15 to 20 degrees of abduction, 20 to 25 degrees of forward flexion, 40 to 50 degrees of internal rotation
      - Avoid excessive external rotation
  - Other joints
    - Acromioclavicular joint
      - Scapular rotation through the conoid and trapezoid ligaments
      - Scapular motion through the joint itself
    - Sternoclavicular joint
      - Clavicular protraction/retraction in a transverse plane through the coracoclavicular ligament
      - Clavicular elevation and depression in the frontal plane
        - Also through the coracoclavicular ligament
      - Clavicular rotation around the longitudinal axis
- Elbow biomechanics
  - Functions
    - A component joint of the lever arm when the hand is positioned
    - Fulcrum for the forearm lever
    - Weight-bearing joint in patients using crutches
    - Activities of daily living

- Kinematics
  - Flexion and extension
    - 0 to 150 degrees
    - Functional ROM: 30 to 130 degrees
    - Axis of rotation: the center of the trochlea
  - Pronation and supination
    - Pronation: 80 degrees
    - Supination: 85 degrees
    - Functional pronation and supination: 50 degrees each
    - Axis: capitellum through radial head to ulnar head (forms a cone)
  - Carrying angle
    - Valgus angle at the elbow
    - For boys and men: 7 degrees; for girls and women: 13 degrees
    - Decreases with flexion
- Kinetics
  - Forces at the elbow have short lever arms and are relatively inefficient (Figure 1-90):

$$\Sigma M_y = 0$$

$$-5B + 15Wt = 0$$

$$B = 3Wt$$

  - Results in large joint reaction forces
  - Subject the joint to degenerative changes
  - Flexion is accomplished primarily by the brachialis and biceps.
  - Extension is accomplished by the triceps.
  - Pronation is accomplished by pronators (teres and quadratus).
  - Supination is accomplished by the biceps and supinator.
  - Static loads approach, and dynamic loads exceed, body weight.
- Stability
  - Provided partially by articular congruity
  - Three necessary and sufficient constraints for stability:

- Coronoid
- Lateral (ulnar) collateral ligament (LCL)
- Anterior band of the medial collateral ligament
  - Most important: anterior oblique fibers
  - Stabilizes against both valgus angulation and distractional force at 90 degrees
- Most important secondary stabilizer against valgus stress: radial head
  - About 30% of valgus stability
  - Important at 0 to 30 degrees of flexion and pronation
- In extension, capsule is the primary restraint to distractional forces
- Lateral stability is provided by lateral collateral ligament, anconeus, and joint capsule.
- Unilateral arthrodesis: 90 degrees of flexion
- Bilateral arthrodesis:
  - One elbow at 110 degrees of flexion for the hand to reach the mouth
  - Other at 65 degrees of flexion for perineal hygiene
- Arthrodesis is difficult to perform and (fortunately) rarely required.
- Forearm
  - Ulna transmits 17% of the axial load
  - Line of the center of rotation runs from radial head to distal ulna
- Wrist and hand biomechanics
  - Wrist
    - Part of an intercalated link system
    - Kinematics
      - Normal ROM
        - Flexion: 65 degrees
          - Functional: 10 degrees
        - Extension: 55 degrees
          - Functional: 35 degrees
        - Radial deviation: 15 degrees
          - Functional: 10 degrees
        - Ulnar deviation: 35 degrees
          - Functional: 15 degrees
      - Flexion and extension
        - Two thirds radiocarpal
        - One third intercarpal
      - Radial deviation
        - Primarily intercarpal movement
      - Ulnar deviation
        - Relies on radiocarpal and intercarpal motion
      - Instant center is usually the head of the capitate, but it varies.
    - Columns (Table 1-54)
    - Link system
      - A system of three links in a "chain":
        - Radius, lunate, and capitate
      - Less motion is required at each link.
        - However, it adds to instability of the chain.

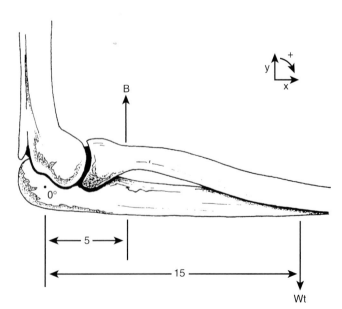

FIGURE 1-90 Free-body diagram of elbow flexion (see text for explanation). *B,* Biceps force; *Wt,* weight of forearm.

Table 1-54	Columns of the Wrist	
COLUMN	**FUNCTION**	**COMMENTS**
Central	Flexion-extension	Distal carpal row and lunate (link)
Medial	Rotation	Triquetrum
Lateral	Mobile	Scaphoid

- Stability is enhanced by strong volar ligaments.
  - Also by the scaphoid, which bridges both carpal rows
- Relationships
  - Carpal collapse
    - Ratio of carpal height to third metacarpal height: normally 0.54
  - Ulnar translation
    - Ratio of ulna-to-capitate length to third metacarpal height
    - Normal is 0.30
  - Distal radius normally bears about 80% of distal radioulnar joint load
    - Distal ulna bears 20%
    - Ulnar load bearing increases with ulnar lengthening and decreases with ulnar shortening.
  - Wrist arthrodesis is relatively common.
    - Dorsiflexion of 10 to 20 degrees is good for unilateral fusion.
    - Bilateral fusion:
      - Avoid if possible
      - If necessary, fuse other wrist at 0 to 10 degrees of palmar flexion
- Hand
  - Kinematics
    - ROM
      - Metacarpophalangeal (MCP) joint
        - Universal joint, 2 degrees of freedom
        - Flexion: 100 degrees
        - Abduction-adduction: 60 degrees
      - Proximal interphalangeal (PIP) joints
        - Flexion: 110 degrees
      - Distal interphalangeal (DIP) joints
        - Flexion: 80 degrees
  - Arches
    - Two transverse arches
      - Proximal through carpus
      - Distal through metacarpal heads
    - Five longitudinal arches
      - Through each of the rays
  - Stability
    - MCP joint
      - Volar plate and the collateral ligaments
      - Collateral ligaments: taut in flexion, lax in extension
    - PIP and DIP joints
      - Rely more on joint congruity
      - Large ratio of ligament to articular surface
  - Other concepts
    - Hand pulleys prevent bowstringing and decrease tendon excursion.
      - Bowstringing increases moment arms.

	Table 1-55	Recommended Positions of Flexion for Arthrodesis of the Joints of the Hand
JOINT	**DEGREES OF FLEXION**	**OTHER FACTORS**
MCP	20-30	
PIP	40-50	Less radial than ulnar
DIP	15-20	
Thumb CMC		
Thumb MCP	25	MC in opposition
Thumb IP	20	

CMC, Carpometacarpal; DIP, distal interphalangeal; MC, metacarpal; MCP, metacarpophalangeal; PIP, proximal interphalangeal.

- Sagittal bands allow MCP extension.
- With hyperextension of the MCP, the intrinsic muscles must function to produce PIP extension, because the extension tendon is lax.
- Normal grasp
  - For boys and men: 50 kg
  - For girls and women: 25 kg
  - Only 4 kg needed for daily function
- Normal pinch
  - For boys and men: 8 kg
  - For girls and women: 4 kg
  - Only 1 kg needed for daily activities
- Kinetics
  - Joint loading with pinch mostly in MCP
    - Because they have large surface area, however, contact pressures (joint load/contact area) are lower.
  - DIP joints have the most contact pressure.
    - Subsequently develop the most degenerative changes with time (Heberden nodes)
  - Grasping contact pressures are decreased, focused on MCP
    - Patients with MCP arthritis often had occupations in which grasping was required.
  - Compressive loads occur at the thumb with pinching.
    - At interphalangeal joint: 3 kg
    - At MCP joint: 5 kg
    - At carpometacarpal joint: 12 kg
      - An unstable joint
      - Frequently leads to degeneration
- Arthrodesis (Table 1-55)

SELECTED BIBLIOGRAPHY

The selected bibliography for this chapter can be found on www.expertconsult.com.

TESTABLE CONCEPTS

SECTION 1 ORTHOPAEDIC TISSUES

I. Bone

A. Histologic Features of Bone

- Osteoblasts are derived from undifferentiated mesenchymal stem cells, and RUNX2 is the multifunctional transcription factor that directs this process.
- Osteoblasts produce type I collagen (i.e., bone), alkaline phosphatase, osteocalcin, bone sialoprotein, and RANKL.
- Osteocytes are former osteoblasts surrounded by newly formed matrix. They constitute 90% of the cells in the mature skeleton, are important for control of extracellular calcium and phosphorous concentration, and are less active in matrix production than are osteoblasts.
- Osteoclasts are derived from hematopoietic cells in the macrophage lineage. RANKL is produced by osteoblasts, binds to immature osteoclasts, and stimulates differentiation into active, mature osteoclasts that result in an increase in bone resorption. Osteoprotegerin inhibits bone resorption by binding and inactivating RANKL.
- Osteoclasts bind to bone surfaces by means of integrins (vitronectin receptor), effectively sealing the space below, and then create a ruffled border and remove bone matrix by proteolytic digestion through the lysosomal enzyme cathepsin K.
- Bisphosphonates directly inhibit osteoclastic bone resorption. Nitrogen-containing bisphosphonates are up to 1000-fold more potent than non–nitrogen-containing bisphosphonates. Bisphosphonates function by inhibiting farnesyl pyrophosphate synthase in the mevalonate pathway. They are associated with osteonecrosis of the jaw, and in animal models, they have reduced the rate of spinal fusion.
- Bone matrix is 60% inorganic (mineral) components and 40% organic components. Calcium hydroxyapatite $Ca_{10}(PO_4)_6(OH)_2$ constitutes the majority of the inorganic matrix. Type I collagen is 90% of the organic component, and osteocalcin is the most abundant noncollagenous protein in bone.
- Wolff's law: Remodeling occurs in response to mechanical stress. Hueter-Volkmann law: Compressive forces inhibit growth, whereas tension stimulates it.
- There are three major types of bone formation. In enchondral formation, bone replaces a cartilage model. Intramembranous formation occurs without a cartilage model; aggregates of undifferentiated mesenchymal differentiate into osteoblasts, which form bone. In appositional formation, osteoblasts lay down new bone on existing bone; the groove of Ranvier supplies the chondrocytes.

B. Bone Injury and Repair

- There are three stages of fracture repair: inflammation, repair, and remodeling. Fracture healing type varies with treatment method. Closed treatment is through periosteal bridging callus and interfragmentary enchondral ossification. Compression plate treatment is through primary cortical healing.
- BMP-2 is used for acute open tibia fractures; BMP-7 is used for tibial nonunions. BMP-3 has no osteogenic activity. Increased BMP-4 is associated with the pathologic condition of fibrodysplasia ossificans progressiva.
  - NSAIDs adversely affect fracture healing and healing of lumbar spinal fusions. COX-2 activity is required for normal enchondral ossification during fracture healing.
- Bone grafts have three properties. Osteoconduction acts as a scaffold for bone growth; osteoinduction involves growth factors that stimulate bone formation; osteogenic grafts contain primitive mesenchymal cells, osteoblasts, and osteocytes.
- Calcium phosphate–based grafts are capable of osseoconduction and osseointegration. They have the highest compressive strength of any graft material. Calcium sulfate is osteoconductive but rapidly resorbed.

C. Normal Bone Metabolism

- The primary homeostatic regulators of serum calcium are PTH and $1,25(OH)_2$-vitamin D_3. PTH results in increased serum Ca^{2+} level and decreased inorganic phosphate level.
- Bone mass peaks between 16 and 25 years of age. Physiologic bone loss affects trabecular bone more than cortical bone.
- Both urinary hydroxyproline and pyridinoline cross-links are elevated when there is bone resorption.
- Serum alkaline phosphatase increases when bone formation increases.

D. Conditions of Bone Mineralization

- The most common cause of hypercalcemia is malignancy. Initial treatment is with hydration, which causes a saline diuresis, along with loop diuretics.
- Renal osteodystrophy is a spectrum of disorders observed in chronic renal disease. The majority of cases are caused by phosphorous retention and secondary hyperparathyroidism.
- Rickets (in children) and osteomalacia (in adults) are caused by a failure of mineralization. In rickets, the width of the zone of provisional calcification is increased, which causes physeal widening and cupping.

E. Conditions of Bone Mineral Density

- Osteoporosis is a quantitative defect in bone. It is defined as a lumbar bone density of 2.5 or more standard deviations less than the peak bone mass of a healthy 25-year-old (T-score).
- Treatment of osteoporosis includes calcium supplements of 1000 to 1500 mg/day, as well as bisphosphonates.
- Scurvy results from ascorbic acid deficiency, which causes a decrease in chondroitin sulfate synthesis and ultimately defective collagen growth and repair. Widening in the zone of provisional calcification is observed.
- Osteogenesis imperfecta is caused primarily by a mutation in genes responsible for metabolism and synthesis of type I collagen.

F. Conditions of Bone Viability

- The causes of osteonecrosis are unclear, but there are numerous risk factors. Bone is weakest during the resorptive and remodeling phases. MRI provides the earliest positive findings and has the highest sensitivity and specificity.

II. Joints

A. Hyaline Cartilage Structure and Function

- Articular cartilage is composed of water (65%-80% of wet weight), collagen (10%-20% of dry weight but more than 50% of dry weight), proteoglycans (10%-15% of wet weight), and chondrocytes (5% of wet weight). Collagen is 95% type II, contains hydroxyproline, and provides tensile strength. Proteoglycans are composed of glycosaminoglycans and include chondroitin sulfate and keratin sulfate; these provide compressive and elastic strength.
- Chondrocytes are derived from mesenchymal precursors; the SOX-9 transcriptional factor is considered the "master switch."

TESTABLE CONCEPTS

Mechanotransduction describes how metabolism is regulated by mechanical stimulation. Chondrocytes produce both the precursors of the matrix and the enzymes that maintain and destroy the matrix metalloproteinases.

- The effects of aging and osteoarthritis on cartilage are generally opposite except for proteoglycan content, which decreases in both conditions. Aging is a lack of anabolic response. Osteoarthritis results from chondrocytes reacting to cytokines and producing enzymes that degrade matrix. In osteoarthritis, the water content is increased, proteoglycan content decreased, keratin sulfate concentration decreased, and proteoglycan degradation significantly increased.
- Synovial tissue lacks a basement membrane but allows nutrition via capillary-rich connective tissue. Type A synovial cells act like macrophages while type B cells make the synovial non-newtonian ultrafiltrate fluid containing lubricin known as a boundary lubricant.

B. Arthritis

- Charcot arthropathy from disturbed sensory innervation is an extreme form of noninflammatory arthritis characterized by radiographic finds worse than clinical complaints and fragments of bone in soft tissue. Diabetes is the most common overall cause and the most common cause of Charcot disease in foot and ankle joints. Syringomyelia is the most common cause in the upper extremity joints, followed by Hansen disease.
- Ochronosis is black cartilage arthritis from alkaptonuria.
- Hemochromatosis often presents first as arthritis with chondrocalcinosis. The cirrhosis and skin "bronzing" develop later.
- Rheumatoid arthritis (RA) affects synovium and soft tissue first. Late synovial changes include hyperplastic cells, increased blood vessels, and abundant lymphocytes. Pannus ingrowth denudes articular cartilage. There are no lymphocytes in pannus.
- DMARDs are increasingly being used in the treatment of RA and most, such as infliximab and etanercept, target TNF-α.
- Systemic lupus erythematosus (SLE) is an autoimmune disease (against nucleic acids and nuclear proteins, hence almost always ANA positive) characterized by immune complex deposition with familiar changes in the skin and kidney.
- Seronegative spondylarthritides have many overlapping findings but are distinguished by their negative RF titer and usually negative ANA. They are named by common extraarticular characteristics: ankylosing spondylitis has fused sacroiliac joints and frequent back involvement that leads to stiffness (positive Schober flexion test). Reactive arthritis is a syndrome where the immune system is reactive to external infections, often of the mucosa, and often has swelling of a knee, along with eye and urologic symptoms. Psoriatic arthritis has nail and skin changes and the unusual inflammatory arthritis involvement of the DIP joints. Enteropathic arthritis is associated with inflammatory bowel disease.
- Gout results in deposition of monosodium urate crystals in joints. The classical radiographic finding is the appearance of punched-out periarticular erosions. Indomethacin is the initial treatment; allopurinol lowers serum acid levels chronically, and colchicine is used for prophylaxis.
- CPPD (pseudogout) is characterized by positively birefringent crystals and is a common cause of chondrocalcinosis.
- Hemophilic arthropathy is most commonly caused by factor VIII deficiency and most commonly involves the knee. Treatment is through correction of factor levels.
- Unusual arthritides that are likely reactive to infections are acute rheumatic fever (group A streptococcus) that causes carditis, erythema marginatum, and chorea; Whipple disease (very rare; *Tropheryma whipplei*) that causes diarrhea and is fatal untreated; and Lyme disease *(Borrelia burgdorferi)* that causes erythema migrans, Bell palsy, and meningitis.

III: Neuromuscular and Connective Tissues

A. Skeletal Muscle

- Myasthenia gravis is an autoimmune disease with defects in transmission of nerve impulses to muscles that result from blocking, altering, or destroying acetylcholine receptors at the neuromuscular junction.
- Botulinum A blocks presynaptic acetylcholine release at the motor end plate.
- Skeletal muscle tension and contractile force are determined by cross-sectional area.
- Skeletal muscle velocity is determined by fiber length.
- There are three types of muscle contractions: isotonic (constant muscle tension), isometric (muscle length remains unchanged), and isokinetic (constant velocity) (see Table 1-26).
- Type I skeletal muscle fibers are slow twitch and fatigue resistant; type II are fast twitch and fatigable (see Table 1-27).
- ATP-creatine phosphate (phosphagen) system is anaerobic, produces no lactate, and is active in muscle activities lasting less than 20 seconds.
- Lactic acid metabolism is also anaerobic and is active in muscle activities of 20 to 120 seconds.
- Strength training increases myofibrils, fiber size, and cross-sectional area, with hypertrophy of type II fibers.
- Muscle tear healing is most reliant upon satellite cells, and TGF-β stimulates proliferation of myofibroblasts and increases fibrosis. In acute muscle injury, the first cells recruited are neutrophils.
- Muscle soreness is due to edema and inflammation within connective tissue.

B. Nervous System

- Preganglionic injuries: normal histamine response test with medial scapular winging due to serratus anterior palsy.
- Post-ganglionic injuries: abnormal histamine response test (with no flare), maintained innervation to cervical paraspinals.
- Axon budding proceeds antegrade, and pain is the first sensation to return.
- SSEPs only monitor dorsal column sensory pathways and are less sensitive to anesthesia.
- MEPs only monitor anterior (ventral and lateral) corticospinal tracts.
- Nerve healing depends on age. Distal injuries recover better, but the longer the wait, the worse the recovery.
- Nerves that are good candidates for grouped fascicular repair are the median and ulnar nerves at the distal third of the forearm, and the sciatic nerve.

C. Connective Tissues

- Decorin has antifibrotic properties.
- Tendons receive blood from the vincular system if they are sheathed and through simple diffusion from the paratenon.
- Surgical tendon repairs are weakest at days 7 to 10.
- Tenocytes are responsible for the ECM generation in tendons.
- Type III collagen is the first collagen produced at sites of tendon injury.
- Achilles tendon is hypovascular 4 to 6 cm proximal to the calcaneal insertion.

TESTABLE CONCEPTS

- Ligaments are composed of type I collagen and elastin. They differ from tendons in that they have less collagen, more proteoglycans (and water), highly cross-linked collagen, and are perfused at insertion sites.
- Ligaments have Sharpey fibers that insert into the periosteum.
- The nucleus pulposus has a low collagen/proteoglycan ratio and dries out/desiccates with age, owing to loss of hydrostatic pressure (from loss of proteoglycans).
- The annulus fibrosis has a high collagen/proteoglycan ratio.
- The dorsal root ganglion gives off the sinuvertebral nerve, which innervates the superficial fibers of the annulus.
- Early degenerative disc disease is an irreversible process, with IL-1β acting on cells.
- Changes due to the aging process are drying out of intervertebral discs, decrease and fragmentation of proteoglycans, and increased keratin sulfate/chondroitin sulfate ratio, but no change in absolute quantity of collagen.
- Osteochondral allografts are used for lesions larger than 2 cm.
- Osteochondral autografts are used for lesions smaller than 2 cm.

SECTION 2 ORTHOPAEDIC BIOLOGY

I. Cellular and Molecular Biology

A. Chromosomes

- Anti-Scl-70 is linked to scleroderma.
- Anti-Jo-1 is linked to polymyositis and dermatomyositis.
- Anti-Sm is linked to SLE (specific but not sensitive—i.e., only present in one fifth of those with SLE).
- Anti-RNP leads to mixed connective tissue disease.
- Anti-ds-DNA is linked to SLE and implicated in SLE nephritis.
- Antihistone is present in drug-induced lupus.
- Anti-Ro and Anti-La are linked to Sjögren syndrome.
- The cell cycle goes from diploid (2N) to tetraploid (4N) during the S phase.
- pRb is implicated in retinoblastoma and osteosarcoma.
- p53 is implicated in osteosarcoma, rhabdomyosarcoma, and chondrosarcoma.
- A plasmid is a small extrachromosomal circular piece of DNA that replicates independently of DNA.
- Blotting
  - Southern—detection of **DNA** sequences in a sample
  - Northern—detection of **RNA** in a sample
  - Western—detection of specific amino-acid sequences in **proteins**
- RT-PCR produces DNA from RNA.

B. Immunology

- The immune system is broadly categorized into two branches: the **innate** and **adaptive,** with interaction and overlap between the two. Excessive immune responses can lead to host tissue damage and are known as *hypersensitivity reactions.*
  - Type II hypersensitivity is antibody mediated. Examples are heparin-induced thrombocytopenia and myasthenia gravis.
  - Type IV hypersensitivity occurs in response to orthopaedic hardware.
  - Pseudotumor hypersensitivity syndrome can occur years after total hip arthroplasty.
- Immunoglobulins
  - Rheumatoid factor is an IgM against IgG.
  - IgA is seen in mucosa-associated lymphoid tissue.
  - IgE mediates type I hypersensitivity reactions.

- Neutrophils are the first cells recruited to the site of injury.
- Macrophages initiate the inflammatory response in osteolysis/aseptic loosening in response to particles smaller than 1 μm.
- Ibuprofen inhibits COX and can be nephrotoxic, depending on the dose.
- Anti-TNF-α medications are associated with opportunistic infections.
- TGF-β promotes fibrosis.
- If unmanaged for more than 20 years, a chronically draining sinus tract in osteomyelitis or burns can undergo malignant degeneration into squamous cell carcinoma.
- Common tumor antigens are as follows:
  - Carcinoembryonic antigen (CEA): colorectal carcinoma
  - Carbohydrate antigen 19-9 (CA-19-9): pancreatic cancer
  - Carbohydrate antigen 125 (CA-125): ovarian cancer
  - Cancer antigen 15-3 (CA-15-3): breast cancer
  - α-Fetoprotein (AFP): hepatocellular carcinoma

C. Genetics

- Classic mendelian inheritance is through one of four modes: autosomal dominant, autosomal recessive, X-linked recessive, and (very rare) X-linked dominant.
- Frequently tested mendelian inheritance patterns and associated genetic defects are as follows:
  - Autosomal dominant:
    - Achondroplasia: FGF receptor 3 *(FGFR3)*
    - Apert Syndrome: *FGFR2*
    - Cleidocranial dysplasia: *CBFA1*
    - Charcot-Marie-Tooth (most common variety): *PMP22*
    - Pseudoachondroplasia: *COMP*
      - SED congenital: *COL2A1* for type II collagen
      - Kniest syndrome: type II collagen
      - MED type 1: *COMP*
      - MED type 2: type IX collagen
      - Jansen metaphyseal chondrodysplasia: PTHrP
      - Schmid metaphyseal chondrodysplasia: type X collagen
    - Ehlers-Danlos (most common variety): *COL*
    - Hereditary multiple exostoses: *EXT1/EXT2/EXT3*
    - Neurofibromatosis: *NF1, NF2*
    - Marfan syndrome: *FBN1*
    - Osteopetrosis (tarda form)
    - Osteogenesis imperfecta (types I and IV): *COL1A1/COL1A2*
  - Autosomal recessive:
    - Diastrophic dysplasia: DTD-ST (sulfate transport protein)
    - Friedreich ataxia: frataxin
    - Gaucher disease: lysosomal glucocerebrosidase
    - Sickle cell disease: HbSS
    - Osteopetrosis (malignant form)
    - Osteogenesis imperfecta (types II and III): *COL1A1/COL1A2*
    - Thrombocytopenia-aplasia of radius (TAR) syndrome
    - Charcot Marie Tooth (rare form): connexin gene
  - X-linked recessive:
    - Duchenne and Becker muscular dystrophy: dystrophin
    - Hemophilia: factors VIII or IX
    - SED tarda: *COL2A1*
  - X-linked dominant:
    - Hypophosphatemic rickets: *PHEX*
    - Léri-Weill dyschondrosteosis: *SHOX*
  - Sporadic

TESTABLE CONCEPTS

- McCune-Albright syndrome: Gsα subunit of the receptor/adenylyl cyclase–coupling G proteins
- Common translocations tested:
  - t(X:18) in synovial sarcoma
  - t(11:22) in Ewing sarcoma
  - t(2:13) in rhabdomyosarcoma
  - t(12:16) in myxoid liposarcoma
  - t(12:22) in clear cell sarcoma
  - t(9,22) in myxoid chondrosarcoma

II. Infections and Microbiology

A. Musculoskeletal Infections Overview

- Necrotizing fasciitis involves subcutaneous fat and deep fascia. Diabetes is the most common risk factor. Polymicrobial infection is the most common cause; group A β-hemolytic streptococcal infections are most common in healthy individuals.
- Community-acquired methicillin-resistant *Staphylococcus aureus* (MRSA) is increasingly prevalent among athletes, military recruits, and prison populations.
- C-reactive protein is the most sensitive monitor of the course of infection; it has a short half-life and dissipates about 1 week after effective treatment.
- The most common causes of osteomyelitis by age or disease are as follows:
  - Age 0 to 4 months: *S. aureus*, gram-negative bacilli, group B streptococcus
  - Age 4 months to 21 years: *S. aureus*, group A streptococci
  - Epiphyseal osteomyelitis: *S. aureus*
  - Age older than 21 years: *S. aureus*, coagulase-negative staphylococci
  - Patients with sickle cell disease: *S. aureus* and *Salmonella* organisms
  - Patients with open fracture: *S. aureus*, *P. aeruginosa*, and gram-negative bacilli
  - Diabetic patients: polymicrobial (both aerobic and anaerobic)
  - Intravenous drug abusers: *S. aureus*, *Serratia* spp., *Pseudomonas* spp.
  - Meat handlers: *Brucella* spp.
  - Fishermen: *Mycobacterium* spp.
- Radiographic changes of osteomyelitis include sequestrum (dead bone with surrounding granulation tissue) and involucrum (periosteal new bone).
- Except for sexually active adults, in whom the most common causative organism is *Neisseria gonorrhoeae*, the most common cause of septic arthritis is *S. aureus*.
- In non–sexually active adults, *S. aureus* and streptococci are the most common causative organisms.
- Tetanus immune globulin is administered only when tetanus status is unknown or the patient has received fewer than three immunizations. Tetanus toxoid is given if the wound is severe or occurred more than 24 hours previously and if the patient has received no booster vaccination within the previous 5 years.
- The risk of acquiring disease from a needlestick from contaminated source is as follows: hepatitis B, 30% in unvaccinated persons; hepatitis C, 3%; HIV, 0.3%.

D. Antibiotics

- Frequently tested antibiotic mechanisms of action are as follows:
  - β-Lactam antibiotics (penicillin and cephalosporins): inhibit cross-linking of polysaccharides in the cell wall by blocking transpeptidase enzyme

- Vancomycin: interferes with the insertion of glycan subunits into the cell wall
- Rifampin: inhibits RNA polymerase F
- Clindamycin: binds to 50S ribosomal subunits and inhibits protein synthesis
- Quinolones (ciprofloxacin): inhibit DNA gyrase
- Antibiotic resistance is mediated by plasmids and transposons. MRSA has the *mecA* gene that produces the enzyme penicillin-binding protein 2a, which prevents the normal enzymatic acylation of antibiotics.

SECTION 3 PERIOPERATIVE AND ORTHOPAEDIC MEDICINE

I. Perioperative Problems

- Pathophysiologic effects of DVT are caused by the Virchow triad: endothelial damage, venous stasis, and hypercoagulability. Tissue factor (thromboplastin) is released in large amounts during orthopaedic procedures, triggering the coagulation cascade.
- Warfarin (Coumadin) inhibits posttranslational modification of vitamin K–dependent clotting factors (factors II, VII, IX, and X; proteins C and S).
- Fat embolism is characterized by the triad of hypoxemia, CNS depression, and petechiae. Early skeletal stabilization decreases the incidence.

C. Shock

- There are four types of shock:
  - Hypovolemic: volume loss
  - Cardiogenic: ineffective pumping
  - Septic: blood pooling from vasodialation
  - Neurogenic: blood pooling and bradycardia

M. Special Anesthesia Issues

- **Malignant hyperthermia** is an autosomal dominant condition. It is triggered by "-ane" inhalational agents, depolarizing muscle relaxants (succinylcholine), and amide-based local anesthetics. The first signs are increased end-tidal CO_2 and tachycardia. Treatment is with dantrolene sodium, which blocks calcium release by stabilizing the sarcoplasmic reticulum.

II. Orthopaedic Pharmacology

- NSAIDs inhibit COX, which is involved in forming prostaglandins from arachidonic acid. Gastrointestinal complications are common, and concurrent anticoagulant use is the most important risk factor, followed by age older than 60 and a history of previous gastrointestinal disease. COX-2 inhibitors do not inhibit COX-1, which maintains gastric mucosa.
- The most common transfusion adverse event is a clerical error that leads to a transfusion reaction.
- Garlic, *Ginkgo biloba*, and ginseng increase the risk of bleeding in the perioperative period.

SECTION 4 OTHER BASIC PRINCIPLES

I. Imaging and Special Studies

A. Radiation Safety

- Basic radiation safety principles are decreased radiation exposure with increased distance between surgeon and radiation beam, limiting fluoroscopic time, using the mini c-arm, orienting the beam in a position inverted to the patient, use of protective shielding, and collimation.

D. Magnetic Resonance Imaging

- MRI basic principles are as follows:
  - T1 weighting: fat best demonstrates anatomic structure.
  - T2 weighting: water is best for contrasting normal and abnormal tissues.
  - The following appear dark on T1-weighted images and bright on T2-weighted images: water, cerebrospinal fluid, acute hemorrhage, and soft tissue tumors.

II. Biomaterials and Biomechanics

A. Basic Concepts

- Force is a mechanical push or pull (load) causing external (acceleration) and internal (strain) effects.
- Moment is the rotational effect of a force. The mass moment of inertia is the resistance to rotation.
- The human body's center of gravity is just anterior to S2.

B. Biomaterials

- Stress is the intensity of internal force. Stress = force/area. Unit of measure: pascal (N/m^2).
- Strain is a measure of deformation resulting from loading. Strain is the change in length/original length. There is no standard unit of measure.
- Young's modulus of elasticity (*E*) is a measure of material stiffness (ability to resist deformation in tension): E = stress/strain. Materials with higher *E* withstand greater forces. The following materials are listed in order of high to low modulus: ceramic, cobalt-chrome, stainless steel, titanium, cortical bone, PMMA, polyethylene, cancellous bone, tendon/ligament, and cartilage.
- Strain energy (toughness) is the capacity of material to absorb energy before failure.
- Material types include the following:
  - Brittle: linear stress-strain curve with limited capacity for plastic deformation
    - PMMA
  - Ductile: large plastic deformation before failure
    - Metal
  - Viscoelastic: have time- and rate-dependent stress-strain behavior and exhibit hysteresis (loading and unloading curves differ)
    - Bone, ligaments, and most biological tissues

- Isotropic: mechanical properties are the same for all directions of applied load
  - Golf ball
- Anisotropic: mechanical properties vary with direction of applied load
  - Bone is stronger with axial load than with radial load.
- Galvanic corrosion occurs when dissimilar metals are in direct contact and result in corrosion products (metal oxides and chlorides). Risk of galvanic corrosion is highest between 316 L stainless steel and cobalt-chromium (Co-Cr) alloy.
- There are three major types of orthopaedically important alloys:
- 316 L stainless steel: iron-carbon, chromium, nickel, molybdenum, and manganese
- Cobalt: cobalt, chromium, molybdenum, and nickel
- Titanium: titanium, aluminum, and vanadium
- PMMA bone cement acts as a grout, not an adhesive. It is strongest in compression and has poor tensile and shear strength.

C. Biomechanics

- *Joint reaction force* is the force generated within a joint in response to external force. Muscle contraction is the major contributing factor.
- *Friction* is the resistance between two objects as one slides over the other. Lubrication decreases resistance between surfaces. Elastohydrodynamic lubrication is the primary lubrication mechanism for articular cartilage during dynamic function.
- Principles of arthrodesis (Figure 1-91) are as follows:
  - Hip: 25 to 30 degrees of flexion, 0 degrees of abduction and rotation
  - Knee: 0 to 7 degrees of valgus angulation, 10 to 15 degrees of flexion
  - Ankle: neutral dorsiflexion, 5 to 10 degrees of external rotation, 5 degrees of hindfoot valgus angulation
  - Shoulder: 15 to 20 degrees of abduction, 20 to 25 degrees of forward flexion, 40 to 50 degrees of internal rotation
  - Elbow: 90 degrees of flexion if arthrodesis is unilateral. If it is bilateral: one elbow at 110 degrees of flexion for the hand to reach the mouth and the other at 65 degrees of flexion for perineal hygiene.
  - Wrist: 10 to 20 degrees of dorsiflexion for unilateral fusion. If arthrodesis is bilateral, fuse the other side at 0 to 10 degrees of palmar flexion.

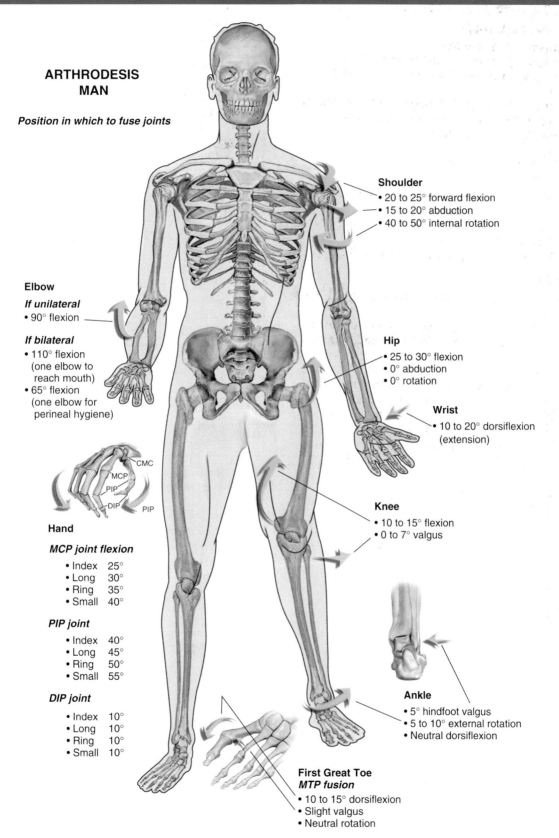

ARTHRODESIS MAN

Position in which to fuse joints

Shoulder
- 20 to 25° forward flexion
- 15 to 20° abduction
- 40 to 50° internal rotation

Elbow

If unilateral
- 90° flexion

If bilateral
- 110° flexion
  (one elbow to
  reach mouth)
- 65° flexion
  (one elbow for
  perineal hygiene)

Hip
- 25 to 30° flexion
- 0° abduction
- 0° rotation

Wrist
- 10 to 20° dorsiflexion
  (extension)

CMC
MCP
PIP
DIP
PIP

Hand

MCP joint flexion
- Index   25°
- Long   30°
- Ring   35°
- Small   40°

PIP joint
- Index   40°
- Long   45°
- Ring   50°
- Small   55°

DIP joint
- Index   10°
- Long   10°
- Ring   10°
- Small   10°

Knee
- 10 to 15° flexion
- 0 to 7° valgus

Ankle
- 5° hindfoot valgus
- 5 to 10° external rotation
- Neutral dorsiflexion

First Great Toe
MTP fusion
- 10 to 15° dorsiflexion
- Slight valgus
- Neutral rotation

FIGURE 1-91 Recommended positions for arthrodesis of common joints. *CMC,* Carpometacarpal; *DIP,* distal interphalangeal; *MCP,* metacarpophalangeal; *MTP,* metatarsophalangeal; *PIP,* proximal interphalangeal.

CHAPTER 2

ANATOMY

F. Winston Gwathmey, Jr., and M. Tyrrell Burrus

CONTENTS

SECTION 1 INTRODUCTION

OVERVIEW

- **Osteology: 206 bones in the human skeleton—80 in the axial skeleton and 126 in the appendicular skeleton**
- Ossification:
  - Intramembranous (direct laying down of bone without a cartilage model [skull]) or enchondral (with a cartilage precursor [most bones]).
  - Enchondral growth begins in the diaphyses of long bones at primary ossification centers, most of which are present at birth (Table 2-1).
- Secondary ossification centers usually develop at proximal or distal ends of bones and are important for growth.
  - Frequently the site of pediatric physeal fractures
- Heterotopic ossification: formation of bone tissue in an atypical extraskeletal location
- **Arthrology: joints are commonly classified into three types on the basis of their freedom of movement.**
- Synarthroses: joining of two bony elements with no motion during maturity (e.g., skull sutures)
- Amphiarthroses: have hyaline cartilage and intervening discs with limited motion (e.g., symphysis pubis)
- Diarthroses: characterized by hyaline cartilage, synovial membranes, capsules, and ligaments
- **Myology: classification based on the arrangement of muscle fibers**
- Parallel (e.g., rhomboids)
- Fusiform (e.g., biceps brachii)
- Oblique (with tendinous interdigitation): further classified as pennate, bipennate, multipennate
- Triangular (e.g., pectoralis minor)
- Spiral (e.g., latissimus dorsi)
- **Nerves**
- Peripheral nerves
  - Originate from the ventral rami of spinal nerves and are distributed via several plexuses (cervical, brachial, lumbosacral)
  - The mnemonic "SAME" can be used to help understand the function of nerves: sensory = afferent; motor = efferent.
  - Efferent (motor) fibers carry impulses from the central nervous system (CNS) to muscles.
  - Afferent (sensory) fibers carry information toward the CNS.
- Autonomic nerves
  - Control visceral structures
  - Consist of parasympathetic (craniosacral) and sympathetic (thoracolumbar) divisions
    - Preganglionic neurons of parasympathetic nerves:
      - Arise in the nuclei of cranial nerves III, VII, IX, and X and in the S2, S3, and S4 segments of the spinal cord
      - Synapse in peripheral ganglia
    - Preganglionic neurons in the sympathetic system
      - Located in the spinal cord (T1-L3)
      - Synapse in chain ganglia adjacent to spine and collateral ganglia along major abdominal blood vessels
- **Vessels: arteries, veins, and lymphatic vessels**
- Courses and relationships are important and are highlighted in this chapter.

Table 2-1	Summary of Ossification Patterns		
BONE	**OSSIFICATION CENTER**	**AGE AT APPEARANCE**	**AGE AT FUSION**
Scapula	Body (primary)	8 wk (fetal)	
	Coracoid (tip)	1 yr	
	Coracoid	15 yr	
	Acromion	15 yr	
	Acromion	16 yr	
	Inferior angle	16 yr	
	Medial border	16 yr	
Clavicle	Medial (primary)	5 wk (fetal)	25 yr
	Lateral (primary)	5 wk (fetal)	
	Sternal	19 yr	
Humerus	Body (primary)	8 wk (fetal)	Blends at 6 yr and unites at 20 yr
	Head	1 yr	
	Greater tuberosity	3 yr	
	Lesser tuberosity	5 yr	
	Capitellum	2 yr	Blends and unites with body at 16-18 yr
	Medial epicondyles	5 yr	
	Trochlea	9 yr	
	Lateral epicondyles	13 yr	
Ulna	Body (primary)	8 wk (fetal)	
	Distal ulna	5 yr	20 yr
	Olecranon	10 yr	16 yr
Radius	Body (primary)	8 wk (fetal)	
	Distal radius	2 yr	17-20 yr
	Proximal radius	5 yr	15-18 yr
Pelvis	Ilium (primary)	2 mo	15 yr
	Ischium (primary)	4 mo	15 yr
	Pubis (primary)	6 mo	15 yr
	Acetabulum	12 yr	15 yr
Tibia	Body (primary)	7 wk (fetal)	
	Proximal (secondary)	Birth	20 yr
	Distal (secondary)	2 yr	18 yr
Fibula	Body (primary)	8 wk (fetal)	
	Proximal (secondary)	3 yr	25 yr
	Distal (secondary)	2 yr	20 yr

SECTION 2 UPPER EXTREMITY

SHOULDER

- **Osteology:** shoulder girdle consists of the scapula and clavicle (which articulate with chest wall) and the proximal humerus (which articulates with scapula at glenohumeral joint).
- Scapula
  - Spans second through seventh ribs and serves as an attachment for 17 muscles
  - Anteverted on chest wall approximately 30 degrees relative to the body
  - **Glenoid retroverted approximately 5 degrees relative to scapular body**
  - Scapular spine: separates supraspinatus from infraspinatus
  - Acromion: continuation of scapular spine
    - Os acromiale: incomplete fusion of secondary ossification centers, most commonly between meso- and metaacromion
  - Coracoid: attachments to coracoid include coracoacromial ligament, coracoclavicular ligaments (conoid [medial] and trapezoid [lateral]), conjoined tendon (coracobrachialis and short head of biceps), and pectoralis minor.
  - Suprascapular notch: superior transverse scapular ligament separates suprascapular artery (superior) from suprascapular nerve (inferior). Mnemonic: "Army over Navy" for artery over nerve

- Spinoglenoid notch: both the artery and nerve inferior to the inferior transverse scapular ligament
- Coracoacromial ligament
  - Contributes to anterosuperior stability in rotator cuff deficiency
  - **Should be preserved with irreparable cuff tears to prevent anterosuperior escape**
  - Acromial branch of the thoracoacromial artery runs on medial aspect of the coracoacromial ligament.
- Clavicle
  - Strut for lateral movement of the arm
  - Double curvature (sternal-ventral, acromial-dorsal)
  - **First bone in the body to ossify (at 5 weeks' gestation) and last to fuse (medial epiphysis at 25 years of age)**
  - Fracture of clavicle is the most common musculoskeletal birth injury.
- Proximal humerus
  - Humeral head retroverted 30 degrees relative to transepicondylar axis of humerus
    - **Head height approximately 5.6 cm above superior border of pectoralis major tendon (important for arthroplasty)**
  - Anatomic neck, directly below humeral head, serves as an attachment for the shoulder capsule.
  - Surgical neck more distal and more often involved in fractures

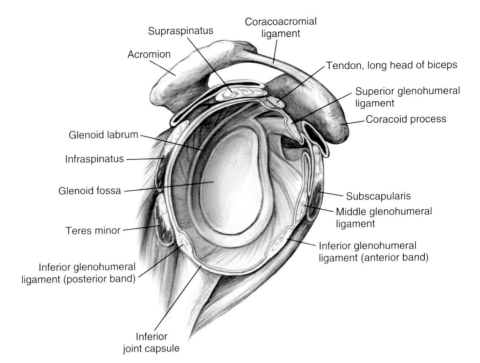

FIGURE 2-1 Glenohumeral ligaments and rotator cuff muscles. The rotator interval is between the anterior border of the supraspinatus and the superior border of the subscapularis. This interval helps limit flexion and external rotation of the shoulder. Within the rotator interval is the superior glenohumeral ligament, the primary restraint both in inferior translation of the adducted shoulder and in external rotation of the adducted or slightly abducted arm. The middle glenohumeral ligament, absent in up to 30% of shoulders, is the primary stabilizer in anterior translation with the arm slightly abducted (45 degrees). The inferior glenohumeral ligament complex is the primary stabilizer for anterior and inferior instability in abduction. The inferior glenohumeral ligament complex is composed of the anterior and posterior bands of the inferior glenohumeral ligament. (From Miller MD et al: *Orthopaedic surgical approaches,* Philadelphia, 2008, Saunders, Figure SA-4.)

- Greater tuberosity lateral to humeral head
  - Serves as attachment for supraspinatus, infraspinatus, and teres minor muscles (anterior to posterior, respectively)
- Lesser tuberosity, located anteriorly, has only one muscular insertion, the subscapularis.
- Bicipital groove (for tendon of long head of biceps brachii) is a bony groove between the two tuberosities.
- **Transverse humeral ligament is an important stabilizer of the biceps tendon.**
- ■ **Arthrology:** one major articulation (glenohumeral joint) and several minor articulations (sternoclavicular, acromioclavicular, scapulothoracic joints)
- Glenohumeral joint (Figure 2-1): ball and socket; greatest joint range of motion in body; motion is at the expense of stability which is provided by static and dynamic restraints
  - Static restraints: articular anatomy, glenoid labrum, glenohumeral ligaments, capsule, and negative intraarticular pressure
  - Dynamic stabilizers: rotator cuff and biceps tendon; scapulothoracic mechanics contribute to stability
  - Important glenohumeral stabilizers summarized in Table 2-2
  - Fibrocartilaginous glenoid labrum deepens socket 50% and provides bumper to translation
    - Labral anatomic variants include sublabral foramen (anterosuperior) and Buford complex (absence of anterosuperior labrum and cordlike middle glenohumeral ligament). **Use caution repairing anterosuperior labral variant—may cause loss of external rotation.**

Table 2-2	Glenohumeral Stabilizers
STRUCTURE	**FUNCTION**
Glenoid labrum	Increases surface area, deepens socket, static stabilizer
Coracohumeral ligament	Restrains inferior translation and external rotation of adducted arm
Superior glenohumeral ligament	Restrains external rotation and inferior translation of adducted or slightly abducted arm
Middle glenohumeral ligament (absent in up to 30% of shoulders)	Restrains anterior translation with arm abducted to 45 degrees
Inferior glenohumeral ligament, anterior band	Restrains anterior and inferior translation with arm externally rotated and abducted to 90 degrees (position of apprehension)
Inferior glenohumeral ligament, posterior band	Restrains posterior and inferior translation with arm internally rotated and abducted to 90 degrees

- ■ Sternoclavicular joint: (Figure 2-2)
  - Double gliding with an articular disc
  - **Only true joint connecting upper extremity with axial skeleton**
  - Anterior and posterior sternoclavicular ligaments, an interclavicular ligament, and a costoclavicular ligament. Posterior sternoclavicular ligament strongest and primary restraint to anteroposterior instability.
  - Rotates 30 degrees with shoulder motion

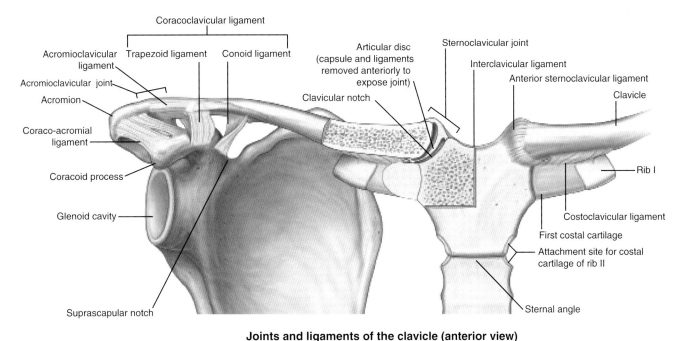

Joints and ligaments of the clavicle (anterior view)

FIGURE 2-2 Joints and ligaments of the clavicle (anterior view). (From Drake RL et al, editors: *Gray's atlas of anatomy,* ed 2, Philadelphia, 2015, Churchill Livingstone.)

- Acromioclavicular (AC) joint:
  - Plane/gliding joint with a fibrocartilaginous disc
  - Ligaments (see Figure 2-2):
    - **AC ligaments: prevent anteroposterior displacement**
    - Coracoclavicular ligaments: prevent superior displacement of distal clavicle
      - **Trapezoid (anterolateral): approximately 25 mm from AC joint**
      - **Conoid (posteromedial and stronger): approximately 45 mm from AC joint**
  - When the arm is maximally elevated, about 5 to 8 degrees of rotation is possible at the AC joint, although the clavicle rotates approximately 40 to 50 degrees.
- Scapulothoracic joint:
  - Though not a true joint, this attachment allows scapular movement against the posterior rib cage and contributes to glenohumeral joint positioning and mechanics.
  - Fixed primarily by the scapular muscular attachments
  - Positions the glenoid for glenohumeral motion. **Glenohumeral motion in comparison with scapulothoracic motion is in a 2:1 ratio.**
- **Muscles of the shoulder girdle (Figure 2-3, Table 2-3)**
- Muscles connecting the upper limb to the vertebral column: trapezius, latissimus, both rhomboid muscles, and levator scapulae
- Muscles connecting the upper limb to the thoracic wall: both pectoralis muscles, subclavius, and serratus anterior
- Muscles acting on the shoulder joint itself: deltoid, teres major, and the four rotator cuff muscles (supraspinatus, infraspinatus, teres minor, subscapularis)
  - **Rotator cuff muscles depress and stabilize the humeral head against the glenoid; all insert on the greater tuberosity except the subscapularis, which inserts on the lesser tuberosity insertion (shoulder internal rotator).**

- Shoulder internal rotators (pectoralis major, latissimus dorsi, teres major, and subscapularis) are stronger than external rotators (teres minor and infraspinatus), which is why posterior shoulder dislocations may occur with electric shock and seizures (Figure 2-4).
- Three important (and testable) spaces formed by muscles around the posteromedial shoulder (Figure 2-5, Table 2-4)
  - **Quadrangular space**
    - Borders: teres minor (superior), teres major (inferior), long head of triceps (medial), humerus (lateral)
    - Contents: axillary nerve and posterior humeral circumflex vessels
  - **Triangular space:** medial to quadrangular space
    - Borders: teres minor (superior), teres major (inferior), long head of triceps (lateral)
    - Contents: circumflex scapular vessels
  - **Triangular interval:** inferior to the quadrangular space (mnemonic: intervAL is distAL)
    - Borders: teres major (superior), long head of triceps (medial), lateral head of triceps/humerus (lateral)
    - Contents: radial nerve and profunda brachii artery

ARM

■ Osteology
- Humerus
  - Humeral shaft has a posterior spiral groove (for radial nerve) adjacent to the deltoid tuberosity that runs obliquely from proximal medial to distal lateral.
  - Distal humerus flares into medial and lateral epicondyles.
    - Trochlea: medial spool-shaped structure; articulates with olecranon of the ulna

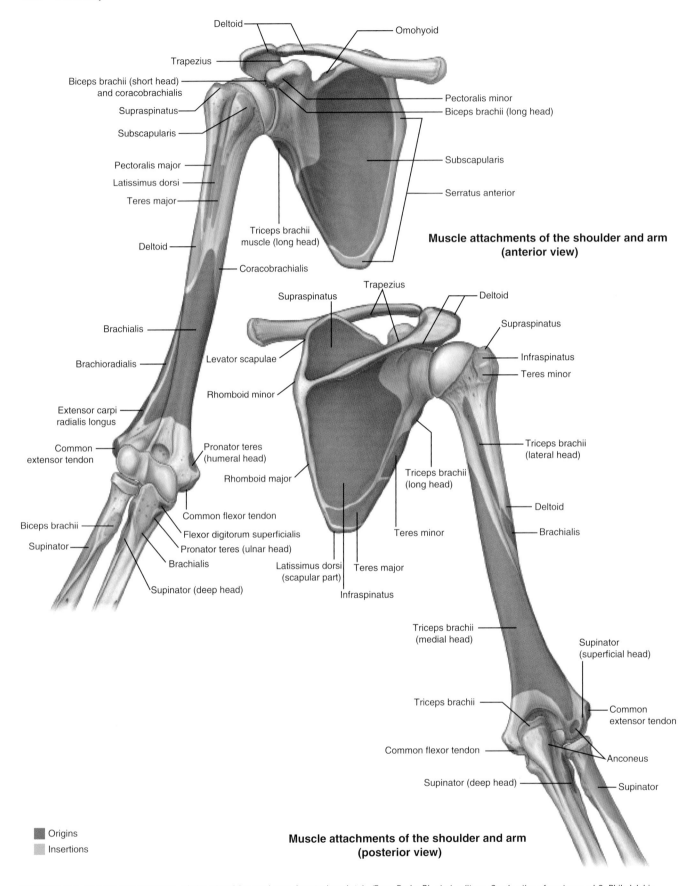

Deltoid — Omohyoid

Trapezius

Biceps brachii (short head) and coracobrachialis

Supraspinatus

Subscapularis

Pectoralis minor
Biceps brachii (long head)

Pectoralis major
Latissimus dorsi
Teres major

Subscapularis

Serratus anterior

Triceps brachii muscle (long head)

Deltoid

Coracobrachialis

Muscle attachments of the shoulder and arm (anterior view)

Supraspinatus
Trapezius
Deltoid
Supraspinatus

Brachialis

Levator scapulae

Infraspinatus
Teres minor

Brachioradialis

Rhomboid minor

Extensor carpi radialis longus

Common extensor tendon

Pronator teres (humeral head)

Rhomboid major

Triceps brachii (lateral head)

Triceps brachii (long head)

Deltoid

Biceps brachii

Supinator

Common flexor tendon
Flexor digitorum superficialis
Pronator teres (ulnar head)
Brachialis
Supinator (deep head)

Teres minor

Brachialis

Latissimus dorsi (scapular part)
Teres major
Infraspinatus

Triceps brachii (medial head)

Supinator (superficial head)

Triceps brachii

Common extensor tendon

Common flexor tendon

Anconeus

Supinator (deep head)

Supinator

Origins
Insertions

Muscle attachments of the shoulder and arm (posterior view)

FIGURE 2-3 Muscle attachments of the shoulder and arm (posterior view). (From Drake RL et al, editors: *Gray's atlas of anatomy,* ed 2, Philadelphia, 2015, Churchill Livingstone.)

Table 2-3	Muscles of the Shoulder			
MUSCLE	**ORIGIN**	**INSERTION**	**ACTION**	**INNERVATION**
Trapezius	SP C7-T12	Clavicle, scapula (acromion, SP)	Rotating scapula	Cranial nerve XI
Latissimus dorsi	SP T6-S5, ilium	Humerus (ITG)	Extending, adducting, internally rotating humerus	Thoracodorsal nerve
Rhomboid major	SP T2-T5	Scapula (medial border)	Adducting scapula	Dorsal scapular nerve
Rhomboid minor	SP C7-T1	Scapula (medial spine)	Adducting scapula	Dorsal scapular nerve
Levator scapulae	Transverse process C1-C4	Scapula (superior medial)	Elevating, rotating scapula	C3, C4 nerves
Pectoralis major	Sternum, ribs, clavicle	Humerus (lateral ITG)	Adducting, internally rotating arm	Medial and lateral pectoral nerves
Pectoralis minor	Ribs 3-5	Scapula (coracoid)	Protracting scapula	Medial pectoral nerve
Subclavius	Rib 1	Inferior clavicle	Depressing clavicle	Upper trunk nerves
Serratus anterior	Ribs 1-9	Scapula (ventral medial)	Preventing winging	Long thoracic nerve
Deltoid	Lateral clavicle, scapula	Humerus (deltoid tuberosity)	Abducting arm	Axillary nerve
Teres major	Inferior scapula	Humerus (medial ITG)	Adducting, internally rotating, extending arm	Lower subscapular nerve
Subscapularis	Ventral scapula	Humerus (lesser tuberosity)	Internally rotating arm, providing anterior stability	Upper and lower subscapular nerves
Supraspinatus	Superior scapula	Humerus (GT)	Abducting and externally rotating arm, providing stability	Suprascapular nerve
Infraspinatus	Dorsal scapula	Humerus (GT)	Providing stability, externally rotating arm	Suprascapular nerve
Teres minor	Scapula (dorsolateral)	Humerus (GT)	Providing stability, externally rotating arm	Axillary nerve

GT, Greater tuberosity; *ITG,* intertubercular groove; *SP,* spinous process.

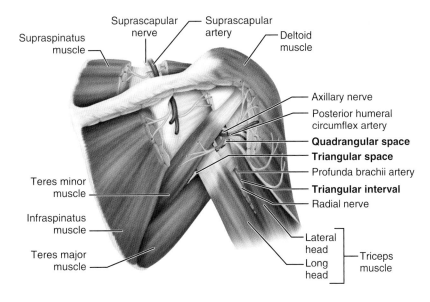

FIGURE 2-4 Borders of the key spaces and intervals, including the suprascapular nerve course as well as the quadrangular space and triangular space/interval.

- Capitellum: lateral globe-shaped structure; opposes radial head
- Articular surface of distal humerus has 7-degree valgus tilt relative to shaft (carrying angle of elbow).

■ **Arthrology**

▣ Elbow: hinge joint (humeroulnar articulation) and pivot joint (radiocapitellar articulation) (Table 2-5)

- Axis of rotation for the elbow is centered through the trochlea and capitellum and passes through a point anteroinferior on the medial epicondyle.
- **Radial head should line up with capitellum at all arm positions with all radiographic views.**
- **Tensile forces at medial elbow, compressive forces at lateral elbow**

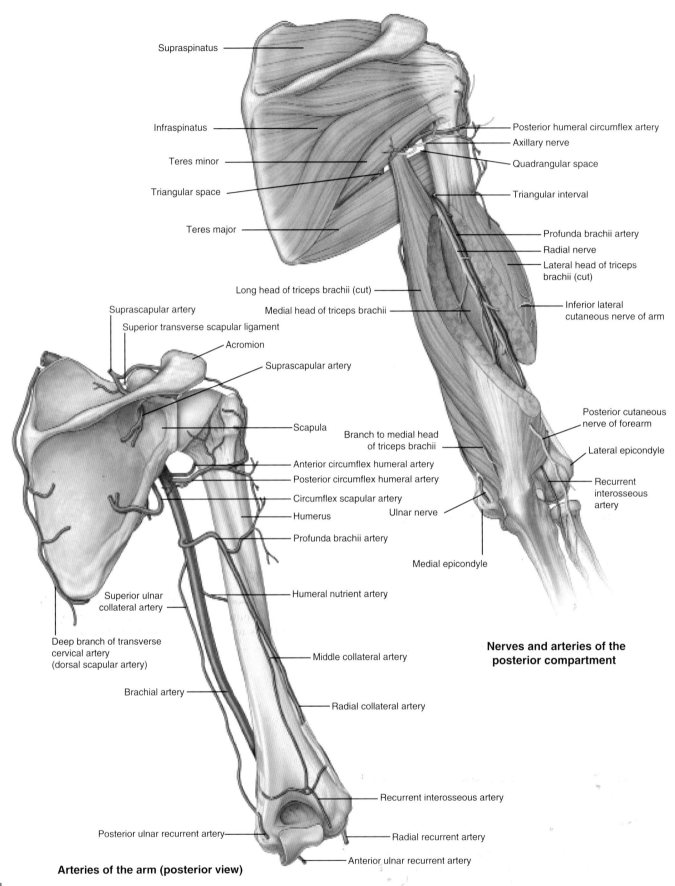

Supraspinatus

Infraspinatus

Teres minor

Triangular space

Teres major

Posterior humeral circumflex artery

Axillary nerve

Quadrangular space

Triangular interval

Profunda brachii artery

Radial nerve

Lateral head of triceps brachii (cut)

Long head of triceps brachii (cut)

Medial head of triceps brachii

Inferior lateral cutaneous nerve of arm

Suprascapular artery

Superior transverse scapular ligament

Acromion

Suprascapular artery

Scapula

Branch to medial head of triceps brachii

Anterior circumflex humeral artery

Posterior circumflex humeral artery

Circumflex scapular artery

Humerus

Profunda brachii artery

Ulnar nerve

Posterior cutaneous nerve of forearm

Lateral epicondyle

Recurrent interosseous artery

Medial epicondyle

Humeral nutrient artery

Superior ulnar collateral artery

Deep branch of transverse cervical artery (dorsal scapular artery)

Brachial artery

Middle collateral artery

Radial collateral artery

Nerves and arteries of the posterior compartment

Recurrent interosseous artery

Posterior ulnar recurrent artery

Radial recurrent artery

Anterior ulnar recurrent artery

Arteries of the arm (posterior view)

FIGURE 2-5 Nerves and arteries of the arm (posterior and compartment). (From Drake RL et al, editors: *Gray's atlas of anatomy,* ed 2, Philadelphia, 2015, Churchill Livingstone.)

Table 2-4   Shoulder Spaces and Intervals

SPACE	BORDERS	NERVE	ARTERY
Quadrangular (quadrilateral) space	Superior: lower border of teres minor Inferior: upper border of teres major Medial: long head of triceps Lateral: surgical neck of humerus	Axillary	Posterior humeral circumflex
Triangular space	Superior: lower border of teres minor Inferior: upper border of teres major Lateral: long head of triceps		Circumflex scapular
Triangular interval	Superior: lower border of teres major Medial: long head of triceps Lateral: shaft of humerus	Radial	Profunda brachii

Table 2-5   Elbow Joint Articulations

ARTICULATION	COMPONENTS
Humeroulnar	Trochlea and trochlear notch
Humeroradial	Capitellum and radial head
Proximal radioulnar	Radial notch and radial head

- Capsuloligamentous structures of elbow are a key source of testable material (Figure 2-6).
  - Capsule allows maximum distension at approximately 70 to 80 degrees of flexion, which is why patients with effusion hold their arms in this position, which is most comfortable.
  - Anterior capsule attaches at a point approximately 6 mm distal to the tip of the coronoid.
    - Coronoid tip is an intraarticular structure that is visualized during elbow arthroscopy.
  - Ligaments (Table 2-6)
  - **Medial or ulnar collateral ligament (MCL or UCL) (anterior, posterior, and transverse bundles) arises from the anteroinferior portion of the medial humeral epicondyle and is the primary static stabilizer to valgus stress.**
    - Anterior bundle is the most important in helping resist valgus forces and attaches 18 mm distal to the coronoid tip at the sublime tubercle. Reconstructed in UCL reconstruction (Tommy John surgery).
    - Valgus stability with the arm in pronation suggests that the anterior bundle of the UCL is intact.
    - Posterior bundle: greatest change in length from flexion to extension
  - Lateral collateral ligament (annular, radial, and ulnar parts) originates on the lateral humeral epicondyle near the axis of elbow rotation.
    - Lateral ulnar collateral ligament (LUCL) attaches distally at the ulna crista supinatoris (supinator crest).
    - **LUCL deficiency is manifested as posterolateral rotatory instability (PLRI) of the elbow** (see Figure 2-6).
  - Osborne ligament—stabilizes ulnar nerve in cubital tunnel
  - **Ligament of Struthers—variant anatomy attaching a supracondylar process to the medial epicondyle; potential site of median nerve compression**
- **Muscles of the arm/elbow** (Table 2-7)
  - Primary elbow flexors (biceps, brachialis)
    - Brachialis attaches to the coronoid 11 mm distal to the tip.

- Biceps brachii inserts at ulnar margin radial tuberosity (long head proximal, short head distal); also a powerful supinator of forearm.
- Primary elbow extensor (triceps) inserts on olecranon process.
- Mobile wad: brachioradialis, extensor carpi radialis longus (ECRL), extensor carpi radialis brevis (ECRB)
- Flexor-pronator mass: pronator teres, flexor carpi radialis, palmaris longus, flexor carpi ulnaris (FCU), flexor digitorum superficialis (FDS)

FOREARM

- **Osteology: includes ulna and radius, which articulate with humerus (principally ulna) and carpi (principally radius)**
- Ulna
  - Proximally, the ulna is composed of two curved processes, the olecranon and the coronoid processes, with an intervening trochlear notch.
  - Distally, the ulna tapers and ends in a lateral head and a medial styloid process.
- Radius
  - Proximally, the radius is composed of a head with a central fovea, neck, and proximal medial radial tuberosity (for insertion of biceps tendon).
  - Gradual bend (convex laterally) and increase in size distally; **restoration of the radial bow (and length) is paramount in the fixation of radial shaft fractures to maintain arc of pronation and supination.**
  - Distally, the radius is composed of the carpal articular surface, an ulnar notch, a dorsal tubercle (Lister tubercle, which is at the level of the scapholunate joint), and a lateral styloid process.
- **Arthrology: proximally includes the elbow joint (discussed earlier) and distally includes the wrist joint (discussed in IV. Wrist and Hand)**
- Radius and ulna connected by interosseous membrane/ligament
- **Muscles** (Figure 2-7, Table 2-8): arranged according to both location and function
- Volar flexors (superficial and deep) Figure 2-8
- Dorsal extensors (superficial and deep)

WRIST AND HAND

- **Osteology** (Figure 2-9)
- Carpal bones
  - **Ossification begins at the capitate (usually present at 1 year of age) and proceeds in a**

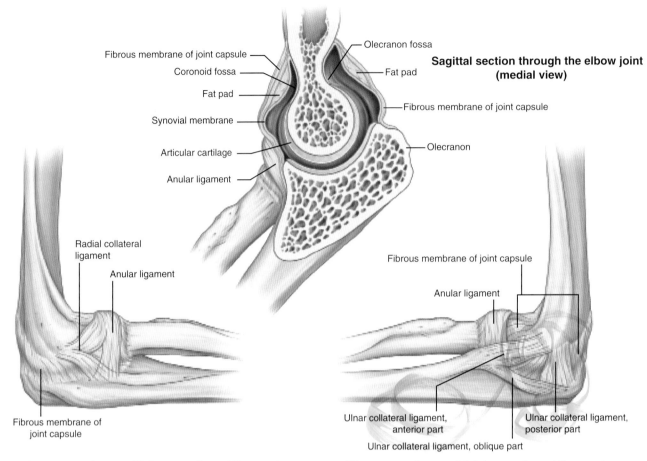

Fibrous membrane of joint capsule

Coronoid fossa

Fat pad

Synovial membrane

Articular cartilage

Anular ligament

Olecranon fossa

Fat pad

Sagittal section through the elbow joint (medial view)

Fibrous membrane of joint capsule

Olecranon

Radial collateral ligament

Anular ligament

Fibrous membrane of joint capsule

Fibrous membrane of joint capsule

Anular ligament

Ulnar collateral ligament, anterior part

Ulnar collateral ligament, posterior part

Ulnar collateral ligament, oblique part

Fibrous membrane of joint capsule and ligaments of the elbow joint (lateral view)

Fibrous membrane of joint capsule and ligaments of the elbow joint (medial view)

 FIGURE 2-6 Elbow joint including fibrous membranes of joint capsule and ligaments. (From Drake RL et al, editors: *Gray's atlas of anatomy,* ed 2, Philadelphia, 2015, Churchill Livingstone.)

Table 2-6	Elbow Ligaments	
LIGAMENT	**COMPONENTS**	**COMMENTS**
Medial collateral	Anterior bundle of MCL (ulnar collateral), posterior bundle, transverse bundle (Cooper ligament)	Anterior bundle (strongest of all elbow ligaments); anterior band taut from 60 degrees of flexion to full extension, posterior band taut from 60-120 degrees of flexion
Lateral collateral	LUCL, annular ligament, quadrate (annular ligament to radial neck), and oblique cord	Deficiency of LUCL results in posterolateral rotator instability.

LUCL, Lateral ulnar collateral ligament; *MCL,* medial collateral ligament.

Table 2-7	Muscles of the Arm			
MUSCLE	**ORIGIN**	**INSERTION**	**ACTION**	**INNERVATION**
Coracobrachialis	Coracoid	Midhumerus (medial)	Flexion, adduction	Musculocutaneous
Biceps brachii	Coracoid (short head) Supraglenoid (long head)	Radial tuberosity	Supination, flexion	Musculocutaneous
Brachialis	Anterior humerus	Ulnar tuberosity (anterior)	Flexing forearm	Musculocutaneous, radial
Triceps brachii	Infraglenoid (long head) Posterior humerus (lateral head) Posterior humerus (medial head)	Olecranon	Extending forearm	Radial

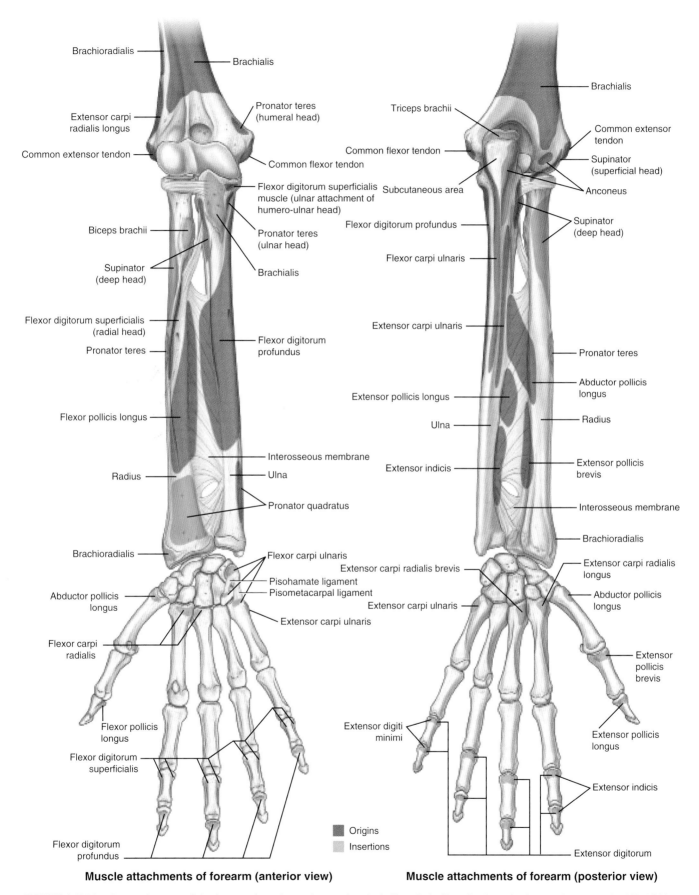

Muscle attachments of forearm (anterior view)

Muscle attachments of forearm (posterior view)

FIGURE 2-7 Muscle attachments of the forearm (anterior and posterior view). (From Drake RL et al, editors: *Gray's atlas of anatomy,* ed 2, Philadelphia, 2015, Churchill Livingstone.)

Table 2-8	Muscles of the Forearm			
MUSCLE	**ORIGIN**	**INSERTION**	**ACTION**	**INNERVATION**
SUPERFICIAL FLEXORS				
Pronator teres	Medial epicondyle and coronoid	Midlateral radius	Pronating, flexing forearm	Median nerve
Flexor carpi radialis	Medial epicondyle	Second and third metacarpal bases	Flexing wrist	Median nerve
Palmaris longus	Medial epicondyle	Palmar aponeurosis	Flexing wrist	Median nerve
Flexor carpi ulnaris	Medial epicondyle and posterior ulna	Pisiform	Flexing wrist	Ulnar nerve
Flexor digitorum superficialis	Medial epicondyle, proximal anterior ulna and anterior radius	Base of middle phalanges	Flexing PIP joint	Median nerve
DEEP FLEXORS				
Flexor digitorum profundus	Anterior and medial ulna	Base of distal phalanges	Flexing DIP joint	Median–anterior interosseous/ulnar nerves
Flexor pollicis longus	Anterior and lateral radius	Base of distal phalanges	Flexing IP joint, thumb	Median–anterior interosseous nerve
Pronator quadratus	Distal ulna	Volar radius	Pronating hand	Median–anterior interosseous nerve
SUPERFICIAL EXTENSORS				
Brachioradialis	Lateral supracondylar humerus	Lateral distal radius	Flexing forearm	Radial nerve
Extensor carpi radialis longus	Lateral supracondylar humerus	Second metacarpal base	Extending wrist	Radial nerve
Extensor carpi radialis brevis	Lateral epicondyle of humerus	Third metacarpal base	Extending wrist	Radial nerve
Anconeus	Lateral epicondyle of humerus	Proximal dorsal ulna	Extending forearm	Radial nerve
Extensor digitorum	Lateral epicondyle of humerus	Extensor aponeurosis	Extending digits	Radial–posterior interosseous nerve
Extensor digiti minimi	Common extensor tendon	Small finger extensor expansion over P1	Extending small finger	Radial–posterior interosseous nerve
Extensor carpi ulnaris	Lateral epicondyle of humerus	Fifth metacarpal base	Extending/adducting hand	Radial–posterior interosseous nerve
DEEP EXTENSORS				
Supinator	Lateral epicondyle of humerus, ulna	Dorsolateral radius	Supinating forearm	Radial–posterior interosseous nerve
Abductor pollicis longus	Dorsal ulna/radius	First metacarpal base	Abducting/extending thumb	Radial–posterior interosseous nerve
Extensor pollicis brevis	Dorsal radius	Thumb proximal phalanx base	Extending thumb MCP joint	Radial–posterior interosseous nerve
Extensor pollicis longus	Dorsolateral ulna	Thumb dorsal phalanx base	Extending thumb IP joint	Radial–posterior interosseous nerve
Extensor indicis proprius	Dorsolateral ulna	Index finger extensor apparatus (ulnarly)	Extending index finger	Radial–posterior interosseous nerve

DIP, Distal interphalangeal joint; *IP,* interphalangeal joint; *MCP,* metacarpophalangeal joint; *PIP,* proximal interphalangeal joint.

counterclockwise direction, according to posteroanterior radiographs of the right hand.
- Several key features are important to recognize in the individual carpal bones (Table 2-9).
- Metacarpals
  - Two ossification centers:
    - One for the body (primary center of ossification), which ossifies at 8 weeks' gestation (like most long bones)
    - One distally at the neck, which usually appears before 3 years of age
  - First metacarpal is a primordial phalanx, and its secondary ossification center is located at the base (like those of phalanges).
  - Several characteristics allow identification of individual metacarpals (Table 2-10).
- Phalanges
  - Each hand has 14 phalanges (three for each finger and two for the thumb), which are similar.
  - All have secondary ossification centers proximally at their bases that appear at ages 3 years (proximal), 4 years (middle), and 5 years (distal).

- Bases of the proximal phalanges are oval and concave, with the smaller heads ending in two condyles.
- Middle phalanges have two concave facets at their bases and pulley-shaped heads.
- Distal phalanges are smaller and have palmar ungual tuberosities distally.

■ **Arthrology**
- Distal radioulnar joint (DRUJ) articulation (most stable in supination)
- Radiocarpal (wrist) joint
  - Ellipsoid shape involving distal radius and the scaphoid, lunate, and triquetrum
  - Located at the level of the crease of proximal wrist flexion
  - **Ligaments** (Table 2-11; see Figure 2-9)
    - Palmar/volar radiocarpal ligaments are the strongest supporting structures.
    - **Space of Poirier: central weak area in floor of carpal tunnel; implicated in volar dislocation of lunate in perilunate dislocation**

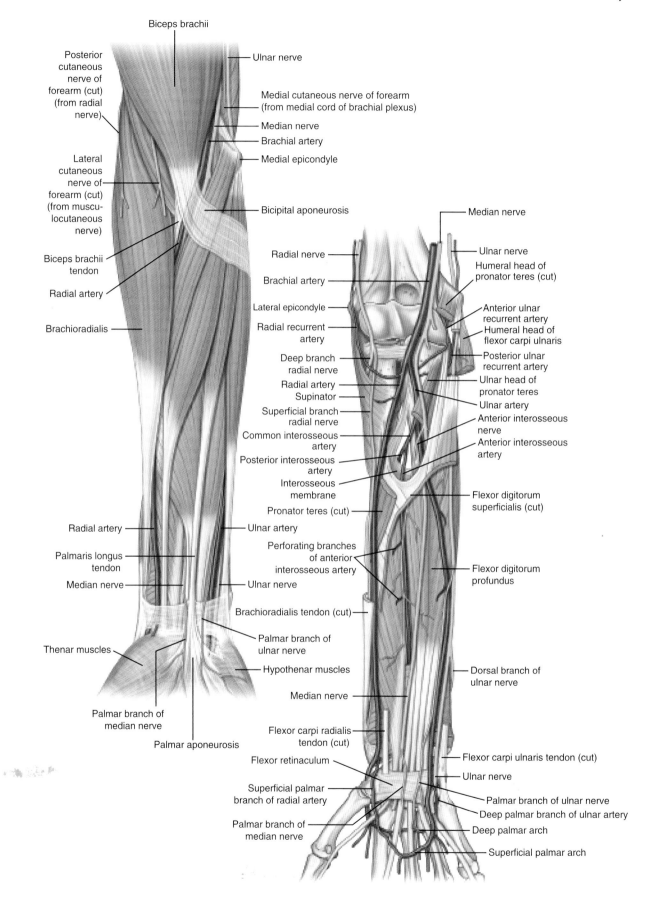

FIGURE 2-8 Volar flexors (superficial and deep). (From Drake RL et al, editors: *Gray's atlas of anatomy,* ed 2, Philadelphia, 2015, Churchill Livingstone.)

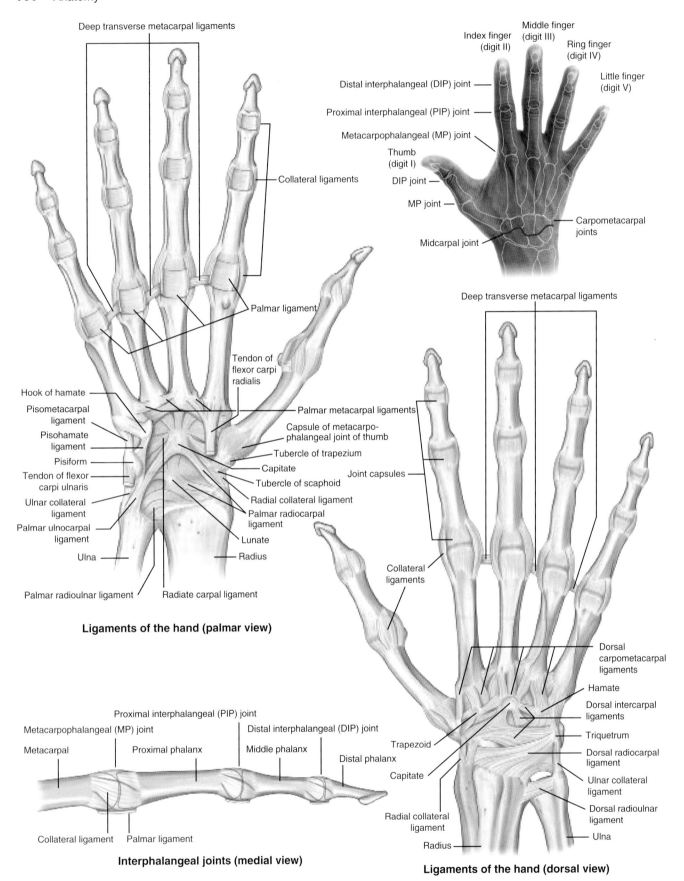

Deep transverse metacarpal ligaments

Index finger (digit II)

Middle finger (digit III)

Ring finger (digit IV)

Little finger (digit V)

Distal interphalangeal (DIP) joint

Proximal interphalangeal (PIP) joint

Metacarpophalangeal (MP) joint

Thumb (digit I)

DIP joint

MP joint

Carpometacarpal joints

Midcarpal joint

Collateral ligaments

Palmar ligament

Tendon of flexor carpi radialis

Hook of hamate

Pisometacarpal ligament

Pisohamate ligament

Pisiform

Tendon of flexor carpi ulnaris

Ulnar collateral ligament

Palmar ulnocarpal ligament

Ulna

Palmar radioulnar ligament

Palmar metacarpal ligaments

Capsule of metacarpo-phalangeal joint of thumb

Tubercle of trapezium

Capitate

Tubercle of scaphoid

Radial collateral ligament

Palmar radiocarpal ligament

Lunate

Radius

Radiate carpal ligament

Ligaments of the hand (palmar view)

Deep transverse metacarpal ligaments

Joint capsules

Collateral ligaments

Dorsal carpometacarpal ligaments

Hamate

Dorsal intercarpal ligaments

Triquetrum

Dorsal radiocarpal ligament

Ulnar collateral ligament

Dorsal radioulnar ligament

Ulna

Trapezoid

Capitate

Radial collateral ligament

Radius

Ligaments of the hand (dorsal view)

Proximal interphalangeal (PIP) joint

Metacarpophalangeal (MP) joint

Distal interphalangeal (DIP) joint

Metacarpal

Proximal phalanx

Middle phalanx

Distal phalanx

Collateral ligament

Palmar ligament

Interphalangeal joints (medial view)

FIGURE 2-9 Ligaments of the hand and interphalangeal joints (medial view). (From Drake RL et al, editors: *Gray's atlas of anatomy*, ed 2, Philadelphia, 2015, Churchill Livingstone.)

Table 2-9 | Carpal Features

CARPAL BONE	DISTINCTIVE FEATURES	NUMBER OF ARTICULATIONS
Scaphoid	Tubercle (TCL, APB), distal vascular supply	5
Lunate	Half-moon–shaped	5
Triquetrum	Pyramid-shaped	3
Pisiform	Spheroidal (TCL, FCU)	1
Trapezium	FCR groove, tubercle (opponens, APB, flexor pollicis brevis, TCL)	4
Trapezoid	Wedge-shaped	4
Capitate	Largest bone, central location	7
Hamate	Hook (TCL)	5

APB, Abductor pollicis brevis; *FCR,* flexor carpi radialis; *FCU,* flexor carpi ulnaris; *TCL,* transverse carpal ligament.

Table 2-10 | Metacarpal Features

METACARPAL	DISTINCTIVE FEATURES
I (Thumb)	Short, stout; base is saddle-shaped
II (Index)	Longest, largest base; medial at base
III (Middle)	Styloid process
IV (Ring)	Small quadrilateral base, narrow shaft
V (Small)	Tubercle at base (extensor carpi ulnaris)

- Ligament of Testut (radioscapholunate ligament) functions as a neurovascular conduit.
- Triangular fibrocartilage complex (TFCC) (Figure 2-10, Table 2-12): vascular supply from periphery (central portion avascular)

■ Intercarpal joints
- **Extrinsic ligaments bridge carpal bones to radius or metacarpals (i.e., radioscaphocapitate); intrinsic ligaments attach carpal bones together (i.e., scapholunate).**

Table 2-11 | Radiocarpal Wrist Ligaments

STRUCTURE	ATTACHMENTS	DISTINCTIVE FEATURES
Articular capsule	Surrounds joint	Reinforced by volar and dorsal radiocarpal ligament
Volar (radiocarpal ligament)	Radius, ulna, scaphoid, lunate, triquetrum, capitate	Oblique ulnar, strong
Dorsal radiocarpal ligament	Radius, scaphoid, lunate, triquetrum	Oblique radial, weak
Ulnar collateral ligament	Ulna, triquetrum, pisiform, transverse carpal ligament	Fan-shaped, two fascicles
Radial collateral ligament	Radius, scaphoid, trapezium, transverse carpal ligament	Radial artery adjacent

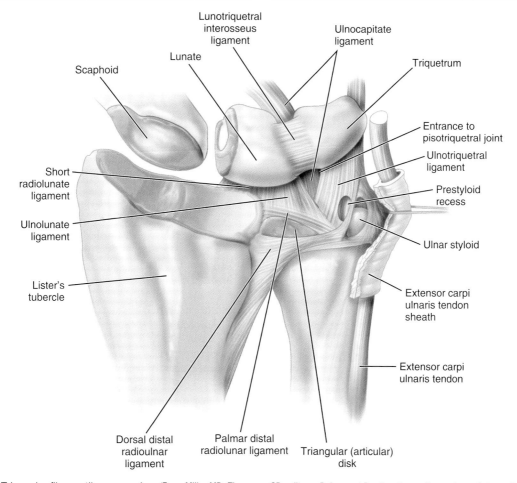

FIGURE 2-10 Triangular fibrocartilage complex. (From Miller MD, Thompson SR, editors: *DeLee and Drez's orthopaedic sports medicine: principles and practice,* ed 4, Philadelphia, 2014, Saunders.)

Table 2-12	Components of the Triangular Fibrocartilage Complex	
COMPONENT	**ORIGIN**	**INSERTION**
Dorsal and volar radioulnar ligament	Ulnar radius	Caput ulnae
Articular disc	Radius/ulna	Triquetrum
Prestyloid recess	Disc	Meniscus homolog
Meniscus homolog	Ulna/disc	Triquetrum/ulnar collateral ligament
Ulnar collateral ligament	Ulna	Fifth metacarpal

- Proximal row
  - Scaphoid, lunate, and triquetrum form gliding joints. Connected by dorsal and palmar intercarpal ligaments.
  - Dorsal intercarpal ligaments are stronger.
  - Interosseous ligaments are narrow bundles connecting the scaphoid and lunate and the lunate and triquetrum.
- Pisiform articulation
  - Pisotriquetral joint has a thin articular capsule.
  - Ulnar collateral and palmar radiocarpal ligaments also connect the pisiform proximally.
  - Pisohamate and pisometacarpal ligaments help extend the pull of the FCU.
- Distal row
  - Trapezium, trapezoid, capitate, and hamate gliding joints
  - Dorsal and palmar intercarpal ligaments connect trapezium with trapezoid, trapezoid with capitate, and capitate with hamate.
  - Interosseous ligaments are much thicker in the distal row, connecting capitate and hamate (strongest), capitate and trapezoid, and trapezium and trapezoid (weakest).
- Midcarpal joint
  - Transverse articulations between proximal and distal rows are reinforced by palmar and dorsal intercarpal ligaments and carpal collateral ligaments.
  - The radial ligament is stronger.
- Carpometacarpal (CMC) joints
  - Thumb CMC joint
    - Highly mobile saddle-shaped joint
    - Supported by a capsule and radial, palmar, and dorsal CMC ligaments
  - Finger CMC joints
    - Gliding joints with capsules, dorsal CMC ligaments (strongest), palmar CMC ligaments, and interosseous CMC ligaments
- Metacarpophalangeal (MCP) joints
  - Ellipsoid and covered by palmar (volar plate), collateral, and deep transverse metacarpal ligaments
  - Cam mechanism (collateral ligaments tighten with MCP joint flexion)
- Interphalangeal joints
  - Hinge joints with capsules and obliquely oriented collateral ligaments
- **Muscles (Figure 2-11, Table 2-13)**
- Extensor tendon anatomy
  - Extensor compartments of wrist: formed by the extensor retinaculum over dorsal wrist (Figure 2-12, Table 2-14)

- First dorsal compartment contains the abductor pollicis longus (APL) and extensor pollicis brevis (EPB).
- EPB tendon is ulnar to APL tendon (APL frequently has multiple tendon slips, which should be addressed during release for de Quervain tenosynovitis).
- Second dorsal compartment: ECRL tendon is radial to ECRB tendon; extensor pollicis longus (EPL) tendon is ulnar to ECRB tendon at the wrist level.
- Anatomic snuffbox is bordered by tendons of the first and third dorsal wrist compartments; EPB tendon serves as the radial snuffbox border, EPL tendon serves as the ulnar border.
- Extensor mechanism anatomy/intrinsic apparatus
  - Complex arrangement of structures that surround digits (Figure 2-13, Table 2-15)
- Flexor tendon anatomy
  - **Carpal tunnel** (Figures 2-14 and 2-15)
    - Transverse carpal ligament (TCL): component of flexor retinaculum; serves as roof of carpal tunnel. Attached radially to the scaphoid tuberosity and trapezial ridge and ulnarly to the hook of the hamate and pisiform.
    - Contains the median nerve and nine tendons (one flexor pollicis longus [FPL], four FDS, and four flexor digitorum profundus [FDP]).
    - FDS to the middle and ring fingers are volar to FDS to index and small fingers.
    - Decreases in volume with wrist flexion
  - **Guyon canal: contains ulnar nerve and artery. Borders: flexor retinaculum (deep), volar carpal ligament (superficial), pisiform (ulnar/proximal), hook of hamate (radial/distal).**
  - Flexor tendon sheath (Figure 2-16)
    - Covers flexor tendons, protecting and nourishing tendons (vincula)
    - Five annular pulleys (A1-A5) with three intervening cruciate attachments (C1-C3)
    - A2 and A4 pulleys originate from bone, whereas A1, A3, and A5 pulleys originate from the palmar plates of the metacarpal, proximal interphalangeal, and distal interphalangeal joints.
    - **A2 pulley, overlying the proximal phalanx, is the most critical to function, followed by A4, which covers the middle phalanx.**
    - A1 pulley is involved in trigger digits.
- **Nerves of the upper extremity**
- Brachial plexus (Figure 2-17)
  - Formed from the ventral primary rami of C5 to T1
  - Exits neck between the anterior and middle scalene muscles
  - Dorsal rami of C5 to T1 innervate the dorsal neck musculature and skin.
  - **From proximal to distal: roots, trunks, divisions, cords, and branches (mnemonic: "Real Texans Drink Cold Beer").**
    - Five roots (C5-T1, although contributions from C4 (pre-fixed) and T2 (post-fixed) can be small)
      - Dorsal scapular nerve (C5)—to levator scapula, rhomboid major/minor
      - Long thoracic nerve (C5, 6, 7)—to serratus anterior

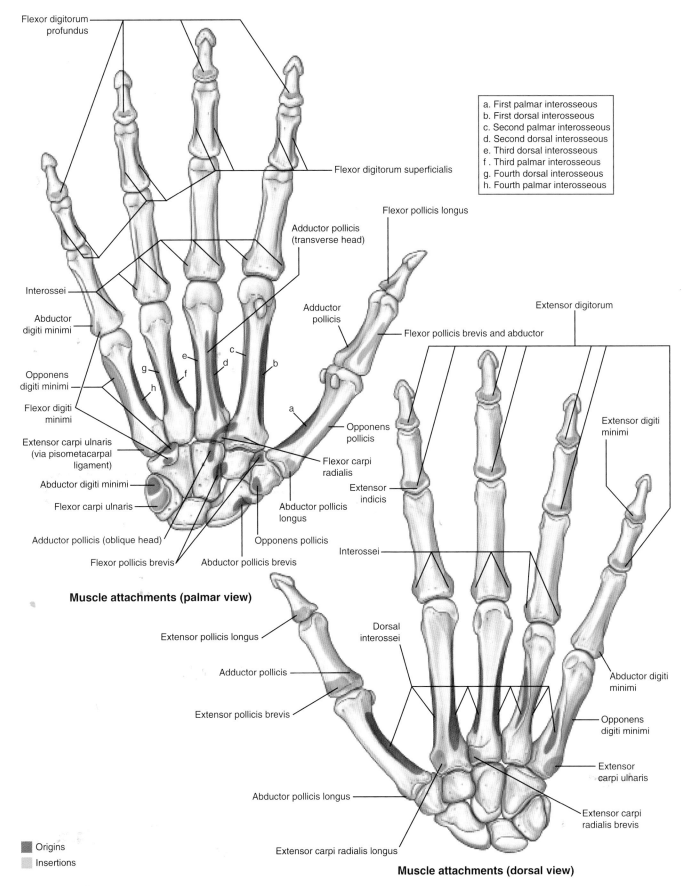

a. First palmar interosseous
b. First dorsal interosseous
c. Second palmar interosseous
d. Second dorsal interosseous
e. Third dorsal interosseous
f . Third palmar interosseous
g. Fourth dorsal interosseous
h. Fourth palmar interosseous

Flexor digitorum profundus

Flexor digitorum superficialis

Flexor pollicis longus

Adductor pollicis (transverse head)

Interossei

Adductor pollicis

Flexor pollicis brevis and abductor

Extensor digitorum

Abductor digiti minimi

Opponens digiti minimi

Flexor digiti minimi

Extensor digiti minimi

Extensor carpi ulnaris (via pisometacarpal ligament)

Opponens pollicis

Flexor carpi radialis

Abductor digiti minimi

Extensor indicis

Flexor carpi ulnaris

Adductor pollicis (oblique head)

Abductor pollicis longus

Opponens pollicis

Flexor pollicis brevis

Abductor pollicis brevis

Interossei

Muscle attachments (palmar view)

Opponens digiti minimi

Extensor pollicis longus

Dorsal interossei

Adductor pollicis

Extensor pollicis brevis

Abductor digiti minimi

Opponens digiti minimi

Extensor carpi ulnaris

Abductor pollicis longus

Extensor carpi radialis brevis

Extensor carpi radialis longus

Origins

Insertions

Muscle attachments (dorsal view)

FIGURE 2-11 Muscle attachments (planar and dorsal view). (From Drake RL et al, editors: *Gray's atlas of anatomy,* ed 2, Philadelphia, 2015, Churchill Livingstone.)

Table 2-13	Muscles of the Hand and Wrist			
MUSCLE	**ORIGIN**	**INSERTION**	**ACTION**	**INNERVATION**
THENAR MUSCLES				
Abductor pollicis brevis	Scaphoid, trapezoid	Base of proximal phalanx, radial side	Abducting thumb	Median nerve
Opponens pollicis	Trapezium	Thumb metacarpal	Abducting, flexing, rotating (medially)	Median nerve
Flexor pollicis brevis	Trapezium, capitate	Base of proximal phalanx, radial side	Flexing MCP joint	Median, ulnar nerves
Adductor pollicis	Capitate, second and third metacarpals	Base of proximal phalanx, ulnar side	Adducting thumb	Ulnar nerve
HYPOTHENAR MUSCLES				
Palmaris brevis	TCL, palmar aponeurosis	Ulnar palm	Retracting skin	Ulnar nerve
Abductor digiti minimi	Pisiform	Base of proximal phalanx, ulnar side	Abducting small finger	Ulnar nerve
Flexor digiti minimi brevis	Hamate, TCL	Base of proximal phalanx, ulnar side	Flexing MCP joint	Ulnar nerve
Opponens digiti minimi	Hamate, TCL	Small-finger metacarpal	Abducting, flexing, rotating (laterally)	Ulnar nerve
INTRINSIC MUSCLES				
Lumbrical	Flexor digitorum profundus	Lateral bands (radial)	Extending proximal interphalangeal joint	Median, ulnar nerves
Dorsal interosseous	Adjacent metacarpals	Proximal phalanx base/extensor apparatus	Abducting, flexing MCP joint	Ulnar nerve
Volar interosseous	Adjacent metacarpals	Proximal phalanx base/extensor apparatus	Adducting, flexing MCP joint	Ulnar nerve

MCP, Metacarpophalangeal; *TCL,* transverse carpal ligament.

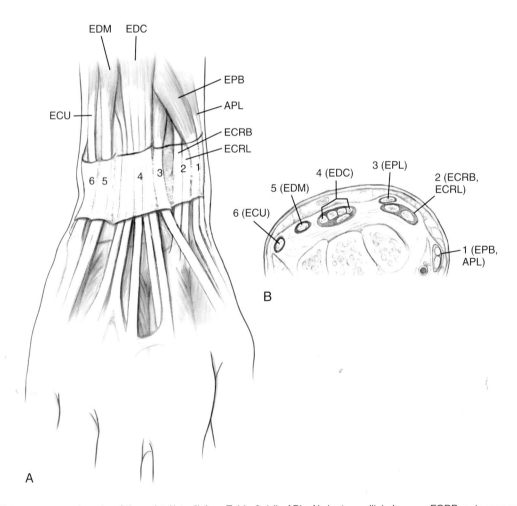

 FIGURE 2-12 Extensor compartments of the wrist (1 to 6) (see Table 2-14). *APL,* Abductor pollicis longus; *ECRB,* extensor carpi radialis brevis; *ECRL,* extensor carpi radialis longus; *ECU,* extensor carpi ulnaris; *EDC,* extensor digitorum communis; *EDM,* extensor digiti minimi; *EPB,* extensor pollicis brevis; *EPL,* extensor pollicis longus. (Modified from Miller MD et al: *Orthopaedic surgical approaches,* Philadelphia, 2008, Saunders, Figure HW-6.)

Table 2-14	Dorsal Wrist Compartments	
COMPARTMENT	**CONTENTS**	**PATHOLOGIC CONDITION**
I	Abductor pollicis longus, extensor pollicis brevis	De Quervain tenosynovitis
II	Extensor carpi radialis longus, brevis	Extensor tendinitis (intersection syndrome)
III	Extensor pollicis longus	Rupture at Lister tubercle (after wrist fractures)
		Drummer's tendinitis of the wrist
IV	Extensor digitorum communis, extensor indicis proprius	Extensor tenosynovitis
V	Extensor digiti minimi	Rupture (rheumatoid arthritis: Vaughn-Jackson syndrome)
VI	Extensor carpi ulnaris	Snapping at ulnar styloid

Table 2-15	Intrinsic Apparatus	
STRUCTURE	**ATTACHMENTS**	**SIGNIFICANCE**
Sagittal bands	Covers MCP joint	Allows MCP extension
Transverse (sagittal)	Volar plate fibers	Allows MCP flexion (interossei)
Lateral bands	Covers PIP joint	Allows PIP extension (lumbrical muscles)
Oblique retinacular ligament (Landsmeer)	A4 pulley, terminal tendon	Allows DIP extension (passive)

A4, Annular 4; *DIP,* distal interphalangeal; *MCP,* metacarpophalangeal; *PIP,* proximal interphalangeal; *TCL,* transverse carpal ligament.

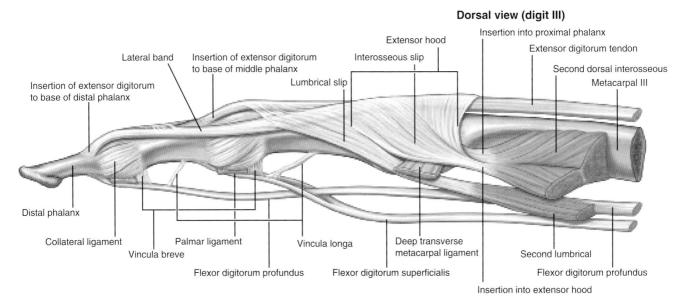

FIGURE 2-13 Dorsal view of digit III. (From Drake RL et al, editors: *Gray's atlas of anatomy,* ed 2, Philadelphia, 2015, Churchill Livingstone.)

- Three trunks (upper, middle, lower)
  - Suprascapular nerve (upper trunk, C5, 6)
  - Nerve to subclavius (upper trunk, C5, 6)
- Six divisions (anterior and posterior; two limbs from each trunk)
  - **No terminal branches at this level**
- Three cords (lateral, medial, and posterior) named for their anatomic relationship to the axillary artery (Table 2-16)
  - Main terminal branches (musculocutaneous, axillary, radial, median, ulnar)
  - Other terminal branches
    - Lateral cord
      - Lateral pectoral nerve (C5, 6, 7)—to pectoralis major

- Posterior cord
  - Upper subscapular nerve (C5, 6)—to subscapularis
  - Lower subscapular nerve (C5, 6)—to subscapularis, teres major
  - Thoracodorsal nerve (C6, 7, 8)—to latissimus dorsi
- Medial cord
  - Medial pectoral nerve (C8, T1)—to pectoralis minor/major
  - Medial brachial cutaneous nerve (T1)
  - Medial antebrachial cutaneous nerve (C8, T1)
- **Preclavicular branches (from roots and upper trunk):**
  - **Dorsal scapular nerve**

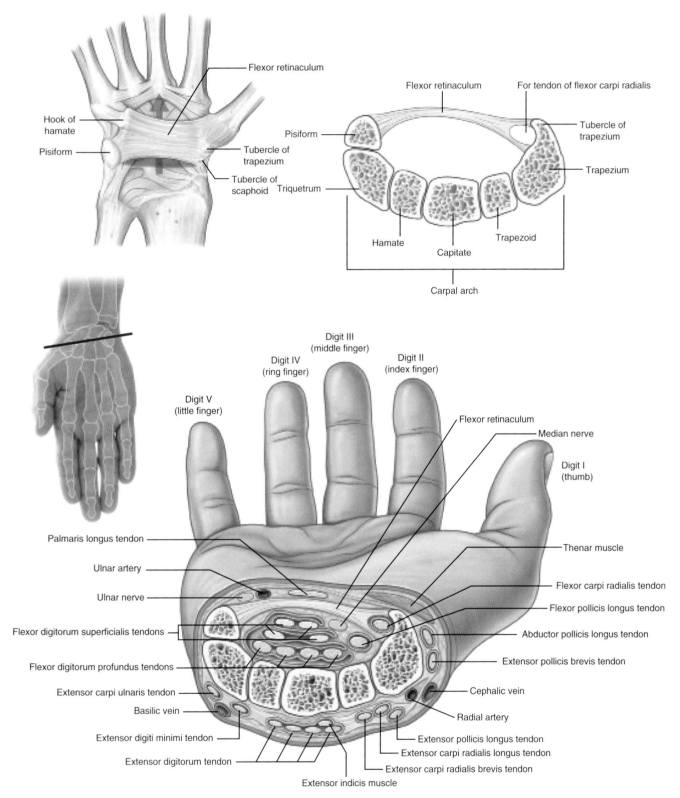

FIGURE 2-14 Anatomy of hand. (From Drake RL et al, editors: *Gray's atlas of anatomy,* ed 2, Philadelphia, 2015, Churchill Livingstone.)

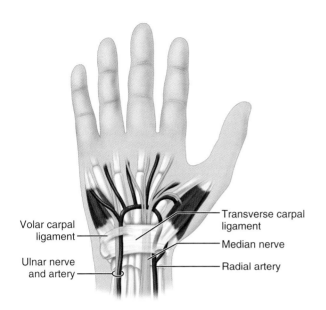

FIGURE 2-15 Hand with carpal tunnel syndrome.

Table 2-16	Brachial Plexus Cord Terminations
CORD	**TERMINATION**
Lateral	Musculocutaneous nerve*
	Lateral pectoral nerve
Posterior	Radial and axillary nerve*
	Upper and lower subscapular nerve
	Thoracodorsal nerve
Medial	Ulnar nerve*
	Medial pectoral nerve
	Medial brachial cutaneous nerve
	Medial antebrachial cutaneous nerve
Medial and lateral	Median nerve*

*Major branches.

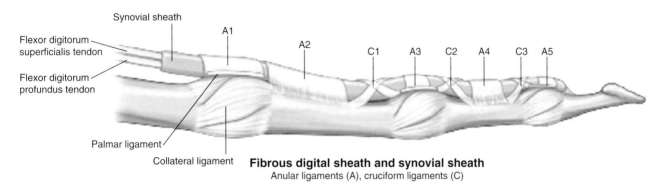

Fibrous digital sheath and synovial sheath
Anular ligaments (A), cruciform ligaments (C)

FIGURE 2-16 Tendons and ligaments of the finger. (From Drake RL et al, editors: *Gray's atlas of anatomy,* ed 2, Philadelphia, 2015, Churchill Livingstone.)

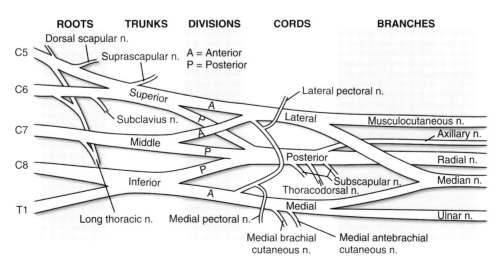

FIGURE 2-17 Brachial plexus. There are four preclavicular/supraclavicular branches: the long thoracic nerve (serratus anterior muscle), dorsal scapular nerve (rhomboid muscle), suprascapular nerve (supraspinatus and infraspinatus muscles), and nerve to the subclavius. (From Miller MD et al: *Orthopaedic surgical approaches,* Philadelphia, 2008, Saunders, Figure SA-7.)

Table 2-17	Rotator Cuff Muscle Innervation: All C5 and C6 Muscle Innervation
MUSCLES INNERVATED	**NERVES**
EXTERNAL ROTATORS	
Supraspinatus	Suprascapular nerve (C5, C6)
Infraspinatus	Suprascapular nerve (C5, C6)
Teres minor	Axillary nerve (C5, C6)
INTERNAL ROTATOR	
Subscapularis	Upper (C5) and lower (C5, C6) subscapular nerve

Table 2-18	Obstetric Brachial Plexus Palsies		
PALSY TYPE	**ROOTS**	**DEFICIT**	**PROGNOSIS**
Erb-Duchenne	C5, C6	Weakness of deltoid, rotator cuff, elbow flexors, and wrist and hand extensors "Waiter's tip"	Best
Klumpke	C8, T1	Weakness of wrist flexors and intrinsic apparatus, Horner syndrome	Poor
Total plexus	C5-T1	Flaccid arm	Worst

- **Long thoracic nerve**
- **Suprascapular nerve**
- **Nerve to the subclavius**
- **Innervation of all rotator cuff muscles derived from C5 and C6 of the brachial plexus** (Table 2-17)
- Brachial plexus injury
  - Preganglionic brachial plexus injuries
    - Proximal to dorsal root ganglion—**CNS injury with little potential for recovery**
    - Characteristics: medial scapular winging (long thoracic nerve to serratus anterior), rhomboid paralysis (dorsal scapular nerve), Horner syndrome (disruption of stellate ganglion/sympathetic chain at C8-T1), rotator cuff dysfunction (suprascapular nerve to supra-/infraspinatus), latissimus dorsi paralysis (thoracodorsal nerve), elevated hemidiaphragm (phrenic nerve)
  - Postganglionic brachial plexus injuries
    - Less preclavicular nerve involvement (no scapular winging, rhomboid paralysis, etc.)
    - Characteristic obstetric brachial plexus palsies (Table 2-18)

- Scapular winging
  - **Medial winging: long thoracic nerve (C5-C7) injury leading to serratus anterior dysfunction**
    - Superior elevation with scapular translation medially and the inferior angle rotated medially
  - **Lateral winging: spinal accessory nerve (cranial nerve XI) injury leading to trapezius dysfunction**
    - Shoulder depression with scapular translation laterally and the inferior angle rotated laterally because of the unopposed pull of the serratus anterior
- Major brachial plexus branches (Figure 2-18; Tables 2-19 and 2-20)

- Suprascapular nerve (upper trunk, C5, 6)
  - Passes through scapular notch beneath superior transverse scapular ligament, sending a branch to the supraspinatus before traveling through the spinoglenoid notch to innervate the infraspinatus
- Musculocutaneous nerve (lateral cord, C5, 6, 7) (Figure 2-19)
  - **Pierces the coracobrachialis 5 to 8 cm distal to the coracoid**
  - Branches supply the coracobrachialis, biceps, and brachialis.
  - Gives off a sensory branch to the elbow joint before it becomes the lateral antebrachial cutaneous nerve of the forearm, which is located deep to the cephalic vein
- Axillary nerve (posterior cord, C5, 6)
  - Passes anterior to subscapularis muscle and inferior to shoulder capsule, traveling from anterior to posterior through quadrangular space
  - **Anterior branch supplying deltoid and skin over lateral shoulder passes around humerus in deep deltoid fascia approximately 5 to 7 cm distal to acromion.**
  - Posterior branch supplies teres minor and posterior deltoid.
- Radial nerve (posterior cord, C5-T1) (Figure 2-20)
  - Passes through triangular interval and then spirals around the humerus (medial to lateral) in the spiral groove. **Approximately 20 cm from medial epicondyle and 14 cm from lateral epicondyle.**
  - Emerges on the lateral side of the arm after piercing the lateral intermuscular septum approximately 7.5 cm above the trochlea between the brachialis and brachioradialis anterior to the lateral epicondyle (where it supplies the anconeus muscle)
  - Passes anterior to the lateral epicondyle between the brachialis and brachioradialis and divides into the superficial and deep (posterior interosseous nerve [PIN]) branches approximately 1 to 3 cm distal to lateral epicondyle
    - **PIN splits the supinator and supplies all of the extensor muscles except the mobile wad (brachioradialis, ECRB, ECRL).**
    - Terminal sensory branch to dorsal wrist joint in floor of fourth extensor compartment
    - Superficial branch of the radial nerve emerges through antebrachial fascia approximately 6 to 9 cm proximal to the radial styloid. Runs between the brachioradialis and ERCL to supply sensation to the dorsal radial surface distal forearm and hand.
- Median nerve (medial and lateral cords, C5-T1) (Figure 2-21)
  - Accompanies brachial artery in the arm, crossing it during its course (lateral to medial) approximately 15 cm from the medial epicondyle
  - **Supplies some branches to the elbow joint but has no branches in the arm itself**
  - Medial to brachial artery and superficial to brachialis muscle as it passes
  - In forearm, the median nerve splits the two heads of the pronator teres and then runs between the FDS and FDP. Supplies all the superficial flexor muscles of the forearm except the FCU.

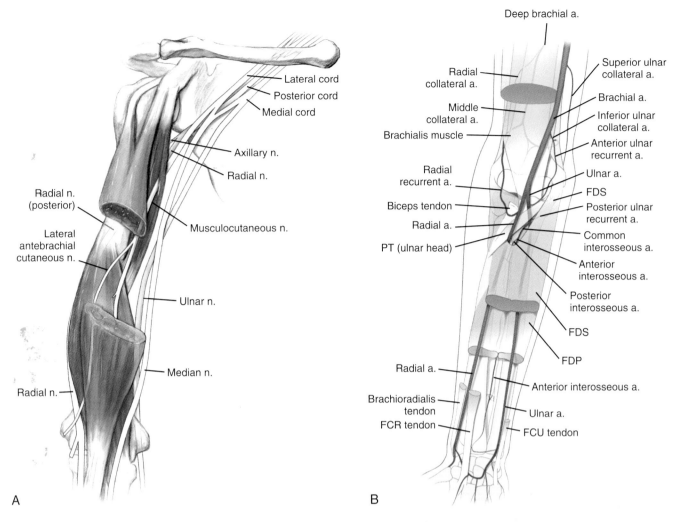

FIGURE 2-18 Principal nerves **(A)** and arteries **(B)** of the upper extremity. *FCR,* Flexor carpi radialis; *FCU,* flexor carpi ulnaris; *FDP,* flexor digitorum profundus; *FDS,* flexor digitorum superficialis; *PT,* pronator teres. (From Miller MD et al: *Orthopaedic surgical approaches,* Philadelphia, 2008, Saunders, Figures SA-8 and EF-12.)

Table 2-19	Summary of Upper Extremity Innervation
NERVES	**MUSCLES INNERVATED**
Musculocutaneous (lateral cord)	Coracobrachialis, biceps, brachialis
Axillary (posterior cord)	Deltoid, teres minor
Radial (posterior cord)	Triceps, brachioradialis, extensor carpi radialis longus and brevis
Posterior interosseous	Supinator, extensor carpi ulnaris, extensor digitorum, extensor digiti minimi, abductor pollicis longus, extensor pollicis longus and brevis, extensor indicis proprius
Median (medial and lateral cord)	Pronator teres, flexor carpi radialis, palmaris longus, flexor digitorum superficialis, abductor pollicis brevis, supinator head of flexor pollicis brevis, opponens pollicis, first and second lumbrical muscles
Anterior interosseous	Flexor digitorum profundus (first and second), flexor pollicis longus, pronator quadratus
Ulnar (medial cord)	Flexor carpi ulnaris, flexor digitorum profundus (third and fourth), palmaris brevis, abductor digiti minimi, opponens digiti minimi, flexor digiti minimi, third and fourth lumbrical muscles, interossei, adductor pollicis, deep head of flexor pollicis brevis

Table 2-20	Innervation of the Forearm
NERVES	**MUSCLES INNERVATED**
RADIAL NERVE	
Radial (posterior cord)	Triceps, brachioradialis, extensor carpi radialis longus, extensor carpi radialis brevis
Posterior interosseous	Supinator, extensor carpi ulnaris, extensor digitorum, extensor digiti minimi, abductor pollicis longus, extensor pollicis longus, extensor pollicis brevis, extensor indicis proprius
MEDIAN NERVE	
Median (medial and lateral cord)	Pronator teres, flexor carpi radialis, palmaris longus, flexor digitorum superficialis, abductor pollicis brevis, superficial head of flexor pollicis brevis, opponens pollicis, first and second lumbrical muscles
Anterior interosseous	Flexor digitorum profundus (first and second), flexor pollicis longus, pronator quadratus
ULNAR NERVE	
Ulnar (medial cord)	Flexor carpi ulnaris, flexor digitorum profundus (third and fourth), pollicis brevis, abductor digiti minimi, opponens digiti minimi, flexor digiti minimi, third and fourth lumbrical muscles, interossei, adductor pollicis, deep head of flexor pollicis brevis

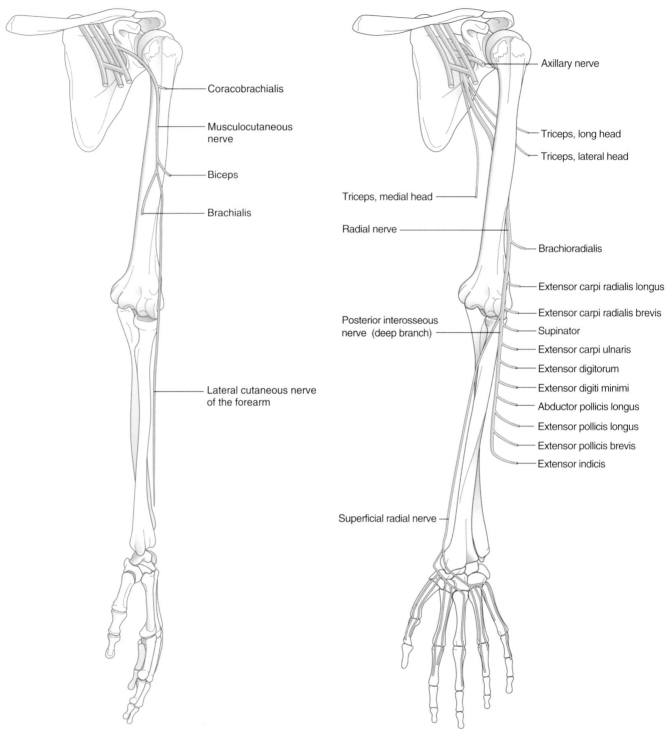

FIGURE 2-19 Nerves in shoulder and arm (lateral cord). (From Drake RL et al, editors: *Gray's atlas of anatomy,* ed 2, Philadelphia, 2015, Churchill Livingstone.)

FIGURE 2-20 Nerves in shoulder and arm (posterior cord). (From Drake RL et al, editors: *Gray's atlas of anatomy,* ed 2, Philadelphia, 2015, Churchill Livingstone.)

- Anterior interosseous nerve branches 4 cm distal to elbow and runs between the FPL and FDP, supplies all the deep flexors except the ulnar half of the FDP. Terminates in the pronator quadratus (PQ).
- **Palmar cutaneous branch arises approximately 6 cm proximal to radial styloid and passes superficial to the flexor retinaculum to innervate the thenar skin.**
- Median nerve passes through the carpal tunnel between FDS and flexor carpi radialis (FCR) to

supply the radial lumbricals, thenar musculature via a deep recurrent branch, and sensation to the volar aspect of thumb, index, long, and radial half of the ring fingers.
- Ulnar nerve (medial cord, C8, T1) (Figure 2-22)
  - **Posteromedial to brachial artery in upper arm and then passes posterior to the medial intermuscular septum at the arcade of Struthers (8-10 cm from medial epicondyle)**

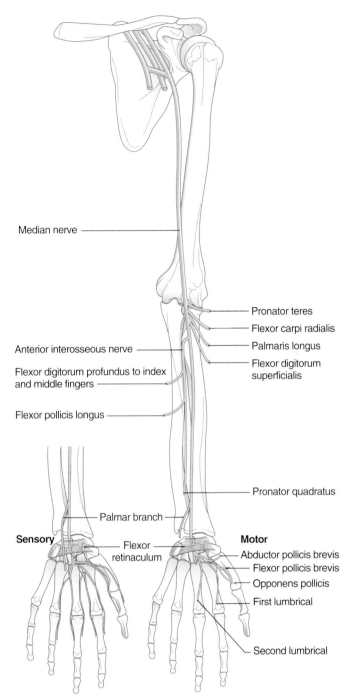

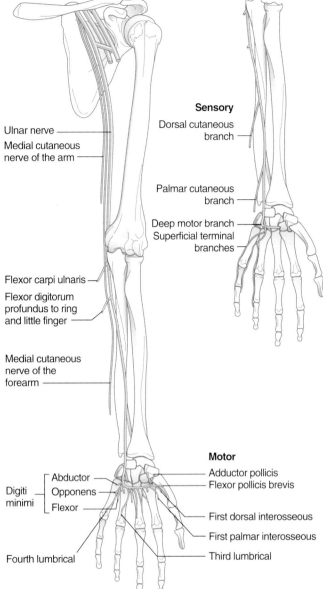

FIGURE 2-22 Nerves in shoulder and arm (medial cord). (From Drake RL et al, editors: *Gray's atlas of anatomy,* ed 2, Philadelphia, 2015, Churchill Livingstone.)

FIGURE 2-21 Nerves in shoulder and arm (medial and lateral cord). (From Drake RL et al, editors: *Gray's atlas of anatomy,* ed 2, Philadelphia, 2015, Churchill Livingstone.)

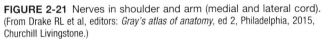

- Crosses elbow posterior to medial epicondyle at elbow through the cubital tunnel
  - Cubital tunnel: Osborne ligament (roof), MCL (floor)
- No branches in arm, but supplies articular branch to elbow joint
- Enters the forearm between the two heads of the FCU (humeral and ulnar)
- Runs between the FCU and FDP, innervating the ulnar half of this muscle (FDP to ring and small fingers)
- Runs radial to FCU at distal forearm and wrist

- Dorsal cutaneous nerve branches approximately 7 cm proximal to ulnar styloid and provides sensation to dorsoulnar forearm and wrist.
- Ulnar nerve enters hand superficial to TCL through Guyon canal. Divides into a superficial sensory branch (palmaris brevis and skin) and a deep motor branch.
  - **Deep branch travels around the hook of the hamate between the abductor digiti minimi and flexor digiti minimi brevis, providing motor to intrinsic muscles of hand.**
  - Sensory branch supplies ulnar half of the ring and the small finger.
- Cutaneous innervation to upper extremity (Figures 2-23 through 2-25)
  - Supraclavicular nerve (C3 and C4) supplies the upper shoulder.

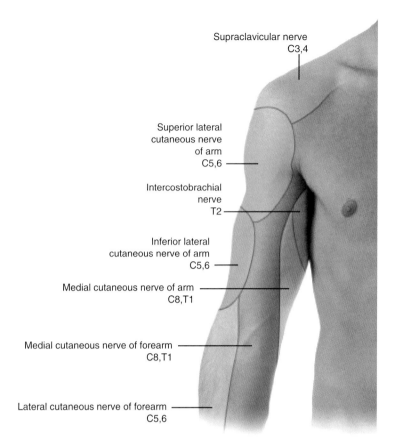

Supraclavicular nerve
C3,4

Superior lateral
cutaneous nerve
of arm
C5,6

Intercostobrachial
nerve
T2

Inferior lateral
cutaneous nerve of arm
C5,6

Medial cutaneous nerve of arm
C8,T1

Medial cutaneous nerve of forearm
C8,T1

Lateral cutaneous nerve of forearm
C5,6

FIGURE 2-23 Nerve regions in shoulder and arm. (From Drake RL et al, editors: *Gray's atlas of anatomy,* ed 2, Philadelphia, 2015, Churchill Livingstone.)

- Axillary nerve supplies the shoulder joint and the overlying skin.
- Medial, lateral, and dorsal brachial cutaneous nerves supply the balance of cutaneous innervation of the arm.
- **Lateral antebrachial cutaneous nerve: continuation of the musculocutaneous nerve that passes lateral to the cephalic vein after emerging laterally from between the biceps and brachialis at the elbow**
- **Medial antebrachial cutaneous nerve: a branch from the medial cord of the brachial plexus**
- Posterior antebrachial cutaneous nerve: a branch of the radial nerve given off in the arm
- Sensation to thumb
  - Provided by five branches: lateral antebrachial cutaneous nerve, superficial and dorsal digital branches of the radial nerve, and digital and palmar branches of the median nerve
- Compressive neuropathies of the upper extremity (Table 2-21)
  - Median
    - Pronator syndrome
      - Proximal forearm aching pain, median nerve paresthesias
      - Worse with repetitive pronation
      - Potential sites of compression
        - Between ulnar and humeral heads of pronator teres
        - FDS aponeurotic arch

- Supracondylar process (residual osseous structure on distal humerus present in 1% of population)
- **Ligament of Struthers (travels from tip of supracondylar process to medial epicondyle; not to be confused with arcade of Struthers, which is a site of ulnar compression neuropathy in cubital tunnel syndrome)**
- Accessory head of the FPL (i.e., Gantzer muscle)
- Bicipital aponeurosis (lacertus fibrosus)
- Anterior interosseous nerve (AIN) syndrome
  - **Motor only (weak FPL, FDP to index, long, PQ), no sensory deficits**
  - Potential site of compression
    - Deep head of pronator teres (most common)
    - FDS
    - Edge of lacertus fibrosus
    - Aberrant vessels
    - Accessory muscles (i.e., Gantzer muscles)
- Carpal tunnel syndrome
  - Pain and paresthesias in the radial 3½ digits, night pain, hand clumsiness (Table 2-22)
  - Site of compression: carpal tunnel/TCL
- Ulnar
  - Cubital tunnel syndrome
    - Paresthesias in ulnar side of ring and small fingers, night pain, hand intrinsic muscle atrophy, ulnar clawing in chronic cases
    - Potential sites of compression

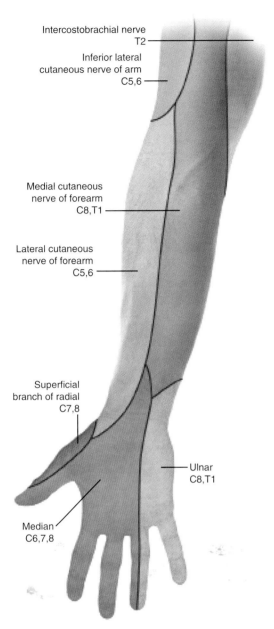

Intercostobrachial nerve
T2

Inferior lateral
cutaneous nerve of arm
C5,6

Medial cutaneous
nerve of forearm
C8,T1

Lateral cutaneous
nerve of forearm
C5,6

Superficial
branch of radial
C7,8

Median
C6,7,8

Ulnar
C8,T1

FIGURE 2-24 Nerve regions in arm and hand. (From Drake RL et al, editors: *Gray's atlas of anatomy*, ed 2, Philadelphia, 2015, Churchill Livingstone.)

- Arcade of Struthers (hiatus in medial intermuscular septum, thickened fascia from intermuscular septum to triceps)
- Medial intermuscular septum
- **Between Osborne ligament and MCL**
- Medial epicondyle
- Between the two heads of FCU (most common site)
- Less common causes of compression include:
  - Fibers within the FCU
  - Anconeus epitrochlearis muscle
  - Cubitus valgus deformity
  - Elbow contracture release
  - Tumor and ganglions cysts
- Ulnar tunnel/Guyon canal compression
  - Presentation variable based on location of compression

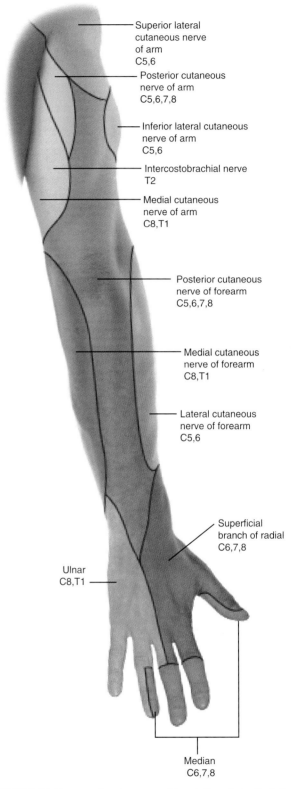

Superior lateral
cutaneous nerve
of arm
C5,6

Posterior cutaneous
nerve of arm
C5,6,7,8

Inferior lateral cutaneous
nerve of arm
C5,6

Intercostobrachial nerve
T2

Medial cutaneous
nerve of arm
C8,T1

Posterior cutaneous
nerve of forearm
C5,6,7,8

Medial cutaneous
nerve of forearm
C8,T1

Lateral cutaneous
nerve of forearm
C5,6

Superficial
branch of radial
C6,7,8

Ulnar
C8,T1

Median
C6,7,8

FIGURE 2-25 Nerve regions in arm and hand. (From Drake RL et al, editors: *Gray's atlas of anatomy*, ed 2, Philadelphia, 2015, Churchill Livingstone.)

- Zone 1 (proximal to nerve bifurcation)—mixed motor and sensory
- Zone 2 (deep motor branch)—motor only
- Zone 3 (superficial sensory branch)—sensory only

Table 2-21	Neuroanatomic Relationships in the Forearm
NERVE	**RELATIONSHIPS**
Radial	Between brachialis and brachioradialis
Posterior interosseous	Splits supinator
Superficial radial	Between brachioradialis and extensor carpi radialis longus
Median	Medial to brachial artery at elbow
Anterior interosseous	Splits pronator teres and runs between flexor digitorum superficialis and flexor digitorum profundus
	Between flexor pollicis longus and flexor digitorum profundus
Ulnar	Between flexor carpi ulnaris and flexor digitorum profundus

Table 2-22	Innervation of the Wrist and Hand
NERVE	**MUSCLES INNERVATED**
Median (medial and lateral cord)	Abductor pollicis brevis, superficial head of flexor pollicis brevis, opponens pollicis, first and second lumbrical muscles
Ulnar (medial cord)	Abductor digiti minimi, opponens digiti minimi, flexor digiti minimi, third and fourth lumbrical muscles, interossei, adductor pollicis, deep head of flexor pollicis brevis

- Cause of compression
  - Ganglion cyst (most cases) (zone 1, 2)
  - Hook of hamate fracture (zone 1, 2)
  - Ulnar artery thrombosis/aneurysm (zone 3)
- Proximal (cubital tunnel) versus distal (Guyon canal) ulnar nerve compression
  - **More clawing with distal compression (FDP to ring and small fingers remain intact); dorsal hand sensory deficit with proximal compression (dorsal cutaneous branch of ulnar nerve)**
- Radial
  - Compression prior to branching
    - Radial + PIN symptoms
  - Potential site of compression
    - Fibrous arch of the long head of triceps
    - Lateral head of triceps
  - PIN syndrome
    - Weakness in wrist, finger, and thumb extension. ECRL function may remain owing to radial nerve innervation, leading to radial deviation with wrist extension.
    - Potential sites of compression
      - Fibrous bands overlying elbow joint capsule between brachialis and brachioradialis
      - **Leash of Henry (recurrent radial artery vessels)**
      - ECRB
      - Arcade of Frohse (proximal edge of superficial head of supinator)
      - Supinator distal margin or muscle belly
      - Lipomas or peri-elbow synovitis associated with rheumatoid arthritis

- Radial tunnel syndrome
  - Mobile wad and lateral forearm pain; discomfort with writing/typing
  - Potential sites of compression
    - Same as in PIN syndrome
    - Controversy over whether this is even a compressive neuropathy
- Superficial branch of radial nerve (**Wartenberg syndrome** or cheiralgia paresthetica)
  - Paresthesias over dorsoradial hand; symptoms at rest
  - Site of compression
    - Between brachioradialis and ECRL (6-9 cm proximal to radial styloid)
    - Handcuffs, tight wristwatch, bracelets, closed reduction of forearm fracture

■ **Vascularity of the upper extremity (Figures 2-26 and 2-27)**

▦ Subclavian artery
  - Left subclavian artery arises directly from the aorta; right subclavian artery arises from the brachiocephalic trunk.
  - Emerges between anterior and middle scalene muscles and becomes the axillary artery at outer border of the first rib

▦ Axillary artery
  - Divided into three parts on the basis of its physical relationship to pectoralis minor muscle (first part is medial to it, second is under it, and third is lateral to it).
  - **Each part of the artery has as many branches as the number of that portion (e.g., the second part has two branches: thoracoacromial and lateral thoracic)** (Table 2-23).
  - Third part, at the origin of the anterior and posterior humeral circumflex arteries, is the most vulnerable to traumatic vascular injury.

▦ Brachial artery
  - Originates at the lower border of the tendon of the teres major and runs with the median nerve in the medial arm anterior to the intermuscular septum
  - **Deep muscular branch (also known as the *profunda brachii*) accompanies the radial nerve posteriorly in the triangular interval).**
  - Radial collateral and superior/inferior ulnar collateral branches around the elbow
  - Supratrochlear branch is least flexible branch.
  - Enters antecubital fossa (bordered by the two epicondyles, the brachioradialis laterally, and the pronator teres medially), passing anterior to brachialis and supinator muscles
  - Divides at the level of the radial neck into the radial and ulnar arteries (Table 2-24)

▦ Radial artery
  - Initially runs on the pronator teres, deep to the brachioradialis
  - Continues to the wrist between this muscle and the FCR
  - Forearm branches include the recurrent radial (which anastomoses with radial collateral artery) and muscular branches.
  - **At the wrist, the radial artery reaches the dorsum of the carpus by passing between the FCR and the APL and EPB tendons (snuffbox).**

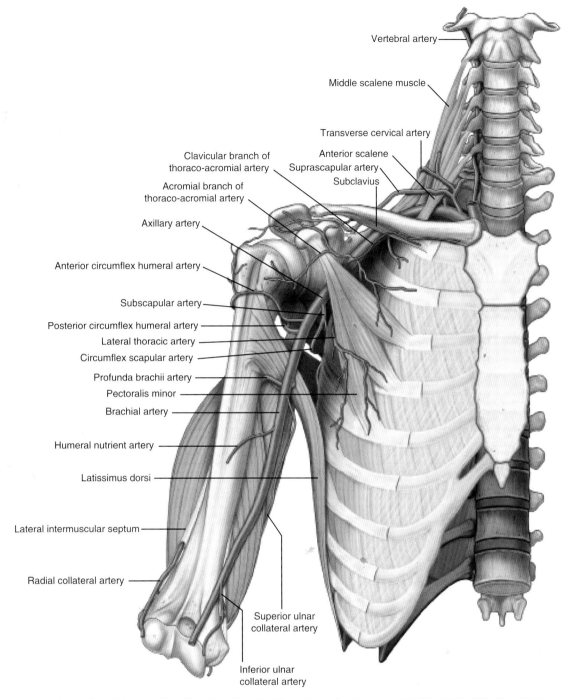

Vertebral artery

Middle scalene muscle

Transverse cervical artery

Clavicular branch of
thoraco-acromial artery

Anterior scalene

Suprascapular artery

Subclavius

Acromial branch of
thoraco-acromial artery

Axillary artery

Anterior circumflex humeral artery

Subscapular artery

Posterior circumflex humeral artery

Lateral thoracic artery

Circumflex scapular artery

Profunda brachii artery

Pectoralis minor

Brachial artery

Humeral nutrient artery

Latissimus dorsi

Lateral intermuscular septum

Radial collateral artery

Superior ulnar
collateral artery

Inferior ulnar
collateral artery

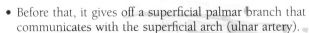

FIGURE 2-26 Arteries of the shoulder. (From Drake RL et al, editors: *Gray's atlas of anatomy,* ed 2, Philadelphia, 2015, Churchill Livingstone.)

- Before that, it gives off a superficial palmar branch that communicates with the superficial arch (ulnar artery).
- **It forms the deep palmar arch in the hand.**
- The dorsal carpal branch of the radial artery enters the scaphoid dorsally and distally.
- Ulnar artery: larger of the two branches
  - Covered by the superficial flexors proximally (between FDS and FDP)
  - Distally the artery lies on the FDP between the tendons of the FCU and FDS.
  - Forearm branches include the anterior and posterior recurrent ulnar (which anastomose with inferior and superior ulnar collateral arteries, respectively), the

common interosseous (with anterior and posterior branches), and several muscular and nutrient arteries.
- At the wrist, ulnar artery lies on the TCL.
- **Gives off a deep palmar branch (which anastomoses with the deep arch) and then forms the superficial palmar arch**
- Digital arteries arise from superficial palmar arch and run dorsal to digital nerves.
- **Approaches to the upper extremity** (Table 2-25)
  - Surgical approaches to the shoulder (Figure 2-28)
    - Anterior (deltopectoral) approach (Figure 2-29)
      - Interval: deltoid (**axillary nerve**) and pectoralis major (**medial and lateral pectoral nerves**); can be extended

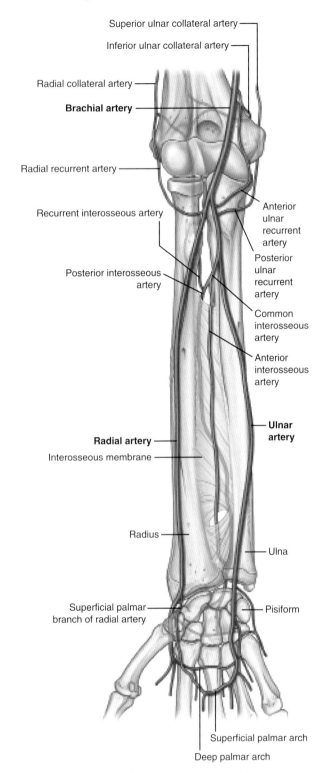

Table 2-23 | **Axillary Artery Branches**

PART	BRANCH	COURSE
I	Supreme thoracic	Medial to serratus anterior and pectoral muscles
II	Thoracoacromial	Four branches: deltoid, acromial, pectoralis, clavicular
	Lateral thoracic	Descends to serratus anterior
III	Subscapular	Two branches: thoracodorsal and circumflex scapular (triangular space)
	Anterior humeral circumflex	Blood supply to humeral head: arcuate artery lateral to bicipital groove
	Posterior humeral circumflex	Branch in the quadrangular space accompanying axillary nerve

Table 2-24 | **Vascular Anatomic Relationships in the Forearm**

ARTERY	RELATIONSHIPS
Radial	On pronator teres deep to brachioradialis
	Enters wrist between brachioradialis and flexor carpi radialis
Ulnar	Proximally between FDS and FDP
	Distally on FDP between flexor carpi ulnaris and FDS

FDP, Flexor digitorum profundus; *FDS,* flexor digitorum superficialis.

- Incise clavipectoral fascia lateral to the conjoint tendon to expose the subscapularis and proximal humerus. Retract deltoid laterally. Shoulder abduction relaxes deltoid to improve access.
- To access shoulder joint, subscapularis may be divided longitudinally, detached from the lesser tuberosity, or taken off with a lesser tuberosity osteotomy.
- **A leash of three vessels (one artery and the superior and inferior venae comitantes) marks the lower border of the subscapularis.**
- Anterior shoulder capsule closely associated with subscapularis tendon
- Layers of the anterior shoulder are summarized in Table 2-26.
- Risks:
  - Musculocutaneous nerve
    - Penetrates posterior aspect of conjoint tendon approximately 5 cm distal to coracoid (may be more proximal in 30% of shoulders)
    - Protect by staying lateral to conjoint tendon and avoiding vigorous retraction medially.
    - Musculocutaneous palsy would affect coracobrachialis, biceps brachii, and brachialis muscles, and sensation in the lateral antebrachial cutaneous nerve (termination of musculocutaneous nerve).
  - Axillary nerve
    - Passes anterior to posterior through quadrangular space just inferior to the shoulder capsule
    - Shoulder adduction and external rotation reduces tension on the nerve.

 FIGURE 2-27 Arteries of the arm. (From Drake RL et al, editors: *Gray's atlas of anatomy,* ed 2, Philadelphia, 2015, Churchill Livingstone.)

distally along lateral border of biceps into anterolateral approach to humerus
- Dissection:
  - Interval marked by cephalic vein. Develop plane between deltoid and pectoralis major to expose the clavipectoral fascia. Cephalic vein is mobilized either laterally or medially based on surgeon preference.

Table 2-25	Standard Orthopaedic Approaches to the Upper Extremity		
APPROACH	**SUPERFICIAL INTERVAL (NERVE)**	**DEEP INTERVAL (NERVE)**	**STRUCTURES AT RISK**
SHOULDER			
Anterior (deltopectoral)	Deltoid (axillary) AND pectoralis major (medial/lateral pectoral)		Cephalic vein Musculocutaneous nerve Axillary nerve AHCA
Lateral (deltoid-splitting)	Split deltoid (axillary)		Axillary nerve
Posterior	Split deltoid (axillary)	Infraspinatus (suprascapular) AND teres minor (axillary)	Axillary nerve PHCA Suprascapular nerve
HUMERUS			
Anterolateral (proximal)	Deltoid (axillary) AND pectoralis major (medial/lateral pectoral)		Cephalic vein Musculocutaneous nerve
Anterolateral (middle/distal)	Lateral to biceps (musculocutaneous)	Split brachialis (radial and musculocutaneous)	Cephalic vein Musculocutaneous nerve
Anterolateral (distal)	Brachialis (musculocutaneous) AND brachioradialis (radial)		Radial nerve LABCN
Posterior (triceps-splitting)	Lateral and long head of triceps (distal to branching of radial nerve)	Split medial (deep) head of triceps (radial)	Radial nerve Ulnar nerve
Posterior (triceps-slide)	Triceps (radial) AND medial intermuscular septum		Radial nerve Ulnar nerve
ELBOW			
Anterior (antecubital fossa)	Biceps (musculocutaneous) AND brachioradialis (radial)	Pronator teres (median) AND supinator (PIN)	Cephalic vein basilic vein LABCN Brachial artery Recurrent radial artery Median nerve SBRN PIN
Medial (Hotchkiss)	Brachialis (musculocutaneous) AND triceps (radial) or pronator teres (median)	Split or elevation of flexor-pronator mass (median)	Ulnar nerve MABCN
Lateral (Kaplan)	ECRB (radial/PIN) AND EDC (PIN)		PIN LUCL
Posterolateral (Kocher)	Anconeus (radial) AND ECU (PIN)		PIN LUCL
Posterior	Multiple options (olecranon osteotomy, triceps-sparing (Bryan-Morrey), triceps splitting) but none with a true internervous plane		Ulnar nerve Radial nerve
FOREARM			
Anterior (Henry)	Brachioradialis (radial) AND pronator teres/FCR (median)		PIN Recurrent radial artery Radial artery SBRN
Posterior (Thompson)	ECRB (radial/PIN) AND EDC/EPL (PIN)		PIN
Posterior ulna	ECU (radial) AND FCU (ulnar)		Ulnar artery Ulnar nerve
WRIST			
Dorsal	Third and fourth extensor compartments (no internervous plane)		PIN
Volar (distal Henry)	Median nerve and radial artery		Median nerve as well as motor branch and PCB Radial artery
Carpal tunnel	Median nerve and ulnar nerve	Transverse carpal ligament	Median nerve as well as motor branch and PCB

AHCA, Anterior humeral circumflex artery; *ECRB,* extensor carpi radialis brevis; *EDC,* extensor digitorum communis; *FCR,* flexor carpi radialis; *FCU,* flexor carpi ulnaris; *LABCN,* lateral antebrachial cutaneous nerve; *LUCL,* lateral ulnar collateral ligament; *MABCN,* medial antebrachial cutaneous nerve; *PCB,* palmar cutaneous branch of median nerve; *PHCA,* posterior humeral circumflex artery; *PIN,* posterior interosseous branch of radial nerve; *SBRN,* superficial branch of radial nerve.

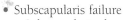

- Subscapularis failure
  - Subscapularis should be securely repaired when closing.
  - **Protect subscapularis repair postoperatively with passive external rotation restrictions.**
- Lateral (deltoid-splitting) approach
  - Interval: none; often split is made through the anterior raphe.
  - Dissection:

- Either split the deltoid muscle or detach it subperiosteally from the acromion.
- Supraspinatus tendon is exposed, which allows for repairs of the rotator cuff.
- Risks:
  - Axillary nerve
    - **Courses from posterior to anterior around shoulder in deep fascia of deltoid approximately 5 to 7 cm distal to acromion**

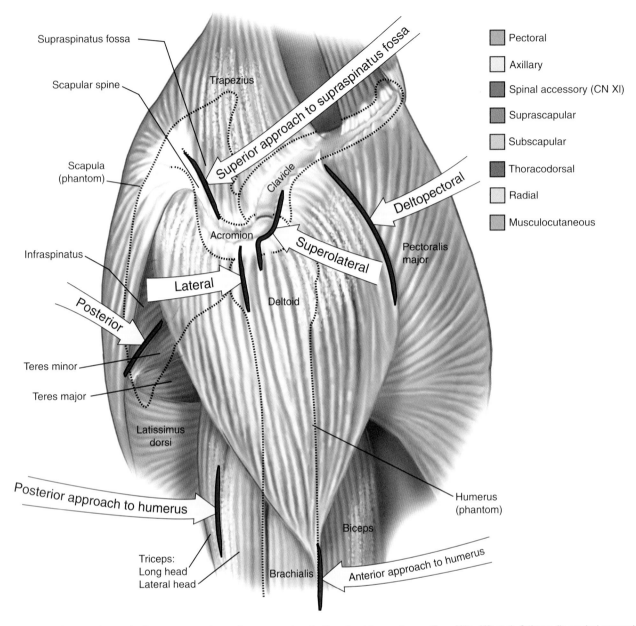

Pectoral

Axillary

Spinal accessory (CN XI)

Suprascapular

Subscapular

Thoracodorsal

Radial

Musculocutaneous

FIGURE 2-28 Surgical intervals. Internervous planes for approaches to the shoulder and arm. (From Miller MD et al: *Orthopaedic surgical approaches,* ed 2, Philadelphia, 2014, Saunders, Figure 2-11.)

- Damage to axillary nerve may denervate anterior deltoid.
- Place a stich at the inferior border of the muscle split so it will not accidentally propagate distally during the case.
- Posterior approach
  - **Interval: infraspinatus (suprascapular nerve) and teres minor (axillary nerve)**
  - Dissection:
    - Split the posterior deltoid, thereby exposing the interval between the infraspinatus and teres minor.
    - Posterior capsule lies immediately deep to the interval.
  - Risks:
    - Quadrangular space (axillary nerve and posterior humeral circumflex artery): stay above the teres minor.

- Suprascapular nerve
  - May be damaged with excessive medial retraction of the infraspinatus
- Surgical approaches to the humerus
  - Anterolateral approach
    - Interval: deltoid (axillary nerve) and pectoralis major (medial and lateral pectoral nerves) and along lateral biceps proximally, **between the fibers of the brachialis (radial and musculocutaneous nerves)** midhumerus, and between the brachialis (radial and musculocutaneous nerves) and brachioradialis (radial nerve) distally
    - Dissection:
      - Proximal approach:
        - Interval marked by the cephalic vein. Retract the pectoralis major medially and the deltoid laterally.

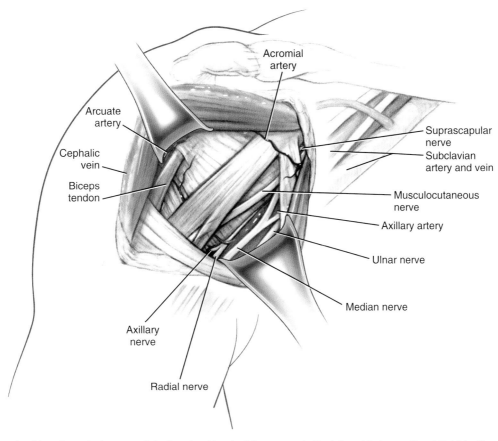

FIGURE 2-29 Anterior (Henry) surgical approach to the shoulder. In this approach, the interval between the deltoid (axillary nerve) and the pectoralis major (medial and lateral pectoral nerves) is explored. To prevent injury to the musculocutaneous nerve, avoid excessive medial retraction (see medial retractor) on the coracobrachialis or avoid dissection medial to this muscle. Also avoid the axillary nerve, which is inferior to the shoulder capsule. Positioning the arm in adduction and external rotation helps displace the axillary nerve from the surgical field. (From Miller MD et al: *Orthopaedic surgical approaches,* Philadelphia, 2008, Saunders, Figure SA-12.)

Table 2-26	Shoulder-Supporting Anatomic Layers
LAYER	**STRUCTURES**
I	Deltoid, pectoralis major, trapezius
II	Clavipectoral fascia, conjoined tendon, short head of biceps, and coracobrachialis
III	Deep layer of subdeltoid bursa, rotator cuff muscles (supraspinatus, infraspinatus, teres minor, subscapularis [SITS])
IV	Glenohumeral joint capsule, coracohumeral ligament

- Anterior circumflex humeral vessels may need to be ligated.
- Middle approach:
  - Split the brachialis fibers longitudinally.
  - Alternatively, the humerus may be exposed between the brachialis and biceps, but this approach is not extensile distally.
- Distal approach:
  - Retract the brachialis muscle medially and the brachioradialis laterally.
  - May be extended distally to the forearm when combined with a volar Henry approach
- Risks:
  - Radial and axillary nerves are at risk for injury mainly because of forceful retraction. Radial nerve can also be injured by screw penetration or retraction compression as it courses within the spiral groove.
  - For distal exposure, be wary of the lateral antebrachial cutaneous nerve entering the field (coursing medially to lateral under the biceps tendon) and the radial nerve (traveling under the brachioradialis muscle).
- Posterior approach to the humerus:
  - Interval: none
  - Dissection:
    - Triceps-splitting
      - Superficial approach: dissect between lateral and long heads of the triceps (triceps-splitting).
      - Deep approach: split the medial head of the triceps (triceps-splitting).
    - Lateral triceps slide
      - Mobilize the entire triceps complex medially by dissecting the lateral head off the lateral intermuscular septum.
  - Risks:
    - Radial nerve: limits proximal extension of approach
      - **Identify and protect the radial nerve as it passes from medial to lateral in the proximal part of the exposure.**
    - With the triceps-splitting approach, can increase access to posterior humerus from 55% to 76% by mobilizing the radial nerve.

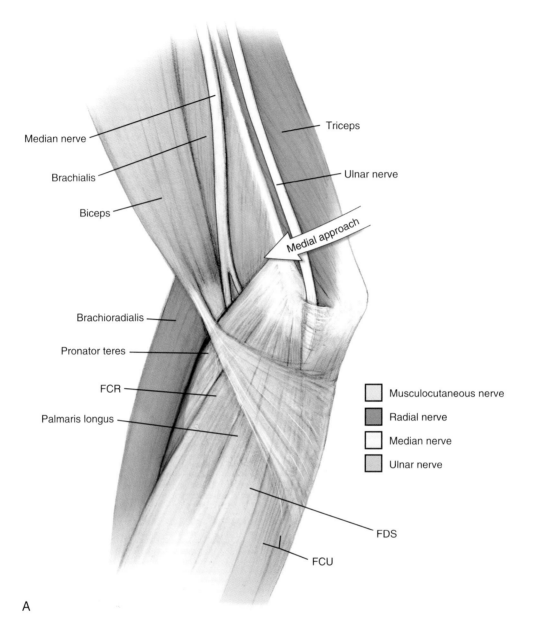

Median nerve

Brachialis

Biceps

Triceps

Ulnar nerve

Medial approach

Brachioradialis

Pronator teres

FCR

Palmaris longus

☐ Musculocutaneous nerve

■ Radial nerve

☐ Median nerve

▨ Ulnar nerve

FDS

FCU

A

FIGURE 2-30 Internervous planes for medial **(A)** and lateral **(B)** approaches to the elbow. (From Miller MD et al: *Orthopaedic surgical approaches,* ed 2, Philadelphia, 2014, Saunders, Figures 3-8 and 3-9.)

- Ulnar nerve: jeopardized unless subperiosteal dissection of the humerus is performed meticulously
- Axillary nerve: seen in the proximal exposure of the lateral triceps slide
■ Surgical approaches to the elbow (Figure 2-30)
- Anterior approach to the antecubital fossa
  - Interval: biceps, brachioradialis, and pronator teres (Figure 2-31)
  - Dissection:
    - Curved incision from medial border of biceps transversely across the flexion crease and distally along radial border of brachioradialis
      - Avoid 90-degree angle across flexion crease.

- Brachioradialis retracted laterally, pronator teres retracted medially
- Dissect supinator from radius to expose elbow capsule and anterior radius.
- Risks:
  - Multiple veins, including cephalic and basilic vein, anastomose in antecubital fossa.
  - Lateral antebrachial cutaneous nerve emerges from beneath the biceps tendon.
  - Brachial artery lies directly deep to biceps aponeurosis.
  - Recurrent branches of radial artery
  - Median nerve most medial major neurovascular structure in antecubital fossa
  - PIN (supinate forearm to protect)

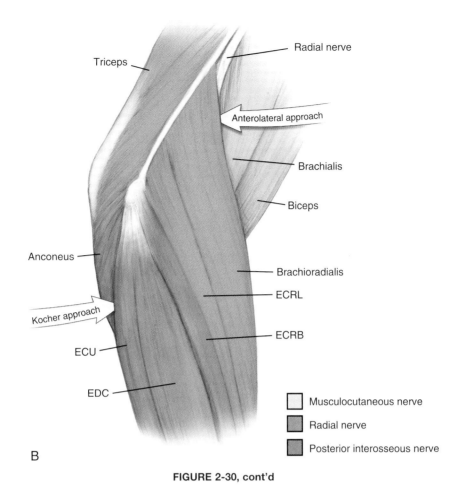

Triceps

Radial nerve

Anterolateral approach

Brachialis

Biceps

Anconeus

Brachioradialis

ECRL

Kocher approach

ECRB

ECU

EDC

☐ Musculocutaneous nerve

▨ Radial nerve

▨ Posterior interosseous nerve

B

FIGURE 2-30, cont'd

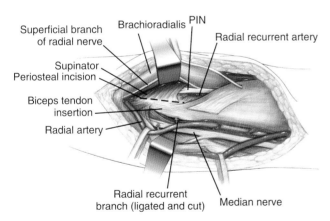

Superficial branch of radial nerve

Brachioradialis PIN

Radial recurrent artery

Supinator
Periosteal incision

Biceps tendon insertion

Radial artery

Radial recurrent branch (ligated and cut)

Median nerve

FIGURE 2-31 Anterior approach to the elbow. Deep dissection and ligation of the recurrent radial artery branches. Subperiosteally reflect the supinator muscle, protecting the posterior interosseous nerve (PIN), to expose the anterior joint capsule. (From Miller MD et al: *Orthopaedic surgical approaches,* ed 2, Philadelphia, 2014, Saunders, Figure 3-19.)

- Medial approach to the elbow (Hotchkiss) (Figure 2-32)
  - Interval: between the brachialis (musculocutaneous nerve) and triceps (radial nerve) proximally and between the brachialis and pronator teres (median nerve) distally

- Dissection: incise anterior third of the flexor pronator mass to reach the anterior elbow capsule.
- Risks:
  - **Medial antebrachial cutaneous nerves cross field and must be protected.**
  - Ulnar nerve
- Lateral (Kaplan) approach to the elbow
  - **Interval: between the ECRB (radial/PIN) and extensor digitorum communis (EDC) (PIN)** (Note: uses the same muscular interval as the more distal dorsal Thompson approach.)
  - Dissection: split the annular ligament while remaining anterior to the LUCL. **Pronate the arm to move the PIN anteriorly and radially.**
  - Risks: PIN, LUCL
- Posterolateral (Kocher) approach to the elbow (Figure 2-33)
  - Interval: between the anconeus (radial nerve) and the origin of the main extensor (extensor carpi ulnaris [ECU], PIN)
  - Dissection: **pronate the arm to move the PIN anteriorly and radially, and approach the radial head through the proximal supinator fibers.**
  - Risks: extending this approach distal to annular ligament increases risk for injury to PIN.
- Proximal extension of lateral approach
  - Interval: along lateral intercondylar ridge, between triceps and ECRL (brachioradialis nerve)

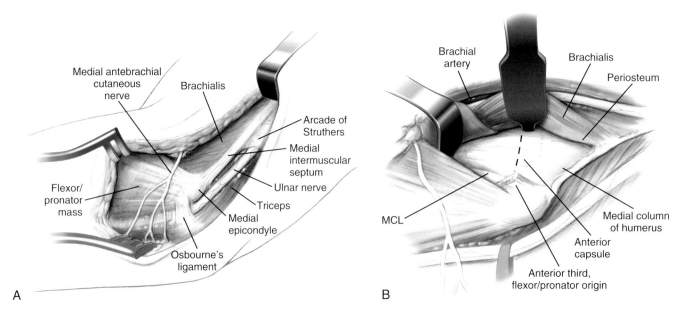

A

B

FIGURE 2-32 Medial approach to the elbow. **A,** Superficial exposure. **B,** Deep exposure. The interval between the brachialis (musculocutaneous nerve) and triceps (radial nerve) can be used to access the anterior distal humerus. *MCL,* Medial collateral ligament. (From Miller MD et al: *Orthopaedic surgical approaches,* Philadelphia, 2008, Saunders, Figures EF-23 and EF 26.)

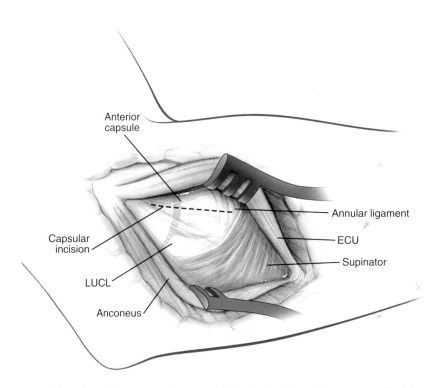

FIGURE 2-33 Lateral approach to the elbow. This approach explores the interval between the anconeus (radial nerve) and the extensor carpi ulnaris (ECU) (posterior interosseous nerve [PIN]). Arm pronation helps move the PIN away from the surgical field. *LUCL,* Lateral ulnar collateral ligament. (From Miller MD et al: *Orthopaedic surgical approaches,* Philadelphia, 2008, Saunders, Figure EF-32.)

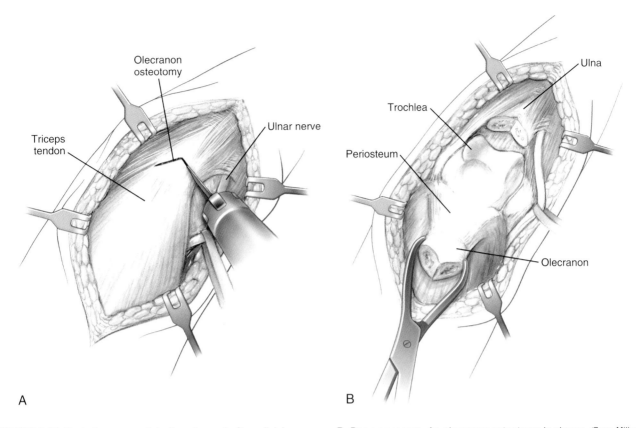

FIGURE 2-34 Posterior approach to the elbow. **A,** Superficial exposure. **B,** Deep exposure. An olecranon osteotomy is shown. (From Miller MD et al: *Orthopaedic surgical approaches,* Philadelphia, 2008, Saunders, Figures EF-46 and EF-47.)

- Dissection: subperiosteally expose the anterior humerus and lateral column.
- Risks: retractor placed under brachialis anteriorly to protect radial nerve, distally limited by PIN
- Posterior approach to the elbow:
  - Interval: none
  - Dissection:
    - Olecranon osteotomy: predrill the olecranon osteotomy (best done with a chevron cut 2 cm distal to the tip), and protect the ulnar nerve (Figure 2-34).
    - Triceps-sparing (Bryan-Morrey): elevate the triceps insertion subperiosteally off the olecranon and retract laterally. Repair triceps mechanism with transosseous sutures.
    - Triceps splitting: in an alternative approach, split the triceps and leave the olecranon intact.
    - Paratricipital (triceps slide): triceps is elevated off the medial and lateral intermuscular septa so the tendon may be mobilized in either direction to access the humerus. The triceps insertion is undisturbed.
  - Risks:
    - Ulnar nerve can be injured with dissection or excessive retraction.
    - **Radial nerve limits the proximal extension along the humerus.**
    - Do not divide triceps transversely in the triceps-sparing approach.
- Surgical approaches to the forearm
  - Anterior (Henry) approach (Figures 2-35 and 2-36)

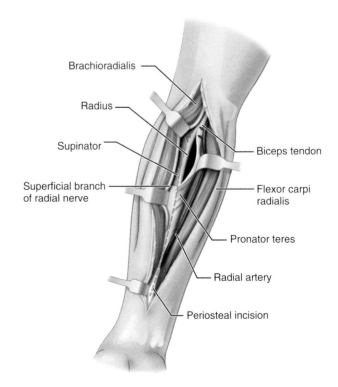

FIGURE 2-35 Internervous planes for volar approaches to the forearm. (From Miller MD et al: *Orthopaedic surgical approaches,* ed 2, Philadelphia, 2014, Saunders, Figure 3-10.)

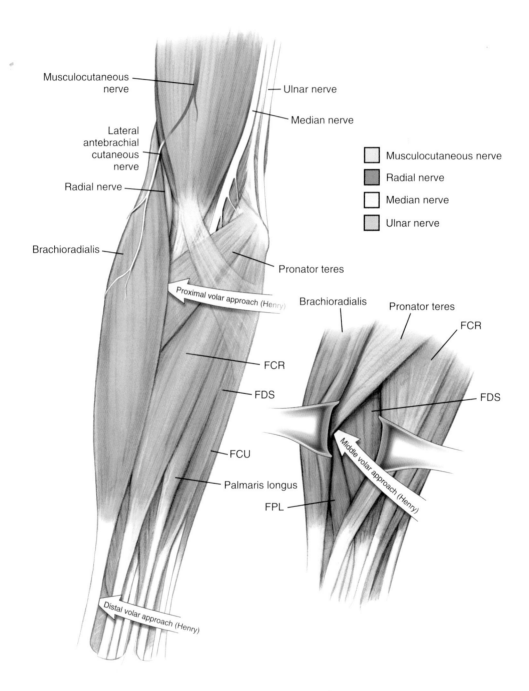

Musculocutaneous nerve

Ulnar nerve

Median nerve

Lateral antebrachial cutaneous nerve

Radial nerve

Brachioradialis

Pronator teres

Proximal volar approach (Henry)

Brachioradialis

Pronator teres

FCR

FCR

FDS

FDS

FCU

Palmaris longus

FPL

Middle volar approach (Henry)

Distal volar approach (Henry)

Musculocutaneous nerve

Radial nerve

Median nerve

Ulnar nerve

FIGURE 2-36 Henry approach.

- Interval: between the brachioradialis (radial nerve) and pronator teres proximally or FCR distally (median nerve)
- Dissection:
  - Proximally: isolate and ligate the leash of Henry (radial artery branches) proximally, and strip the supinator from its insertion subperiosteally. **Supination of the forearm displaces the PIN ulnarly (i.e., laterally and posteriorly).**
  - Middle third: pronate forearm and incise the insertion of the pronator teres subperiosteally.
  - Distally: dissect off the FPL and PQ.
- Risks:
  - Superficial branch of the radial nerve must be protected (retract laterally) with the brachioradialis.
  - Radial artery is at risk for injury proximally because it courses medial to the biceps tendon and distally with retraction of the brachioradialis.

- PIN can be injured during deep dissection of proximal exposure (fully supinate to move laterally).
- Posterior (Thompson) approach (Figure 2-37)
  - Interval: **between ECRB (radial nerve/PIN) and EDC or EPL distally (PIN)**
  - Dissection:
    - Identify PIN as it exits the supinator before the forearm is supinated, and reflect the supinator off the anterior surface of the proximal radius (Figure 2-38).
    - Distally, retract the APL and EPB to gain access to the middle and distal portions of the radius.
  - Risks: PIN must be identified and protected.
- Exposure of the ulna (ECU/FCU approach)
  - Interval: between the ECU (PIN) and the FCU (ulnar nerve)
  - Dissection: strip muscles from the ulna subperiosteally.
  - Risks: FCU stripped subperiosteally to protect ulnar nerve and artery

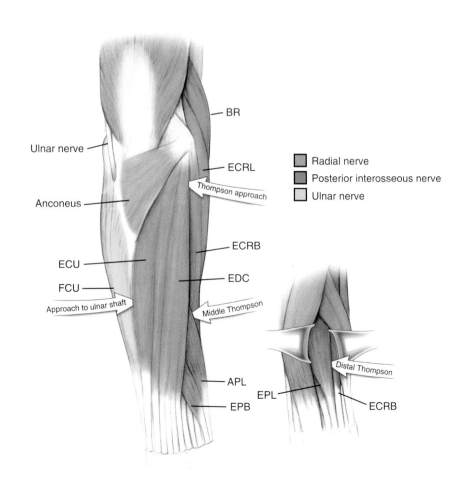

■ Radial nerve
■ Posterior interosseous nerve
□ Ulnar nerve

FIGURE 2-37 Internervous planes for dorsal approaches to the forearm. (From Miller MD et al: *Orthopaedic surgical approaches,* ed 2, Philadelphia, 2014, Saunders, Figure 3-11.)

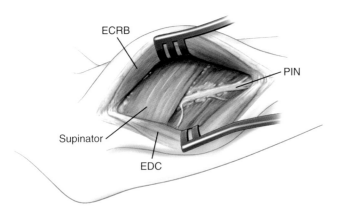

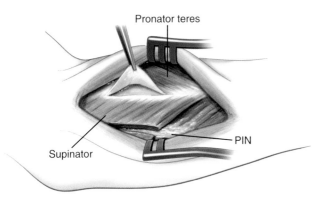

FIGURE 2-38 Dorsal (posterior [Thompson]) approach to the forearm. In this approach, the interval between the extensor carpi radialis brevis (radial nerve) and the extensor digitorum communis (posterior interosseous nerve [PIN]) is explored. *ECRB,* Extensor carpi radialis brevis; *EDC,* extensor digitorum communis. (From Miller MD et al: *Orthopaedic surgical approaches,* Philadelphia, 2008, Saunders, Figures EF-65 and EF-68.)

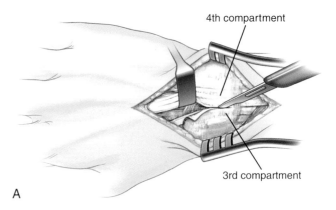

A

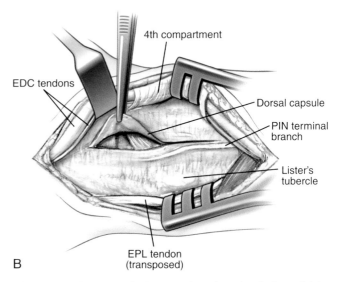

B

FIGURE 2-39 Dorsal surgical approach to the wrist. **A,** Superficial exposure. **B,** Deep exposure. In this approach, the interval between the third (extensor pollicis longus) and fourth (extensor digitorum communis) dorsal wrist compartments is explored. *EDC,* Extensor digitorum communis; *EPL,* extensor pollicis longus; *PIN,* posterior interosseous nerve. (From Miller MD et al: *Orthopaedic surgical approaches,* Philadelphia, 2008, Saunders, Figures HW-13 and HW-14.)

■ Surgical approaches to the wrist and hand
  • Dorsal approach to the wrist (Figure 2-39)
    • Interval: between the third and fourth extensor compartments (EPL and extensor digitorum)
    • Dissection:
      • Incise the extensor retinaculum between the third and fourth compartments.
      • Protect and retract these tendons to allow access to the distal radius and the dorsal radiocarpal joint.
      • Transpose the EPL and incise the dorsal capsule.
    • Risks: do not violate the interosseous scapholunate ligament.
  • Carpal tunnel release
    • Incision is usually made in line with the fourth ray to avoid the palmar cutaneous branch of the median nerve.
    • Dissection through the TCL must be performed carefully to avoid injury to median nerve or its motor branch.
  • Volar (Russé) approach to the scaphoid
    • Interval: between FCR and radial artery

  • An approach through the radial aspect of the FCR sheath: often easier and protects the radial artery
• Dorsolateral approach to the scaphoid
  • Using an incision within the anatomic snuffbox (first and third dorsal wrist compartment) helps protect the superficial radial nerve and radial artery (deep).
• Volar approach to the flexor tendons (Bunnell)
  • Zigzag incisions across the flexor creases help to expose the flexor sheaths.
  • Digital sheaths should be avoided.
• Midlateral approach to the digits
  • Good for stabilization of fractures and neurovascular exposure
  • Requires a laterally placed incision at the dorsal extent of the interphalangeal creases
  • Exposure of the digital neurovascular bundle: volar to the incision

■ Cross-sectional diagrams of the upper extremity with MRI are demonstrated in Figures 2-40 through 2-44

Text continued on p. 193

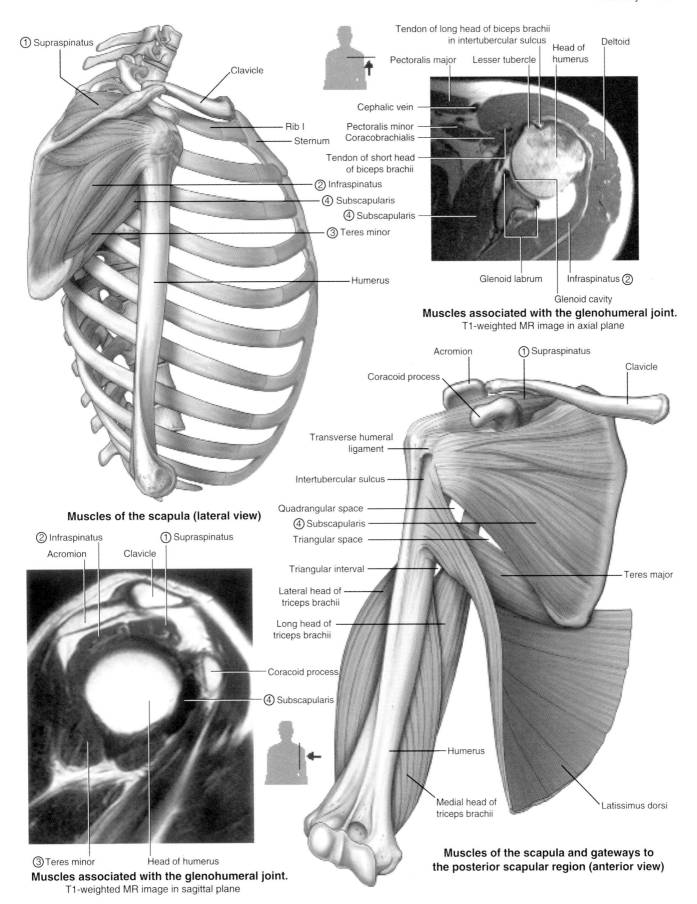

① Supraspinatus

Clavicle

Rib I

Sternum

② Infraspinatus

④ Subscapularis

④ Subscapularis

③ Teres minor

Humerus

Muscles of the scapula (lateral view)

Tendon of long head of biceps brachii
in intertubercular sulcus

Head of humerus

Deltoid

Pectoralis major   Lesser tubercle

Cephalic vein

Pectoralis minor
Coracobrachialis

Tendon of short head
of biceps brachii

Glenoid labrum   Infraspinatus ②

Glenoid cavity

Muscles associated with the glenohumeral joint.
T1-weighted MR image in axial plane

Acromion   ① Supraspinatus

Coracoid process

Clavicle

Transverse humeral
ligament

Intertubercular sulcus

Quadrangular space

④ Subscapularis

Triangular space

Triangular interval

Lateral head of
triceps brachii

Long head of
triceps brachii

Coracoid process

④ Subscapularis

Teres major

Humerus

Medial head of
triceps brachii

Latissimus dorsi

**Muscles of the scapula and gateways to
the posterior scapular region (anterior view)**

② Infraspinatus   ① Supraspinatus

Acromion   Clavicle

③ Teres minor   Head of humerus

Muscles associated with the glenohumeral joint.
T1-weighted MR image in sagittal plane

FIGURE 2-40 Muscles of the scapula and glenohumeral joint. (From Drake RL et al, editors: *Gray's atlas of anatomy,* ed 2, Philadelphia, 2015, Churchill Livingstone.)

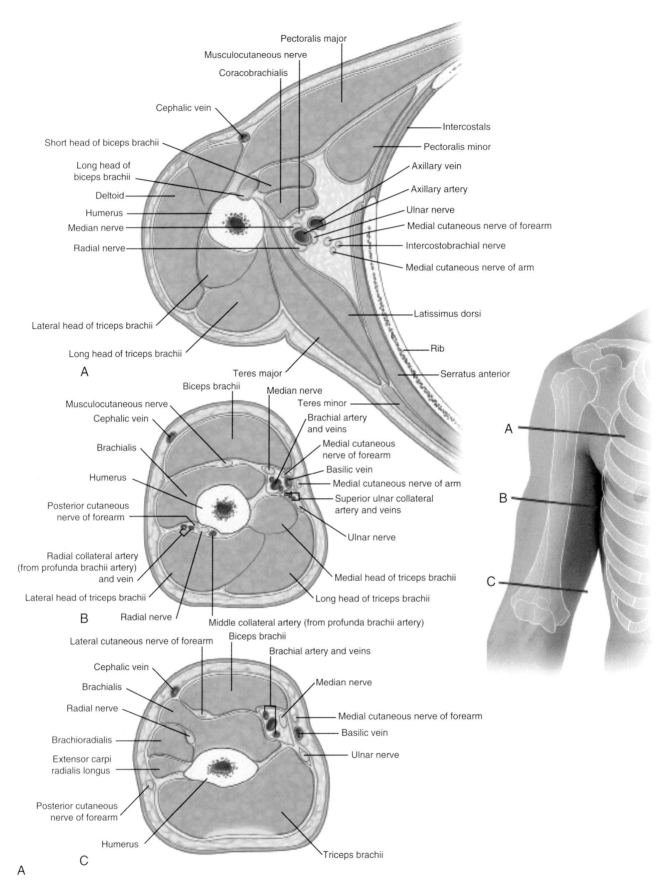

FIGURE 2-41 Illustration **(A)** and imaging **(B)** of nerves surrounding the humerus. (From Drake RL et al, editors: *Gray's atlas of anatomy,* ed 2, Philadelphia, 2015, Churchill Livingstone.)

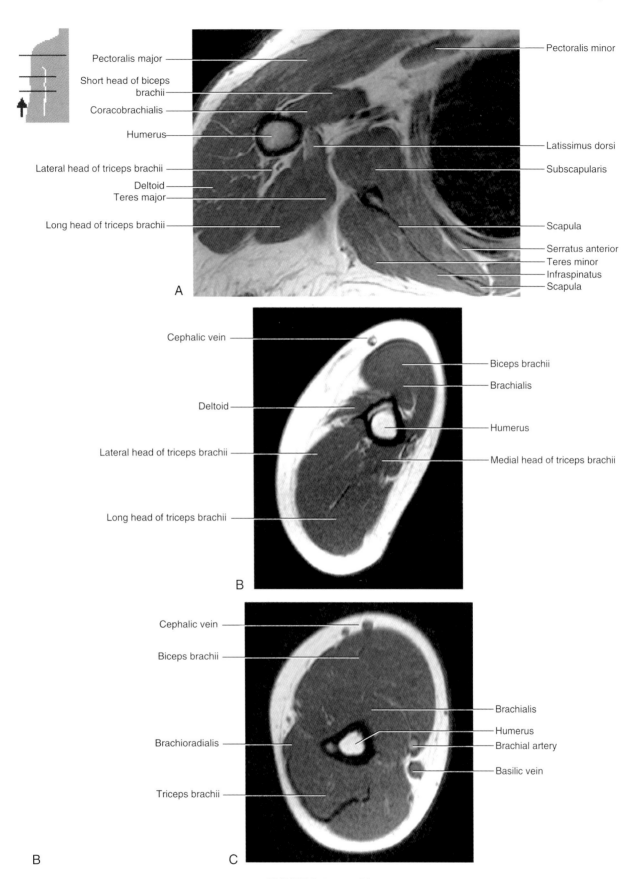

FIGURE 2-41, cont'd

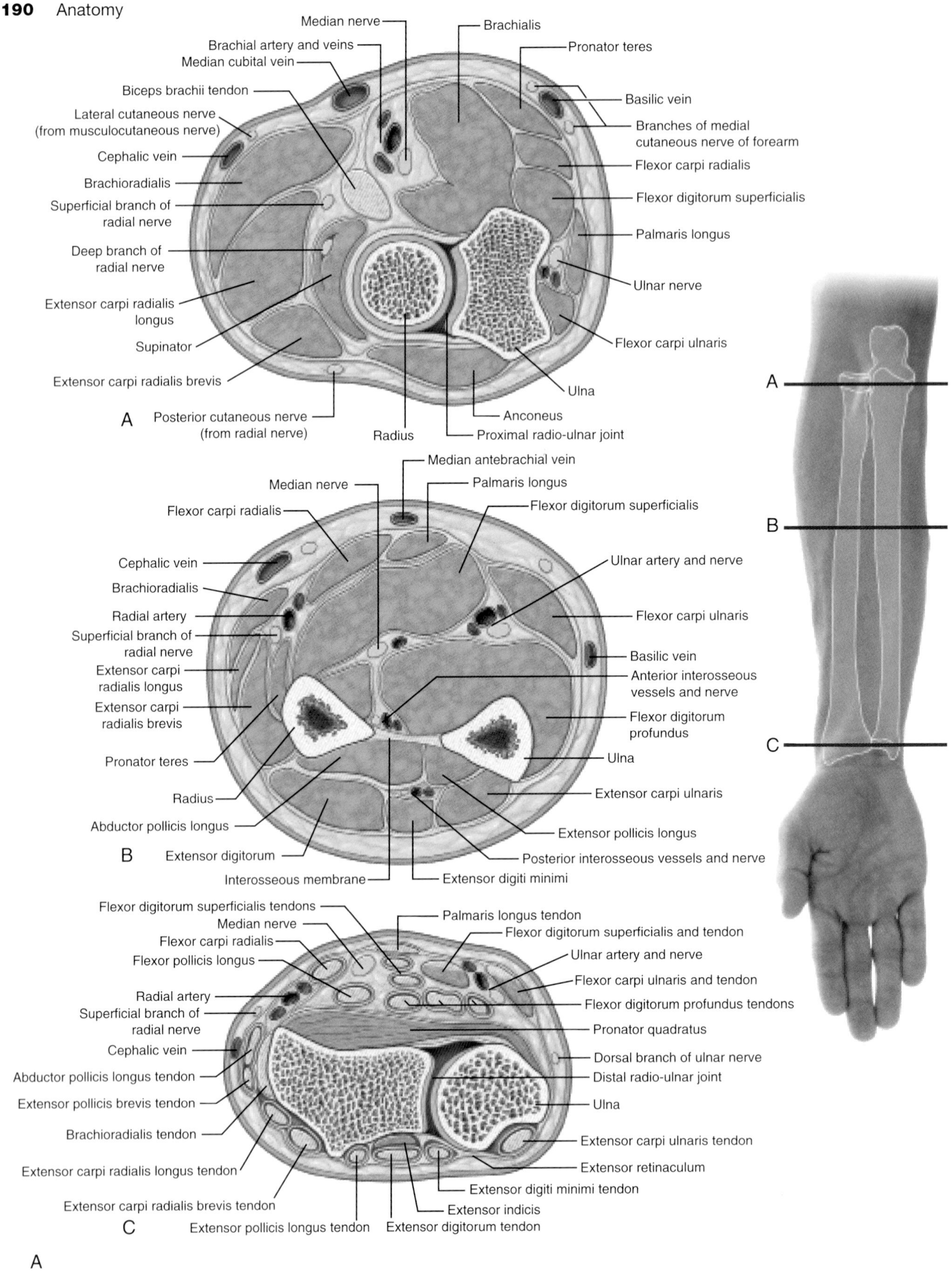

FIGURE 2-42 Illustration **(A)** and imaging **(B)** of anatomy of the forearm. (From Drake RL et al, editors: *Gray's atlas of anatomy,* ed 2, Philadelphia, 2015, Churchill Livingstone.)

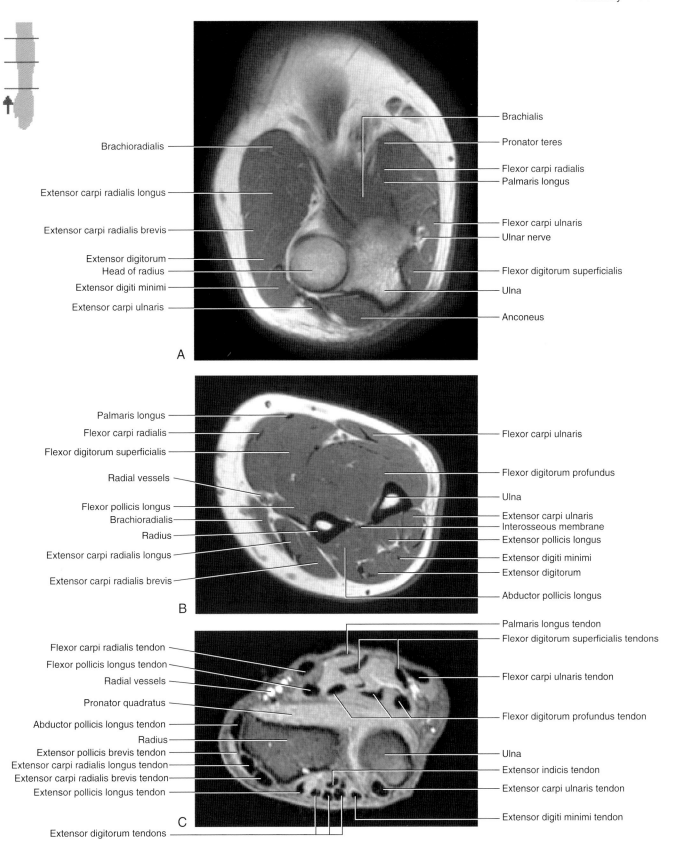

Brachioradialis

Extensor carpi radialis longus

Extensor carpi radialis brevis

Extensor digitorum
Head of radius
Extensor digiti minimi
Extensor carpi ulnaris

Brachialis
Pronator teres
Flexor carpi radialis
Palmaris longus

Flexor carpi ulnaris
Ulnar nerve

Flexor digitorum superficialis
Ulna

Anconeus

A

Palmaris longus
Flexor carpi radialis
Flexor digitorum superficialis
Radial vessels
Flexor pollicis longus
Brachioradialis
Radius
Extensor carpi radialis longus
Extensor carpi radialis brevis

Flexor carpi ulnaris

Flexor digitorum profundus

Ulna
Extensor carpi ulnaris
Interosseous membrane
Extensor pollicis longus
Extensor digiti minimi
Extensor digitorum

Abductor pollicis longus

B

Flexor carpi radialis tendon
Flexor pollicis longus tendon
Radial vessels
Pronator quadratus
Abductor pollicis longus tendon
Radius
Extensor pollicis brevis tendon
Extensor carpi radialis longus tendon
Extensor carpi radialis brevis tendon
Extensor pollicis longus tendon
Extensor digitorum tendons

Palmaris longus tendon
Flexor digitorum superficialis tendons

Flexor carpi ulnaris tendon

Flexor digitorum profundus tendon

Ulna
Extensor indicis tendon
Extensor carpi ulnaris tendon

Extensor digiti minimi tendon

C

B

FIGURE 2-42, cont'd

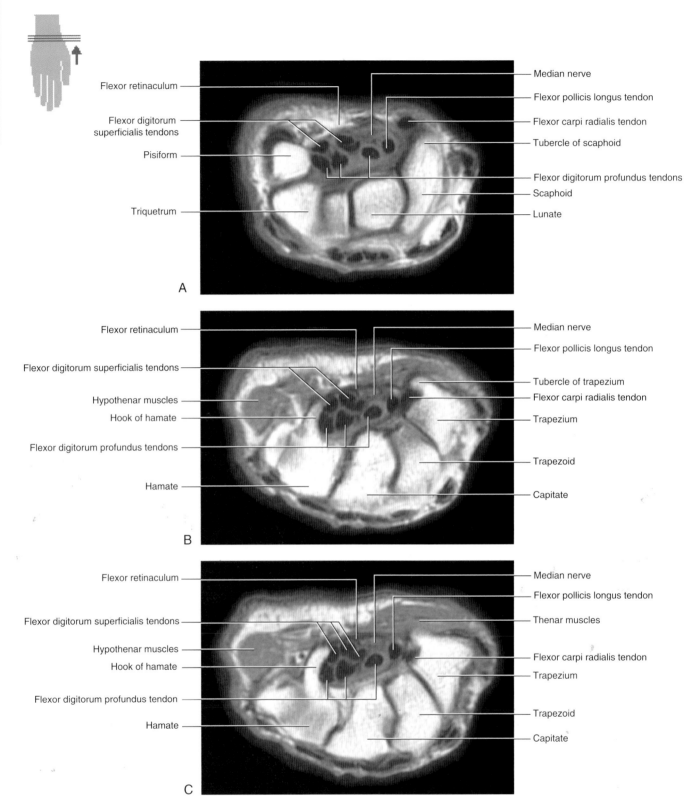

FIGURE 2-43 Imaging of carpal region anatomy. (From Drake RL et al, editors: *Gray's atlas of anatomy,* ed 2, Philadelphia, 2015, Churchill Livingstone.)

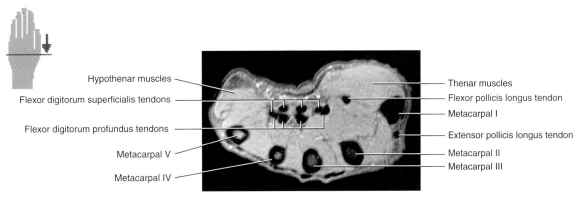

FIGURE 2-44 Imaging of the anatomy of the hand. (From Drake RL et al, editors: *Gray's atlas of anatomy,* ed 2, Philadelphia, 2015, Churchill Livingstone.)

SECTION 3 LOWER EXTREMITY

PELVIS, HIP, AND THIGH

■ Osteology

▦ Pelvic girdle is composed of two innominate (coxal) bones that articulate with the sacrum and proximal femora.

▦ Each innominate bone is composed of three united bones: ilium, ischium, and pubis. (Figure 2-45, *A* and *B*)
  • Converge in the acetabular fossa at the triradiate fusion center

▦ Ilium: important landmarks include iliac crest, anterior-superior iliac spine (ASIS), anterior-inferior iliac spine (AIIS), and posterior-superior iliac spine (PSIS)
  • Iliac crest—palpable rim of ilium, important site for bone graft harvest (iliac tubercle 5 cm posterior to ASIS)
  • **ASIS: palpable at lateral edge of inguinal ligament; origin of sartorius muscle and transverse and internal abdominal muscles**
  • **AIIS: less prominent; origin of direct head of the rectus femoris and iliofemoral ligament (Y ligament of Bigelow)**
  • PSIS: 4 to 5 cm lateral to S2 spinous process; important landmark for posterior iliac crest bone graft harvest

▦ Ischium: posterior column of acetabulum
  • **Iliac spine separates greater and lesser sciatic notch; sacrospinous ligament (anterior sacrum to ischial spine) separates greater and lesser sciatic foramina.**
  • Greater sciatic notch: posterior and superior to acetabulum
  • Ischial tuberosity: origin of hamstrings; sacrotuberous ligament (posterolateral sacrum to ischial tuberosity) inferior border of lesser sciatic foramen

▦ Pubis: anterior pelvic ring, bilateral pubic rami articulate at pubic symphysis
  • Iliopectineal eminence: anterior pelvic rim prominence at the union of the ilium and pubis
  • Iliopsoas muscle/tendon traverses a groove between iliopectineal eminence and AIIS.

▦ Acetabulum: normally anteverted (15 degrees) and obliquely oriented in coronal plane (45 degrees caudally)
  • Posterosuperior articular surface thickened to accommodate weight bearing
  • Inferior surface contains the acetabular (cotyloid) notch, which is bound by the transverse acetabular ligament.

▦ Femur
  • Proximal femur: femoral head, femoral neck, and greater and lesser trochanters
    • Femoral head blood supply changes with age (Table 2-27).
    • **Pediatric femoral nail insertion: piriformis starting point threatens the posterosuperior retinacular vessels (potential for femoral head avascular necrosis [AVN]).**
    • **Adult posterior hip approach: do not completely transect the quadratus femoris muscle (to prevent damage to medial femoral circumflex artery).**
    • Femoral neck normally anteverted approximately 14 degrees in relation to femoral condyles (range 1-40 degrees)
    • Femoral neck shaft angle averages 127 degrees (begins at 141 degrees in the fetus).
    • Proximal femoral trabecular architecture is illustrated in Figure 2-46.
  • Femoral shaft: anterior bow
  • Ossification: important areas of femoral ossification include the head and the distal femur.
    • Femoral head is usually not present at birth but appears as one large physis that includes both trochanters at about the age of 11 months and fuses at age 18 years.
    • **Slipped capital femoral epiphysis occurs through the femoral head physis (zone of hypertrophy).**
    • Distal femoral epiphysis is present at birth and fuses at age 19 years.

■ Arthrology

▦ Hip (Figure 2-47)
  • Ball-and-socket diarthrodial joint
  • Stability is based primarily on the bony architecture.
  • **Fibrocartilaginous labrum deepens acetabulum, enhancing stability. Labral functions include load transmission, maintenance of vacuum seal, regulation of synovial fluid hydrodynamics, and joint lubrication.**

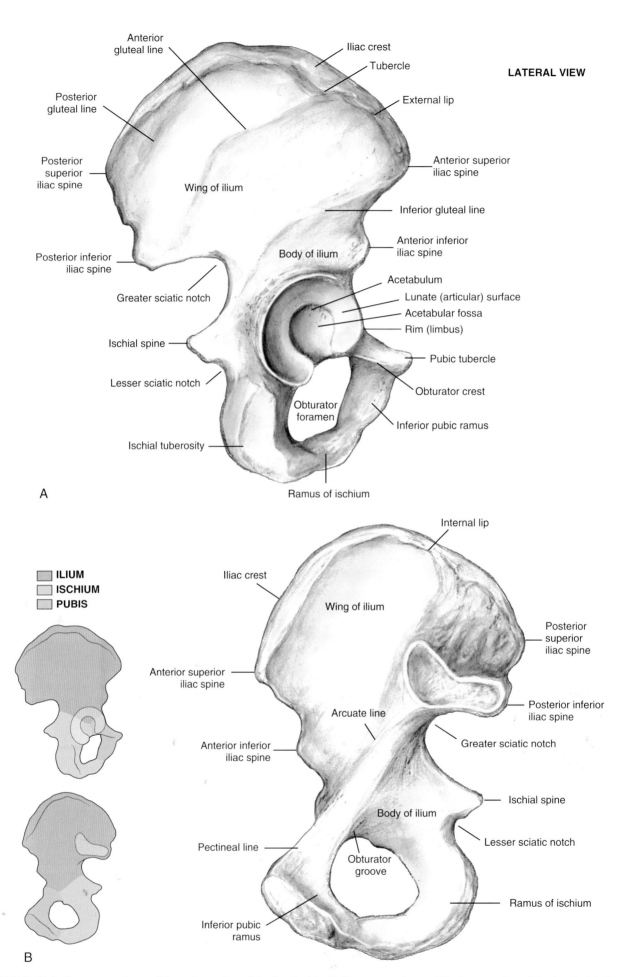

FIGURE 2-45 A, Osseous anatomy of the outer portion of the hemipelvis. **B,** Osseous anatomy of the inner portion of the hemipelvis from the sacroiliac joint to the pubic symphysis. (From Miller MD et al: *Orthopaedic surgical approaches,* ed 2, Philadelphia, 2014, Saunders, Figures 6-1 and 6-2.)

Table 2-27	Age-Dependent Changes to Blood Supply to Femoral Head
AGE	**BLOOD SUPPLY**
Birth to 4 yr	Primary medial and lateral circumflex arteries (from deep femoral artery) Ligamentum teres with posterior division of obturator artery
4 yr to adult	Negligible amount from lateral circumflex artery Minimal amount from ligamentum teres Posterosuperior and posteroinferior retinacular from medial femoral circumflex artery
Adult	Medial femoral circumflex to lateral epiphyseal artery

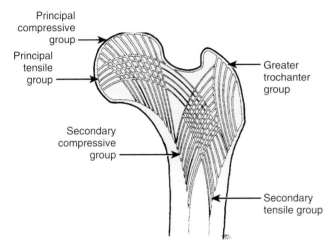

FIGURE 2-46 Hip trabeculae. Trabecular patterns help determine the presence of osteopenia and displacement of femoral neck fractures. (From DeLee JC: Fractures and dislocations of the hip. In Rockwood CA Jr et al, editors: *Fractures in adults*, ed 3, Philadelphia, 1991, JB Lippincott, p 1488.)

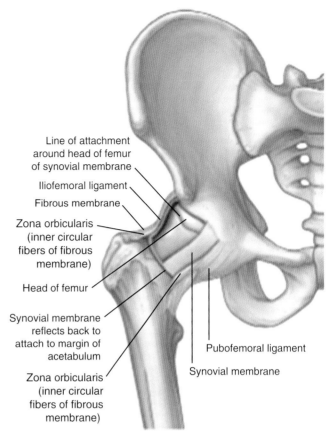

FIGURE 2-47 Ligaments and membranes of the hip joint. (From Drake RL et al, editors: *Gray's atlas of anatomy*, ed 2, Philadelphia, 2015, Churchill Livingstone.)

- Hip joint capsule: extends anteriorly to intertrochanteric crest but posteriorly only partially across femoral neck
  - **Basicervical and intertrochanteric crest regions are extracapsular.**
  - Capsular ligaments
    - **Iliofemoral ligament (Y ligament of Bigelow) is the strongest ligament in the body and attaches AIIS to intertrochanteric line in an inverted Y manner.**
    - Ischiofemoral and pubofemoral ligaments are weaker but provide additional stability.
    - Capsule tight in extension, relaxed in flexion
- Ligamentum teres: arises from apex of cotyloid notch and attaches to fovea of femoral head
  - Transmits an arterial branch of the posterior division of the obturator artery to femoral head (less significant in adults)
- Sacroiliac joint
  - Stabilized by posterior and anterior sacroiliac ligaments and interosseous ligaments
- Symphysis pubis
  - Stabilized by superior and arcuate pubic ligaments and contains fibrocartilaginous disc

- ■ **Muscles that act on the hip joint** (Figures 2-48 and 2-49; Table 2-28)
  - ▦ Hip flexion: iliopsoas, rectus femoris, and sartorius
  - ▦ Hip extension: gluteus maximus and hamstrings (semitendinosus, semimembranosus, and long head of biceps femoris)
  - ▦ Hip abduction: gluteus medius and minimus (primary); tensor fasciae latae (TFL) helps with abduction in a flexed hip.
  - ▦ Hip adduction: adductors brevis, longus, and magnus, pectineus, and gracilis
  - ▦ Hip external rotation: obturator internus, obturator externus, superior and inferior gemellus, quadratus femoris, and piriformis
  - ▦ Hip internal rotation: secondary actions of anterior fibers of gluteus medius and gluteus minimus, TFL, semimembranosus, semitendinosus, pectineus, and posterior part of adductor magnus
- ■ **Muscles of the thigh that do not cross the hip joint are listed in Table 2-29.**
- ■ **Muscles with dual innervation**
  - ▦ Pectineus (obturator and femoral)
  - ▦ Adductor magnus (obturator and tibial)
  - ▦ **Biceps femoris (long head, tibial nerve; short head, peroneal nerve)**
- ■ **Muscles that cross the hip and knee** (more prone to strain injury)
  - ▦ Rectus femoris (hip flexion, knee extension)
  - ▦ Sartorius (hip flexion, knee flexion)

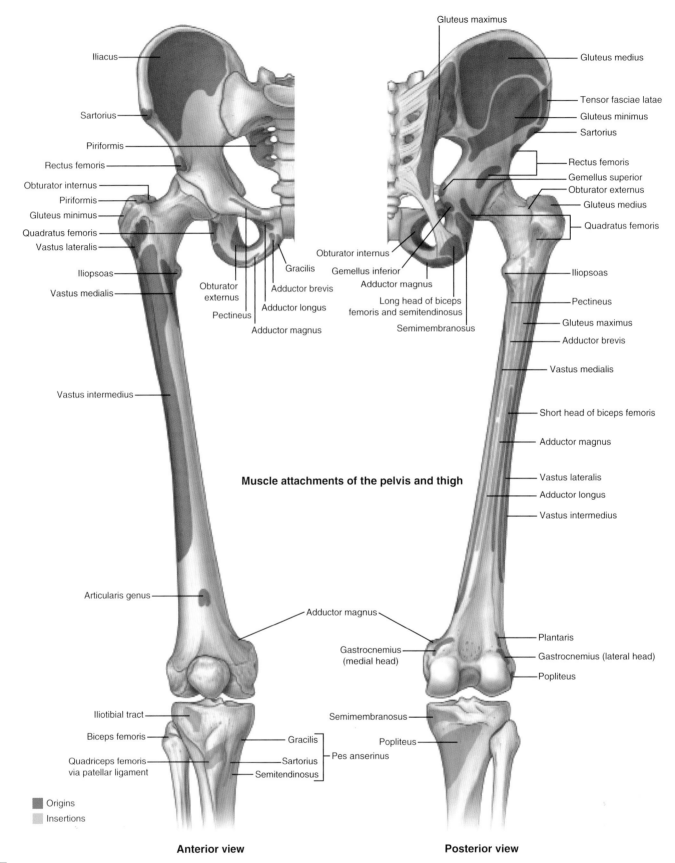

Muscle attachments of the pelvis and thigh

Anterior view

Posterior view

FIGURE 2-48 Muscle attachments of the pelvis and thigh. (From Drake RL et al, editors: *Gray's atlas of anatomy,* ed 2, Philadelphia, 2015, Churchill Livingstone.)

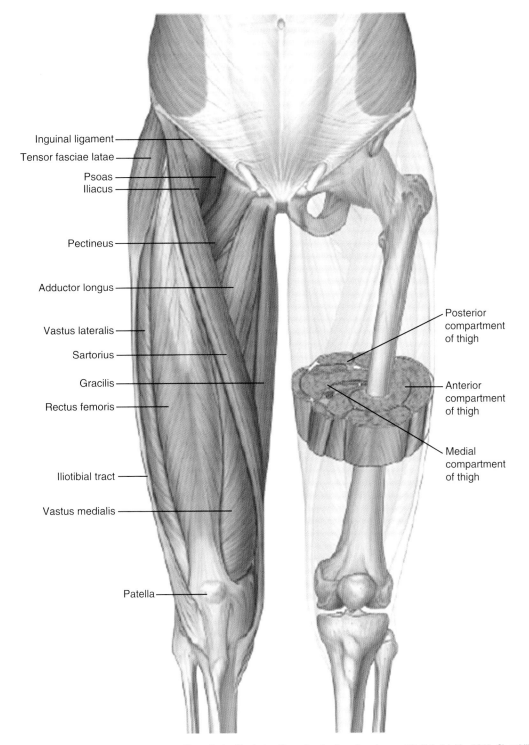

FIGURE 2-49 Thigh muscles and compartments. (From Drake RL et al, editors: *Gray's atlas of anatomy,* ed 2, Philadelphia, 2015, Churchill Livingstone.)

- Gracilis (hip adduction, knee flexion)
- Biceps femoris, long head (hip extension, knee flexion)
- Semimembranosus (hip extension, knee flexion)
- Semitendinosus (hip extension, knee flexion)

KNEE AND LEG

Osteology
- Distal femur
  - Two femoral condyles (**medial condyle is larger**)
  - More prominent medial epicondyle supports the adductor tubercle.
  - Sulcus terminalis on lateral femoral condyle
- Tibia
  - **Proximal medial facet (oval and concave) and lateral facet (circular and convex)**
  - Gerdy tubercle on lateral side of the proximal tibia is the insertion of the iliotibial (IT) tract.
  - Tibial shaft is triangular in cross section and tapers to its thinnest point at the junction of the middle and distal thirds before widening again to form the tibial plafond.
- Fibula
  - Fibular head attachment point for lateral collateral ligament and insertion point for biceps femoris

Table 2-28	Muscles That Act on the Hip			
MUSCLE	**ORIGIN**	**INSERTION**	**NERVE**	**SEGMENT**
FLEXORS				
Iliacus	Iliac fossa	Lesser trochanter	Femoral	L2-L4 (P)
Psoas	Transverse processes of L1-L5	Lesser trochanter	Femoral	L2-L4 (P)
Pectineus	Pectineal line of pubis	Pectineal line of femur	Femoral and obturator	L2-L4 (P)
Rectus femoris	Anterior inferior iliac spine, acetabular rim	Patella and tibial tubercle	Femoral	L2-L4 (P)
Sartorius	Anterior superior iliac spine	Proximal medial tibia	Femoral	L2-L4 (P)
EXTENSORS				
Biceps femoris (long head)	Medial ischial tuberosity	Fibular head/lateral tibia	Tibial	L5-S2 (A)
Semitendinosus	Distal medial ischial tuberosity	Anterior tibial crest	Tibial	L5-S2 (A)
Semimembranosus	Proximal lateral ischial tuberosity	Oblique popliteal ligament Posterior capsule Posterior/medial tibia Popliteus Medial meniscus	Tibial	L4-S3 (A)
ADDUCTORS				
Adductor magnus	Inferior pubic ramus/ischial tuberosity	Linea aspera/adductor tubercle	Obturator (P) and tibial	L2-L4 (A)
Adductor brevis	Inferior pubic ramus	Linea aspera/pectineal line	Obturator (P)	L2-L4 (A)
Adductor longus	Anterior pubic ramus	Linea aspera	Obturator (A)	L2-L4 (A)
Gracilis	Inferior symphysis/pubic arch	Proximal medial tibia	Obturator (A)	L2-L4 (A)
EXTERNAL ROTATORS				
Gluteus maximus	Ilium, posterior gluteal line	Iliotibial band/gluteal sling (femur)	Inferior gluteal	L5-S2 (P)
Piriformis	Anterior sacrum/sciatic notch	Proximal greater trochanter	Piriformis	S2 (P)
Obturator externus	Ischiopubic rami/obturator	Trochanteric fossa	Obturator	L2-L4 (A)
Obturator internus	Ischiopubic rami/obturator membrane	Medial greater trochanter	Obturator internus	L5-S2 (A)
Superior gemellus	Outer ischial spine	Medial greater trochanter	Obturator internus	L5-S2 (A)
Inferior gemellus	Ischial tuberosity	Medial greater trochanter	Quadratus femoris	L5-S1 (A)
Quadratus femoris	Ischial tuberosity	Quadrate line of femur	Quadratus femoris	L5-S1 (A)
ABDUCTORS				
Gluteus medius	Ilium between posterior and anterior gluteal lines	Greater trochanter	Superior gluteal	L4-S1 (P)
Gluteus minimus	Ilium between anterior and inferior gluteal lines	Anterior border of greater trochanter	Superior gluteal	L4-S1 (P)
Tensor fasciae latae (tensor fasciae femoris)	Anterior iliac crest	Iliotibial band	Superior gluteal	L4-S1 (P)

A, Anterior; *P*, posterior.

Table 2-29	Muscles of the Thigh		
MUSCLE	**ORIGIN**	**INSERTION**	**INNERVATION**
ANTERIOR THIGH			
Vastus lateralis	Iliotibial line/greater trochanter/lateral linea aspera	Lateral patella	Femoral
Vastus medialis	Iliotibial line/medial linea aspera/supracondylar line	Medial patella	Femoral
Vastus intermedius	Proximal anterior femoral shaft	Patella	Femoral
POSTERIOR THIGH			
Biceps femoris (long head)	Medial ischial tuberosity	Fibular head/lateral tibia	Tibia
Biceps (short head)	Lateral linea aspera/lateral intermuscular septum	Lateral tibial condyle	Peroneal
Semitendinosus	Distal medial ischial tuberosity	Anterior tibial crest	Tibial
Semimembranosus	Proximal lateral ischial tuberosity	Oblique popliteal ligament Posterior capsule Posterior/medial tibia Popliteus Medial meniscus	Tibial

tendon; popliteofibular ligament attaches to fibular styloid process.
- Fibular neck has a groove for the common peroneal nerve.
- Patella: the largest sesamoid bone
  - Serves three functions:
    - Fulcrum for quadriceps to facilitate knee extension
    - Protects knee joint
    - Enhances lubrication and nutrition of knee
  - **Accessory or "bipartite" patella may represent failure of fusion of the superolateral corner of the**

patella and is commonly confused with patellar fractures.

■ **Arthrology**

▦ Knee (Figure 2-50)
- Enclosed in a capsule that has posteromedial and posterolateral recesses extending 15 mm distal to the subchondral surface of the tibial plateau (be careful to avoid intraarticular pin placement).
- **Medial and lateral femoral condyles articulate with corresponding tibial facets. Shape of tibial plateau confers greater articular congruity medially than**

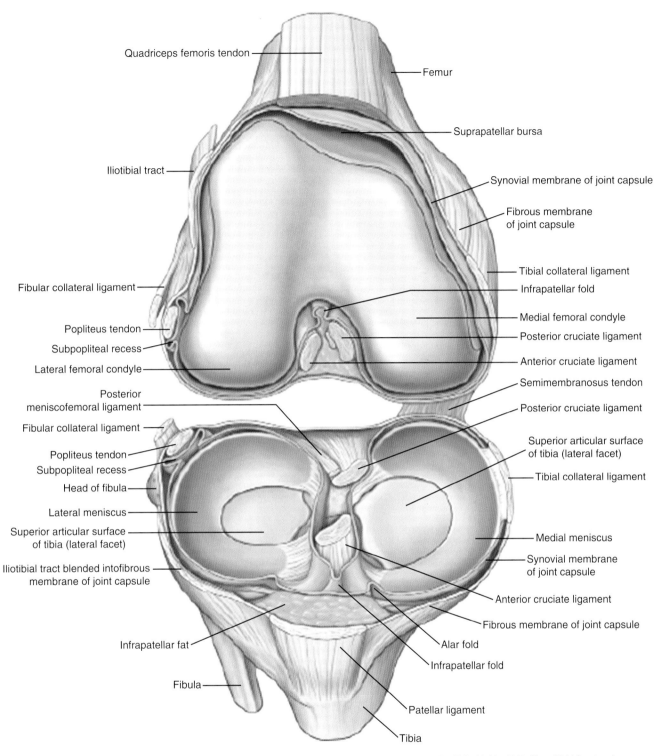

FIGURE 2-50 Anatomy of the Knee. (From Drake RL et al, editors: *Gray's atlas of anatomy*, ed 2, Philadelphia, 2015, Churchill Livingstone.)

laterally (important when considering consequences of meniscectomy).

- Menisci
  - Serve to deepen concavity of facets, help protect the articular surface, and assist in rotation of the knee
  - **Peripheral third of menisci are vascular and can be repaired (red zone); inner two thirds are nourished by synovial fluid (white zone) and have limited healing capacity.**

- Medial meniscus tears three times more often than the more mobile lateral meniscus.
  - **Must protect saphenous nerve during medial meniscus repair**
- Lateral meniscus is associated with meniscal cysts and discoid menisci; most common site of tears in acute injuries to the anterior cruciate ligament (ACL).
  - Protect peroneal nerve during lateral meniscus repair.

Table 2-30	Ligaments of the Knee		
LIGAMENT	**PROXIMAL ATTACHMENT**	**DISTAL ATTACHMENT**	**FUNCTION**
ANTERIOR KNEE			
Retinacular	Vastus medialis and vastus lateralis , tibial condyles	Medial and lateral patella	Forms anterior capsule
Medial patellofemoral	Between adductor tubercle and medial femoral epicondyle (Schottle point)	Superomedial patella	Resists lateral translation of patella
POSTERIOR KNEE			
Posterior fibers	Femoral condyles	Tibial condyles	Forms posterior capsule
Oblique popliteal	Semimembranosus tendon	Lateral femoral condyle/ posterior capsule	Strengthens capsule
MEDIAL KNEE			
Superficial MCL	Medial femoral epicondyle	Medial tibial metaphysis	Resists valgus force
Deep MCL	Medial femoral epicondyle/ medial meniscus	Medial tibial condyle/ medial meniscus	Resists valgus force, stabilizes medial meniscus
Posterior oblique	Adductor tubercle	Posteromedial tibia	Resists valgus force, internal rotation
LATERAL KNEE			
Lateral collateral	Lateral epicondyle	Lateral fibular head	Resists varus force
Popliteofibular ligament	Popliteus tendon	Fibular styloid process	Resists external rotation
Arcuate ligament	Lateral femoral condyle, over popliteus	Posterior tibia/fibular head	Posterior support
CRUCIATES/INTRAARTICULAR LIGAMENTS			
Anterior cruciate	Posteromedial lateral femoral condyle	Anterior intercondylar tibia	Resists anterior translation, hyperextension
Posterior cruciate	Anteromedial femoral condyle	Posterior sulcus of tibia	Resists posterior translation, hyperflexion
Humphrey	Medial femoral condyle (anterior to PCL)	Posterolateral meniscus	Stabilizes lateral meniscus
Wrisberg	Medial femoral condyle (posterior to PCL)	Posterolateral meniscus	Stabilizes lateral meniscus
Transverse meniscal	Anteromedial meniscus	Anterolateral meniscus	Stabilizes menisci

MCL, Medial collateral ligament; *PCL,* posterior collateral ligament.

- Ligaments
  - Stability of the knee is enhanced by a complex arrangement of ligaments (Table 2-30).
  - Cruciate ligaments are crucial for anteroposterior stability; collateral ligaments provide varus and valgus stability.
  - Each cruciate ligament is made up of two portions, or bundles. Anterior bundles of each cruciate tight in flexion.
  - **ACL has anteromedial (tight in flexion) and posterolateral (tight in extension) bundles; PL bundle tested with pivot shift exam.**
    - Mnemonic: "AMPLe" (AnteroMedial and PosteroLateral bundle, PL tight in Extension)
  - PCL has anterolateral (tight in flexion) and posteromedial (tight in extension) bundles.
    - Mnemonic: "PAL" (PCL has anterolateral bundle)
  - Ligament of Humphrey (anterior to PCL) and the Wrisberg ligament (posterior to PCL). Mnemonic: *H* comes before *W* in alphabet; Humphrey is anterior, Wrisberg posterior.
  - MCL has superficial and deep component; superficial MCL attaches 5 to 7 cm distal to joint (Figure 2-51)
  - Posterior oblique ligament resists internal rotation with knee in full extension.
  - **Posterolateral corner (PLC): fibular collateral ligament, popliteus tendon, and popliteofibular ligament; other PLC structures include biceps femoris tendon, lateral head of gastrocnemius, biceps femoris, arcuate ligament, and posterolateral capsule** (Figure 2-52, *A* and *B*).

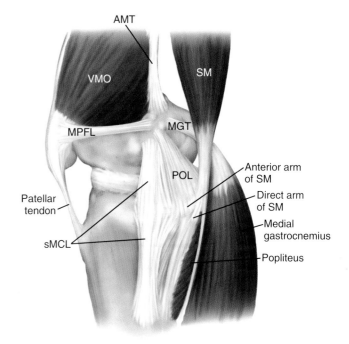

FIGURE 2-51 Illustration of the main medial knee structures (right knee). (From Scott WN: *Insall & Scott surgery of the knee,* ed 5, Philadelphia, 2012, Elsevier, Figure 39-3.)

- Isolated injuries to the PCL cause the greatest instability at 90 degrees of knee flexion.
- Combined injuries of the PCL and PLC result in increasing instability as the knee is flexed from 30 to 90 degrees.

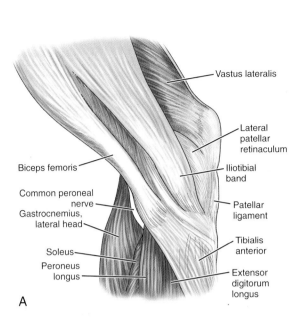

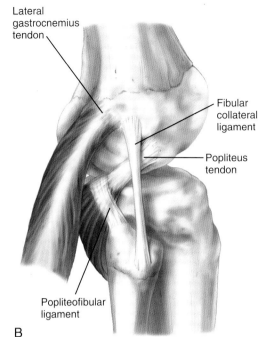

A — Vastus lateralis, Lateral patellar retinaculum, Biceps femoris, Iliotibial band, Common peroneal nerve, Patellar ligament, Gastrocnemius, lateral head, Soleus, Tibialis anterior, Peroneus longus, Extensor digitorum longus

B — Lateral gastrocnemius tendon, Fibular collateral ligament, Popliteus tendon, Popliteofibular ligament

FIGURE 2-52 A, Lateral aspect of the knee, layer 1. **B,** Drawing of lateral knee dissection. (From Scott WN: *Insall & Scott surgery of the knee,* ed 5, Philadelphia, 2012, Elsevier, Figures 1-70 and 40-1.)

- Dial test: rotational instability at **30 degrees** = PLC injury, at 30 and 90 degrees = combined **PLC + PLC injury**
- MPFL runs from proximal third of medial patella to Schottle's point on the femur (between adductor tubercle and medial epicondyle); **just distal to vastus medialis obliquus**
▦ Proximal tibiofibular joint: strengthened by the anterior and posterior ligaments of the head of the fibula

▪ Muscles and tendons around the knee
▦ Several muscles and tendons traverse the knee, giving it dynamic stability.
▦ Popliteal fossa is bordered by the gastrocnemius lateral and medial heads, the semimembranosus, and the biceps; the plantaris muscle makes up the floor of the fossa.
▦ Autograft hamstrings for ACL reconstruction: gracilis and semitendinosus (run deep to the sartorial fascia and superficial to the superficial MCL); saphenous nerve at risk with harvest

▪ Muscles of the leg
▦ Origins and insertions are noted in Figure 2-53.
▦ Divided into compartments (anterior, lateral, superficial posterior, and deep posterior) (Figure 2-54, Table 2-31)
- Anterior and lateral compartments are supplied by the common peroneal nerve (anterior supplied by the deep peroneal nerve, and lateral supplied by the superficial peroneal nerve) and contain postaxial muscles.
- Posterior compartments are supplied by the tibial nerve and contain preaxial muscles.
- **Four compartment releases of the leg are key testable material** and are summarized in Table 2-32. The saphenous nerve (termination of the femoral nerve) is subcutaneous.

ANKLE AND FOOT

▪ Osteology
▦ Ankle
- Distal tibia flares to form an inferior quadrilateral surface for articulation with the talus and the pyramid-shaped medial malleolus.
- Laterally, the fibular notch forms articulation with the fibula.
- Lateral malleolus: distal fibula expansion that extends beyond distal tip of medial malleolus and serves as lateral buttress of ankle joint
▦ Foot
- 26 bones of the foot: 7 tarsal bones, 5 metatarsals, and 14 phalanges
- Divided into the **hindfoot (talus and calcaneus),** midfoot (navicular, cuboid, and three cuneiforms), and forefoot (metatarsals and phalanges)
- Tarsals: includes talus, calcaneus, cuboid, navicular, and three cuneiform
- Talus (Figure 2-55)
  - Trochlea (including surfaces for the malleoli articulations)
  - Posterior and middle calcaneal facets (body)
  - Anterior calcaneal facet (head)
  - Two thirds of the talus is covered with cartilage; no muscular attachments.
  - **Groove posteriorly for the tendon of the FHL. Os trigonum (if present) lateral to FHL.**
  - Posterior process (for posterior talofibular ligament)
  - Talar body wider anteriorly, conferring greater stability with ankle in dorsiflexion
  - Talar neck connects with the head, which in turn articulates with the navicular distally and the calcaneus inferiorly.
  - **Primary blood supply to the talar body is from the artery of the tarsal canal (posterior tibial artery)** (Figure 2-56).

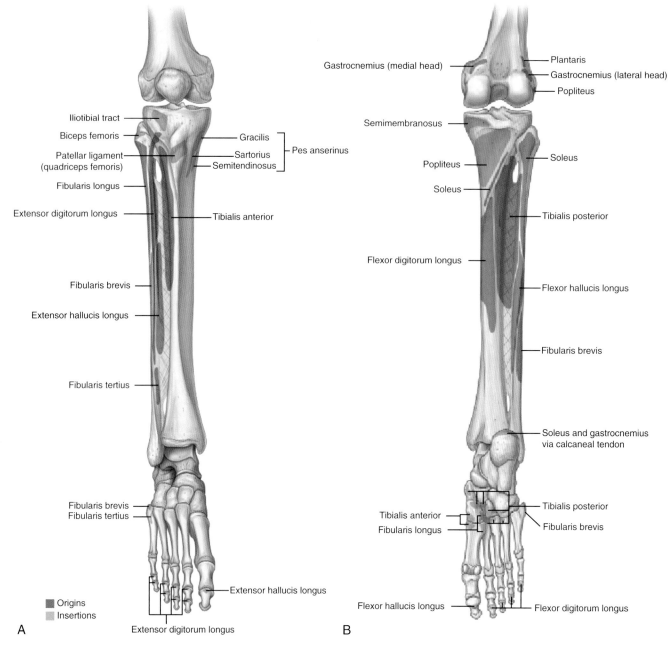

FIGURE 2-53 Origins and insertions of muscles of the leg. (From Drake RL et al, editors: *Gray's atlas of anatomy*, ed 2, Philadelphia, 2015, Churchill Livingstone.)

- Other blood supply is from the superior neck vessels (anterior tibial artery) and the artery of the tarsal sinus (dorsalis pedis).
- Calcaneus
  - Three surfaces that articulate with the talus: a large posterior facet, an anterior facet, and a middle facet
  - Distally, an articular surface receives the cuboid bone.
  - Sustentaculum tali is an overhanging horizontal eminence on the anteromedial surface of the calcaneus.
    - Supports the middle articular surface above it and has an inferior groove for the FHL tendon
- Cuboid
  - **Grooved on the plantar surface by the peroneus longus**
- Four facets for articulation with the calcaneus, the lateral cuneiform, and the fourth and fifth metatarsals
- Navicular
  - Most medial tarsal bone, the navicular lies between the talus and the cuneiforms.
  - Proximally, the surface is oval and concave for its articulation with the head of the talus.
  - Distally, the navicular has three articular surfaces, one for each of the cuneiforms.
  - Medial plantar projection serves as the insertion for the posterior tibial tendon.
- Cuneiforms (Figure 2-57)
  - Three bones (medial, intermediate, and lateral)
  - Articulate with the navicular and posterior cuboid (lateral cuneiform) and the first three metatarsals

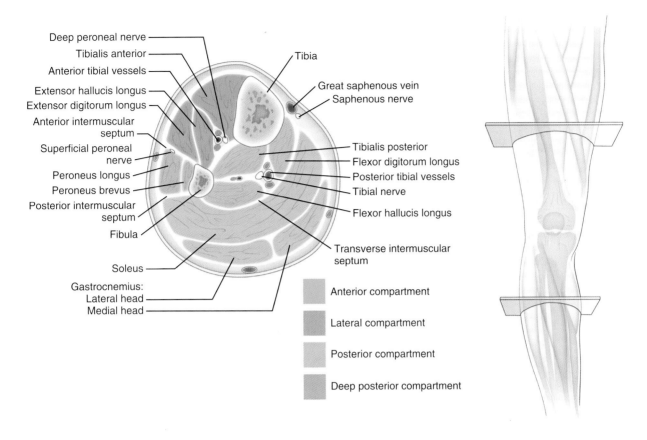

Anterior compartment

Lateral compartment

Posterior compartment

Deep posterior compartment

FIGURE 2-54 Anterior and lateral compartment release. (From DeLee JC, Drez D Jr: *Orthopaedic sports medicine: principles and practice,* Philadelphia, 1994, WB Saunders, p 1618.)

Table 2-31	Muscles of the Leg			
MUSCLE	**ORIGIN**	**INSERTION**	**ACTION**	**INNERVATION**
ANTERIOR COMPARTMENT				
Tibialis anterior	Lateral tibia	Medial cuneiform, first metatarsal	Dorsiflexing, inverting foot	Deep peroneal (L4) nerve
Extensor hallucis longus	Midfibula	Great toe, distal phalanx	Dorsiflexing, extending toe	Deep peroneal (L5) nerve
Extensor digitorum longus	Tibial condyle/fibula	Toe, middle and distal phalanges	Dorsiflexing, extending toe	Deep peroneal (L5) nerve
Peroneus tertius	Fibula and extensor digitorum longus tendon	Fifth metatarsal	Everting, dorsiflexing, abducting foot	Deep peroneal (S1) nerve
LATERAL COMPARTMENT				
Peroneus longus	Proximal fibula	Medial cuneiform, first metatarsal	Everting, plantar flexing, abducting foot	Superficial peroneal (S1) nerve
Peroneus brevis	Distal fibula	Tuberosity of fifth metatarsal	Everting foot	Superficial peroneal (S1) nerve
SUPERFICIAL POSTERIOR COMPARTMENT				
Gastrocnemius	Posterior medial and lateral femoral condyles	Calcaneus	Plantar flexing foot	Tibial (S1) nerve
Soleus	Fibula/tibia	Calcaneus	Plantar flexing foot	Tibial (S1) nerve
Plantaris	Lateral femoral condyle	Calcaneus	Plantar flexing foot	Tibial (S1) nerve
DEEP POSTERIOR COMPARTMENT				
Popliteus	Lateral femoral condyle, fibular head	Proximal tibia	Flexing, internally rotating knee	Tibial (L5, S1) nerve
Flexor hallucis longus	Fibula	Great toe, distal phalanx	Plantar flexing great toe	Tibial (S1) nerve
Flexor digitorum longus	Tibia	Second to fifth toes, distal phalanges	Plantar flexing toes, foot	Tibial (S1, S2) nerve
Tibialis posterior	Tibia, fibula, interosseous membrane	Navicular, medial cuneiform	Inverting/plantar flexing foot	Tibial (L4, L5) nerve

- Intermediate cuneiform does not extend as far distally as the medial cuneiform, which allows the second metatarsal to "key" into place.
- Metatarsals
  - Five bones, numbered from a medial to lateral direction, span the distance between the tarsal bones and phalanges.
  - Shape and function are similar to those of the metacarpals of the hand.
  - First metatarsal has a plantar crista that articulates with the **fibular and tibial sesamoids contained within the flexor hallucis brevis tendon.**

Table 2-32	Compartment Releases of Leg	
COMPARTMENT	**MUSCLES**	**NEUROVASCULAR STRUCTURES RELEASED**
Anterior	Tibialis anterior, extensor hallucis longus, extensor digitorum longus, peroneus tertius	Deep peroneal nerve and anterior tibial artery
Lateral	Peroneus longus and brevis	Superficial peroneal nerve
Superficial posterior	Gastrocnemius-soleus complex, plantaris	Sural nerve
Deep posterior	Popliteus, flexor hallucis longus, flexor digitorum longus, tibialis posterior	Posterior tibial artery and vein, tibial nerve, peroneal artery and vein

- Phalanges
  - Similar to those of the hand. Great toe (analogous to thumb) has two phalanges, and the remaining digits have three.
- Ossification
  - Each tarsal bone has a single ossification center except for the calcaneus, which has a second center posteriorly.
  - Calcaneus, talus, and usually the cuboid are present at birth.
  - Lateral cuneiform appears during the first year, the medial cuneiform during the second year, and the intermediate cuneiform and navicular during the third year.
  - Posterior center for the calcaneus usually appears during the eighth year.
  - The second through fifth metatarsals have two ossification centers:
    - Primary center in the shaft
    - Secondary center for the head, which appears at ages 5 to 8 years
  - Phalanges and first metatarsal have secondary centers at their bases that appear proximally during the third or fourth year and distally during the sixth or seventh year.

■ Arthrology

- Distal tibiofibular joint
  - Formed by the medial distal fibula and the notched lateral distal tibia
  - **Ankle syndesmosis (connection between the tibia and fibula) supported by four ligaments: anterior and posterior inferior tibiofibular ligaments, a**

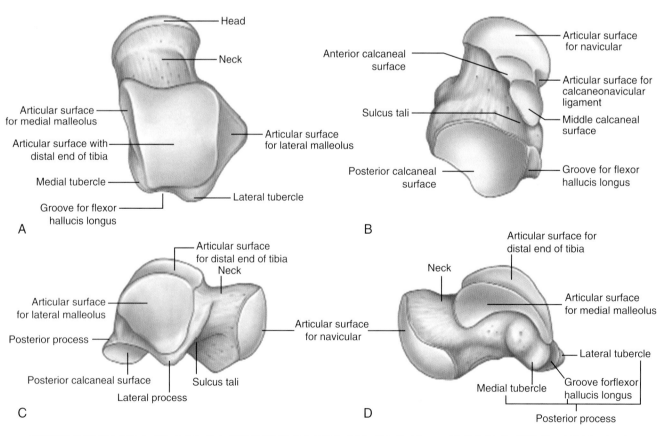

FIGURE 2-55 Talus from different angles. (From Drake RL et al, editors: *Gray's atlas of anatomy,* ed 2, Philadelphia, 2015, Churchill Livingstone.)

transverse tibiofibular ligament, and an interosseous ligament. Syndesmotic injury often referred to as "high-ankle sprain."
- Anteroinferior tibiofibular ligament (AITFL) is an oblique band that connects the bones anteriorly. Bony avulsion of this ligament in adolescents may result in a Tillaux fracture.
- Ankle joint (Table 2-33)
  - Mortise formed by the medial and lateral malleoli, tibial plafond, and talus
  - Deltoid ligament composed of two layers (Figure 2-58)
    - Superficial layer (tibionavicular and tibiocalcaneal) crosses ankle and subtalar joint.
    - Deep layer (anterior and posterior tibiotalar) crosses ankle joint only.
  - Lateral fibular ligaments: anterior talofibular ligament (ATFL), calcaneofibular ligament (CFL), and posterior talofibular ligament (PTFL) (Figure 2-59)
    - ATFL is the weakest and is intracapsular (intracapsular thickening). Injured with lateral ankle sprain.
    - CFL crosses subtalar joint.
    - **Position of the ankle is critical when the lateral ligament complex is tested. Plantar flexion tightens the anterior talofibular ligament, and** inversion with neutral flexion tightens the calcaneofibular ligament.
- Subtalar joint
  - Talar plantar facets articulate with the calcaneus (Figure 2-60).
  - Stability is derived from four ligaments: medial ligament, lateral ligament, interosseous talocalcaneal ligament, and cervical ligament.
  - Intertarsal joints: several ligamentous structures are important (Table 2-34).
    - **Plantar calcaneonavicular ligament (spring ligament) supports head of talus; attenuated in pes planus deformity** (Figure 2-61).
- Other joints
  - Tarsometatarsal joints are gliding joints supported by dorsal, plantar, and interosseous ligaments.
  - Base of first metatarsal is not ligamentously connected to second metatarsal.
  - **Lisfranc ligament connects medial (shortest) cuneiform to second (longest) metatarsal.**
    - Plantar and dorsal structure in about 20% of patients
  - Deep transverse metatarsal ligaments interconnect metatarsal heads.
    - Digital nerve courses in a plantar direction under the transverse metatarsal ligament and is the spot where

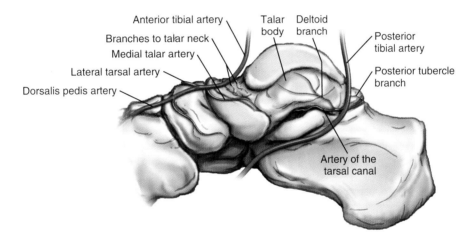

FIGURE 2-56 Arterial supply to the talus. (From Miller MD et al: *Orthopaedic surgical approaches,* Philadelphia, 2008, Saunders, Figure FA-26.)

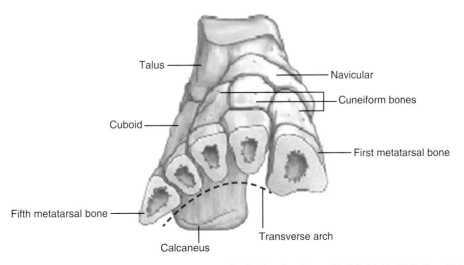

FIGURE 2-57 Bones of the foot. (From Drake RL et al, editors: *Gray's atlas of anatomy,* ed 2, Philadelphia, 2015, Churchill Livingstone.)

Table 2-33	Ankle Joint Ligaments			
LIGAMENT	**PROXIMAL ATTACHMENT**	**DISTAL ATTACHMENT**	**FUNCTION**	
TIBIOFIBULAR (SYNDESMOSIS)				
Anterior inferior tibiofibular	Tibia	Fibula	Stability of ankle mortise	
Interosseous ligament	Tibia	Fibula	Stability of ankle mortise	
Posterior inferior tibiofibular ligament	Tibia	Fibula	Stability of ankle mortise	
MEDIAL ANKLE (DELTOID)				
Tibionavicular	Medial malleolus	Navicular tuberosity	Limits talar external rotation	
Tibiocalcaneal	Medial malleolus	Sustentaculum tali	Limits hindfoot eversion	
Anterior tibiotalar	Medial malleolus	Medial surface of talus	Limits lateral displacement of talus, external rotation	
Posterior tibiotalar	Medial malleolus	Inner side of talus	Limits lateral displacement	
LATERAL ANKLE				
Anterior talofibular	Lateral malleolus	Transversely to talus anteriorly	Limits inversion in plantar flexion	
Calcaneofibular	Lateral malleolus	Obliquely to calcaneus posteriorly	Limits inversion in neutral or dorsiflexion	
Posterior talofibular	Lateral malleolus	Transversely to talus posteriorly	Limits posterior talar displacement and external rotation	

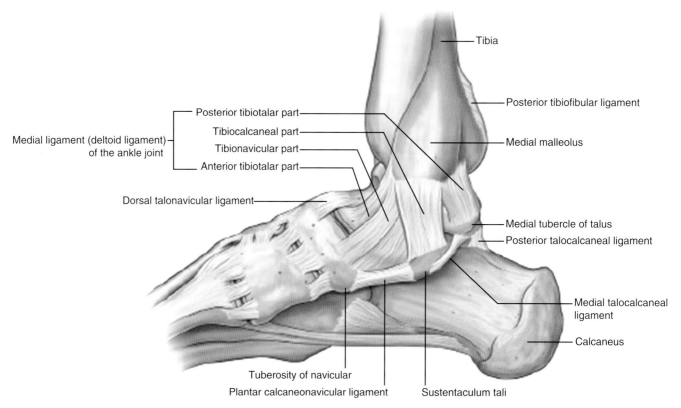

FIGURE 2-58 Ligaments of the foot. (From Drake RL et al, editors: *Gray's atlas of anatomy,* ed 2, Philadelphia, 2015, Churchill Livingstone.)

interdigital neuritis (Morton neuroma, usually the second or third interdigital space) occurs.
- Transverse metatarsal ligament attaches second metatarsal head to fibular sesamoid.
- Holds hallucal sesamoids in place and gives the appearance of sesamoid subluxation when the first metatarsal moves medially in hallux valgus.
  - Plantar and collateral ligaments support the metatarsophalangeal joints.
    - Primary stabilizing structure of the metatarsophalangeal joint is the plantar plate.
- Interphalangeal joints are supported mainly by their capsules.

■ **Muscles**
▦ Origins and insertions of muscles are shown in Figure 2-62.
▦ Major tendons (Figure 2-63) crossing the ankle joint include:
- Anterior (from lateral to medial): peroneus tertius, extensor digitorum longus (EDL), extensor hallucis longus (EHL), tibialis anterior
- **Medial (mnemonic: "Tom, Dick, and Harry": tibialis posterior, flexor digitorum longus, and flexor hallucis longus)**
- Lateral: peroneal tendons with longus (superficial) and brevis (deep)

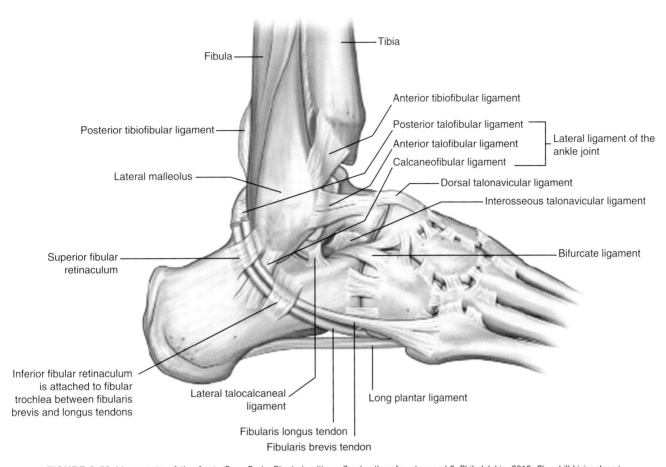

FIGURE 2-59 Ligaments of the foot. (From Drake RL et al, editors: *Gray's atlas of anatomy,* ed 2, Philadelphia, 2015, Churchill Livingstone.)

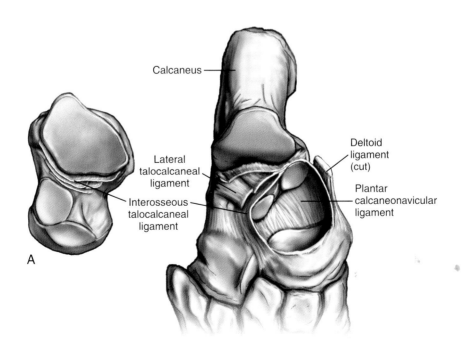

FIGURE 2-60 A, Inferior view of the talus showing the interosseous ligament. **B,** Dorsal view of the hindfoot (after removal of the talus) showing the calcaneal facets with the spring ligaments. (From Miller MD et al: *Orthopaedic surgical approaches,* ed 2, Philadelphia, 2014, Saunders, Figure 8-7.)

Table 2-34	Ligaments of the Intertarsal Joints		
LIGAMENT	**COMMON NAME**	**PROXIMAL ATTACHMENT**	**DISTAL ATTACHMENT**
Interosseous talocalcaneal	Cervical	Talus	Calcaneus
Calcaneocuboid/calcaneonavicular	Bifurcate	Calcaneus	Cuboid and navicular
Calcaneocuboid-metatarsal	Long plantar	Calcaneus	Cuboid and first to fifth metatarsals
Plantar calcaneocuboid	Short plantar	Calcaneus	Cuboid
Plantar calcaneonavicular	Spring	Sustentaculum tali	Navicular
Tarsometatarsal	Lisfranc	Medial cuneiform	Second metatarsal base

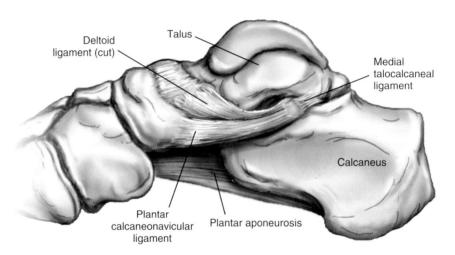

FIGURE 2-61 Ligaments of the hind foot-medial view. (From Miller MD et al: *Orthopaedic surgical approaches,* ed 2, Philadelphia, 2014, Saunders, Figure 8-6.)

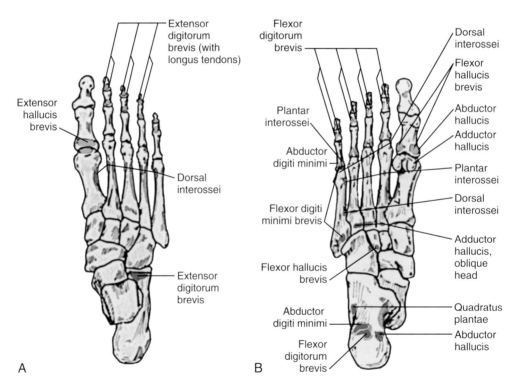

FIGURE 2-62 Origins and insertions of the muscles of the foot. **A,** Dorsal view. **B,** Plantar view. (From Jenkins DB: *Hollinshead's functional anatomy of the limbs and back,* ed 6, Philadelphia, 1991, Saunders, Figure 20-7.)

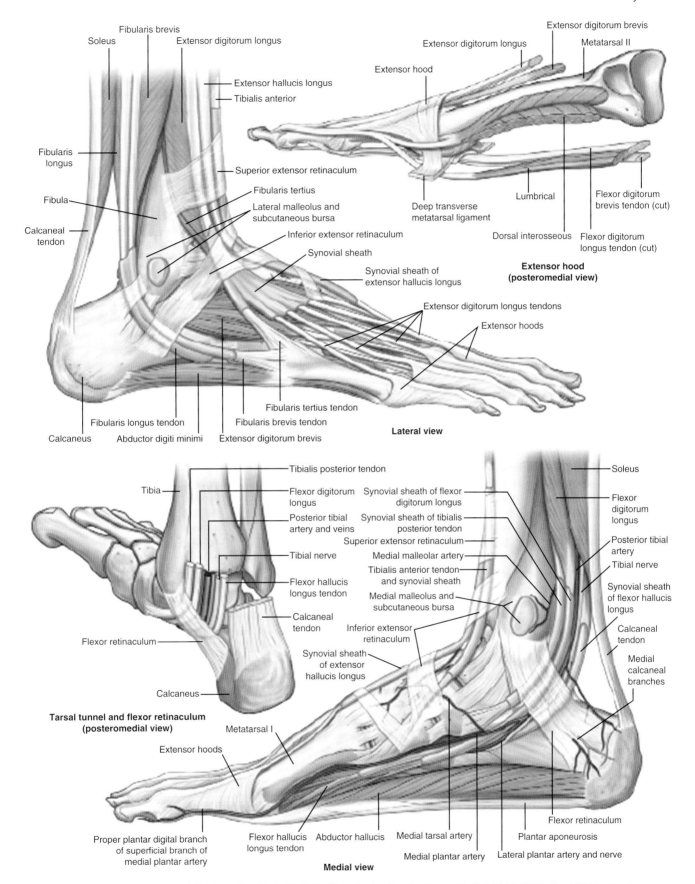

FIGURE 2-63 Anatomy of the foot. (From Drake RL et al, editors: *Gray's atlas of anatomy,* ed 2, Philadelphia, 2015, Churchill Livingstone.)

- Posterior: Achilles
  - Maximum anteroposterior dimension on MRI is 8 mm.
- Only one dorsal intrinsic muscle of the foot: the extensor digitorum brevis (EDB) (innervated by the lateral terminal branch of the deep peroneal nerve)
- Arrangement of muscles and tendons in the foot is best considered in layers (Figure 2-64, Table 2-35).
  - Intrinsic muscles dominate the first and third layers.
  - Extrinsic tendons are more important in the second and fourth layers.
  - Plantar heel spurs originate in the flexor digitorum brevis (medial plantar nerve innervation).
  - Lumbrical muscles are located plantar to the transverse metatarsal ligament, and interosseous tendons are dorsal.
  - The tendons are arranged about the toe as shown in Figure 2-65.
- Neuromuscular interactions (Table 2-36)
- **Nerves of the lower extremity** arise from the lumbosacral plexus (Figure 2-66; Tables 2-37 through 2-39)
- Lumbar plexus
  - Ventral rami of T12-L4; forms part of lumbosacral plexus
  - Anterior and posterior divisions
  - **Anterior surface of quadratus lumborum under (and within) psoas major muscle**
  - **Genitofemoral nerve pierces the psoas and then lies on the anteromedial surface of the psoas.**
- Sacral plexus
  - Ventral rami of L4-S3; lies posterior to psoas muscle
  - Anterior and posterior divisions
  - L5 nerve root on anterior sacrum—at risk with anteriorly placed sacroiliac screw
- Sciatic foramen
  - Piriformis is the "key" to the sciatic foramen—major reference point for sciatic nerve and other neurovascular structures (Figure 2-67).
  - Structures exiting the greater and lesser sciatic foramen are listed in Table 2-40.
  - Superior and inferior gluteal nerve and vessels named for position relative to piriformis muscle (superior exits above muscle and inferior below)
  - Pudendal nerve and vessels and nerve to obturator internus exit the greater sciatic foramen and reenter the pelvis through the lesser sciatic foramen.
  - **Mnemonic: POP'S IQ (nerves exiting below piriformis): Pudendal, nerve to Obturator internus, Posterior femoral cutaneous, Sciatic, Inferior gluteal, nerve to Quadratus femoris**
- **Peripheral nerve anatomy (Figures 2-68 and 2-69)**
- Lateral femoral cutaneous nerve (L2-L3)
  - Travels on the surface of the iliacus muscle and exits the pelvis 1 to 2 cm medial to ASIS under the lateral attachment of the inguinal ligament
  - Supplies the skin and fascia on the surface of the anterolateral thigh from the greater trochanter to the knee
  - Meralgia paresthetica (lateral femoral cutaneous nerve [LFCN] compression)

- Femoral nerve (L2-L4)
  - Largest branch of the lumbar plexus and supplies thigh muscles
  - Femoral nerve lies between the iliacus and psoas muscles. Iliacus hematoma may irritate the femoral nerve because of its proximity.
  - Anteriorly, the great nerves and vessels enter the thigh (and into the femoral triangle) under the inguinal ligament (Figure 2-70).
  - Femoral triangle
    - Borders: sartorius (lateral), pectineus (medial), inguinal ligament (superiorly)
    - Floor: (lateral to medial) iliacus, psoas, pectineus, and adductor longus
    - **Structures: (lateral to medial) femoral Nerve, Artery, Vein and the Lymphatic vessels (mnemonic: "NAVaL").**
- Saphenous nerve (L3, 4)
  - Branches off femoral nerve at apex of femoral triangle and travels under the sartorius muscle
  - Becomes subcutaneous on medial aspect of knee between the sartorius and gracilis; travels with greater saphenous vein
  - At risk with medial meniscus repair, hamstring harvest
  - Sensation to the medial aspect of the leg and foot
  - **Infrapatellar branch supplies skin of the medial side of the front of the knee and patellar ligament and can be damaged during total knee replacement surgery or patella tendon harvest.**
  - Terminal branch supplies sensation to medial ankle and foot.
  - Obturator nerve (L2-L4)
  - Exits the pelvis via the obturator canal
  - Divides into anterior and posterior divisions within the canal
  - Anterior division proceeds anteriorly to the obturator externus and posteriorly to the pectineus, supplying the adductor longus, adductor brevis, and gracilis; it then delivers cutaneous branches to the medial thigh.
  - Posterior division supplies the obturator externus, adductor brevis, and upper part of the adductor magnus, and it delivers other branches to the knee joint.
  - Pain from the hip can be referred to the knee as a result of the continuation of the obturator nerve anteriorly, which can provide sensation to the medial side of the knee.
  - **Retractors placed behind the transverse acetabular ligament or screw placement in anteroinferior quadrant of acetabulum can injure the obturator nerve and artery.**
- Sciatic nerve (L4-S3)
  - **Passes anterior to piriformis and posterior to obturator internus and short external rotators**
  - Passes through the piriformis in 2% of people
  - Descends below gluteus maximus and proceeds posterior to adductor magnus and between the long head of the biceps femoris and semimembranosus
  - Functionally separate tibial and peroneal divisions throughout length
  - Peroneal division more lateral than tibial division, making it more vulnerable to iatrogenic injury (most common nerve injury during total hip arthroplasty)

Text continued on p. 215

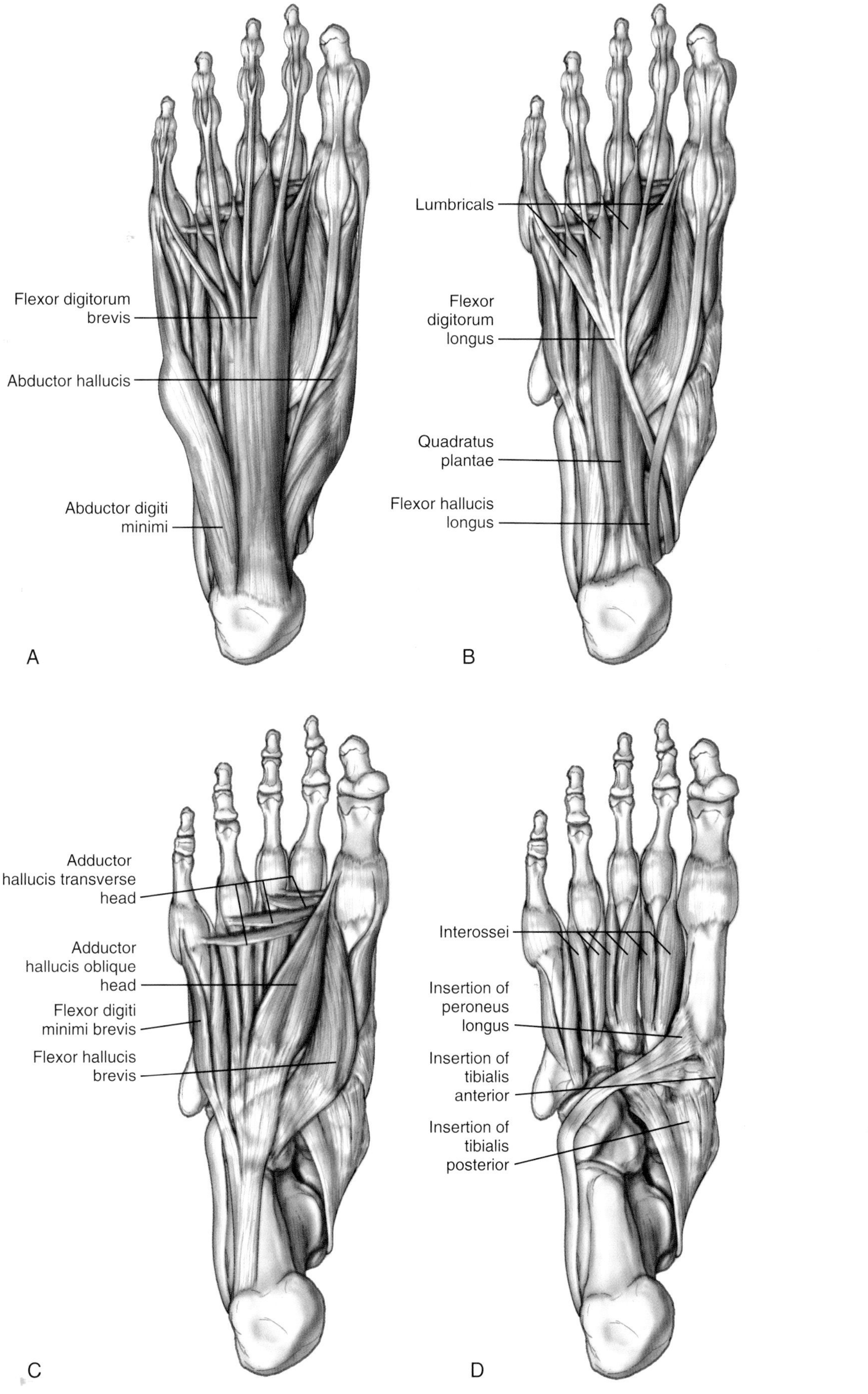

FIGURE 2-64 Four layers of the plantar surface of the foot. **A,** First layer. **B,** Second layer. **C,** Third layer. **D,** Fourth layer. (From Miller MD, et al: *Orthopaedic surgical approaches,* Philadelphia, 2008, Saunders, Figures FA-17 to FA-20.)

Table 2-35	Muscles of the Ankle and Foot			
MUSCLE	**ORIGIN**	**INSERTION**	**ACTION**	**INNERVATION**
DORSAL LAYER				
Extensor digitorum brevis	Superolateral calcaneus	Base of proximal phalanges	Extending	Deep peroneal nerve
FIRST PLANTAR LAYER				
Abductor hallucis	Calcaneal tuberosity	Base of great toe, proximal phalanx	Abducting great toe	Medial plantar nerve
Flexor digitorum brevis	Calcaneal tuberosity	Distal phalanges of second to fifth toes	Flexing toes	Medial plantar nerve
Abductor digiti minimi	Calcaneal tuberosity	Base of small toe	Abducting small toe	Lateral plantar nerve
SECOND PLANTAR LAYER				
Quadratus plantae	Medial and lateral calcaneus	Flexor digitorum longus tendon	Helping flex distal phalanges	Lateral plantar nerve
Lumbrical muscles	Flexor digitorum longus tendon	Extensor digitorum longus tendon	Flexing metatarsophalangeal joint, extending interphalangeal joint	Medial and lateral plantar nerves
Flexor digitorum longus and flexor hallucis longus	Tibia/fibula	Distal phalanges of digits	Flexing toes, inverting foot	Tibial nerve
THIRD PLANTAR LAYER				
Flexor hallucis brevis	Cuboid/lateral cuneiform	Proximal phalanx of great toe	Flexing great toe	Medial plantar nerve
Adductor hallucis	Oblique: second to fourth metatarsals	Proximal phalanx of great toe (lateral)	Adducting great toe	Lateral plantar nerve
Flexor digiti minimi brevis	Base of fifth metatarsal head	Proximal phalanx of small toe	Flexing small toe	Lateral plantar nerve
FOURTH PLANTAR LAYER				
Dorsal interosseous	Metatarsal	Dorsal extensors	Abducting	Lateral plantar nerve
Plantar interosseous (peroneus longus and tibialis posterior)	Third to fifth metatarsals	Proximal phalanges medially	Adducting toes	Lateral plantar nerve
	Fibula/tibia	Medial cuneiform/navicular	Everting/inverting foot	Superficial peroneal/tibial nerve

NOTE: For abduction and adduction in the foot, the second toe serves as the reference.

Table 2-36	Foot Neuromuscular Interactions	
FOOT FUNCTION	**MUSCLE**	**INNERVATION**
Inversion	Tibialis anterior	Deep peroneal nerve (L4)
	Tibialis posterior	Tibial nerve (S1)
Dorsiflexion	Tibialis anterior, extensor digitorum longus, extensor hallucis longus	Deep peroneal nerve: tibialis anterior (L4), extensor digitorum longus, and extensor hallucis longus (L5)
Eversion	Peroneus longus and peroneus brevis	Superficial peroneal nerve (S1)
Plantar flexion	Gastrocnemius-soleus complex, flexor digitorum longus, flexor hallucis longus, tibialis posterior (also hindfoot inverter)	Tibial nerve (S1)

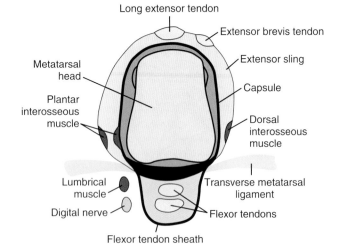

FIGURE 2-65 Cross-sectional view of the toe at the metatarsal head. The lumbrical muscles are plantar to the transverse ligament (with the digital nerve), and the interossei are dorsal to this ligament. The interossei and lumbrical muscles (except the first lumbrical muscle [medial plantar nerve]) are innervated by the lateral plantar nerve. (From Jahss MH: *Disorders of the foot*, Philadelphia, 1982, Saunders, pp 623.)

Labels for figure:
Long extensor tendon
Extensor brevis tendon
Extensor sling
Capsule
Dorsal interosseous muscle
Transverse metatarsal ligament
Flexor tendons
Flexor tendon sheath
Digital nerve
Lumbrical muscle
Plantar interosseous muscle
Metatarsal head

Table 2-37	Lumbosacral Plexus Divisions and Branches	
NERVE		**LEVEL**
LUMBAR PLEXUS, ANTERIOR DIVISION		
Iliohypogastric		T12, L1
Ilioinguinal		L1
Genitofemoral		L1, L2
Obturator		L2-4
LUMBAR PLEXUS, POSTERIOR DIVISION		
Lateral femoral cutaneous nerve		L2, 3
Femoral		L2-4
SACRAL PLEXUS, ANTERIOR DIVISION		
Tibial		L4-S3
Quadratus femoris		L4-S1
Obturator internus		L5-S2
Pudendal		S2-S4
Coccygeus		S4
Levator ani		S3-S4
SACRAL PLEXUS, POSTERIOR DIVISION		
Peroneal		L4-S2
Superior gluteal		L4-S1
Inferior gluteal		L5-S2
Piriformis		S2
Posterior femoral cutaneous		S1-S3

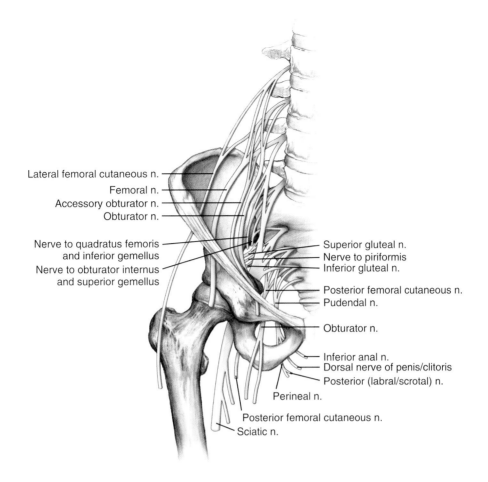

FIGURE 2-66 Divisions of the lumbosacral plexus. (From Miller MD et al: *Orthopaedic surgical approaches,* ed 2, Philadelphia, 2014, Saunders, Figure 6-14.)

Labels on figure:
- Lateral femoral cutaneous n.
- Femoral n.
- Accessory obturator n.
- Obturator n.
- Nerve to quadratus femoris and inferior gemellus
- Nerve to obturator internus and superior gemellus
- Superior gluteal n.
- Nerve to piriformis
- Inferior gluteal n.
- Posterior femoral cutaneous n.
- Pudendal n.
- Obturator n.
- Inferior anal n.
- Dorsal nerve of penis/clitoris
- Posterior (labral/scrotal) n.
- Perineal n.
- Posterior femoral cutaneous n.
- Sciatic n.

Table 2-38	Innervation of Lower Extremity
NERVES	**MUSCLES INNERVATED**
Femoral	Iliacus, psoas, pectineus (along with obturator nerve), sartorius, quadriceps femoris (rectus femoris, vastus lateralis, vastus intermedius, and vastus medialis)
Obturator	Pectineus (along with femoral nerve), adductor brevis, adductor longus, adductor magnus (along with tibial nerve), gracilis
Superior gluteal	Gluteus medius, gluteus minimus, tensor fasciae latae
Inferior gluteal	Gluteus maximus
Sciatic	Semitendinosus, semimembranosus, biceps femoris (long head [tibial division] and short head [peroneal division]), adductor magnus (with obturator nerve)
Tibial	Gastrocnemius, soleus, tibialis posterior, flexor digitorum longus, flexor hallucis longus, foot intrinsic musculature (except EDB) via medial and lateral plantar nerves
Deep peroneal	Tibialis anterior, extensor digitorum longus, extensor hallucis longus, peroneus tertius, extensor digitorum brevis
Superficial peroneal	Peroneus longus, peroneus brevis

Table 2-39	Important Neurologic Features of Lower Extremity	
JOINT	**FUNCTION**	**NEUROLOGIC LEVEL**
Hip	Flexion	T12-L3
	Extension	S1
	Adduction	L2-L4
	Abduction	L5
Knee	Flexion	L5, S1
	Extension	L2-L4
Ankle	Dorsiflexion	L4, L5
	Plantar flexion	S1, S2
	Inversion	L4
	Eversion	S1

Table 2-40	Structures That Exit Greater and Lesser Sciatic Foramen	
FORAMEN		**STRUCTURES EXITING**
Greater sciatic foramen		Piriformis
		Superior and inferior gluteal nerve
		Superior and inferior gluteal vessels
		Sciatic nerve
		Pudendal nerve*
		Internal pudendal vessels*
		Posterior femoral cutaneous nerve
		Nerve to obturator internus*
		Nerve to quadratus femoris
Lesser sciatic foramen		Obturator internus
		Pudendal nerve*
		Nerve to obturator internus*
		Internal pudendal vessels*

*Pudendal nerve, internal pudendal artery and vein, and nerve to obturator internus traverse both foramina.

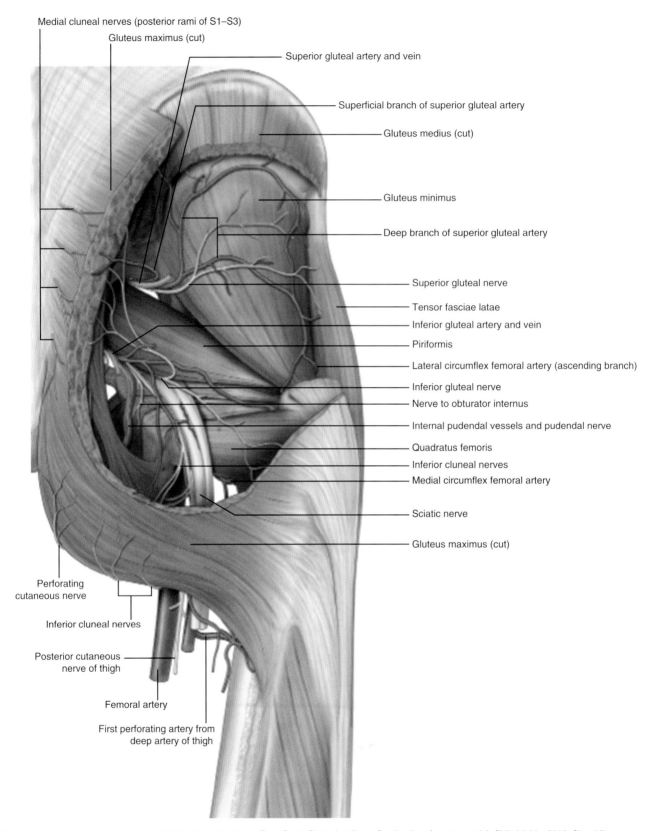

Medial cluneal nerves (posterior rami of S1–S3)

Gluteus maximus (cut)

Superior gluteal artery and vein

Superficial branch of superior gluteal artery

Gluteus medius (cut)

Gluteus minimus

Deep branch of superior gluteal artery

Superior gluteal nerve

Tensor fasciae latae

Inferior gluteal artery and vein

Piriformis

Lateral circumflex femoral artery (ascending branch)

Inferior gluteal nerve

Nerve to obturator internus

Internal pudendal vessels and pudendal nerve

Quadratus femoris

Inferior cluneal nerves

Medial circumflex femoral artery

Sciatic nerve

Gluteus maximus (cut)

Perforating cutaneous nerve

Inferior cluneal nerves

Posterior cutaneous nerve of thigh

Femoral artery

First perforating artery from deep artery of thigh

FIGURE 2-67 Arteries and nerves of the gluteal region. (From Drake RL et al, editors: *Gray's atlas of anatomy,* ed 2, Philadelphia, 2015, Churchill Livingstone.)

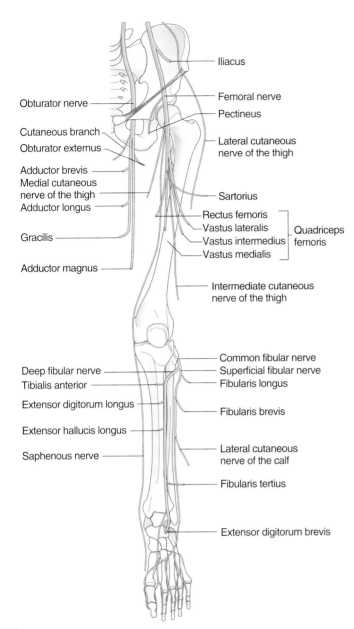

 FIGURE 2-68 Nerves of the hip, leg, and foot. (From Drake RL et al, editors: *Gray's atlas of anatomy,* ed 2, Philadelphia, 2015, Churchill Livingstone.)

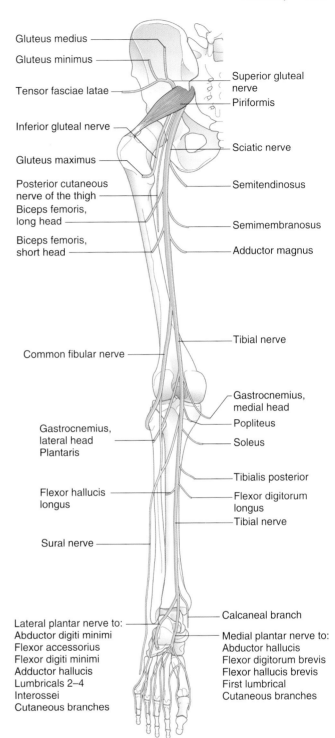

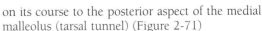

 FIGURE 2-69 Nerves of the hip, leg, and foot. (From Drake RL et al, editors: *Gray's atlas of anatomy,* ed 2, Philadelphia, 2015, Churchill Livingstone.)

- **Tibial division supplies all posterior thigh musculature except short head of biceps femoris (peroneal division).**
- Divides into the common peroneal nerve and the tibial nerve at the popliteal fossa
- All ankle, foot, and toe plantar flexors are supplied by tibial nerve.
- All sensation in foot is supplied by terminal branches of sciatic nerve, except for medial foot (saphenous nerve branch of femoral nerve).
- Tibial nerve (L4-S3)
  - Emerges into popliteal fossa laterally, proceeds posteriorly to the vessel, then descends between the heads of the gastrocnemius
  - Crosses over the popliteus muscle and splits the two heads of the gastrocnemius, passing deep to the soleus

on its course to the posterior aspect of the medial malleolus (tarsal tunnel) (Figure 2-71)
- Muscular branches supply the posterior leg along its course (superficial and deep posterior compartments.
- Supplies all intrinsic foot muscles except the EDB (deep peroneal nerve) and plantar sensation
- Splits into two branches (the medial and lateral plantar nerves) under the flexor retinaculum

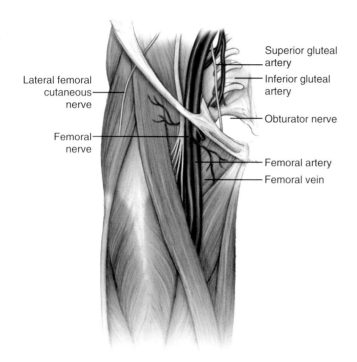

FIGURE 2-70 Femoral triangle. The order of structures of the femoral canal from lateral to medial: iliopsoas/iliacus, femoral nerve, femoral artery, femoral vein, and pectineus. (From Miller MD et al: *Orthopaedic surgical approaches*, Philadelphia, 2008, Saunders, Figure HP-24.)

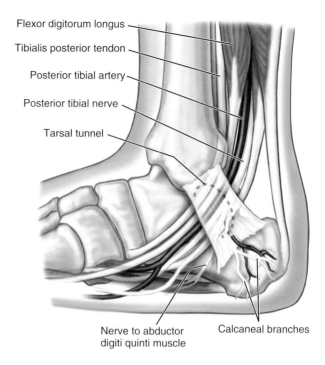

FIGURE 2-71 Tibial nerve anatomy. (From Miller MD, Thompson SR, editors: *DeLee and Drez's orthopaedic sports medicine: principles and practice*, ed 4, Philadelphia, 2014, Saunders.)

- Both of these nerves run in the second layer of the foot.
- Medial plantar nerve runs deep to the abductor hallucis, and the lateral plantar nerve runs obliquely under the cover of the quadratus plantae.
- **Most proximal branch of the lateral plantar nerve is the nerve to the abductor digiti quinti (Baxter nerve).**
- Distribution of the sensory and motor branches of the plantar nerves is similar to that in the hand.
  - Medial plantar nerve (like the median nerve of the hand) supplies plantar sensation to the medial $3\frac{1}{2}$ digits and motor sensation to only a few plantar muscles (flexor hallucis brevis, abductor hallucis, flexor digitorum brevis, and the first lumbrical muscle).
  - Lateral plantar nerve (like the ulnar nerve in the hand) supplies plantar sensation to the lateral $1\frac{1}{2}$ digits and the remaining intrinsic muscles of the foot.
- Digital nerve of the third web space consists of branches from both the medial and lateral plantar nerves.
- Common peroneal nerve (L4-S2)
  - **Diverges laterally and traverses the lateral popliteal fossa deep to the biceps femoris tendon**
  - Winds around fibular neck
  - Runs deep to the peroneus longus, where it divides into the superficial and deep branches
  - Potentially injured with traction and by lateral meniscal repair
- Superficial peroneal nerve
  - Runs along the border between the lateral and anterior compartments in the leg, supplying muscular branches to the peroneus longus and brevis (lateral compartment)
  - Terminates in two cutaneous branches (**medial dorsal and intermediate dorsal cutaneous nerves**) supplying the dorsal foot
  - Medial and intermediate dorsal cutaneous nerves of the superficial peroneal nerve supply the bulk of the remaining sensation to the dorsal aspect of the foot.
  - **Dorsal intermediate branch is at risk for injury during placement of the anterolateral ankle arthroscopy portal.**
  - Supplies dorsal medial sensation to the great toe
  - **Dorsal medial cutaneous nerve (a branch of the superficial peroneal nerve) crosses the EHL in a lateral-to-medial direction and supplies sensation to the dorsomedial aspect of the great toe.**
- Deep peroneal nerve
  - Runs along the anterior surface of the interosseous membrane, supplying the musculature of the anterior compartment: tibialis anterior, EHL, EDL, and peroneus tertius
    - Lateral terminal branch of the deep peroneal nerve ends in the proximal dorsal foot by supplying the EDB muscle.
    - **Medial terminal branch supplies sensation to the first web space.**
- Sural nerve (S1-S2) is formed by cutaneous branches of both the tibial (medial sural cutaneous) and common peroneal (lateral sural cutaneous) nerves.
  - Often used for nerve grafting
  - Inadvertent cutting of this nerve can cause painful neuroma.
  - Traverses lateral aspect of the ankle and foot

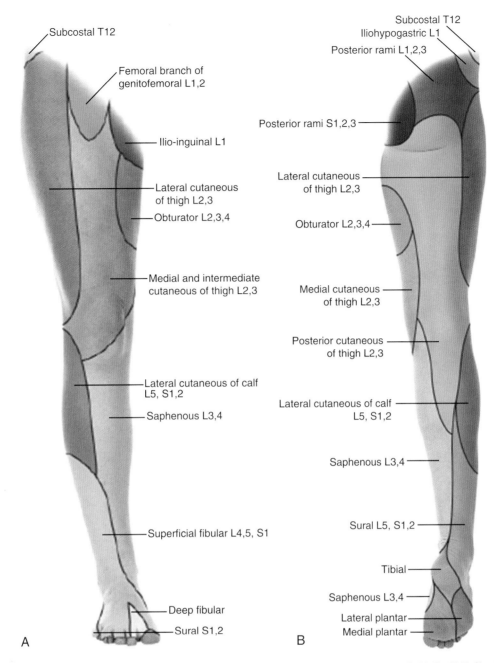

FIGURE 2-72 Regions of the leg and foot. (From Drake RL et al, editors: *Gray's atlas of anatomy*, ed 2, Philadelphia, 2015, Churchill Livingstone.)

- Cutaneous innervation of the thigh and leg are demonstrated in Figure 2-72.
- Nerves around the foot and ankle are demonstrated on Figure 2-73.
- **Vessels (Figure 2-74)**
- Aorta branches into the common iliac arteries anterior to the L4 vertebral body.
- Common iliac vessels in turn divide into the internal (or hypogastric [medial] and external [lateral]) iliac vessels at the S1 level (Figure 2-75).
- Important internal iliac artery branches:
  - Obturator (posterior branch supplies the transverse acetabular ligament)
    - Obturator artery and vein jeopardized by anteroinferior screws and acetabular retractors

- Posterior branch supplies the ligamentum teres acetabular artery. This artery is an important source of blood to the femoral head from birth to age 4.
- Superior gluteal (can be injured in sciatic notch)
- Inferior gluteal (supplies gluteus maximus and short external rotators)
- Internal pudendal (reenters pelvis through lesser sciatic notch)
- **Corona mortis is an anastomotic connection between the inferior epigastric branch of the external iliac vessels and the obturator vessels in the obturator canal.**
  - Can lead to life-threatening bleeding if injured
- External iliac artery continues under the inguinal ligament to become the femoral artery.

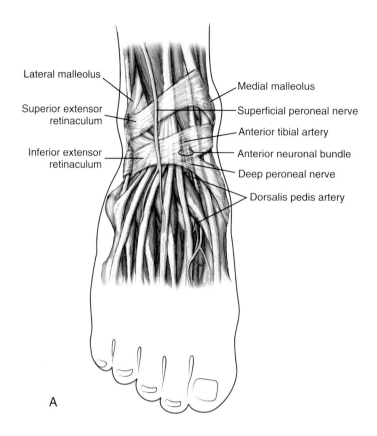

Lateral malleolus

Superior extensor retinaculum

Inferior extensor retinaculum

Medial malleolus

Superficial peroneal nerve

Anterior tibial artery

Anterior neuronal bundle

Deep peroneal nerve

Dorsalis pedis artery

A

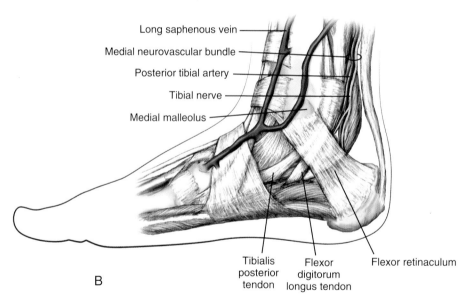

Long saphenous vein

Medial neurovascular bundle

Posterior tibial artery

Tibial nerve

Medial malleolus

Tibialis posterior tendon

Flexor digitorum longus tendon

Flexor retinaculum

B

FIGURE 2-73 Hazards. **A,** Anterior view. **B,** Medial view.

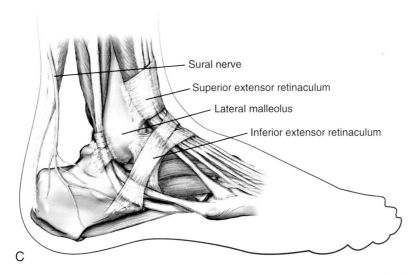

FIGURE 2-73, cont'd C, Lateral view. (From Miller MD et al: *Orthopaedic surgical approaches,* ed 2, Philadelphia, 2014, Saunders, Figures 8-31, 8-32, and 8-33.)

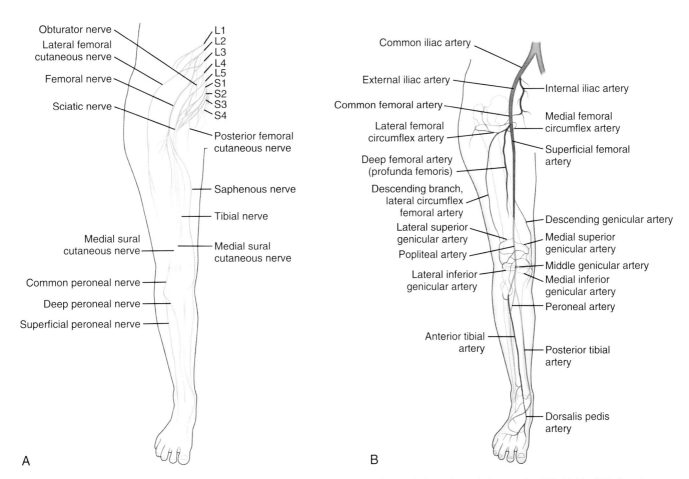

FIGURE 2-74 Nerves **(A)** and vessels **(B)** of the lower extremity. (From Miller MD et al: *Orthopaedic surgical approaches,* Philadelphia, 2008, Saunders, Figures KL-8 and KL-9.)

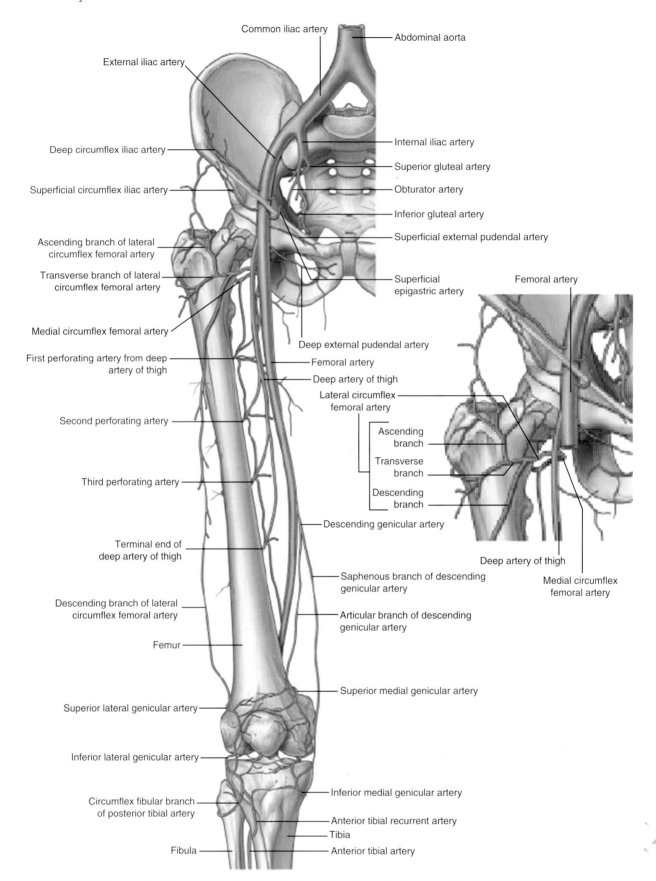

FIGURE 2-75 Arteries of the hip and thigh. (From Drake RL et al, editors: *Gray's atlas of anatomy,* ed 2, Philadelphia, 2015, Churchill Livingstone.)

- **Can be injured by placement of acetabular screws in the anterosuperior quadrant during total hip arthroplasty**
- Cruciate anastomosis: confluence of ascending branch of the first perforating artery, descending branch of the inferior gluteal artery, and transverse branches of the medial and lateral femoral circumflex arteries
- Femoral artery enters the femoral triangle. Two branches: superficial femoral artery and profunda femoris (deep femoral artery).
- Superficial femoral artery supplies the leg and foot.
  - Continues on medial side of thigh (between vastus medialis and adductor longus) toward the adductor (Hunter) canal
  - Becomes popliteal artery when it passes posteriorly into the popliteal fossa
- Profunda femoris supplies the musculature of the thigh.
  - **Key branches (named for location relative to iliopsoas tendon):**
    - Lateral femoral circumflex, which travels obliquely and deep to the sartorius and rectus femoris
      - Ascending branch (at risk for injury during anterolateral approaches), which proceeds to greater trochanteric region
      - Descending branch travels laterally under the rectus femoris.
    - Medial femoral circumflex supplies most of the blood to the femoral head.
      - **Runs between the pectineus and iliopsoas and proceeds distally anterior to the quadratus femoris on its cranial edge just distal to the obturator externus**
      - Particularly at risk for injury during psoas tenotomy during an anteromedial approach for developmental dysplasia of the hip
    - Also gives off the femoral artery perforators; these perforators pierce the lateral intermuscular septum to supply the vastus lateralis muscle.
- Popliteal artery travels posterior to the knee and is the primary blood supply to the leg (Figure 2-76).
  - Enters the popliteal fossa between the biceps and semimembranosus and descends underneath the tibial nerve, terminating between the medial and lateral heads of the gastrocnemius and dividing into the anterior and posterior tibial arteries
  - Vein usually posterior to artery
  - At risk with knee dislocation and trauma about the knee
  - **Several genicular branches are given off in the popliteal fossa, including the medial and lateral geniculate arteries (which supply the menisci) and the middle geniculate artery (which supplies the cruciate ligaments).**
  - Superior lateral geniculate artery can be injured during lateral-release procedures.
  - Descending geniculate artery (branch of femoral artery proximal to Hunter canal) supplies the vastus medialis at the anterior border of the intermuscular septum.
  - Inferior geniculate artery passes between the popliteal tendon and fibular collateral ligament in the posterolateral corner of the knee.
- Anterior tibial artery (Figure 2-77)

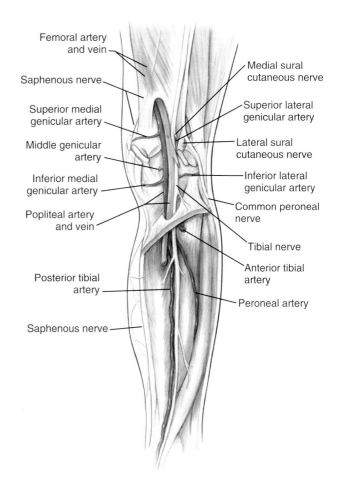

FIGURE 2-76 Hazards of the posterior leg and thigh. (From Miller MD et al: *Orthopaedic surgical approaches*, ed 2, Philadelphia, 2014, Saunders, Figure 7-16.)

- First branch of the popliteal artery
- Passes between the two heads of the tibialis posterior and the interosseous membrane to lie on the anterior surface of that membrane between the tibialis anterior and EHL
- Terminates as the dorsalis pedis artery
- Dorsalis pedis artery provides the blood supply to the dorsum of the foot via its lateral tarsal, medial tarsal, arcuate, and first dorsal metatarsal branches.
  - Its largest branch, the deep plantar artery, runs between the first and second metatarsals and contributes to the plantar arch.
- Posterior tibial artery (Figure 2-78)
  - Continues in the deep posterior compartment of the leg, coursing obliquely to pass behind the medial malleolus
  - Terminates by dividing into the medial and lateral plantar arteries
  - Main branch: peroneal artery
    - Given off 2.5 cm distal to the popliteal fossa and continues in the deep posterior compartment lateral to its parent artery between the tibialis posterior and flexor hallucis longus (FHL)
    - Terminates in the calcaneal branches
  - Terminal branches: medial and lateral plantar branches
    - Divides under the abductor hallucis muscle

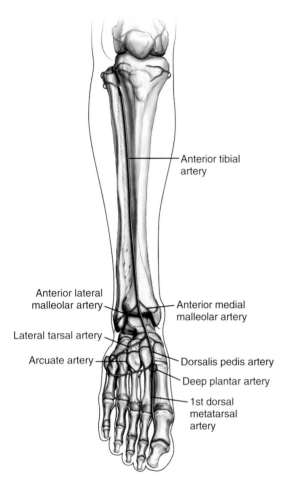

FIGURE 2-77 The arterial system of the anterior leg and dorsum of the foot. (From Miller MD et al: *Orthopaedic surgical approaches,* ed 2, Philadelphia, 2014, Saunders, Figure 8-23.)

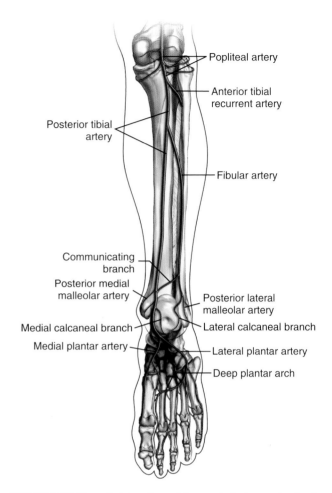

FIGURE 2-78 The arterial system of the posterior leg and sole of the foot. (From Miller MD et al: *Orthopaedic surgical approaches,* ed 2, Philadelphia, 2014, Saunders, Figure 8-24.)

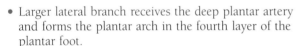

- Larger lateral branch receives the deep plantar artery and forms the plantar arch in the fourth layer of the plantar foot.

■ **Lower-extremity approaches** (Table 2-41)

▩ **Pelvis**

- Iliac crest
  - Iliac crest bone graft (ICBG) may be harvested from anterior or posterior iliac crest
  - Anterior ICBG—LFCN at risk as it runs medial to ASIS
  - Posterior ICBG—**superior cluneal nerves 8 cm lateral to PSIS, sciatic nerve exits pelvis through greater sciatic notch (at risk during osteotomy)** (Figure 2-79)
- Ilioinguinal (anterior) approach to the acetabulum
  - Access to iliac fossa from pubic symphysis to sacroiliac joint, anterior column of acetabulum
  - Relies on mobilization of the rectus abdominis and iliacus
  - Three windows are available with this approach (Figure 2-80):
    - First (lateral) window (lateral to iliopsoas/iliopectineal fascia) provides access to the internal iliac fossa, anterior sacroiliac joint, and upper portion of the anterior column.
    - Second (middle) window (between the iliopectineal fascia and the external iliac vessels) provides access to the pelvic brim from the anterior sacroiliac joint to the lateral portion of the superior pubic ramus.
    - Third (medial) window (below the vessels and spermatic cord) gives access to the symphysis pubis.
  - Stoppa modification uses a more extensive medial window and provides access to pelvic brim and quadrilateral plate.
  - Risks:
    - LFCN: exits pelvis medial to ASIS; injury causes numbness of anterolateral thigh.
    - Spermatic cord: protect as it exits superficial inguinal ring.
    - Femoral nerve: lateral to femoral vessels; injury causes weakness in knee extension, numbness in anterior thigh.
    - Inferior epigastric vessels cross just medial to inguinal ring and should be ligated.
    - Corona mortis: vascular anastomosis between external iliac and obturator vessels that crosses anterior pelvic rim; injury can result in intrapelvic hemorrhage.

Table 2-41	Standard Orthopaedic Surgical Approaches to the Lower Extremity		
APPROACH	**SUPERFICIAL INTERVAL (NERVE)**	**DEEP INTERVAL (NERVE)**	**STRUCTURES AT RISK**
ILIAC CREST			
Anterior	TFL/gluteal muscles (superior/inferior gluteal) AND external oblique (segmental)		LFCN
Posterior	Gluteus maximus (inferior gluteal) AND latissimus dorsi (thoracodorsal), spinal erector muscles		Superior cluneal nerves Sciatic nerve Superior gluteal artery
PELVIS/ACETABULUM			
Anterior (ilioinguinal)	External oblique (segmental) AND inguinal ligament	Divide internal oblique (segmental)	LFCN Spermatic cord Inferior epigastric artery Femoral artery and nerve Corona mortis
Posterior (Kocher-Langenbeck)	Divide gluteus maximus (inferior gluteal), IT band	Piriformis (nerve to piriformis) AND gluteus medius (superior gluteal)	Sciatic nerve Superior and inferior gluteal nerve and artery MFCA
HIP			
Anterior (Smith-Peterson)	Sartorius (femoral) AND TFL (superior gluteal)	Rectus femoris (femoral) AND gluteus medius (superior gluteal)	LFCN Femoral nerve and artery Superficial iliac circumflex artery LFCA (ascending branch)
Anterolateral (Watson-Jones)	TFL (superior gluteal) AND gluteus medius (superior gluteal)	Split gluteus medius (superior gluteal)	Femoral nerve and artery Superior gluteal nerve LFCA (descending branch)
Lateral (Hardinge)	Split IT band	Divide gluteus medius (superior gluteal), divide vastus lateralis (femoral)	Superior gluteal nerve LFCA (transverse branch)
Posterior (Moore, Southern)	Divide gluteus maximus (inferior gluteal), IT band	Piriformis, short external rotators AND femur	Sciatic nerve Inferior gluteal artery MFCA
Medial (Ludloff)	Adductor longus (obturator) AND gracilis (obturator)	Adductor brevis (anterior division of obturator) AND adductor magnus (obturator and tibial)	Obturator nerve MFCA Deep external pudendal artery
THIGH			
Lateral	Divide IT band	Divide or lift vastus lateralis (femoral)	Perforating branches of profunda femoris artery
Posterolateral	Vastus lateralis (femoral) AND biceps femoris (sciatic)		Perforating branches of profunda femoris artery
Anteromedial	Rectus femoris (femoral) AND vastus medialis (femoral)		Medial superior geniculate artery Infrapatellar branch of saphenous nerve
KNEE			
Anterior (medial parapatellar)	Rectus femoris (femoral) AND vastus medialis (femoral), patella AND medial patellar retinaculum		Infrapatellar branch of saphenous nerve
Medial	Medial patellar retinaculum AND sartorius (femoral)		Saphenous nerve MCL
Lateral	Iliotibial band AND biceps femoris (sciatic)		Peroneal nerve Superior and inferior lateral geniculate artery Popliteus tendon LCL
Posterior	Semimembranosus (tibial), biceps femoris (sciatic) AND lateral head gastrocnemius (tibial)		Popliteal artery Tibial nerve Peroneal nerve Medial sural cutaneous nerve
LEG			
Lateral	Gastrocnemius, soleus, FHL (tibial) AND peroneal longus and brevis (superficial peroneal)		Lesser saphenous vein Superficial peroneal nerve Posterior tibial artery
Medial	Gastrocnemius, soleus (tibial) AND tibia		Saphenous nerve and vein
ANKLE			
Anterior	EHL (deep peroneal) AND tibialis anterior (deep peroneal) OR EDL (deep peroneal)		Superficial and deep peroneal nerve Anterior tibial artery
Posteromedial	Tibialis posterior, FDL, FHL (tibial) AND Achilles tendon		Saphenous nerve and vein
Posterolateral	Peroneus brevis (superficial peroneal) AND Achilles tendon	Peroneus brevis (superficial peroneal) AND FHL (tibial)	Sural nerve Small saphenous vein

EDL, Extensor digitorum longus; *EHL,* extensor hallucis longus; *FDL,* flexor digitorum longus; *FHL,* flexor hallucis longus; *IT,* iliotibial; *LFCA,* lateral femoral circumflex artery; *LFCN,* lateral femoral cutaneous nerve; *MFCA,* medial femoral circumflex artery; *TFL,* tensor fasciae latae.

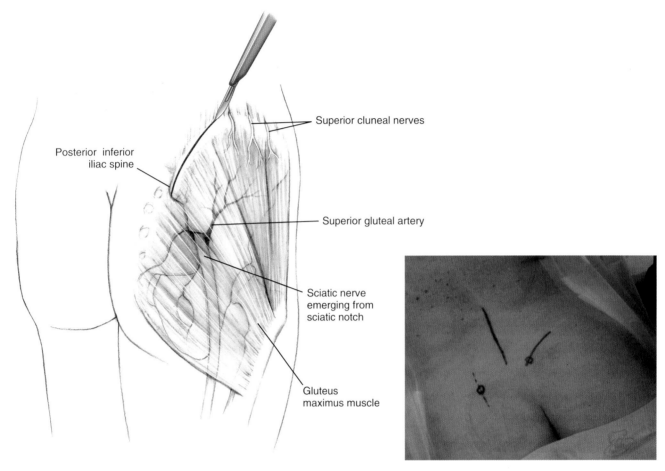

FIGURE 2-79 Incision for exposure of the posterior iliac crest. (From Miller MD et al: *Orthopaedic surgical approaches,* ed 2, Philadelphia, 2014, Saunders, Figure 5-120.)

- Kocher-Langenbeck (posterior) approach to the acetabulum (Figure 2-81)
  - Provides access to the posterior column and wall of the acetabulum
  - Not a true internervous plane—splits the gluteus maximus
  - Risks:
    - Sciatic nerve: anterior to piriformis and posterior to obturator internus
      - Hip extension and knee flexion take tension off sciatic nerve.
    - Superior and inferior gluteal artery: if injured, may retract into pelvis and cause heavy bleeding
    - Superior and inferior gluteal nerve: excessive retraction may damage
    - **Lateral ascending branch of medial femoral circumflex artery: divide short external rotators 1 to 2 cm off bone to protect blood supply to femoral head.**
    - **Damage to gluteus minimus may result in heterotopic ossification.**
- Hip (Figures 2-82 and 2-83)
  - Anterior (Smith-Peterson) approach to the hip (Figure 2-84)
    - Gained increased utilization with minimally invasive anterior total hip replacement
    - Interval: between sartorius and TFL

- Dissection
  - Retract LFCN anteriorly and ligate the ascending branch of the lateral femoral circumflex artery (which lies superficial to the rectus).
  - For deeper dissection, approach the interval between the rectus femoris and gluteus medius.
  - Approach anterior hip capsule between rectus femoris and gluteus medius; may detach both heads of rectus femoris for access.
- Risks:
  - LFCN: several branches anterior or medial to the sartorius muscle, about 6 to 8 cm below ASIS
  - Lateral femoral circumflex artery: ascending branch ligated during approach; descending branch may be injured with excessive distal reflection of the rectus tendon.
  - Superficial iliac circumflex artery: penetrates TFL just anterior to LFCN
  - Femoral nerve and artery: avoid aggressive medial retraction of the sartorius.
- Anterolateral (Watson-Jones) approach to the hip (Figure 2-85)
  - **No true interneural plane, but the intermuscular plane between the TFL and gluteus medius is used.**

Text continued on p. 229

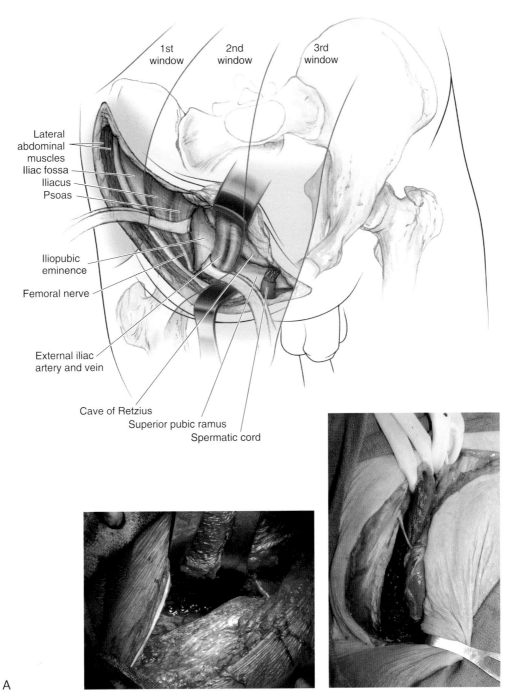

1st
window

2nd
window

3rd
window

Lateral
abdominal
muscles

Iliac fossa

Iliacus

Psoas

Iliopubic
eminence

Femoral nerve

External iliac
artery and vein

Cave of Retzius

Superior pubic ramus

Spermatic cord

A

FIGURE 2-80 Three windows are developed by placing Penrose drains or vessel loops around the femoral nerve and iliopsoas and the femoral artery, vein, and lymphatics. (From Miller MD et al: *Orthopaedic surgical approaches,* ed 2, Philadelphia, 2014, Saunders, Figure 6-39.)

Continued

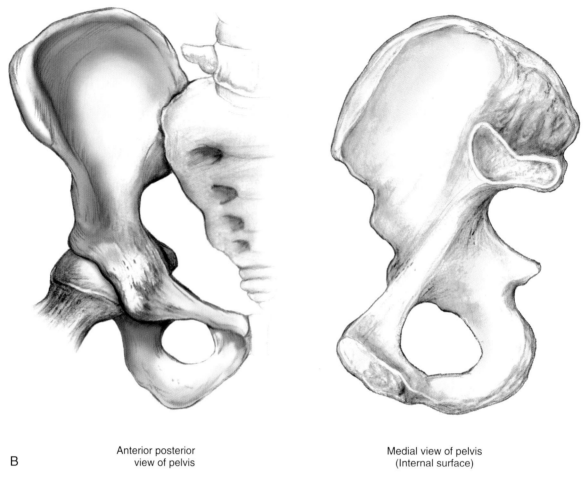

B

Anterior posterior
view of pelvis

Medial view of pelvis
(Internal surface)

FIGURE 2-80, cont'd

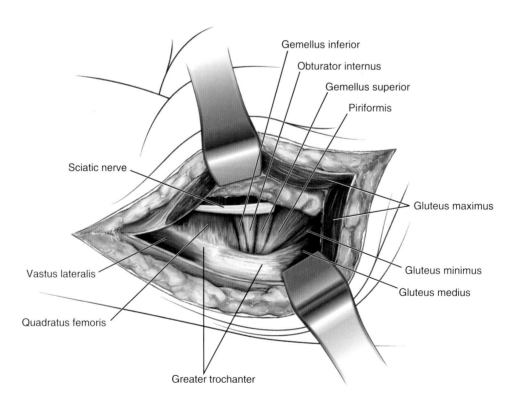

Gemellus inferior

Obturator internus

Gemellus superior

Piriformis

Sciatic nerve

Gluteus maximus

Vastus lateralis

Gluteus minimus

Gluteus medius

Quadratus femoris

Greater trochanter

FIGURE 2-81 The maximus and iliotibial band are retracted to expose the external rotators. (From Miller MD et al: *Orthopaedic surgical approaches,* ed 2, Philadelphia, 2014, Saunders, Figure 6-46.)

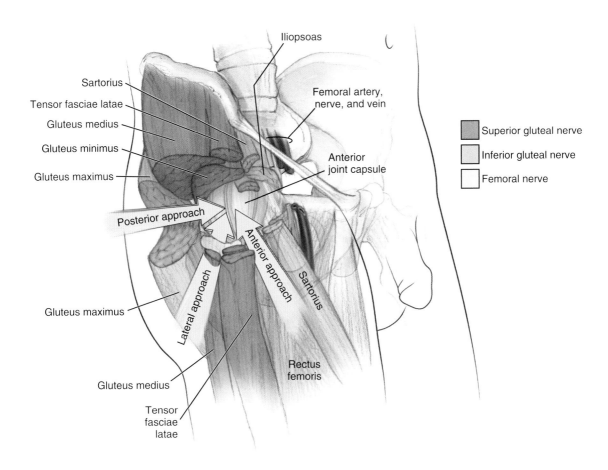

Iliopsoas

Sartorius

Tensor fasciae latae

Gluteus medius

Gluteus minimus

Gluteus maximus

Femoral artery, nerve, and vein

Anterior joint capsule

Posterior approach

Anterior approach

Lateral approach

Sartorius

Gluteus maximus

Gluteus medius

Tensor fasciae latae

Rectus femoris

Superior gluteal nerve

Inferior gluteal nerve

Femoral nerve

FIGURE 2-82 Synopsis of the anterior, lateral, and posterior approaches to the hip joint and the anatomic planes that are exploited for each approach as depicted by the arrows. (From Miller MD et al: *Orthopaedic surgical approaches,* ed 2, Philadelphia, 2014, Saunders, Figure 6-48.)

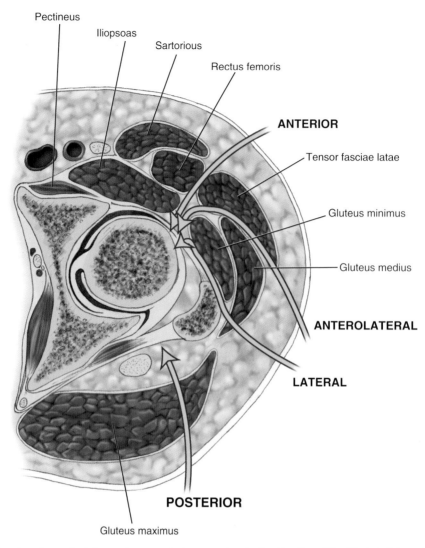

Pectineus
Iliopsoas
Sartorious
Rectus femoris

ANTERIOR

Tensor fasciae latae

Gluteus minimus

Gluteus medius

ANTEROLATERAL

LATERAL

POSTERIOR

Gluteus maximus

FIGURE 2-83 Cross-sectional anatomy depicting various surgical approaches to the hip. (From Miller MD et al: *Orthopaedic surgical approaches,* ed 2, Philadelphia, 2014, Saunders, Figure 6-49.)

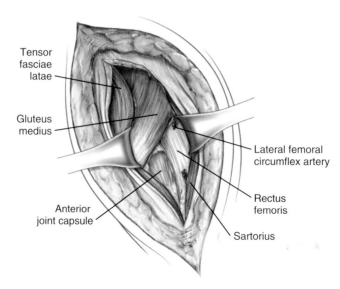

Tensor fasciae latae

Gluteus medius

Anterior joint capsule

Lateral femoral circumflex artery

Rectus femoris

Sartorius

FIGURE 2-84 Anterior (Smith-Peterson) surgical approach to the hip. In this approach, the interval between (1) the sartorius and rectus femoris (femoral nerve) and (2) the tensor fasciae latae and gluteus medius (superior gluteal nerve) is explored. The ascending branch of the lateral femoral circumflex artery is ligated. (From Miller MD et al: *Orthopaedic surgical approaches,* Philadelphia, 2008, Saunders, Figure HP-49.)

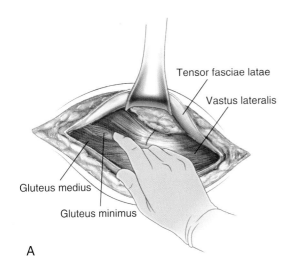

A

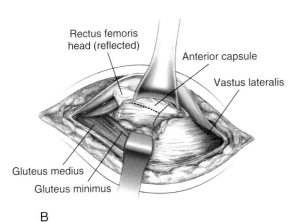

B

FIGURE 2-85 Anterolateral (Watson-Jones) approach to the hip. **A,** Superficial exposure. **B,** Deep exposure. In this approach, the interval between the tensor fasciae latae (superior gluteal nerve) and the gluteus medius (superior gluteal nerve) is explored. (From Miller MD et al: *Orthopaedic surgical approaches,* Philadelphia, 2008, Saunders, Figures HP-80 and HP-81.)

- Dissection:
  - Split the fasciae latae to expose the vastus lateralis.
  - Dissect the reflected head of the rectus femoris (and capsular attachment of the iliopsoas, if necessary), and retract medially to gain access to the capsule.
  - Detach the anterior third of the gluteus medius from the greater trochanter and the entire gluteus minimus.
  - Dissect the reflected head of the rectus femoris (and capsular attachment of the iliopsoas if necessary), and retract medially to gain access to the capsule.
- Risks:
  - Femoral nerve and artery: injured with excessive medial retraction
  - **Superior gluteal nerve: passes about 5 cm above acetabular rim; injury may result in denervation of the TFL.**
  - Lateral femoral circumflex artery: injury to the descending branch with anterior and inferior dissection

- Lateral (Hardinge) approach to the hip (Figure 2-86)
  - Involves splitting of the gluteus medius and vastus lateralis in tandem
  - Dissection:
    - Incise the skin and the fasciae latae to expose the gluteus medius and the vastus lateralis.
    - Incise the gluteus medius from the greater trochanter, leaving a cuff of tissue and the posterior half to two thirds attached.
    - Extend this incision to split the gluteus medius proximally.
    - Split the vastus lateralis distally along its anterior fourth down to the femoral shaft.
    - Detach the gluteus minimus from its insertion to expose hip capsule.
  - Risks:
    - Superior gluteal nerve: may be damaged if the gluteus medius split is too proximal (>5 cm proximal to greater trochanter).
    - Lateral femoral circumflex artery (transverse branch)
- Posterior (Moore or Southern) approach to the hip (Figure 2-87)
  - Distal extension of posterior acetabular approach (Kocher-Langenbeck)
  - Dissection
    - IT band incised over greater trochanter, and fibers of gluteus maximus split bluntly
    - Short external rotators dissected from insertions and reflected laterally to protect sciatic nerve and expose posterior hip capsule
    - Portion of the quadratus femoris may be taken down with the short external rotators, but be aware of the significant bleeding that can come from the inferior portion of this muscle (ascending branches of medial femoral circumflex artery).
  - Risks:
    - Sciatic nerve: neurapraxia (usually peroneal division) may occur with retraction if not protected by the short external rotators; may be stretched with excessive lengthening.
    - Inferior gluteal artery: may be injured during splitting of the gluteus maximus
    - Medial femoral circumflex artery: may be damaged during takedown of external rotators from insertion
- Medial (Ludloff) approach to the hip (Figures 2-88 and 2-89)
  - Used for open reduction of congenital hip dislocation, psoas release
  - Interval: adductor longus and gracilis
  - Risks:
    - **Obturator nerve (anterior division) and medial femoral circumflex artery are between the adductor brevis and adductor magnus/pectineus.**
    - Deep external pudendal artery (anterior to the pectineus near the adductor longus origin) is also at risk proximally for injury.

Text continued on p. 234

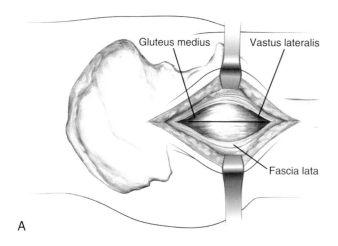

A

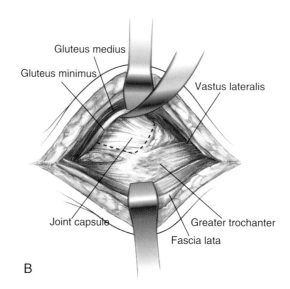

B

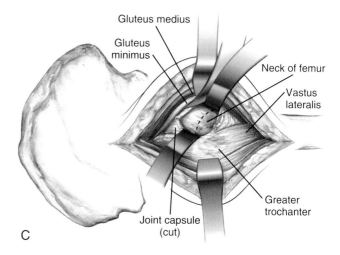

C

FIGURE 2-86 Lateral (Hardinge) approach to the hip. **A,** Superficial exposure. **B,** Deep exposure. **C,** Close-up view of deep exposure. In this approach, the interval between the gluteus medius (superior gluteal nerve) and the vastus lateralis (femoral nerve) is explored. (From Miller MD et al: *Orthopaedic surgical approaches,* Philadelphia, 2008, Saunders, Figures HP-72, HP-73, and HP-74.)

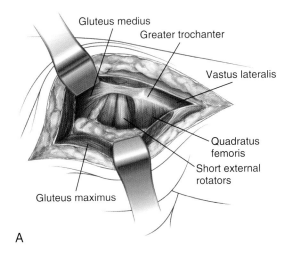

A

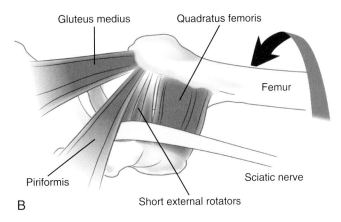

B

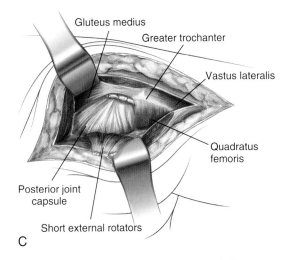

C

FIGURE 2-87 Posterior (Moore or Southern) approach to the hip. **A,** Superficial exposure. **B,** Relationship of muscles to bones. **C,** Deep exposure. In this approach, the interval between the gluteus maximus (inferior gluteal nerve) and the gluteus medius/tensor fascia lata (superior gluteal nerve) is explored. (From Miller MD et al: *Orthopaedic surgical approaches,* Philadelphia, 2008, Saunders, Figures HP-58, HP-59, and HP-60.)

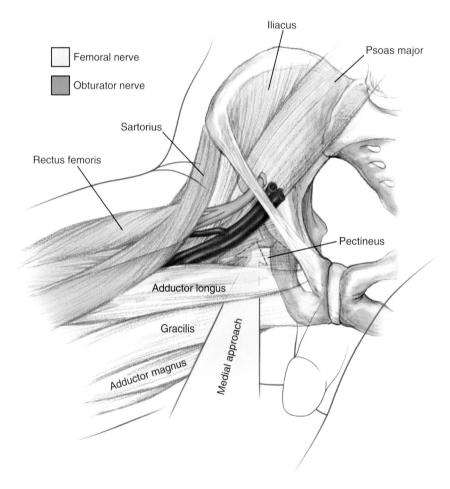

FIGURE 2-88 Characterization of the plane exploited by the medial approach to the hip, represented by the yellow plane. (From Miller MD et al: *Orthopaedic surgical approaches,* ed 2, Philadelphia, 2014, Saunders, Figure 6-50.)

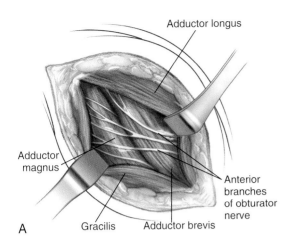

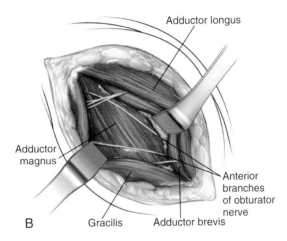

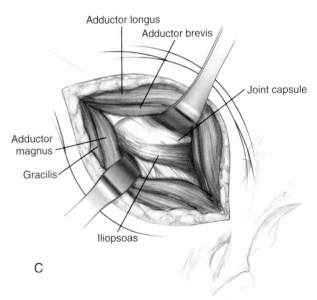

FIGURE 2-89 Medial (Ludloff) approach to the hip. **A,** Superficial exposure. **B,** Deep exposure. **C,** View of the joint capsule. In this approach, the interval between the adductor longus (obturator nerve) and the gracilis (obturator nerve) is explored. (From Miller MD et al: *Orthopaedic surgical approaches,* Philadelphia, 2008, Saunders, Figures HP-65, HP-66, and HP-67.)

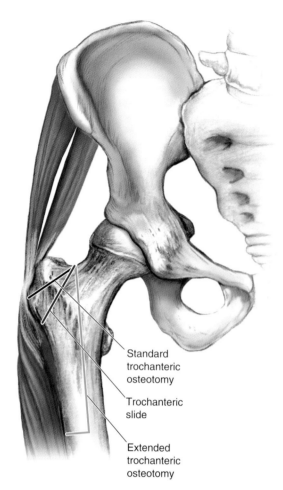

Standard trochanteric osteotomy

Trochanteric slide

Extended trochanteric osteotomy

FIGURE 2-90 Trochanteric osteotomies. (From Miller MD et al: *Orthopaedic surgical approaches,* ed 2, Philadelphia, 2014, Saunders, Figure 6-96.)

- Trochanteric osteotomies are depicted in Figure 2-90.
▓ **Thigh**
- Lateral approach to the thigh
  - Used for open reduction and internal fixation (ORIF) of intertrochanteric and femoral neck fractures; can be extended for access to shaft and supracondylar fractures
  - Dissection:
    - Split the IT band in line with the femoral shaft.
    - If necessary, include part of the TFL.
    - Then bluntly dissect the vastus lateralis in line with its fibers, or dissect the fibers of the intermuscular septum.
  - Risks:
    - Perforators from the profunda femoris should be protected or ligated.
- Posterolateral approach to the thigh
  - Dissection:
    - Incise the fascia under the IT band and retract the vastus superiorly.
    - Continue anteriorly to the lateral intermuscular septum with blunt dissection until the periosteum over the linea aspera is reached.

- Risks:
  - Perforators from the profunda femoris pierce the lateral intermuscular septum to reach the vastus. If they are approached without care, vessels can retract and bleed underneath the septum.
- Anteromedial approach to the distal femur
  - Interval: between the rectus femoris and vastus medialis (femoral nerve) and extending to a point medial to the patella
  - Dissection:
    - Retract the rectus laterally to reveal the vastus intermedius.
    - Split vastus intermedius to expose femur.
    - To open the knee joint, incise the medial patellar retinaculum and split a portion of the quadriceps tendon just lateral to the medial border.
    - After identifying the vastus intermedius, split it along its fibers to expose the femur.
  - Risks:
    - Medial superior geniculate artery and infrapatellar branch of the saphenous nerve can be injured because both cross the site of exposure.
    - Adequate cuff of tissue must be left for a strong patellar retinacular repair; otherwise, there is a risk of lateral subluxation of the patella.
▓ **Knee and leg**
- Anterior approach (medial parapatellar)
  - Dissection: midline skin incision and a medial parapatellar capsular incision.
  - Risks:
    - **Infrapatellar branch of the saphenous nerve is sometimes cut with incisions that stray too far medially, leading to painful neuroma and anterolateral numbness**
    - Medial superior geniculate artery
- Medial approach to the knee (Figure 2-91)
  - Interval: between the sartorius and medial patellar retinaculum
  - **Dissection: three layers are commonly recognized (from superficial to deep): (1) the pes anserinus tendons, (2) the superficial MCL, and (3) the deep MCL and capsule.**
  - Risks
    - Saphenous nerve and vein must be identified and protected.
    - MCL should be protected to prevent valgus instability.
- Lateral approach to the knee (Figure 2-92)
  - **Interval: either split IT band or approach between the IT band and the biceps (sciatic nerve).**
  - Dissection:
    - Develop interval between the IT band and biceps for identification of LCL and popliteus.
    - Develop a second interval within the IT band to identify the lateral femoral epicondyle.
  - Risks:
    - Common peroneal nerve (located near posterior border of biceps) must be isolated and carefully retracted.
    - LCL and popliteus tendon also at risk for injury and should be identified.

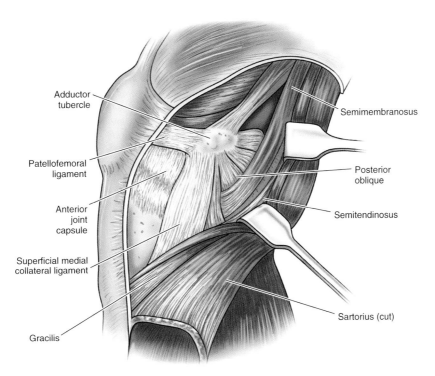

FIGURE 2-91 Medial aspect of the knee. (From Scott WN: *Insall & Scott surgery of the knee,* ed 5, Philadelphia, 2012, Elsevier, Figure 1-64.)

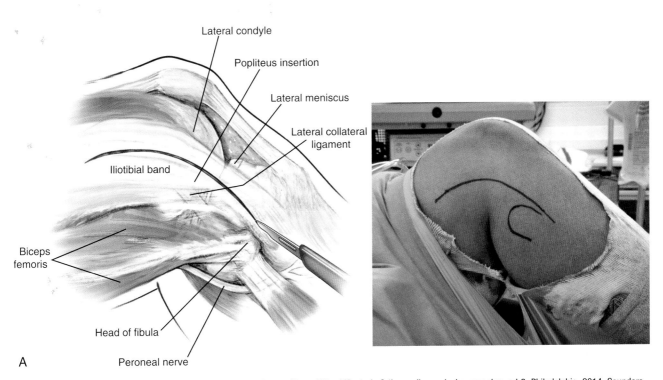

A

FIGURE 2-92 Incisions for the lateral approach to the knee. (From Miller MD et al: *Orthopaedic surgical approaches,* ed 2, Philadelphia, 2014, Saunders, Figure 7-31A.)

Continued

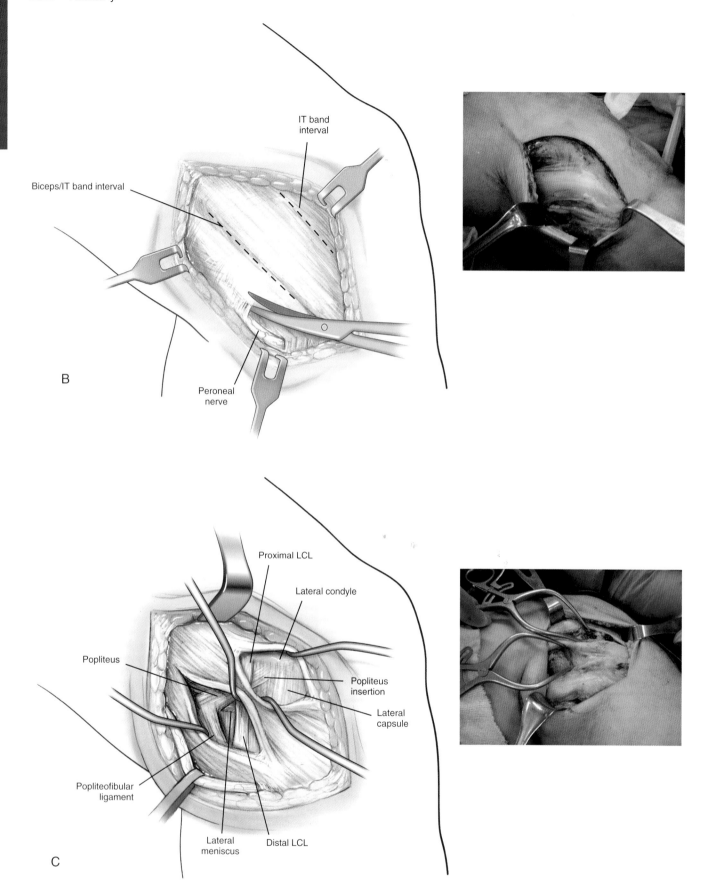

FIGURE 2-92, cont'd

- Superior lateral geniculate artery is located between the femur and vastus lateralis.
- Inferior lateral geniculate artery is posterior to the LCL between the lateral head of the gastrocnemius and the posterolateral capsule.
- Posterior approach to the knee
  - Dissection:
    - S-shaped incision, beginning laterally and ending medially (distally)
    - **Expose the popliteal fossa by using the small saphenous vein and medial sural cutaneous nerves as landmarks.**
    - If greater exposure is necessary, detach the two heads of the gastrocnemius.
    - In an alternative approach, mobilize the medial head of the gastrocnemius (lateral to the semimembranosus) and retract it laterally, using its muscle belly to protect the neurovascular structures.
  - Risks: popliteal vessels and tibial nerve, common peroneal nerve, medial sural cutaneous nerve
- Anterior approach to the tibia
  - ORIF of fractures and bone grafting; it relies on subperiosteal elevation of the tibialis anterior.
- Medial approach
  - Superficial and deep leg compartment release
  - Posterior border of tibia and medial gastrocnemius/soleus
  - Enter deep compartment by incising deep fascia in line with posterior border of tibia.
  - Risk: saphenous vein and nerve
- Posterolateral approach to the tibia (for bone grafting)
  - Interval: between the gastrocnemius/soleus and the FHL (tibial nerve) and the peroneal muscles (superficial peroneal nerve)
  - Dissection: detach the FHL from its origin on the fibula; detach the tibialis posterior from its origin along the interosseous membrane to reach the tibia.
  - Risks: neurovascular structures in the posterior compartment (including the peroneal artery) are protected by the muscle bellies of the tibialis posterior and FHL medially to laterally and between soleus and tibialis posterior anteriorly to posteriorly.
- Approach to the fibula
  - Same interval as the posterolateral approach to the tibia, but it stays more anterior and relies on isolation and protection of the common peroneal nerve in the proximal dissection.

Foot and Ankle
- Anterior approach to the ankle
  - Interval: between the EHL and EDL or tibialis anterior (both deep peroneal nerve)
  - Dissection: before incising the extensor retinaculum, carefully protect the superficial peroneal nerve, which courses superficially.
  - Risks: deep peroneal nerve and anterior tibial artery, which lie directly in this interval, must be retracted medially along with the EHL.

- Approach to the medial malleolus
  - Dissection:
    - Because it is superficial, use an anterior or posterior approach.
    - Posteromedial approach behind the medial malleolus through the tendon sheath of the posterior tibialis
  - Risks:
    - Anterior approach—saphenous nerve and the long saphenous vein
    - Posterior approach—posterior tibial tendon, FDL, posterior tibial vein, posterior tibial artery, tibial nerve, and FHL (mnemonic: "Tom, Dick, and very angry nervous Harry").
- Posteromedial approach to the ankle and foot: used for release of clubfoot in children
  - Dissection:
    - Begin this approach medial to the Achilles tendon, and follow the curve distally along the medial border of the foot.
    - Use the posterior tibialis tendon as a landmark for the location of the subluxated navicular in the clubfoot.
  - Risks: posterior tibial nerve and artery and their branches
- Lateral approach to the ankle
  - Dissection: use a subcutaneous approach for ORIF of distal fibula fractures.
  - Risks: sural nerve (posterolateral) and the superficial peroneal nerve (anterior)
- Posterolateral approach to ankle
  - Interval: between the peroneus brevis and FHL
  - Dissection:
    - Identify the peroneal tendons (brevis more muscular and anterior to longus directly behind the fibula).
    - Incise peroneal retinaculum to mobilize tendons laterally, which exposes the FHL.
    - Retract FHL medially to expose tibia and ankle joint.
  - Risks: lesser saphenous vein and sural nerve posterior to lateral malleolus
- Lateral approach to the hindfoot: used for triple arthrodesis
  - Interval: between the peroneus tertius (deep peroneal nerve) and peroneal tendons (superficial peroneal nerve)
  - Dissection: remove the fat pad covering the sinus tarsi, and reflect the EDB from its origin to expose the joints.
  - Risks:
    - Lateral branch of the deep peroneal nerve (which supplies the EDB) must be protected in this approach.
    - Deep penetration with an instrument used in this approach can injure the FHL.
- Anterolateral approach to the midfoot
  - Dissection: approach commonly used for excision of a calcaneonavicular bar; release the EDB.
  - Risk: calcaneal navicular (spring) ligament may be injured.

■ **Cross-sectional diagrams of the lower extremity with MRI are demonstrated in Figures 2-93 through 2-95.**

Text continued on p. 243

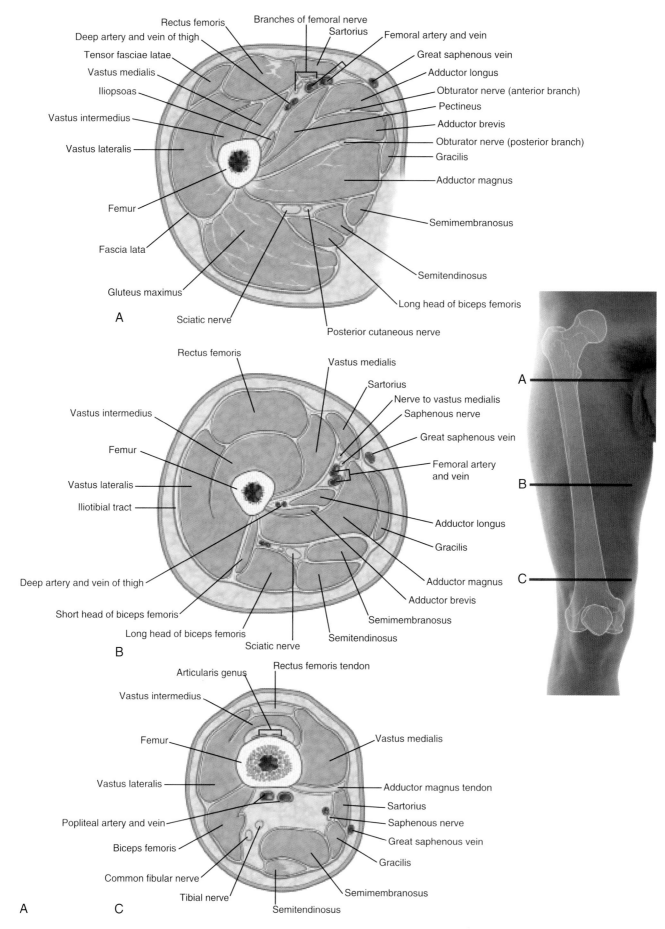

FIGURE 2-93 Illustration **(A)** and imaging **(B)** of the cross sections of the thigh. (From Drake RL et al, editors: *Gray's atlas of anatomy,* ed 2, Philadelphia, 2015, Churchill Livingstone.)

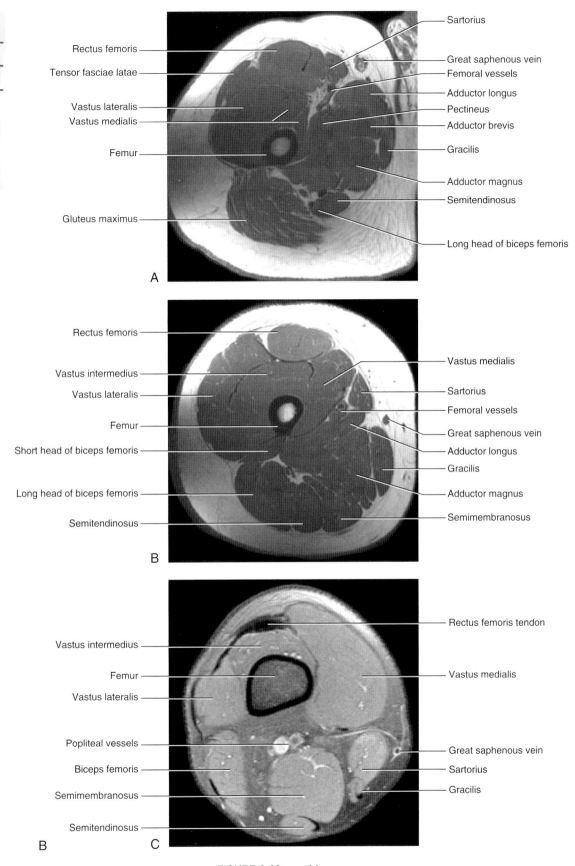

Rectus femoris

Tensor fasciae latae

Vastus lateralis

Vastus medialis

Femur

Gluteus maximus

Sartorius

Great saphenous vein

Femoral vessels

Adductor longus

Pectineus

Adductor brevis

Gracilis

Adductor magnus

Semitendinosus

Long head of biceps femoris

A

Rectus femoris

Vastus intermedius

Vastus lateralis

Femur

Short head of biceps femoris

Long head of biceps femoris

Semitendinosus

Vastus medialis

Sartorius

Femoral vessels

Great saphenous vein

Adductor longus

Gracilis

Adductor magnus

Semimembranosus

B

Vastus intermedius

Femur

Vastus lateralis

Popliteal vessels

Biceps femoris

Semimembranosus

Semitendinosus

Rectus femoris tendon

Vastus medialis

Great saphenous vein

Sartorius

Gracilis

B

C

FIGURE 2-93, cont'd

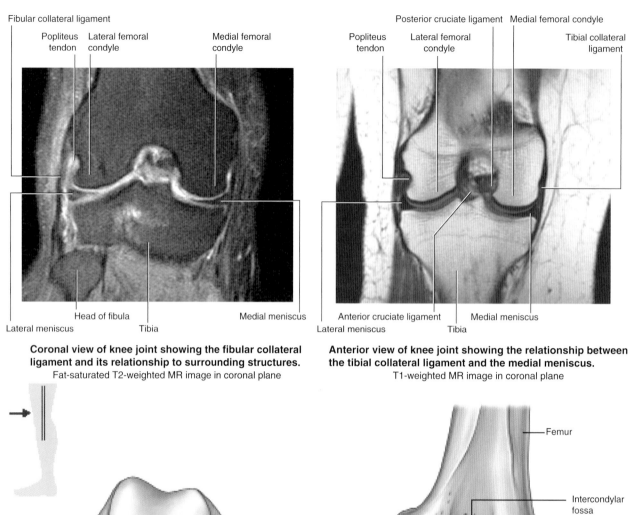

Fibular collateral ligament
Popliteus tendon
Lateral femoral condyle
Medial femoral condyle
Lateral meniscus
Head of fibula
Tibia
Medial meniscus

Coronal view of knee joint showing the fibular collateral ligament and its relationship to surrounding structures.
Fat-saturated T2-weighted MR image in coronal plane

Posterior cruciate ligament
Medial femoral condyle
Popliteus tendon
Lateral femoral condyle
Tibial collateral ligament
Anterior cruciate ligament
Lateral meniscus
Medial meniscus
Tibia

Anterior view of knee joint showing the relationship between the tibial collateral ligament and the medial meniscus.
T1-weighted MR image in coronal plane

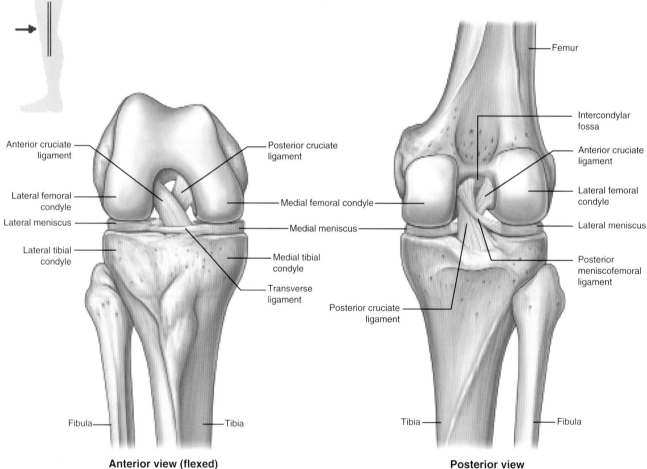

Anterior cruciate ligament
Posterior cruciate ligament
Lateral femoral condyle
Medial femoral condyle
Lateral meniscus
Medial meniscus
Lateral tibial condyle
Medial tibial condyle
Transverse ligament
Fibula
Tibia

Anterior view (flexed)

Femur
Intercondylar fossa
Anterior cruciate ligament
Lateral femoral condyle
Lateral meniscus
Medial meniscus
Posterior meniscofemoral ligament
Posterior cruciate ligament
Tibia
Fibula

Posterior view

FIGURE 2-94 Anterior and posterior views of the knee joint. (From Drake RL et al, editors: *Gray's atlas of anatomy,* ed 2, Philadelphia, 2015, Churchill Livingstone.)

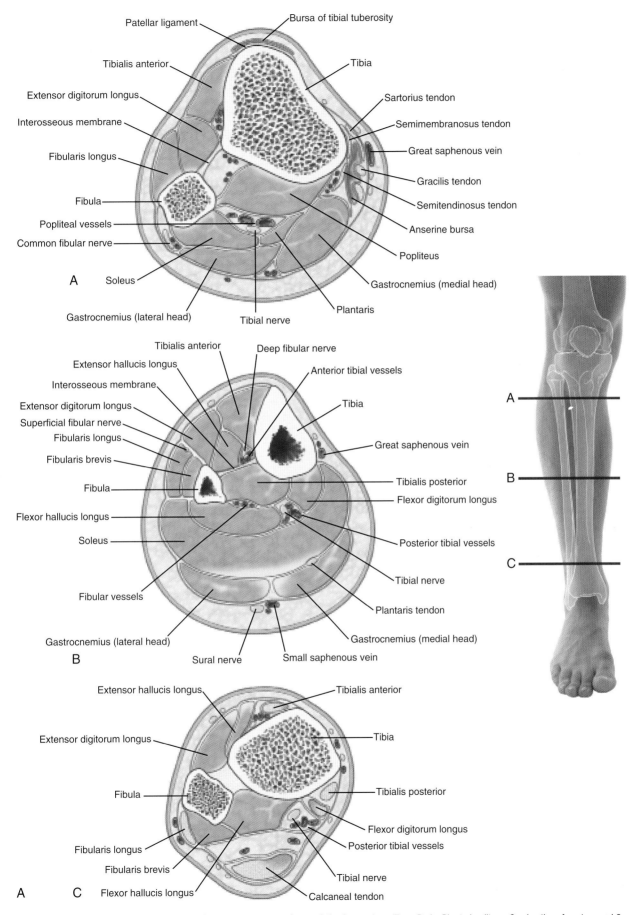

FIGURE 2-95 Illustration **(A)** and imaging **(B)** of the cross sections of the lower leg. (From Drake RL et al, editors: *Gray's atlas of anatomy,* ed 2, Philadelphia, 2015, Churchill Livingstone.)

Continued

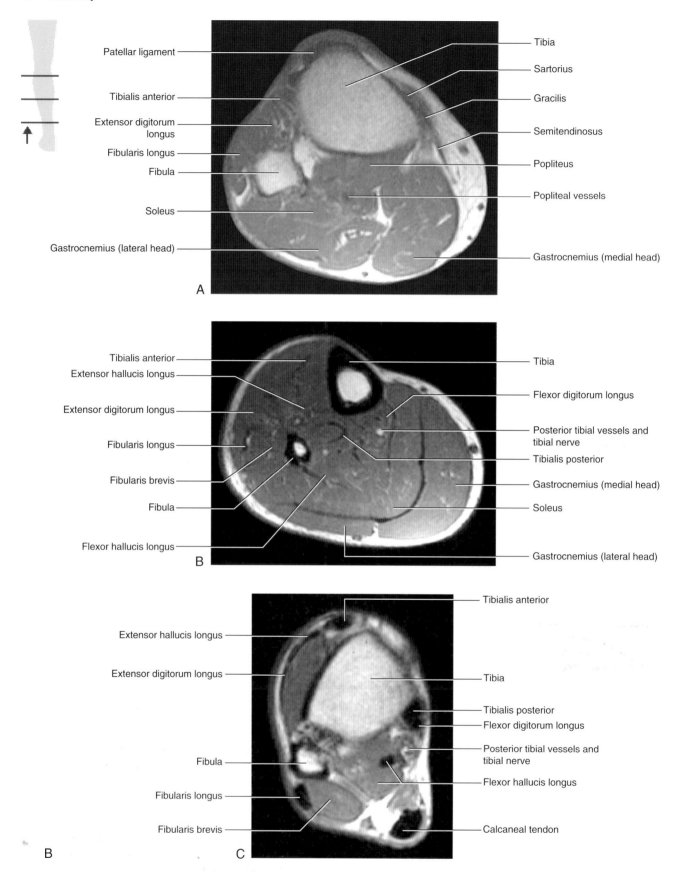

A

Patellar ligament

Tibialis anterior

Extensor digitorum longus

Fibularis longus

Fibula

Soleus

Gastrocnemius (lateral head)

Tibia

Sartorius

Gracilis

Semitendinosus

Popliteus

Popliteal vessels

Gastrocnemius (medial head)

B

Tibialis anterior

Extensor hallucis longus

Extensor digitorum longus

Fibularis longus

Fibularis brevis

Fibula

Flexor hallucis longus

Tibia

Flexor digitorum longus

Posterior tibial vessels and tibial nerve

Tibialis posterior

Gastrocnemius (medial head)

Soleus

Gastrocnemius (lateral head)

C

Extensor hallucis longus

Extensor digitorum longus

Fibula

Fibularis longus

Fibularis brevis

Tibialis anterior

Tibia

Tibialis posterior

Flexor digitorum longus

Posterior tibial vessels and tibial nerve

Flexor hallucis longus

Calcaneal tendon

B

FIGURE 2-95, cont'd

SECTION 4 SPINE

OSTEOLOGY

- **The spine** has 33 vertebrae: 7 cervical, 12 thoracic, 5 lumbar, 5 fused sacral, and 4 fused coccygeal (Figure 2-96).
- Normal curves are cervical lordosis, thoracic kyphosis, lumbar lordosis, and sacral kyphosis.
- Vertebral body width generally increases in a craniocaudad direction, with the exception of T1 to T3.
- Important spine topographic landmarks are listed in Table 2-42.
- **Cervical spine** (Figure 2-97)
- Atlas (C1) has no vertebral body and no spinous process.
  - Two concave superior facets that articulate with the occipital condyles
  - **50% of total neck flexion and extension occurs at occiput-C1 articulation**
- Axis (C2) develops from five ossification centers, with an initial cartilaginous junction between the dens and vertebral body (subdental synchondrosis) that fuses at 7 years of age.
  - Base of the dens narrows because of the transverse ligament.
  - 50% of total neck rotation occurs at atlantoaxial (C1-C2) articulation
  - Atlantoaxial joint is diarthrodial.
    - *Pannus* **in rheumatoid arthritis can affect this articulation and result in instability (see Chapter 8, Spine).**
    - Cervical spine clearance (including radiographs) is recommended for elective orthopaedic procedures in patients with rheumatoid arthritis.
- C2 to C7 vertebrae have foramina in each transverse process and bifid spinous processes (except for the C7 nonbifid posterior spinous process [vertebral prominens]).
- **Vertebral artery travels in the transverse foramina of C6 to C1 (not C7).**
- Carotid (Chassaignac) tubercle is found at C6.
- **Diameter of the cervical spine canal is normally 17 mm, and the cervical cord may become compromised when the diameter is reduced to less than 13 mm (relative stenosis).**
- **Thoracic spine** (Figure 2-98)
- Unique features include costal facets (present on all 12 vertebral bodies and the transverse processes of T1-T9) and a rounded vertebral foramen.
- Thoracic vertebral articulation with the rib cage makes this the most rigid region of the axial skeleton.

Table 2-42	Spine Topographic Landmarks
TOPOGRAPHIC LANDMARK	**SPINAL LEVEL**
Mandible	C2-C3
Hyoid cartilage	C3
Thyroid cartilage	C4-C5
Cricoid cartilage	C6
Vertebra prominens	C7
Scapular spine	T3
Distal tip of scapula	T7
Iliac crest	L4-L5

- Narrowest pedicles at T5
- **Lumbar spine** (Figure 2-99)
- Lumbar vertebrae are the largest vertebrae and are higher anteriorly than posteriorly, significantly contributing to the lumbar lordosis.
- Lumbar lordosis ranges from 55 to 60 degrees, with the apex at L3.
- 66% of lordosis occurs in the region from L4 to the sacrum
- Lumbar vertebrae contain short laminae and pedicles.
- Mammillary processes (separate ossification centers) project posteriorly from the superior articular facet.
- Spondylolysis is a defect in the pars interarticularis and the most common cause of back pain in children and adolescents.
- **Sacrum**
- Formed from the fusion of five spinal elements
- Sacral promontory is an anterosuperior portion that projects into the pelvis.
- Four pairs of pelvic sacral foramina located both anteriorly and posteriorly transmit respective ventral and dorsal branches of the upper four sacral nerves.
- Sacral canal opens caudally into the sacral hiatus.
- **Coccyx**
- Formed from the fusion of the lowest four spinal elements
- Attachments dorsally to the gluteus maximus, external anal sphincter, and coccygeal muscles

ARTHROLOGY

- **Spinal ligaments** (Figure 2-100)
- Anterior longitudinal ligament (ALL)
  - Strong; thickest at center of vertebral body and thinnest at periphery
  - Characterized by separate fibers extending from one to five levels
  - Resists hyperextension
- Posterior longitudinal ligament
  - Weaker than ALL
  - Extends from occiput (tectorial membrane) to posterior sacrum
  - Separated from the center of the vertebral body by a space that allows passage of the dorsal branches of the spinal artery and veins
  - **Hourglass shaped, with the wider (yet thinner) sections located over the discs; ruptured discs tend to be lateral to these expansions.**
- Ligamentum flavum
  - Strong yellow elastic ligament connecting the laminae
  - **Runs from anterior surface of the superior lamina to posterior surface of the inferior lamina and is constantly in tension**
  - Hypertrophy of the ligamentum flavum is said to contribute to nerve root compression.
- Supraspinous, interspinous, and intertransverse ligaments

Text continued on p. 248

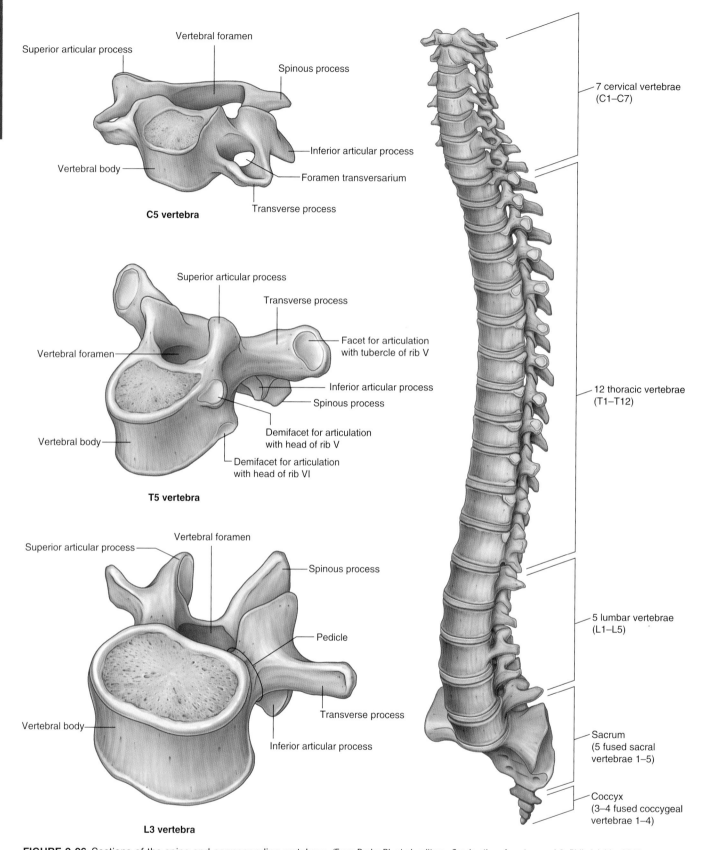

FIGURE 2-96 Sections of the spine and corresponding vertebrae. (From Drake RL et al, editors: *Gray's atlas of anatomy,* ed 2, Philadelphia, 2015, Churchill Livingstone.)

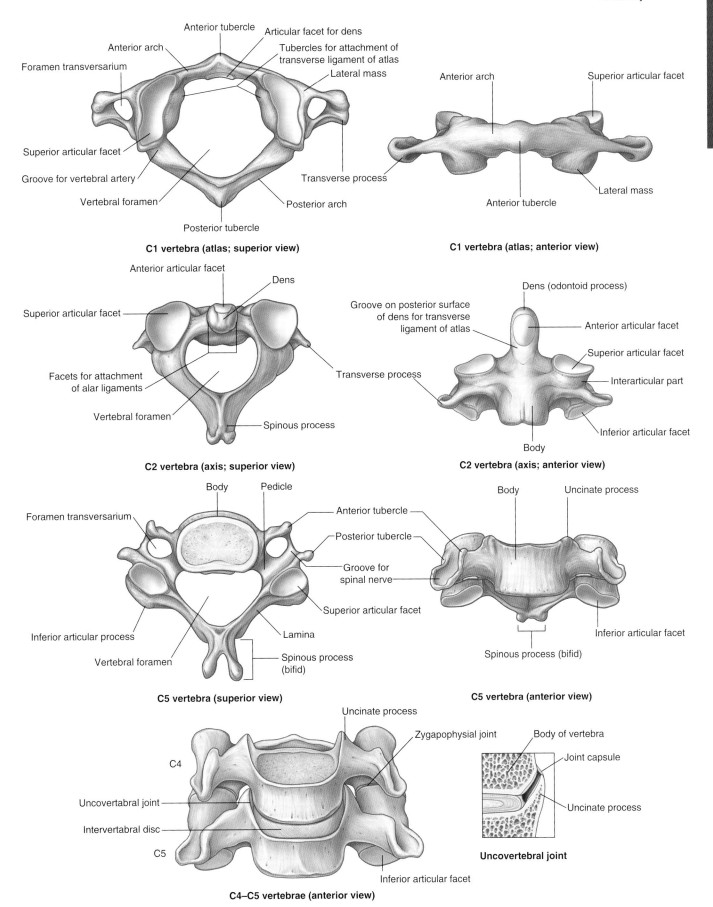

FIGURE 2-97 Cervical vertebral anatomy. (From Drake RL et al, editors: *Gray's atlas of anatomy,* ed 2, Philadelphia, 2015, Churchill Livingstone.)

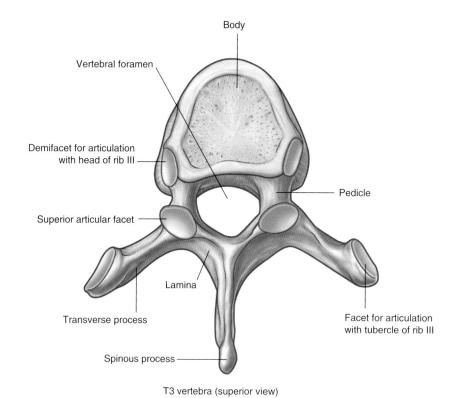

T3 vertebra (superior view)

FIGURE 2-98 Thoracic vertebral anatomy (superior view). (From Drake RL et al, editors: *Gray's atlas of anatomy,* ed 2, Philadelphia, 2015, Churchill Livingstone.)

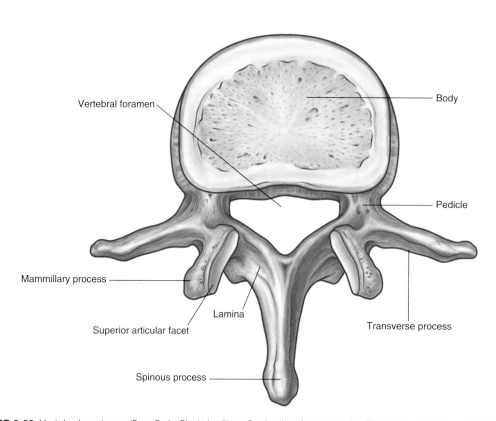

FIGURE 2-99 Vertebral anatomy. (From Drake RL et al, editors: *Gray's atlas of anatomy,* ed 2, Philadelphia, 2015, Churchill Livingstone.)

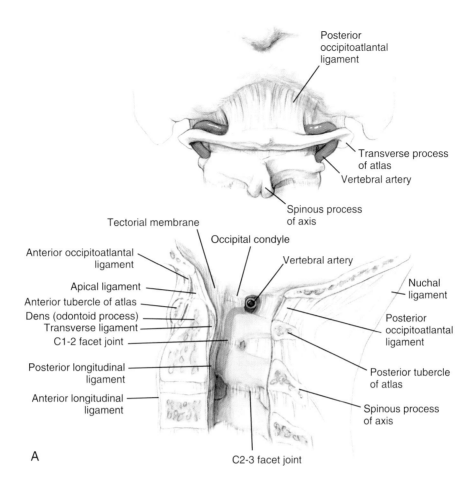

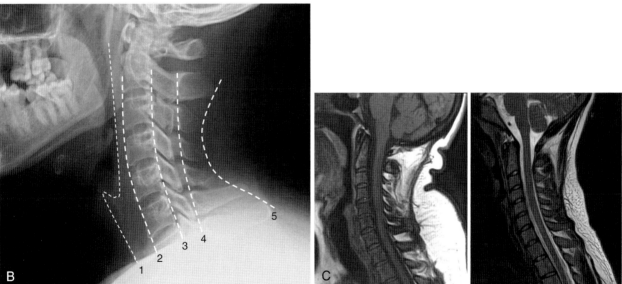

FIGURE 2-100 The occipitocervical junction. Note the location and course of the vertebral artery. (From Miller MD et al: *Orthopaedic surgical approaches,* ed 2, Philadelphia, 2014, Saunders, Figure 5-5A.)

- Ligamentous capsules overlying the zygapophyseal joints; the intertransverse ligaments contribute little to interspinous stability.
- Supraspinous ligament lies dorsal to the spinous processes, and interspinous ligament lies between the spinous processes.
  - Supraspinous ligament begins at C7 and is in continuity with the ligamentum nuchae (which runs from C7 to occiput).
- Spine stability (Denis model): the three-column system (Figure 2-101, Table 2-43)
- Specialized ligaments
  - Atlantooccipital joint
    - Composed of two articular capsules (anterior and posterior) and the tectorial membrane (cephalad extension of the posterior longitudinal ligament)
    - Further stabilization by the ligamentous attachments to the dens
  - Atlantoaxial joint (Figure 2-102)
    - **Transverse ligament is the major stabilizer of the atlantoaxial joint.**
    - Further stabilized by the apical ligament (longitudinal), which together with the transverse ligament, compose the cruciate ligament
    - In addition, a pair of alar ("check") ligaments runs obliquely from the tip of the dens to the occiput.
  - Iliolumbar ligament
    - This stout ligament connects the transverse process of L5 with the ilium.
    - Tension on this ligament in patients with unstable vertical shear pelvic fractures can lead to avulsion fractures of the transverse process.
- Facet (apophyseal) joints
  - Orientation of the facets of the spine dictates the plane of motion at each relative level.
  - Facet orientation varies with the spinal level (Figure 2-103, Table 2-44).

- Cervical spine—superior articular facet is anterior and inferior to the inferior articular process of the vertebra above; the nerve roots exit near the superior articulating process.
- Lumbar spine—the superior articular facet is anterior and lateral to the inferior articular facet.

Table 2-43	Denis Model of Spine Columns
COLUMN	**COMPOSITION**
Anterior	Anterior longitudinal ligament, anterior two thirds of annulus and vertebral body
Middle	Posterior third of body and annulus, posterior longitudinal ligament
Posterior	Pedicles, facets and facet capsules, spinous processes, posterior ligaments that include interspinous and supraspinous ligaments, ligamentum flavum

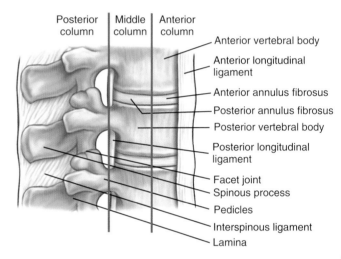

FIGURE 2-101 Three-column system of spine stability (Denis model). (From Miller MD, Thompson SR, editors: *DeLee and Drez's orthopaedic sports medicine: principles and practice,* ed 4, Philadelphia, 2014, Saunders.)

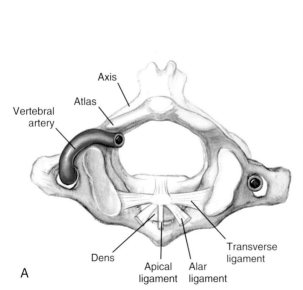

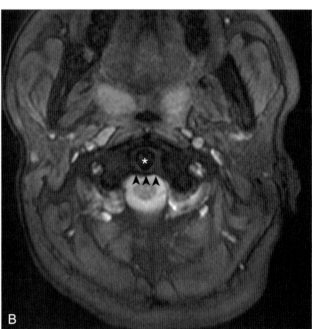

FIGURE 2-102 Superior view of the atlantoaxial articulation. Note the relationship of the transverse ligament to C1-C2. (From Miller MD et al: *Orthopaedic surgical approaches,* ed 2, Philadelphia, 2014, Saunders, Figure 5-6A.)

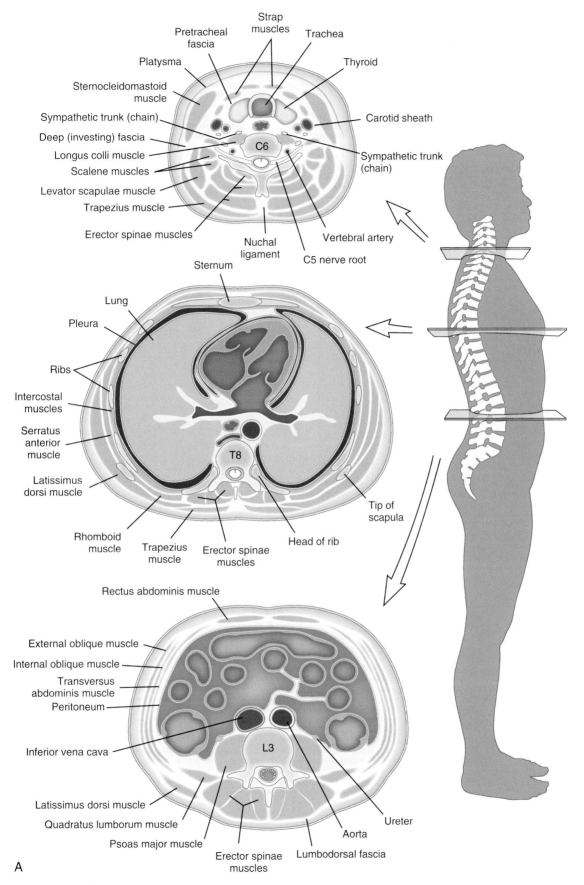

FIGURE 2-103 Cross-sectional anatomy of the cervical, thoracic, and lumbar spine. (From Miller MD et al: *Orthopaedic surgical approaches,* ed 2, Philadelphia, 2014, Saunders, Figure 5-19A.)

Continued

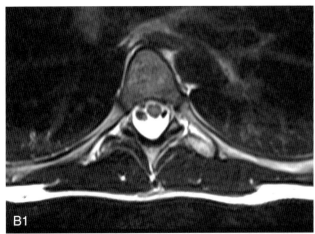

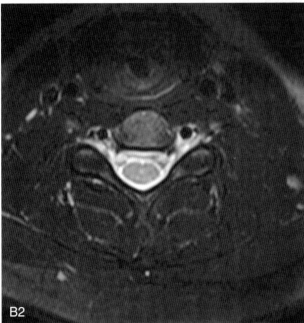

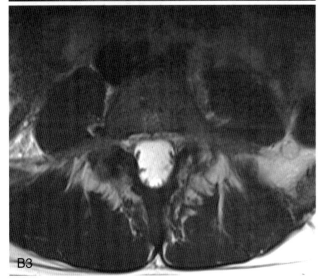

FIGURE 2-103, cont'd

Table 2-44	Orientation of Spine Facets	
SPINAL LEVEL	**ORIENTATION OF SAGITTAL FACET**	**ORIENTATION OF CORONAL FACET**
Cervical	35 Degrees at C2, increasing to 55 degrees at C7	Neutral, 0 degrees
Thoracic	60 Degrees at T1, increasing to 70 degrees at T12	20 Degrees posterior
Lumbar	137 Degrees at L1, decreasing to 118 degrees at L5	45 Degrees anterior

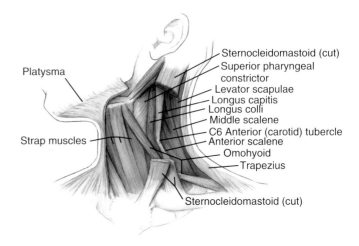

FIGURE 2-104 Muscles of the anterior cervical spine. (From Miller MD et al: *Orthopaedic surgical approaches,* ed 2, Philadelphia, 2014, Saunders, Figure 5-10.)

- Intervertebral discs
  - Fibrocartilaginous
  - **Annulus fibrosus: obliquely oriented, composed of type I collagen**
  - **Central nucleus pulposus: made of type II collagen and softer than the annulus**
  - Nucleus pulposus: high polysaccharide content and approximately 88% water
  - **Aging results in the loss of water and conversion to fibrocartilage.**
  - Intervertebral discs: account for 25% of the total height of the spinal column
  - Attach to the vertebral bodies by hyaline cartilage, which is responsible for the vertical growth of the column
  - Intradisc pressure: position dependent; pressure is lowest in supine position and highest in the sitting position and flexed forward with weights on the hands.
- **Muscles**
- Neck: functional classification (anterior and posterior regions)
  - Anterior neck region (Figure 2-104)
    - Contains the superficial platysma muscle (cranial nerve VII innervated), stylohyoid and digastric muscles (cranial nerve VII innervated) above the hyoid, and "strap" muscles below the hyoid
    - Strap muscles include the sternohyoid and omohyoid in the superficial layer and the thyrohyoid and sternohyoid in the deep layer; all are innervated by the ansa cervicalis (C1-C3).

- Sternocleidomastoid muscle (cranial nerve XI and ansa) runs obliquely across the neck, rotating the head to the contralateral side.
- Anterior triangle (borders: sternocleidomastoid, midline of the neck, and lower border of the mandible) is the largest area.
- Three smaller triangles are as follows:
  - Submandibular
  - Carotid (bordered by posterior aspect of the digastric and omohyoid and used for the anterior approach to C5)
  - Posterior (bordered by the trapezius muscle, sternocleidomastoid muscle, and clavicle)
- Posterior neck region
  - Posterior neck muscles form the borders of the suboccipital triangle.
    - Superior and inferior heads of the obliquus capitis muscle and the rectus capitis posterior major muscle form this triangle.
    - **Vertebral artery and the first cervical nerve are within this triangle; greater occipital nerve (C2) is superficial.**

- Back
  - Blanketed by the trapezius (superiorly) and latissimus dorsi (inferiorly)
  - Rhomboid muscles and levator scapulae are deep to this layer.
  - Deep muscles: the erector spinae and transversospinalis (Figure 2-105)
    - Erector spinae run from the transverse and spinous processes of the inferior vertebrae to the spinous processes of the superior vertebrae.
    - They stabilize and extend the back.
    - All of the deep back musculature is innervated by dorsal primary rami of the spinal nerves.

Nerves

- Spinal cord
  - General anatomy
    - Spinal cord extends from the brainstem to the inferior border of L1, where it terminates as the conus medullaris.
    - Small filum terminale continues distal with the surrounding nerve roots contained within a common dural sac (cauda equina) to its termination in the coccyx.
    - Spinal cord is enclosed within the bony spinal canal, with variable amounts of space (greatest in the upper cervical spine).
    - Cord also varies in diameter (widest at the origin of the plexuses).
    - In cross section, the cord is observed to have both geographic and functional boundaries. It is divided in the midline anteriorly by a fissure and posteriorly by the sulcus.
  - Functional anatomy (Figure 2-106): functions of the ascending (sensory) and descending (motor) tracts are summarized in Table 2-45.
    - Posterior funiculi (**dorsal columns**) are located dorsally and receive ascending fibers, which deliver deep tactile, proprioceptive, and vibratory sensations.
    - Lateral spinothalamic tract are ascending fibers that transmit sensations of pain and temperature.
    - Lateral corticospinal tract are descending fibers for voluntary muscular contraction.

- Sacral structures are the most peripheral in the lateral corticospinal tracts; cervical structures are more medial.
  - This is why central cord syndrome affects the upper extremities more than the lower extremities.
- Ventral (anterior) spinothalamic tract are ascending fibers that transmit light tactile sensation.
- Ventral (anterior) corticospinal tract are descending fibers for voluntary muscular contraction.
- Deficits associated with patterns of incomplete spinal cord injury are predictable from the anatomy of the ascending and descending tracts.
- **Prognosis with incomplete spinal cord injury is unaffected by the presence or absence of the bulbocavernosus reflex.**
  - Incomplete spinal cord injury patterns are summarized in Table 2-46.
  - Spinal cord injury distal to the conus medullaris may permanently interrupt the bulbocavernosus reflex.
- Nerve roots (Figure 2-107)
  - 31 pairs of spinal nerves: 8 cervical, 12 thoracic, 5 lumbar, 5 sacral, and 1 coccygeal
  - Within the subarachnoid space, the dorsal root (and ganglia) and ventral roots converge to form the spinal nerve.
    - Nerve becomes "extradural" as it approaches the intervertebral foramen (the dura becomes epineurium) at all levels above L1.
    - Below this level, the nerves are contained within the cauda equina.
  - After exiting the foramen, the spinal nerve gives off dorsal primary rami, which supply the muscles and skin of the neck and back regions.
  - Innervation of structures within the spinal canal—including the periosteum, meninges, vascular structures, and articular connective tissue—is from the sinuvertebral nerve.
  - Ventral rami supply the anteromedial trunk and limbs.
  - With the exception of the thoracic nerves, the ventral rami are grouped in plexuses before delivering sensorimotor functions to a general region.
  - **In the cervical spine, the numbered nerve exits at a level above the pedicle of the corresponding vertebral level (e.g., the C2 nerve exits at the level of vertebrae C1-C2) (Figure 2-108).**
  - **In the lumbar spine, the nerve root traverses the respective disc space above the named vertebral body and exits the respective foramen under the pedicle (Figure 2-109).**
  - Herniated discs usually impinge on the traversing nerve root and facet joint.
    - Example: a central disc herniation at the level of L4-L5 would cause compression of the traversing L5 nerve root, resulting in a positive tension sign (straight-leg raise) and diminished strength in the hip abductors and EHL and pain and numbness in the lateral leg to the dorsum of the foot.
    - Far lateral disc herniation at the L4-L5 level would compress the exiting L4 nerve root, resulting in a positive tension sign (femoral nerve stretch test) and L4 nerve compromise.
  - **L5 nerve root is relatively fixed to the anterior sacral ala and can be damaged by sacral fractures and errant anteriorly placed iliosacral screws.**

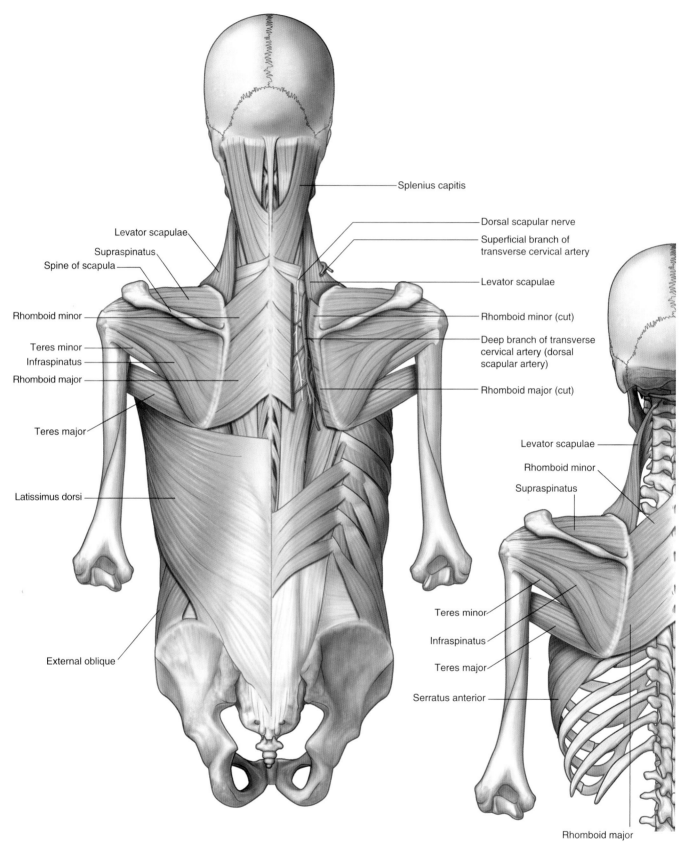

FIGURE 2-105 Muscles of the back and shoulders. (From Drake RL et al, editors: *Gray's atlas of anatomy,* ed 2, Philadelphia, 2015, Churchill Livingstone.)

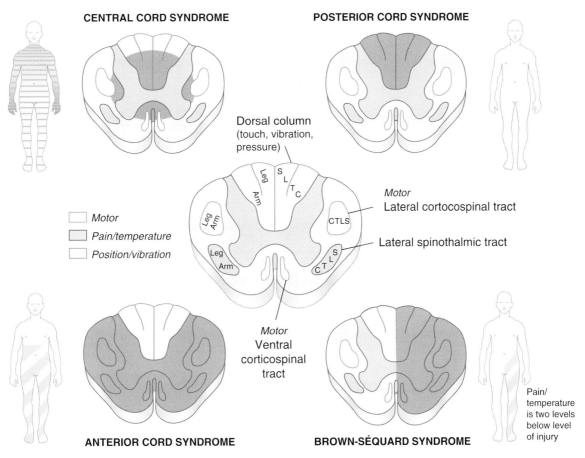

FIGURE 2-106 Incomplete spinal cord injury syndromes.

Table 2-45	Spinal Cord Tracts	
DIRECTION	**TRACTS**	**FUNCTION**
Ascending (sensory)	Dorsal columns	Deep touch, proprioception, vibratory
	Lateral spinothalamic	Pain and temperature
	Anterior spinothalamic	Light touch
Descending (motor)	Lateral corticospinal	Voluntary motor
	Anterior corticospinal	Voluntary motor

Table 2-46	Patterns of Incomplete Spinal Cord Injury	
PATTERN OF INJURY	**FUNCTIONAL DEFICIT**	**RECOVERY**
Central (most common)	Upper extremity affected more than lower extremity, usually quadriparetic with sacral sparing; flaccid paralysis of upper extremity and spastic paralysis of lower extremity	75%
Anterior	Complete motor deficit	**10% (worst prognosis)**
Brown-Séquard	Unilateral cord injury with ipsilateral motor deficit, contralateral pain, and temperature deficit (two levels below injury)	>90% recovery

- Dermatomal patterns are depicted in Figure 2-110.
- **Key testable neurologic levels** are listed in Table 2-47.
- Nerve root compression: summary of nerve root compression is highlighted in Chapter 8, Spine.
- Sympathetic chain
  - Cervical sympathetic chain posterior and medial to the carotid sheath
    - Anterior to the longus capitis muscle
    - Cross-sectional relationships in the carotid sheath are key testable material; contents include the internal carotid artery, common carotid artery, internal jugular vein, and cranial nerve X (vagus nerve).
  - Three ganglia of cervical sympathetic chain: superior, middle, and inferior (Table 2-48)
    - Disruption of the inferior ganglia can lead to Horner syndrome (ptosis, miosis [pupillary constriction], and anhidrosis).
    - Can be seen with preganglionic brachial plexus lesions
  - Sympathetic ganglia: 11 in thoracic region, 4 in lumbar region, 4 in sacral region
- **Vessels (Figure 2-111)**
- Spinal blood supply from segmental arteries
  - Located at vertebral midbodies via the aorta (which lies on left side of vertebral column; inferior vena cava and azygos vein are on the right).
  - Primary supply to the dura and posterior elements is from the dorsal branches.
  - Ventral branches supply the vertebral bodies via the ascending and descending branches, which are

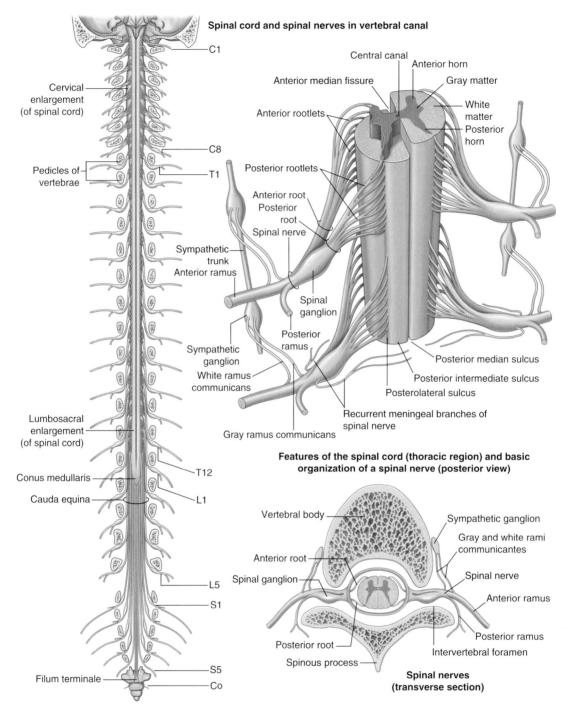

Spinal cord and spinal nerves in vertebral canal

C1

Cervical enlargement (of spinal cord)

C8

Pedicles of vertebrae

T1

Central canal

Anterior horn

Anterior median fissure

Gray matter

Anterior rootlets

White matter

Posterior rootlets

Posterior horn

Anterior root

Posterior root

Spinal nerve

Sympathetic trunk

Anterior ramus

Spinal ganglion

Sympathetic ganglion

Posterior ramus

White ramus communicans

Posterior median sulcus

Posterior intermediate sulcus

Posterolateral sulcus

Recurrent meningeal branches of spinal nerve

Gray ramus communicans

Lumbosacral enlargement (of spinal cord)

T12

Conus medullaris

Cauda equina

L1

Features of the spinal cord (thoracic region) and basic organization of a spinal nerve (posterior view)

Vertebral body

Sympathetic ganglion

Gray and white rami communicantes

Anterior root

Spinal ganglion

Spinal nerve

Anterior ramus

L5

S1

Posterior ramus

Intervertebral foramen

Posterior root

Spinous process

S5

Co

Filum terminale

Spinal nerves (transverse section)

FIGURE 2-107 Features of the spinal cord and basic organization of spinal nerves. (From Drake RL et al, editors: *Gray's atlas of anatomy,* ed 2, Philadelphia, 2015, Churchill Livingstone.)

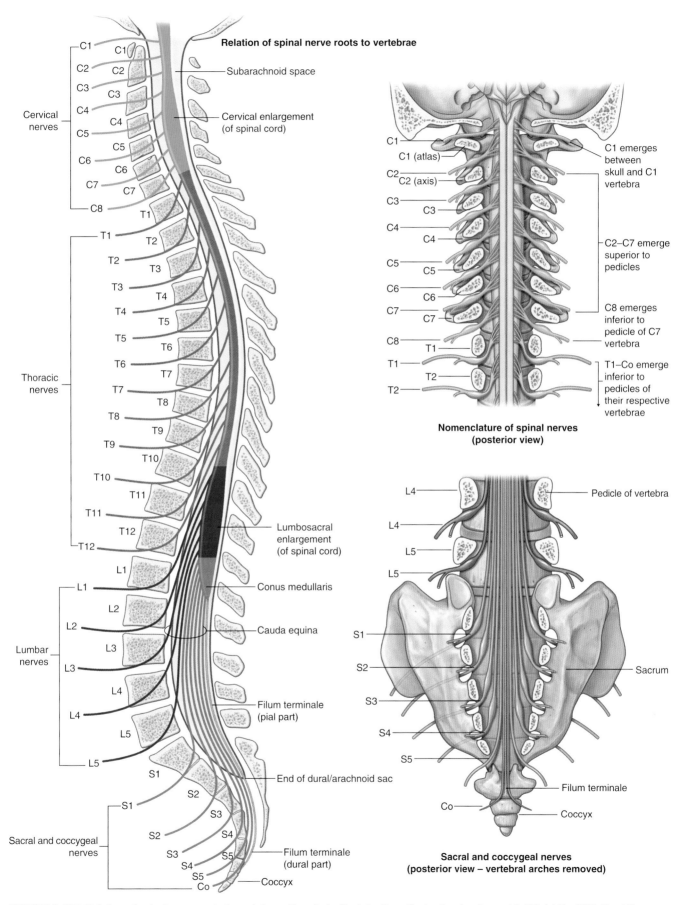

FIGURE 2-108 Relation of spinal nerve roots to vertebrae. (From Drake RL et al, editors: *Gray's atlas of anatomy,* ed 2, Philadelphia, 2015, Churchill Livingstone.)

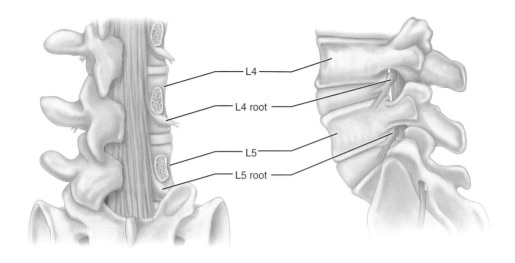

FIGURE 2-109 Lumbar spine nerve roots.

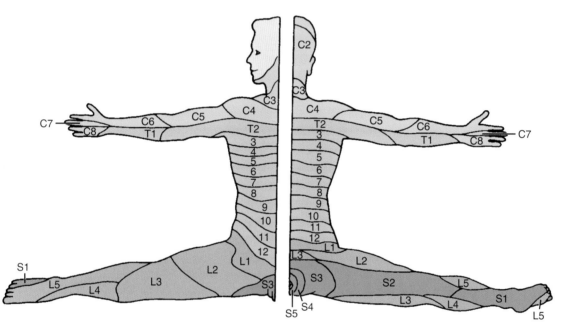

FIGURE 2-110 Dermatome patterns.

Table 2-47	Key Testable Neurologic Levels	
NEUROLOGIC LEVEL	**REPRESENTATIVE MUSCLE**	**REFLEX**
C5	Deltoid	Biceps
C6	Wrist extension	Brachioradialis
C7	Wrist flexion	Triceps
C8	Finger flexion	
T1	Interossei	
L4	Tibialis anterior	Patellar
L5	Toe extensors	
S1	Peroneal	Achilles

Table 2-48	Cervical Sympathetic Ganglia	
GANGLION	**LOCATION**	**COMMENTS**
Superior	C2-C3	Largest
Middle	C6	Variable
Inferior	C7-T1	Stellate

delivered underneath the posterior longitudinal ligament in four separate ostia.

▪ Vertebral artery (a branch of the subclavian artery)
  ● Ascends through the transverse foramina of C1 to C6 (anterior to and not through C7) posterior to the longus colli muscle and then posterior to the lateral masses; courses along the cephalic surface of the posterior arch of C1 (atlas); and passes ventromedially around the spinal cord and through the foramen magnum before uniting at the midline basilar artery
  ● The distance from the spinous process of C1 laterally to the vertebral artery is 2 cm (a safe distance for dissections would therefore be less than 2 cm).

▪ **Artery of Adamkiewicz (great anterior medullary artery)**
  ● Enters through the left intervertebral foramen in the lower thoracic spine from T8 to T12; supplies the interior two thirds of the anterior cord

▪ Spinal cord arterial supply
  ● From the anterior and posterior spinal arteries and segmental branches of the vertebral artery and dorsal

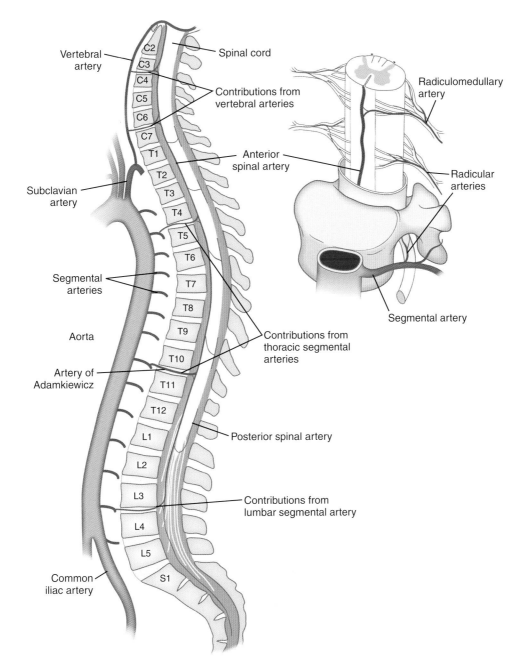

FIGURE 2-111 Vascular anatomy of the spinal column. (From Miller MD et al: *Orthopaedic surgical approaches,* ed 2, Philadelphia, 2014, Saunders, Figure 5-18.)

arteries, which travel via the dorsal and ventral rootlets to the respective dorsal and anterolateral portions of the cord
- Disruption of the anterior longitudinal artery can result in loss of function of the anterior two thirds of the cord.
▤ Venous drainage of the vertebral bodies
- Primarily through the central sinusoid located on the dorsum of each vertebral body

SURGICAL APPROACHES TO THE SPINE (TABLE 2-49)

■ **Cervical spine (see Figure 2-111)**
▤ Anterior approach to the cervical spine
- Surface landmarks demonstrated in Figure 2-112

- Incision: transverse and based on the desired level (e.g., for C5, the carotid triangle should be entered)
- Dissection
  - Retract the platysma with the skin.
  - Expose the pretracheal fascia to explore the interval between the carotid sheath—which contains the internal and common carotid arteries, the internal jugular vein, and the vagus nerve (cranial nerve X)—and the trachea.
  - Incise the prevertebral fascia sharply, and then retract the longus colli muscle gently (protecting the recurrent laryngeal nerve, a branch of the vagus nerve that lies outside the sheath) to expose the vertebral body. The anterior surface of the vertebral body is exposed.

Table 2-49	**Surgical Approaches to the Spine**	
APPROACH	**INTERVAL**	**STRUCTURES AT RISK**
Anterior cervical	Carotid sheath and the trachea	Recurrent laryngeal nerve
		Sympathetic ganglion
Posterior cervical	Midline approach between paracervical muscle	Vertebral artery
Anterior thoracic	Transverse between ribs two levels above surgical site	Intercostal neurovascular bundle; to avoid, dissect over top of rib
Posterior thoracolumbar	Midline approach over spinous processes	Posterior primary rami and segmental vessels; protect nerve root
Anterior lumbar (transperitoneal)	Between segmentally innervated rectus abdominis	Presacral plexus of parasympathetic nerve

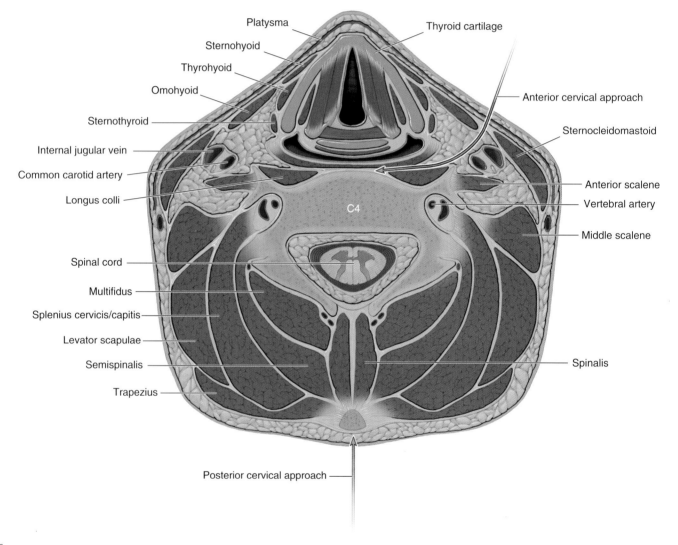

FIGURE 2-112 Cervical spine surgical intervals. (From Miller MD et al: *Orthopaedic surgical approaches,* ed 2, Philadelphia, 2014, Saunders, Figure 5-16.)

- Risks:
  - **Injury to the recurrent laryngeal nerve with right-sided approaches (paralysis is identified by a hoarse, scratchy voice caused by unilateral vocal cord paralysis, visualized with direct laryngoscopy).**
  - **Recurrent laryngeal nerve arises from the vagus at the level of the subclavian artery on the right; the left arises at the level of the aortic arch.**

- Anterior cervical approaches from the lower left side increase the risk for injury to the thoracic duct, which is posterior to the carotid sheath.
- When the longus muscles are dissected subperiosteally, the stellate ganglion is also protected (avoiding Horner syndrome).
- Postoperatively, the upper airway is at risk for edema, vocal cord paralysis, and hematoma.

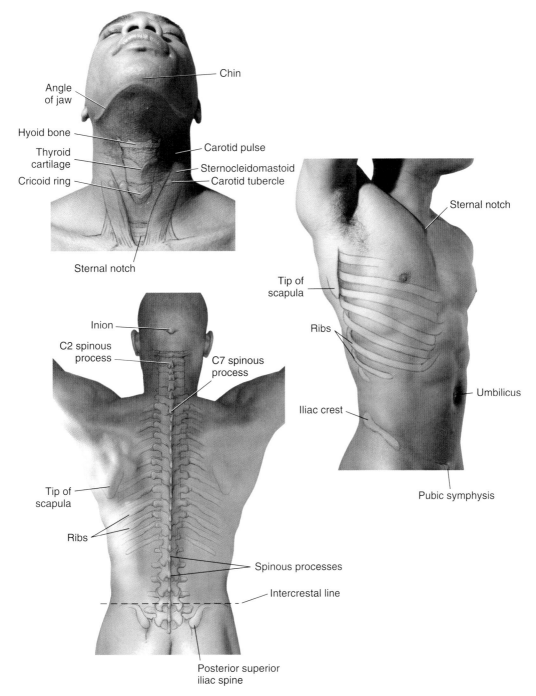

FIGURE 2-113 Surface landmarks. (From Miller MD et al: *Orthopaedic surgical approaches,* ed 2, Philadelphia, 2014, Saunders, Figure 5-20.)

▓ Posterior approach to the cervical spine
- Incision: midline
- Dissection:
  - After a midline approach through the ligamentum nuchae, reflect the superficial (trapezius) and intermediate (splenius, semispinalis, longissimus capitis) layers laterally; the vertebrae are exposed.
  - Access to the spinal canal is through laminectomy or facetectomy.
- Risks:
  - The vertebral artery is especially vulnerable as it leaves the foramen transversarium and travels superiorly and medially to pierce the atlantooccipital membrane at its lateral angle.

- The greater occipital nerve (C2) and the third occipital nerve (C3) should also be protected in the suboccipital region.
- **Postoperative C5 palsy is the most common complication with a posterior approach.**

▓ **Thoracic spine (Figure 2-113)**
▓ Anterior (transthoracic) approach to the thoracic spine
- Incision: transverse, made approximately two ribs above the level of interest
- Dissection:
  - Dissect over the top of the rib to avoid injuring the intercostal neurovascular bundle (which lies on the inferior internal surface of the rib).

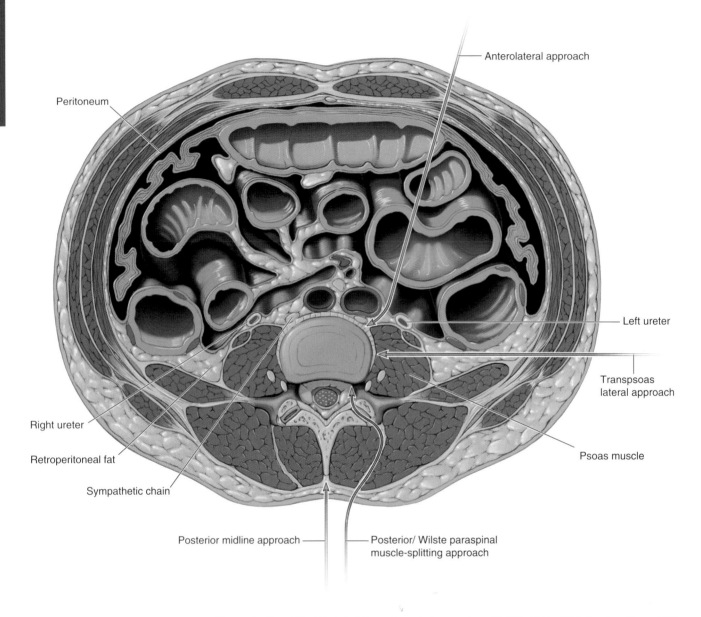

Peritoneum

Anterolateral approach

Left ureter

Transpsoas
lateral approach

Psoas muscle

Right ureter

Retroperitoneal fat

Sympathetic chain

Posterior midline approach

Posterior/ Wilste paraspinal
muscle-splitting approach

FIGURE 2-114 Lumbar spine surgical intervals. (From Miller MD et al: *Orthopaedic surgical approaches,* ed 2, Philadelphia, 2014, Saunders, Figure 5-17.)

- Further dissect the rib and remove it from the surgical field.
- The right-sided approach is favored to avoid the aorta, segmental arteries, artery of Adamkiewicz, and thoracic duct (in the upper thoracic spine on the left side of the esophagus and behind the carotid sheath).
- Risks:
  - The esophagus, aorta, venae cavae, and pleura of the lungs should be identified and protected.
  - Intercostal neuralgia is the most common complication.
- Posterior approach to the thoracolumbar spine
  - Incision: straight, midline, over the spinous processes and carried down through the thoracolumbar fascia
  - Dissection:
    - Use the plane between the two segmentally innervated erector spinae muscles.

- Subperiosteally dissect the paraspinal musculature from the attached spinous processes, thereby exposing the posterior elements.
- Perform partial laminectomy to allow greater exposure of the cord and discs.
- Place pedicle screws at the junction of the lateral border of the superior facet and the middle of the transverse process.
- Angle these screws 15 degrees medially and in line with the slope of the vertebra, as seen on lateral radiographs.
- Risks: injury to the posterior primary rami (near the facet joints) and segmental vessels (anterior to the plane connecting the transverse processes)

■ **Lumbar spine**

▨ Anterior approach to the lumbar spine (transperitoneal)
  - Incision: longitudinal, from below the umbilicus to just above the pubic symphysis (Figure 2-114)

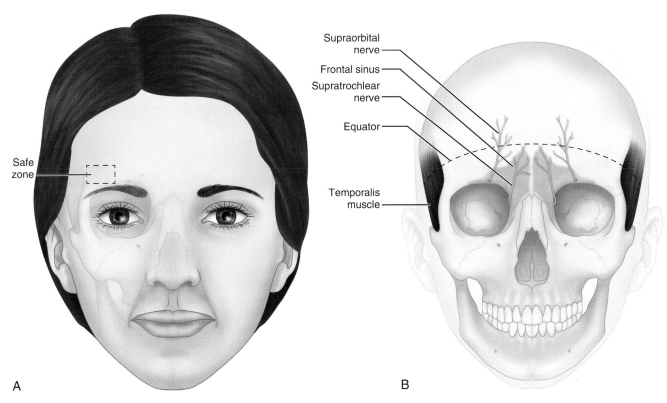

Supraorbital nerve

Frontal sinus

Supratrochlear nerve

Equator

Temporalis muscle

A

B

FIGURE 2-115 Safe zone and surrounding nerves of Halo pin placement.

- Dissection:
  - Split the rectus abdominis muscles and incise the peritoneum.
  - Protect and retract the bladder distally and the bowel cephalad; incise the posterior peritoneum longitudinally over the sacral promontory.
  - The aortic bifurcation is revealed; ligate the middle sacral artery.
  - The L5-S1 disc space is exposed.
- **Risks: injury to the lumbar plexus (particularly the superior hypogastric plexus of the sympathetic plexus that lies over the L5 vertebral body) can cause sexual dysfunction and retrograde ejaculation.** (Ejaculation is predominantly a sympathetic nervous system function and erection predominantly a parasympathetic nervous system function.)
- Anterolateral approach to the lumbar spine (retroperitoneal)
  - Incision: oblique, centered over the twelfth rib to the lateral border of the rectus abdominis muscle
  - Dissection:
    - Incise the external oblique, internal oblique, and transversus abdominis muscles in line with the skin incision.
    - Elevate the retroperitoneal fat, thereby revealing the psoas major muscle and genitofemoral nerve.

- Ligate the segmental lumbar vessels; mobilize the aorta and venae cavae to expose the desired vertebral level.
- **The great vessels typically bifurcate at the L4-L5 disc level;** therefore, use a larger area of dissection than would be used for operating on the L5-S1 disc level, which lies below the bifurcation of the aorta.
- Risks: injury to the sympathetic chain (medial to the psoas and lateral to the vertebral body) and ureters (between the peritoneum and psoas fascia)
- Halo pin placement
  - **Safe zone for anterolateral halo pins is approximately 1 cm superior to the orbital rim in the outer two thirds of the orbit below the equator of the skull** (Figure 2-115)
  - With this pin position, the temporal fossa and temporalis muscle are situated laterally, and the supraorbital nerve, supratrochlear nerve, and frontal sinus are situated medially.
  - Supraorbital nerve is lateral to the supratrochlear nerve, which lies anterior to the frontal sinus.
  - Most commonly injured cranial nerve with halo traction is the abducens (cranial nerve VI); injury is recognized from the loss of lateral gaze.

TESTABLE CONCEPTS

SECTION 2 UPPER EXTREMITY

- Glenoid retroverted approximately 5 degrees relative to scapular body. Suprascapular notch: superior transverse scapular ligament separates suprascapular artery (superior) from the suprascapular nerve (inferior). mnemonic: "Army over Navy" for artery over nerve).
- Coracoacromial ligament is an important anterosuperior restraint and should be preserved with irreparable cuff tears to prevent anterosuperior escape.
- Clavicle first bone to ossify (at 5 weeks' gestation) and the last to fuse (medial epiphysis at 25 years of age)
- Do not repair anterosuperior glenoid labral variants; loss of external rotation can result.
- Humeral head height is approximately 5.6 cm above superior border of pectoralis major tendon (important for arthroplasty).
- Trapezoid ligament (anterolateral) and conoid ligament (posteromedial) approximately 25 and 45 mm, respectively, from AC joint
- Approximately 2:1 ratio between glenohumeral and scapulothoracic motion with arm elevation
- Rotator cuff depresses and stabilizes the humeral head against the glenoid.
- Radial head should line up with capitellum at all arm positions with all radiographic views.
- Tensile forces at medial elbow, compressive forces at lateral elbow
- Ulnar collateral ligament (especially anterior band) is primary static stabilizer to valgus stress at the elbow.
- Posterolateral rotatory instability (PLRI) of elbow with lateral ulnar collateral (LUCL) injury
- Restoration of radial bow is paramount in fixation of radial shaft fractures to prevent pronation and supination loss.
- Space of Poirier is a central weak area in the floor of carpal tunnel that is implicated in lunate volar dislocation in perilunate injuries of the wrist.
- Guyon canal: contains ulnar nerve and artery; borders are flexor retinaculum (deep), volar carpal ligament (superficial), pisiform (ulnar/proximal), hook of hamate (radial/distal).
- A2 pulley, overlying the proximal phalanx, is the most critical to function, followed by A4, which covers the middle phalanx.
- Medial winging: long thoracic nerve (C5-C7) injury leading to serratus anterior dysfunction
- Lateral winging: spinal accessory nerve (cranial nerve XI) injury leading to trapezius dysfunction
- Preclavicular brachial plexus branches: dorsal scapular nerve, long thoracic nerve, suprascapular nerve, nerve to subclavius
- The radial nerve traverses the radial groove in the posterior humerus approximately 20 cm from medial epicondyle and 14 cm from lateral epicondyle.
- The ulnar nerve is posteromedial to brachial artery in upper arm and then passes posterior to the medial intermuscular septum at the arcade of Struthers (8-10 cm from the medial epicondyle).
- The ulnar nerve splits the two heads of the FCU as it enters the forearm, and the median nerve splits the two heads of the pronator teres.
- Lateral antebrachial cutaneous nerve: continuation of the musculocutaneous nerve that passes lateral to the cephalic vein after emerging laterally from between the biceps and brachialis at the elbow
- Digital arteries arise from superficial palmar arch and run dorsal to the digital nerves.
- Median nerve sites of potential compression: ligament of Struthers, pronator teres, FDS aponeurosis, bicipital aponeurosis, accessory head of FPL, carpal tunnel

- AIN syndrome is motor only with no sensory symptoms.
- Ulnar nerve sites of potential compression: arcade of Struthers, medial intermuscular septum, cubital tunnel, medial epicondyle, two heads of FCU, anconeus epitrochlearis, Guyon canal
- More clawing with distal ulnar nerve compression as FDP function to ring and small maintained
- Radial nerve sites of potential compression: fibrous bands at elbow joint, recurrent leash of Henry, ECRB, arcade of Frohse, supinator
- Pronate the forearm during lateral approach to elbow/posterior approach to forearm to move the PIN anteriorly and radially.
- Supinate the forearm during anterior approach to forearm to move PIN posteriorly and laterally.

SECTION 3 LOWER EXTREMITY

- Iliac spine separates greater and lesser sciatic notch; sacrospinous ligament (anterior sacrum to ischial spine) separates greater and lesser sciatic foramina.
- Pediatric femoral nail insertion: piriformis starting point threatens the posterosuperior retinacular vessels (potential for femoral head avascular necrosis [AVN]).
- Slipped capital femoral epiphysis occurs through the femoral head physis (zone of hypertrophy).
- Fibrocartilaginous labrum deepens acetabulum, enhancing stability. Labral functions include load transmission, maintenance of vacuum seal, regulation of synovial fluid hydrodynamics, and joint lubrication.
- Iliofemoral ligament (Y ligament of Bigelow) is the strongest ligament in the body and attaches the AIIS to the intertrochanteric line in an inverted Y manner.
- At the knee joint, the medial tibial plateau is concave and the lateral plateau is convex. This results in a joint with greater osseous congruity medially than laterally.
- Accessory or "bipartite" patella may represent failure of fusion of the superolateral corner of the patella and is commonly confused with patellar fractures.
- Peripheral one third of the menisci are vascular and are amenable to repair (red zone); the inner two thirds are nourished by synovial fluid (white zone) and have limited healing capacity.
- ACL has anteromedial (tight in flexion) and posterolateral (tight in extension) bundles; PL bundle tested with pivot shift exam.
- PCL has anterolateral (tight in flexion) and posteromedial (tight in extension) bundles.
- Posterolateral corner (PLC): fibular collateral ligament, popliteus tendon, and popliteofibular ligament; other PLC structures include biceps femoris tendon, lateral head of gastrocnemius, biceps femoris, arcuate ligament, and posterolateral capsule.
- Dial test: rotational instability at 30 degrees = PLC injury, at 30 and 90 degrees = combined PLC + PLC injury
- Primary blood supply to the talar body is from the artery of the tarsal canal (posterior tibial artery).
- Position of the ankle is critical when the lateral ligament complex is tested. Plantar flexion tightens the anterior talofibular ligament, and inversion with neutral flexion tightens the calcaneofibular ligament.
- Ankle syndesmosis (connection between the tibia and fibula) supported by four ligaments: anterior and posterior inferior tibiofibular ligaments, a transverse tibiofibular ligament, and an interosseous ligament. Syndesmotic injury often referred to as "high-ankle sprain."
- Plantar calcaneonavicular ligament (spring ligament) supports head of talus; attenuated in pes planus deformity.
- Position of the ankle is critical when the lateral ligament complex is tested. Plantar flexion tightens the anterior talofibular ligament, and inversion with neutral flexion tightens the calcaneofibular ligament.

TESTABLE CONCEPTS

- The Lisfranc ligament connects the medial (shortest) cuneiform to the second (longest) metatarsal.
- Use the mnemonic "Tom, Dick, and Harry" to remember the order of the structures coursing along the posterior border of the medial malleolus (tibialis posterior, flexor digitorum longus, and flexor hallucis longus).
- Use the mnemonic "POP'S IQ" to remember the nerves exiting the pelvis below the piriformis (pudendal, nerve to obturator internus, posterior femoral cutaneous, sciatic, inferior gluteal, nerve to quadratus femoris).
- Infrapatellar branch supplies the skin of the medial side of the front of the knee and patellar ligament and can be damaged during total knee replacement surgery or patella tendon harvest.
- Retractors placed behind the transverse acetabular ligament or screw placement in anteroinferior quadrant of acetabulum can injure the obturator nerve and artery.
- Most proximal branch of the lateral plantar nerve is the nerve to the abductor digiti quinti (Baxter nerve).
- The dorsal medial cutaneous nerve (a branch of the superficial peroneal nerve) crosses the EHL in a lateral-to-medial direction and supplies sensation to the dorsomedial aspect of the great toe.
- Corona mortis is an anastomotic connection between the inferior epigastric branch of the external iliac vessels and the obturator vessels in the obturator canal.
- Medial and lateral femoral circumflex vessels are named for location relative to iliopsoas tendon.
- Several genicular branches are given off in the popliteal fossa, including the medial and lateral geniculate arteries (which supply the menisci) and the middle geniculate artery (which supplies the cruciate ligaments).
- Stoppa modification uses more extensive medial window and provides access to pelvic brim and quadrilateral plate.
- Superior gluteal nerve passes between gluteus medius and minimus approximately 5 cm proximal to tip of greater trochanter.

SECTION 4 SPINE

- 50% of total neck flexion and extension occurs at the occiput-C1 articulation; 50% of total neck rotation occurs at C1-C2.

- Vertebral artery travels in the transverse foramina of C6 to C1 (not C7).
- Diameter of the cervical spine canal is normally 17 mm, and the cervical cord may become compromised when the diameter is reduced to less than 13 mm (relative stenosis).
- Narrowest pedicles at T5
- Transverse ligament is the major stabilizer of the atlantoaxial joint.
- Annulus fibrosus: obliquely oriented, composed of type I collagen
- Central nucleus pulposus: made of type II collagen and softer than the annulus
- In the cervical spine, the numbered nerve exits at a level above the pedicle of the corresponding vertebral level (e.g., the C2 nerve exits at the level of vertebrae C1-C2) (see Figure 2-108).
- In the lumbar spine, the nerve root traverses the respective disc space above the named vertebral body and exits the respective foramen under the pedicle.
- Central disc herniation impinges upon the traversing nerve root; lateral disc herniation impinges on the exiting nerve root.
- L5 nerve root is relatively fixed to the anterior sacral ala and can be damaged by sacral fractures and errant anteriorly placed iliosacral screws.
- Disruption of the inferior cervical ganglia can lead to Horner syndrome (ptosis, miosis [pupillary constriction], and anhidrosis).
- Injury to the recurrent laryngeal nerve can occur with right-sided anterior cervical approaches; paralysis is identified by a hoarse, scratchy voice caused by unilateral vocal cord paralysis, visualized with direct laryngoscopy.
- Recurrent laryngeal nerve arises from the vagus at the level of the subclavian artery on the right; the left arises at the level of the aortic arch.
- Postoperative C5 palsy is the most common complication with a posterior cervical approach.
- Injury to the lumbar plexus, particularly the superior hypogastric plexus of the sympathetic plexus that lies over the L5 vertebral body, can cause sexual dysfunction and retrograde ejaculation.
- Great vessels bifurcate at the L4-L5 disc.
- Safe zone for anterolateral halo pins is approximately 1 cm superior to the orbital rim in the outer two thirds of the orbit below the equator of the skull.

CHAPTER 3

PEDIATRIC ORTHOPAEDICS

Matthew R. Schmitz, Jeremy K. Rush, and Todd A. Milbrandt

CONTENTS

SECTION 1 UPPER EXTREMITY PROBLEMS*

BRACHIAL PLEXUS PALSY

- **Clinical features**
- In 2 per 1000 births, an injury is still associated with stretching or contusion of the brachial plexus.
- Typically present with internal rotation shoulder contracture and elbow and wrist flexion contractures
  - Progressive glenoid hypoplasia occurs in 70% of children with significant internal rotation contracture.
- Hand function varies with level of brachial plexus deformity.
- Three types commonly recognized (Table 3-1):
  - Erb-Duchenne (C5, C6)—best prognosis, most common
  - Klumpke (C8, T1)—poor prognosis
  - Total plexus palsy—worse prognosis
- **Causes**
- Large size of neonate, shoulder dystocia, forceps delivery, breech position, prolonged labor
- **Radiologic studies**
- Investigations have focused on the position of the humeral head within the glenoid.
  - Posterior subluxation with erosion of the glenoid should be prevented.
- Axillary lateral view of the shoulder should be obtained to evaluate position of humeral head.
- Consider computed tomographic (CT) scanning instead of magnetic resonance imaging (MRI) of the shoulder if surgical reconstruction is planned.
- **Treatment**
- Key to success of therapy is maintaining passive ROM and awaiting return of motor function (up to 18 months)
  - Parents should focus on passive elbow motion and shoulder elevation, abduction, and external rotation.
- More than 90% of cases eventually resolve without intervention.
  - Lack of biceps function 6 months after injury and the presence of Horner syndrome carry a poor prognosis.

- Options: early surgery to address nerve function, late surgery to address deformities
  - Microsurgical nerve grafting
  - Latissimus and teres major transfer to shoulder external rotators (L'Episcopo)
  - Tendon transfers for elbow flexion (Clark pectoral transfer and Steindler flexorplasty)
  - Pectoral and subscapularis release for internal rotation contracture and secondary glenoid hypoplasia (<5 years old)
  - Proximal humerus rotational osteotomy (>5 years old)
- Release of the subscapularis tendon for internal rotation contracture, if performed by age 2 years, may result in improved active external rotation of the shoulder, with muscle transfer to assist in active external rotation.

SPRENGEL DEFORMITY

- **Clinical features**
- Undescended scapula often associated with winging, hypoplasia, and omovertebral connections (30% of cases; Figure 3-1)
- Most common congenital anomaly of the shoulder in children
- Affected scapulae are usually small, relatively wide, and medially rotated.
- Associated diseases:
  - Klippel-Feil syndrome (one third have Sprengel deformity)
  - Kidney disease
  - Scoliosis
  - Diastematomyelia
- **Treatment**
- Surgery for cosmetic or functional deformities (decreased abduction)
  - Distal advancement of associated muscles and scapula (Woodward procedure) or
  - Detachment and movement of scapula (Schrock and Green procedures)
  - Both can improve abduction by 40 to 50 degrees
- Clavicular osteotomy is often needed to avoid brachial plexus injury caused by stretch.

---

*See Chapter 7, Hand, Upper Extremity, and Microvascular Surgery.

Table 3-1	Brachial Plexus Palsy		
TYPE	**ROOTS**	**DEFICIT**	**PROGNOSIS**
Erb-Duchenne palsy	C5, C6	Deltoid, cuff, elbow flexors, wrist and hand dorsiflexors; "waiter's tip" deformity	Best
Total plexus	C5, T1	Sensory and motor; flaccid arm	Worst
Klumpke palsy	C8, T1	Wrist flexors, intrinsic muscles; Horner syndrome	Poor

AR, Autosomal recessive; *XR,* X-linked recessive.

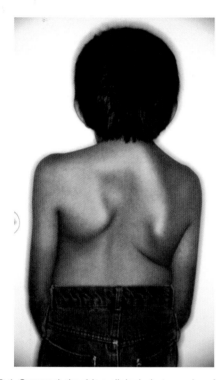

FIGURE 3-1 Sprengel shoulder: clinical photographs of a child affected with Sprengel deformity on the left side. Note the elevation and rotation of the scapula. (From Jones KL: *Smith's recognizable patterns of human malformation,* Philadelphia, 2006, Elsevier Saunders, p 716.)

▥ Surgery is best done when patients are 3 to 8 years of age.

FIBROTIC DELTOID PROBLEMS

■ **Clinical features**
▥ Short fibrous bands replace the deltoid muscle and cause abduction contractures at the shoulder, with elevation and winging of the scapula when the arms are adducted.
■ **Treatment**
▥ Surgical resection of these bands is often required.

CONGENITAL PSEUDARTHROSIS OF THE CLAVICLE

■ **Clinical features**
▥ Failure of union of medial and lateral ossification centers of right clavicle
   • Bilateral in less than 10%; left side if situs inversus
▥ Manifests as an enlarging, painless, nontender mass
■ **Causes**
▥ May be related to pulsations of the underlying subclavian artery
■ **Radiologic findings**
▥ Anteroposterior (AP) view of the clavicle reveals rounded sclerotic bone at the pseudarthrosis site.
■ **Treatment**
▥ Surgery (open reduction and internal fixation [ORIF] with bone grafting) is indicated for unacceptable cosmetic deformities or significant functional symptoms (mobility of fragments and winging of scapula) at age 3 to 6 years.
▥ Successful union is predictable (in contrast to congenital pseudarthrosis of tibia).

POLAND SYNDROME

■ **Clinical features**
▥ **Unilateral chest wall hypoplasia (sternocostal head of pectoralis major absent)**
▥ **Hypoplasia of hand and forearm**
▥ **Symbrachydactyly and shortening of middle fingers—simple syndactyly of ulnar digits, absence of shortening of middle digits**
■ **Cause: thought to be linked to subclavian artery hypoplasia**
■ **Exam**
▥ Chest deformities: chest wall hypoplasia, Sprengel deformity, scoliosis
▥ Hand deformities
   • Absence or hypoplasia of metacarpals and phalanges
   • Carpal bone abnormalities
   • Absence of flexor and extensor tendons
   • Can be associated with radioulnar synostosis
■ **Treatment: syndactyly release; caution with lack of soft tissue coverage requiring full thickness skin graft**

APERT SYNDROME

■ **Introduction**
▥ **Autosomal dominant due to mutation in *FGFr2* gene**
▥ Syndrome characteristics
   • Bilateral complex syndactyly of hands and feet
   • **Craniosynostosis—premature closure of cranial sutures—flattened skull with broad forehead**
   • Ankylosis of interphalangeal joints (symphalangism)
   • Radioulnar synostosis
   • Glenoid hypoplasia
   • Decreased mental capabilities
■ **Treatment**
▥ Surgical release of border digits done at 1 year of life
▥ Digital reconstruction of middle digits to turn 3 digits into 2 digits done at 2 years old

SECTION 2 LOWER EXTREMITY PROBLEMS: GENERAL

ROTATIONAL PROBLEMS OF THE LOWER EXTREMITIES

▪ Introduction
▦ In-toeing usually attributable to metatarsus adductus (in infants), internal tibial torsion (in toddlers), and femoral anteversion (in children < 10 years)
▦ **Out-toeing typically a result of external rotation hip contracture (in infants) and external tibial torsion and external femoral torsion (in older children and adolescents)**
▦ All these problems may be a result of intrauterine positioning.
▦ Deformities usually bilateral; clinician should be wary of asymmetric findings
▦ Evaluation should include measurements noted in Table 3-2 and illustrated in Figure 3-2.

▪ Metatarsus adductus
▦ Clinical features
  • Forefoot adducted at tarsal-metatarsal joint
  • Lateral border of foot is convex instead of straight
  • Usually seen during first year of life
  • May be associated with hip dysplasia (10%-15% of cases)
  • Approximately 85% of cases resolve spontaneously.

▦ Treatment
  • Nonoperative
    • Feet that can be actively corrected to neutral position require no treatment.
    • Stretching exercises are used for feet that can be passively corrected to neutral position (heel bisector line aligns with second metatarsal).
    • Feet that cannot be passively corrected (rare situation) usually respond to serial casting, with mixed results.
  • Surgery
    • Lateral column shortening and medial column lengthening
    • Results with osteotomies are best when surgery is performed after 5 years of age (mixed results).

▪ Internal tibial torsion
▦ Clinical features
  • Most common cause of inward turning of toes
  • Usually seen during second year of life and can be associated with metatarsus adductus and developmental dysplasia of the hip (DDH)
  • Often bilateral and may be secondary to excessive medial ligamentous tightness
  • Internal rotation of tibia causes pigeon-toed gait.

Table 3-2	Evaluation of Rotational Problems of the Lower Extremities		
MEASUREMENT	**TECHNIQUE**	**NORMAL VALUES (degrees)**	**SIGNIFICANCE**
Foot-progression angle	Foot vs. straight line	–5 to +20	Nonspecific rotation
Medial rotation	Prone hip ROM	20-60	>70 degrees: femoral anteversion
Lateral rotation	Prone hip ROM	30-60	<20 degrees: femoral anteversion
Thigh-foot angle	Knee bent; foot up	0-20	<–10 degrees: tibial torsion
Foot lateral border	Convex; medial crease	Straight; flexible	Metatarsus adductus

ROM, Range of motion.

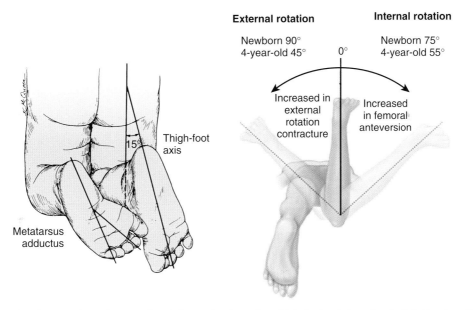

FIGURE 3-2 Hip internal and external rotation to estimate femoral anteversion; thigh-foot axis to estimate tibial torsion. (From Herring JA, editor: *Tachdjian's pediatric orthopaedics*, ed 5, Philadelphia, 2014, Elsevier Saunders, Figure 4-5.)

- Transmalleolar axis is internal.
- Thigh-foot axis of −10
- Treatment
  - Resolves spontaneously with growth
  - Operative correction is rarely necessary except in severe cases, which are addressed with a supramalleolar osteotomy when child is between 7 and 10 years of age.

External tibial torsion

- Clinical features
  - Cause of out-toeing; may cause disability and decrease physical performance
  - Can worsen with growth as tibia normally externally rotates with growth
  - Associated with increased femoral anteversion (miserable malalignment syndrome), early degenerative joint disease, neuromuscular conditions
  - Presents with knee pain due to patellofemoral malalignment
  - Thigh-foot axis greater than 40
- Treatment
  - Rest, rehabilitation
  - Supramalleolar osteotomy if age older than 8 to 10 years and external tibial torsion more than 40 degrees

Femoral anteversion

- Clinical features
  - Internal rotation of femur; seen in 3- to 6-year-olds
  - Children with this problem classically sit with the legs in a W-shaped position.
  - If associated with external tibial torsion, femoral anteversion may lead to patellofemoral problems.
- Treatment
  - Disorder usually corrects spontaneously by age 10
  - Special shoes, therapy, and derotational braces have never been shown to improve rates of remodeling.
  - In older children with less than 10 degrees of external rotation, femoral derotational osteotomy (intertrochanteric is best) may be considered for cosmesis, although this is not a functional problem.

LEG LENGTH DISCREPANCY

Clinical features

- Many potential causes:
  - Congenital disorders (e.g., hemihypertrophy, dysplasias, proximal femoral focal deficiency [PFFD], DDH)
  - Paralytic disorders (e.g., spasticity, polio)
  - Infection (disruption of physis)
  - Tumors
  - Trauma
- Long-term problems associated with leg length discrepancy include inefficient gait, equinus contractures of ankle, postural scoliosis and low back pain, possible hip osteoarthritis with uncovering of the femoral head of the long leg.
- Discrepancy must be measured accurately (e.g., with blocks of set height under affected side; with scanography).
  - Lateral CT scanography—more accurate than conventional scanography if there are soft tissue contractures of hip, knee, or ankle

- Can be tracked with Green-Anderson data, Moseley graph (with serial leg length radiographs or CT scanograms and with bone age determinations) or the Paley multiplier method (most accurate for congenital deformities)
- **A gross estimation of leg length discrepancy can be made under the following assumption of growth per year up to age 16 in boys and age 14 in girls** (Figure 3-3):
  - Distal femur: ⅜ inch (9 mm) per year
  - Proximal tibia: ¼ inch (6 mm) per year
  - Proximal femur: ⅛ inch (3 mm) per year
    - More accurate results with Moseley data

Treatment

- In general, projected discrepancies at maturity of less than 2 cm are observed or treated with shoe lifts.
  - Over 50% of population will have up to 2 cm of leg length discrepancy and be asymptomatic
- Discrepancies of 2 to 5 cm:
  - Epiphysiodesis of the long side
  - Shortening of the long side (ostectomy)
  - Lengthening of the short side
- Discrepancies of more than 5 cm are generally treated with lengthening.
- Lengthening:
  - With use of standard techniques, lengthening of 1 mm a day is typical.
  - Ilizarov principles are followed, including metaphyseal corticotomy (preserving medullary canal and blood supply) followed by gradual distraction
  - On rare occasions, physeal distraction (chondrodiastasis) can be considered.
    - This procedure must be performed in patients near skeletal maturity, because the physis almost always closes after this type of limb lengthening.

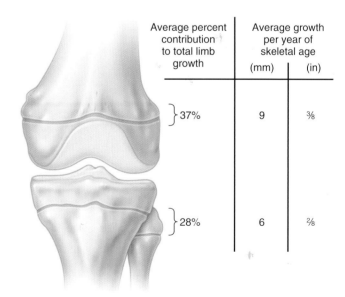

	Average percent contribution to total limb growth	Average growth per year of skeletal age	
		(mm)	(in)
	37%	9	⅜
	28%	6	¼

FIGURE 3-3 Approximate percentage of contribution to total leg length increase and average growth per skeletal year of maturation (in millimeters and inches) of the distal femoral and proximal tibial physes. (From Herring JA, editor: *Tachdjian's pediatric orthopaedics,* ed 4, Philadelphia, 2008, Saunders, Figure 24-16.)

SECTION 3 HIP AND FEMUR

DEVELOPMENTAL DYSPLASIA OF THE HIP

- **Introduction**
- Previously called *congenital dysplasia of the hip*
- Represents abnormal development or dislocation of the hip secondary to capsular laxity and mechanical factors (e.g., intrauterine positioning)
- Spectrum of disease
  - Dysplasia—shallow acetabulum
  - Subluxation
  - Dislocation
  - Teratologic—dislocated in utero and irreducible; associated with neuromuscular conditions and genetic abnormalities
  - Late dysplasia (adolescent and adult)
- **Risk factors**
- Breech positioning, positive family history (ligamentous laxity), female sex, and being a firstborn child are risk factors (in that order).
- Less intrauterine space accounts for increased incidence of DDH in firstborn children.
- DDH is observed most often in the **left hip** (67% of cases), in **girls** (85%), in infants with a positive family history (≥20%), in the presence of increased maternal estrogens, and in **breech births** (30% to 50%).
- Also associated with postnatal positioning such as swaddling with the hips in extension
- **Clinical features**
- Associated with other problems related to intrauterine positioning, such as torticollis (20% of cases) and metatarsus adductus (10%); no association with clubfoot
- If left untreated, muscles about the hip become contracted, and the acetabulum becomes more dysplastic and filled with fibrofatty tissue (pulvinar).
- Potential obstructions to obtaining a concentric reduction in DDH:
  - Iliopsoas tendon
  - Pulvinar
  - Contracted inferomedial hip capsule
  - Transverse acetabular ligament
  - Inverted labrum
- The teratologic form is most severe and usually necessitates early surgery.
  - A pseudoacetabulum is present at or near birth.
  - Teratologic hip dislocations commonly manifest in association with syndromes such as arthrogryposis and Larsen syndrome.
- **Diagnosis**
- Physical examination
  - Early diagnosis possible with **Ortolani test** (elevation and abduction of femur relocates a dislocated hip) and **Barlow test** (adduction and depression of femur dislocates a dislocatable hip)
  - All children should have screening done via physical examination.
    - Advanced screening is controversial, but many authors agree that children with significant risk factors (breech position, family history) should undergo screening ultrasound.

- Three phases are commonly recognized:
  - *Dislocated* (positive result of Ortolani test early; negative result of Ortolani test late, when femoral head cannot be reduced)
  - *Dislocatable* (positive result of Barlow test)
  - *Subluxatable* (suggestive result of Barlow test)
- Subsequent diagnosis is made with limitation of hip abduction in the affected hip as the laxity resolves and stiffness becomes more clinically evident.
  - Caution: abduction may be decreased symmetrically with bilateral dislocations.
- Another sign of dislocation includes the **Galeazzi sign**, demonstrated by the clinical appearance of foreshortening of the femur on the affected side.
  - This clinical test is performed with the feet held together and knees flexed (a congenitally short femur can also cause the Galeazzi sign).
- Other clinical findings associated with DDH include asymmetric gluteal folds (less reliable) and Trendelenburg stance (in older children), increased lumbar lordosis, and pelvic obliquity.
- Repeated examination, especially in an infant, is important because a child's irritability can prevent proper evaluation.
- Radiography
  - Dynamic ultrasonography is useful for making the diagnosis in young children before ossification of the femoral head (which occurs at age 4-6 months) (Figure 3-4).
    - Also useful for assessing reduction in a Pavlik harness and diagnosing acetabular dysplasia or capsular laxity
    - Success dependent on operator's skill
    - On the coronal view, the normal α angle is greater than 60 degrees, and the femoral head is bisected by the line drawn down the ilium.
  - Radiographic studies and findings (Figure 3-5)
    - Used in older children (after age 3 months)
    - Measurement of the acetabular index (normal, <25 degrees)
    - Measurement of the Perkin line (normally the ossific nucleus of the femoral head is medial to this line)
    - Evaluation of the Shenton line useful
    - Later, delayed ossification of the femoral head on the affected side may be visible **(femoral head ossification begins to show between 4 and 6 months old).**
    - Arthrography used to help judge closed reduction and possible blocks to reduction
    - Advanced imaging (CT, MRI) helpful after closed reduction to determine concentric reduction
- **Treatment (Figure 3-6)**
  Based on achieving and maintaining early "concentric reduction" to prevent future degenerative joint disease. Specific therapy is based on the child's age.
- Birth to 6 months:
  - In hips that have normal exam but abnormal ultrasound findings, treatment recommendations are uncertain
    - Children should have close follow-up.

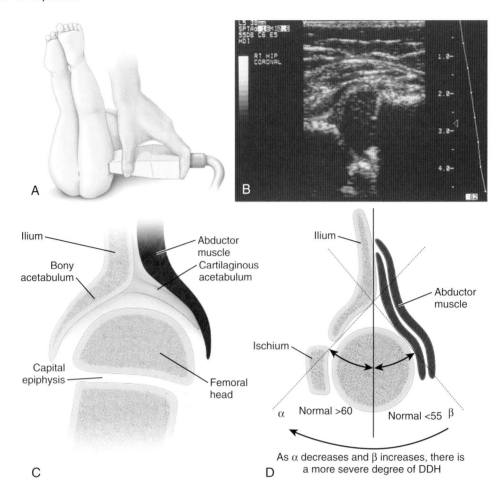

Ilium
Abductor muscle
Bony acetabulum
Cartilaginous acetabulum
Capital epiphysis
Femoral head

Ilium
Abductor muscle
Ischium
α Normal >60
Normal <55 β
As α decreases and β increases, there is a more severe degree of DDH

FIGURE 3-4 Ultrasound evaluation of the neonate's hip. **A,** Positioning of ultrasound transducer on a normal hip. **B,** Ultrasonogram. **C,** Illustration of ultrasound findings of a dislocated hip with poor bony roof. **D,** Graphic illustration of the dislocated hip. *DDH,* Developmental dysplasia of the hip. (From Herring JA, editor: *Tachdjian's pediatric orthopaedics,* ed 4, Philadelphia, 2008, Saunders.)

- Most authors recommend repeat ultrasound at age 6 weeks, with treatment if continued signs of dysplasia
- Pavlik harness
  - All Ortolani-positive hips (dislocated but reducible) should be treated with Pavlik.
  - Barlow-positive hips (reduced but dislocatable) may stabilize without treatment but should be watched closely; many authors advocate treating with Pavlik while observing.
- If dislocated, check reduction after 3 weeks on ultrasonography.
  - Not reduced: consider transition to rigid abduction orthosis vs. closed reduction, arthrography, and spica casting.
  - Reduced: continue harness until findings of examination and ultrasonography are normal.
- 6 to 18 months:
  - Hip arthrography, percutaneous adductor tenotomy, closed reduction, and spica casting
  - Postreduction CT or MRI scan used to confirm concentric reduction
  - If closed reduction fails: open reduction
- 18 months to 3 years:
  - Open reduction
- 3 to 8 years:
  - Osteotomy
    - Salter, Dega, Pemberton, or Staheli procedures

- Older than 8 years:
  - Osteotomy
    - Growth plate open: triple (Steele), double pelvic (Southerland), Staheli procedure
    - Growth plate closed: Ganz and Chiari procedures
  - Wait until the child is an adult to perform total hip arthroplasty.
- **Specific treatment modalities**
- Pavlik harness
  - Designed to maintain reduction in infants (<6 months) in about 100 degrees of flexion and mild abduction (the "human position" [Salter procedure])
  - Reduction should be confirmed by radiographs or ultrasound after placement in the harness and brace adjustment.
  - **Position of the hip should be within the "safe zone" of Ramsey (between maximum adduction before redislocation and excessive abduction, which increases risk of avascular necrosis [AVN]).**
  - Impingement of the **posterosuperior retinacular** branch of the medial femoral circumflex artery has been implicated in osteonecrosis associated with DDH treated in an abduction orthosis.
  - Pavlik harness treatment is contraindicated in teratologic hip dislocations.
  - A patient with a narrow safe zone (<40 degrees) should be considered for an adductor tenotomy.

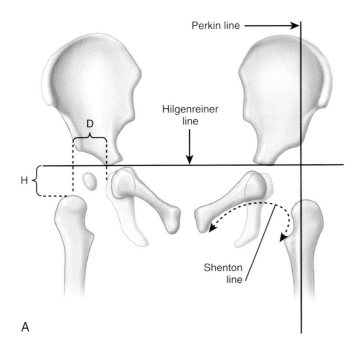

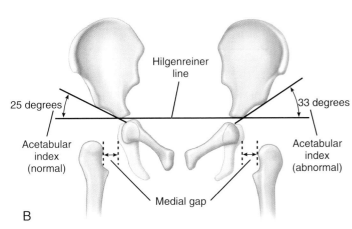

FIGURE 3-5 Common measurements used to evaluate developmental dysplasia of the hip, anterior view. Note the delayed ossification, disruption of the Shenton line, and increased acetabular index on the left hip, which is dislocated. (From Herring JA, editor: *Tachdjian's pediatric orthopaedics,* ed 4, Philadelphia, 2008, Saunders.)

- **Excessive flexion may result in transient femoral nerve palsy.**
- If attempts to reduce a hip do not succeed in 3 weeks, the Pavlik harness should be discontinued to prevent "Pavlik disease"—erosion of the pelvis superior to the acetabulum and subsequent difficulty with closed reduction and casting.
- The Pavlik harness is usually worn 23 hours a day for at least 6 weeks after a reduction has been achieved and then an additional 6 to 8 weeks part time (nights and during naps).
- **Risk factors for Pavlik failure:**
  - Patient older than age 7 weeks at initiation of treatment
  - Bilateral dislocations
  - Absent Ortolani sign
- Closed and open reduction
  - Closed reduction

- In general, performed for patients for whom Pavlik treatment fails and for patients 6 to 18 months of age
- Performed with patient under general anesthesia; procedure includes a physical examination, arthrography to assess reduction (look for "thorn sign" on arthrogram, indicating normal labral position), and hip spica casting with the legs flexed to at least 90 degrees and in the stable zone of abduction
- CT or MRI often performed to confirm that hip is well reduced, especially in questionable cases
- Open reduction
  - Reserved for children 6 to 18 months old in whom closed reduction fails, who have an obstructive limbus, or have an unstable safe zone
  - Open reduction is also the initial treatment for children 18 months of age and older.
  - Usually done through an anterior approach, especially for patients older than 12 months (less risk to medial femoral circumflex artery) and includes capsulorrhaphy, adductor tenotomy, femoral shortening to take tension off the reduction, and an acetabular procedure if severe dysplasia is present
  - **Five obstacles to reduction: transverse acetabular ligament, pulvinar, in-folded labrum, inferior capsular restriction, and psoas tendon**
  - Medial open reduction can be performed in children up to 12 months of age, results in less blood loss, directly addresses obstacles to reduction but does not provide access for a capsulorrhaphy, and is more often associated with osteonecrosis.
  - Surgical risks:
    - **Osteonecrosis**—the major risk associated with both open and closed reductions; caused by direct vascular injury or impingement vs. disruption of circulation from osteotomies
    - **Damage to medial femoral circumflex** can occur with medial approach to hip; close association to psoas, which undergoes a tenotomy because it is a block to reduction
    - Failure of open reduction is difficult to treat surgically because of the high complication rate of revision surgery (osteonecrosis in 50% and pain and stiffness in 33% according to one study)
    - Diagnosis after age 8 (younger in patients with bilateral DDH) may contraindicate reduction because the acetabulum has little chance to remodel, although reduction may be indicated in conjunction with salvage procedures.
- Osteotomy
  - Indications
    - May be required in toddlers and school-age children, usually for residual and persistent acetabular dysplasia
    - Osteotomies should be performed only after a congruent reduction is confirmed on an abduction–internal rotation view, with satisfactory range of motion (ROM), and after reasonable femoral sphericity is achieved by closed or open methods.
    - The choice of femoral versus pelvic osteotomy (Figure 3-7) is sometimes a matter of the surgeon's preference.

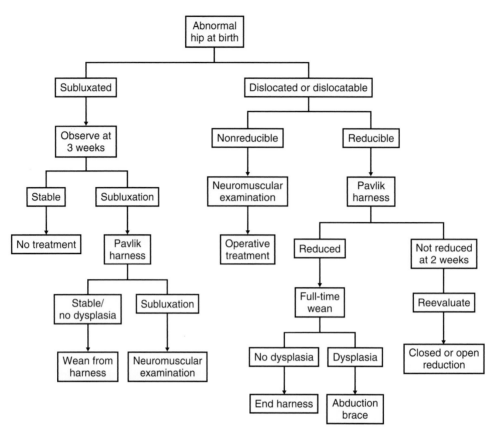

FIGURE 3-6 Algorithm for the treatment of developmental dysplasia of the hip. (Redrawn from Guille JT et al: Developmental dysplasia of the hip from birth to 6 months, *J Am Acad Orthop Surg* 8:232–242, 2000.)

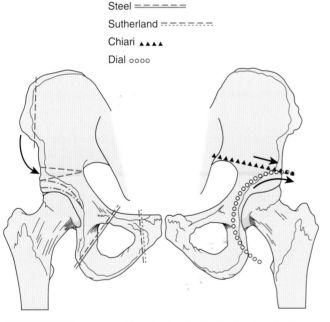

FIGURE 3-7 Common pelvic osteotomies for the treatment of developmental dysplasia of the hip. Both the Steel and Sutherland cuts use the Salter cut in addition to another cut.

- Pelvic osteotomies should be performed when severe dysplasia is accompanied by significant radiographic changes on the acetabular side (i.e., increased acetabular index, failure of lateral acetabular ossification), whereas changes on the

femoral side (e.g., marked anteversion, coxa valga) are best treated by femoral osteotomies.
- Osteotomies rarely correct hip dysplasia successfully after the age of 5 years. Table 3-3 lists common reconstructive osteotomies.
- Procedures
  - Salter osteotomy: redirectional; may lengthen the affected leg up to 1 cm
  - Pemberton acetabuloplasty: volume reducing; good choice for residual dysplasia (bends on triradiate cartilage)
  - Acetabular reorientation procedures in older patients include the triple innominate osteotomy (Steel or Tönnis procedure)
  - Dega-type osteotomies: volume reducing; often favored for paralytic dislocations and in patients with posterior acetabular deficiency
  - Ganz periacetabular osteotomy: redirectional; provides improved three-dimensional correction because the cuts are close to the acetabulum, allow immediate weight bearing, spare stripping of the abductor muscles, allow for a capsulotomy to inspect the joint, and are performed through a single incision. However, the triradiate cartilage must be closed.
  - Chiari osteotomy: salvage procedure when a concentric reduction of the femoral head within the acetabulum cannot be achieved. This osteotomy shortens the affected leg and requires periarticular soft tissue metaplasia for success. It depends on metaplastic tissue (fibrocartilage) for a successful result.

Table 3-3	Common Pelvic Osteotomies, Procedures, Requirements, and Indications		
OSTEOTOMY	PROCEDURE	REQUIREMENT	INDICATIONS
WITH CONCENTRIC REDUCTION			
Femoral	Intertrochanteric osteotomy (VDRO)	Concentric reduction before the age of 8 years	High neck-shaft angle, hip subluxation; usually performed in patients with cerebral palsy
Salter	Open-wedge osteotomy through ileum	Concentric reduction before the age of 8 years	Acetabular dysplasia without posterior wall loss; redirection osteotomy
Pemberton	Through acetabular roof to triradiate cartilage; does not enter sciatic notch	Concentric reduction before the age of 8 years	Acetabular dysplasia with a patulous cup; volume-reducing osteotomy
Dega	Through lateral ilium above acetabulum to triradiate cartilage; incomplete cuts through innominate bone	Concentric reduction; favored in those with posterior acetabular deficiency	Acetabular dysplasia with patulous cup; volume-reducing; favored in neuromuscular dislocations with posterior deficiency
Sutherland (double)	Salter and pubic osteotomy	Concentric reduction Open triradiate cartilage	More severe acetabular dysplasia; redirection procedure
Steel (triple)	Salter and osteotomy of both rami	Concentric reduction Open triradiate cartilage	Most severe acetabular dysplasia; redirection procedure
Ganz	Periacetabular osteotomy	Surgeon's experience Closed triradiate cartilage	Acetabular dysplasia in a skeletally mature patient
WITHOUT CONCENTRIC REDUCTION			
Chiari	Through ilium above acetabulum (makes new roof)	Nonreconstructable acetabulum	Salvage procedure for asymmetric incongruity
Shelf	Slotted lateral acetabular augmentation	Nonreconstructable acetabulum	Salvage procedure for asymmetric incongruity

VDRO, Varus derotation osteotomy.

- Lateral shelf acetabular augmentation procedure: for patients older than 8 years with inadequate lateral coverage or trochanteric advancement and increased trochanteric overgrowth (improves hip abductor biomechanics). It does not require concentric reduction. Success of this procedure depends on metaplastic tissue (fibrocartilage).

CONGENITAL COXA VARA

■ **Clinical features**
■ Bilateral in one third to half of cases
■ Coxa vara can be congenital (noted at birth and differentiated from DDH by MRI), developmental (autosomal dominant, progressive), acquired (e.g., trauma, Legg-Calvé-Perthes, slipped capital femoral epiphysis [SCFE]), or associated with skeletal dysplasia (cleidocranial dysplasia, spondyloepiphyseal dysplasia, metaphyseal dysplasia)
■ May manifest with waddling gait (bilateral) or painless limp (unilateral)
■ **Radiographic findings**
■ Triangular ossification defect in the inferomedial femoral neck in developmental coxa vara is common.
■ Neck-shaft angle is decreased as a result of a defect in ossification of the femoral neck.
■ Evaluation of the Hilgenreiner epiphyseal angle (angle between Hilgenreiner line and a line through proximal femoral physis) is the key to treatment (Figure 3-8).
■ **Treatment**
■ Based on Hilgenreiner epiphyseal angle (normal, < 25 degrees)
  - Less than 45 degrees spontaneously corrects
  - 45 to 60 degrees requires close observation
  - More than 60 degrees (with neck-shaft angle < 110 degrees) usually necessitates surgery
■ Surgical treatment is a corrective valgus osteotomy of the proximal femur.

▨ Subtrochanteric valgus osteotomy with or without derotation (Pauwels) is indicated for a neck-shaft angle of less than 90 degrees, a vertically oriented physeal plate, progressive deformities, or significant gait abnormalities.
▨ Concomitant distal/lateral transfer of the greater trochanter may also be indicated to restore more normal hip abductor mechanics.

LEGG-CALVÉ-PERTHES DISEASE (COXA PLANA)

■ **Clinical features**
▨ Noninflammatory deformity of proximal femur secondary to vascular insult of unknown origin, leading to osteonecrosis of proximal femoral epiphysis
▨ Pathologically, osteonecrosis is followed by revascularization and resorption through creeping substitution that eventually allows remodeling and fragmentation.
▨ Most common in boys 4 to 8 years of age with delayed skeletal maturation who are very active
▨ Increased incidence with a positive family history, low birth weight, and abnormal birth presentation (associated with delayed bone age and attention deficit hyperactivity disorder [ADHD])
▨ Symptoms include pain (often knee pain), effusion (from synovitis), and a limp.
▨ Decreased hip ROM (especially abduction and internal rotation) and a Trendelenburg gait are also common.
▨ Bilateral involvement may be seen in 12% to 15% of cases.
  - However, in bilateral cases the involvement is asymmetric and virtually never simultaneous.
  - Bilateral involvement may mimic multiple epiphyseal dysplasia (MED) and warrants a skeletal survey.
▨ Differential diagnosis includes septic arthritis, blood dyscrasias, hypothyroidism, and epiphyseal dysplasia.

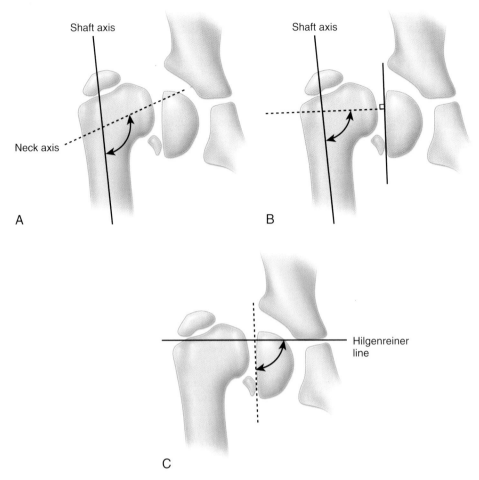

FIGURE 3-8 Quantification of the extent of radiographic deformity of the proximal femur in developmental coxa vara. **A,** The neck-shaft angle is the angle between the axis of the femoral shaft and the axis of the femoral neck. **B,** The head-shaft angle is the angle between the axis of the femoral shaft and an imaginary perpendicular line to the base of the capital femoral epiphysis. **C,** The Hilgenreiner–epiphyseal angle is the angle between the Hilgenreiner line and an imaginary line parallel to the capital femoral physis. (From Herring JA, editor: *Tachdjian's pediatric orthopaedics,* ed 3, Philadelphia, 2002, WB Saunders, p 767.)

- ■ **Radiographic findings**
- ▦ Vary with stage of disease but include cessation of growth of the ossific nucleus, medial joint space widening, and development of a "crescent sign" that represents subchondral fracture
- ▦ Classification
  - • Waldenström classification determines the four stages all cases follow:
    - • Initial—sclerotic epiphysis with joint widening (x-rays may not show changes for 4-6 months)
    - • Fragmentation—due to bone resorption and collapse (lateral pillar classification based on this stage)
    - • Reossification—new bone appears (may last up to 18 months)
    - • Healed or reossified—continued remodeling until maturity
  - • Most prognostic classification is Herring classification, or lateral pillar classification
    - • Based on involvement of lateral pillar of capital femoral epiphysis during the fragmentation stage (Figure 3-9, Table 3-4)
- ■ **Prognosis**
- ▦ Maintaining sphericity of femoral head is the most important factor in achieving a good result.

- ▦ Early degenerative hip joint disease results from aspherical femoral heads.
- ▦ Poor prognosis is associated with older age at onset (bone age > 6 years), female sex, lateral column C classification (regardless of age), and decreased hip ROM (decreased abduction).
- ▦ Radiographic findings associated with poor prognosis (Catterall "head at risk" signs):
  - • Lateral calcification
  - • Gage sign (V-shaped defect at lateral physis)
  - • Lateral subluxation
  - • Metaphyseal cyst formation
  - • Horizontal growth plate
- ■ **Treatment**
- ▦ Goals: relief of symptoms, restoration of ROM, and containment of the hip
- ▦ Use of outpatient or inpatient traction, antiinflammatory medications, and partial weight bearing with crutches for periods of 1 to 2 days to several weeks is helpful for relieving symptoms.
- ▦ ROM is maintained with traction, muscle release, exercise, use of a Petrie cast, or a combination of these measures.
- ▦ Herring described a treatment plan based on age and the lateral pillar classification of disease involvement.

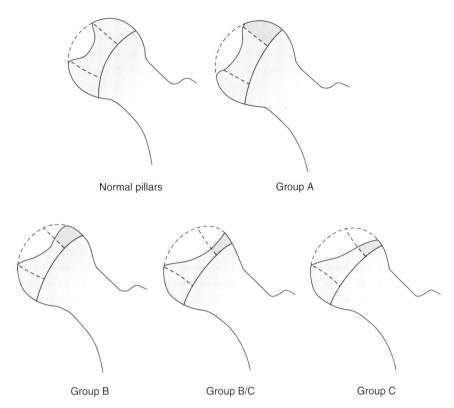

FIGURE 3-9 Lateral pillar classification of Legg-Calvé-Perthes disease. The definition of normal pillars was derived by noting the lines of demarcation between the central sequestrum and the remainder of the epiphysis on the anteroposterior radiograph. In group A, normal height of lateral pillar is maintained. In group B, more than 50% of height of lateral pillar is maintained. In group B/C (borderline), lateral pillar is 50% or less in height, but (1) it is very narrow (2 to 3 mm wide), (2) it has very little ossification, or (3) it has depressions in comparison with the central pillar. In group C, less than 50% of height of lateral pillar is maintained. (Adapted from Herring JA et al: The lateral pillar classification of Legg-Calvé-Perthes disease, *J Pediatr Orthop* 12:143–150, 1992.)

Table 3-4	Lateral Pillar Classification	
GROUP	**PILLAR INVOLVEMENT**	**PROGNOSIS**
A	Little or no involvement of the lateral pillar	Uniformly good outcome
B	>50% of lateral pillar height maintained	Good outcome in younger patients (bone age < 6 yr) but poorer outcome in older patients
C	<50% of lateral pillar height maintained	Poor prognosis in all age groups

- Surgical treatment may improve radiographic outcome at skeletal maturity for older patients (chronologic age > 8 years or bone age > 6 years) with lateral pillar groups B and B/C hips
- Containment
  - Femoral osteotomy—proximal femoral varus osteotomy
  - Pelvic osteotomy—Salter, triple, Dega, Pemberton
    - Shelf osteotomy to prevent lateral subluxation and lateral epiphyseal overgrowth
- Salvage
  - Valgus femoral osteotomy for hinge abduction
  - Chiari and/or shelf pelvic osteotomies for hips that can no longer be contained

SLIPPED CAPITAL FEMORAL EPIPHYSIS

Clinical features
- Disorder of proximal femoral epiphysis caused by weakness of perichondrial ring and slippage through hypertrophic zone of the growth plate

- Epiphysis remains in the acetabulum, and the neck is displaced anteriorly and rotates externally.
- SCFE is seen most often in obese adolescent African American boys during their rapid growth spurt (10-16 years of age); occasional patients have a positive family history.
- From 17% to 50% of cases are bilateral (25% is safe estimate).
- Patients presenting when younger than age 10 should have an endocrine workup.
- SCFE may be associated with hormonal disorders in young children, such as hypothyroidism (most common), growth hormone deficiency, or renal osteodystrophy.
- Patients present with a coxalgic externally rotated gait, decreased internal rotation, thigh atrophy, and hip, thigh, or knee pain.
  - Diagnosis is missed when patients present with knee pain with pain activation of the medial obturator nerve.
- In all patients, physical examination reveals obligate external rotation with flexion of the hip.

Classification
- Stability
  - Developed by Loder, is prognostic for the severe complication of osteonecrosis of the femoral head
  - Stable: weight bearing with or without crutches possible
  - Unstable: weight bearing not possible because of severe pain
  - No patients with stable slippages develop osteonecrosis, whereas 47% of patients with unstable slips develop it.

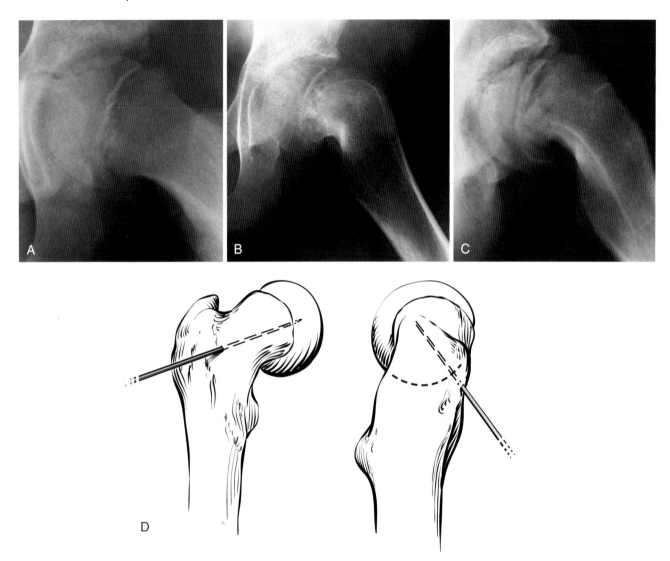

FIGURE 3-10 Slipped capital femoral epiphysis (SCFE). **A,** Acute SCFE with no remodeling present. **B,** Chronic SCFE showing adaptive changes including callus in the junction of the metaphysis and epiphysis. **C,** Acute-on-chronic changes with both sequelae of chronic SCFE (callus) but acute worsening displacement of the epiphysis. **D,** Correct pin placement for guiding of percutaneous in situ screw fixation of SCFE; note that the starting point is anterior on the femoral neck to account for the posteriorly displaced epiphysis. (From Herring JA, editor: *Tachdjian's pediatric orthopaedics,* ed 5, Philadelphia, 2014, Elsevier Saunders, Figure 18-1 and Plate 18-1.)

■ Temporal: no prognostic information
  • Acute: symptoms less than 3 weeks
  • Chronic: symptoms more than 3 weeks
  • Acute on chronic: exacerbation of chronic symptoms
■ **Radiographic studies**
■ AP and frog-leg pelvic views are needed for comparison.
■ If the slippage is unstable, a cross-table lateral view is required.
■ SCFE can be graded on the basis of the percentage of slippage:
  • Grade I: 0% to 33% slippage
  • Grade II: 34% to 50% slippage
  • Grade III: more than 50% slippage
■ In mild cases, loss of the lateral overhang of the femoral ossific nucleus (Klein line) and blurring of the proximal femoral metaphysis may be all that is visible on the AP radiograph.
■ **Treatment**
■ **Recommended treatment for stable and unstable slippages is pinning in situ.**

■ Positioning on the table may partially reduce the acute component of an unstable slippage.
  • Forceful reduction before pinning is not indicated— can cause AVN.
■ **A single pin can be placed percutaneously** (Figure 3-10).
■ The pin should be started anteriorly on the femoral neck, ending in the central portion of the femoral head.
■ Goal of treatment: stabilize epiphysis and promote closure of proximal femoral physis
■ Prophylactic pinning of the opposite hip is controversial but is generally recommended in patients with an endocrinopathy or in young children (<10 years) or with an open triradiate cartilage.
■ Emerging techniques for unstable severe SCFE include surgical hip dislocation with modified Dunn technique (Figure 3-11).
  • Protection of femoral head blood supply via surgical dislocation technique and creating periosteal flaps on the femoral neck

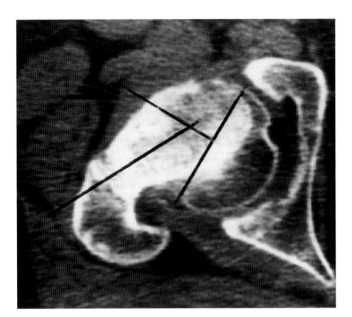

FIGURE 3-11 Unstable slipped capital femoral epiphysis can be treated with a surgical hip dislocation and acute correction of the proximal epiphyseal displacement by creating periosteal flaps that protect the blood supply to the epiphysis while the femoral neck is shortened. (From Herring JA, editor: *Tachdjian's pediatric orthopaedics*, ed 5, Philadelphia, 2014, Elsevier Saunders, Plate 18-3.)

- Allows acute correction of deformity with femoral neck shortening and reorientation of proximal femoral epiphysis
- Initial results with low rates of AVN; follow-up results show AVN rates approaching 25%, still lower than Loder's initial 47% AVN rate with unstable SCFE.

■ **Prognosis and complications**

▦ In severe SCFE, the residual proximal femoral deformity may partially remodel with the patient's remaining growth.

▦ Intertrochanteric (Kramer) or subtrochanteric (Southwick) osteotomies may be useful in treating the deformities caused by SCFE that fail to remodel.

▦ Cuneiform osteotomy at the femoral neck has the potential to correct severe deformity but remains controversial because of the high reported rates of osteonecrosis (37% of cases) and future osteoarthritis (37%).

▦ Complications associated with SCFE:
  - Osteonecrosis
    - Unstable slippage is the most accurate predictor.
  - Chondrolysis
    - Characterized by narrowed joint space, pain, and decreased motion
    - Pin placement into the anterior superior quadrant of the femoral head has the highest rate of joint penetration.
    - Associated with inadvertent pin penetration into the joint
  - Degenerative joint disease
    - Pistol-grip deformity of the proximal femur
    - Slip progression—occurs in up to 2% of cases treated with in situ pinning

BLADDER EXSTROPHY

■ **Introduction**

▦ Congenital disorder involving both musculoskeletal and genitourinary systems

▦ Altered migration of sclerotomes that make up the pubis

■ **Presentation**

▦ Exposed bladder

▦ Acetabuli are externally rotated.

▦ Can present with an externally rotated foot progression

■ **Treatment involves stated multidisciplinary approach.**

▦ Closure of bladder in newborn

▦ Genitourinary repair in males during years 1 to 2

▦ Bladder neck reconstructions (4 years old)

▦ Pelvic osteotomies may be performed at any stage of process but are most commonly performed during bladder reconstruction as a newborn.

PROXIMAL FEMORAL FOCAL DEFICIENCY

■ **Clinical features**

▦ Developmental defect of the proximal femur recognizable at birth

▦ Patients with PFFD have a short, bulky thigh that is flexed, abducted, and externally rotated.

▦ PFFD often associated with coxa vara or fibular hemimelia (50% of cases)

▦ Congenital knee ligamentous deficiency (anterior cruciate ligament [ACL] deficiency) and contracture also common

▦ Bilateral in 50% of cases

▦ Associated with sonic hedgehog gene

■ **Classification**

▦ A: femoral head present with normal acetabulum

▦ B: femoral head present with dysplastic acetabulum

▦ C: femoral head absent with markedly dysplastic acetabulum

▦ D: both femoral head and acetabulum absent

■ **Treatment**

▦ Individualized based on:
  - Leg length discrepancy
  - Adequacy of musculature
  - Proximal joint stability
  - Presence or absence of foot deformities

▦ In general, prosthetic management with foot amputation is used when femoral length is less than 50% that of the opposite side, whereas lengthening with or without contralateral epiphysiodesis is used when the femoral length is more than 50% that of the opposite side.

▦ Percentage of shortening remains constant during growth

▦ Aiken classification
  - In PFFD classes A and B, the femoral head is present, which potentially allows for reconstructive procedures that include limb lengthening.
  - In PFFD classes C and D, the femoral head is absent; treatment includes amputation, femoral-pelvic fusion (Brown procedure), Van Ness rotationplasty, and limb lengthening.

CONGENITAL DISLOCATION OF THE KNEE

■ **Introduction**

▦ Spectrum of disease including positional contractures to rigid dislocations

▦ Quad contracture, anterior subluxation of hamstrings, tight collateral ligaments

▦ Associated with myelomeningocele, arthrogryposis, Larsen syndrome

■ **Treatment**

▦ Nonoperative—reduction with serial casting

- If both hip and knee dislocated first, treat knee
- Pavlik cannot be used if knee dislocated

■ Operative
- Soft tissue release—if failure to gain 30 degrees of knee flexion after 3 to 4 months of serial casting
- Goal of surgery to gain 90 degrees of knee flexion with:
  - Quadriceps lengthening
  - Anterior capsular release
  - Hamstring transposition
  - Mobilization of collateral ligaments

LOWER EXTREMITY INFLAMMATION AND INFECTION (SEE CHAPTER 1, BASIC SCIENCES.) (TABLE 3-5)

■ **Transient synovitis**
■ Clinical features
- Most common cause of pain in hips during childhood, but the diagnosis is one of exclusion. In many cases, a septic arthritis should be considered.
- Can be related to viral infection, allergic reaction, or trauma; true cause unknown
- Onset can be acute or insidious.
- Symptoms, which are self-limiting, include muscle spasm and voluntary limitation of motion.
- With transient synovitis, erythrocyte sedimentation rate (ESR) is usually less than 20 mm/hr.
- See "Septic arthritis" for Kocher criteria that suggest an infectious etiology.

■ Imaging studies
- Entire limb
- Consider spine radiographs.
- Hip ultrasonography
- Consider MRI to evaluate persistent pain.

■ Treatment
- If Kocher criteria not met then can consider no aspiration
- Aspiration required if any doubt or with mixed findings
- If findings are negative, observe the patient with a trial of nonsteroidal antiinflammatory drugs (NSAIDs).
- Symptoms should improve within 24 to 48 hours with NSAIDs

■ **Osteomyelitis**
■ Clinical features
- Occurs more often in children because of their rich metaphyseal blood supply and thick periosteum
- More common in boys
- Pathology:
  - Most common organism is *Staphylococcus aureus*
  - With the advent of the *Haemophilus influenzae* vaccination, *H. influenzae* is now much less commonly found in musculoskeletal sepsis.
  - *Kingella kingae* infection is becoming more common in younger age groups and is thought to be potential cause of culture negative infections—difficult to isolate; **need blood culture medium**.
- History of trauma common in children with osteomyelitis

Table 3-5	Causative Organisms for Musculoskeletal Infections and Empirical Antibiotic Regimens Based on Patient Age and Risk Factors	
PATIENT CHARACTERISTICS	**CAUSATIVE ORGANISMS**	**EMPIRICAL ANTIBIOTICS**
AGE GROUP		
Neonatal (birth to 8 wk)		
Nosocomial infection	*Staphylococcus aureus, Streptococcus* spp., *Enterobacteriaceae, Candida* spp.	Nafcillin or oxacillin plus gentamicin **or** Cefotaxime (or ceftriaxone) plus gentamicin
Community-acquired infection	*S. aureus,* group B streptococci, *Escherichia coli, Klebsiella* spp.	Nafcillin or oxacillin plus gentamicin **or** Cefotaxime (or ceftriaxone) plus gentamicin
Infantile (2-18 mo)	*S. aureus, Kingella kingae, Streptococcus pneumoniae, Neisseria meningitidis Haemophilus influenzae* type b (nonimmunized)	Immunized: nafcillin, oxacillin, or cefazolin Nonimmunized: nafcillin or oxacillin plus cefotaxime, or cefuroxime
Early childhood (18 mo-3 yr)	*S. aureus, K. kingae, S. pneumoniae, N. meningitidis H. influenzae* type b (nonimmunized)	Immunized: nafcillin, oxacillin, or cefazolin Nonimmunized: nafcillin or oxacillin plus cefotaxime, or cefuroxime
Childhood (3-12 yr)	*S. aureus,* GABHS	Nafcillin, oxacillin, or cefazolin
Adolescent (12-18 yr)	*S. aureus,* GABHS, *Neisseria gonorrhoeae*	Nafcillin, oxacillin, or cefazolin; ceftriaxone and doxycycline for disseminated gonococcal infection
RISK FACTOR		
Sickle cell disease	*Salmonella* spp., *S. aureus, S. pneumoniae*	Ceftriaxone
Foot puncture wound	*Pseudomonas aeruginosa, S. aureus*	Ceftazidime or piperacillin-tazobactam and gentamicin
HIV	*S. aureus, Streptococcus* spp., *Salmonella* spp., *Nocardia asteroides, N. gonorrhoeae,* cytomegalovirus, *Aspergillus, Toxoplasma gondii, Torulopsis glabrata, Cryptococcus neoformans, Coccidioides immitis*	Broad-spectrum antibiotics per infectious disease recommendations
CGD	*Aspergillus* spp., *Staphylococcus* spp., *Burkholderia cepacia, Nocardia* spp., *Mycobacterium* spp.	Nafcillin, oxacillin, or cefazolin

From Herring JA, editor: *Tachdjian's pediatric orthopaedics,* ed 4, Philadelphia, 2008, Saunders, Table 35-2.
CGD, Chronic granulomatous disease; *GABHS,* group A beta-hemolytic streptococci; *HIV,* human immunodeficiency virus.

- Osteomyelitis in children usually begins with hematogenous seeding of a bony metaphysis.
  - Small arterioles just beyond the physis
  - Blood flow becomes sluggish and phagocytosis is poor.
  - Bone abscess can be created (Figure 3-12).
- Pus lifts the thick periosteum and puts pressure on the cortex, causing coagulation.
- Chronic bone abscesses may become surrounded by thick fibrous tissue and sclerotic bone (Brodie abscess).
- Manifests with a tender, warm, sometimes swollen area over a long-bone metaphysis
- Fever may or may not be present.
- Methicillin-resistant *S. aureus* (MRSA) is associated with deep venous thrombosis and septic emboli.
- Diagnosis
  - Laboratory tests may be helpful (blood cultures, white blood cell [WBC] count, ESR, C-reactive protein [CRP]).
  - Imaging studies
    - Radiographs show soft tissue edema early, metaphyseal rarefaction late.
    - Periosteal new bone appears at 5 to 7 days.
    - Osteolysis—30% to 50% loss of bone mineral—may not appear until 10 to 14 days.
    - MRI examination is key to evaluate for abscess (either intraosseous vs. subperiosteal).
  - **Definitive diagnosis is made with aspiration or positive clinical picture with convincing MRI (50%+ of affected patients have positive blood cultures).**

- Treatment
  - Intravenous antibiotics are the best initial treatment if osteomyelitis is diagnosed early.
    - If no subperiosteal abscess or abscess within the bone
  - Broad-spectrum antibiotics are initially chosen, followed by antibiotics specific for the organism cultured from percutaneous aspiration/biopsy.
    - CRP measurements can be used to monitor the therapeutic response to antibiotics.
    - Failure to decline within 48 to 72 hours warrants alteration in treatment.
  - Failure to respond to antibiotics, appearance of frank pus on MRI, or presence of a sequestered abscess (not accessible to antibiotics) necessitates operative drainage and débridement.
    - Drilling the metaphysis can assist in draining some of the infection.
  - Specimens should be sent for histologic study and culture.
  - Antibiotics should be continued until the ESR (or CRP level) returns to normal, usually at 4 to 6 weeks.

- **Septic arthritis**
- Clinical features
  - Can develop from osteomyelitis
    - Especially in neonates, in whom transphyseal vessels allow proximal spread into the joint in joints with an intraarticular metaphysis (hip, elbow, shoulder, ankle) (Figure 3-13)
  - Septic arthritis can also occur as a result of hematogenous spread of infection.
  - Because pus is chondrolytic, septic arthritis in children is an acute surgical emergency.
  - **Most frequently occurs in children younger than 2 years**

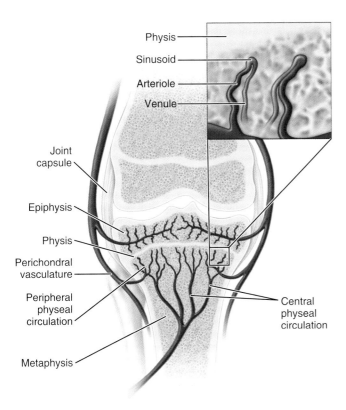

FIGURE 3-12 Metaphyseal sinusoids, where sluggish blood flow increases susceptibility to osteomyelitis. (From Herring JA, editor: *Tachdjian's pediatric orthopaedics,* ed 4, Philadelphia, 2008, Saunders.)

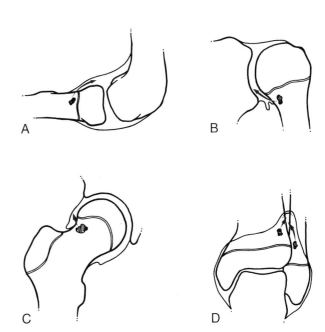

FIGURE 3-13 Metaphyses of the proximal radius **(A),** proximal humerus **(B),** proximal femur **(C),** and distal tibia and fibula **(D)** are intraarticular. Osteomyelitis in these locations may decompress into the joint and produce concomitant septic arthritis. (From Herring JA, editor: *Tachdjian's pediatric orthopaedics,* ed 5, Philadelphia, 2014, Elsevier Saunders, Figure 27-23)

Table 3-6	Common Organisms in Septic Arthritis, by Age	
AGE	**COMMON ORGANISMS**	**EMPIRICAL ANTIBIOTICS**
<12 mo	*Staphylococcus* spp., group B streptococci	First-generation cephalosporin
6 mo-5 yr	*Staphylococcus* spp., *Haemophilus influenzae*	Second- or third-generation cephalosporin
5-12 yr	*Staphylococcus aureus*	First-generation cephalosporin
12-18 yr	*S. aureus, Neisseria gonorrhoeae*	Oxacillin/cephalosporin

- Infecting organisms vary with age (Table 3-6).
- Septic arthritis manifests as a much more acute process than osteomyelitis.
- Decreased ROM and severe pain with passive motion may be accompanied by systemic symptoms of infection.
- Diagnosis and radiographic findings:
  - Radiographs may show a widened joint space or even dislocation.
  - Joint fluid aspirate shows a high WBC count (>50,000/mm^3); glucose level may be 50 mg/dL lower than in serum; and in patients with gram-positive cocci or gram-negative rods, lactic acid level may be high.

- Distinguishing septic arthritis of the hip from transient synovitis is a common problem; however, when three of four of the following criteria are present, the diagnosis of septic arthritis is made in more than 90% of cases: WBC count higher than 12,000 cells/mL, ESR higher than 40, inability to bear weight, temperature higher than 101.5° F (38.6° C) (Kocher criteria).
- Ultrasonography can be helpful in identifying the presence of an effusion.
- Lumbar puncture should be considered in a joint when sepsis is caused by *H. influenzae*, because of the increased incidence of meningitis
- Prognosis is usually good except in patients with a delayed diagnosis.
- *Neisseria gonorrhoeae* septic arthritis is usually preceded by migratory polyarthralgia, small red papules, and multiple joint involvement.
  - This organism typically elicits less WBC response (<50,000 cells/mL) and usually does not necessitate surgical drainage.
  - Large doses of penicillin are required to eliminate this organism.
- Treatment: aspiration should be followed by irrigation and débridement in major joints (especially in the hip; a culture of synovium is also recommended).

SECTION 4   KNEE AND LEG

LEG

■ Introduction
- Genu varum (bowed legs) normally evolves naturally to genu valgum ("knock-knees") by age 2.5 years, with a gradual transition to physiologic valgus angulation by age 4 years (Figure 3-14).
■ Physiologic genu varum (bowed legs)
- Normal in children younger than 2 years
- Radiographs in physiologic bowing typically show flaring of the tibia and femur in a symmetric manner.
- Pathologic conditions that can cause genu varum include osteogenesis imperfecta, osteochondromas, trauma, various dysplasias, and (most commonly) Blount disease.
■ Infantile Blount disease (age 0-4 years)
- Clinical features
  - Abnormal tibia vara
  - More common and usually affects both extremities
  - Classic presentation is in a child who is overweight and who begins walking before 1 year of age; disease is associated with internal tibial torsion.
- Radiographic findings
  - Metaphyseal-diaphyseal angle abnormality and metaphyseal beaking
  - A Drennan metaphyseal-diaphyseal angle of more than 16 degrees is considered abnormal and is formed between the metaphyseal beaks (demonstrated in Figure 3-15).
  - Langenskiöld classification is based on degree of metaphyseal-epiphyseal changes (Figure 3-16)
- Treatment
  - Based on age and correlated with stage of disease

- Stage I or II: bracing in patients younger than 3 years
  - Better outcomes if unilateral or nonobese patients
  - Very difficult to ensure compliance
- Stage II (if patient > 3 years) and stage III: proximal osteotomy for tibia/fibula valgus angulation to overcorrect the deformity (because medial physeal growth abnormalities persist)
- Stages IV to VI are complex, and multiple procedures may be required.
  - Epiphysiolysis is also needed for stages V and VI disease
■ Adolescent Blount disease
- Clinical features
  - Less severe than infantile forms and more often unilateral
  - Epiphysis appears relatively normal and does not have the beaking seen in infantile forms
  - Most characteristic radiographic finding is widening of the proximal medial physis
  - Thought to be from mechanical overload in genetically susceptible patients (obese, African American)
- Treatment
  - Initial treatment is proximal tibial and fibular lateral hemiepiphysiodesis when growth remains.
  - Larger plates are usually required because of incidence of plate failure.
  - If residual deformity exists or physes are closed proximally, tibial and fibular osteotomy is performed.
  - When significant leg length discrepancy is present, the Ilizarov technique allows for deformity correction and lengthening.

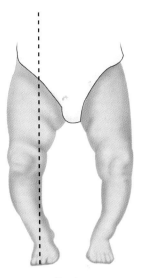 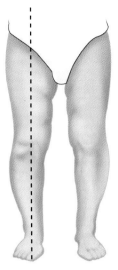 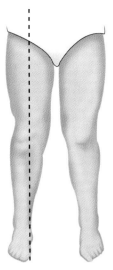 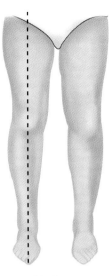

Newborn
Moderate genu varum

11/2 to 2 years
Legs straight

2 1/2 years
Physiologic genu valgum

4 to 6 years
Legs straight

FIGURE 3-14 In children with physiologic genu varum, the bowing begins to slowly improve at approximately 18 months of age and continues as the child grows. By age 3 to 4, the bowing has corrected and the legs typically have a normal appearance.

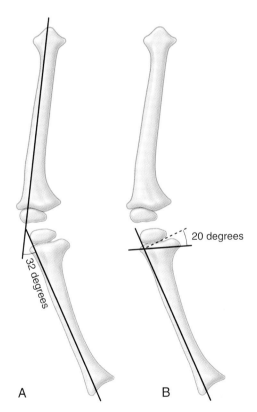

FIGURE 3-15 Comparison of tibiofemoral angle with the Drennan metaphyseal-diaphyseal angle in tibia vara. **A,** Lines are drawn along the longitudinal axes of the tibia and femur; the angle between the lines is the tibiofemoral angle (32 degrees). **B,** The metaphyseal-diaphyseal angle method is used to determine the metaphyseal-diaphyseal angle in the same extremity. A line is drawn perpendicular to the longitudinal axis of the tibia, and another is drawn through the two beaks of the metaphysis to determine the transverse axis of the tibial metaphysis. The metaphyseal-diaphyseal angle (20 degrees) is the angle bisected by the two lines. (From Herring JA, editor: *Tachdjian's pediatric orthopaedics,* ed 4, Philadelphia, 2008, Saunders.)

■ **Genu valgum ("knock-knees")**
▨ Clinical features
  • Up to 15 degrees at the knee is common in children 2 to 6 years of age.
    • Maximum valgus between ages 3 and 4
  • Patients within this physiologic range do not require treatment.
  • Differential diagnosis includes renal osteodystrophy (most common cause if condition is bilateral), tumors (e.g., osteochondromas), infections (may stimulate proximal asymmetric tibial growth), and trauma.
▨ Treatment
  • Conservative treatment is ineffective in pathologic genu valgum.
  • Consider surgery at the site of the deformity in children older than 10 years with more than 10 cm between the medial malleoli or more than 15 degrees of valgus angulation.
  • Hemiepiphysiodesis (temporary or timed) of the medial side is effective before the end of growth for severe deformities.

TIBIAL BOWING

Tibial bowing is classified in three types (Table 3-7) on the basis of the apex of the curve.

■ **Posteromedial tibial bowing**
▨ Physiologic—thought to be due to intrauterine positioning. Posteromedial (PM) bowing is *Probably Mild.*
▨ Usually of the middle and distal thirds of the tibia (Figure 3-17)
▨ Commonly associated with leg length discrepancy, calcaneovalgus feet, and tight anterior structures
▨ Spontaneous correction is the rule, but patient should be monitored to evaluate leg length discrepancy.

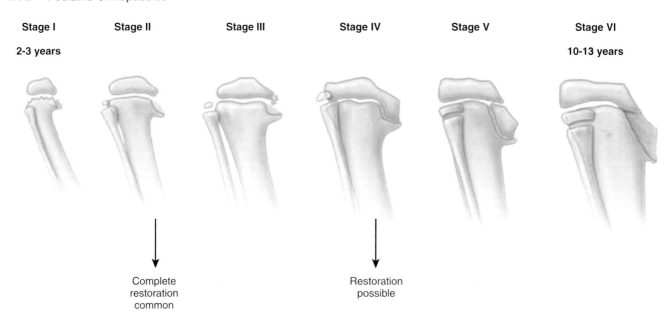

FIGURE 3-16 Langenskiöld classification of infantile tibia vara in six progressive stages with increasing age. (From Herring JA, editor: *Tachdjian's pediatric orthopaedics,* ed 4, Philadelphia, 2008, Saunders, Figure 22-8.)

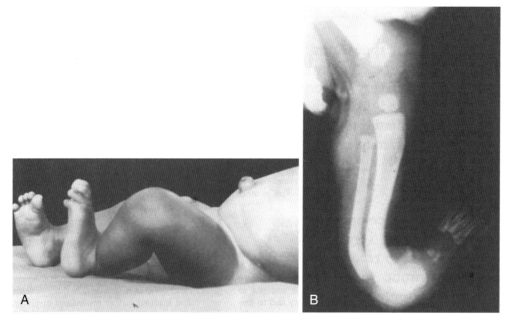

FIGURE 3-17 Posterior medial angulation of the tibia. **A,** Clinical photograph of an affected 5-month-old. **B,** Lateral radiograph of the same patient. The appearance is dramatic, but these deformities are best treated with stretching and splinting into equinus position. (From Herring JA, editor: *Tachdjian's pediatric orthopaedics,* ed 4, Philadelphia, 2008, Saunders, Figures 22-46 and 22-47.)

Table 3-7	Tibial Bowing	
TYPE	**CAUSE**	**TREATMENT**
Posteromedial	Physiologic/ intrauterine positioning	Observation; monitor for significant limb length discrepancy
Anteromedial	Fibular hemimelia	Bracing vs. amputation for severe deformities
Anterolateral	Congenital pseudarthrosis	Total-contact brace, intramedullary fixation, vascularized bone graft, or amputation of leg and foot

▦ Most common sequela of posteromedial bowing is an average leg length discrepancy of 3 to 4 cm, which may necessitate an age-appropriate epiphysiodesis of the long limb.

▦ Tibial osteotomies not indicated

■ **Anteromedial tibial bowing**

▦ Commonly caused by fibular hemimelia (a congenital longitudinal deficiency of fibula, which is the most common long-bone deficiency)

▦ In addition to anteromedial bowing, fibular hemimelia is associated with:
  - Ankle instability due to ball-and-socket joint
  - Equinovarus foot (with or without lateral rays)
  - Tarsal coalition

- Femoral shortening (coxa vara, PFFD)
- ACL insufficiency
▧ Significant leg length discrepancy often results from this disorder.
▧ Classically, skin dimpling is seen over the tibia.
▧ The fibular deficiency can be intercalary, which involves the whole bone (fibula is absent), or terminal.
▧ **Fibular hemimelia is linked to the sonic hedgehog (SHH) gene.**
▧ Radiographic findings:
  - Complete or partial absence of fibula, a ball-and-socket ankle joint (secondary to tarsal coalitions), and deficient lateral rays in the foot
▧ Treatment:
  - Varies from a simple shoe lift or bracing to Syme amputation
  - Decisions are based on the degree of foot deformity, the number of rays, and the degree of shortening of the limb.
  - Amputation is usually performed in limbs with severe shortening or a stiff, nonfunctional foot at about 10 months of age.
  - For less severe cases, reconstructive procedures, including lengthening, may be an alternative.
  - This procedure should include resection of the fibular remnant to avoid future foot problems.

■ **Anterolateral tibial bowing**
▧ Clinical features
  - Congenital pseudarthrosis of the tibia is the most common cause of anterolateral bowing. Rarely is anterolateral (AL) bowing physiologic, so you should *Always Look.*
  - Often accompanied by neurofibromatosis
    - About 50% of patients with anterolateral tibial bowing have neurofibromatosis.
    - Only 10% of patients with neurofibromatosis have tibial bowing.
▧ Radiographic findings
  - Classification (Boyd) is based on bowing and the presence of cystic changes, sclerosis, or dysplasia.
▧ Treatment
  - Initial management/workup should include genetic consultation to check for possibility of neurofibromatosis.
  - Initial treatment includes a total-contact brace to protect the patient from fractures.
  - Intramedullary fixation with excision of hamartomatous tissue and autogenous bone grafting are options for nonhealing fractures.
  - A vascularized fibular graft or the Ilizarov method should also be considered if bracing fails.
  - Osteotomies to correct the anterolateral bowing are contraindicated.
  - Amputation (Syme) and prosthetic fitting are indicated after two or three failed surgical attempts or as primary treatment.
    - Syme amputation is preferred to below-knee amputation in these patients because the soft tissue available at the heel pad is superior to that in the calf as a weight-bearing stump.
    - The soft tissue in the calf in these patients is often scarred and atrophic.

■ **Other lower limb deficiencies**
▧ Tibial hemimelia
  - Congenital longitudinal deficiency of the tibia

- Tibial hemimelia is the only long-bone deficiency with a known inheritance pattern (autosomal dominant).
- It is much less common than fibular hemimelia and is often associated with other bone abnormalities (especially a lobster-claw hand).
- Also associated with insufficient extensor mechanism, clubfoot deformity
- Clinically, the extremity is shortened and bowed anterolaterally with a prominent fibular head and an equinovarus foot, with the sole of the foot facing the perineum.
- Treatment for severe deformities with an entirely absent tibia is a knee disarticulation.
- Fibular transposition (Brown) has been unsuccessful, especially when quadriceps function is absent and when the proximal tibia is absent.
- When the proximal tibia and quadriceps functions are present, the fibula can be transposed to the residual tibia and create a functional below-knee amputation.

OSTEOCHONDRITIS DISSECANS (SEE CHAPTER 4, SPORTS MEDICINE.)

■ **Clinical features**
▧ An intraarticular condition common in children 10 to 15 years of age that can affect many joints, especially the knee and elbow (capitellum)
▧ Lesion thought to be secondary to trauma, ischemia, or abnormal epiphyseal ossification
▧ Posterolateral portion of medial femoral condyle is most frequently involved
▧ Symptoms include activity-related pain, localized tenderness, stiffness, and swelling, with or without mechanical symptoms.
▧ Differential diagnosis includes anomalous ossification centers.
■ **Radiographic studies**
▧ Tunnel (notch) view to evaluate condyles
▧ MRI can determine whether there is synovial fluid behind the lesion (the worst prognosis for nonoperative healing).
■ **Treatment**
▧ Nonoperative:
  - Bracing and restricted weight bearing if the potential for growth remains significant (highest healing rates with open physes)
▧ Operative:
  - Surgical therapy is reserved for the adolescent with minimal growth left or a loose lesion.
  - Operative treatment includes drilling with multiple holes, fixation of large fragments, and bone grafting of large lesions.
  - Osteochondritis dissecans is commonly treated arthroscopically.
  - Poor prognosis is associated with lesions in the lateral femoral condyle and patella.

OSGOOD-SCHLATTER DISEASE (SEE CHAPTER 4, SPORTS MEDICINE.)

■ **Clinical features**
▧ An osteochondrosis, or fatigue failure, of the tibial tubercle apophysis caused by stress from the extensor mechanism in a growing child (tibial tubercle apophysitis)

- Pain over tibial tubercle, especially with direct pressure
- Seen in active children
- **Radiographic findings**
- Irregularity and fragmentation of the tibial tubercle
- **Treatment**
- **Usually self-limiting; activity modification may be required.**
- **Ice and quadriceps stretching also alleviate symptoms.**
- Condition usually does not resolve until growth has halted.
- Late excision of separate ossicles is rarely needed.

DISCOID MENISCUS (SEE CHAPTER 4, SPORTS MEDICINE.)

- **Clinical features**
- Abnormal development of the lateral meniscus leads to formation of a disc-shaped (or hypertrophic) meniscus rather than the normal crescent-shaped meniscus.
- Symptoms include mechanical block and pain with catching and palpable click at knee
- **Radiographic findings**
- Widening of the cartilage space on the affected side (up to 11 mm)
- Squaring of condyles may be visible.
- MRI yields three successive sagittal images with the meniscal body present.
- **Classification**
- Complete covering of tibial plateau
- Incomplete covering of tibial plateau
- Wrisberg variant—lacks posterior meniscotibial attachment; unstable
- **Treatment**
- If symptomatic and torn, the discoid meniscus can be arthroscopically débrided and undergo saucerization to resemble normal appearing meniscus.

- If not torn, it should be observed.
- Repair meniscus if detached (Wrisberg variant)

CONGENITAL DISLOCATION OF THE KNEE

- **Clinical features**
- Spectrum of disease including rigid dislocation to mild contractures
- Classical position is knee hyperextension
- Often occurs in patients with myelodysplasia, arthrogryposis, Larsen syndrome
- Structural components
  - Quadriceps contracture
  - Tight collateral ligaments and anterior subluxation of hamstring tendons
- **Associations**
- Developmental hip dysplasia (50% of patients will have concomitant DDH)
- Clubfoot
- Metatarsus adductus
- **Treatment**
- Nonoperative
  - **Reduction with manipulation and serial casting**
  - **Weekly casting**
  - **Reduce and cast knees before treating with Pavlik harness for DDH**
- Operative
  - If failure to achieve 30 degrees of knee flexion after 3 months of casting
  - Goal is to achieve 90 degrees of knee flexion.
  - Quadriceps lengthening (V-Y-plasty or Z-plasty)
  - Hamstring tendon transposition posteriorly
  - Collateral ligament mobilization

SECTION 5 FOOT

Figure 3-18 depicts common childhood foot disorders.

CLUBFOOT (CONGENITAL TALIPES EQUINOVARUS)

- **Clinical features**
- Mnemonic: **CAVE—cavus, adduction of forefoot, varus of hindfoot, equinus**
- Talar neck deformity (medial and plantar deviation) with medial rotation of calcaneus and medial displacement of navicular and cuboid
- Shortening or contraction of muscles (intrinsic muscles, Achilles tendon, tibialis posterior, flexor hallucis longus, flexor digitorum longus), joint capsules, ligaments, and fascia, which leads to the associated deformities
- **Epidemiology**
- Boys affected twice as often as girls
- 50% of cases bilateral
- Genetic cause strongly suggested in idiopathic cases
- **Causes**
- Majority of cases idiopathic
- Can be associated with **arthrogryposis,** myelomeningocele, hand anomalies (Streeter dysplasia),

diastrophic dwarfism, prune-belly syndrome, tibial hemimelia, and other neuromuscular and syndromic conditions
- **Radiographic studies and findings**
- Diagnosis in infants based on physical examination; minimal ossification of foot in the infant, thus radiographs rarely used
- **"Parallelism" of calcaneus and talus seen on radiographs**
- On the dorsiflexion lateral view (Turco) the talocalcaneal angle will be less than normal (35 degrees).
- On the AP view the talocalcaneal (Kite) angle will also be less than normal (20-40 degrees). The talus–first metatarsal angle will be negative (normally 0-20 degrees) (Figure 3-19).
- **Treatment**
- Ponseti casting
  - First-line treatment
  - Serial weekly manipulation and casting using long-leg plaster casts
  - **Sequence of correction—remember the mnemonic CAVE: cavus, adductus, varus, equinus**

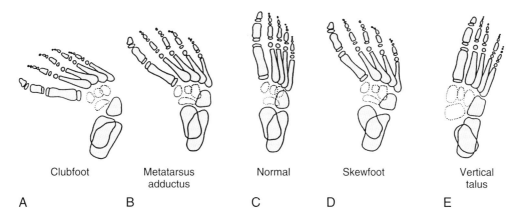

| Clubfoot | Metatarsus adductus | Normal | Skewfoot | Vertical talus |
| A | B | C | D | E |

FIGURE 3-18 Skeletal illustrations of common childhood foot disorders: anteroposterior view. **A,** Varus position of hindfoot and adducted forefoot in clubfoot. **B,** Normal hindfoot and adducted forefoot in metatarsus adductus. **C,** Normal foot. **D,** Valgus hindfoot (with increased talocalcaneal angle) and adducted forefoot in skewfoot. **E,** Increased talocalcaneal angle and lateral deviation of the calcaneus in congenital vertical talus.

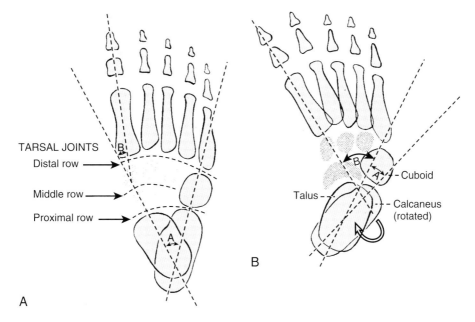

FIGURE 3-19 Skeletal illustrations of the radiographic evaluation of the foot. **A,** Normal foot. **B,** Clubfoot. Note the "parallelism" of the talus and calcaneus, with a talocalcaneal angle (angle A) of less than 20 degrees and a negative talus–first metatarsal angle (angle B) on the clubfoot side. (From Simons GW: Analytical radiology of club feet, *J Bone Joint Surg Br* 59:485–489, 1977.)

- First cast corrects cavus by supinating the forefoot and dorsiflexing the first ray; must be done initially.
- Subsequent casts correct adduction and varus using lateral pressure on the distal talar head as a fulcrum.
- Most patients undergo percutaneous Achilles lengthening at the end of casting to address hindfoot equinus (up to 90% of patients).
- **Last cast placed in 70 degrees of abduction.**
- Post-casting bracing with foot-abduction brace is imperative. Typically used fulltime for 3 months, followed by use during naps and nighttime for 3 years.
- Complications
  - Recurrence or undercorrection
  - Rocker bottom deformity: attempting to dorsiflex hindfoot before varus corrected
  - Flat-top talus: aggressive dorsiflexion causing flattening of talar dome

- Operative treatment
  - Posteromedial release (Table 3-8)
    - Reserved for resistant or refractory clubfeet (only 5% of presenting idiopathic clubfeet)
    - Tendon lengthening, capsular release, and realignment
    - Posterior tibial artery must be carefully protected; dorsalis pedis artery often insufficient
    - Casting for several months usually required postoperatively
    - In older patients (3-10 years of age), a medial opening or lateral column–shortening osteotomy or cuboidal decancellation is used to treat adductus.
  - Triple arthrodesis for children presenting late
    - Contraindicated in patients with insensate feet; causes rigidity of the foot, which may lead to ulceration
  - Talectomy can be used in salvage operations.

Table 3-8	Structures to Be Addressed in the Surgical Correction of Clubfoot
STRUCTURE	**PROCEDURE**
Achilles tendon	Z-lengthening
Calcaneal-fibular ligament	Release
Posterior talofibular ligament	Release
Posterior tibialis tendon	Z-lengthening
Flexor digitorum longus tendon	Z-lengthening
Superficial deltoid	Release
Flexor hallucis longus tendon	Z-lengthening
Tibiotalar, subtalar capsule	Complete release
Talonavicular capsule	Release

Table 3-9	Metatarsus Adductus (MTA)	
TYPE*	**FEATURES**	
Simple MTA	MTA alone	
Complex MTA	MTA + lateral shift of midfoot	
Skewfoot	MTA + valgus hindfoot	
Complex skewfoot	MTA, lateral shift, valgus hindfoot	

*Based on Berg classification.

- Dorsal bunion can occur after clubfoot surgery.
  - **Strong tibialis anterior and flexor hallucis brevis/abductor hallucis contribute**
  - **May be iatrogenic if peroneus longus divided**
  - **Treatment is with capsulotomy, flexor hallucis longus lengthening, and transfer of the flexor hallucis brevis to become a metatarsophalangeal extensor.**
- Dynamic supination
  - Common deformity after clubfoot treatment; occurs in up to 15% to 20% of patients
  - Proposed causes:
    - Overpull of the anterior tibialis, with a weak peroneus longus
    - Undercorrection of forefoot supination
  - Treated with transfer of the tibialis anterior laterally

METATARSUS ADDUCTUS AND SKEWFOOT

- **Clinical features**
- Forefoot adduction with the hindfoot in normal alignment
- Skewfoot:
  - Adductus with hindfoot valgus and lateral subluxation of the navicular on the talus
  - More significant and rigid deformities than simple metatarsus adductus
- Grading:
  - Based on the heel bisector line (Bleck method)
  - Normally, the heel bisector should align with the web space between the second and third toes.
  - Four subtypes (Berg) have been identified (Table 3-9).
- **Treatment**
- If peroneal muscle stimulation corrects metatarsus adductus, the condition usually responds to stretching.
- Otherwise, manipulation and off-the-shelf orthoses or serial casting may be required.
- Surgical for refractory cases in older children
  - Abductor hallucis longus recession (for an atavistic first toe)

- Osteotomies include lateral column shortening osteotomies of the calcaneus or cuboid and opening wedge osteotomies of the medial cuneiform.
- Include calcaneal osteotomy for hindfoot valgus in skewfoot

PES CAVUS (CAVUS FOOT)

- **Cavus deformity of the foot (elevated longitudinal arch) with calcaneus or varus hindfoot**
- **Causes**
- Up to 67% of cases due to neurologic disorder:
  - **Charcot-Marie-Tooth disease (CMT) (most commonly): defect in gene responsible for peripheral myelin protein 22 (PMP22)**
  - Also polio, cerebral palsy, Friedreich ataxia, myelomeningocele, and spinal cord injury, tumor, or abnormality
- Muscle imbalance:
  - **CMT: strong peroneus longus and posterior tibialis overpower tibialis anterior and peroneus brevis, resulting in hindfoot varus and a depressed first metatarsal head.**
  - **In addition, recruitment of the extensor hallucis longus for dorsiflexion of the foot over time causes shortening of plantar fascia and resultant cavus.**
- **Evaluation**
- Full neurologic examination
- MRI of the neuraxis (especially for unilateral cavus foot)
- Consider genetics/neurology referral (DNA testing for CMT)
- **The lateral block (Coleman) test is used to assess hindfoot flexibility of the cavovarus foot (a flexible hindfoot corrects to neutral with a lift placed under the lateral aspect of the foot) (Figure 3-20).**
- **Treatment (Figure 3-21)**
- Nonoperative management rarely successful once deformity has developed
- Operative management (see Figure 3-21)
  - Options include soft tissue procedures (plantar fascia release, tendon transfer), osteotomies, and triple arthrodesis.
  - Generally, if hindfoot is fixed in varus (Coleman block test) add calcaneal osteotomy.
  - Triple arthrodesis has been used for rigid deformity in skeletally mature patients.

CONGENITAL VERTICAL TALUS

- **Also called *congenital convex pes valgus***
- **Clinical features**
- Irreducible dorsal dislocation of the navicular on the talus
- Fixed equinus hindfoot deformity
- Talar head is prominent medially, the sole is convex, the forefoot is abducted and in dorsiflexion, and the hindfoot is in equinovalgus (Persian slipper foot).
- Patients may demonstrate a "peg-leg" gait (awkward gait with limited forefoot push-off).
- Often associated with neuromuscular and syndromic conditions: myelomeningocele, arthrogryposis, prune-belly syndrome, spinal muscular atrophy, neurofibromatosis, and trisomies
- Less severe form is termed *oblique talus*
  - **Navicular reduced with plantar flexion**

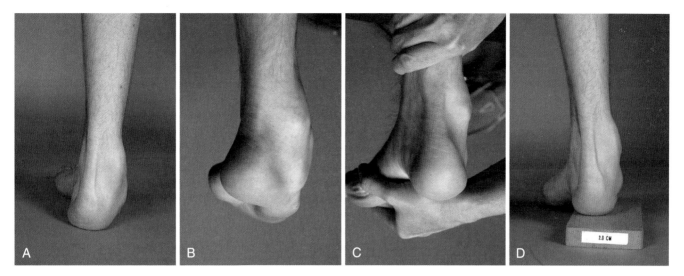

FIGURE 3-20 A, Varus foot in adolescent boy with cerebral palsy. **B,** Hindfoot varus is present, and there is a callus beneath his fifth metatarsal base. **C,** The hindfoot varus is passively correctable to neutral. **D,** The Coleman block test shows partial correction of the varus. (From Herring JA, editor: *Tachdjian's pediatric orthopaedics,* ed 5, Philadelphia, 2014, Elsevier Saunders, Figure 23-97.)

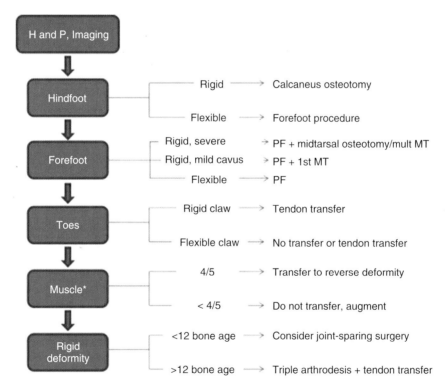

FIGURE 3-21 Algorithm for surgical decision making in the treatment of cavovarus feet. Each section of the foot is considered separately, and appropriate treatments are planned depending on clinical and radiographic findings. (From Lee MC: Pediatric issues with cavovarus foot deformities, *Foot Ankle Clin* 13:199–219, 2008.)

- Radiographic findings (Figure 3-22)
  - Lateral radiograph
    - **Talus appears nearly vertical, calcaneus is in equinus, navicular is dorsally dislocated, and talocalcaneal angle is increased.**
    - **Can infer position of navicular (not ossified in children < 3) by looking at first metatarsal and medial cuneiform**
    - **Navicular does not reduce on forced plantar flexion lateral**
  - AP radiograph
    - Increased talocalcaneal angle (normal, 20-40 degrees)
- Treatment
  - Recent reports have advocated less invasive approach.
    - Serial manipulation and casting followed by limited surgery consisting of percutaneous Achilles tenotomy and minimal talonavicular capsulotomies and pin fixation
  - If casting fails then surgery at 6 to 12 months of age
    - Soft tissue release with lengthening of the extensor tendons, peroneal muscles, and Achilles tendon and

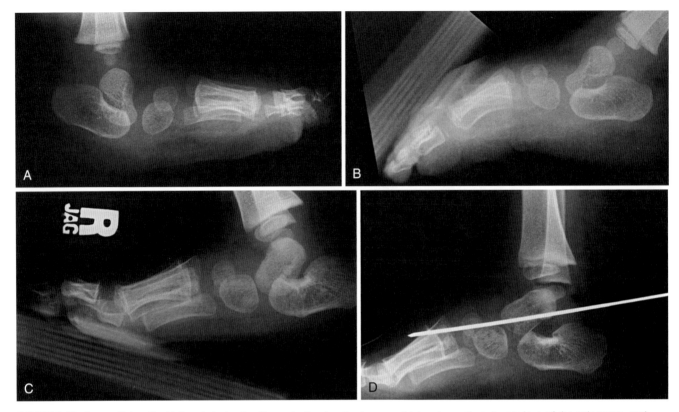

FIGURE 3-22 Congenital vertical talus. **A,** Lateral radiograph showing the increased talocalcaneal angle, equinus of the calcaneus, and dorsal dislocation of the navicular. The bone ossified over the talus is the medial cuneiform; it indicates the position of the navicular, which is not yet ossified in this child. **B,** Plantar flexion lateral radiograph. The navicular is still dorsally displaced over the talar neck. **C,** Dorsiflexion lateral radiograph. The hindfoot remains in neutral position and lacks true dorsiflexion. **D,** Lateral radiograph after open reduction of the dislocated navicular and soft tissue release. (From Herring JA, editor: *Tachdjian's pediatric orthopaedics,* ed 5, Philadelphia, 2014, Elsevier Saunders, Figure 23-74.)

reduction of the talonavicular joint with reconstruction of the spring ligament
▧ Oblique talus
  • Treatment consists of observation and occasionally a UCBL orthotic (University of California Biomechanics Laboratory).
  • Some patients require pinning of the talonavicular joint in the reduced position and Achilles tendon lengthening.

TARSAL COALITIONS (FIGURE 3-23)

■ **Clinical features**
▧ A disorder of mesenchymal segmentation that leads to fusion of tarsal bones and rigid flatfoot
▧ Occurs primarily as a talocalcaneal or calcaneonavicular coalition and is the leading cause of peroneal spastic flatfoot
▧ Symptoms include calf and sinus tarsi pain caused by peroneal spasticity, flatfoot, and limited subtalar motion.
▧ Coalitions may be fibrous, cartilaginous, or osseous.
▧ **Calcaneonavicular coalition is most common in children 9 to 12 years of age, and talocalcaneal coalition is more common in children 12 to 14 years of age.**
■ **Radiographic findings**
▧ **Lateral radiographs may demonstrate an elongated anterior process of the calcaneus ("anteater" sign).**
▧ Talocalcaneal coalitions may demonstrate talar beaking on the lateral view (does not denote degenerative joint

disease) or an irregular middle facet on the Harris axial view.
▧ **The best study for identifying and measuring the cross-sectional area of a talocalcaneal coalition is a CT scan, which can also reveal multiple coalitions (20% of cases).**
■ **Treatment**
▧ Nonoperative
  • Initial treatment for either type involves immobilization (casting) or orthoses.
  • Observation is reasonable for asymptomatic bars in young children.
▧ Surgery
  • Calcaneonavicular coalitions:
    • Resection with interposition of muscle (extensor digitorum brevis) or fat
  • Talocalcaneal coalitions:
    • Involving less than 50% of the middle facet: resection and interposition
    • If more than 50% of the middle facet is involved: subtalar arthrodesis preferred
  • In advanced case, failed resections, and patients with multiple coalitions, triple arthrodesis is often required.

CALCANEOVALGUS FOOT

■ **Clinical features**
▧ Neonatal condition associated with intrauterine positioning
▧ Common in firstborn children

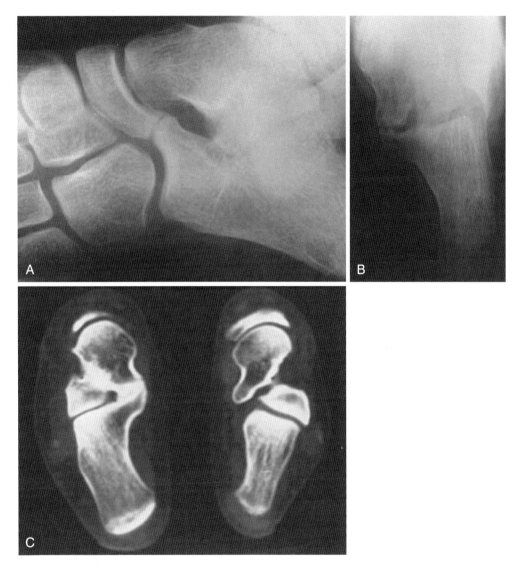

FIGURE 3-23 Tarsal coalition. **A,** Oblique radiograph demonstrating a calcaneonavicular coalition. **B,** Harris view showing irregular surfaces and narrowing of the medial facet, suggestive of a talocalcaneal coalition. **C,** Computed tomographic scan showing a large bar across the medial facet of the subtalar joint, which confirms the subtalar coalition. (From Herring JA, editor: *Tachdjian's pediatric orthopaedics,* ed 4, Philadelphia, 2008, Saunders, Figure 23-83.)

▓ Manifests with a dorsiflexed hindfoot and eversion and abduction of the hindfoot that is passively correctable to neutral positioning

▓ Also seen with myelomeningocele at the L5 level as a result of muscular imbalance between foot dorsiflexors/evertors (L4 and L5 roots) and plantar flexors/inverters (S1 and S2 roots)

■ **Treatment**

▓ Passive stretching and observation

JUVENILE BUNIONS

■ **Clinical features**

▓ Often bilateral and familial

▓ Less common and usually less severe than adult form

▓ May be associated with ligamentous laxity, hypermobile first ray, and metatarsus primus varus

▓ Usually occurs in adolescent girls

■ **Treatment**

▓ Nonoperative
 • Modification of shoe wear with a wide toe box and arch supports

▓ Surgical
 • Should be avoided because recurrence is frequent in growing patients
 • Symptomatic patients with an intermetatarsal angle of more than 10 degrees (metatarsus primus varus) and a hallux valgus angle of more than 20 degrees may need proximal metatarsal osteotomy, distal capsular reefing, and adductor tenotomy with a bunionectomy (modified McBride procedure).
 • Complications include **recurrence**, overcorrection, and hallux varus.

KOHLER DISEASE

■ **Clinical features**

▓ Osteonecrosis of the tarsal navicular bone

▓ Manifests at the age of about 5 years

▓ Pain is the typical presenting complaint.

▓ Radiographs show sclerosis of the navicular bone.

■ **Treatment**

▓ Resolves spontaneously with decreased activity, with or without immobilization

FLEXIBLE PES PLANUS

- **Clinical features**
- Foot is flat only when standing and not with toe walking or foot hanging.
- **If arch does not reconstitute upon toes standing, consider tarsal coalition**
- This condition is frequently familial and almost always bilateral.
- Commonly associated with mild lower extremity rotational problems and ligamentous laxity
- Symptoms can include an aching midfoot or pretibial pain.
- **Radiographic findings**
- Lateral radiograph: broken Meary angle with plantar-directed sag, hindfoot equinus
- AP radiograph: talar head uncoverage
- **Treatment**
- **Asymptomatic patients should be monitored with observation.**
- Symptomatic patients: arch supports and shoes with stiffer soles may offer pain relief but do not result in deformity correction.
- Thorough evaluation should be completed to rule out tight heel cords and decreased subtalar motion.
- UCBL heel cups are sometimes indicated for advanced cases with pain (symptomatic treatment only).
- Surgical treatment
  - **Indicated with failure of nonoperative treatment**
  - **Calcaneal lengthening osteotomy with or without medial soft tissue tightening may provide pain relief at the expense of inversion/eversion.**
  - Sliding calcaneal osteotomy, opening-wedge cuboid osteotomy, and a plantar flexion closing-wedge osteotomy of the medial cuneiform (3C) is another option.

HABITUAL TOE WALKING

- **Clinical features**
- Can be associated with many neurologic diagnoses, such as autism
- Other diagnoses (muscular dystrophy, cerebral palsy, CMT) must be ruled out with neurologic evaluation
- Contracture of the Achilles tendon may be present.
- **Treatment**
- Nonoperative
  - Stretching and night splints
  - Serial casting
- Operative treatment
  - Surgical lengthening if nonoperative treatment fails

ACCESSORY NAVICULAR

- **Clinical features**
- Normal variant that is present in up to 12% of the general population
- Posterior tibial tendon typically inserts into accessory navicular
- Commonly associated with flat feet
- Symptoms usually include medial arch pain with overuse, which usually resolve with activity restriction or immobilization.
- **Radiographic studies**

- External oblique radiographic views often helpful in the diagnosis
- **Treatment**
- **Most cases resolve spontaneously and can be treated with activity restriction and shoe modification and occasionally a course of casting.**
- If nonoperative treatment fails, the accessory bone can be excised with repair and advancement of the posterior tibial tendon.

BALL-AND-SOCKET ANKLE

- **Clinical features**
- Abnormal formation with a spherical talus (ball) and a cup-shaped tibiofibular articulation (socket)
- Usually necessitates no treatment but should be recognized because of high association with **tarsal coalition (50% of cases)**, absence of lateral rays (50% of cases), fibular deficiency, and leg length discrepancy

CONGENITAL TOE DISORDERS

- **Syndactyly**
- Fusion of the soft tissues (simple) and sometimes bones (complex) of the toes
- Simple syndactyly usually does not necessitate treatment; complex syndactyly is treated in the same way as it is in the hand.
- **Polydactyly (extra digits)**
- May be autosomal dominant and usually involves the lateral ray in patients with a positive family history
- Treatment includes ablation of the extra digit and any bony protrusion of the common metatarsal (the border digit is typically excised).
- Procedure usually done at ages 9 to 12 months, but some rudimentary digits can be ligated in the newborn nursery
- **Oligodactyly**
- Congenital absence of the toes
- May be associated with more proximal agenesis (i.e., fibular hemimelia) and tarsal coalition
- Usually necessitates no treatment
- **Atavistic great toe (congenital hallux varus)**
- Deformity involving great-toe adduction that is often associated with polydactyly
- Must be differentiated from metatarsus adductus
- Deformity usually occurs at metatarsophalangeal joint and includes a short, thick first metatarsal and a firm band (abductor hallucis longus muscle) that may be responsible for the disorder
- Surgery sometimes required and includes release of abductor hallucis longus muscle
- **Overlapping toe**
- Fifth toe overlaps fourth (usually bilaterally) and may cause problems with footwear.
- Initial treatment includes passive stretching and "buddy" taping, but usually the overlapping toes resolve with time.
- Surgical options include tenotomy, dorsal capsulotomy, and syndactylization to the fourth toe (McFarland procedure).
- **Underlapping toe (congenital curly toe)**
- Usually involves the lateral three toes and is rarely symptomatic
- Surgery (flexor tenotomies) occasionally indicated

SECTION 6 PEDIATRIC SPINE

ADOLESCENT IDIOPATHIC SCOLIOSIS

■ General

- Onset after 10 years of age
- Unknown and likely multifactorial cause
  - May be related to a hormonal, brainstem, or proprioception disorder
  - Most patients have a positive family history but variable expression.

■ Diagnosis

- Referral from two main sources: school screening and pediatrician
  - School screening: mandated by several states
- Rotational deformities noted on the Adams forward bend test, with the use of a scoliometer
  - **Threshold level of 7 degrees is thought to be an acceptable compromise between over-referral and a false-negative diagnosis and correlates with a 20-degree coronal curve.**
- Physical findings
  - Shoulder elevation, waistline asymmetry, trunk shift, limb-length inequality, rib rotational deformity (rib hump), and prominent scapula
  - Neurologic examination:
    - Findings should be normal.
    - **Abnormal findings, especially asymmetric abdominal reflexes, should prompt an MRI study.**
  - Examination of the lower extremities: look for cavus deformities; if present, obtain an MRI to assess for intraspinal abnormalities.
- Imaging studies
  - Standing full-length posteroanterior radiograph
    - Cobb method used to measure magnitude of curves (Figure 3-24)
    - Assess Risser sign (ossification of the iliac crest apophysis).
    - Assess overall balance.
    - Look for congenital abnormalities.
  - Lateral radiograph
    - Hypokyphosis of thoracic spine and hypolordosis of lumbar spine typically seen
    - If hyperkyphosis of the thoracic spine is observed, consider MRI.
    - Look for spondylolisthesis at the level of L5 to S1.
  - MRI:
    - Indications
      - Left thoracic curves
      - Painful or rapidly progressing scoliosis
      - Apical kyphosis of the thoracic curve
      - Juvenile-onset scoliosis (onset before age 10 years)
      - Neurologic signs or symptoms
      - Congenital abnormalities

■ Classification

- Lenke classification: six curve types, three lumbar modifiers, three thoracic sagittal modifiers (Figure 3-25)
  - Helps determine fusion levels during surgery
  - Structural curves: (1) the largest curve, (2) additional curves that fail to bend to less than 25 degrees
  - Curve type:
    - Type I: single thoracic curve
    - Type II: double thoracic curve

- Type III: double major curve
- Type IV: triple major curve
- Type V: single thoracolumbar/lumbar curve
- Type VI: primary thoracolumbar/lumbar curve and structural (but smaller) thoracic curve
- Lumbar modifier: based on position of the center sacral vertical line (CSVL) in relation to the apical vertebra of the thoracolumbar/lumbar curve
  - Type A: CSVL is between the pedicles of the apical vertebra
  - Type B: CSVL touches between the concave pedicle and the lateral body
  - Type C: CSVL falls outside of apical vertebral body

■ Risk factors for curve progression

- **Risk of progression is related to curve size and remaining skeletal growth, which can be difficult to assess** (Table 3-10).
- Curves greater than 20 degrees in very young patients
- **Thoracic curves greater than 45 to 50 degrees at skeletal maturity are likely to progress during adulthood.**
- Lumbar curves may progress at a lower threshold.
- Peak height velocity (PHV) (Figure 3-26)
  - **Best predictor for progression**
  - **Occurs during Risser 0, which makes the Risser sign less useful**

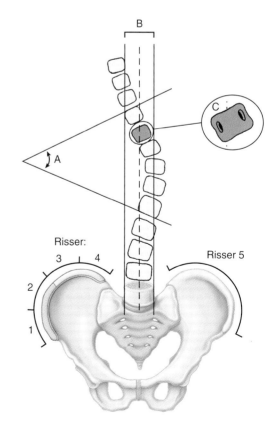

FIGURE 3-24 Measurements for idiopathic scoliosis: Cobb angle (A); Harrington stable zone (B); Moe neutral vertebra (C); and grading of Risser sign (1 to 5). (Modified from Herring JA, editor: *Tachdjian's pediatric orthopaedics,* ed 4, Philadelphia, 2008, Saunders.)

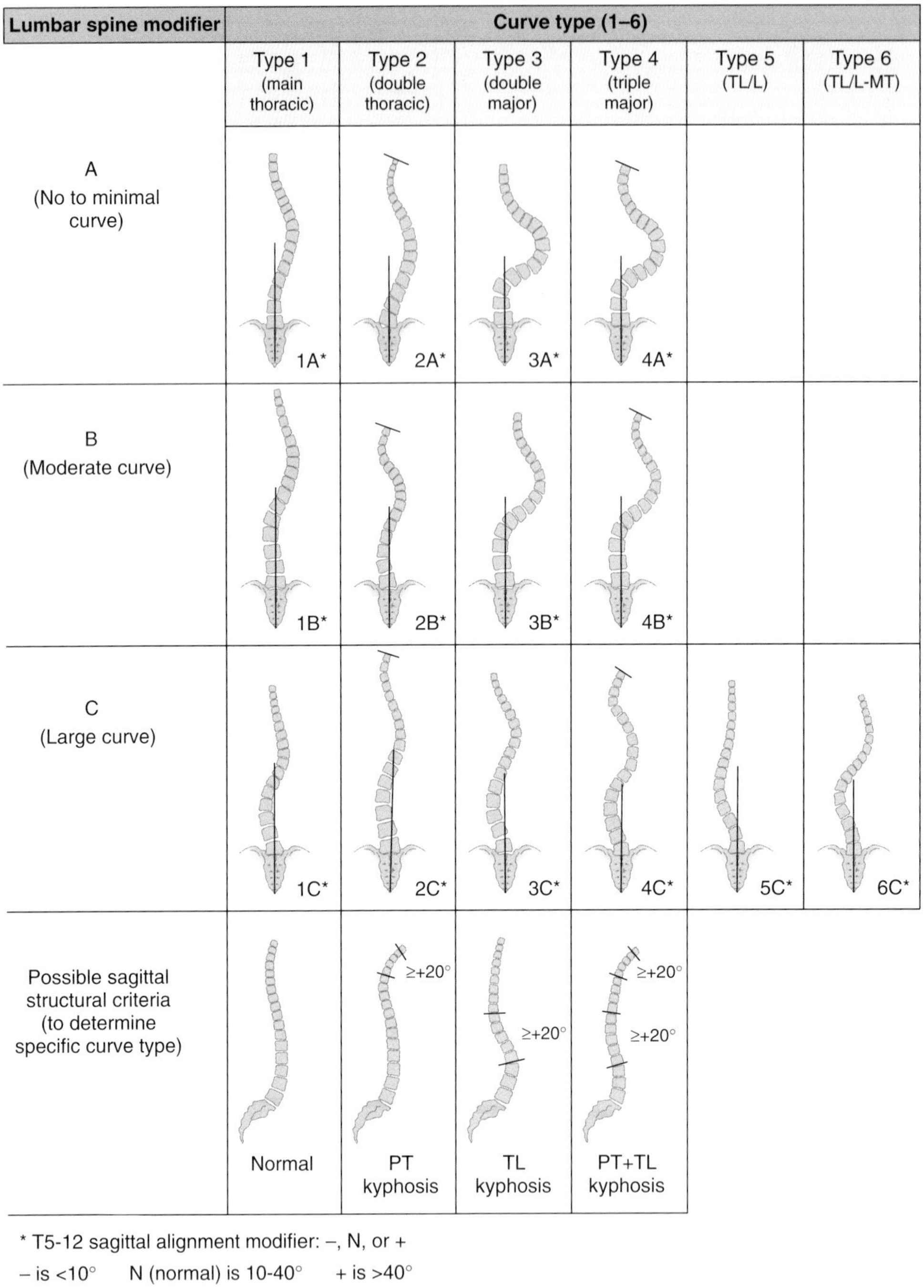

Lumbar spine modifier	Curve type (1–6)					
	Type 1 (main thoracic)	Type 2 (double thoracic)	Type 3 (double major)	Type 4 (triple major)	Type 5 (TL/L)	Type 6 (TL/L-MT)
A (No to minimal curve)	1A*	2A*	3A*	4A*		
B (Moderate curve)	1B*	2B*	3B*	4B*		
C (Large curve)	1C*	2C*	3C*	4C*	5C*	6C*
Possible sagittal structural criteria (to determine specific curve type)	Normal	PT kyphosis ≥+20°	TL kyphosis ≥+20°	PT+TL kyphosis ≥+20° ≥+20°		

* T5-12 sagittal alignment modifier: −, N, or +

− is <10°   N (normal) is 10-40°   + is >40°

A

FIGURE 3-25 Lenke classification. **A,** Schematic drawings of the curve types, lumbar modifiers, and sagittal structural criteria that determine specific curve patterns. *MT,* Main thoracic; *PT,* proximal thoracic; *TL,* thoracolumbar; *TL/L,* thoracolumbar/lumbar.

Lumbar spine modifier A, B, C rules

1. Examine upright coronal radiograph.

2. Accept pelvic obliquity <2 cm. If >2 cm, must block out leg length inequality to level pelvis.

3. Draw CSVL with a fine-tip pencil or marker. Bisects proximal sacrum and line drawn vertical to parallel lateral edge of radiograph.

4. Stable vertebra—most proximal lower thoracic or lumbar vertebra most closely bisected by CSVL. If a disc is most closely bisected, then choose next caudal vertebra as stable.

5. Apex of curve is the most horizontal and laterally placed vertebral body or disc.

6. SRS definitions:

Curves	Apex
Thoracic	T2 to T11-12
Thoracolumbar	T12-L1
Lumbar	L1-2 to L4

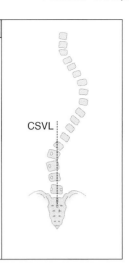

Lumbar modifier A

- CSVL falls between lumbar pedicles up to stable vertebra

- Must have a thoracic apex

- If in doubt whether CSVL touches medial aspect of lumbar apical pedicle, *choose type B*

- Includes King types III, IV, and V

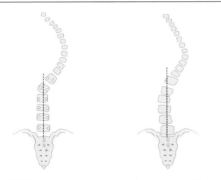

CSVL between pedicles up to stable vertebra, no to minimal scoliosis and rotation of L-spine

Lumbar modifier B

- CSVL falls between medial border of lumbar concave pedicle and lateral margin of apical vertebral body or bodies (if apex is a disc)

- Must have a thoracic apex

- If in doubt whether CSVL touches lateral margin of apical vertebral body or bodies, *choose type B*

- Includes King types II, III, and V

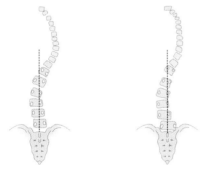

CSVL touches apical vertebral bodies or pedicles, minimal to moderate L-spine rotation

Lumbar modifier C

- CSVL falls medial to lateral aspect of lumbar apical vertebral body or bodies (if apex is a disc)

- May have a thoracic, thoracolumbar, and/or lumbar apex

- If in doubt whether CSVL actually touches lateral aspect of vertebral body or bodies, *choose type B*

- Includes King types I, II, V, double major, triple major thoracolumbar, and lumbar curves

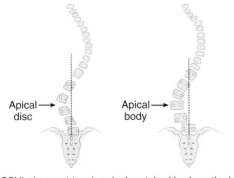

Apical disc

Apical body

CSVL does not touch apical vertebral body or the bodies immediately above and below the apical disc

B

FIGURE 3-25, cont'd B, Rules and definitions for determining the lumbar spine modifiers A, B, and C. (From Herring JA, editor: *Tachdjian's pediatric orthopaedics,* ed 5, Philadelphia, 2014, Elsevier Saunders, Figures 12-26 and 12-27.)

- Occurs before menarche
- Closure of the olecranon apophysis correlates with PHV.
- Modified Tanner-Whitehouse RUS Score of 3 (the majority of digits are capped and the metacarpal epiphyses are wider than their metaphyses) correlates with PHV. Patients with a curve of 30 degrees at this stage have a nearly 100% chance of progressing to a surgical range.

Table 3-10	Incidence of Curve Progression as Related to the Magnitude of the Curve and Risser Stage	
	PERCENTAGE OF CURVES THAT PROGRESSED	
RISSER STAGE	**5 TO 19 DEGREES (CURVES)**	**20 TO 29 DEGREES (CURVES)**
0, 1	22%	68%
2, 3, 4	1.6%	23%

From Lonstein JE, Carlson JM: The prediction of curve progression in untreated idiopathic scoliosis during growth, *J Bone Joint Surg Am* 66:1067, 1984.

■ **Treatment (Table 3-11)**
▥ Depends on the likelihood of curve progression
▥ Observation
- Skeletally immature patients with curves less than 20 to 25 degrees
- Skeletally mature patients with curves less than 45 degrees
▥ Bracing
- Goal: to halt or slow curve progression in skeletally immature patients (Risser 0 to 2); however, bracing does not reverse the curve.
- Indications: curves of more than 25 degrees or 20 degrees with documented progression
- Types of braces:
  - Milwaukee brace (cervicothoracolumbosacral (CTLSO) orthosis); *rarely* used
  - Boston underarm thoracolumbosacral (TLSO) orthosis
    - For curves with the apex at T8 or below
    - Thoracic lordosis or hypokyphosis is a relative contraindication.
  - **Bracing has been shown to be less effective in boys and overweight patients.**

Table 3-11	Guidelines for Treating Patients with Idiopathic Scoliosis		
	RISSER SIGN		
CURVE MAGNITUDE (degrees)	**GRADE 0/PREMENARCHAL**	**GRADE 1 OR 2**	**GRADE 3, 4, OR 5**
<25	Observation	Observation	Observation
25-45	Brace therapy (begin when curve is > 25 degrees)	Brace therapy	Observation
>45	Surgery	Surgery	Surgery (when curve is > 50 degrees)

From Herring JA, editor: *Tachdjian's pediatric orthopaedics,* ed 4. Philadelphia, 2008, Saunders, Table 12-2.

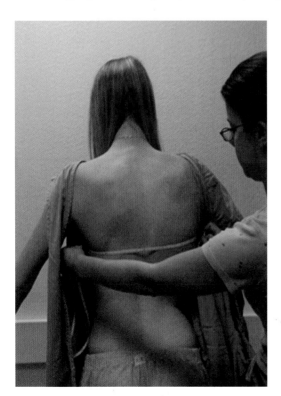
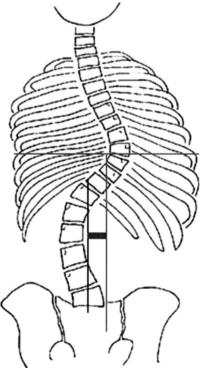
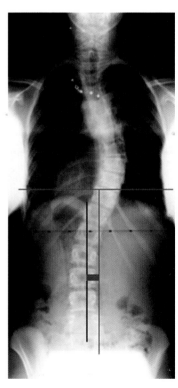

FIGURE 3-26 Schematic drawing of height velocity. Closure of the triradiate cartilage (TRC) occurs after the period of peak height velocity (PHV) and before Risser grade 1 and menarche are attained. (From Herring JA, editor: *Tachdjian's pediatric orthopaedics,* ed 5, Philadelphia, 2014, Elsevier Saunders, Figure 12-3.)

- **Effectiveness of bracing patients with idiopathic scoliosis is "dose dependent"; effective when worn more than 12 hours a day.**
- Surgery
  - Goals
    - To prevent curve progression and obtain a fusion
    - To obtain and maintain correction in the coronal, axial, and sagittal planes while avoiding complications
  - Posterior instrumentation and fusion
    - Segmental instrumentation with pedicle screws (most common), hooks, or wires connected to rods
    - Correction of coronal deformity and sagittal deformities and rotation
    - Arthrodesis (fusion) using autograft and allograft
  - Anterior instrumentation and fusion
    - Uncommon as single approach but useful in two cases:
      - Single thoracic fusion: especially if hypokyphosis is present and if fusion levels can be saved
      - Single thoracolumbar/lumbar fusion
  - Indications for use in combination with posterior approach:
    - Very young patients: triradiate cartilage open; used to prevent crankshaft phenomenon
    - Large or stiff curves: to improve flexibility, usually for curves of more than 75 degrees. However, the use of pedicle screws and posterior osteotomies may obviate this.
  - Fusion levels
    - Determining levels is complex and based on many factors.
    - Main goal: to minimize the number of fusion levels while achieving good coronal and sagittal balance
    - Definitions
      - Stable vertebra: most proximal vertebra that is the most closely bisected by CSVL
      - End vertebrae: the most tilted vertebrae
      - Neutral vertebra: the vertebra that has no rotation in the axial plane
    - Generally:
      - Include structural curves
      - Include nonstructural lumbar curves that are:
        - Greater than 45 degrees
        - Associated with significant rotation or translation
      - Fuse to T2 proximally when:
        - Left shoulder is elevated
        - T1 tilt is greater than 5 degrees
        - Proximal thoracic curve has significant rotation
      - Lenke 1 and 2 curves:
        - A modifier: fuse distally to vertebra touched by CSVL unless L4 is tilted to the right (fuse one or two levels distally)
        - B modifier: fuse distally to stable vertebra
      - Lenke 3 through 6 curves:
        - Fuse to distal end vertebra
  - Complications
    - Infection
      - Overall rate in idiopathic scoliosis: 1.2% to 1.3%
      - Acute
        - **S. aureus most common**
        - **Incision and drainage and antibiotic suppression usually required until fusion if deep infection**
      - Delayed
        - Slow-growing organisms: *Propionibacterium acnes, Staphylococcus epidermidis*
        - **Treatment: removal of implants, check for pseudarthrosis, and a short course of antibiotics**
    - Pseudarthrosis: present in 1% to 3% of cases
      - Manifests with pain, fractured rod
      - Difficult to visualize with imaging studies
      - Treatment: compression instrumentation bone grafting
    - Neurologic deficits
      - Rare: present in 0.5% to 0.7% of cases
      - Usually nerve root or incomplete spinal cord injury
      - Implant related: with anchors placed in the canal
      - Vascular related: during correction
      - Intraoperative spinal cord monitoring is crucial.
        - If changes occur intraoperatively: check leads, raise blood pressure, transfuse, reverse steps of surgery, and reassess
        - If neurologic responses still diminished: complete removal of implants
    - Crankshaft phenomenon
      - Continued anterior spinal growth after posterior fusion in skeletally immature patients
      - Increased rotation and deformity of the spine
      - Can be avoided by anterior discectomy and fusion coupled with posterior spinal fusion
    - Miscellaneous
      - Postoperative drains
        - Have not been shown to decrease infection, wound, or overall complication rate
        - Increase transfusion rate
      - Postoperative intensive care unit (ICU) versus hospital floor
        - Patients treated on hospital floor have lower overall costs, fewer lab draws, less medication usage, and earlier discharge

EARLY-ONSET SCOLIOSIS (EOS)

- **The Scoliosis Research Society defines EOS as scoliosis diagnosed before the age of 10.**
- **Heterogeneous group including congenital scoliosis and infantile and juvenile idiopathic scoliosis; see individual sections for treatment options.**
- **Thoracic insufficiency syndrome**
- Inability of the thorax to support normal respiration or lung growth
- Causes
  - Severe congenital scoliosis with rib fusions
  - Jarcho-Levin syndrome: extensive vertebral and rib fusions
  - Jeune syndrome or asphyxiating thoracic dystrophy: rib dysplasia causing a shortened and narrow thorax
- Diagnosis
  - Clinical signs of respiratory insufficiency
  - Loss of chest wall mobility as demonstrated by the thumb excursion test
  - Worsening indices of three-dimensional thoracic deformity
    - Radiographic studies: measurement of T1-T12 height
    - CT scans: lung volumes

- Relative decline in percentage of predicted vital capacity as a result of thoracic failure to thrive, as demonstrated by pulmonary function tests
- Treatment
  - Vertical Expandable Prosthetic Titanium Rib (VEPTR) with expansion thoracoplasty
    - Can use ribs, posterior spinal elements, or pelvis as anchor points
    - High rate of complications

JUVENILE IDIOPATHIC SCOLIOSIS

- **Definition: idiopathic scoliosis that presents between 4 and 10 years of age**
- **Presentation: similar to that of adolescent scoliosis in terms of manifestations and treatment**
- **Right thoracic curve most common**
- **Differences from adolescent idiopathic scoliosis**
- Higher risk of progression, up to 95% in one study
- Less likely to respond to bracing
- More likely to require surgical treatment
- **Rate of spinal cord abnormality: 25%**
- **MRI should routinely be obtained.**
- **Treatment**
- Observation: curves less than 25 degrees
- Nonoperative treatment: curves between 25 and 45 degrees
  - Bracing
  - Stiff, inflexible curves may require initial casting.
- Growing rods for patients younger than 8 to 10 years with large progressive curves
- Definitive fusion for patients older than 10 years
  - Anterior and posterior fusion often required

INFANTILE IDIOPATHIC SCOLIOSIS

- **Definition: idiopathic scoliosis that presents before the age of 4**
- **Differences from adolescent idiopathic scoliosis:**
- Left thoracic curve most common
- More common in boys
- Plagiocephaly (skull flattening) often present
- Other congenital defects frequent
- **Natural history**
- **Significant number of curves will resolve spontaneously; up to 90% in one study.**
- Risk for curve progression
  - Phase of the ribs: position of the medial rib relative to the apical vertebra
    - Phase I: *no* rib overlap
      - Measure the rib-vertebral angle difference with Mehta classification:
        - Less than 20 degrees: low risk for progression (80% chance of no progression)
        - More than 20 degrees: high risk for progression (80% chance of progression)
    - Phase II: rib overlaps the apical vertebra
      - Very high risk for curve progression
- **Evaluation**
- Clinical: look for plagiocephaly, perform complete neurologic examination, ask about developmental milestones.
- MRI: progressive infantile idiopathic scoliosis should be evaluated with MRI of the spinal cord.
  - The incidence of neural axis abnormalities is 20%.

- **Treatment**
- Observation: curves less than 25 degrees with rib-vertebra angle difference (RVAD) less than 20 degrees
- Bracing
  - Used for modest and/or flexible deformity
  - Milwaukee brace frequently used
- Mehta or derotational casting
  - Indications: progressive deformity (progression of 10 degrees or past 25 degrees)
  - Changed every 2 to 4 months
  - Goals
    - May be definitive treatment when initiated in very young patients
    - May delay surgical treatment in other patients
- Surgery
  - Distraction-based techniques
    - Growing rods or VEPTR
    - Serial lengthening every 4 to 6 months
    - High rate of complications, both implant related and wound related
  - Definitive fusion when patient is older than 10 years, if possible

CONGENITAL SPINAL DEFORMITIES

- **Congenital scoliosis**
- Caused by a developmental defect in formation of the spine during fifth to eighth week of gestation
- **High incidence of associated abnormalities**
  - **Intraspinal abnormality: 20 to 40%; obtain MRI**
  - **Cardiac system: 12% to 26%**
  - **Genitourinary system: 20%**
- Three basic types of defects (Figure 3-27)
  - Failure of segmentation (i.e., vertebral bar)
  - Failure of formation (i.e., hemivertebrae)
  - Mixed
- Risk for progression (Table 3-12)
  - Dependent on:
    - Type of anomaly
    - Remaining growth: worsens most rapidly during first 2 years of life and during adolescent growth spurt
  - From most likely to progress to least likely:
    - Unilateral bar with contralateral fully segmented hemivertebra(e): rapid and severe progression
    - Unilateral bar: most common congenital deformity
    - Multiple unilateral fully segmented hemivertebrae
    - Single fully segmented hemivertebra
    - Unsegmented or incarcerated hemivertebra (fused above and below)
    - Block vertebrae: best prognosis
- Treatment
  - Nonoperative
    - Bracing generally ineffective
    - May be useful for controlling compensatory curves and delaying surgery
  - Operative
    - Surgical options are varied and somewhat controversial.
    - In situ spinal fusion
      - Posterior in older patients or anterior/posterior spinal fusion in younger patients to avoid crankshaft phenomenon
      - For smaller deformities with high likelihood of progression

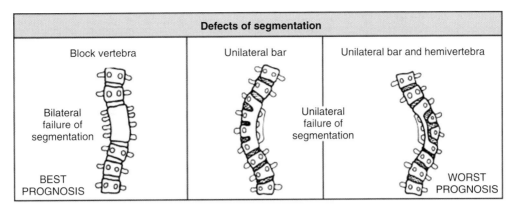

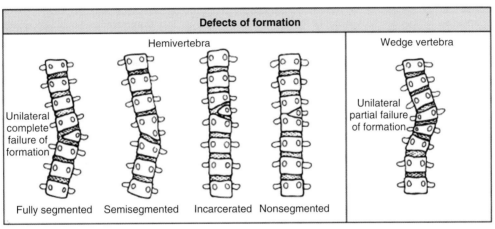

 FIGURE 3-27 Vertebral anomalies that lead to congenital scoliosis. (Adapted from Herring JA, editor: *Tachdjian's pediatric orthopaedics,* ed 4, Philadelphia, 2008, Saunders, Figure 12-57.)

Table 3-12	Progression of Congenital Scoliosis Patterns and Treatment Options	
RISK FOR PROGRESSION (highest to lowest)	**CHARACTER OF CURVE PROGRESSION**	**TREATMENT OPTIONS**
Unilateral unsegmented bar with contralateral hemivertebra	Rapid and relentless	Posterior spinal fusion (add anterior fusion for girls < 10 yr, boys < 12 yr)
Unilateral unsegmented bar	Rapid	Posterior spinal fusion (add anterior fusion for girls < 10 yr, boys < 12 yr)
Fully segmented hemivertebra	Steady	Anterior spinal fusion Hemivertebra excision
Partially segmented hemivertebra	Less rapid; curve usually < 40 degrees at maturity	Observation, hemivertebra excision
Incarcerated hemivertebra	May slowly progress	Observation
Nonsegmented hemivertebra	Little progression	Observation

- Convex hemiepiphysiodesis
  - For smaller deformities with high likelihood of progression
- "Growth friendly" techniques
  - Growing rods
  - VEPTR
  - Shilla technique
    - Apical fusion with pedicle screws placed at proximal and distal extent of curve
    - Rods slide along pedicle screws, promoting guided growth
  - Designed to allow thorax to continue to grow and delay definitive treatment
- Hemivertebra resection
  - May be indicated for lumbosacral hemivertebrae associated with progressive curves and an oblique takeoff (severe truncal imbalance)

- Isolated hemivertebra excision should be accompanied by anterior/posterior arthrodesis with instrumentation to stabilize the adjacent vertebrae.

■ **Congenital kyphosis (Figure 3-28)**
▦ Types
  - Failure of formation (type I)
    - Most common
    - Worse prognosis
    - Highest risk for neurologic complications
    - When severe: immediate indication for surgery
  - Failure of segmentation (type II)
  - Mixed abnormalities (type III)
▦ Treatment
  - Posterior fusion:
    - Favored in young children (<5 years) with curves of less than 50 degrees and normal findings on neurologic examination

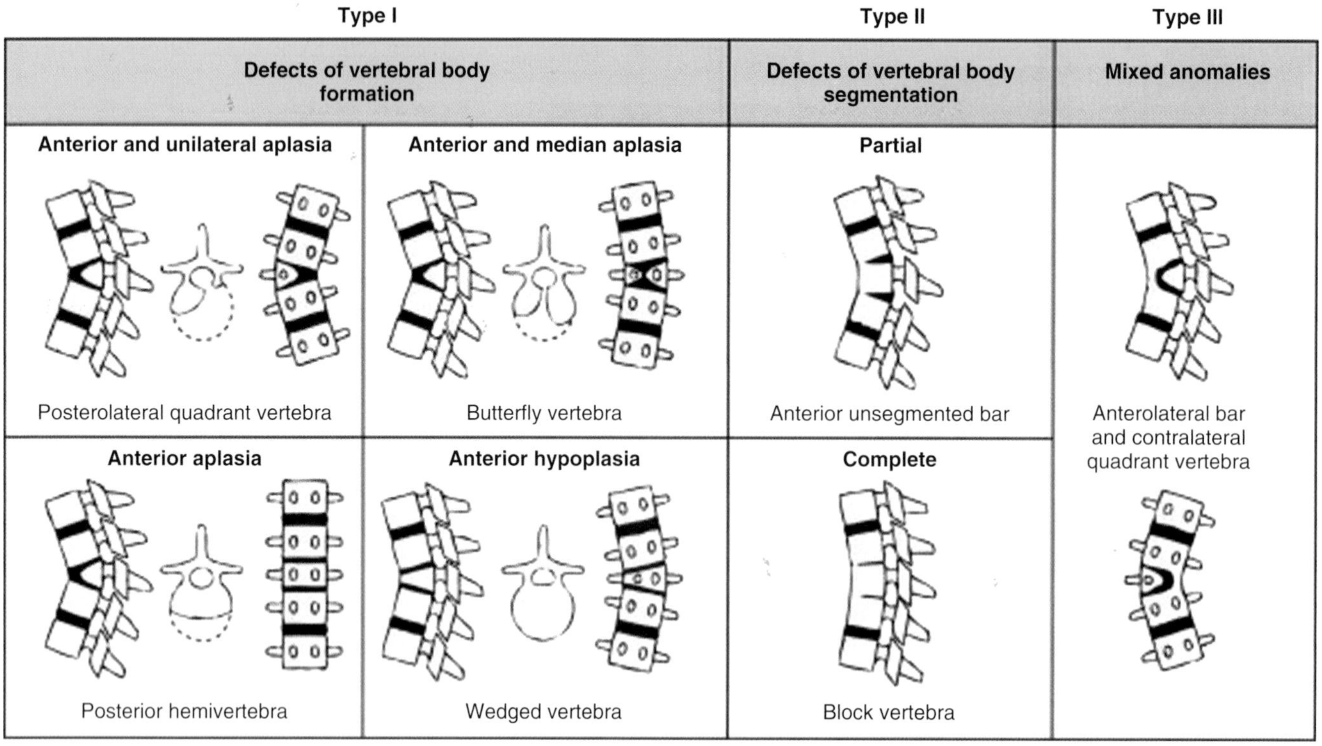

	Type I		Type II	Type III
	Defects of vertebral body formation		**Defects of vertebral body segmentation**	**Mixed anomalies**
	Anterior and unilateral aplasia	**Anterior and median aplasia**	**Partial**	
	Posterolateral quadrant vertebra	Butterfly vertebra	Anterior unsegmented bar	Anterolateral bar and contralateral quadrant vertebra
	Anterior aplasia	**Anterior hypoplasia**	**Complete**	
	Posterior hemivertebra	Wedged vertebra	Block vertebra	

FIGURE 3-28 Vertebral anomalies leading to congenital kyphosis. (Adapted from Herring JA, editor: *Tachdjian's pediatric orthopaedics,* ed 4, Philadelphia, 2008, Saunders, Figure 12-69.)

Table 3-13	**Treatment in Neuromuscular Scoliosis**	
CONDITION	**BRACING**	**OPERATIVE**
Duchenne muscular dystrophy	Ineffective	Early; 25-30 degrees to delay pulmonary function deterioration
Friedrich ataxia	Ineffective	Fusion if > 50 degrees or progressive
Spinal muscular atrophy	Useful to delay fusion in young patients with curves between 25 and 45 degrees	Fusion if > 50 degrees or progressive
Spina bifida (myelomeningocele)	Useful to delay fusion in young patients with curves between 25 and 45 degrees	Fusion if > 50 degrees or progressive
Cerebral palsy	Ineffective	>50 degrees in ambulatory patients Progressive curves > 50 degrees in communicative and aware patients Curve interfering with seating and nursing, with family desire for surgery
Neurofibromatosis	Nondystrophic curves between 25 and 40 degrees	Fusion if > 40 degrees or progressive
Arthrogryposis	Ineffective	Fusion if > 50 degrees or progressive

- Functions as a posterior (convex) hemiepiphysiodesis
- Anterior/posterior fusion:
  - Reserved for older children or more severe curves
- Anterior vertebrectomy, spinal cord decompression, and anterior fusion followed by posterior fusion are indicated for curves associated with neurologic deficits.
- Vertebral column resection: hemivertebra causing coronal or sagittal plane deformity and/or large fixed spinal deformity
- A type II congenital kyphosis can be monitored to document progression, but progressive curves should be fused posteriorly.

NEUROMUSCULAR SCOLIOSIS (TABLE 3-13)

- Spine deformity is common with neuromuscular conditions.
- Typical underlying neuromuscular conditions associated with scoliosis:

- Traumatic paralysis
- Duchenne muscular dystrophy
- Friedrich ataxia
- Spinal muscular atrophy
- Myelomeningocele
- Cerebral palsy
- Neurofibromatosis
- Arthrogryposis
- Curve characteristics:
- Long, sweeping C-shaped curves
- Associated pelvic obliquity
- Can be rapidly progressive, especially for patients who are in a wheelchair
- Associated characteristics
- Pulmonary issues
  - Most affected patients have some involvement secondary to the underlying condition (Duchenne muscular dystrophy) and detrimental contribution from the scoliosis.

- Cardiac issues
  - Duchenne muscular dystrophy and other conditions
- **Evaluation**
- Pulmonary: bilevel positive airway pressure (BiPAP) may be required before and after surgery.
- Cardiac: for patients with Duchenne muscular dystrophy
- Nutritional lab markers:
  - **Patients with leukocyte count less than 1500 leukocytes/μL and albumin less than 3.5 g/dL have a higher infection rate and longer hospital stay**
  - **Consider supplemental nutrition or gastrostomy tube feeding**
- **Nonoperative treatment**
- Wheelchair modifications
  - For patients in a wheelchair, trunk support can be modified to provide better truncal balance.
- **Corticosteroids in boys with Duchenne muscular dystrophy have been shown to reduce incidence and delay development of scoliosis.**
- Brace
  - Controversial and not typically used
  - May be used to delay surgical treatment
- **Surgical treatment**
- Indications: vary with diagnosis and somewhat controversial
  - Duchenne muscular dystrophy
    - Surgery indicated when curve is progressive and over 25 to 30 degrees in patients whose forced vital capacity (FVC) is greater than 40% of normal.
    - Surgery is best tolerated before the patient's FVC is less than 35% of age-matched normal values.
    - Curve progression is rapid, and pulmonary and cardiac conditions worsen with time, precluding surgery.
  - Cerebral palsy
    - Ambulatory patients: curve exceeding 50 degrees
    - Nonambulatory patients: dependent on sitting balance and whether there are challenges with caring for the child. Curve magnitudes may be very large before surgical treatment.
- Fusion levels
  - Nonambulatory patients:
    - Usually from T2 to pelvis
    - Pelvic fixation with unit rods, Dunn-McCarthy rods, or iliac screws
    - Segmental spinal fixation with wires or pedicle screws
- Goal of surgery
  - To center the trunk over the pelvis and achieve a balanced spine
- High complication rate
  - Infection: up to 15% in one study; pelvic instrumentation a risk factor

NEUROFIBROMATOSIS

- **Most patients with orthopedic manifestations have type 1 neurofibromatosis (NF1)**
- **Autosomal dominant disorder affecting *NF1* gene (neurofibromin 1) on chromosome 17**
- **Diagnosis—two of the following criteria:**

- More than six café au lait spots
- Two or more neurofibromas of any type or one plexiform neurofibroma
- Freckling in the axillae or inguinal regions
- Optic glioma
- Two or more Lisch nodules (iris hamartomas)
- A distinctive bone lesion, such as thinning of the cortex of a long bone
- A first-degree relative (parent, sibling, or offspring) with neurofibromatosis
- **The spine is the most common site of skeletal involvement; up to 10% of patients.**
- **Curve classification:**
- Nondystrophic (similar to idiopathic scoliosis): can modulate into dystrophic pattern
- Dystrophic
  - Characteristic radiographic abnormalities:
    - Short segment curves with tight apex
    - Vertebral scalloping
    - Enlarged foramina
    - Penciling of transverse processes
    - Penciling of ribs
    - Severe apical rotation
    - Can have severe kyphoscoliosis
- Evaluation
  - Plain radiographic findings
    - Penciling of three or more ribs is a prognostic factor for impending rapid progression of spinal deformity.
  - MRI
    - Neurologic involvement is common in neurofibromatosis and may be caused by the deformity itself, an intraspinal tumor, a soft tissue mass, or dural ectasia.
  - CT scan
    - Especially when surgery is planned
    - To assess the bony anatomy
      - Pedicle sizes and posterior body are small and eroded secondary to the dural ectasia.
- Treatment
  - Nondystrophic scoliosis: treatment is similar to that of idiopathic scoliosis.
  - Dystrophic deformities:
    - More aggressively treated, especially when kyphosis is present; surgical treatment is indicated for any progression and when curves reach 40 degrees.
    - Anterior/posterior surgery:
      - In young patients, especially when deformities are associated with kyphosis
      - To prevent crankshaft phenomenon
      - To improve fusion rates
    - Isolated kyphosis of the thoracic spine is treated with anterior decompression of the kyphotic angular cord compression, followed by anterior and posterior fusion or vertebral column resection from the posterior approach.
    - Cervical spine involvement includes kyphosis or atlantoaxial instability.
      - Treatment: posterior fusion with autologous grafting and halo immobilization is recommended for severe cervical spine deformity with instability.

KYPHOSIS

▥ Scheuermann disease

▥ Definition: increased thoracic kyphosis (>45 degrees) with 5 degrees or more anterior wedging at three sequential vertebrae (Figure 3-29)

▥ Cause unknown

▥ Other radiographic findings
- Disc space narrowing
- End plate irregularities
- Spondylolysis (30% to 50% of cases)
- Scoliosis (33% of cases)
- Schmorl nodes

▥ Clinical characteristics
- More common in boys
- Affected patients usually overweight
- Kyphosis is not postural—does not completely correct with hyperextension.
- Neurologic changes are rare; MRI indicated if they are present.

▥ Treatment
- Bracing
  - Progressive curve in a patient with 1 year or more of skeletal growth remaining (Risser stage 2 or below)
  - Indicated for kyphotic curvature of 50 to 75 degrees
  - A modified Milwaukee brace is used but often not well tolerated.
- Surgery
  - Indications: progressive or severe (>75 degrees) curve, continued pain despite physical therapy (PT), skeletal maturity

- Technique
  - All posterior: nearly always enough
  - Multiple Ponte osteotomies
  - Fusion levels
    - Proximal: for thoracic Scheuermann disease, T2; for thoracolumbar Scheuermann disease, T3 or T4
    - Distal: always include the first lordotic disc and the vertebra touched by the posterior sacral vertical line (vertical line extending from the posterior edge of S1).

▥ Thoracolumbar or lumbar Scheuermann disease
- Less common than thoracic form
- Causes more back pain
- End plates may be more irregular
- Not associated with vertebral wedging

▥ Postural kyphosis or round back

▥ Does not demonstrate vertebral body changes

▥ No sharp angulation as in Scheuermann disease

▥ Correction with backward bending and prone hyperextension is typical.

▥ Treatment includes a hyperextension exercise program.

▥ Other causes of kyphosis:

▥ Trauma

▥ Infection

▥ Spondylitis

▥ Bone dysplasias (mucopolysaccharidoses, Kniest syndrome, diastrophic dysplasia), and neoplasms

▥ Postlaminectomy kyphosis (most often for spinal cord abnormalities)
- Can be severe and necessitates anterior and posterior fusion

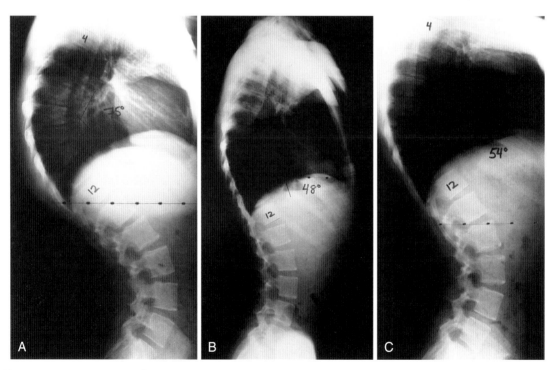

FIGURE 3-29 A, A 16-year-old boy with Scheuermann kyphosis measuring 75 degrees. **B,** After 6 months of serial Risser casting, the deformity was reduced to 48 degrees. **C,** At 18 years of age, the kyphosis measured 54 degrees. (From Herring JA, editor: *Tachdjian's pediatric orthopaedics,* ed 5, Philadelphia, 2014, Elsevier Saunders, Figure 13-7.)

- Total laminectomy in immature patients without stabilization is contraindicated because of this.

CERVICAL SPINE DISORDERS

▪ Klippel-Feil syndrome
- Abnormalities in multiple cervical segments as a result of failure of normal segmentation or formation of cervical somites at 3 to 8 weeks of gestation
- Associations
  - Congenital scoliosis
  - **Renal disease (aplasia: 33% of cases)**
  - Synkinesis (mirror motions)
  - Sprengel deformity (30% of cases)
  - **Congenital heart disease (14%-29% of cases)**
  - Brainstem abnormalities
  - Congenital cervical stenosis
  - **MRI required to rule out intraspinal cord abnormalities**
  - **Renal and cardiac evaluation is mandatory.**
- The classic triad (seen in < 50% of cases)
  - Low posterior hairline
  - Short "webbed" neck
  - Limited cervical ROM
- Disc degeneration: almost 100% of cases
- Treatment
  - Avoid collision sports
  - Conservative (most commonly)
  - Surgery for chronic pain with myelopathy

▪ Atlantoaxial instability
- Associated with:
  - Down syndrome (trisomy 21)
    - If normal neurologic picture: avoid contact sports
    - If neurologic symptoms or atlanto-dens interval (ADI) greater than 10 mm: posterior fusion (associated with high rate of complications)
  - Juvenile rheumatoid arthritis
  - Skeletal dysplasias such as spondyloepiphyseal dysplasia, diastrophic dysplasia, and Kniest dysplasia among others
  - Os odontoideum and other abnormalities

▪ Atlantoaxial rotatory displacement or subluxation
- May manifest with torticollis
- Causes

- Ligamentous laxity (Down syndrome)
- Retropharyngeal inflammation (Grisel disease)
- Trauma
- Diagnosis:
  - CT scans at the C1-C2 level with the head straight forward, then in maximum rotation to the right, and then in maximum rotation to the left
- Treatment
  - **Symptoms for less than 1 week: C-collar, analgesics, heat**
  - **Symptoms for between 1 and 4 weeks: Halter or Halo traction**
  - **Symptoms for greater than 1 month: surgical reduction and fusion often needed**

▪ Os odontoideum
- Previously thought to result from failure of fusion of the base of the odontoid (**usually fuses between ages 4 and 6**)
- May represent the residue of an old traumatic process
- Two types
  - Orthotopic type: in place of the normal odontoid process
  - Dystopic type: may fuse to the clivus (more often seen with neurologic compromise)
- Treatment
  - Conservative except in the following cases:
    - Instability (>10 mm of the atlanto-dens interval or <13 mm space available for the cord)
    - Presence of neurologic symptoms, which necessitate a posterior C1-C2 fusion

▪ Pseudosubluxation of the cervical spine
- Subluxation of C2 on C3 (and occasionally of C3 on C4) of up to 40%, or 4 mm
- Can be a normal finding in children younger than 8 years because of the orientation of the facets
- Rapid resolution of pain, relatively minor trauma, lack of anterior swelling
- Continued alignment of the posterior interspinous distances and the posterior spinolaminar line (Swischuk line) on radiographs (Figure 3-30)
- The fact that the subluxation can be reduced with neck extension helps differentiate this entity from more serious disorders.

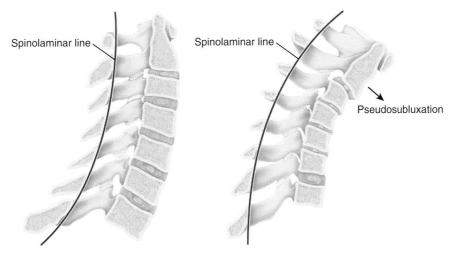

FIGURE 3-30 Pseudosubluxation of C2-C3 (most common). Actual subluxation is not possible because of the intact spinolaminar line at C2-C3. (From Herring JA, editor: *Tachdjian's pediatric orthopaedics,* ed 4, Philadelphia, 2008, Saunders, Figure 11-4.)

■ **Intervertebral disc calcification syndrome**

▥ Pain, decreased ROM

▥ Low-grade fevers

▥ Increased ESR

▥ Characteristic radiographic finding: disc calcification (within the annulus) without erosion

▥ Usually involves the cervical spine

▥ Conservative treatment indicated for this self-limiting condition

■ **Basilar impression/invagination**

▥ Deformity at the base of the skull causes odontoid migration into the foramen magnum

▥ Sagittal MRI scan best demonstrates impingement of the dens on the brainstem.

▥ Clinical presentation: weakness, paresthesias, and hydrocephalus may result.

▥ Treatment is often operative and may include transoral resection of the dens, occipital laminectomy, and occipitocervical fusion and wiring.

SPONDYLOLYSIS AND SPONDYLOLISTHESIS

■ **Spondylolysis: stress fracture at the pars interarticularis**

▥ Common in athletes who use hyperextension (gymnasts, football linemen, wrestlers, divers)

▥ Imaging
  • Plain radiographs: classically, oblique views were obtained, but recent studies question their utility (more radiation).
  • MRI: high sensitivity, shows early stress fractures
  • CT scan: best bony detail

▥ Treatment
  • Skeletally mature patients with incidental finding of spondylolysis require no follow-up.
  • Nonoperative for symptomatic spondylolysis:

• Rest
• Bracing in the acute period with an antilordotic brace (TLSO with thigh extension)
• PT: core strengthening and hamstring stretch
• Operative:
  • Indications: continued pain or neurologic symptoms despite conservative treatment
  • Direct pars repair
    • Useful in young patients with "hot" bone scan indicating healing potential
    • MRI mandatory to ensure no disc degeneration (contraindication)
    • Multiple techniques including lag screw fixation (Buck technique), compression wiring, and hybrid pedicle constructs
  • L5-S1 fusion: for defects at L5

■ **Spondylolisthesis: forward slippage of the proximal vertebra on the distal vertebra**

▥ Most commonly seen at L5-S1

▥ Types (Wiltse classification)
  • Isthmic (from spondylolysis)
  • Dysplastic (congenital absence or dysplasia of the facets)
    • Greater risk for progression

▥ Radiographs (Figure 3-31)
  • Translation: Meyerding grading system (low: grades 1 and 2; high: grades 3 and 4)
  • Slip angle
    • Most important determinant for nonunion and pain
    • Measured from the bottom end plate of L5 and a perpendicular to the line on the posterior sacrum
    • **Angle greater than 45 to 50 degrees associated with greater risk of slip progression, instability, and development of postoperative pseudarthrosis**
  • Pelvic incidence (PI) (Figure 3-32)

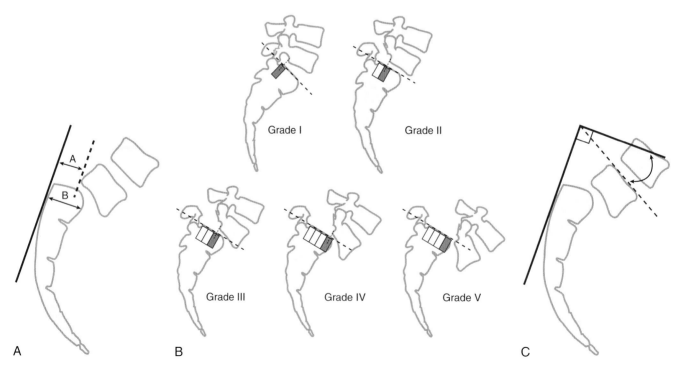

FIGURE 3-31 Spondylolisthesis. **A,** Percentage of forward slippage (A/B) described by Taillard. **B,** Meyerding grades I to V. The degree of spondylolisthesis is determined by dividing the sacral body into four segments. Grade V is complete spondyloptosis. **C,** The slip angle is measured from the superior border of L5, and a line is drawn perpendicular to the posterior edge of the sacrum. (From Herring JA, editor: *Tachdjian's pediatric orthopaedics,* ed 5, Philadelphia, 2014, Elsevier Saunders, Figure 14-7.)

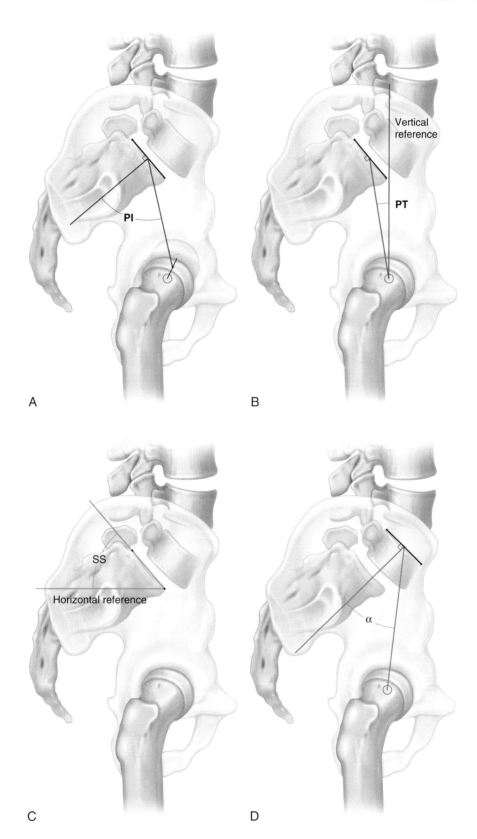

FIGURE 3-32 Pelvic incidence (PI). A line perpendicular to the midpoint of the sacral end plate is drawn. A second line connecting the same sacral midpoint and the center of the femoral heads is drawn. The angle subtended by these lines is the PI. (From Herring JA, editor: *Tachdjian's pediatric orthopaedics*, ed 5, Philadelphia, 2014, Elsevier Saunders, Figure 14-9A.)

- Angle created by a line from the midpoint of the sacral end plate to the center of the femoral heads and a line perpendicular to the sacral end plate (normal, ≈50 degrees)
- Unaffected by posture
- **Increased PI may predispose to spondylolisthesis.**
- Clinical manifestation
  - Low-grade slippage may manifest with low back pain and normal examination findings
  - High-grade slippage (>50%) may be accompanied by a flexed hip and knee posture with equinus, sacral prominence, and proximal hyperlordosis.
- Treatment
  - Asymptomatic low-grade spondylolisthesis
    - No treatment; monitor younger patients for progression
  - Symptomatic low-grade spondylolisthesis
    - Similar to spondylolysis (rest, PT, activity modification, brace)
    - If continued pain: arthrodesis with or without instrumentation
  - High-grade spondylolisthesis
    - In general, surgery indicated because high risk for progression
    - Surgery:
      - Multiple techniques, controversial
      - In general, L4-S1 fusion required
      - Neurologic decompression with high-grade slippage or neurologic symptoms
      - Anterior fusion through posterior approach should be considered.
      - Correction of slip angle and reduction (controversial because it may increase risk of neurologic deficits). **L5 root injury is the most common neurologic complication.**

OTHER SPINAL CONDITIONS

- **Infectious spondylitis (discitis and vertebral osteomyelitis)**
- Epidemiology
  - Patients with discitis often younger (mean age, 2.8 vs. 7.5 years)
  - Most commonly seen at L3-L4 and L4-L5 disc spaces
  - *S. aureus* most commonly seen, though *K. kingae, Mycobacterium tuberculosis, Bartonella henselae,* and *Salmonella* also seen
- Presentation and evaluation
  - Acute back pain, refusal to sit or bear weight
  - Radiographic changes usually lag behind clinical findings.
    - Loss of lumbar lordosis, disc space narrowing, and end plate changes in that order
  - MRI also highly sensitive and specific
- Treatment
  - Cultures positive in only 60% of cases; routine disc cultures not necessary
  - Intravenous antibiotic treatment with coverage for *S. aureus*
  - Surgery indications include abscess or failure of nonoperative management.
- **Low back pain (Table 3-14)**
- Low back pain and especially painful scoliosis should be taken seriously in children.

- However, up to 75% to 80% of children with low back pain will not have a diagnosis.
- Additional etiologies not discussed
  - Discitis and osteomyelitis
    - Manifestations
      - Acute back pain
      - Refusal to sit or walk
      - Increased ESR
    - Radiographic findings
      - Loss of normal lumbar lordosis (earliest radiographic finding)
      - Disc space narrowing but preservation of end plates (develops over a period of 3 weeks after loss of lumbar lordosis)
    - Treatment
      - Antibiotics
  - Herniated nucleus pulposus (can also be a herniated end plate in adolescence)
    - Uncommon in children
    - Manifestations
      - Back pain
      - Pain radiating down the leg
    - Treatment
      - Pain management
      - Rest in the acute period
      - PT when symptoms allow
- **Diastematomyelia**
- Fibrous, cartilaginous, or osseous bar creating a longitudinal cleft in the spinal cord

Table 3-14	Differential Diagnosis for Low Back Pain in Children
CATEGORY	**DISEASE**
Musculoskeletal	Nonspecific back pain or sprain/strain
	Spondylolysis/spondylolisthesis
	Fracture
	Intervertebral disc degeneration or herniation
	Scoliosis
	Scheuermann kyphosis
Infectious	Discitis
	Vertebral osteomyelitis
	Epidural abscess
	Sacroiliac septic arthritis
	Paraspinal abscess
	Nonspinal infection (pneumonia, pyelonephritis, appendicitis)
Inflammatory	Ankylosing spondylitis
	Psoriatic arthritis
	Reactive arthritis
Neoplastic	Osteoid osteoma or osteoblastoma
	Aneurysmal bone cyst
	Neurofibroma
	Eosinophilic granuloma
	Leukemia/lymphoma
	Solid malignancy (Ewing sarcoma, osteosarcoma)
	Primary spinal cord tumors (astrocytoma, ependymoma)
	Metastatic disease
Miscellaneous	Sickle cell crisis
	Syringomyelia or tethered cord
	Idiopathic juvenile osteoporosis
	Chronic multifocal recurrent osteomyelitis (CMRO)
	Conversion disorder

- More commonly occurs in the lumbar spine: can lead to tethering of the cord, with associated neurologic deficits
- Intrapedicular widening on plain radiographs is suggestive.
- CT or MRI is necessary to fully define the disorder.
- Must be resected before correction of a spinal deformity, otherwise if asymptomatic it may monitored without surgery
- **Sacral agenesis**
- Partial or complete absence of the sacrum and lower lumbar spine

- **Strongly associated with maternal diabetes**
- Often accompanied by gastrointestinal, genitourinary, and cardiovascular abnormalities
- Presentation:
  - Prominent lower lumbar spine and atrophic lower extremities
  - May sit in a "Buddha" position
  - Motor impairment is at the level of the agenesis, but sensory innervation is largely spared
- Management may include amputation of the legs or spinal-pelvic fusion.

SECTION 7 CEREBRAL PALSY

INTRODUCTION

- **Nonprogressive neuromuscular disorder**
- Onset before age 2 years
- Results from injury to the immature brain
- **Cause is usually not identifiable but can include:**
- Prematurity (most common)
- Prenatal intrauterine factors
- Perinatal infections (TORCH—*t*oxoplasmosis, *o*ther infections, *r*ubella, *c*ytomegalovirus infection, and *h*erpes simplex)
- Anoxic injuries
- Meningitis
- **This upper motor neuron disease results in a mixture of muscle weakness and spasticity.**
- **Initially the abnormal muscle forces cause dynamic deformity at joints.**

- Persistent spasticity can lead to contractures, bony deformity, and ultimately joint subluxation/dislocation.
- **MRI of the brain commonly reveals periventricular leukomalacia.**

CLASSIFICATION

- **Cerebral palsy can be classified on the basis of physiology (according to the movement disorder), anatomy (according to geographic distribution), or function.**
- **Physiologic classification (Figure 3-33):**
- Spastic
  - Increased muscle tone and hyperreflexia with slow, restricted movements because of simultaneous contraction of agonist and antagonist

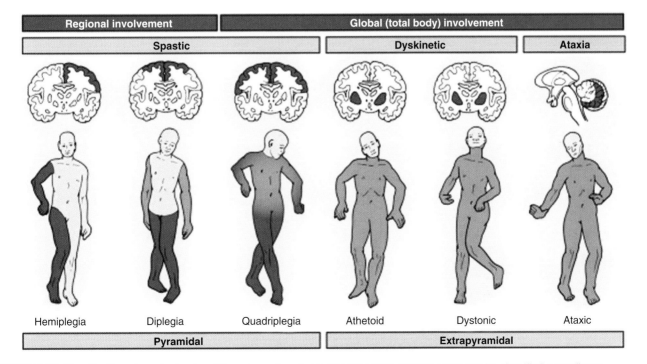

FIGURE 3-33 Classification of cerebral palsy. Although overlaps in terminology exist, cerebral palsy can be classified according to distribution (regional versus global involvement; hemiplegic, diplegic, quadriplegic), physiologic type (spastic, dyskinetic/dystonic, dyskinetic/athetoid, ataxic), or presumed neurologic substrate (pyramidal, extrapyramidal). (Redrawn from Pellegrino L: Cerebral palsy. In Batshaw ML, editor: *Children with disabilities,* ed 4, Baltimore, 1997, Paul H. Brookes.)

- Most common and is most amenable to improvement of musculoskeletal function by operative intervention
- Athetosis
  - Constant succession of slow, writhing, involuntary movements
  - Less common and more difficult to treat
- Ataxia
  - Inability to coordinate muscles for voluntary movement, resulting in unbalanced wide-based gait
  - Less amenable to orthopaedic treatment
- Mixed
  - Typically involves a combination of spasticity and athetosis with total body involvement
- **Anatomic classification (see Figure 3-33):**
- Hemiplegia
  - Involves upper and lower extremities on the same side, usually with spasticity
  - "Handedness" often develops early
  - All children with hemiplegia are eventually able to walk, regardless of treatment
- Diplegia
  - Lower extremity involved more extensively than upper extremity
  - Most diplegic patients eventually walk
  - IQ may be normal; strabismus is common.
  - Total involvement (quadriplegia)
  - Extensive involvement, low IQ, and a high mortality rate
  - Affected patients usually unable to walk
- **Functional classification**
- Gross motor and functional classification system (GMFCS) (Figure 3-34)
  - Classification is based on walking ability and need for assistive devices.
  - Functional loss over time or after surgery can be monitored with GMFCS.

ORTHOPAEDIC ASSESSMENT

- **Examination**
- Based on examination and thorough birth and developmental history
- A patient's locomotor profile is based on the persistence of primitive reflexes; the presence of two or more usually means the child will not be able to ambulate.
  - Commonly tested reflexes include the Moro startle reflex (normally disappears by age 6 months) and the parachute reflex (normally disappears by age 12 months).
  - The ability to sit independently by age 2 years is highly prognostic of ability to walk.

SPASTICITY TREATMENT

- **Botulinum toxin**
- Intramuscular botulinum A toxin can temporarily decrease dynamic spasticity.
- **Mechanism of action of botulinum toxin is a presynaptic blockade at the neuromuscular junction.**
- Effectiveness of botulinum toxin is limited to 3 to 6 months; therefore, it is not a permanent cure for spasticity.
- It is used to maintain joint motion during rapid growth when a child is too young for surgery.
- **Dorsal rhizotomy**

- Selective dorsal root rhizotomy is a neurosurgical procedure designed to decrease lower extremity spasticity.
- Includes resection of dorsal rootlets that do not exhibit a myographic or clinical response to stimulation
- Performed primarily in ambulatory patients (age 4-8) with spastic diplegia to help reduce spasticity and complement orthopaedic management
- Requires multilevel laminoplasty, which may lead to late spinal instability and deformity
- Contraindicated in athetoid patients and nonambulatory patients with spastic quadriplegia (increased spinal deformities)
- **Systemic medication**
- Oral baclofen used as adjunct therapy to control overall tone
  - Provides decreased tone in all extremities by inhibiting signals through the γ-aminobutyric acid (GABA) pathway
  - Negative effects include increased somnolence and decreased alertness during the day
- **Baclofen pump**
- Surgical implantation of a pump that provides only local delivery of baclofen to an area of the spinal cord
  - Pump then delivers a much lower dose of baclofen.
  - Pump is then refilled when empty.
- No systemic delivery; thus less somnolence
- May exacerbate scoliosis progression
- Wound problems common in thin children

GAIT DISORDERS

- **Evaluation**
- Findings are usually the impetus for the orthopaedic consultation.
- In many hemiplegic patients, toe walking is the only manifestation.
- Three-dimensional computerized gait analysis with dynamic electromyography and force-plate studies have allowed a more scientific approach to preoperative decision making and postoperative analysis of the results of surgery for cerebral palsy.
- **Types**
- Toe-walking—contracted heel cords
  - Treat with ankle foot orthosis (AFO) if passively correctable
  - Posterior leaf spring orthotic used if excessive ankle plantar flexion in swing phase of gate
  - Surgical treatment includes gastrocnemius recession verses tendo Achilles lengthening
- Crouched gait
  - Usually due to hamstring contracture
  - Resultant deformity includes hip flexion, knee flexion, ankle equinus
  - Treat with lengthenings at hip, knee, and ankle.
    - Caution with isolated heel cord lengthening—will worsen crouched gait secondary to worsening hip and knee flexion
- Stiff knee gait
  - Common in spastic diplegia with rectus femoris firing out of phase
  - Treat with transfer of distal rectus transfer to the hamstrings

GMFCS FOR CHILDREN AGED 6–12 YEARS: DESCRIPTORS AND ILLUSTRATIONS

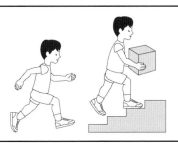

GMFCS level I

Children walk indoors and outdoors and climb stairs without limitation. Children perform gross motor skills including running and jumping, but speed, balance, and coordination are impaired.

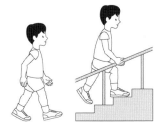

GMFCS level II

Children walk indoors and outdoors and climb stairs holding onto a railing but experience limitations walking on uneven surfaces and inclines and walking in crowds or confined spaces and with long distances.

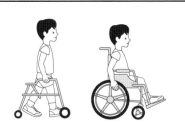

GMFCS level III

Children walk indoors or outdoors on a level surface with an assistive mobility device and may climb stairs holding onto a railing. Children may use wheelchair mobility when traveling for long distances or outdoors on uneven terrain.

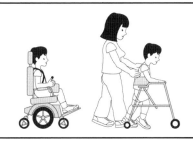

GMFCS level IV

Children use methods of mobility that usually require adult assistance. They may continue to walk for short distances with physical assistance at home but rely more on wheeled mobility (pushed by an adult or operate a powered chair) outdoors, at school, and in the community.

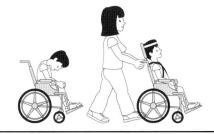

GMFCS level V

Physical impairment restricts voluntary control of movement and the ability to maintain antigravity head and trunk postures. All areas of motor function are limited. Children have no means of independent mobility and are transported by an adult.

FIGURE 3-34 Gross motor and functional classification system (GMFCS) for children ages 6 to 12 years: descriptors and illustrations. (Illustrations copyrighted by Kerr Graham, Bill Reid, and Adrienne Harvey, The Royal Children's Hospital, Melbourne Eastern Resource Centre, Melbourne, Australia.)

■ **Treatment**
▦ Lengthening of continuously active muscles and transfer of muscles out of phase are often helpful.
▦ Surgeries should usually be done at multiple levels to best correct the problem.
▦ In general, surgery is performed at age 4 to 5 years. A few generalized guidelines are given in Table 3-15.

SPINAL DISORDERS

■ **Evaluation**
▦ Scoliosis can be severe, making proper wheelchair sitting difficult.

▦ Risk for scoliosis highest in children with total body involvement (spastic quadriplegic)
▦ Surgical indications include curves greater than 45 to 50 degrees, worsening pelvic obliquity, or wheelchair seating problems.
▦ Scoliosis more likely to progress than in idiopathic scoliosis
  • 1 to 2 degrees per year starting at age 8 to 10 years
  • Bracing is less effective.
■ **Treatment**
▦ Treatment is tailored to the needs of the patient and must involve all caregivers.

Table 3-15	Surgical Options for Gait Disorders	
PROBLEM	**DIAGNOSTIC FINDINGS**	**SURGICAL OPTION**
Hip flexion	Positive result of Thomas test	Psoas tenotomy or recession
Spastic hip	Decreased abduction, uncovered femoral head	Adductor release, osteotomy (late)
Hip adduction	Scissoring gait	Adductor release
Femoral anteversion	Prone internal rotation increased	Osteotomy, VDRO, hamstring lengthening
Knee flexion	Increased popliteal angle	Hamstring lengthening
Knee hypertension	Recurvatum	Rectus femoris lengthening
Stiff-leg gait	Electromyographic study of hamstring and quadriceps; continuous passive knee flexion decreased with hip extension	Distal rectus transfer to hamstrings
Talipes equinus	Toe walking	Achilles tendon lengthening
Talipes varus	Appearance in standing position	Split–anterior or split–posterior tibialis transfer (on the basis of EMG findings)
Talipes valgus	Appearance in standing position	Peroneal lengthening, Grice subtalar fusion, calcaneal lengthening osteotomy
Hallux valgus	Appearance on examination and radiographs	Osteotomy, metatarsophalangeal fusion

EMG, Electromyographic; *VDRO,* varus derotation osteotomy.

- Small curves with no loss of function or large curves in severely involved patients may necessitate only observation.
- Curves in ambulatory patients are treated as idiopathic scoliosis with posterior fusion and instrumentation.
- Curves in nonambulatory and those with pelvic obliquity may necessitate posterior fusion with segmental posterior instrumentation from the upper thoracic spine to the pelvis (Luque-Galveston technique), with or without anterior fusion.
- Kyphosis is also common and may necessitate fusion and instrumentation.
- It is important to assess nutritional status (albumin < 3.5 g/dL and WBC count < 1500/μL) preoperatively and to consider gastrostomy tube placement before spinal surgery if indicated.
- Much higher complication rate than with idiopathic scoliosis
  - Wound infection (3%-5%)
  - Pulmonary complications
  - Implant failure
  - Increased rate of fatality (as high as 7% in some series)

HIP SUBLUXATION AND DISLOCATION

■ Evaluation
- In many children, pathologic processes of the hip are asymptomatic.
- Caregivers may describe a pain response.
- Difficulty with abduction for peroneal care is the most common problem.

■ Treatment
- Initial treatment is with a soft tissue release (adductor/psoas) plus abduction bracing.
- Later, hip subluxation or dislocation may necessitate femoral or acetabular osteotomies (Dega) or both to maintain hip stability.
- The goal is to keep the hip reduced.
- This entity is characterized by four stages:
  - Hip at risk: abduction of less than 45 degrees, with partial uncovering of the femoral head on radiographs. This situation is the only exception to the general rule

of avoiding surgery in patients with cerebral palsy during the first 3 years of life.
  - Patient may benefit from adductor and psoas release.
- Hip subluxation: best treated with adductor tenotomy in children with abduction of less than 20 degrees, sometimes with psoas release or recession
  - Femoral or pelvic osteotomies may be considered in cases of femoral coxa valga and acetabular dysplasia, which is usually lateral and posterior.
- Spastic dislocation: patients may benefit from open reduction, femoral shortening, varus derotation osteotomy, Dega osteotomy (Figure 3-35), triple osteotomy, or Chiari osteotomy.
  - The type of pelvic osteotomy indicated is best determined in a three-dimensional CT scan, which demonstrates the area of acetabular deficiency (anterior, lateral, or posterior) and the congruency of the joint surfaces.
  - Addressing both hips can prevent dislocation of opposite hip.
  - **Late dislocations may best be left untreated or treated with a Schanz abduction osteotomy or a modified Girdlestone resection arthroplasty (resection below the lesser trochanter).**
- Windswept hips: characterized by abduction of one hip and adduction of the contralateral hip
  - Bilateral femoral osteotomies to achieve a more varus angle can assist in maintaining reduction.

KNEE ABNORMALITIES

■ Evaluation
- Usually includes hamstring contractures and decreased ROM
- Crouch gait in spastic diplegia patients

■ Treatment
- Hamstring lengthening is often helpful (sometimes increases lumbar lordosis).
  - To prevent peroneal nerve injury, be careful not to overextend the knee in the operating room.
- Distal transfer of an out-of-phase rectus femoris muscle to the semitendinosus or gracilis muscle is indicated

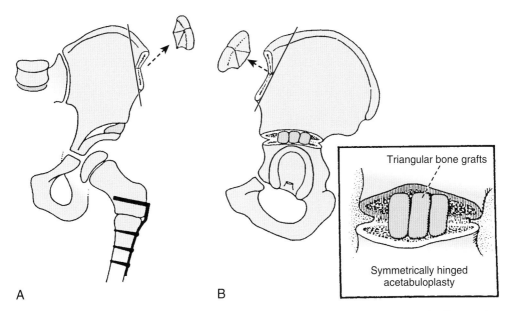

A   B

Triangular bone grafts

Symmetrically hinged
acetabuloplasty

FIGURE 3-35 Placement of graft for Dega acetabuloplasty. **A,** Bone graft is obtained from the anterosuperior iliac crest and shaped into three small triangles whose bases are 1 cm long. **B,** The grafts are placed in the osteotomy site; the largest is placed in the area where maximal improvement of coverage is desired. The triangular wedges are packed close to each other to prevent collapse, turning, or dislodgment; the result is a symmetric hinging on the **triradiate cartilage** *(inset).* With the medial wall of the pelvis maintained, the elasticity of the osteotomy keeps the wedges in place. No pins are necessary to maintain the osteotomy. (Adapted from Mubarak SJ et al: One-stage reconstruction of the spastic hip, *J Bone Joint Surg Am* 74:1352, 1992.)

when there is loss of knee flexion during the swing phase of gait (stiff knee gait).

FOOT AND ANKLE ABNORMALITIES

■ **Goal of treatment is to obtain a plantigrade, painless, braceable foot**
■ **Equinovalgus foot**
▦ Most common in spastic diplegia; also in quadriplegic
▦ Causes
  • Caused by spastic peroneal muscles, contracted heel cords, and ligamentous laxity
▦ Treatment
  • Peroneus brevis lengthening is often helpful in correcting moderate valgus angulation. Lateral column-lengthening calcaneal osteotomy is used to correct hindfoot valgus angulation.
■ **Equinovarus foot**
▦ Most common in spastic hemiplegia
▦ Causes
  • Overpull of the posterior or anterior tibialis tendons (or both)
▦ Treatment
  • Lengthening of the posterior tibialis is rarely sufficient.
  • Transfers
    • Likewise, transfer of an entire muscle (posterior or anterior tibialis) is rarely recommended.
    • Split-muscle transfers are helpful when the affected muscle is spastic during both the stance and swing phases of gait.
    • Split–posterior tibialis transfer (rerouting half of the tendon dorsally to the peroneus brevis) is used in cases with spasticity of the muscle, flexible varus foot, and weak peroneal muscles.
    • Complications include decreased foot dorsiflexion.
    • Split–anterior tibialis transfer (rerouting half of its tendon laterally to the cuboid) is used in patients

with spasticity of the muscle and a flexible varus deformity.
  • Often coupled with Achilles tendon lengthening and posterior tibial tendon intramuscular lengthening (Rancho procedure) to treat the fixed equinus contracture.
■ **Hallux valgus**
▦ Treatment includes first metatarsophalangeal (MTP) joint fusion
  • Recurrence rate unacceptably high, with bunion deformity correction without fusion
▦ Proximal phalanx (Akin) osteotomy
  • Used for hallux valgus interphalangeus in association with hallux valgus and can be done at same time as first MTP fusion

UPPER EXTREMITY MANAGEMENT

■ **Overview**
▦ Treatment divided into procedures to increase hygiene and those to produce better function
■ **Functional procedures indicated for patients with voluntary control and better sensibility**
■ **Shoulder contracture**
▦ Internal rotation contracture of the glenohumeral joint
▦ Treated with proximal humerus derotational osteotomy
  • May need subscapularis and pectoralis lengthening in addition to biceps/brachialis lengthening and capsulotomy
  • Indications include contractures greater than 30 degrees interfering with hand function.
■ **Elbow contracture**
▦ Flexion contracture
  • Treat with lacertus fibrosis release.
  • Biceps and brachialis lengthening
  • Brachioradialis origin release

- Pronation deformity
  - Treat with pronator teres release.
  - Caution with PT transfer to an anterolateral position—can lead to a supination deformity
- **Wrist flexion deformity**
- Wrist typically presents with flexion and ulnar deviation contracture.
- **May be treated early with flexor carpi ulnaris (FCU) to extensor carpi radialis brevis (ECRB) tendon transfer or FCU to extensor digitorum communis (EDC) transfer in functional patients with voluntary control**
  - Concomitant proximal row carpectomy may improve wrist position and severe digital finger tightness.
- Wrist arthrodesis for severe deformity or for hygienic procedure

- **Thumb in palm deformity**
- Flexed thump prevents grasping and can interfere with hygiene.
- Treatment with lengthening of adductor pollicis, first dorsal interosseous, flexor pollicis brevis, and flexor pollicis longus muscles
  - Combine with first web space Z-plasty and tendon transfer to augment thumb extension and abduction
- **Finger flexion deformity**
- Swan neck deformities can sometimes be corrected with correction of wrist flexion deformity.
- Fractional or Z-lengthening of tendon (with or without ulnar motor neurectomy) may improve digital flexor tightness and intrinsic spasticity in patients with a clenched fist.

SECTION 8 NEUROMUSCULAR DISORDERS

ARTHROGRYPOTIC SYNDROMES

- **Arthrogryposis multiplex congenita (amyoplasia):**
- Overview
  - Nonprogressive disorder with multiple joints that are congenitally rigid (Figure 3-36)
  - Can be myopathic, neuropathic, or both
  - Associated with a decrease in anterior horn cells and other neural elements of the spinal cord
  - Intelligence is normal.

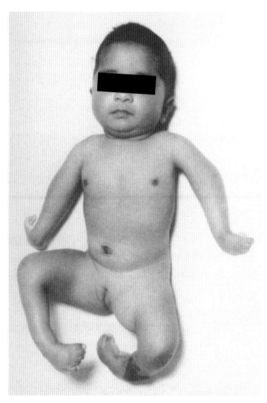

FIGURE 3-36 Arthrogryposis. Typical appearance of a child in whom all four limbs are affected. Note the lack of creases at the elbows, the flexion contractures at the knees, and the severe clubfoot deformities. (From Benson M et al: *Children's orthopaedics and fractures*, New York, 1994, Churchill Livingstone, p 321.)

- Evaluation
  - Evaluation should include neurologic studies, enzyme tests, and muscle biopsy (at 3 to 4 months of age).
  - Affected patients typically have normal facies, normal intelligence, multiple joint contractures, and no visceral abnormalities.
  - Upper extremity involvement
    - Adduction and internal rotation of the shoulder
    - Extension of the elbow—no appreciable elbow crease
    - Flexion and ulnar deviation of the wrist
  - Lower extremity involvement
    - Teratologic hip dislocations
    - Knee contractures (extended is classical, flexed is more common)
    - Resistant clubfeet
    - Vertical talus
  - The spine may be involved, with characteristic C-shaped (neuromuscular) scoliosis (33% of cases).
- Treatment
  - Upper extremity
    - Passive manipulation and serial casting to achieve some motion
    - Posterior elbow release with tricepsplasty to improve motion
    - Active elbow flexion achieved through one of:
      - Anterior transfer of long head of triceps
      - Bipolar transfer of latissimus or pectoralis major
      - Steindler flexorplasty—transfer origin of flexor pronator to the anterior humerus (rarely indicated because unopposed wrist flexion produces deformity in patients without active extension)
    - Osteotomies are also considered after 4 years of age to allow independent eating.
    - One upper extremity should be left in extension at the elbow for positioning and perineal care and the other elbow in flexion for feeding.
  - Lower extremity
    - Hip dislocation:
      - Unilateral: medial open reduction with possible femoral shortening
      - Bilateral: typically left unreduced because ambulation is often preserved
      - Pavlik harness contraindicated

- Knee contractures are treated with early (age 6-9 months) soft tissue releases (especially hamstrings).
- Foot deformities (clubfoot and vertical talus) are initially treated with a soft tissue release, but later recurrences may necessitate bone procedures (talectomy).
  - The goal is for the foot to be stiff and plantigrade to wear shoes and possibly ambulate.
- Knee contractures should be corrected before hip reduction to maintain the reduction.
- Spine
  - Fusion if curve is large (>50 degrees) or progressive
  - May impede function and ambulatory ability

■ **Distal arthrogryposis syndrome**
▥ Evaluation
- Autosomal dominant disorder that affects predominantly hands and feet
- Ulnarly deviated fingers (at metacarpal joints), metacarpal and proximal interphalangeal flexion contractures, and adducted thumbs with web space thickening are common.
- Clubfoot and vertical talus deformities are common in the feet.
▥ Treatment
- Comprehensive releases are more often required, combined with bony surgery.

■ **Larsen syndrome**
▥ Evaluation
- Similar to arthrogryposis in clinical appearance, but joints are less rigid
- Characterized primarily by multiple joint dislocations (including bilateral congenital knee dislocations), flattened facies, scoliosis, and clubfeet
- **Cervical kyphosis** (watch for late myelopathy) is important to recognize early.
- Affected patients have normal intelligence.
- Autosomal dominant form linked to mutation of gene encoding filamin B
- Autosomal recessive form linked to carbohydrate sulfotransferase 3 deficiency
▥ Treatment
- Posterior cervical fusion for progressive cervical kyphosis
- Knee reduction may necessitate femoral shortening and excision of collateral ligaments; closed reduction often unsuccessful.
- Open hip reduction is required; closed reduction unsuccessful.

■ **Multiple pterygium syndrome**
▥ Evaluation

- Autosomal recessive disorder whose name means "little wing" in Greek
- Characterized by cutaneous flexor surface webs (knee and elbow), congenital vertical talus, and scoliosis
▥ Treatment
- Care must be taken when the webs are elongated because of the superficial nature of the neurovascular bundle.

MYELODYSPLASIA (SPINA BIFIDA)

■ **Introduction**
▥ Causes
- Disorder of incomplete spinal cord closure or rupture of the developing cord secondary to hydrocephalus
▥ Classification:
- Spina bifida occulta: defect in the vertebral arch, with confined cord and meninges
- Meningocele: sac without neural elements protruding through the defect
- Myelomeningocele: in spina bifida, sac with neural elements protrudes through the skin
- Rachischisis: neural elements exposed, with no covering
- Function is related primarily to the level of the defect and the associated congenital abnormalities.
  - Myelodysplasia level based on lowest functional level (Table 3-16)
  - L4 is a key level because the quadriceps can function and allow independent ambulation around the community (Figure 3-37).

■ **Evaluation**
▥ Diagnosis
- Can be diagnosed in utero (increased levels of α-fetoprotein)
- Related to a folate deficiency in utero
- Type II Arnold-Chiari malformation is the most common comorbid condition.
▥ Central axis
- Sudden changes in function (rapid increase of scoliotic curvature, spasticity, new neurologic deficit, or increase in urinary tract infections) can be associated with tethered cord, hydrocephalus (most common), or syringomyelia.
- Head CT scans (70% of myelodysplastic patients have hydrocephalus) and myelography or spinal MRI are required.
▥ Fractures
- Fractures are also common in myelodysplasia, most often about the knee and hip in children 3 to 7 years

Table 3-16	Levels of Myelodysplasia				
	CHARACTERISTICS				
LEVEL	**HIP**	**KNEE**	**FEET**	**ORTHOSIS**	**EXTENT OF AMBULATION**
L1	External rotation/flexed	—	Equinovarus	HKAFO	Nonfunctional
L2	Adduction/flexed	Flexed	Equinovarus	HKAFO	Nonfunctional
L3	Adduction/flexed	Recurvatum	Equinovarus	KAFO	Household
L4	Adduction/flexed	Extended	Cavovarus	AFO	Household, some community
L5	Flexed	Limited flexion	Calcaneal valgus	AFO	Community
S1	—	—	Foot deformities	Shoes	Near normal

AFO, Ankle-foot orthosis; *HKAFO*, hip-knee-ankle-foot orthosis; *KAFO*, knee-ankle-foot orthosis.

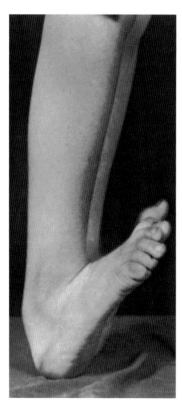

FIGURE 3-37 Myelodysplasia below L5. Typical posture of a leg and foot in an affected child. The feet assume a progressive calcaneus posture that necessitates surgical correction. (From Herring JA, editor: *Tachdjian's pediatric orthopaedics*, ed 4, Philadelphia, 2008, Saunders.)

Table 3-17	Milestones in Myelodysplasia	
AGE (months)	**FUNCTION**	**TREATMENT**
4-6	Head control	Positioning
6-10	Sitting	Supports/orthoses
10-12	Prone mobility	Prone board
12-15	Upright stance	Standing orthosis
15-18	Upright mobility	Trunk/extremity orthosis

of age, and can frequently be diagnosed only by noting redness, warmth, and swelling.
- Fractures are commonly misdiagnosed as infection in these patients.
- Fractures are treated conservatively with a well-padded splint.
- Fractures usually heal with abundant callus.

■ **Treatment principles**
■ Careful observation of patients with myelodysplasia is important. Several myelodysplasia "milestones" have been developed to assess progress (Table 3-17).
■ Treatment involves a team approach (urologist, orthopaedist, neurosurgeon, and developmental pediatrician) to allow maximal function consistent with the patient's level and other abnormalities.
■ Proper use of orthoses is essential in patients with myelodysplasia.
■ Determination of ambulation potential is based on the level of the deficit and motivation of the child.
■ Surgery for myelodysplasia focuses on balancing of muscles and correction of deformities.

■ Increased attention has been focused on latex sensitivity in myelodysplastic patients (immunoglobulin [Ig]E-mediated allergy).
- A latex-free environment is necessary to prevent life-threatening allergic reactions.

■ **Hip pathology**
■ Wide spectrum of hip disease:
- Flexion contractures
- Hip subluxation and dislocation
- DDH
- Abduction or external rotation contracture
- Management of the hip in patients with myelomeningocele is controversial.
■ Flexion contractures:
- Occur in patients with thoracic/high lumbar myelomeningocele as a result of unopposed hip flexors or in patients who sit most of the time
- Treatment
  - Anterior hip release with tenotomy of the iliopsoas, sartorius, rectus femoris, and tensor fasciae latae
  - For patients with lesions at the low lumbar level, the psoas should be preserved for independent ambulation.
  - Hip abduction contracture can cause pelvic obliquity and scoliosis; it is treated with proximal division of the tensor fasciae latae and distal iliotibial band release (Ober-Yount procedure).
  - Adduction contractures are treated with adductor myotomy
■ Hip dislocation
- Caused by paralysis of the hip abductors and extensors with unopposed hip flexors and adductors
  - Hip dislocation is most common at the level of L3-L4.
- Treatment
  - Containment is controversial, but in general, it is considered essential only in patients with a functioning quadriceps.
  - Redislocation may occur no matter what treatment is used to maintain the reduction.
  - Principles of treatment should follow those for any paralytic hip dislocation:
    - Concentric reduction
    - Bony abnormality correction (femoral anteversion with valgus, posterior acetabular insufficiency)
    - Muscle balance correction by means of transfer or release (flexor-adductor, extensor-abductor balance)
  - Late dislocation at the low lumbar level may be caused by a tethered cord, which must be released before the hip is reduced.
  - The functional outcome of thoracic-level myelomeningocele is independent of whether the hips are in proper position or dislocated.
    - Management should focus on limiting soft tissue contractures.

■ **Knee problems**
■ Usually include quadriceps weakness (usually treated with knee-ankle-foot orthoses)
■ Flexion deformities are not problematic in patients who use wheelchairs but can be treated with hamstring release and posterior capsular release.
■ Recurvatum is rarely a problem and can be treated early with serial casting and knee-ankle-foot orthoses.

- Tenotomies (quadriceps lengthening) are sometimes required.
- Valgus deformities are usually not a problem.
  - Occasionally, iliotibial band release, guided growth, or osteotomies are needed.

Ankle and foot deformities
- Objectives: (1) for feet to be braceable and plantigrade and (2) muscle balance
- Calcaneal deformity (see Figure 3-37)
  - Often caused by unopposed action of the tibialis anterior in patients with paralysis at the lower lumbar level
  - Predisposes to heel ulcers that can result in osteomyelitis of the calcaneus
  - Passive stretching is initial treatment, but tibialis anterior transfer to calcaneus often required
    - At time of transfer, do not fix foot in equinus position; this predisposes to distal tibial metaphyseal fracture
- Valgus foot and ankle
  - Valgus ankle deformity is common in ambulatory patients with the deformity in the distal tibia or subtalar joint (or both).
    - Surgical correction is warranted when pressure sores are present and orthotics fail to hold correction.
  - For skeletally immature patients: distal tibial hemiepiphysiodesis or Achilles tendon–fibular tenodesis
  - For skeletally mature patients: distal tibial osteotomy
  - In subtalar region valgus, ankle-foot orthoses are often helpful, but tendon release (anterior tibialis, Achilles), posterior tibialis lengthening, and other procedures may be required.
    - Triple arthrodesis should be avoided in most myelodysplastic patients and is used only for severe deformities with sensate feet.
- Rigid clubfoot
  - Secondary to retained activity or contracture of the tibialis posterior and tibialis anterior; common in patients with L4-level lesions
  - Treatment consists of complete subtalar release through a transverse (Cincinnati) incision, lengthening of the tibialis posterior and Achilles tendons, and transfer of the tibialis anterior tendon to the dorsal midfoot.
  - Talectomy may be appropriate for refractory clubfoot.

Spine problems
- Lumbar kyphosis or other congenital malformation of the spine as a result of a lack of segmentation or formation (i.e., hemivertebrae, diastematomyelia, unsegmented bars)
  - Treatment of kyphosis is based on problems with skin breakdown or necessity of using upper extremities to hold up their torso.
  - Resection of the kyphosis (kyphectomy) with local fusion or fusion to the pelvis with instrumentation is required in severe cases (Figure 3-38).
- Scoliosis can also occur with severe lordosis as a result of muscular imbalance that is caused by thoracic-level paraplegia.
  - Nearly all patients with thoracic-level paraplegia develop scoliosis.

- Bracing is generally unsuccessful in treating these spinal deformities.
- Rapid curve progression can be associated with hydrocephalus or a tethered cord, which may be manifested as lower extremity spasticity or an increase in urinary tract infections.
- Severe progressive curves necessitate surgical treatment.
  - Segmental Luque sublaminar wiring with fixation to the pelvis (Galveston technique) or fixation to the front of the sacrum (Dunn technique) may be used (see Figure 3-38).
  - Infection rates are high because of frequent septicemia and poor skin quality over the lumbar spine.

Pelvic obliquity
- Result of prolonged unilateral hip contractures or scoliosis
- Treatment
  - Custom seat cushions, thoracolumbosacral orthosis, spinal fusion, and ultimately pelvic osteotomies may be required.

MYOPATHIES (MUSCULAR DYSTROPHIES)

Introduction
- These noninflammatory inherited disorders are characterized by progressive muscle weakness.
- Treatment focuses on PT, orthoses, genetic counseling, and surgery.
- Several types of muscular dystrophy are classified on the basis of their inheritance patterns.

Duchenne muscular dystrophy
- Caused by absence of dystrophin protein
  - **Markedly elevated creatine phosphokinase level and absence of dystrophin protein on muscle biopsy and DNA testing**
  - A muscle biopsy sample shows foci of necrosis and connective tissue infiltration.
  - Dystrophin absence leads to poor muscle fiber regeneration and progressive replacement of muscle tissue with fibrofatty tissue.
  - **X-linked recessive inheritance (Xp21.2 dystrophin gene mutation; one third of cases are from spontaneous mutation)**
  - Occurs in young boys
- Physical findings
  - Manifested as muscle weakness (proximal groups weaker than distal)
  - Clumsy walking
  - Decreased motor skills
  - Lumbar lordosis
  - Calf pseudohypertrophy
  - Positive Gowers sign (rises by walking the hands up the legs to compensate for gluteus maximus and quadriceps weakness) (Figure 3-39)
  - Hip extensors are typically the first muscle group affected.
  - Also associated with low IQ, megacolon, volvulus, malabsorption
- Treatment
  - Goals are to keep patients ambulatory as long as possible.
  - Patients lose independent ambulation by age 10.

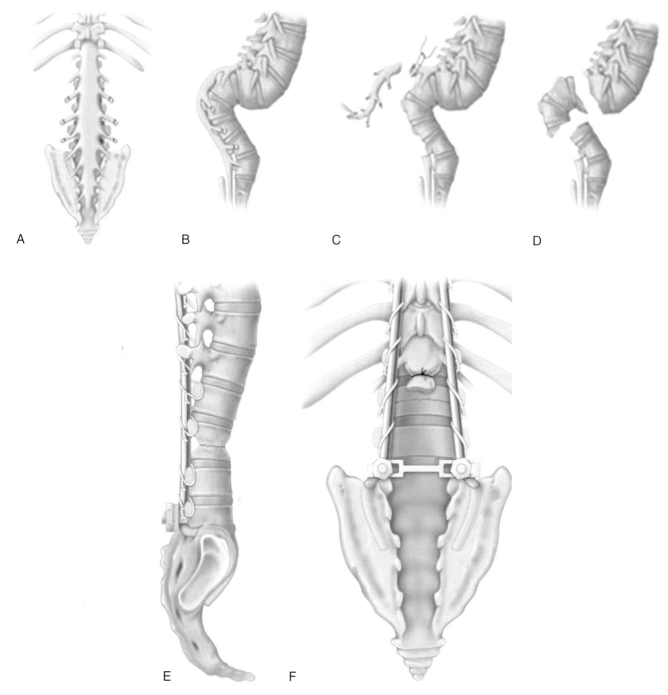

A B C D

E F

FIGURE 3-38 Lumbar kyphectomy in patients with myelomeningocele. Fixation to the pelvis is accomplished with the Dunn-McCarthy technique. (From Herring JA, editor: *Tachdjian's pediatric orthopaedics,* ed 5, Philadelphia, 2014, Elsevier Saunders., Plate 36-3.)

- Although controversial, the use of knee-ankle-foot orthoses and release of contractures can extend walking ability for 2 to 3 years.
- Patients are usually wheelchair dependent by age 15 years.
- Patients usually die of cardiorespiratory complications before age 20.
- Newer medical treatment includes high-dose steroids (prednisone 0.75 mg/kg/day), which have been shown to prevent scoliosis formation and prolong walking ability.
- Foot deformities:

- Treat with tendo Achilles lengthening (TAL), split posterior tibialis tendon transfer into peroneus brevis (if tibialis posterior active in both stance and swing phase).
- Rancho procedure: TAL, tibialis posterior lengthening, split anterior tibialis transfer into dorsal cuboid
- Scoliosis:
  - With no muscle support, scoliosis rapidly progresses in virtually all patients by age 14 years.
  - Patients can become bedridden by age 16 as a result of spinal deformity and are unable to sit for more than 8 hours.

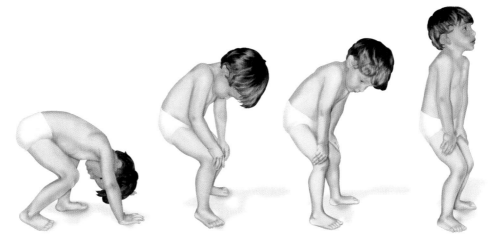

FIGURE 3-39 Gowers sign. The child rises from the floor by "walking up" the thighs with his hands—a functional test for quadriceps muscle weakness. Note the bulky calf. (Redrawn from Herring JA, editor: *Tachdjian's pediatric orthopaedics,* ed 3, Philadelphia, 2002, WB Saunders, p 85.)

- FVC decreases by 4% each year and another 4% for every 10 degrees of thoracic scoliosis.
- Scoliosis should be treated early (at 25 to 30 degrees of curvature) before pulmonary and cardiac function deteriorate.
- Surgical approach includes posterior spinal fusion with segmental instrumentation to include the pelvis.
- Differential diagnosis
  - Becker muscular dystrophy (also sex-linked recessive with a decrease in dystrophin)
    - Found in boys with red/green color-blindness, with a similar but less severe picture
    - Diagnosis of Becker muscular dystrophy applies to patients with the same examination findings but who live beyond 22 years without respiratory support.

■ **Facioscapulohumeral muscular dystrophy**
- Causes and findings
  - Autosomal dominant disorder typically observed in patients 6 to 20 years of age
  - Slow progression of muscle weakness involving muscles of facial expression and proximal upper extremity
  - Normal creatine phosphokinase level
  - Winging of the scapula
  - Inability to whistle
- Treated with stabilization by means of scapulothoracic fusion

■ **Limb-girdle muscular dystrophy**
- Causes and findings
  - Autosomal recessive disorder seen in patients 10 to 30 years of age
  - Pelvic or shoulder girdle involvement
  - Increased creatine phosphokinase levels

■ **Other muscular dystrophies**
- Gowers (distal involvement; high incidence in Sweden); ocular, oculopharyngeal (high incidence among French Canadians)

POLYMYOSITIS AND DERMATOMYOSITIS

■ **Causes/findings**
- Manifest with a febrile illness that may be acute or insidious

- Females predominate and typically exhibit photosensitivity and increased creatine phosphokinase and ESR values.
- Muscles are tender, brawny, and indurated.
- Biopsy findings demonstrate the pathognomonic inflammatory response.

■ **Treatment**
- Anti–tumor necrosis factor medication can decrease symptoms and control flares.

HEREDITARY NEUROPATHIES

■ **Disorders associated with multiple central nervous system lesions**

■ **Friedreich ataxia**
- Causes and findings
  - **Autosomal recessive disorder with problems with the frataxin gene (GAA repeat at 9q13)**
  - Spinocerebellar degenerative disease with mean onset between 7 and 15 years of age
  - Manifests with staggering wide-based gait, nystagmus, cardiomyopathy, a cavus foot, and scoliosis
  - Involves motor and sensory defects, with an increase in polyphasic potentials on electromyograms
  - Use of a wheelchair is needed by age 15; death occurs between ages 40 and 50, usually from cardiomyopathy.
- Treatment
  - Foot deformities treated with plantar release with or without metatarsal and calcaneal osteotomies early, and triple arthrodesis later
  - Spine fusion when curves progress to 50 degrees, and number of levels should be interpreted as if a curve is a neuromuscular curve
  - Bracing ineffective for treatment of scoliosis

■ **Hereditary sensory motor neuropathies: a group of inherited neuropathic disorders with similar characteristics (Table 3-18)**

■ **Charcot-Marie-Tooth disease (peroneal muscular atrophy)**
- Causes and findings
  - Autosomal dominant sensory motor demyelinating neuropathy
  - Two forms are described: a hypertrophic form with onset during the second decade of life, and a neuronal

Table 3-18	Major Hereditary Motor Sensory Neuropathies		
TYPE	**TERMINOLOGY**	**INHERITANCE**	**DESCRIPTION**
I	Charcot-Marie-Tooth syndrome (hypertrophic form)	Autosomal dominant	Peroneal weakness, slow nerve conduction, absence of reflexes
II	Charcot-Marie-Tooth syndrome (neuronal form)	Variable	Peroneal weakness, normal nerve conduction, and normal reflexes
III	Dejerine-Sottas disease	Autosomal recessive	Begins in infancy and more severe

form with onset during the third or fourth decade but with more extensive foot involvement.

- Orthopaedic manifestations include pes cavus, hammer toes with frequent corns and calluses, peroneal weakness, and muscular atrophy usually distal to the knees ("stork legs").
- Involves motor defects much more than sensory defects
- Low nerve conduction velocities with prolonged distal latencies are noted in peroneal, ulnar, and median nerves.
- Diagnosis is made most reliably by DNA testing for a duplication of a genomic fragment that encompasses the **peripheral myelin protein-22 (PMP22) gene on chromosome 17.**
- Intrinsic wasting is noted in the hands.
- Most common cause of pes cavus
- The most severely affected muscles are the tibialis anterior, peroneus longus, and peroneus brevis.
  - Plantar flexion of the first ray is the foot deformity that occurs first, as a result of a weakened tibialis anterior muscle.
- Treatment for feet
  - Plantar release, posterior tibial tendon transfer (if hindfoot varus is flexible); hindfoot flexibility tested via Coleman block test
  - Triple arthrodesis (poor long-term results) versus calcaneal and metatarsal osteotomies (if heel varus is fixed and the foot not too short)
  - The Jones procedure for hammer toes, and intrinsic procedures for hand deformity
  - The Coleman block test—block placed under lateral rays, allowing first ray to plantar flex
    - Flexible hindfoot will correct to neutral.
    - Rigid hindfoot will not correct to neutral.

- **Dejerine-Sottas disease**
- Causes and findings
  - Autosomal recessive hypertrophic neuropathy of infancy
  - Delayed ambulation, pes cavus foot, foot drop, stocking-glove dysesthesia, and spinal deformities are common.
  - The patient is wheelchair dependent by the third or fourth decade.
- **Riley-Day syndrome (dysautonomia)**
- Causes and findings
  - One of five inherited (autosomal recessive) sensory and autonomic neuropathies
  - This disease is found only in patients of Ashkenazi Jewish ancestry.
  - Clinical presentation includes dysphagia, alacrima, pneumonia, excessive sweating, postural hypotension, and sensory loss.

Table 3-19	Spinal Muscular Atrophy		
TYPE	**DESCRIPTION**	**AGE AT ONSET**	**PROGNOSIS**
I	Acute Werdnig-Hoffman disease	<6 mo	Poor
II	Chronic Werdnig-Hoffman disease	6-24 mo	May live into fifth decade
III	Kugelberg-Welander disease	2-10 yr	Good: may need respiratory support

MYASTHENIA GRAVIS

- **Causes and findings**
- Chronic disease with insidious development of easy muscle fatigability after exercise
- Caused by competitive inhibition of acetylcholine receptors at the motor end plate by antibodies produced in the thymus gland
- **Treatment consists of cyclosporine, anti-acetylcholinesterase agents, or thymectomy.**

ANTERIOR HORN CELL DISORDERS

- **Poliomyelitis**
- Causes and findings
  - Viral destruction of anterior horn cells in the spinal cord and brainstem motor nuclei
    - This disease all but disappeared in the United States after a vaccine was developed.
    - Still occurs in underdeveloped countries and in locales where vaccination is unpopular
  - *Postpolio syndrome* is an aging phenomenon where more nerve cells become inactive with time.
    - Patients should exercise at subexhaustion levels to tone muscles but prevent muscle breakdown.
  - Many surgical procedures in current use were originally developed for the treatment of polio.
  - The hallmark of polio is muscle weakness with normal sensation.
- **Spinal muscular atrophy**
- Causes and findings
  - Autosomal recessive, associated with survival motor neuron gene (SMN) causing lack of SMN-1 protein in all types
  - Loss of anterior horn cells from the spinal cord. Three types (Table 3-19):
    - Type I—acute Werdnig-Hoffman: presents earlier than age 6 months, absent deep tendon reflexes, tongue fasciculations, usually deceased by age 2

- Type II—chronic Werdnig-Hoffman: presents at 6 to 12 months, muscle weakness worse in lower extremities, able to sit, cannot walk, may live into fifth decade
- Type III—Kugelberg-Welander disease: presents in adolescence, walk as children, wheelchair as adults, proximal muscle weakness
- Patients have symmetric paresis with more involvement of the lower extremity and proximal muscles.
- All three types lose SMN-1; disease severity depends on the amount of SMN-2 remaining, with type I having the least amount of SMN-2.
- Hip subluxation or dislocation is common and treated nonoperatively.
- Scoliosis is treated surgically, like Duchenne muscular dystrophy curves, except that fusion may be required while patient is still ambulatory (may result in loss of ambulatory ability).
  - Upper extremity function may decrease after spinal fusion, but this decrease may be temporary.
  - Before fusion, ensure that the patient does not have lower extremity muscle contractures that could interfere with sitting balance.

ACUTE IDIOPATHIC POSTINFECTIOUS POLYNEUROPATHY (GUILLAIN-BARRÉ SYNDROME)

- **Causes and findings**
- Symmetric ascending motor paresis caused by demyelination after viral infection
- Cerebrospinal fluid protein level typically elevated
- Usually self-limiting; better prognosis with the acute form

OVERGROWTH SYNDROMES

- **Proteus syndrome**
- Causes and findings
  - Overgrowth of hands and feet, with bizarre facial disfigurement
  - Scoliosis, genu valgum, hemangiomas, lipomas, and nevi also common
  - Must be differentiated from neurofibromatosis and McCune-Albright syndrome
- **Klippel-Trénaunay syndrome**
- Causes
  - Overgrowth caused by underlying arteriovenous malformations
  - Associated with cutaneous hemangiomas and varicosities
- Treatment
  - Embolization of vascular abnormalities in selected patients
  - Severely hypertrophied extremities often must be amputated.
  - Epiphysiodesis is mainstay for treatment of deformities of limb length
- **Hemihypertrophy**
- Causes
  - Can be caused by various syndromes, but most cases are idiopathic
  - Most commonly known cause is neurofibromatosis
  - Disorder is often associated with renal abnormalities (especially Wilms tumor)
    - Best evaluated with serial ultrasonography until age 5 years
- Treatment
  - Epiphysiodesis versus lengthening to correct leg length discrepancies
  - Length can be manipulated, but the girth of the limb will always be asymmetric.

SECTION 9 BONE DYSPLASIAS

INTRODUCTION

- **Definition: *dysplasia* means abnormal development.**
- Shortening of the involved bones affects specific portions of the growing bone (Figure 3-40), hence the term *dwarfism*. Most forms of dwarfism are related to genetic defects (single or multiple genes [Table 3-20]).
- ***Proportionate dwarfism:* symmetric decrease in both trunk and limb length (e.g., as occurs with mucopolysaccharidoses)**
- **Disproportionate dwarfism:**
- Short-trunk variety (e.g., Kniest syndrome–spondyloepiphyseal)
- Short-limb variety (e.g., achondroplasia, diastrophic dysplasia)
  - Short-limb dwarfism can be subclassified by the region of the limb that is short (e.g., rhizomelic-proximal, mesomelic-middle, acromelic-distal).
  - All types of dwarfism are summarized in Table 3-21.

ACHONDROPLASIA

- **Introduction and etiology**
- Achondroplasia is the most common form of disproportionate short-limbed dwarfism.
- **Autosomal dominant condition; 80% of cases caused by a spontaneous mutation in the fibroblast growth factor receptor 3 (FGFR3)**
- Abnormal endochondral bone formation that is more affected than appositional growth
- **Achondroplasia is categorized as a physeal dysplasia (cartilaginous proliferative zone)**
- Quantitative, not a qualitative, cartilage defect
- May be associated with advanced paternal age
- **Signs and symptoms**
- Normal trunk and short limbs (rhizomelic) with hypotonia
- Frontal bossing, button noses, small nasal bridges, trident hands (inability to approximate extended middle and ring fingers) (Figure 3-41)

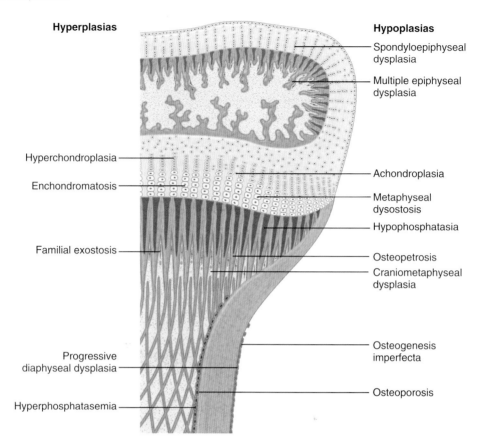

FIGURE 3-40 Locations of abnormalities that lead to dysplasias. (Adapted from Rubin P: *Dynamic classification of bone dysplasias,* Chicago, 1964, Year Book Medical Publishers.)

Table 3-20	Pediatric Congenital Disorders and Associated Genetic Defects		
DISORDER	**GENETIC DEFECT**	**DISORDER**	**GENETIC DEFECT**
Achondroplasia	FGFR3	Osteogenesis imperfecta	Collagen type I
Hypochondroplasia	FGFR3	Ehlers-Danlos syndrome	
Thanatophoric dysplasia	FGFR3	Types I and II	Collagen type V
Pseudoachondroplasia	COMP	Type IV	Collagen type IV
Multiple epiphyseal dysplasia type I	COMP	Types VI and VII	Collagen type I
Multiple epiphyseal dysplasia type II	Collagen type IX	Duchenne/Becker muscular dystrophies	Dystrophin
Spondyloepiphyseal dysplasia congenita	Collagen type II	Limb-girdle dystrophies	Sarcoglycan and dystroglycan complex
Kniest syndrome	Collagen type II	Charcot-Marie-Tooth disease	PMP22
Stickler syndrome (hereditary arthro-ophthalmopathy)	Collagen type II	Spinal muscular atrophy	Survival motor neuron protein
Diastrophic dysplasia	Sulfate transporter gene	Myotonic dystrophy	Myotonin
Schmid metaphyseal chondrodysplasia	Collagen type X	Friedreich ataxia	Frataxin
Jansen metaphyseal chondrodysplasia	PTHRP	Neurofibromatosis	Neurofibromin
Craniosynostosis	FGFR2	McCune-Albright syndrome	cAMP
Cleidocranial dysplasia	CBFA1		
Hypophosphatemic rickets	PEX		
Marfan syndrome	Fibrillin-1		

cAMP, Cyclic adenosine monophosphate; *CBFA1,* transcription factor for osteocalcin; *COMP,* cartilage oligomeric matrix protein; *FGFR3* and *FGFR2,* fibroblast growth factor receptors 3 and 2; *PEX,* period-extender gene; *PMP22,* peripheral myelin protein-22; *PTHRP,* parathyroid hormone–related peptide.

■ Thoracolumbar kyphosis (which usually resolves around the age at ambulation)

■ **Lumbar stenosis (most likely to cause disability) and excessive lordosis (short pedicles with decreased interpedicular distances)**

　• Neurologic symptoms are usually related to nerve root or spinal cord compression.

• Compression at foramen magnum may cause periods of apnea.

■ Radial head subluxation

■ Shows normal intelligence but delayed motor milestones

■ Although sitting height may be normal, standing height is below the third percentile.

Table 3-21	Summary of Major Types of Dwarfism		
DWARFISM TYPE	**GENETIC DEFECT**	**INHERITANCE**	**PATHOGNOMONIC FEATURE**
Achondroplasia	*FGFR3*	AD	Trident hands and lumbar kyphosis
Pseudoachondroplasia	*COMP*	AD	Normal facies and cervical instability
Spondyloepiphyseal dysplasia	Type II collagen	Congenita: AD Tarda: X-linked recessive	Epiphyseal fragmentation with spine involvement
Kniest syndrome	Type II collagen	AD	Retinal detachment and dumbbell-shaped bone
Jansen metaphyseal chondroplasia	*PTHRP*	AD	Hypercalcemia with metaphyseal expansion
Schmid metaphyseal chondroplasia	Type X collagen	AD	Coxa vara with proximal femur involvement
McKusick metaphyseal chondroplasia	Unknown *COMP*	AR	Odontoid hypoplasia
Multiple epiphyseal dysplasia	Type II collagen	AD	Bilateral hip involvement
Mucopolysaccharidosis (see Table 3-22)			
Diastrophic dysplasia	Sulfate transport protein	AR	Cauliflower ears and kyphoscoliosis
Cleidocranial dysplasia	*CBFA1*	AD	Aplasia of clavicles and coxa vara

AD, Autosomal dominant; *AR,* autosomal recessive; *CBFA1,* transcription factor for osteocalcin; *COMP,* cartilage oligomeric matrix protein; *FGFR3,* fibroblast growth factor receptor 3; *PTHRP,* parathyroid hormone–related peptide.

■ Radiographic findings
▓ Spine: narrowed interpedicular distance in the distal spine (L1-S1), T12/L1 wedging, generalized posterior vertebral scalloping
▓ Pelvis: wider than it is deep ("champagne glass" pelvic outlet)
■ Treatment
▓ Lumbar stenosis: decompression and fusion of the spine for a developing neurologic deficit (usually in children > age 10)
▓ Foramen magnum stenosis: decompression
▓ Progressive kyphosis: if fail bracing, anterior and posterior fusion are indicated for residual kyphosis greater than 60 degrees by age 5
▓ Genu varum: tibial osteotomies or hemiepiphysiodesis
▓ Limb lengthening through callodiastasis (lengthening through a metaphyseal corticotomy)
  • High rate of complications
  • Controversial

PSEUDOACHONDROPLASIA

■ **Clinically similar to achondroplasia**
■ **Autosomal dominant**
■ **Defect of cartilage oligometric matrix protein (COMP) on chromosome 19.**
■ **Signs and symptoms:**
▓ Normal facies
▓ Cervical instability and scoliosis with increased lumbar lordosis
▓ Significant lower extremity bowing
▓ Hip, knee, and elbow flexion contractures with precocious osteoarthritis
■ **Radiographic findings: metaphyseal flaring and delayed epiphyseal ossification**

MULTIPLE EPIPHYSEAL DYSPLASIA (MED)

■ **Clinical features**
▓ Short-limbed, disproportionate dwarfism that often is not manifested until between the ages of 5 and 14
▓ Must be differentiated from spondyloepiphyseal dysplasia
▓ A mild form (Ribbing) and a more severe form (Fairbanks) exist.

■ Causes
■ **Most common gene mutation is in COMP but also type IX collagen.**
■ Radiologic findings
▓ MED is characterized by irregular delayed ossification at multiple epiphyses (Figure 3-42).
▓ Short, stunted metacarpals and metatarsals, irregular proximal femora, abnormal ossification (tibial "slant sign" and flattened femoral condyles, patella with double layer), valgus knees (early osteotomy should be considered), waddling gait, and early hip arthritis are common.
■ **Proximal femoral involvement can be confused with Perthes disease.**
  • **MED is bilateral and symmetric, characterized by early acetabular changes, and not accompanied by metaphyseal cysts.**
■ Treatment
■ **Obtain bone survey to differentiate between MED and single epiphyseal dysplasia, as well as to identify all areas of involvement.**
▓ Treat limb alignment and perform early joint replacement.

SPONDYLOEPIPHYSEAL DYSPLASIA (SED)

■ Clinical features
▓ Must be differentiated from MED
▓ MED and SED involve abnormal epiphyseal development in the upper and lower extremities.
■ **Distinguishing feature of SED is the added spine involvement**
  • Scoliosis: typically with a sharp curve over a small number of vertebrae
  • Atlantoaxial instability with cervical myelopathy
▓ Retinal detachment and respiratory problems are common.
■ **Cause: genetic defect is within the gene encoding type II collagen.**

CHONDRODYSPLASIA PUNCTATA

■ Clinical features
▓ Characterized by multiple punctate calcifications seen on radiographs during infancy

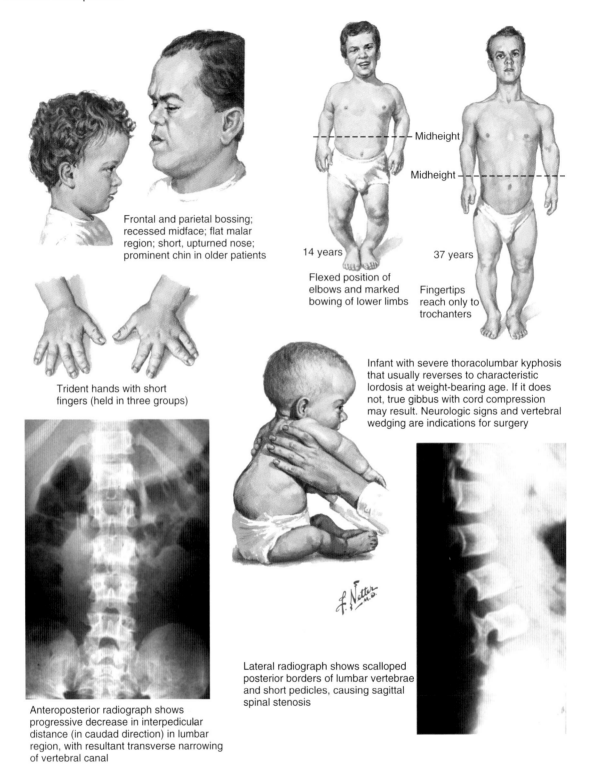

Frontal and parietal bossing; recessed midface; flat malar region; short, upturned nose; prominent chin in older patients

Midheight

Midheight

14 years

Flexed position of elbows and marked bowing of lower limbs

37 years

Fingertips reach only to trochanters

Trident hands with short fingers (held in three groups)

Infant with severe thoracolumbar kyphosis that usually reverses to characteristic lordosis at weight-bearing age. If it does not, true gibbus with cord compression may result. Neurologic signs and vertebral wedging are indications for surgery

Anteroposterior radiograph shows progressive decrease in interpedicular distance (in caudad direction) in lumbar region, with resultant transverse narrowing of vertebral canal

Lateral radiograph shows scalloped posterior borders of lumbar vertebrae and short pedicles, causing sagittal spinal stenosis

FIGURE 3-41 Clinical features of achondroplasia. Note the space between the middle and ring fingers. (From Greene WB: *Netter's orthopaedics,* Philadelphia, 2005, WB Saunders, Figure 3-6.)

▦ Autosomal dominant form (Conradi-Hünermann) has a wide variation of clinical expression
▦ Autosomal recessive rhizomelic form usually fatal during first year of life
  ● Cataracts, asymmetric limb shortening that may necessitate surgical correction, and spinal deformities are common.

KNIEST SYNDROME

■ Clinical features
▦ Autosomal dominant
▦ Short-trunked, disproportionate dwarfism
▦ Joint stiffness/contractures, scoliosis, kyphosis, dumbbell-shaped femora, and hypoplastic pelvis and spine

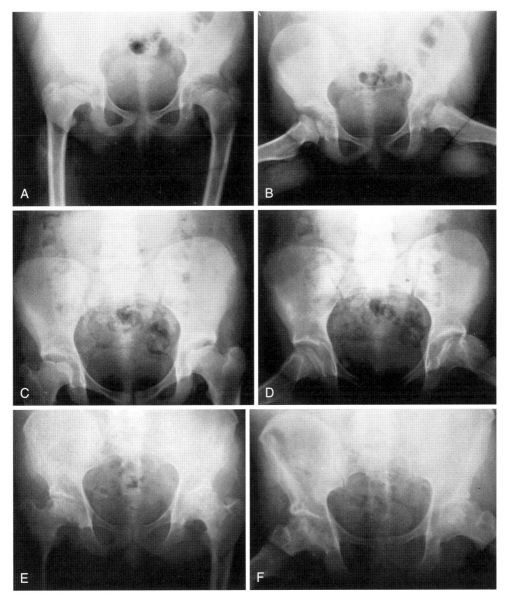

FIGURE 3-42 Multiple epiphyseal dysplasia in two sisters and their 40-year-old father. Anteroposterior (AP) **(A)** and frog-leg lateral **(B)** radiographs of both hips of a 12-year-old girl. Note the irregularity and flattening of the capital femoral epiphyses. Involvement is bilateral. AP **(C)** and lateral **(D)** views of both hips of the 14-year-old sister showing similar changes. AP **(E)** and lateral **(F)** radiographs of the father's hips. Note the irregularity of the femoral heads and marked degenerative arthritis in both hips. (From Herring JA, editor: *Tachdjian's pediatric orthopaedics,* ed 5, Philadelphia, 2014, Elsevier Saunders, Figure 40-41.)

▓ Otitis media and hearing loss are frequent.
▪ **Cause: defect within type II collagen**
▪ **Radiographic findings: osteopenia and dumbbell-shaped bones**
▪ **Treatment**
▓ Early therapy for joint contractures is required.
▓ Reconstructive procedures may be required for early hip degenerative arthritis.

METAPHYSEAL CHONDRODYSPLASIA

▪ **Clinical features**
▓ Heterogeneous group of disorders characterized by metaphyseal changes of tubular bones with normal epiphyses
▪ **Causes**
▓ Defect appears to be in proliferative and hypertrophic zones of the physis
▪ **Types**

▓ Jansen (rare): most severe form
  • **Genetic defect in parathyroid hormone–related peptide**
  • Autosomal dominant inheritance
  • Mental retardation, markedly short-limbed dwarfism with wide eyes, monkey-like stance, and hypercalcemia
  • Striking bulbous metaphyseal expansion of long bones is a distinctive radiographic finding.
▓ Schmid type
  • More common, less severe form
  • Genetic defect is in **type X collagen,** transmitted by autosomal dominant inheritance; short-limbed dwarfism not diagnosed until patient is older, as a result of coxa vara and genu varum
  • Predominantly involves proximal femur. Gait is often Trendelenburg, and patients have increased lumbar lordosis.

- Condition often confused with rickets, but laboratory test results normal
- McKusick type
  - Autosomal recessive inheritance; cartilage-hair dysplasia (hypoplasia of cartilage and small diameter of hair) is observed most commonly among the Amish population and in Finland.
  - Atlantoaxial instability is common (odontoid hypoplasia).
  - Ankle deformity develops as a result of fibular overgrowth distally.
  - Affected patients may have abnormal immunocompetence and have an increased risk for malignancies, intestinal malabsorption, and megacolon.

DYSPLASIA EPIPHYSEALIS HEMIMELICA (TREVOR DISEASE)

- **Clinical features**
- Epiphyseal osteochondroma
- Most commonly seen at the knee and ankle
- Usually affects only one joint
- Caused by a defect in groove of Ranvier
- **Radiologic findings**
- Calcifications are seen within the joint
- **Treatment**
- Excision of the prominent overgrowth (if symptomatic) and later osteotomies may be required.
- Recurrence is a common complication.

PROGRESSIVE DIAPHYSEAL DYSPLASIA (CAMURATI-ENGELMANN DISEASE)

- **Clinical features**
- Autosomal dominant inheritance
- Affected children are often "late walkers" (because of associated muscle weakness).
- Symmetric cortical thickening of long bones
- Tibia, femur, and humerus are most often involved (in that order), affecting only the diaphyseal portion of bone.
- Watch for leg length inequality.
- **Radiographic findings**
- Widened fusiform diaphyses with increased bone formation and sclerosis
- **Treatment**
- Salicylates, NSAIDs, and steroids for refractory cases

MUCOPOLYSACCHARIDOSIS

- **Introduction**
- Easily differentiated on the basis of the presence of complex sugars in the urine
- Accumulation of mucopolysaccharides, as a result of a hydrolase enzyme deficiency
- Produces a proportionate dwarfism
- **Types (Table 3-22)**

- Morquio syndrome (autosomal recessive inheritance)
  - **Most common form;** manifests by age 18 months to 2 years
  - Waddling gait, genu valgum ("knock-knees"), thoracic kyphosis, cloudy corneas, and normal intelligence
  - **Urinary excretion of keratan sulfate**
  - Bony changes include a thickening skull, wide ribs, anterior beaking of vertebrae, a wide, flat pelvis, coxa vara with unossified femoral heads, and bullet-shaped metacarpals.
  - **C1-C2 instability (caused by odontoid hypoplasia) can be seen, manifesting with myelopathy and necessitating decompression and cervical fusion.**
- Hurler syndrome (autosomal recessive inheritance)
  - Most severe form
  - **Urinary excretion of dermatan/heparan sulfate**
  - Mental retardation
  - Bone marrow transplantation has increased the lifespan for patients with this disorder.
- Hunter syndrome (sex-linked recessive inheritance)
  - Urinary excretion of dermatan/heparan sulfate
  - Mental retardation
  - Bone marrow transplantation has increased the lifespan for patients.
- Sanfilippo syndrome (autosomal recessive inheritance)
  - Urinary excretion of heparan sulfate
  - Associated with mental retardation
  - Bone marrow transplantation has increased the lifespan for patients.

DIASTROPHIC DYSPLASIA

- **Clinical features**
- **Autosomal recessive inheritance**; severe short-limbed dwarfism
- Cleft palate (59% of cases)
- Severe joint contractures (especially hip and knee)
- **Cauliflower ears (80% of cases), hitchhiker's thumb**
- **Rigid clubfeet**
- **Causes**
- **Deficiency in *DTDST* gene, which codes for sulfate transport protein**
- **Radiologic findings**
- Spine radiographs reveal cervical kyphosis (often severe, necessitating immediate treatment), thoracolumbar kyphoscoliosis (83% of cases), spina bifida occulta, and atlantoaxial instability
- **Treatment**
- Quadriplegia is a major concern with deformities of the cervical spine.
  - Must fuse early
- Surgical release of clubfoot deformities
- Osteotomies for contractures
- Spinal fusion often required

Table 3-22	Mucopolysaccharidoses				
SYNDROME	**INHERITANCE**	**INTELLIGENCE**	**CORNEA**	**URINARY EXCRETION**	**OTHER**
Hurler	AR	Below normal	Cloudy	Dermatan/heparan sulfate	Worst prognosis
Hunter	XR	Below normal	Clear	Dermatan/heparan sulfate	
Sanfilippo	AR	Below normal	Clear	Heparin sulfate	Normal development until 2 yr of age
Morquio	AR	Normal	Cloudy	Keratan sulfate	Most common

CLEIDOCRANIAL DYSPLASIA (DYSOSTOSIS)

- ■ Clinical features
- ▥ Autosomal dominant inheritance
- ▥ Proportionate dwarfism that affects bones formed by intramembranous ossification (clavicles, cranium, pelvis)
- ■ Causes
- ▥ **Defect in transcription factor for osteocalcin (*CBFA1*)**
- ■ Radiologic findings
- ▥ Hypoplasia or aplasia of the clavicle (no intervention necessary) (Figure 3-43)
- ▥ Delayed closure of skull sutures
- ▥ Frontal bossing
- ▥ Coxa vara
- ▥ Delayed ossification of the pubis
- ▥ Small iliac wings
- ▥ Wormian-type bone
- ■ Treatment
- ▥ Intertrochanteric valgus osteotomy if neck-shaft angle is less than 100 degrees

OSTEOPETROSIS

- ■ Clinical features
- ▥ Bone pain
- ▥ **Loss of the medullary canal can cause anemias and encroachment on the optic and oculomotor nerve and blindness.**
- ■ Causes
- ▥ Failure of osteoclastic resorption, probably secondary to a defect in the thymus, leading to dense bone (so-called marble bone)
- ▥ The mild form is autosomal dominant; the "malignant" form is autosomal recessive.

- ▥ **Due to defect in carbonic anhydrase II gene when associated with renal tubular acidosis and cerebral calcifications**
- ■ Radiologic findings (Figure 3-44)
- ▥ "Rugger jersey" spine

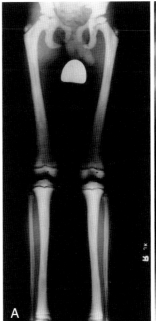
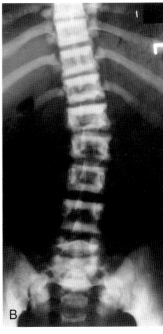

FIGURE 3-44 Osteopetrosis. **A,** Five-year-old child. The intramedullary canals have been filled with bone. There is no distinction between cortical and cancellous bone. **B,** "Rugger jersey" spine in a 16-year-old patient. (From Herring JA, editor: *Tachdjian's pediatric orthopaedics,* ed 5, Philadelphia, 2014, Elsevier Saunders, Figures 40-77 and 40-79.)

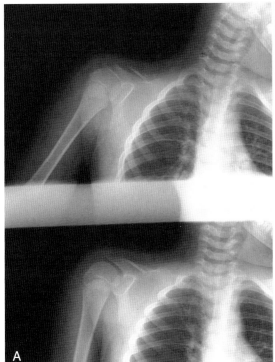
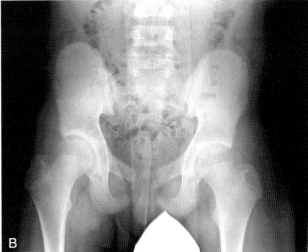

FIGURE 3-43 Cleidocranial dysplasia. **A,** Anteroposterior (AP) shoulder radiographs show hypoplasia of the clavicle. **B,** AP pelvic radiograph shows a lack of ossification of the symphysis pubis. (From Herring JA, editor: *Tachdjian's pediatric orthopaedics,* ed 5, Philadelphia, 2014, Elsevier Saunders, Figure 40-100.)

- Marble bone
- **Erlenmeyer flask deformity of proximal humerus and distal femur**
- Treatment
- Healing is normal, but amount of time for healing may be prolonged.
- Bone marrow transplantation may be helpful for treating the malignant form.

INFANTILE CORTICAL HYPEROSTOSIS (CAFFEY DISEASE)

- **Clinical features**
- Soft tissue swelling and bony cortical thickening (especially jaw and ulna) that follow a febrile illness in infants 0 to 9 months old
- This disorder may be differentiated from trauma (and child abuse) on the basis of single-bone involvement.
- Infection, scurvy, tumor, and progressive diaphyseal dysplasia may be included in the differential diagnosis.
- **Radiologic findings**
- Characteristic periosteal reaction
- **Treatment**
- The condition is benign and self-limiting.

HOMOCYSTINURIA

- **Clinical features**
- Osteoporosis
- Marfanoid-like habitus (but with stiffening joints)
- Inferior lens dislocation
- **Differentiated from Marfan syndrome on the basis of the direction of lens dislocation and the presence of osteoporosis in homocystinuria**
- Central nervous system effects, including mental retardation, are common in this disorder.
- **Causes**
- Autosomal recessive inborn error of methionine metabolism (decreased enzyme cystathionine β-synthase).
- Accumulation of the intermediate metabolite homocysteine
- Diagnosis is made by demonstrating increased homocysteine in urine (cyanide-nitroprusside test).
- **Treatment**
- Early treatment with vitamin B_6 and a diet with decreased amounts of methionine are often successful.

DYSPLASIAS ASSOCIATED WITH BENIGN BONE GROWTH

- **Conditions include multiple hereditary exostosis (osteochondromatosis), fibrous dysplasia, Ollier disease (enchondromatosis), and Maffucci syndrome (enchondromatosis and hemangiomas). These entities are discussed in Chapter 9, Orthopaedic Pathology.**

SECTION 10 ORTHOPAEDIC-RELATED SYNDROMES

DOWN SYNDROME (TRISOMY 21)

- **Clinical features**
- Orthopaedic problems
  - Metatarsus primus varus and pes planus
  - Spinal abnormalities (**atlantoaxial instability** [Figure 3-45], scoliosis [50% of cases], spondylolisthesis [6% of cases])
  - **Hip instability** (open reduction with or without osteotomy usually required)
  - SCFE (hypothyroidism should be sought)
  - **Patellar dislocation**
  - Generalized ligamentous laxity
- Associated problems
  - Hypotonia and mental retardation
  - **Heart disease with atrial septal defect (50% of cases)**
  - Endocrine disorders (hypothyroidism and diabetes) and premature aging
- **Causes**
- Trisomy 21 is the most common chromosomal abnormality; its incidence increases with maternal age.
- Chromosome 21 is the location of genes that encode for type VI collagen (*COL6A1* and *COL6A2*)
  - Abnormal type VI collagen is thought to be cause for generalized joint laxity and other orthopaedic problems
- **Radiologic studies**
- Lower extremity radiographs needed to evaluate for patella dislocations and genu valgum
- AP and frog-leg pelvic views to evaluate for SCFE

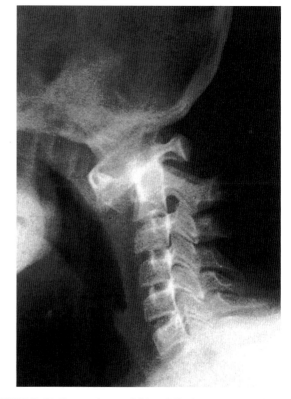

FIGURE 3-45 Gross atlantoaxial instability in an 11-year-old with Down syndrome. His gait was clumsy, and he had poor coordination of his extremities. Therefore, he underwent posterior stabilization. (From Benson M et al: *Children's orthopaedics and fractures,* New York, 1994, Churchill Livingstone, p 590.)

- Flexion-extension radiographs of the cervical spine to evaluate atlantoaxial instability
- **Treatment**
- Cervical spine instability:
  - Usefulness of screening controversial, with exception of preoperative assessment before administration of anesthetic
  - Special Olympics requires cervical spine x-ray screening for participation in selected sports.
  - **Children with asymptomatic instability should avoid contact sports, diving, and gymnastics.**
  - Children with symptomatic instability often require surgery, but the rate of wound healing problems and infection is high.
  - Cervical instability with neurologic symptoms: fusion with autologous bone graft and instrumentation
- Scoliosis
  - Bracing for 25- to 30-degree curves
  - Surgery for 50- to 60-degree curves
- Hip: initially may be treated with closed reduction, but capsulorrhaphy, pelvis osteotomy, and femoral osteotomy may be required
- Patellar instability: if symptomatic, then lateral release, medial reefing, or bony realignment of the patellar tendon should be considered.

TURNER SYNDROME

- **Clinical features**
- Affected patients are female
- Short stature, lack of sexual development, webbed neck, and cubitus valgus
- Idiopathic scoliosis is common. **Growth hormone therapy can exacerbate scoliosis.**
- Malignant hyperthermia is common with anesthetic use.
- Must be differentiated from Noonan syndrome (same appearance except for normal gonadal development, mental retardation, and more severe scoliosis)
- Osteoporosis is common.
- **Causes**
- 45 XO genotype
- **Radiologic findings**
- Genu valgum and shortening of fourth and fifth metacarpals, which usually necessitate no treatment

PRADER-WILLI SYNDROME

- **Clinical features**
- Floppy, hypotonic infant
- Intellectual impairment
- Insatiable appetite resulting in significant obesity
- Growth retardation
- Hypoplastic genitalia
- **Causes**
- Partial chromosome 15 deletion (missing portion from father)
- **Radiologic findings**
- Hip dysplasia and juvenile-onset scoliosis

MARFAN SYNDROME

- **Clinical features**
- Arachnodactyly (long, slender fingers; "peeking thumb sign")

- **Pectus deformities**
- **Scoliosis (50% of cases)**
- Acetabular protrusio (15% to 25%)
- **Cardiac abnormalities (aortic dilation)**
- **Ocular abnormalities (superior lens dislocation in 60%)**
- **Dural ectasia and meningocele**
- Joint laxity
- **Causes**
- **Defect in fibrillin-1 (FBN1)**
- **Autosomal dominant inheritance**
- **Treatment**
- Joint laxity is treated conservatively.
- Bracing for scoliosis is ineffective.
- Curves may necessitate anterior and posterior fusion.
- **Echocardiographic and cardiologic evaluation are required before surgery.**
- Acetabular protrusio should be observed unless the patient has severe symptoms.

EHLERS-DANLOS SYNDROME

- **Clinical features**
- Hyperextensibility and "cigarette paper" skin
- Joint hypermobility and dislocation
- Soft tissue and bone fragility, and soft tissue calcification
- **Classification**
- Of types I to XI, types II and III are the most common and least disabling
- **Causes**
- Autosomal dominant disorder of collagen V (coexpressed with collagen I)
- **Radiologic findings**
- Dislocations may be shown.
- Kyphoscoliosis
- **Treatment**
- PT and orthosis
- Arthrodesis when soft tissue procedures fail

FIBRODYSPLASIA OSSIFICANS PROGRESSIVA

- **Clinical features**
- Congenital malformation of the great toe (short, valgus position, and have an abnormally shaped proximal phalanx)
- Progressive heterotopic ossification of tendons, ligaments, fascia, and skeletal muscle, which ultimately eliminates motion of the jaw, neck, spine, shoulders, hips, and more distal joints
- Any form of trauma may precipitate new ossification.
- Also called *myositis ossificans progressiva* or *stone man syndrome*
- **Causes**
- **Defect in the gene encoding activin receptor type IA/ activin-like kinase 2 (ACVR1/ALK2), a BMP type 1 receptor**
- **Also linked to overproduction of BMP-4**
- **Treatment**
- No clearly effective medical treatment
- Minimize the risk of injury without compromising the patient's functional level and independence.
- Surgical excision not indicated; may precipitate new ossification

MENKES SYNDROME

- **Clinical features**
- Characteristic "kinky" hair
- May be differentiated from occipital horn syndrome (which also affects copper transport) in that the latter is characterized by bony projections from the occiput of the skull
- **Causes**
- Sex-linked recessive disorder of copper transport
- **Radiologic findings**
- Skull (wormian bones), long bones (metaphyseal spurring), and ribs (anterior flaring and multiple fractures)

RETT SYNDROME

- **Clinical features**
- Progressive impairment and stereotaxic abnormal hand movements (like those in autism)
- Manifests in girls at 6 to 18 months of age
- Loss of developmental milestones that is rapid and then stabilizes
- **Causes**
- Family of deletion mutations of the X-linked gene encoding a protein called **methyl-CpG-binding protein 2 (*MECP2*)**
- **Radiologic findings**
- Scoliosis with a C-shaped curve that is unresponsive to bracing
- **Treatment**
- Spinal instrumentation must include all of the kyphosis and the scoliosis.
- Spasticity results in joint contractures, which are treated as they are in cerebral palsy.

BECKWITH-WIEDEMANN SYNDROME

- **Clinical features**
- Organomegaly, omphalocele, and a large tongue
- **Orthopaedic manifestations include hemihypertrophy with spasticity**
- **Predisposition to Wilms tumor (patient must be screened regularly with kidney ultrasonography)**
- **Causes**

- Spasticity is thought to be the result of infantile hypoglycemic episodes secondary to pancreatic islet cell hypertrophy
- **Treatment**
- Growth arrest may be necessary in large limb

NAIL-PATELLA SYNDROME (HEREDITARY ONYCHOOSTEODYSPLASIA)

- **Clinical features**
- Nail deformity (present in 98% of patients) is greatest in the thumbnails and becomes less severe in the more ulnar digits.
- Absent or hypoplastic patella, hypoplastic lateral femoral condyle, and genu valgum may all contribute to patellar instability.
- Hypoplasia of the lateral side of the elbow, cubitus valgus
- Iliac horns (conical bony projections on posterior ilia)
- Nephropathy present in up to 40% of patients
- **Causes**
- Autosomal dominant
- The gene for nail-patella syndrome is *LMX1B*, located on chromosome 9
- **Treatment**
- There is no specific treatment for the disorder.
- The iliac horns do not affect gait and should not be resected.
- Recurrent dislocation of the patella is treated by proximal or distal realignment.

TERATOGEN-INDUCED DISORDERS

- **Fetal alcohol syndrome**
- Growth disturbances
- Central nervous system dysfunction
- Dysmorphic facies
- Hip dislocation
- Cervical spine congenital scoliosis and myelodysplasia
- Contractures respond to PT.
- **Maternal diabetes**
- Heart defects
- Sacral agenesis and anencephaly
- **Other teratogens include drugs (e.g., aminopterin, phenytoin, thalidomide), trace metals, maternal conditions, infections, and intrauterine factors; may also lead to orthopaedic manifestations in affected children**

SECTION 11 HEMATOPOIETIC AND METABOLIC DISORDERS AND ARTHRITIDES

GAUCHER DISEASE

- **Clinical features**
- Osteopenia
- Bone pain (Gaucher crisis) and bleeding abnormalities
- Hepatosplenomegaly (characteristic finding)
- Types
  - Type I: most commonly in persons of Ashkenazi Jewish descent

  - Type II: infantile
  - Type III: chronic neuropathic
- **Causes**
- Autosomal recessive lysosomal storage disease
- **Deficiency of the enzyme β-glucocerebrosidase**
- Results in accumulation of cerebroside in the reticuloendothelial system
- **Radiologic findings**
- Metaphyseal enlargement (failure of remodeling)

- **Femoral head necrosis (may be confused with Perthes disease or MED)**
- "Moth-eaten" trabeculae, patchy sclerosis, and Erlenmeyer flask deformity of the distal femora (70% of cases)
- **Treatment**
- Treatment is supportive; new enzyme therapy is available but extremely expensive.

NIEMANN-PICK DISEASE

- Autosomal recessive disorder
- Accumulation of sphingomyelin in reticuloendothelial system cells
- Occurs commonly in Jews of eastern European descent
- Marrow expansion and cortical thinning common in long bones; coxa valga also seen

SICKLE CELL ANEMIA

- **Clinical features**
- Sickle cell disease affects 1% of African Americans.
- More severe but less common than sickle cell trait (8% prevalence)
- Bone infarction is more common than acute osteomyelitis in children who present with acute musculoskeletal pain.
- *Salmonella* infection is more commonly seen in children with sickle cell disease, but *Staphylococcus aureus* is still the most common infection.
- Dactylitis (acute hand/foot swelling) also common
- **Causes**
- Mutation in the β-globin gene, resulting in sickle hemoglobin (HbS)
- When the cell becomes deoxygenated, HbS molecules assemble into fibers that produce a sickle-shaped red blood cell.
- Crises usually begin at ages 2 to 3 years, are caused by substance P, and may lead to characteristic bone infarctions.
- **Radiologic findings**
- Growth retardation or skeletal immaturity
- **Osteonecrosis of femoral and humeral heads**
- Biconcave "fish" vertebrae
- Acetabular protrusio
- **Treatment**
- Differentiating bone infarction and osteomyelitis:
  - **Sequential bone marrow tests and bone scans within 24 hours of hospital admission**
  - Gadolinium-enhanced T1-weighted MRI sequences
  - Aspiration and culture may be necessary to differentiate infarction from osteomyelitis.
- Preoperative oxygenation and exchange transfusion are helpful for affected patients requiring surgery.
- Hydroxyurea has produced dramatic relief of pain in bone crises.

THALASSEMIA

- **Similar to sickle cell anemia in manifestation**
- **Most commonly observed in people of Mediterranean descent**
- **Common symptoms include bone pain and leg ulceration.**
- **Radiographic findings**
- Long-bone thinning, metaphyseal expansion, osteopenia, and premature physeal closure

HEMOPHILIA

- **Clinical features**
- Hemarthrosis manifests with painful swelling and decreased ROM of affected joints
- Knee most commonly affected
- Deep intramuscular bleeding is also common and can lead to formation of a pseudotumor (blood cyst).
  - **Intramuscular hematomas can lead to compression of adjacent nerves.**
  - The classic scenario is an iliacus hematoma that causes femoral nerve paralysis and mimics bleeding into the hip joint.
- **Causes**
- X-linked recessive disorder
- Decreased amounts of factor VIII (hemophilia A)
- Abnormal factor VIII with platelet dysfunction (von Willebrand disease)
- Decreased amounts of factor IX (hemophilia B, Leyden, or Christmas disease)
- Can be mild (5%-25% of normal amounts of factor present), moderate (1%-5% available), or severe (<1% present)
- **Radiologic findings**
- Squaring of patellae and condyles, epiphyseal overgrowth with leg length discrepancy
- Generalized osteopenia with resulting fractures
- Cartilage atrophy resulting from enzymatic matrix degeneration and chondrocyte death
- **Treatment**
- Acute treatment of hemarthrosis is crucial and should begin immediately with administration of factor VIII or factor IX
  - Administration should continue for 3 to 7 days after cessation of bleeding and should be followed by PT.
- Home transfusion therapy has reduced the severity of the arthropathy, with the advantage of immediate treatment when bleeding occurs.
- Aspiration of a hemarthrosis is controversial.
- Treatment of sequelae
  - Synovectomy
    - Indicated for hemarthroses that recur despite optimal medical management
    - Arthroscopy has better results with motion and duration of hospitalization than does open synovectomy.
    - Radiation synovectomy: useful in patients with antibody inhibitors and poor medical management
  - Contracture release and osteotomies
  - Total joint arthroplasty for hemophilic arthropathy
- **Factor VIII levels should be increased for prophylaxis in the following situations:**
  - **Vigorous PT (20%)**
  - **Treatment of hematoma (30%)**
  - **Acute hemarthrosis or soft tissue surgery (>50%)**
  - **Skeletal surgery (approaching 100% preoperatively and maintained at > 50% for 10 days postoperatively)**
- IgG antibody inhibitors are present in 4% to 20% of hemophiliac patients; their presence is a relative contraindication to surgery.
- **Large percentage of older hemophiliac patients are HIV positive because of large amount of blood component therapy given prior to screening**

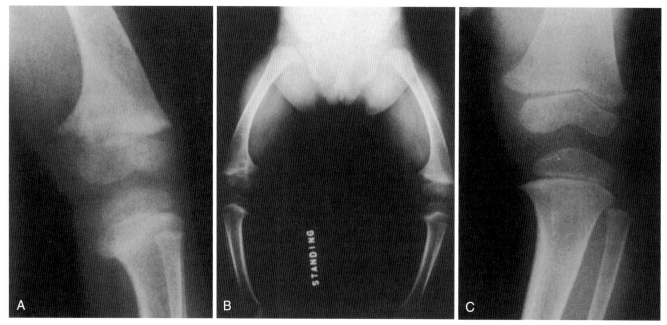

FIGURE 3-46 Rickets. **A,** Hazy metaphysis with cupping in a young boy with rickets. **B,** Accentuated genu varum is present. **C,** With vitamin D replacement therapy, the bony lesions healed in 6 months. (From Herring JA, editor: *Tachdjian's pediatric orthopaedics*, ed 5, Philadelphia, 2014, Elsevier Saunders, Figure 42-4.)

LEUKEMIA

■ **Clinical features**
▥ Most common malignancy of childhood
▥ Acute lymphocytic leukemia represents 80% of cases of leukemia.
▥ Incidence peaks at 4 years of age.
▥ **One fourth to one third of affected children have musculoskeletal complaints (back, pelvic, leg pains).**
■ **Radiologic findings**
▥ Demineralization of bones, periostitis, and occasionally lytic lesions
▥ Radiolucent "leukemia" lines may be seen in the metaphyses of affected bones in older affected children.
■ **Treatment**
▥ Management of leukemia includes chemotherapy, which may predispose the patient to pathologic fractures.

RICKETS

■ **Clinical features**
▥ Short stature
▥ Limb angulation (usually varus)
▥ Bone pain
■ **Causes**
▥ Deficiency of calcium (and sometimes phosphorus) affecting mineralization at the epiphyses of long bones
▥ Histologic findings: widened osteoid seams and "Swiss cheese" trabeculae are characteristic in bone.
▥ **Growth plate abnormalities include enlarged and distorted maturation zone (zone of hypertrophy) and a poorly defined zone of provisional calcification.**
■ **Radiologic findings**
▥ **Brittle bones with physeal cupping/widening, bowing of long bones, transverse radiolucent Looser lines, ligamentous laxity, flattening of the skull, enlargement of costal cartilages (rachitic rosary), and dorsal kyphosis (cat back)** (Figure 3-46)

■ **Treatment**
▥ Based on the underlying abnormality (e.g., gastrointestinal, kidney, diet, and organ); they are discussed in detail in Chapter 1, Basic Sciences, Section 1.

OSTEOGENESIS IMPERFECTA

■ **Clinical features**
▥ Bone fragility (brittle "wormian" bone), short stature
▥ Scoliosis
▥ Tooth defects (dentinogenesis imperfecta)
▥ Hearing defects
▥ Blue sclerae in types I and II
▥ Ligamentous laxity
▥ **Basilar invagination is common in more severe clinical phenotypes.**
▥ Fractures are common:
 • Healing is normal, but bone typically does not remodel.
 • Fractures occur less frequently with advancing age (usually cease at puberty).
 • Compression fractures (codfish vertebrae) are also common.
▥ Bowing results from multiple transverse fractures of the long bones and muscle contraction across the weakened diaphysis.
 • Typically an anterolateral bow or proximal varus deformity of the femur develops.
 • An anterior or anteromedial bow of the tibia may develop.
■ **Causes**
▥ **Defect in type I collagen (*COL1A2* gene) that causes abnormal cross-linking and leads to decreased collagen secretion**
▥ Histologic findings: increased diameters of haversian canals and osteocyte lacunae, increased numbers of cells, and replicated cement lines, which result in the thin cortices seen on radiographs

Table 3-23	Osteogenesis Imperfecta		
TYPE	**INHERITANCE**	**SCLERAE**	**FEATURES**
IA, IB	AD	Blue	Onset at preschool age (tarda); hearing loss; involvement of teeth (type IA only)
II	AR	Blue	Lethal; concertina femur, beaded ribs
III	AR	Normal	Fractures at birth, progressively short stature
IVA, IVB	AD	Normal	Milder form; normal hearing, involvement of teeth (type IVA only)

AD, Autosomal dominant; *AR,* autosomal recessive.

- Classification
  - Four types have been identified (Sillence, 1981)
  - Disorder probably best considered as a continuum with different inheritance patterns and severity (Table 3-23)
- **Radiologic findings**
- Thin cortices and generalized osteopenia
- **Treatment**
- Fracture management and long-term rehabilitation
- Bracing of extremities early to prevent deformity and minimize fractures
- Sofield osteotomies—"shish kebab" multiple long-bone osteotomies with either fixed-length Rush rods or telescoping (Bailey-Dubow or Fassier-Duval) intramedullary rods—are sometimes required for progressive bowing of long bones.
- Fractures:
  - In children younger than 2 years are treated similarly to those in children without osteogenesis imperfecta
  - After age 2, telescoping intramedullary rods can be considered.
- Bisphosphonates have been shown to decrease the number of fractures in these patients.
  - **Characteristic dense parallel metaphyseal bands may be seen on x-ray. Distance between bands corresponds to time between treatment.**
  - **Iatrogenic osteopetrosis can occur with high-dose, long-term use of bisphosphonates**
- **Scoliosis is common, and bracing is ineffective treatment. Surgery is necessary for scoliosis deformities exceeding 50 degrees, and a large blood loss is to be expected.**

IDIOPATHIC JUVENILE OSTEOPOROSIS

- **Clinical features**
- Rare self-limiting disorder that appears between age 8 and 14 years, with osteopenia, growth arrest, and bone and joint pain
- Must be differentiated from other causes of osteopenia (e.g., osteogenesis imperfecta, malignancy, Cushing disease)
- **Causes**
- Remains unknown, serum calcium and phosphorus levels normal
- **Radiologic findings**
- Diffuse generalized osteoporosis
- Possible multiple vertebral body microfractures
- **Treatment**
- Bracing for vertebral body fractures
- Disorder resolves spontaneously 2 to 4 years after onset of puberty

JUVENILE IDIOPATHIC ARTHRITIS

- **Includes both juvenile rheumatoid arthritis and juvenile chronic arthritis**
- **Clinical features**
- Persistent noninfectious arthritis lasting 6 weeks to 3 months and diagnosed after other possible causes have been ruled out
- Affects girls more than boys and typically manifests before age 4 years
- Commonly involves the knee, wrist (flexed and ulnar deviated), and hand (fingers extended, swollen, radially deviated)
- To confirm the diagnosis, one of the following must be present: rash, presence of rheumatoid factor, iridocyclitis, cervical spine involvement, pericarditis, tenosynovitis, intermittent fever, or morning stiffness.
- In 50% of affected patients, symptoms resolve without sequelae; 25% of patients are slightly disabled, and 20% to 25% have crippling arthritis, blindness, or both.
- **Radiologic findings**
- **Cervical spine involvement can lead to kyphosis, facet ankylosis, and atlantoaxial subluxation.**
- Lower extremity problems include flexion contractures (hip and knee flexed, ankle dorsiflexed), subluxation, and other deformities (hip protrusio, valgus knees, equinovarus feet)
- **Treatment**
- Medical therapy involves less high-dose steroids and salicylates and immunomodulating drugs (infliximab).
- Surgical interventions:
  - Joint injections and (rarely) synovectomy (for chronic swelling refractory to medical management)
  - Arthrodesis and arthroplasty may be required for severe juvenile idiopathic arthritis.
- Slit-lamp examination is required twice yearly because progressive iridocyclitis can lead to rapid loss of vision if left untreated.

ANKYLOSING SPONDYLITIS

- **Clinical features**
- Typically affects adolescent boys
- Asymmetric, lower extremity, large-joint arthritis
- Heel pain
- Hip and back pain (cardinal symptoms) may develop later.
- **Limitation of chest wall expansion is a more specific finding than is a positive HLA-B27 test result.**
- Sometimes eye symptoms
- **Causes**
- The HLA-B27 test yields positive results in 90% to 95% of patients with ankylosing spondylitis or Reiter syndrome.

The result is also positive in 4% to 8% of all white Americans; thus its usefulness as a screening tool is limited.

■ **Radiologic findings**

▥ Bilateral symmetric sacroiliac erosion followed by joint space narrowing, subsequent ankylosis, and late vertebral scalloping (bamboo spine). Radiographs typically lack sensitivity in early stages of the condition.

▥ Early sacroiliitis evident on MRI may allow for diagnosis far earlier than was previously possible.

■ **Treatment**

▥ NSAIDs and PT

▥ Tumor necrosis factor antagonists such as etanercept, infliximab, and adalimumab are used if NSAIDs are ineffective.

SELECTED BIBLIOGRAPHY

The selected bibliography for this chapter can be found on https://expertconsult.inkling.com.

TESTABLE CONCEPTS

SECTION 1 UPPER EXTREMITY PROBLEMS

- Brachial plexus palsy can be classified on the basis of root involvement.
  - Erb-Duchenne palsy (C5, C6): "waiter's tip" deformity with shoulder adducted and internally rotated, elbow extended, forearm pronated, and wrist and fingers flexed
  - Klumpke palsy (C8, T1): elbow flexion and forearm supination contracture
  - Total plexus palsy (C5-T1): complete sensory and motor deficits
  - Progressive glenoid dysplasia occurs in 70% of children with significant internal rotation contracture.
  - Lack of biceps function 6 months after injury and Horner syndrome carry a poor prognosis.
  - Treatment includes latissimus and teres major transfer to the shoulder external rotators.

SECTION 2 LOWER EXTREMITY PROBLEMS: GENERAL

I. Rotational Problems of the Lower Extremities

- In-toeing is usually attributable to metatarsus adductus (in infants), internal tibial torsion (in toddlers), and femoral anteversion (in children < 10 years).
  - Metatarsus adductus: inward deviation of lateral board of foot from base of fourth metatarsal
  - Internal tibial torsion: inward (negative) thigh-foot angle
  - Femoral anteversion: increased internal rotation and decreased external rotation
- Out-toeing is typically caused by external rotation hip contracture in infants.
- Most of these cases are treated nonoperatively.

VI. Leg Length Discrepancy

- A gross estimation of leg length discrepancy can be made under the following assumption of growth per year up to age 16 in boys and age 14 in girls:
  - Distal femur: 9 mm
  - Proximal tibia: 6 mm
  - Proximal femur: 3 mm
- Discrepancies of 2 to 5 cm can be treated with epiphysiodesis of the long side, shortening of the long side (ostectomy), or lengthening of the short side. Discrepancies of more than 5 cm are generally treated with lengthening.

SECTION 3 HIP AND FEMUR

I. Developmental Dysplasia of the Hip

- Risk factors (in order): breech positioning, positive family history, female sex, and being a firstborn child
- Early diagnosis is possible with the Ortolani test (elevation and abduction of femur relocates a dislocated hip) and the Barlow test (adduction and depression of femur dislocates a dislocatable hip).

- Subsequent diagnosis is made with limitation of hip abduction in the affected hip as the laxity resolves and stiffness becomes more clinically evident.
- Dynamic ultrasonography is used for diagnosis before ossification of the femoral head at age 4 to 6 months.
  - Radiographic signs of DDH: broken Shenton line, metaphysis lateral to the Perkin line, increased acetabular index
- Therapy is based on child's age:
  - Birth to 6 months: Pavlik harness
  - Check reduction with ultrasonography after 3 weeks.
  - Not reduced: closed reduction, arthrogram and spica casting
  - Reduced: continue harness until examination and ultrasound findings are normal.
  - Ages 6 to 18 months: hip arthrography, percutaneous adductor tenotomy, closed reduction and spica casting; if closed reduction fails, perform open reduction.
  - Ages 18 months to 3 years: open reduction
  - Ages 3 to 8 years: osteotomy
- Pavlik harness complications include avascular necrosis (AVN; caused by excessive abduction) and femoral nerve palsy (hyperflexion). If attempts to reduce a hip in 3 weeks fail, the Pavlik harness should be discontinued to prevent "Pavlik disease" (erosion of the pelvis superior to the acetabulum) and subsequent difficulty with closed reduction and casting.
- Open reductions are typically performed through an anterior approach (less risk to the medial femoral circumflex artery than in the medial approach).
- Osteotomies should be performed only after a congruent reduction is confirmed on an abduction–internal rotation radiograph, with satisfactory ROM, and after reasonable femoral sphericity is achieved by closed- or open-reduction methods.
  - The Chiari osteotomy is a salvage procedure when a concentric reduction of the femoral head within the acetabulum cannot be achieved.
  - The lateral shelf acetabular augmentation procedure also does not require concentric reduction. A successful result depends on fibrocartilage.

II. Congenital Coxa Vara

- When to observe:
  - Bilateral arthrogryposis
  - Myelomeningocele if no functional quadriceps
  - Spinal muscular atrophy
- When to treat or operate:
  - Down syndrome
  - Cerebral palsy, unless chronic

III. Legg-Calvé-Perthes Disease

- Bilateral involvement occurs in 15% of cases, but it is virtually never synchronous and may mimic MED.

TESTABLE CONCEPTS

- The Herring lateral pillar classification, which is most prognostic, is based on involvement of the lateral pillar of the capital femoral epiphysis during the fragmentation stage.
  - Group A has a uniformly good outcome.
  - Group B and a bone age of less than 6 years has a good prognosis.
  - Group C has a poor prognosis.
- Poor prognosis is also associated with older age (bone age > 6), female sex, and decreased hip abduction.
- Early degenerative hip disease results from aspherical femoral heads.
- Treatment is somewhat controversial. Symptoms may be relieved with traction, antiinflammatory medications, and partial weight bearing.
  - Surgical treatment improves radiographic outcome at skeletal maturity for older patients (chronologic age > 8 years or bone age > 6 years) with lateral pillar group B and B/C hips.

IV. Slipped Capital Femoral Epiphysis

- Disorder of the proximal femoral epiphysis caused by weakness of the perichondrial ring and slippage through the hypertrophic zone of the growth plate
- Associated with hormonal disorders in young children, such as hypothyroidism (most common), growth hormone deficiency, or renal osteodystrophy
- Diagnosis is missed most often because patients present with knee pain.
- On physical examination, all patients have obligate external rotation with flexion of the hip.
- Classification of SCFE is based on ability to bear weight at time of presentation.
  - Stable: weight bearing possible; AVN is rare.
  - Unstable: weight bearing not possible; rate of AVN is 50%.
- Treatment: in situ pinning. Prophylactic pinning of the contralateral hip is controversial but generally recommended in patients with an endocrinopathy, those younger than 10 years, or those with open triradiate cartilage.
  - Pin placement into the anterior superior quadrant of the femoral head has the highest rate of joint penetration.

VIII. Lower Extremity Inflammation and Infection

- Transient synovitis is the most common cause of painful hips during childhood. However, the patient must be evaluated for septic hip with aspiration (especially in children with fever, leukocytosis, or elevated ESR). If findings are negative, observe the patient with a trial of NSAIDs, and symptoms should improve within 24 to 48 hours.
- Acute hematogenous osteomyelitis is most commonly caused by *S. aureus*, regardless of age.
  - Methicillin-resistant *S. aureus* (MRSA) is associated with deep venous thrombosis and septic emboli.
  - Treatment is with intravenous antibiotics.
  - C-reactive protein measurements can be used to monitor the therapeutic response to antibiotics; failure to decline within 48 to 72 hours warrants alteration in treatment.
  - Failure to respond to antibiotics, frank pus on MRI, or the presence of a sequestered abscess (not accessible to antibiotics) necessitates operative drainage and débridement.
- Septic arthritis is most commonly caused by hematogenous seeding of the synovium. It also occurs through direct contact with osteomyelitis in joints with intracapsular metaphyses (hip, elbow, shoulder, ankle).
  - Distinguishing septic arthritis of the hip from transient synovitis is a common problem; however, when three of four of the following criteria are present, the diagnosis of septic arthritis is made in more than 90% of cases: WBC > 12,000 cells/mL, ESR > 40, inability to bear weight, and fever higher than 101.5° F.
- Radiographs may show a widened joint space or even dislocation.
- Because pus is chondrolytic, septic arthritis in children is an acute surgical emergency.

SECTION 4 KNEE AND LEG

- Blount disease occurs in infantile (more common) and adolescent forms.
  - Infantile Blount disease: treatment based on age and correlated with stage of disease
    - Stage I or stage II in children younger than 3 years: bracing
    - Stage II (in children < 3 years) or stage III: proximal osteotomy with valgus overcorrection
    - Stages IV to VI: multiple complex procedures; epiphysiolysis may be required.
  - Adolescent Blount disease: manifests with a relatively normal-appearing physis that shows widening of the proximal medial physeal plate. Beaking is not seen.
- Tibial bowing is classified into three types, according to the apex of the curve:
  - Posteromedial
    - Physiologic; commonly associated with leg length discrepancy, calcaneovalgus feet, and tight anterior structures. Spontaneous correction is the rule, but monitor the patient to evaluate leg length discrepancy.
  - Anteromedial
    - Fibular hemimelia
  - Anterolateral
    - Congenital pseudarthrosis is the most common cause and often accompanied by neurofibromatosis.
    - Initial treatment with total-contact brace to prevent fracture
- Osteochondritis dissecans most frequently involves the lateral portion of the medial femoral condyle. If growth plates are open, treat with bracing and restricted weight bearing.
- Discoid meniscus appears on MRI in three successive sagittal images with the meniscal body present. Saucerization or débridement should be performed.

SECTION 5 FOOT

- Clubfoot deformity is forefoot adductus and supination in combination with hindfoot equinus and varus.
  - Radiographs demonstrate "parallelism" of the calcaneus and talus.
  - Ponseti method is primarily used. A mnemonic for the sequence of correction is "CAVE": *c*avus, *a*dductus, *v*arus, *e*quinus.
  - A dynamic forefoot adduction/supination may develop after clubfoot treatment as a result of overpull of the anterior tibialis. This necessitates transfer of the anterior tibialis tendon laterally.
  - Clubfoot surgery is reserved for resistant or refractory clubfeet.
    - Development of a dorsal bunion can follow operative treatment. Treatment is with capsulotomy, flexor hallucis longus lengthening, and transfer of the flexor hallucis brevis to become a metatarsophalangeal extensor.
- Congenital vertical talus is an irreducible dorsal dislocation of the navicular bone on the talus, with a fixed equinus hindfoot deformity.
  - Plantar-flexion lateral radiographs show a line along the long axis of the talus that passes below the first metatarsal–cuneiform axis.
  - Initial treatment is with corrective casting. Surgery when the patient is 6 to 12 months of age includes soft tissue releases and

reduction of the talonavicular joint with reconstruction of the spring ligament.

- Tarsal coalitions are most commonly calcaneonavicular (in children 10-12 years of age) and talocalcaneal (in children 12-14 years of age).
  - Radiographs may show talar beaking on the lateral view and an irregular middle facet on the Harris axial view.
  - CT scan reliably demonstrates the coalition.
  - Initial treatment is with immobilization.
  - Subtalar coalition involving less than 50% of the joint should be resected and the extensor digitorum brevis interposed. If involvement is more than 50%, performing a subtalar arthrodesis is recommended.
- Köhler disease manifests with sclerosis of the navicular. It is self-limiting.
- Flexible pes planus should be observed if asymptomatic. Surgical treatment is with calcaneal lengthening osteotomy or 3C (calcaneus, cuneiform, cuboid) osteotomy.
- An accessory navicular manifests with medial arch pain and is typically self-limiting. Excision of the accessory bone with reconstruction of the posterior tibial tendon is performed in refractory cases. However, it does not correct the flatfoot.

SECTION 6 PEDIATRIC SPINE

I. Adolescent Idiopathic Scoliosis

- Indications for an MRI: left thoracic curves, painful scoliosis, apical kyphosis of the thoracic curve, juvenile-onset scoliosis (before the age of 11 years), rapid curve progression, associated syndromes, neurologic signs/symptoms, congenital abnormalities
- Risk factors for curve progression:
  - Skeletal immaturity (Risser stages 0 to 2)
  - Curve magnitude before or during peak height velocity. Peak height velocity is the best predictor of progression; it occurs before the onset of menarche and during Risser stage 0.
- Treatment:
  - <25 degrees: observation
  - 25-45 degrees and skeletally immature: bracing
  - 25-45 degrees and skeletally mature: observation
  - >45 to 50 degrees: surgery

III. Juvenile Idiopathic Scoliosis

- Manifestations are generally similar to those of adolescent idiopathic scoliosis, but risk for progression is higher: 70% require treatment (of those who do, 50% need bracing and 50% require surgery).
- Rate of spinal cord abnormality is 25%, and MRI should be routinely obtained.

IV. Infantile Idiopathic Scoliosis

- Manifests in children younger than 3 years
- Differences from adolescent idiopathic scoliosis: left curves, more common in boys, plagiocephaly (skull flattening), congenital defects
- In general, most curves resolve spontaneously.
- Risk for progression is calculated according to rib-vertebral angle difference; 20 degrees is the cutoff between low and high risk for progression.

V. Congenital Spinal Deformities

- Congenital scoliosis
  - A block vertebra has the best prognosis; a unilateral bar with hemivertebra has the worst prognosis.
  - Associated abnormalities are common. MRI should be ordered (reveals abnormalities in 35% of cases), along with renal (25%) and cardiac (10%) ultrasonography.

VIII. Kyphosis

- Scheuermann disease defined as increased thoracic kyphosis (>45 degrees curvature) with 5 degrees or more of anterior wedging at three sequential vertebrae
- Consider a CTLSO brace for skeletal immature patients with kyphotic curvature of 50 to 75 degrees.
- Operative indications include kyphotic curvature of more than 70 to 75 degrees, rigid deformity, progressive curve with failure of 6-month nonoperative management.

IX. Cervical Spine Disorders

- Rotatory atlantoaxial subluxation often manifests with torticollis. It can be caused by retropharyngeal inflammation.
  - Present less than 1 week: soft collar, heat, analgesics
  - Present more than 1 week without resolution: Halter traction, muscle relaxants; halo traction may be required
  - Present more than 1 month: attempt traction (typically halo); if no resolution after 1 week, closed versus open reduction and posterior C1-C2 fusion
- Os odontoideum is either congenital or an unrecognized odontoid fracture that has resulted in nonunion. Instability or presence of neurologic symptoms necessitates posterior C1-C2 fusion.
- Torticollis is a symptom and a sign but not a disease. Congenital muscular torticollis is a diagnosis of exclusion, and the affected patient should be evaluated for infection, congenital spinal deformity, rotatory subluxation of cervical spine, hearing loss, and optic dysfunction.
  - Of patients with congenital muscular torticollis, 90% respond to passive stretching within the first year. The chin should be rotated toward the affected side with a lateral head tilt away from the affected side.
  - Ultrasound demonstration of severe fibrosis of the sternocleidomastoid muscle is associated with failure of nonoperative management.

X. Spondylolysis and Spondylolisthesis

- Spondylolysis is classically seen in athletes who perform repetitive hyperextension (gymnastics, football linebacker, wrestler).
- Increased pelvic incidence may place patient at risk for spondylolisthesis.
- Slip angle > 45-50 degrees is associated with greater risk of slip progression, instability, and development of postoperative pseudarthrosis.
- L5 root injury is the most common neurologic complication in the surgical treatment of high-grade spondylolisthesis.

SECTION 7 CEREBRAL PALSY

- Cerebral palsy can be classified on the basis of physiology, anatomy, or function.
  - Anatomic classification divides cerebral palsy into three types:
  - Hemiplegia: one side of body, both upper and lower extremities
  - Diplegia: lower half involved more than upper half
  - Quadriplegia: both sides, both halves involved
  - A patient's locomotor profile is based on the persistence of primitive reflexes; the presence of two or more usually means that the child will be unable to walk.
    - Moro startle reflex: normally disappears by age 6 months
    - Parachute reflex: normally disappears by age 12 months
- The ability to sit independently by age 2 years is highly prognostic of walking.
- Intramuscular botulinum A toxin can temporarily decrease dynamic spasticity by means of a presynaptic blockade at the neuromuscular junction.

TESTABLE CONCEPTS

- Dorsal rhizotomy is primarily performed in ambulatory spastic diplegic patients to help reduce spasticity and complement orthopaedic management.
- Baclofen is used to control overall tone in the extremities by inhibiting signals through the GABA pathway.
- In general, surgery should be avoided in the first 3 years of life.
- The risk for scoliosis is highest in children with total body involvement (spastic quadriplegic). Surgical indications include curves greater than 45 to 50 degrees, worsening pelvic obliquity, and wheelchair seating problems.
- Hip subluxation and dislocation is a common problem, but in many children, hip disease is asymptomatic. Treatment can be based on four stages:
  - Hip at risk: significant adduction and flexion contractures but minimal subluxation. Adductor and psoas release should be performed before the child is 5 years of age.
  - Hip subluxation: adductor tenotomy in children with abduction of less than 20 degrees, sometimes with psoas release/recession. Femoral or pelvic osteotomies may be considered in femoral coxa valga and acetabular dysplasia.
  - Spastic dislocation: patients may benefit from open reduction, femoral shortening, varus derotation osteotomy, Dega osteotomy, triple osteotomy, or Chiari osteotomy. Addressing both hips can prevent dislocation of the opposite hip.
  - Windswept hips: characterized by abduction of one hip and adduction of the contralateral hip. Bilateral femoral osteotomies to more varus positioning can assist in maintaining reduction.
- Equinovarus foot is more common in spastic hemiplegia and is caused by overpull of either the posterior or anterior tibialis tendon.
  - Split-muscle transfers are helpful when the affected muscle is spastic during both the stance and swing phases of gait. The split–posterior tibialis transfer (rerouting half of the tendon dorsally to the peroneus brevis) is used in cases of spasticity of the muscle, flexible varus foot, and weak peroneal muscles.

SECTION 8 NEUROMUSCULAR DISORDERS

- Arthrogryposis is a nonprogressive disorder in which multiple joints are congenitally rigid.
  - Active elbow flexion achieved via anterior triceps transfer and posterior soft tissue release
  - Hip dislocation, unilateral: medial open reduction with possible femoral shortening
  - Hip dislocation, bilateral: typically left unreduced because ambulation is often preserved
  - Knee: contractures treated with early (age 6-9 months) soft tissue releases (especially hamstrings). To maintain reduction, knee contractures should be corrected before hip reduction.
  - Foot: clubfoot and vertical talus are initially treated with a soft tissue release, but later recurrences may necessitate bone procedures (talectomy). The goal is for the foot to be stiff and plantigrade to wear shoes and possibly ambulate.
- Myelodysplasia (spina bifida) is a spectrum of disorders caused by incomplete spinal cord closure or rupture of the developing cord secondary to hydrocephalus. In myelomeningocele, the sac with the neural elements protrudes through the skin.
  - It can be diagnosed in utero through increased levels of α-fetoprotein and is related to folate deficiency.
  - The myelodysplasia level is based on the lowest functional level. L4 is a key level because the quadriceps can function and allow independent ambulation in the community.
  - Fractures are common, occurring most often about the knee and hip in children 3 to 7 years of age, and can frequently be

diagnosed only by noting redness, warmth, and swelling that is caused by pain insensitivity.
- A significant proportion of patients with spina bifida have a serious allergy to latex. A latex-free environment is required in all cases involving spina bifida.
- Hip dislocation: treatment is controversial; in general, containment is considered essential only in patients with functioning quadriceps. Redislocation may occur regardless of treatment type. The functional outcome of thoracic-level myelomeningocele is independent of whether the hips are located or dislocated. Management should focus on limiting soft tissue contractures.
- Ankle and foot:
  - Calcaneal deformity is most common. Treat with tibialis anterior transfer to the calcaneus.
  - Valgus tibia or subtalar joint: skeletally immature patients should have hemiepiphysiodesis or Achilles tendon–fibular tenodesis. Skeletally mature patients should undergo distal tibial osteotomy.
  - Rigid clubfoot: treatment consists of complete subtalar release through a transverse (Cincinnati) incision, lengthening of the tibialis posterior and Achilles tendons, and transfer of the tibialis anterior tendon to the dorsal midfoot.
- Myopathies (muscular dystrophies) are inherited disorders with progressive weakness. Several types exist and are classified on the basis of their inheritance patterns.
  - Duchenne: X-linked recessive; absence of dystrophin protein; proximal muscle groups weaker than distal groups
  - Becker: X-linked recessive; decreased dystrophin protein
  - Hereditary sensory motor neuropathies are a group of inherited neuropathic disorders with similar characteristics. Charcot-Marie-Tooth (CMT) disease is the most common.
  - Two types of CMT disease; type I shows autosomal dominant inheritance. Diagnosis is made most reliably by DNA testing for a duplication of a genomic fragment that encompasses the peripheral myelin protein-22 (PMP22) gene on chromosome 17.
  - The most severely affected muscles are the tibialis anterior, peroneus longus, and peroneus brevis. Plantar flexion of the first ray is the first foot deformity to appear as a result of a weakened tibialis anterior muscle.
  - If the varus limb is flexible, plantar release and posterior tibial tendon transfer is performed.
- Spinal muscular atrophy is an anterior horn cell disorder. It is caused by a loss of anterior horn cells from the spinal cord.
  - Characterized by autosomal recessive inheritance and associated with survival motor neuron gene (SMN)
  - Scoliosis should be treated early. Upper extremity function may decrease after spinal fusion, but this decrease may be temporary. Before fusion, ensure that the patient does not have lower extremity muscle contractures that could interfere with sitting balance.
  - Hip subluxation or dislocation is common and is treated nonoperatively.

SECTION 9 BONE DYSPLASIAS

- Majority of dwarfisms not associated with mucopolysaccharidosis are autosomal dominant.
  - Autosomal recessive: diastrophic dysplasia, McKusick metaphyseal chondroplasia
  - X-linked recessive: spondyloepiphyseal dysplasia tarda
- Major mucopolysaccharidoses are autosomal recessive disorders, except Hunter syndrome, which is X-linked recessive.

- Common genetic associations:
  - Achondroplasia: *FGFR3*
  - Pseudoachondroplasia: *COMP*
  - Diastrophic dysplasia: sulfate transport protein
  - MED: type II collagen genes
  - Cleidocranial dysplasia: *CBFA1*
- Achondroplasia, the most common form of disproportional dwarfism, is autosomal dominant and caused by a mutation in FGFR3 that results in a failure in the proliferative zone of the physis.
  - Spine: lumbar stenosis; excessive lordosis (short pedicles with decreased interpedicular distances); foramen magnum stenosis
  - Pelvis: wider than it is deep ("champagne glass")
  - Legs: genu varum, tibia vara
  - Elbow: radial head subluxation
  - Growth plates: U- or V-shaped
- MED is characterized by irregular delayed ossification at multiple epiphyses.
  - The proximal femoral involvement can be confused with Perthes disease. MED is bilateral and symmetric and is characterized by early acetabular changes and not by metaphyseal cysts. Perform a bone survey to differentiate between Perthes disease, spondyloepiphyseal dysplasia (MED plus spine involvement), and MED.
- Morquio syndrome is the most common form of mucopolysaccharidosis and is a proportionate dwarfism characterized by urinary excretion of keratan sulfate.
  - C1-C2 instability (resulting from odontoid hypoplasia) can be seen with Morquio syndrome, manifesting with myelopathy and necessitating decompression and cervical fusion.
- Diastrophic dysplasia is autosomal recessive disorder of the sulfate transport protein; it manifests with cauliflower ears, rigid clubfeet, hitchhiker's thumb, and cleft palate. Cervical kyphosis may be severe and necessitate early fusion to prevent quadriplegia.
- Cleidocranial dysplasia affects bone formed by intramembranous ossification. It is characterized by hypoplasia or aplasia of the clavicle with delayed ossification of the symphysis pubis.
- Osteopetrosis is a failure of osteoclastic resorption, probably secondary to a defect in the thymus, and leads to dense bone.
  - Loss of the medullary canal can cause anemias and encroachment on the optic and oculomotor nerves, which lead to blindness.
  - Radiographic features include "marble bone," "rugger jersey spine," and an Erlenmeyer flask deformity of the proximal humerus and distal femur.
  - Bone marrow transplantation may be helpful in treating the malignant form.

SECTION 10 ORTHOPAEDIC-RELATED SYNDROMES

- Down syndrome (trisomy 21) is associated with atlantoaxial instability, hip instability, patellar dislocation, scoliosis, SCFE, and spondylolisthesis. The pathogenesis of generalized laxity is thought to be abnormal type VI collagen, whose genes COL6A1 and COL6A2 are located on chromosome 21.
  - Screening for cervical spine instability is somewhat controversial but is absolutely mandatory before induction of anesthesia.
  - Hip instability initially may be treated with closed reduction, but capsulorrhaphy, pelvis osteotomy, and femoral osteotomies may be required.
    - Scoliosis: bracing for 25- to 30-degree curves, surgery for 50- to 60-degree curves
- Marfan syndrome is an autosomal dominant disorder of fibrillin-1, an important component of elastic and nonelastic connective tissues.

- Nonorthopaedic manifestations are most important; aortic dilation is the major cause of death.
  - Scoliosis is common; bracing is ineffective, so both anterior and posterior fusion are often necessary.
  - Acetabular protrusion rarely causes severe hip dysfunction, and prophylactic surgical closure of the triradiate cartilage is not recommended.
- Beckwith-Wiedemann syndrome is associated with hemihypertrophy and spastic cerebral palsy. There is a predisposition to Wilms tumor (affected patients must be screened regularly by kidney ultrasonography).

SECTION 11 HEMATOPOIETIC AND METABOLIC DISORDERS AND ARTHRITIDES

- Sickle cell anemia is a condition of hemolysis and microvascular occlusion. Consequently, bone infarction, osteomyelitis, osteonecrosis of the femoral and humeral heads and septic arthritis are common.
  - Bone infarction is differentiated from osteomyelitis with sequential bone marrow tests and bone scans within 24 hours, as well as gadolinium-enhanced T1-weighted MRI sequences.
  - *S. aureus* and *Salmonella* infections are the most common cause of osteomyelitis. Empirical antibiotic therapy is with ceftriaxone.
- Hemophilia is an X-linked recessive disorder. Orthopaedic manifestations are secondary to repeated episodes of hemorrhage.
  - Recurrent hemarthroses result in hemophilic arthropathy.
  - Synovectomy is indicated for hemarthroses that recur despite optimal medical management.
  - Iliacus hematoma can result in femoral nerve neurapraxia.
  - Factor VIII levels should be increased for prophylaxis in the following situations: vigorous physical therapy (20% of cases), treatment of hematoma (30%), acute hemarthrosis or soft tissue surgery (>50%), and skeletal surgery (approaching 100% of cases preoperatively and maintained in more than 50% for 10 days postoperatively).
- Rickets manifests with physeal widening and metaphyseal cupping. Growth plate abnormalities include enlarged and distorted maturation zone (zone of hypertrophy) and a poorly defined zone of provisional calcification.
- Osteogenesis imperfecta is caused by a defect in type I collagen (COL1A2 gene) that causes abnormal cross-linking and leads to decreased secretion of collagen.
  - Fractures are ubiquitous, with normal healing but abnormal remodeling.
  - Basilar invagination is common in more severe types.
  - Bisphosphonates have been shown to decrease the number of fractures in affected patients. Iatrogenic osteopetrosis can occur with long-term use of high-dose bisphosphonates.
  - Scoliosis is common; bracing is ineffective, so segmental instrumentation is often necessary.
- Juvenile idiopathic arthritis typically manifests before the age of 4 years and commonly involves the knee, wrist, and hand. Cervical spine involvement can lead to kyphosis, facet ankylosis, and atlantoaxial subluxation.
  - Slit-lamp examination is required twice yearly because progressive iridocyclitis can lead to rapid loss of vision if left untreated.
- Ankylosing spondylitis is associated with HLA-B27, but the HLA-B27 test is not useful as a screening tool. Limitation of chest wall expansion is more specific.

CHAPTER **4**

SPORTS MEDICINE

Stephen R. Thompson and Mark D. Miller

CONTENTS

SECTION 1 KNEE

ANATOMY (FIGURE 4-1) (SEE CHAPTER 2, ANATOMY, FOR A THOROUGH DISCUSSION OF KNEE ANATOMY.)

■ Hinge joint that also incorporates both gliding and rolling, which are essential to its kinematics
■ Ligaments (Table 4-1)

■ Anterior cruciate ligament (ACL)
  • Femoral attachment: semicircular area on the posteromedial aspect of the lateral femoral condyle; divided by the bifurcate ridge and bordered by the intercondylar ridge
  • Tibial insertion: broad, irregular, oval area immediately lateral to the attachment of the anterior horn of the lateral meniscus and posterior to the tubercle of the anterior horn of medial meniscus (Figures 4-2 and 4-3)
• Has two bundles named on the basis of tibial insertion:
  • Anteromedial: originates proximal to the bifurcate ridge; tight in flexion; **primarily an anterior restraint;** evaluated by Lachman and anterior drawer tests
  • Posterolateral: originates distal to the bifurcate ridge; tight in extension; **primarily a rotatory restraint;** evaluated by pivot shift test
• Length 30 mm; diameter 11 mm
• Composition: 90% type I collagen and 10% type III collagen
• Blood supply: both cruciate ligaments receive their blood supply via branches of the middle genicular artery and the fat pad. The inferior genicular artery may play a role in hamstring graft revascularization.

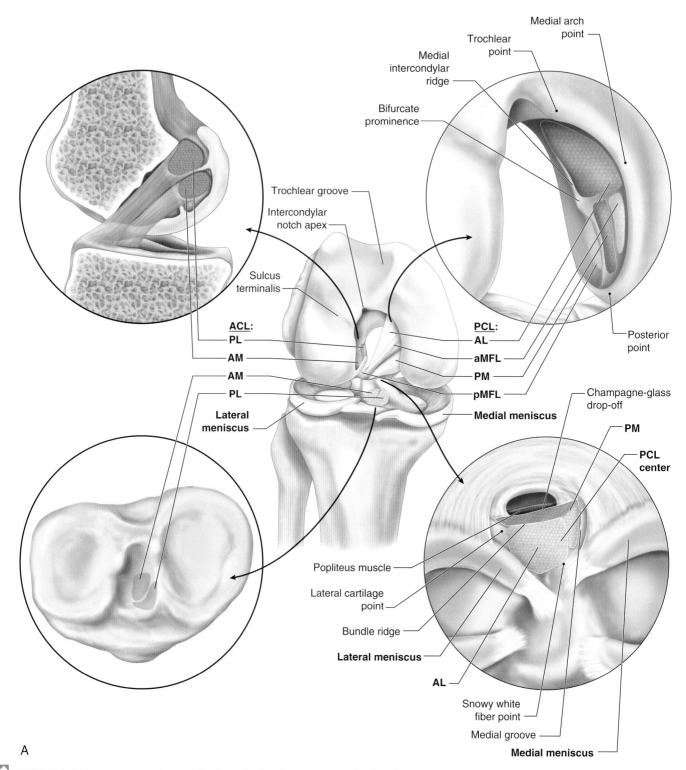

FIGURE 4-1 Ligamentous anatomy of the knee. **A,** Cruciate anatomy. *ACL,* Anterior cruciate ligament; *AL,* anterolateral; *AM,* anteromedial; *aMFL,* anterior meniscofemoral ligament; *PCL,* posterior cruciate ligament; *PL,* posterolateral; *PM,* posteromedial; *pMFL,* posterior meniscofemoral ligament.

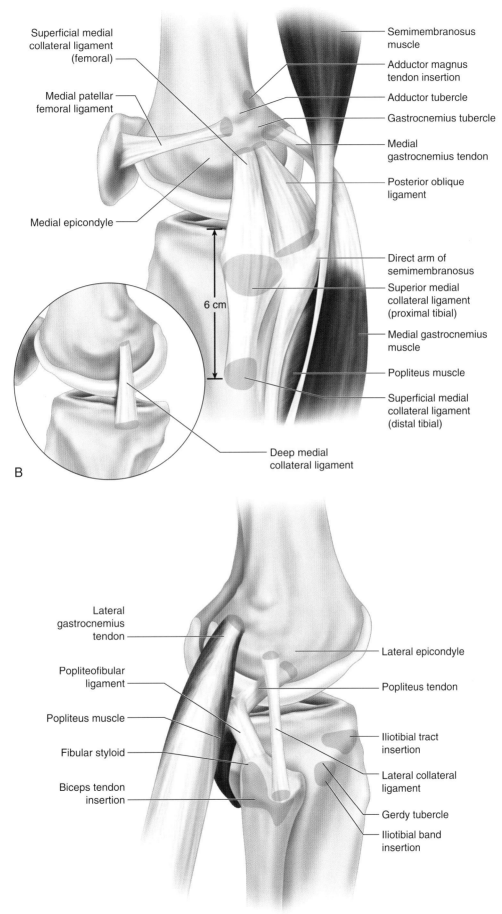

FIGURE 4-1, cont'd B, Medial view. **C,** Lateral view.

Continued

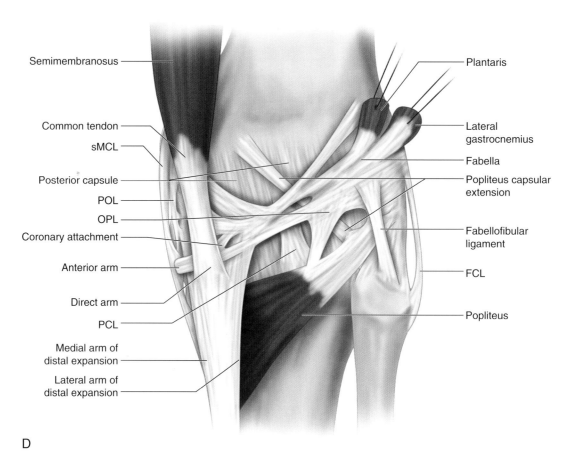

FIGURE 4-1, cont'd D, Posterior view. *FCL,* Fibular collateral ligament; *OPL,* oblique popliteal ligament; *PCL,* posterior cruciate ligament; *sMCL,* superior medial collateral ligament.

Table 4-1	Stabilizing Functions of the Ligaments of the Knee	
LIGAMENT	**PRIMARY FUNCTION**	**SECONDARY FUNCTION**
Anterior cruciate ligament		
Anteromedial bundle	Resists anterior tibial translation in knee flexion	Resists varus translation in knee extension
Posterolateral bundle	Resists rotatory loads in knee extension	Resists varus translation in knee extension
Posterior cruciate ligament (AL and PM bundles codominant)	Resists posterior tibial translation at all degrees of knee flexion	Resists tibial internal and external rotation beyond 90 degrees of knee flexion; resists varus translation
Medial collateral ligament (MCL)		
sMCL (proximal division from femur to proximal tibial attachment)	Resists valgus tibial translation	Resists tibial external rotation
sMCL (distal division from proximal tibial attachment to distal tibial attachment)	Resists tibial external rotation in knee extension	Resists tibial internal rotation
Deep MCL	Resists valgus translation	Resists tibial internal and external rotation
Posterior oblique ligament	Resists tibial internal rotation (especially in knee extension)	Resists tibial external rotation
Lateral collateral ligament	Resists varus tibial translation	Resists tibial external rotation (especially at 30 degrees of knee flexion)
Popliteus tendon	Resists tibial external rotation (especially in knee flexion)	Resists varus tibial translation
Popliteofibular ligament	Resists tibial external rotation (especially in knee flexion)	Resists posterior tibial displacement
Oblique popliteal ligament	Resists knee hyperextension	Resists varus tibial translation

AL, Anterolateral; *PM,* posteromedial; *sMCL,* superficial MCL.

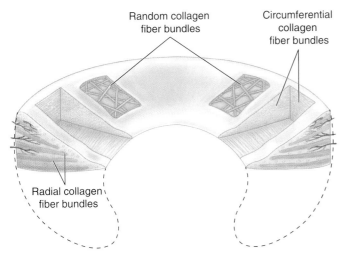

FIGURE 4-2 Meniscus anatomy.

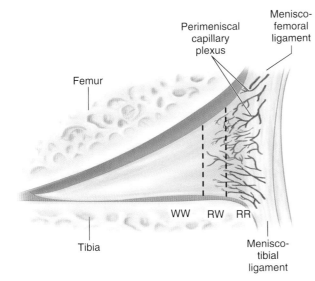

FIGURE 4-3 Meniscus blood supply. *RR,* Red-red; *RW,* red-white; *WW,* white-white.

- Mechanoreceptor nerve fibers have been found within the ACL and may have a proprioceptive role.
▨ Posterior cruciate ligament
  - Femoral attachment: broad crescent-shaped area on the anterolateral medial femoral condyle. Divided by the bifurcate prominence and bordered by the medial intercondylar ridge.
  - Tibial insertion: tibial sulcus below articular surface. Center of insertion is inline with the posterior attachment of medial meniscus.
  - Has two bundles named on the basis of tibial insertion:
    - Anterolateral: originates anterior to the bifurcate prominence; tight in flexion
    - Posteromedial: originates posterior to the bifurcate prominence; tight in extension
  - Both bundles are codominant and function to resist posterior tibial translation at all degrees of knee flexion.
  - Length 38 mm; diameter 13 mm
  - Neurovascular supply similar to ACL
  - Meniscofemoral ligaments

- Variably present
- Insert on the posterior horn of the lateral meniscus and originate on either side of the posteromedial bundle
- Humphrey: anterior
- Wrisberg: posterior
▨ Medial collateral ligament (MCL)
  - Superficial and deep components
  - Superficial (sMCL) (tibial collateral ligament)
    - Lies deep to the superficial sartorial fascia, gracilis tendon, and semitendinosus tendon
    - **Femoral origin: proximal and posterior to the medial epicondyle of the femur. Radiographically, originates slightly anterior to the junction of the posterior femoral cortex reference line and Blumensaat line.**
    - Tibial insertion: has two separate attachments. Proximally inserts onto soft tissue overlying anterior arm of semimembranosus. Distally inserts directly to bone, 6 cm distal to the joint line.
    - Length: 100 to 120 mm
    - Anterior fibers tighten during first 90 degrees of motion; posterior fibers tighten during extension.
  - Deep (mid-third medial capsular ligament)
    - Thickening of the medial joint capsule
    - Distinct meniscofemoral and meniscotibial components
    - Intimately associated with the medial meniscus
▨ Posteromedial corner
  - Structures between the posterior border of the superficial MCL and medial border of the PCL
  - Four important structures:
    - Capsular thickenings of the multiple insertions of semimembranosus
    - Posterior horn of the medial meniscus
    - Posterior oblique ligament (POL)
    - Oblique popliteal ligament
  - POL:
    - Three components: superficial, central, and capsular arms
    - Central arm most important
    - Originates proximal and posterior to the origin of the superficial MCL, as well as distal and posterior to the adductor tubercle
    - Central arm inserts onto posteromedial tibia
    - **Primary stabilizer against internal rotation and valgus between 0 and 30 degrees of knee flexion**
    - Increasingly important factor in the treatment of medial-sided knee injuries
▨ Medial patellofemoral ligament (MPFL)
  - Femoral attachment: anterior and distal to the adductor tubercle; or proximal to the attachment of the superficial medial collateral ligament; or proximal and posterior to the medial epicondyle. Radiographically, originates slightly anterior to the posterior femoral cortex reference line and immediately posterior to the most posterior aspect of the Blumensaat line (Schottle point).
  - Patellar attachment: junction of proximal and middle third on the medial border of the patella as well as the undersurface of the vastus medialis oblique muscle
  - Length: 53 to 55 mm
  - Primary passive restraint to lateral patellar translation; contributes 50% to 60% of restraint at 0 to 30 degrees of knee flexion

- Lateral collateral ligament (LCL) (fibular collateral ligament)
  - Femoral origin: proximal and posterior to the lateral femoral epicondyle; or posterior and proximal to the insertion of the popliteus tendon
  - Tibial insertion: anterior to the midpoint of the lateral aspect of the fibular head. Most anterior structure inserting on the proximal fibula.
  - Length: 63 to 71 mm
  - Tight in extension and lax in flexion because of its location behind the axis of knee rotation
  - Primary restraint to varus stress in all degrees of knee flexion
- Anterolateral ligament (ALL) (lateral capsular ligament)
  - Recently described structure located anterior to the LCL
  - Femoral origin: immediately anterior to popliteus tendon insertion
  - Tibial insertion: posterior to Gerdy tubercle; firm attachments to lateral meniscus
  - Role uncertain; clinical significance currently under investigation. Thought to be a stabilizer against internal tibial rotation.
- Posterolateral corner (PLC)
  - Primary structures:
    - Lateral collateral ligament
    - Popliteus tendon
    - Popliteofibular ligament
  - Additionally cited structures:
    - Iliotibial band
    - Biceps femoris
    - Fabellofibular ligament
    - Arcuate ligament complex (variably present)
    - Lateral gastrocnemius tendon
    - Mid-third lateral capsular ligament
    - Coronary ligament of the lateral meniscus
  - Primary stabilizer of external tibial rotation; also resists varus stress and posterior tibial translation
  - Popliteus tendon
    - Muscle originates on posterior tibia above soleal line
    - **Femoral insertion is distal, anterior, and deep to the LCL**
    - **Internally rotates the tibia**
  - Popliteofibular ligament
    - Originates from musculotendinous junction of popliteus muscle
    - Inserts on medial aspect of fibular head and styloid, posterior to LCL and anterior to biceps femoris
    - Role remains debated in the literature.
  - Order of insertion of structures on the proximal fibula is, from anterior to posterior: LCL, popliteofibular ligament, and biceps femoris

- **Menisci**
- Crescent-shaped fibrocartilaginous structures; triangular-shaped in cross section
- Composed primarily of type 1 collagen
- Collagen fibers are arranged in a variety of patterns
  - Circumferentially to disperse hoop stresses
  - Radially to resist longitudinal tearing
  - Randomly at the surface to disperse sheer stresses caused by knee flexion
- The two menisci are connected anteriorly by the transverse (intermeniscal) ligament
- They are attached peripherally by coronary ligaments

- Only the peripheral 20% to 30% of the medial meniscus and 10% to 25% of the lateral meniscus are vascularized; blood supply is from the medial and lateral genicular arteries, respectively.
  - Three vascular zones:
    - Red-Red
      - Completely within the vascular zone
      - Tears within this zone have the highest healing potential
    - Red-White
      - Intermediate vascularity
      - Less predictable healing
        - Red-Red and Red-White comprise the outer 4 mm of the meniscus
    - White-White
      - Avascular
      - Nutrition solely derived from synovial fluid via passive diffusion
      - Poor healing response
- 50% of medial tibial plateau covered by medial meniscus, 59% of lateral tibial plateau covered by lateral meniscus
- Role: to deepen the articular surfaces of the tibial plateau and function in stability, lubrication, and joint nutrition
- The menisci move anteriorly in extension and posteriorly with flexion. The lateral meniscus has fewer soft tissue attachments and is more mobile than the medial meniscus.
- **Joint relationships**
- Femoral condyles
  - Lateral
    - Greater anteroposterior dimensions than medial condyle
    - Relatively straight in comparison with medial condyle
    - Has a terminal sulcus and groove of the popliteus insertion
  - Medial
    - More curved than lateral condyle, allowing medial tibial plateau to rotate externally in full extension (the "screw-home mechanism")
- Femorotibial joint
  - Medial compartment
    - Convex-concave articulation
  - Lateral compartment
    - Convex-convex articulation
    - Meniscus is thus more important laterally to provide congruency to joint
- Patellofemoral joint
  - Articulation between the patella and femoral trochlea
  - Patella has variably sized medial and lateral facets.
  - Articular surface of the patella is the thickest in the body.
  - The patella can withstand forces several times those of body weight.
  - The patella is restrained in trochlea by the valgus axis of the quadriceps mechanism (Q angle), the oblique fibers of the vastus medialis oblique and lateralis muscles (and their extensions, all of which constitute the patella retinaculum), the bony and cartilaginous anatomy of the trochlea, and the patellofemoral ligaments.
- Vascular structures
  - Popliteal artery is lateral and posterior to the PCL
    - Closest to the knee joint at the PCL insertion of the tibia

BIOMECHANICS

- **Ligamentous biomechanics: role of ligaments of the knee is to provide passive restraints against abnormal motion**
- Structural properties of ligaments: tensile strength of a ligament, or maximal stress a ligament can sustain before failure, has been characterized for all knee ligaments. However, it is important to consider age, ligament orientation, preparation of the specimen, and other factors before determining which graft to use.
  - ACL: approximately 2200 N and up to 2500 N in young individuals
    - Tensile strength of a 10-mm patellar tendon graft (young specimen) is more than 2900 N and is about 30% stronger when it is rotated 90 degrees. However, this strength quickly diminishes in vivo.
    - Studies suggest that the quadrupled hamstring graft has even greater tensile strength but is dependent on graft fixation.
  - PCL: approximately 2500 to 3000 N, but this has been disputed
  - MCL: approximately 5000 N
    - sMCL: approximately 550 N
    - dMCL: approximately 100 N
    - POL: approximately 250 N
  - LCL: approximately 750 N
- Kinematics: motion of knee joint and interplay of ligaments have been described as a four-bar cruciate linkage system
  - As the knee flexes, the center of joint rotation (intersection of the cruciate ligaments) moves posteriorly, causing rolling and gliding at the articulating surfaces.
  - The concept of ligament "isometry" remains controversial.
  - Reconstructed ligaments should approximate normal anatomy and lie within the flexion axis in all positions of knee motion.
  - As the joint flexes, ligaments anterior to the flexion axis stretch and ligaments posterior to the axis shorten.
  - Although many instruments have been designed to achieve isometry, other considerations, such as graft impingement and avoiding flexion contractures, may be of more importance for ligament reconstructions.
- **Meniscal biomechanics:**
- The menisci transmit 50% to 75% of axial loads across the knee in full extension.
  - 85% of axial loads in 90 degrees of knee flexion
  - Medial meniscus bears 40% of the tibiofemoral load.
  - Lateral meniscus bears 70% of the load.
- Decrease peak contact stresses at the articular surface by 100% to 200%
  - Resection of 75% of the radial width results in an increase in peak contact stresses equivalent to those after a segmental or total meniscectomy
  - Posterior and peripheral zones are the most important in decreasing contact stresses
- Lateral meniscus has twice the excursion of the medial meniscus during range of motion (ROM) and rotation of the knee.
- Studies have shown that an ACL deficiency may result in abnormal meniscal strain, particularly in the posterior horn of the medial meniscus.

- Posterior horn of the medial meniscus is a major secondary stabilizer against anterior tibial translation in an ACL-deficient knee
- Meniscal root tears completely disrupt the circumferential fibers of the meniscus, leading to meniscal extrusion.
- Biomechanical studies have shown similar load patterns between posterior root tear and complete meniscectomy.

DIAGNOSTIC TECHNIQUES

- **History**
- Important key historical points (Table 4-2)
- **Physical examination**
- Important physical examination points (Table 4-3)
- **Opening to varus or valgus stress testing at only 30 degrees of knee flexion indicates an isolated collateral injury. Opening in full extension indicates a combined cruciate and collateral injury.**
- **Instrumented measurement of knee laxity**
- KT-1000 and KT-2000 arthrometers are the devices most commonly used for standardized laxity measurement.
- A difference of more than 3 mm between sides is considered significant.
- **Radiographs**
- Standard views:
  - Anteroposterior view
  - Weight-bearing 45-degree knee flexion posteroanterior view
    - Most sensitive view for revealing early osteoarthrosis
  - Lateral view
  - Merchant/Laurin/Sunrise view of the patella
- Additional views include lower extremity hip-to-ankle views, oblique views, stress radiographs.
  - Lower extremity hip-to-ankle views are required to calculate the mechanical axis.
    - A line from the center of the femoral head to the center of the ankle
    - In a neutrally aligned limb, this line should pass through the middle of the knee

Table 4-2	Key Historical Points That Indicate Mechanism of Injury
HISTORY	**SIGNIFICANCE**
Pain after sitting or climbing stairs	Patellofemoral cause
Locking or pain with squatting	Meniscal tear
Noncontact injury with "popping" sound/sensation	ACL tear, patellar dislocation
Contact injury with "popping" sound	Collateral ligament tear, meniscal tear, fracture
Acute swelling	ACL tear, peripheral meniscal tear, osteochondral fracture, capsule tear
Knee "gives way"	Ligamentous laxity, patellar instability
Anterior force: **dorsiflexed foot**	Patellar injury
Anterior force: **plantar-flexed foot**	PCL injury
Dashboard injury	PCL or patellar injury
Hyperextension, varus angulation, and tibial external rotation	Posterolateral corner injury

Table 4-3	Knee: Key Examination Points	
EXAMINATION OR TEST	**METHOD OR APPEARANCE**	**SIGNIFICANCE**
Standing and gait deformity	Observe gait	Based on pathologic process
	Observe patient standing	Based on pathologic process; check valgus/varus deformity
Effusion	Patella: ballottement/milking	Ligament/meniscal injury (acute), arthritis (chronic)
Point of maximal tenderness	Palpate for tenderness	Based on location (joint line tenderness indicates meniscal tear)
ROM	Active and passive	Block indicates meniscal (bucket handle) injury, loose body, impingement of ACL tear
Patellar crepitus	Passive ROM	Patellofemoral pathologic process
Patellar grind	Push patella with quadriceps contraction	Patellofemoral pathologic process
Patellar apprehension	Push patella laterally at 20 to 30 degrees of flexion	Patellar subluxation or dislocation
Q angle	ASIS-patella–tibial tubercle	Increased with patellar malalignment (normal <15 degrees); most pronounced in flexion
Flexion Q angle	ASIS-patella–tibial tubercle	Increased with patellar malalignment
J sign	Lateral deviation of the patella in extension	Patella instability
Patellar tilt	Tilt up laterally	>15 degrees indicates laxity; <0 degrees indicates tight lateral constraint
Patellar glide	Push patella laterally at 20 to 30 degrees of flexion	>50 degrees indicates increased medial constraint laxity
Active glide	Lateral excursion with quadriceps contraction	Lateral excursion > proximate excursion indicates increased functional Q angle of quadriceps
Quadriceps circumference	10 cm (VMO), 15 cm (quadriceps)	Atrophy from inactivity
Symmetric extension	Difference in distance of back of knee from ground or in prone heel height	Contracture, displaced meniscal tear, or other mechanical block
Varus/valgus stress	Laxity of 30 degrees	MCL/LCL laxity (grade I: opening = 1 to 5 mm; grade II: opening = 6 to 10 mm; grade III [complete]: opening > 10 mm)
	Deformity of 0 degrees	MCL/LCL and PCL laxity
Apley	Prone-flexion compression	DJD, meniscal disease
Lachman	Tibia forward at 30 degrees of flexion	ACL injury (most sensitive test)
Finacetto	Lachman test with tibia subluxation beyond posterior horns of menisci	ACL injury (severe)
Anterior drawer	Tibia forward at 90 degrees of flexion	ACL injury
Internal rotation drawer	Foot internally rotated with drawer	Tighter is normal; looser indicates ACL injury
External rotation drawer	Foot externally rotated with drawer	Loose is normal; looser indicates ACL/MCL injury
McMurray	Internal and external tibial rotation while moving from a starting point of maximal flexion into extension of the knee	Meniscal pathologic process
Pivot shift*	Flexion with internal rotation and valgus angulation	ACL injury
Pivot jerk*	Extension with internal rotation and valgus angulation	ACL injury
Posterior drawer	Tibia backward at 90 degrees of flexion	PCL injury
Tibial sag	Flex 90 degrees, observe	PCL injury
90-degree quadriceps active test	Extend flexed knee	PCL injury
Asymmetric external rotation	"Dial" feet externally at 30 and 90 degrees of flexion	Asymmetric increased external rotation of > 10 to 15 degrees indicates injury of posterolateral corner if difference is 30 degrees only; difference at both 30 and 90 degrees indicates injury of PCL and posterolateral corner
External rotation recurvatum	Pick up great toes	PCL injury, PLC injury
Reversed pivot	Extension with external rotation and valgus	PCL injury
Posterolateral drawer	Posterior drawer, lateral > medial	PCL injury

*Examination performed with the patient under anesthesia.

- Stress radiographs
  - Used in pediatric patients for evaluating injuries to the femoral physis and differentiating from an MCL injury
  - Increasingly being used to characterize PCL, MCL, LCL, and PLC injuries
- Several findings and their significance are listed in Table 4-4 and illustrated in Figure 4-4.
- Evaluation of patella height is accomplished by one of three commonly used methods (Figure 4-5).

- The Caton-Deschamps method may be the most reliable, but this is controversial.

■ **Nuclear imaging**
- Technetium 99m bone scans are useful in diagnosing stress fractures, early degenerative joint disease, and complex regional pain syndrome.

■ **Magnetic resonance imaging (MRI)**
- Imaging modality of choice for diagnosis of ligament injuries, meniscal disease, avascular necrosis, spontaneous osteonecrosis of the knee, and articular cartilage defects

Table 4-4	Knee Injuries: Radiographic Findings	
VIEW/SIGN	**FINDINGS**	**SIGNIFICANCE**
Lateral-high patella	Patella alta	Patellofemoral pathologic process
Congruence angle	μ = −6 degrees; SD = 11 degrees	Patellofemoral pathologic process
Tooth sign	Irregular anterior patella	Patellofemoral chondrosis
Varus/valgus stress view	Opening	Collateral ligament injury; Salter-Harris fracture
Lateral capsule (Segond) sign	Small tibial avulsion off lateral tibia	ACL tear
Arcuate sign	Small fibular avulsion	PLC injury
Pellegrini-Stieda lesion	Avulsion of medial femoral condyle	Chronic MCL injury
Lateral-stress view: stress to anterior tibia with knee flexed 70 degrees	Asymmetric posterior tibial displacement	PCL injury
Weight-bearing flexion posteroanterior view	Fairbank changes: square condyle, peak eminences, ridging, narrowing	Early DJD, OCD, notch evaluation
		Early DJD (postmeniscectomy)
Square lateral condyle	Thickened joint space	Discoid meniscus

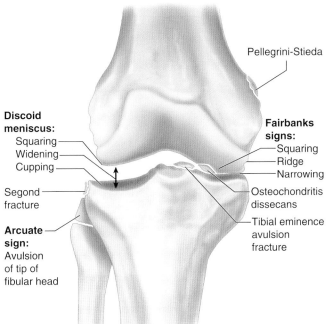

FIGURE 4-4 Common findings visualized on knee radiographs.

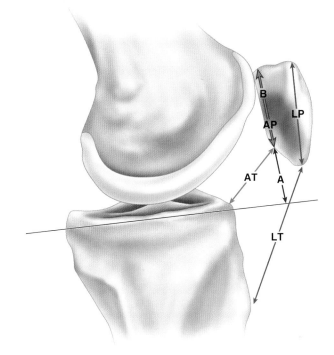

FIGURE 4-5 Three common methods for calculating patellar height. The **Caton-Deschamps index (AT/AP)** is the ratio between the distance from the lower edge of the patella's articular surface to the anterosuperior angle of the tibia outline (AT) and the length of the articular surface of the patella (AP). The **Insall-Salvati index (LT/LP)** is the ratio between the length of the patellar tendon (LT) and the longest sagittal diameter of the patella (LP). The **Blackburne-Peel index (A/B)** is the ratio between the length of the perpendicular line drawn from the tangent to the tibial plateau until the inferior pole of the articular surface of the patella (A) and the length of the articular surface of the patella (B).

- Occult fractures of the knee can be identified by a double fluid-fluid layer, which signifies lipohemarthrosis.

■ Magnetic resonance arthrography

▥ Intraarticular MR arthrography is the most accurate imaging method for confirming the diagnosis of repeated meniscal tears after repair.

▥ A variety of classic MRI findings are shown in Figure 4-6.

■ Computed tomography (CT)

▥ CT has been replaced largely by MRI, but it is still useful in the evaluation of bony tumors, patellar tilt, and fractures.

▥ CT has been advocated as a tool to assist in operative planning for patellar instability and realignment by allowing measurement of the tibial tuberosity–trochlear groove (TT-TG) distance.

- A tibial tubercle osteotomy (distal realignment procedure) is recommended for a TT-TG distance exceeding 20 mm.
- MRI can also be used to measure TT-TG distance.

■ Arthrography

▥ Useful historically for diagnosis of MCL tears; has been supplanted by MRI. However, it can be useful when MRI is not available or tolerated by the patient, and it can be combined with CT.

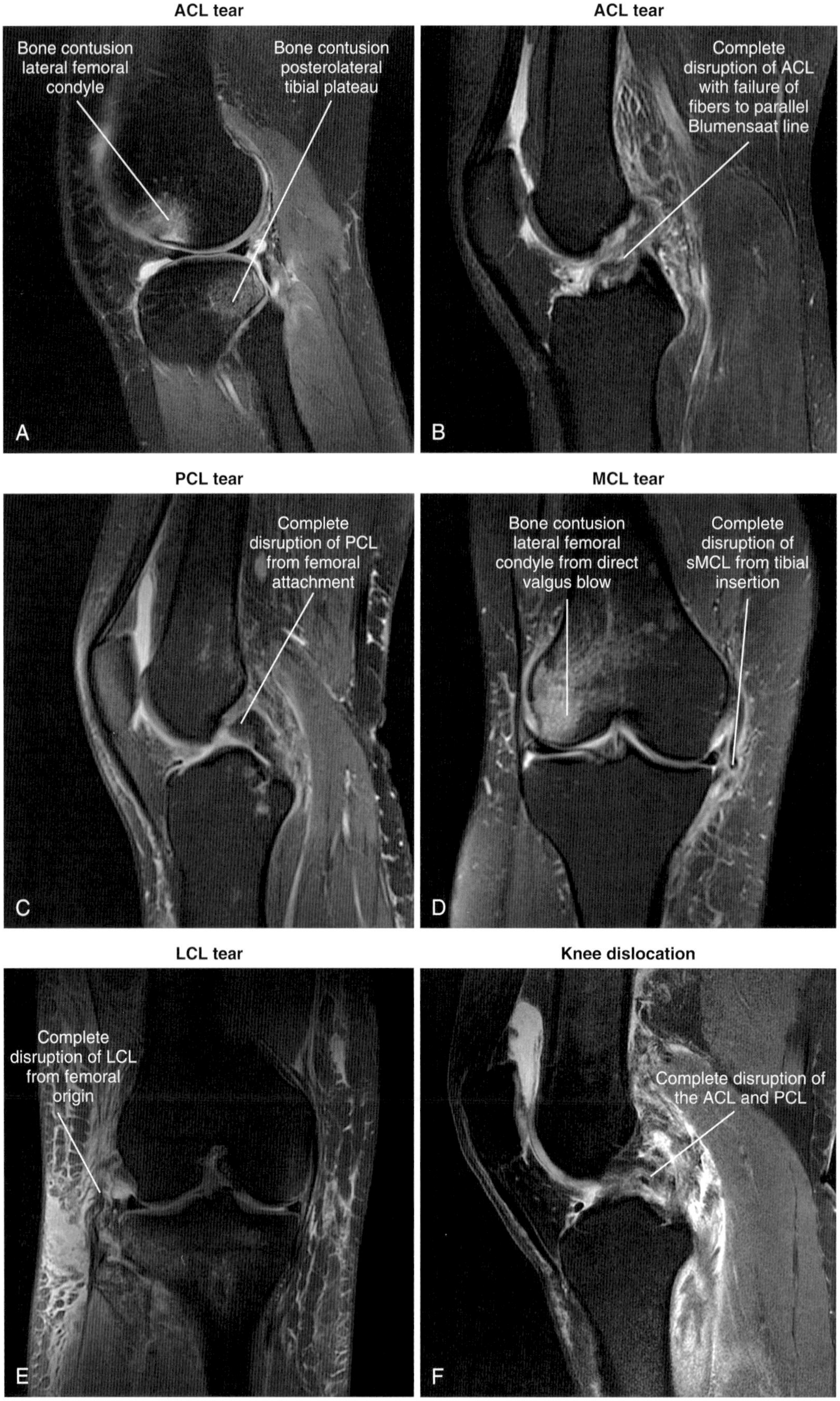

ACL tear

Bone contusion
lateral femoral
condyle

Bone contusion
posterolateral
tibial plateau

A

ACL tear

Complete
disruption of ACL
with failure of
fibers to parallel
Blumensaat line

B

PCL tear

Complete
disruption of PCL
from femoral
attachment

C

MCL tear

Bone contusion
lateral femoral
condyle from direct
valgus blow

Complete
disruption of
sMCL from tibial
insertion

D

LCL tear

Complete
disruption of LCL
from femoral
origin

E

Knee dislocation

Complete disruption of
the ACL and PCL

F

FIGURE 4-6 Magnetic resonance imaging of the knee. **A,** Anterior cruciate ligament (ACL) tear with bone contusion. **B,** ACL tear with complete disruption. **C,** Posterior cruciate ligament tear with complete disruption. **D,** Medial collateral ligament (MCL) tear. **E,** Lateral collateral ligament (LCL) tear. **F,** Knee dislocation with ACL and PCL tear.

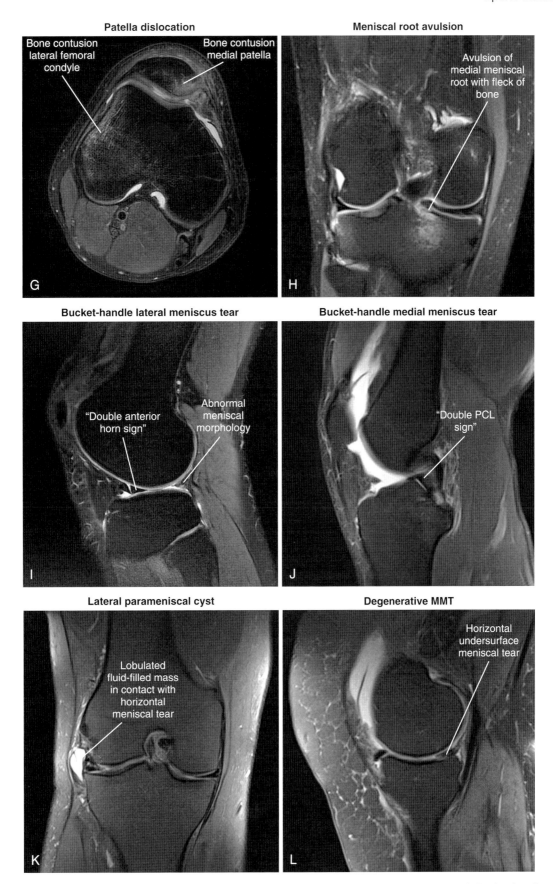

FIGURE 4-6, cont'd G, Patella dislocation. **H,** Meniscal root avulsion. **I,** Bucket-handle lateral meniscus tear. **J,** Bucket-handle medial meniscus tear (MMT). **K,** Lateral parameniscal cyst. **L,** Degenerative MMT.

Ultrasonography

This technique is useful for detecting soft tissue lesions about the knee, including patellar tendinitis, hematomas, and extensor mechanism ruptures.

Arthrocentesis and intraarticular knee injection

Most accurately administered with the knee in extension; a lateral entry point that is in the middle to upper portion of the patella is used

KNEE ARTHROSCOPY

Portals

Standard portals
- Inferomedial and inferolateral portals
  - Made with the knee in flexion; for instrument placement and the arthroscope, respectively (Figure 4-7)
- Superomedial and superolateral outflow portals
  - Made with the knee in extension but may not be necessary with newer pump systems

Accessory portals
- Sometimes helpful for visualizing the posterior horns of the menisci and PCL
- Posteromedial portal
  - 1 cm above the joint line behind the MCL (be careful to avoid saphenous nerve branches)
- Posterolateral portal
  - 1 cm above the joint line between the LCL and biceps tendon (avoiding the common peroneal nerve)
- Transpatellar portal
  - 1 cm distal to the patella, splitting the patellar tendon fibers
  - Can be used for central viewing or grabbing but should be avoided in patients who require subsequent harvesting of autogenous patellar tendon

Less commonly used portals
- Medial and lateral midpatellar portals
- Proximal superomedial and superolateral portals (4 cm proximal to patella)
  - Used for patellofemoral compartment visualization
- Far medial and far lateral portals
  - Used for accessory instrument placement (loose-body removal)

Technique

Each knee arthroscopy should include an evaluation of the suprapatellar pouch; patellofemoral joint and tracking; medial and lateral gutters; medial compartment, including the medial meniscus and the articular surface; the lateral compartment, including the lateral meniscus and the articular surface; and the intercondylar notch to visualize the ACL and PCL.

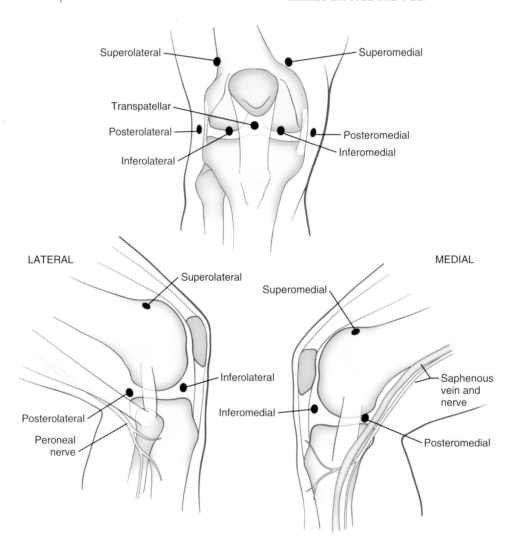

FIGURE 4-7 Knee arthroscopy portals. (From Miller MD, et al: *Orthopaedic surgical approaches, Philadelphia,* 2008, Elsevier.)

- The posteromedial compartment can be best visualized with a 70-degree arthroscope placed through the interval of the PCL and medial femoral condyle (modified Gillquist view) or a posteromedial portal.
- The posterolateral compartment can be best visualized by placing the arthroscope through the interval of the ACL and lateral femoral condyle or a posterolateral portal.

- **Arthroscopic complications**
- Most common arthroscopic complication: iatrogenic articular cartilage damage
- Additional complications: instrument breakage, hemarthrosis, infection, arthrofibrosis, deep venous thrombosis (DVT), neurovascular injury (especially injury to infrapatellar branches of saphenous nerve)

MENISCAL INJURIES

- **Meniscal tears**
- Overview
  - Meniscal tears are the most common injury to the knee that necessitates surgery.
  - The medial meniscus is torn approximately three times more often than the lateral meniscus.
    - However, lateral meniscus tears occur more commonly with concomitant ACL tear.
  - There is an increased rate of osteoarthritis in knees after both meniscal tears and meniscectomy.
  - Traumatic meniscal tears are common in young patients with sports-related injuries.
  - Degenerative tears usually occur in older patients and can have an insidious onset.
  - Meniscal tears can be classified according to:
    - Location in relation to the vascular supply (see Figure 4-2)
    - Position (anterior, middle, or posterior third)
    - Appearance and orientation (Figure 4-8)
  - Meniscal root tears
    - Defined as a radial tear or avulsion of the meniscal root from the tibial plateau
    - Completely disrupt the circumferential fibers of the meniscus
    - Biomechanically, result in a loss of hoop stresses and increase in contact forces
    - Functionally equivalent to a total meniscectomy
    - Lateral root tears are associated with ACL tears.
    - Medial root tears are associated with chondral injuries.
    - Repair should be attempted wherever possible except in the presence of grade III to IV chondral change.

- The vascular supply of the meniscus is a primary determinant of healing potential.
  - Tears in the peripheral third have the highest potential for healing.
- Treatment
  - In the absence of intermittent swelling, catching, locking, or giving way, meniscal tears—particularly those degenerative in nature—may be treated conservatively.
  - Younger patients with acute tears, patients with tears causing mechanical symptoms, and patients with tears that fail to improve with conservative measures may benefit from operative treatment.
- Partial meniscectomy:
  - Tears that are not amenable to repair (e.g., peripheral, longitudinal tears)—excluding those that do not necessitate any treatment (e.g., partial-thickness tears, those < 5-10 mm in length, and those that cannot be displaced > 1-2 mm)—are best treated by partial meniscectomy.
  - In general, complex, degenerative, and central/radial tears are treated with resection of a minimal amount of normal meniscus. A motorized shaver is helpful for creating a smooth transition zone.
  - **Partial meniscectomy increases peak stresses in the affected compartment**
- Meniscal repair
  - Indications:
    - Tear between 1 and 4 cm
    - Vertical tear
    - Red-Red tear
    - Meniscal root tear
    - Age younger than 40 years
  - Concomitant ACL reconstruction may extend the indications because results are typically better.
  - Augmentation techniques (fibrin clot, platelet-rich plasma clot, vascular access channels, synovial rasping) may extend the indications for repair.
  - Four techniques are commonly used: open, "outside-in," "inside-out," and "all-inside" (Figure 4-9).

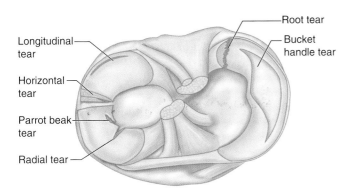

FIGURE 4-8 Types of meniscal tears.

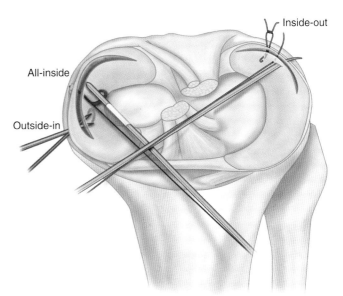

FIGURE 4-9 Meniscal repair techniques.

- Newer techniques for all-inside repairs (e.g., arrows, darts, staples, screws) are popular because of their ease of use; however, they are probably not as reliable as vertical mattress sutures.
- The latest generation of "all-inside" devices allows tensioning of the construct.
- **The gold standard for meniscal repair remains the inside-out technique with vertical mattress sutures**.
- Regardless of the technique used, it is essential to protect the saphenous nerve branches (anterior to both the semitendinosis and gracilis muscles and posterior to the inferior border of the sartorius muscle) during medial repairs and to protect the peroneal nerve (posterior to the biceps femoris) during lateral repairs (Figure 4-10).
- Rehabilitation following meniscus repair should involve avoidance of knee flexion beyond 90 degrees. The degree of allowed weight bearing is controversial.
- Results of meniscal repair
  - In several studies, 80% to 90% success rates with meniscal repairs have been reported. However, success depends on location, type of tear, and chronicity.
- It is generally accepted that the results of meniscal repair are best with acute peripheral tears in young patients with concurrent ACL reconstruction.
- In general, success rates are 90% when meniscal repair is performed in conjunction with an ACL reconstruction, 60% with a repair in which the ACL is intact, and 30% with a repair in which the ACL is deficient.

■ Meniscal cysts

- Occur primarily in conjunction with horizontal cleavage tears of the lateral meniscus
- Operative treatment consisting of arthroscopic partial meniscectomy and decompression through the tear (sometimes including "needling" of the cyst) has been shown to be effective.
- En bloc excision no longer favored for most meniscal cysts
- Popliteal (Baker) cysts are commonly related to meniscal disorders and usually resolve with treatment of the primary disorder.

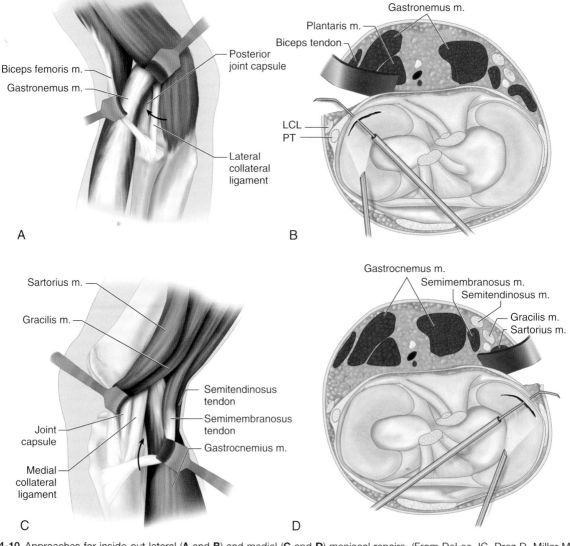

FIGURE 4-10 Approaches for inside-out lateral (**A** and **B**) and medial (**C** and **D**) meniscal repairs. (From DeLee JC, Drez D, Miller MD, editors: *DeLee and Drez's orthopaedic sports medicine,* ed 3, Philadelphia, 2009, Elsevier.)

- Usually located between the semimembranosus and medial head of the gastrocnemius
- ■ **Discoid menisci ("Popping knee syndrome")**
- Can be classified as (I) incomplete, (II) complete, or (III) the Wrisberg variant
- Patients may develop mechanical symptoms or "popping" with the knee in extension.
- Plain radiographs may demonstrate a widened joint space, squaring of the lateral femoral condyle, cupping of the lateral tibial plateau, and a hypoplastic lateral intercondylar spine.
- Appearance of a contiguous lateral meniscus on three consecutive sagittal images on MRI is diagnostic; MRI may also demonstrate associated tears.
- Treatment
  - Observation if asymptomatic
  - Partial meniscectomy (saucerization) for tears
  - Meniscal repair for peripheral detachments (Wrisberg variant)
- ■ **Meniscal transplantation**
- Controversial and all nonoperative management modalities should be exhausted prior to considering meniscal transplantation.
- Indications:
  - Prior total or near-total meniscectomy (especially lateral)
  - Pain in the involved compartment
  - Body mass index (BMI) less than 30
  - Age younger than 50
  - No evidence of advanced arthrosis
  - Normal alignment
  - Ligamentous stability
- Ligamentous deficiency and limb alignment must be addressed to increase success rates of meniscal transplantation.
- Full-thickness cartilage lesions no longer considered a contraindication
- Contraindications:
  - Diffuse grades III and IV chondral lesions
  - Kissing lesions
    - Chondral lesions adjacent to each other on the femur and tibia
  - Advanced age
  - **Inflammatory arthritis**
  - Synovial disease
  - **Radiographic evidence of significant arthrosis**
- Graft size accurate to within 5% of the native meniscus is crucial for success. Sizing is typically done using radiographs but may also be accomplished using MRI.
  - Undersized grafts result in poor congruity and increased load transmission.
  - Oversized grafts result in meniscal extrusion and impaired ability to transmit compressive loads.
- Techniques for implantation include use of individual bone plugs for the anterior and posterior horns and use of a bone bridge, especially laterally.
- Pain relief is the most consistent benefit; most studies have short-term to 5-year data available.
  - Meniscal allograft tissue often remains hypocellular or acellular, particularly at the core.
- The chondroprotective effect of meniscal transplantation has yet to be demonstrated clinically.
- ■ **Meniscal allograft tear is the most common complication.**

- Collagen meniscal implantation has yielded promising initial results for irreparable medial meniscal tears with new meniscus-like matrix formation, in comparison with partial meniscectomy. However, long-term results, especially by independent sources, have not been reported.

LIGAMENT INJURIES

■ **ACL injury**

- Introduction
  - Common injury comprising between 40% and 50% of all knee ligament injuries
  - **Female athletes have a 2 to 8 times higher risk of ACL tear compared to male athletes**
    - Thought to occur because women have different landing biomechanics
      - Women have a greater total valgus knee loading in landing.
      - Women land more erect.
      - Women have increased quadriceps-to-hamstring strength, causing increased anterior sheer.
    - Smaller notches, smaller ligaments (reduced area in cross section), increased generalized ligament laxity, and increased knee laxity are additional proposed factors.
  - Skiing, soccer, basketball, and football are the highest-risk sports.
  - Mechanism of injury is typically a valgus load with internal tibial rotation and anterior tibial translation while the knee is in almost full extension.
  - The in situ force of the ACL is highest at 30 degrees of flexion in response to anterior tibial load. Associated injuries are common.
    - Acute lateral meniscal tears are more common than acute medial tears, whereas medial tears occur more often with chronic ACL deficiency.
    - MCL injuries occur in approximately 25% of cases.
      - MCL typically treated nonoperatively
    - Posterolateral corner (PLC) injuries occur in approximately 10% of cases.
      - Lack of recognition of a PLC injury has been cited as a common cause of ACL reconstruction failure.
  - Chronic ACL deficiency is associated with a higher incidence of complex meniscal tears not amenable to repair and chondral injury.
  - Controversy continues with regard to development of late arthritis in ACL-deficient versus reconstructed knees.
    - Currently there is no high-level evidence to suggest that ACL reconstruction reduces the risk of developing arthritis.
    - Chondral and meniscal injuries that occur at the time of initial ACL rupture have been demonstrated to be the main predictors of arthritic change.
  - ACL injury prevention programs emphasize proprioceptive training and the strengthening of knee flexors.
  - The most common reasons for failure to return to play after ACL reconstruction are pain and fear of reinjury.
- History and physical examination
  - ACL injuries are often the result of noncontact pivoting injuries.
    - Only 30% are the result of direct contact.

- They are commonly associated with an audible "pop" and a hemarthrosis that begins within 12 hours of injury.
- Instability and inability to return to sport are the most frequent complaints.
- The Lachman test is the most sensitive examination for acute ACL injuries.
- Performance on the pivot shift test is most closely correlated with outcome after ACL reconstruction.
  - The pivot shift is a reduction of the subluxated lateral tibial plateau by the iliotibial band when moving from full extension to flexion.
  - This test is also helpful in evaluating an ACL-deficient knee, especially in an examination with the patient under anesthesia.
- The KT-1000 and KT-2000 Knee Ligament Arthrometers are useful in quantifying laxity but unnecessary in diagnosis.
- Imaging
  - Plain radiographs are essential in evaluating ACL injuries.
    - A Segond fracture may be present and may represent an avulsion of the anterolateral ligament or avulsion of the lateral capsule.
    - Lateral radiographs should be carefully scrutinized for the degree of posterior tibial slope. Values greater than 13 degrees have been associated with ACL failure.
  - MRI is useful in confirming the diagnosis.
    - On sagittal imaging, fibers of an intact ACL should parallel the Blumensaat line.
    - Signs of an ACL tear:
      - Disruption of ACL fibers
      - Fibers no longer parallel to Blumensaat line
      - Inability to visualize fibers of ACL
      - "Empty lateral wall" or "empty notch" sign indicating avulsion of ACL from the femoral origin
    - Bone bruises (trabecular microfractures) occur in more than half of acute ACL injuries.
    - **Bone bruises are typically located near the sulcus terminalis on the lateral femoral condyle and the posterolateral aspect of the tibia.**
      - Although the long-term significance of these injuries is unknown, they may be related to late cartilage degeneration.
- Treatment
  - Initial management consists of physical therapy for mobilization. Immobilization is avoided.
    - Full ROM and good quadriceps control should be achieved prior to surgery.
  - Treatment decisions should be individualized on the basis of age, activity level, instability, associated injuries, and other medical factors.
  - Primary repair of ACL tears is not currently recommended.
    - Myofibroblasts "coat" the end of the ACL stumps, making primary healing impossible.
- Surgical technique
  - Single-bundle reconstruction is still the most commonly performed reconstruction. Significant controversy exists regarding the double-bundle ACL reconstruction.
    - Currently there is no difference in patient-reported outcomes between single-bundle and double-bundle techniques.

- Studies have demonstrated that the double-bundle technique results in superior laxity measurements.
- Placement of a more horizontal femoral tunnel (10 or 2 o'clock position, or "anatomic ACL reconstruction") to center the graft in the middle of the femoral ACL footprint has been the focus of newer anteromedial or "far medial" portal drilling techniques (in contrast to traditional transtibial-femoral drilling techniques).
- **A more horizontal graft position may reduce rotational instability.**
- Graft selection depends on patient factors and surgeon's preference and usually includes (1) a bone-patella, tendon-bone (BPTB) autograft, (2) a four-strand hamstring autograft, (3) a quadriceps tendon autograft, and (4) an allograft.
  - BPTB demonstrates faster incorporation into the bone tunnels than does hamstring autograft and, for the authors, is often the graft of choice for patients who desire an early return to sports activity.
  - Several studies have, however, demonstrated a higher incidence of arthritis associated with the use of BPTB autograft than with hamstring autograft 5 to 7 years after ACL reconstruction.
  - BPTB autograft harvest carries the risk of anterior knee pain, pain with kneeling, loss of extension, and poorer recovery of quadriceps strength.
  - Hamstring autograft has similar strength to the native ACL but is less stiff than the native ACL.
    - The ultimate tensile load (UTL) of a quadrupled hamstring autograft is highest of all graft options at 4000 N.
    - The UTL of a BPTB is 3000 N and the native ACL is 2100 N.
  - Hamstring autograft harvest carries the risk of weakness of knee flexion and internal rotation, along with injury to branches of the saphenous nerve.
    - Use of an oblique incision at the harvest site decreases the risk of damaging the infrapatellar branch of the saphenous nerve.
  - Both BPTB and quadriceps tendon with bone block grafts carry the risk of patellar fracture
  - Use of allograft with ACL reconstruction in younger, more active patients may be associated with a higher rate of rerupture.
    - Chemical-processed or irradiated allografts have demonstrated increased rates of failure compared to fresh-frozen allografts.
    - Allografts have been demonstrated to incorporate into bone tunnels more slowly.
  - Allograft risk also includes infection risk (e.g., with *Clostridium* species and human immunodeficiency virus [HIV]), although rates are low (1:1.6 million).
    - Preimplantation culture of allografts not widely recommended
    - In the absence of clinical infection, positive preimplanation allograft culture results do not warrant antibiotic treatment.
- Postoperative rehabilitation
  - Rehabilitation has evolved, and early motion (emphasis on extension) and weight bearing are encouraged in most protocols.
  - **Exercises that do not endanger the ACL graft:**
    - Exercises dominated by the hamstrings (isometric hamstrings)

- Exercises that result in quadriceps activity with the knee flexed beyond 60 degrees
- Exercises involving active knee ROM between 35 and 90 degrees of flexion
- Closed-chain rehabilitation (fixation of terminal segment of extremity [i.e., foot planted]) and compressive loading have been emphasized because they allow physiologic cocontraction of the muscles around the knee.
- Open-chain extension exercises place increased stress on the reconstructed ACL and should be avoided for the first 6 weeks.
  - In summary, avoid open-chain quadriceps-activating exercises from 0 to 30 degrees of knee flexion (i.e., exercises that reproduce a Lachman maneuver).
- No difference in outcome has been found between accelerated and nonaccelerated rehabilitation programs.

- Postoperative bracing has not proved beneficial after ACL reconstruction *except* in downhill skiers.
- Early progressive eccentric exercise has yielded good initial results in terms of quadriceps and gluteus maximus muscle size and function after ACL reconstruction.
- Complications (Figure 4-11)
  - Complications in ACL surgery are usually a result of aberrant tunnel placement.
  - The most common technical error is tunnel malposition.
    - Vertical graft placement results in decreased rotational stability.
    - Anterior placement of the femoral tunnel results in limited flexion.
  - Arthrofibrosis is the most common complication following ACL reconstruction and often occurs with reconstruction for acute ACL tears.

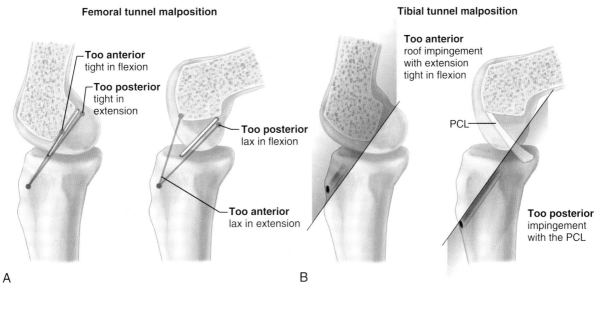

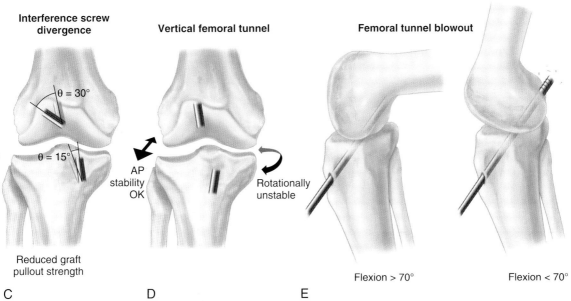

FIGURE 4-11 Common complications of ACL reconstruction. **A,** Femoral tunnel malposition. **B,** Tibial tunnel malposition. **C,** Interference screw divergence. **D,** Vertical femoral tunnel. **E,** Femoral tunnel blowout.

- Risk is minimized by ensuring full ROM prior to surgery.
  - **Associated with loss of patellar translation**
- Aberrant hardware placement (interference screw divergence of > 30 degrees [for endoscopic femoral tunnels] and > 15 degrees [for tibial tunnels]) can also result in complications.
- Infection occurs in less than 1% of cases.
  - Irrigation and débridement with graft retention is successful in up to 85% of cases.
- Graft contamination
  - Graft contamination by dropping on the floor is rare.
  - A survey of surgeons found that the majority favored retention of the graft with disinfection rather than harvesting a new autograft or switching to allograft.
  - A combination of chlorhexidine gluconate and triple antibiotic solution (gentamicin, clindamycin, polymyxin) in sterile saline appears to be the most effective disinfecting regime.
- ▦ Partial ACL tears
  - The existence and treatment of "partial" ACL tears are controversial, although clinical examination and functional stability remain the most important considerations in determining the need for reconstruction.
  - Single-bundle tears can occur and may be addressed with reconstruction of the injured bundle and preservation of the intact bundle.
  - In situations where a single bundle of the ACL is found torn at surgery, ACL remnant preservation compared to removal and standard reconstruction demonstrate equivalent clinical outcomes.
- ■ **PCL injury**
- ▦ History
  - Injuries occur most commonly as a result of a direct blow to the anterior tibia with the knee flexed (the "dashboard injury"), with hyperflexion, or with hyperextension.
  - **A fall onto the ground with a plantar-flexed foot is also a mechanism of injury for PCL tears.**
- ▦ Physical examination and classification
  - Key examination is the posterior drawer test; diagnostic results are an absent or posteriorly directed tibial step-off.
    - Grade I injury: an isolated PCL injury in which the tibia remains anterior to the femoral condyles
    - Grade II injury: an isolated complete PCL injury in which the anterior tibia becomes flush with the femoral condyles
    - Grade III injury: an injury in which the tibia is posterior to the femoral condyles; usually indicative of associated ACL or PLC injuries or both
- ▦ Imaging
  - Plain radiographs should be obtained to evaluate for avulsion injuries (acute) and arthrosis of the medial and patellofemoral compartments (chronic).
  - Stress radiographs are becoming the standard for evaluation and grading of PCL injuries; side-to-side differences of more than 12 mm on stress radiographs are suggestive of a combined PCL and PLC injury.
  - MRI is a confirmatory study.
- ▦ Treatment (Figure 4-12)
  - Nonoperative treatment is favored for most grade I and II (isolated) PCL injuries.

- Rehabilitation should focus on strengthening the knee extensors.
- Grade III injuries are indicative of a combined injury, usually to the posterolateral corner.
- Bony avulsion fractures can be repaired primarily with good results, although primary repair of midsubstance PCL (and ACL) injuries has not been successful.
- Chronic PCL deficiency can result in late chondrosis of the patellofemoral compartment or medial femoral condyle, or both.
- PCL reconstruction is recommended for functionally unstable or combined injuries.
- In general, the results of PCL reconstruction are not as good as those of ACL reconstruction, and some residual posterior laxity often remains.
- For successful reconstruction, concomitant ligament injuries must be addressed.
- A biplanar high tibial osteotomy can be used to treat combined malalignment and PCL insufficiency.
  - Increasing posterior tibial slope results in an anterior shift of the resting position of the tibia and thus minimizes posterior tibial sag.
- ▦ Surgical technique
  - Many techniques for PCL reconstruction have been published, and they can generally be divided into tibial inlay versus transtibial methods and single-bundle versus double-bundle methods.
  - Single-bundle reconstructions should be tensioned in 90 degrees of flexion.
  - **Tibial inlay has biomechanical advantages such as a decrease in the "killer turn" and decreased attenuation of the graft.**
  - In the tibial inlay technique, the average distance from screws used for fixation to the popliteal artery is 20 mm.
  - Double-bundle techniques may improve biomechanical function in both extension and flexion, but a clinical advantage to those techniques has not yet been shown.
  - The anterolateral bundle is the most important for posterior stability at 90 degrees of flexion and should be tensioned in flexion.
  - The posteromedial bundle has a reciprocal function and should be tensioned in extension.
- ▦ Rehabilitation
  - Quadriceps strengthening and open-chain knee extension exercises protect the graft by resulting in an anterior-directed force.
  - Open-chain knee flexion caused by hamstring contraction should be avoided because it causes posterior-directed force across the graft.
- ■ **MCL injury**
- ▦ History and physical examination
  - MCL injury occurs as a result of valgus stress to the knee.
  - Pain and instability with valgus stress testing at 30 degrees of flexion (and not in full extension) is diagnostic.
  - Opening in full extension usually signifies other concurrent injuries (ACL and PCL).
  - Injuries most commonly occur at the femoral origin of the ligament.
- ▦ Treatment (Figure 4-13).
  - Nonoperative treatment (hinged knee brace) is highly successful in alleviating isolated MCL injuries.

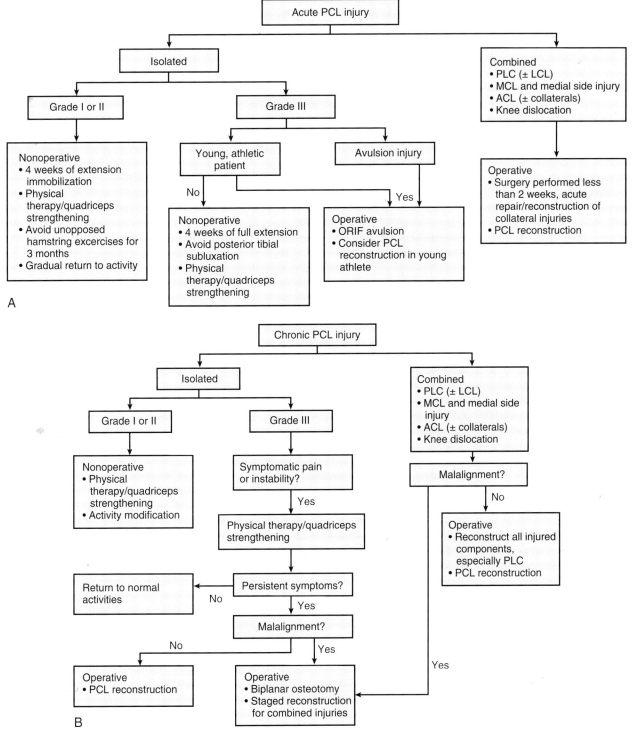

FIGURE 4-12 Algorithm for management of PCL injuries. **A,** Acute. **B,** Chronic.

- Clinical work has shown the advantage of nonoperative treatment (bracing) of an associated MCL injury in patients receiving an ACL reconstruction.
- Distal (tibial-sided) injuries have less healing potential than do proximal (femoral-sided) injuries.
- Prophylactic bracing may be helpful for football players, especially interior linemen.

- Advancement and reinforcement of the ligament are rarely necessary for chronic injuries that do not respond to conservative treatment.
- In chronic injuries, calcification may be present at the medial femoral condyle insertion (Pellegrini-Stieda sign).
- Pellegrini-Stieda syndrome, which can occur with chronic MCL injury, usually responds to a brief period of immobilization followed by progressive motion.

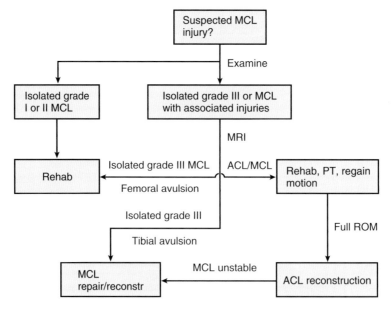

FIGURE 4-13 Algorithm for management of MCL injuries.

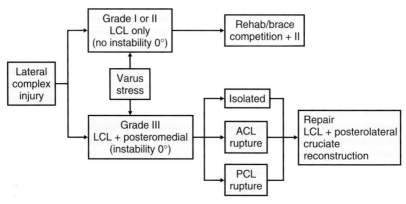

 FIGURE 4-14 Algorithm for management of lateral complex injuries. (From Spindler KP, Walker RN: General approach to ligament surgery. In Fu FH, Harner CD, Vince KG, editors: *Knee surgery,* Baltimore, 1994, Williams & Wilkins.)

- ■ **LCL injury**
- ■ Varus instability in 30 degrees of flexion is diagnostic only for an isolated LCL ligament injury.
- ■ Isolated injuries to the LCL ligament are uncommon and should be managed nonoperatively if laxity is mild (Figure 4-14).
- ■ **Posterolateral corner injury**
- ■ History
  - • Rarely isolated and are usually associated with other ligamentous injuries (especially those of the PCL)
- ■ Physical examination
  - • Examination for increased external rotation (dial test), the external rotation recurvatum test, the posterolateral drawer test, and the reverse pivot shift test are important (see Table 4-5).
  - • Careful evaluation of the peroneal nerve should be performed because approximately 10% of PLC injuries are associated with a peroneal nerve palsy.
  - • Varus alignment is associated with higher rates of PLC reconstruction failure. Evaluation for triple varus alignment should always be performed.

- • Primary varus alignment: tibiofemoral malalignment
- • Secondary varus alignment: LCL deficiency contributing to increased lateral opening
- • Triple varus alignment: deficiency of the remaining PLC with overall varus recurvatum alignment
- • Long-leg standing radiographs are necessary, especially with chronic injuries, to determine mechanical axis and whether a proximal tibial osteotomy is necessary for varus correction.
- ■ Treatment
  - • Recent studies have demonstrated up to a 40% failure rate of acute isolated repairs of PLC injuries.
  - • A hybrid approach has been recommended, with repair of avulsions and reconstruction of midsubstance injuries.
    - • Repair of the LCL, popliteus tendon, or popliteofibular ligament should be performed when the structure can be anatomically reduced to its attachment site with the knee in full extension.
  - • Reconstruction techniques include posterolateral corner advancement (only if structures are attenuated

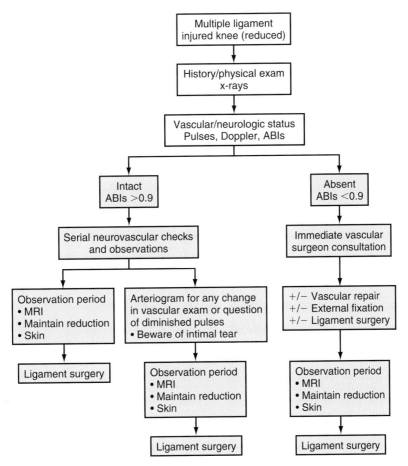

FIGURE 4-15 Multiple ligament injury neurovascular examination algorithm. *ABI,* Ankle-brachial index.

but intact), popliteal bypass (not currently favored), two- and three-tailed reconstruction, biceps tenodesis, and (more recent) "split" grafts and anatomic reconstructions, which are used to reconstruct both the LCL and the popliteal/posterolateral corner.
- Treatment of choice for chronic PLC injuries is often a valgus opening wedge osteotomy.

■ **Multiple ligament injury (MLI)**

▦ Introduction
- Combined ligamentous injuries (especially ACL-PCL injuries) can be a result of a knee dislocation.
- Knee dislocations most frequently occur as a result of high-velocity trauma.
- However, "ultra-low-velocity" multiple ligament injury (ULV-MLI) has recently been described.
  - In the largest series to date, ULV-MLI patients substantially differ from MLI patients.
    - Typically morbidly or super-morbidly obese
    - More frequently female
    - Higher rates of vascular injury
    - Higher rates of neurologic injury
    - Rarely the result of sporting injury
    - Higher rates of postoperative complications
▦ History and physical examination
- Dislocations classified on the basis of direction of tibial displacement
  - Anterior dislocations most common (40%)
  - Vascular injury occurs at 50 degrees of knee hyperextension.

- The incidence of vascular injury knee dislocation is approximately 20% to 30%.
- Initial evaluation should include a neurovascular examination (Figure 4-15).
  - Vascular consultation should be obtained on any patient with absent pulses or an ankle-brachial index (ABI) less than 0.9.
▦ Treatment
- Initial management involves immediate reduction and repeat neurovascular examination.
- Definitive treatment is usually operative.
- Emergency surgical indications include popliteal artery injury, compartment syndrome, open dislocations, and irreducible dislocations.
  - Posterolateral rotatory knee dislocations are the most common irreducible knee dislocation.
    - The medial femoral condyle buttonholes through the medial capsule.
- Most surgeons recommend delaying surgery 1 to 2 weeks to ensure no vascular injury occurs.
- Use of the arthroscope, especially with a pump, must be limited during these procedures because of the risk of fluid extravasation. Avulsion injuries can be repaired primarily; however, interstitial injuries must be reconstructed.
- Incidence of stiff knee after these combined procedures is high; early motion is crucial for avoiding it.
- According to a meta-analysis, staged treatment might have produced better subjective outcomes but, like

acute treatment, was associated with additional procedures to treat joint stiffness. Early mobility was associated with better subjective outcomes than was immobilization after acute surgical treatment.

OSTEOCHONDRAL LESIONS

■ Osteochondritis dissecans
■ Introduction
  - Involves subchondral bone and overlying cartilage separation, probably as a result of occult trauma
  - Most often involves the lateral aspect of the medial femoral condyle
  - The lateral femoral condyle is involved in 15% to 20% of cases; the patella is rarely involved.
  - The condition resolves spontaneously in the majority of the juvenile cases, in about 50% of adolescents, and rarely in adults.
■ Diagnosis
  - Patients usually have poorly localized vague complaints.
  - Radiographs, nuclear imaging, and MRI can be helpful in determining the size, location, and characteristics of the lesion.
■ Treatment and prognosis
  - Children with open growth plates have the best prognosis, and often these lesions can be simply observed.
  - In situ lesions can be treated with retrograde drilling.
  - Detached lesions may necessitate abrasion chondroplasty or newer, more aggressive techniques.
  - Osteochondritis dissecans in adults is usually symptomatic and leads to arthritis if left untreated.

■ Articular cartilage injury
■ Overview
  - The distinction between articular cartilage injury and osteochondritis dissecans is not often clear, but articular cartilage injury occurs as a result of rotational forces in direct trauma.
  - It usually occurs on the medial femoral condyle.
  - MRI has been found to underestimate the size of articular cartilage defects in approximately 75% of cases.
  - The lesions are classified according to their arthroscopic appearance.
■ Treatment
  - Débridement and chondroplasty are currently recommended for symptomatic lesions.
  - Displaced osteochondral fragments can sometimes be replaced and secured with small recessed screws or absorbable pins.
  - For discrete, isolated, full-thickness cartilage injuries, several treatment options are in clinical use: microfracture, chondrocyte implantation, and osteochondral transfer (plugs), including autograft and allograft options (Figure 4-16).
    - Particulated juvenile cartilage allograft remains highly investigational.
  - Diffuse chondral damage is a relative contraindication to these procedures.
  - Donor-site problems and creation of true articular cartilage at the recipient site are still challenges.
  - Age, lesion size, patient's desired activity level, alignment, meniscal integrity, and ligamentous stability must all be taken into consideration in selecting the appropriate treatment option. An algorithm is presented in Figure 4-17.
■ Surgical techniques
  - Marrow-stimulating techniques
    - Include microfracture, drilling, and abrasion arthroplasty
    - Involve perforation of the subchondral bone after removal of the "tidemark" cartilage, with eventual clot formation and fibrocartilaginous repair tissue
      - Type I collagen with inferior wear characteristics
      - Good clinical results in small defects (<4 cm^2) are obtained in 60% to 80% patients.
  - Osteochondral autografts (i.e., osteochondral autograft transplantation [OATS], mosaicplasty)
    - Can be used to address medium-sized lesions (3 cm^2) that include subchondral bone loss
    - Lateral or medial trochlea are acceptable harvest locations.
    - Complications include donor site morbidity.
  - Osteochondral allografts
    - Can be used for larger lesions, especially with bone loss. Main concerns include the small risk of disease transmission and chondrocyte viability, which has improved with graft preservation techniques (storage at 4° C).
  - Autologous chondrocyte implantation (ACI)
    - Allows for creation of type II–rich hyaline-like cartilage
    - Indicated for medium-sized to larger chondral lesions without bony defects. Multiple surgical procedures are required for biopsy/harvest and then definitive repair.
    - Complications related to autologous chondrocyte implantation include chondrocyte overgrowth and periosteal flap hypertrophy, along with the morbidity of the second surgical procedure.
      - The periosteal flap has largely been abandoned as a result, and type I/III bilayer collagen membrane used instead. This has reduced the need for reoperation by 80%.
■ Results
  - At present, no definitive research has demonstrated superiority of any cartilage restoration procedure.
  - Current best available research suggests that for smaller lesions, microfracture, OATS, and ACI have similar recovery periods and functional results.
  - Initial research suggests that for large lesions (>4 cm^2), ACI may be superior in short- to medium-term periods.

■ Osteonecrosis
■ Atraumatic osteonecrosis is similar to idiopathic osteonecrosis of the hip. Risk factors are similar to those of the hip and are common in elderly women.
■ Spontaneous osteonecrosis of the knee is thought to represent a subchondral insufficiency fracture and is typically a self-limiting condition. This condition can follow knee arthroscopy in middle-aged women. It should be treated with limited weight bearing until it resolves.
■ One hypothesis for the cause of spontaneous osteonecrosis of the knee involves a meniscal root tear.

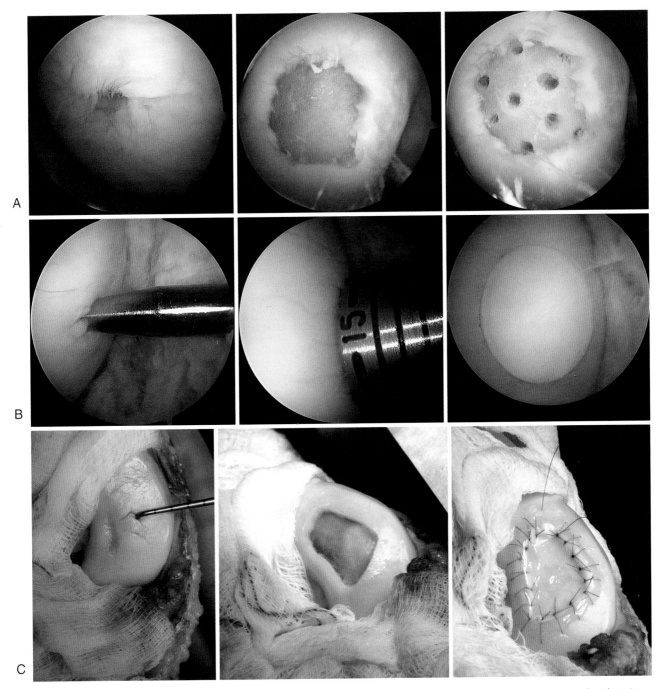

FIGURE 4-16 Surgical treatment of chondral injuries. **A,** Microfracture. **B,** Osteochondral autograft transfer. **C,** Autologous chondrocyte implantation. (Modified from Miller MD, Thompson SR: *DeLee and Drez's orthopaedic sports medicine,* ed 4, Philadelphia, Saunders, 2014, Figures 97-6 to 97-8.)

SYNOVIAL LESIONS

- **Pigmented villonodular synovitis**
  - Affected patients may present with pain and swelling and may have a palpable mass.
  - MRI demonstrates intraarticular nodular masses of low signal intensity on T1- and T2-weighted images.
  - There are nodular and diffuse types.
    - The diffuse type has a higher recurrence rate. Synovectomy is effective, but the recurrence rate is still high.
  - Arthroscopic techniques are as effective as traditional open procedures if a complete synovectomy with multiple portals is performed.

- **Synovial chondromatosis**
  - This proliferative disease of the synovium is associated with cartilaginous metaplasia, which results in multiple intraarticular loose bodies.
  - These often require removal arthroscopically.
- **Plicae**
  - Synovial folds that are embryologic remnants
  - They are occasionally pathologic, particularly the medial patellar plica, which can cause abrasion of the medial femoral condyle and sometimes responds to arthroscopic excision.
- **Other synovial lesions that respond to synovectomy include chondromatosis, osteochondromatosis, pauciarticular juvenile**

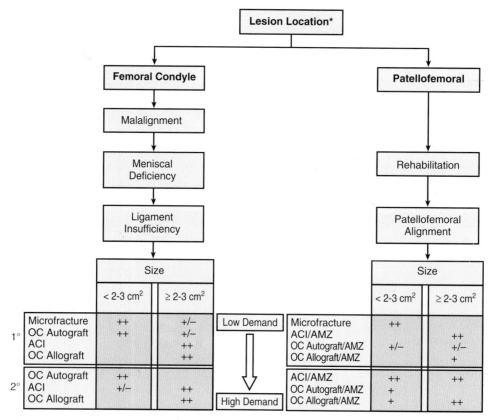

FIGURE 4-17 Algorithm for management of focal cartilaginous lesions of the knee. (Modified from Miller MD, Thompson SR: *DeLee and Drez's orthopaedic sports medicine*, ed 4, Philadelphia, Saunders, 2014, Figure 97-5.)

rheumatoid arthritis, and hemophilia. additional arthroscopic portals are required for complete synovectomy.

PATELLOFEMORAL DISORDERS

■ Introduction

▦ Anterior knee pain is classified based on etiologic factors. The term *chondromalacia* should be replaced with a specific diagnosis.

▦ Abnormalities of patellar height:

• Patella alta (high-riding patella) and patella baja (low-riding patella) are determined on the basis of various measurements made on lateral radiographs of the knee (see Figure 4-5).

• Patella alta can be associated with patellar instability, because the patella may not articulate with the sulcus until higher degrees of knee flexion. Consequently there is reduced contact and stability in knee extension and early flexion.

• Patella baja is often the result of fat pad and tendon fibrosis, and proximal transfer of the tubercle may be required in refractory cases.

■ Trauma

▦ Includes fractures of the patella (discussed in Chapter 11, Trauma) and tendon injuries

▦ Tendon ruptures

• Quadriceps tendon ruptures are more common than patellar tendon ruptures and occur most often with indirect trauma in patients older than 40 years. In younger patients, patellar tendon ruptures occur with direct or indirect trauma (Figure 4-18).

• Both types of tendon rupture are more common in patients with underlying disorders of the tendon.

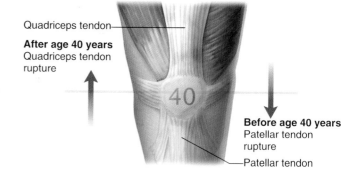

FIGURE 4-18 Patellar tendon ruptures are more common before the age of 40, and quadriceps tendon ruptures are more common after the age of 40.

• A palpable defect and the inability to extend the knee are diagnostic signs.

• Patella alta is a consistent finding with patella tendon rupture.

• Primary repair with temporary stabilization (McLaughlin wire or suture) is indicated.

▦ Repetitive trauma: overuse injuries

• Patellar tendinitis (jumper's knee)

• This condition is perhaps better termed *tendinosis*.

• Most common in athletes who participate in sports such as basketball and volleyball

• **Associated with pain and tenderness near the inferior border of the patella (worse in extension than in flexion)**

- Treatment includes nonsteroidal antiinflammatory drugs (NSAIDs), **physical therapy (strengthening including eccentric exercise and ultrasonography),** and orthoses (patella tendon strap).
  - Surgery involving excision of necrotic tendon fibers is rarely indicated.
- Quadriceps tendinitis
  - Less common than patella tendinosis but just as painful
  - Patients may note painful clicking and localized pain at the superior border of the patella.
  - Operative treatment is occasionally necessary.
- Prepatellar bursitis (housemaid's knee)
  - The most common form of bursitis of the knee and associated with a history of prolonged kneeling
  - Supportive treatment (knee pads, occasional steroid injections) and, in rare cases, bursal excision are recommended.
  - Aspiration is advocated in wrestlers to rule out infection, because wrestling requires kneeling on the flexed knee.
- Iliotibial band friction syndrome
  - Can occur in runners (especially those running hills) and cyclists
  - Result of abrasion between the iliotibial band and the lateral femoral condyle
  - **Localized tenderness at the lateral femoral condyle, worse with the knee flexed 30 degrees, is common.**
  - The Ober test (patient lies in lateral decubitus position with hyperextension of ipsilateral hip; leg can be brought from abduction to adduction to demonstrate tightness of the iliotibial band) is helpful in making the diagnosis.
  - Rehabilitation is usually successful.
  - Surgical excision of an ellipse of the iliotibial band is occasionally necessary.
- Semimembranosus tendinitis
  - Most common in male athletes in their early 30s
  - Can be diagnosed with MRI or nuclear imaging and often responds to stretching and strengthening exercises
  - A steroid injection may be added if no improvement occurs.
- Pes anserinus bursitis
  - Characterized by localized pain, tenderness, and swelling over the proximal anteromedial tibia at the insertion site of the sartorius, gracilis, and semitendinosus (≈6 cm inferior to joint line)
  - Treated conservatively with oral antiinflammatory medication, localized corticosteroid injections, and activity modification
- **Patellar instability**
- Introduction
  - See Knee Anatomy section for important information on MPFL anatomy.
  - Patellar instability, like glenohumeral instability, can fall on the spectrum of frank dislocation to subtle subluxation.
  - Etiology can be multifactorial:
    - Traumatic MPFL rupture
    - Patellar and trochlear dysplasia
    - Patella alta

- Ligamentous laxity
- Muscular imbalance (VMO weakness)
- Dislocation is typically lateral.
- Frequent cause of hemarthrosis
- Recurrence rate following first-time dislocation between 15% and 60%
- Articular cartilage on the medial facet of the patella is most commonly injured after a patellar dislocation.
- If this injury is associated with femoral anteversion, genu valgum, and pronated feet, the symptoms can be exacerbated, especially in adolescents ("miserable malalignment syndrome").
- History and physical examination
  - May be due to external tibial rotation with a planted foot or direct blow to medial aspect of the knee
  - Often a "pop" is felt; do not confuse for an ACL tear
  - Examination may reveal a positive patellar apprehension test, a positive J sign, and three to four quadrants of lateral patellar glide.
- Imaging
  - Radiographs are necessary to identify fracture, loose bodies, arthritis, malalignment and abnormal anatomy.
    - May demonstrate an avulsion fracture of the medial patellofemoral ligament that occurs at the middle third of the patella
    - Trochlea dysplasia can be identified on a lateral radiograph by the presence of a crossing sign.
      - Trochlear groove line normally intersects the anterior femoral cortex.
      - A crossing sign is present when the trochlear groove line intersects the anterior femoral condyle.
      - Crossing sign has been associated with patellar instability.
    - A variety of additional quantitative measurements can be obtained to quantify bony abnormalities.
  - CT scan (Figure 4-19)
    - Most frequently used to obtain patellar tilt and measure the tibial tubercle-trochlear groove distance (TT-TG)
      - A measurement of the lateralization of the tibial tubercle
      - Normal values between 9 and 13 mm
      - TT-TG 15 to 20 mm questionably abnormal

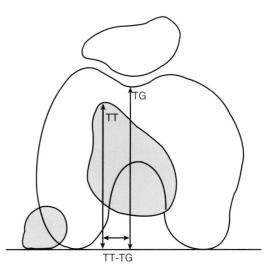

FIGURE 4-19 Tibial tuberosity–trochlear groove (TT-TG) distance.

- TT-TG over 20 mm highly associated with patellar instability
- Utility of dynamic CT scan continues to be examined
- MRI
  - In complete dislocation, a bone bruise pattern involving the lateral femoral condyle and medial patella is often observed.
  - The MPFL is often disrupted, most frequently at its patellar insertion.
  - Useful to diagnose articular cartilage damage on medial patellar facet; typically occurs on reduction
    - Articular cartilage of medial patellar facet is most common donor site
  - May be used to calculate TT-TG distance; often underestimates true TT-TG as calculated on CT scan
- Management
  - Extensive rehabilitation often curative
  - Surgical procedures include proximal and distal realignment.
  - Acute first-time patella dislocations have traditionally been treated nonoperatively
    - However, some surgeons advocate early surgical treatment with arthroscopic evaluation or débridement and acute repair of the medial patellofemoral ligament (usually at the medial epicondyle). This protocol is still somewhat controversial.
  - Occasionally surgery on a first-time patellar dislocation is performed if there is a loose body.
- Surgical techniques
  - Proximal realignment is typically reconstruction of the MPFL.
    - Precise technique is variable but involves use of a gracilis or semitendinous tendon (autograft or allograft) with incorporation into patella and femur
    - **Femoral attachment should be performed at the anatomic origin ("Schottle point") (Figure 4-20).**
    - Several techniques have fallen out of favor:
      - VMO advancement (Green procedure)
      - Medial retinacular plication
      - Isolated lateral release should not be performed for patellar instability.
  - Distal realignment is typically tibial tubercle anterior medialization.
    - Indicated for patients with an increased Q angle or a TT-TG distance exceeding 20 mm.
  - Proximal arthrosis of the medial patellar facet is a contraindication to this procedure.
- Complications
  - Medial patellar instability or medial patellar osteoarthritis from overtightening the MPFL reconstruction
- **Chronic conditions**
- Patellofemoral pain syndrome (idiopathic anterior knee pain)
  - Extremely common cause of anterior knee pain, particularly in the adolescent
  - Typically presents as anterior knee pain made worse by activities that increase compressive loads of the patellofemoral joint
    - Insidious onset, occasionally described as sensation of instability
  - Etiology multifactorial
    - Muscular weakness often present, with weak quadriceps, hip abductors, and core musculature
  - Management is focused on prolonged rehabilitation.

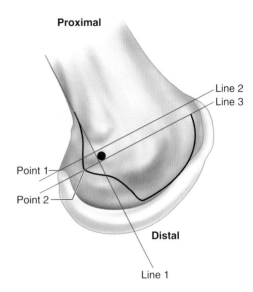

FIGURE 4-20 Schottle's point for radiographically identifying the femoral attachment of the MPFL. This occurs 1 mm anterior to the posterior cortex extension line *(Line 1)*, 2.5 mm distal to the posterior origin of the medial femoral condyle and proximal to the level of the posterior point of the Blumensaat line on a lateral radiograph with both posterior condyles projected in the same plane. To identify this radiographically, two perpendiculars to *Line 1* are drawn, intersecting the contact point of the medial condyle and the posterior cortex *(Point 1, Line 2)* and intersecting the most posterior point of the Blumensaat line *(Point 2, Line 3)*.

- Lateral patellar facet compression syndrome
  - Problem associated with a tight lateral retinaculum and excessive lateral tilt without excessive patellar mobility
  - Lateral tilt is best evaluated by measurement of the lateral patellofemoral angle (Figure 4-21).
  - Treatment includes activity modification, NSAIDs, and strengthening of the vastus medialis oblique muscle.
  - **Arthroscopy and lateral release are occasionally required but indicated only in the setting of objective evidence of lateral tilt that has not responded to extensive nonoperative management.**
  - The best candidates for arthroscopy and lateral release have a neutral or negative tilt with a medial patellar glide of less than one quadrant and a lateral patellar glide of less than three quadrants. Arthroscopic visualization through a superior portal demonstrates that the patella does not articulate medially with 40 degrees of knee flexion.
- Bipartite patella (Figure 4-22)
  - Failure of an ossification center of the patella to coalesce
    - Can result in a bipartite or tripartite patella
  - Most commonly located at the superolateral pole
    - Typically has smooth edges, which differentiates it from a patella fracture
  - Typically asymptomatic and found incidentally on radiographs
  - If symptomatic, presents as anterior knee pain
  - Associated with nail-patella syndrome
  - **Conservative management is the mainstay of symptomatic bipartite patella.**
  - Rarely, surgical excision or arthroscopic lateral release may be performed.
- Patellofemoral arthritis
  - Injury and malalignment can contribute to patellar degenerative joint disease.

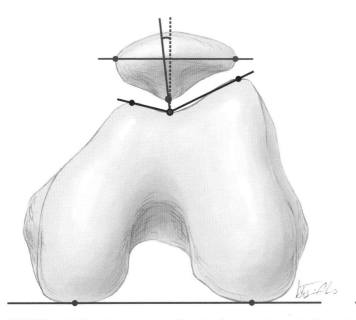
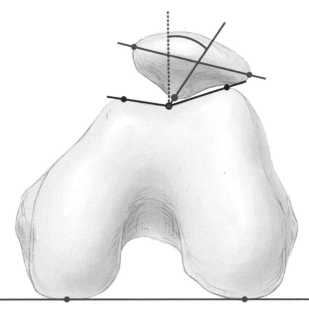

FIGURE 4-21 The sulcus angle *(red lines)* is the angle formed in the axial plane from the highest point on the lateral facet, to the trochlear groove, to the highest point on the medial facet. An angle of 138 degrees represents normal anatomy, with an angle of 150 degrees or greater representing an abnormally shallow groove. The congruence angle *(green lines)* is formed from a line drawn through the apex of the trochlear groove with a line through the lowest point on the articular ridge of the patella. A value of –6 degrees represents normal anatomy, while a value greater than 16 degrees represents an abnormal patellofemoral articulation. Patellar tilt *(blue lines)* is the angle formed by a line drawn parallel to the posterior femoral condyles and a line drawn through the transverse axis of the patella. (Image modified from Sherman SL et al: *Patellofemoral anatomy and biomechanics*, Clin Sports Med 33:389–401.)

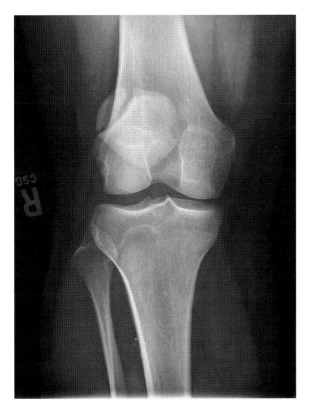

FIGURE 4-22 Radiographic appearance of a bipartite patella.

- Lateral release may be beneficial early only if there is objective evidence of patellar tilting.
- Other procedures may be required for advanced patellar arthritis.
- Options include anterior (Maquet) or anteromedial (Fulkerson) transfer of the tibial tubercle or patellectomy for severe cases.

- Tibial rotational alignment and overall lower extremity alignment should always be assessed in evaluating the cause of patellofemoral disease. Patellofemoral arthroplasty has been introduced as another treatment option but remains controversial.
▓ Anterior fat pad syndrome (Hoffa disease)
- Trauma to the anterior fat pad can lead to fibrous changes and pinching of the fat pad, especially in patients with genu recurvatum.
- Activity modification, ice, knee padding, and injection can be helpful.
- Arthroscopic excision is occasionally beneficial.
▓ Complex regional pain syndrome (formerly known as *reflex sympathetic dystrophy*)
- Characterized by pain out of proportion to physical findings, this condition is an exaggerated response to injury.
- Three stages are typical: (1) swelling, warmth, and hyperhidrosis; (2) brawny edema and trophic changes; and (3) glossy, cool, dry skin and stiffness.
- Patellar osteopenia and a "flamingo gait" are also common.
- Treatment includes nerve stimulation, NSAIDs, and sympathetic or epidural blocks—response to which can be diagnostic.
▓ Idiopathic chondromalacia patellae
- Articular damage and changes to the patella have traditionally been referred to as *idiopathic chondromalacia patellae;* however, this term has fallen into disfavor.
- Treatment is usually symptomatic, and physical therapy is emphasized heavily.
- Débridement procedures are of questionable benefit.
- The Outerbridge classification system is still in common use today.

PEDIATRIC KNEE INJURIES

■ Anterior cruciate ligament injuries
- Historically, tibial spine fractures were thought to be more common than ACL tears. However, more recent data suggest that ACL rupture may be more common.
- History and physical examination similar to adult ACL injuries
- Management remains controversial
  - Proponents of operative management cite an increased risk of meniscal damage, chondral damage, and inability to return to activities with an ACL-deficient knee.
  - Detractors of operative management cite the risk of growth disturbances and angular deformities; most recent meta-analysis suggests a 2% risk of disturbance following ACL reconstruction.
    - BPTB associated with higher risk of physeal disruption
- A variety of surgical techniques have been described. All-epiphyseal, combined intraarticular/extraarticular, hybrid, and traditional transphyseal techniques can be employed.
  - Genu recurvatum has been associated with physeal sparing techniques.

■ Meniscal injuries
- By 10 years of age, the meniscus has developed its adult microvascular structure.
- MRI has lower sensitivity and specificity (compared to adults) for detecting meniscal tears; this is due to increased vascularity of the meniscus.
- Increased vascularity may improve results of meniscal repairs (compared to adults).

■ Osteochondroses
- Also known as a *traction apophysitis*, osteochondroses are due to disordered enchondral ossification of a previous epiphysis.
- Osgood-Schlatter disease
  - Due to repetitive loading of the patella tendon insertion onto the tibial tubercle
  - Pain is isolated to tibial tubercle
  - Responds to nonoperative management, including a period of immobilization
  - Surgical excision of the ossicle is rarely performed.
- Sinding-Larson-Johansson disease
  - Due to repetitive loading of patellar tendon origin at inferior pole of patella
  - Typically occurs in boys who are slightly younger than those with Osgood-Schlatter disease
    - Inferior pole of patella closes prior to the tibial tubercle.
  - Rehabilitation should focus on eccentric quadriceps strengthening.

■ Physeal injuries
- Most often involve Salter-Harris II fractures of the distal femoral physis
- Pain, swelling, and an inability to ambulate are common.
- **Stress radiographs and/or MRI may be necessary to make the diagnosis.**
- Open reduction and internal fixation are indicated for displaced Salter-Harris II, III, and IV fractures and Salter-Harris I that cannot be adequately reduced.
- It is important to counsel the parents that knee physeal injuries, particularly distal femoral physeal injuries, may have a worse prognosis than other physeal fractures.
- **Tibial spine fractures and tibial tubercle fractures are discussed in Chapter 11, Trauma.**

SECTION 2 PELVIS, HIP, AND THIGH

CONTUSIONS

■ Iliac crest contusions ("hip pointer")
- Direct trauma to this area can occur in contact sports.
- An avulsion of the iliac apophysis should be confirmed or ruled out in adolescent athletes.
- Treatment consists of ice, compression, pain control, and placing the affected leg on maximal stretch.
- Corticosteroid injections have occasionally been advocated.
- Additional padding is indicated after the acute phase.

■ Groin contusions
- An avulsion fracture of the lesser trochanter, traumatic phlebitis, thrombosis, athletic pubalgia, or femoral neuropathy must be confirmed or ruled out before supportive treatment is initiated.

■ Quadriceps contusions
- Can result in hemorrhage and late myositis ossificans
- **Acute management includes cold compression and overnight immobilization in 120 degrees of flexion.**
- Close monitoring for compartment syndrome is indicated in the acute phase.

MUSCLE INJURIES

■ Hamstring strain/rupture
- Hamstring strain is a common injury, often the result of sudden stretch on the musculotendinous junction during sprinting.
  - Can occur anywhere in the posterior thigh
  - Treatment is supportive, followed by stretching and strengthening.
  - To prevent recurrence, return to play should be delayed until strength is approximately 90% that of the opposite side.
- Complete rupture much less common
  - Radiographs may demonstrate avulsion from the ischial tuberosity; MRI is important in determining the extent of injury.
  - Nonoperative management is recommended for single tendon ruptures and multiple tendon ruptures with retraction less than 2 cm
  - Operative management of three tendon ruptures entails direct repair to bone

■ Athletic pubalgia ("sports hernia")
- Common in ice hockey, soccer, and rugby, these injuries must be differentiated from subtle hernias.

- Injury to the muscles of the abdominal wall or adductor longus produce anterior pelvis or groin pain (or both) without the classic physical findings of a true inguinal hernia.
- Can result from acute trauma or microtrauma associated with overuse of the affected muscle
- Combination of abdominal hyperextension and thigh hyperabduction
- Confirm or rule out other causes of pain with radiography, bone scan, MRI, or a combination of these.
- Treat nonoperatively for 6 to 8 weeks with rest and therapy.
  - Active strengthening of the core, abductors, and adductors is critical.
- Repair or reinforcement of the anterior abdominal wall is indicated after conservative measures have failed and after other causes have been excluded.
- Decompression of the genital branch of the genitofemoral nerve is also favored by some authors in patients presenting with athletic pubalgia.
- **Rectus femoris strain**
- Acute injuries are usually located more distally on the thigh, but chronic injuries are usually nearer the muscle origin.
- Pain is elicited with resisted hip flexion or extension.
- Treatment includes ice and stretching/strengthening exercises.

BURSITIS

- **Trochanteric bursitis**
- Occurs frequently in female runners and is associated with training on banked surfaces
- Treatment includes oral antiinflammatory drugs, stretching, and rest.
- Corticosteroid injections are occasionally advocated.
- **Iliopsoas bursitis**
- A cause of anterior hip pain in athletes and often associated with mechanical irritation of the iliopsoas tendon
- Also a cause of "snapping" or "clicking" symptoms associated with hip pain
- **Ischial bursitis**
- Caused by direct trauma or prolonged sitting and hard to distinguish from hamstring injuries

NERVE ENTRAPMENT SYNDROMES

- **Ilioinguinal nerve entrapment**
- This nerve can be constricted by hypertrophied abdominal muscles as a result of intensive training.
- Hyperextension of the hip may exacerbate the pain that patients experience, and hyperesthesia symptoms are common. Surgical release is occasionally necessary.
- **Obturator nerve entrapment**
- Can lead to chronic medial thigh pain, especially in athletes with well-developed hip adductor muscles (e.g., skaters)
- Nerve conduction studies are helpful for establishing the diagnosis.
- Treatment is usually supportive.

- **Lateral femoral cutaneous nerve entrapment**
- Can lead to meralgia paresthetica, a painful condition
- Tight belts and prolonged hip flexion may exacerbate symptoms.
- Release of compressive devices, postural exercises, and NSAIDs are usually curative.
- **Sciatic nerve entrapment**
- Can occur anywhere along the course of the nerve, but the two most common locations are at the level of the ischial tuberosity and by the piriformis muscle, known as *piriformis syndrome*

BONE DISORDERS

- **Stress fractures**
- A history of overuse, an insidious onset of pain, and localized tenderness and swelling are typical.
- Stress fractures occur via propagation of a crack.
- Bone scan can be diagnostic, even with normal plain radiographs.
- MRI is the most specific test for detecting stress fractures.
- Treatment includes protected weight bearing, rest, cross-training, analgesics, and therapeutic modalities.
- There are several especially problematic stress fractures:
  - Femoral neck stress fractures
    - Can occur on tension side (superior surface) or compression side (inferior surface)
      - Compression-side fractures are more common and can be treated nonoperatively with rest and protected weight bearing.
      - Tension-side fractures are much more serious and operative stabilization may be required.
  - Femoral shaft stress fractures
    - Usually respond to protected weight bearing but can progress to complete fractures if unrecognized
    - The fulcrum test may be helpful in making this diagnosis.
- **Avascular necrosis**
- Traumatic hip subluxation can disrupt the arterial blood supply to the hip and result in avascular necrosis.
- Early recognition of these injuries, which are seen in football players, is essential.
- With posterior subluxation or dislocation, one study revealed a 25% incidence of avascular necrosis.
- Obturator oblique radiographs (to determine the presence of an avulsion injury) and MRI are recommended.
- Such imaging should be followed by aspiration of the hip if a large hemarthrosis is present, 6 weeks of minimal weight bearing, and a repeat MRI.
- With atraumatic injuries, other causative factors (alcohol, catabolic steroids, and decompression sickness) should be sought.
- **Osteitis pubis**
- Repetitive trauma can cause an inflammation of the symphysis.
- Occurs frequently in soccer players, hockey players, and runners
- Conservative management is usually curative.
- **Tumors**
- Because more than 10% of all musculoskeletal tumors occur in the hip and pelvis, they must be suspected in cases of unexplained pain.

INTRAARTICULAR DISORDERS

- Recent studies have demonstrated a high rate of abnormal MRI findings in asymptomatic patients.
  - 60 to 80% prevalence of labral tears
  - 25% prevalence of chondral defects
  - 20% prevalence of acetabular paralabral cysts
- Loose bodies
  - Often result from trauma or diseases such as synovial chondromatosis
  - Should be removed, either in an open procedure or arthroscopically, to prevent third-body wear
- Labral tears
  - Often a cause of mechanical hip pain manifesting with vague symptoms
  - MR arthrography is the most sensitive and specific test.
  - Incidence of labral tears is highest in patients with acetabular dysplasia.
  - Underlying hip disease should be addressed in addition to the labral tear for the best results.
  - Arthroscopic labral débridement has yielded good short-term and midterm results.
  - Labral repair may yield better results than débridement according to emerging data on new techniques.
- Chondral injuries
  - Articular surface injury is often a cause of mechanical hip pain.
  - Microfracture is effective in the treatment of focal lesions.
- Ruptured ligamentum teres
  - Associated with mechanical hip pain as the ruptured ligament catches within the joint after a hip dislocation.
  - Débridement is often necessary.
- The viability of the femoral head is not in jeopardy with a ruptured ligamentum teres.

FEMOROACETABULAR IMPINGEMENT (FAI)

- Definition
- Abnormal contact between proximal femur and acetabulum that leads to chondral damage and symptoms
- Types (Figure 4-23)
- Cam, pincer, and a combination of cam and pincer; combined form most common
  - Cam impingement
    - Most common in young males
    - Caused by nonspherical femoral head and decreased head-neck offset. Typically located anterolateral on femoral neck
    - In hip flexion, the aspherical head creates a shearing force along the acetabular cartilage, resulting in delamination. Avulsion of the labrum may also occur
  - Pincer impingement
    - Most common in middle-aged females
    - Caused by acetabular overcoverage that results in abnormal contact between the acetabular rim and femoral head-neck junction
      - Overcoverage may be due to protrusio acetabuli, coxa profunda or acetabular retroversion
    - Results in intrasubstance tears of the labrum, typically in the anterosuperior quadrant. The anterosuperior femoral head is levered against the acetabular rim and a contrecoup cartilage lesion may occur in the posteroinferior acetabulum.

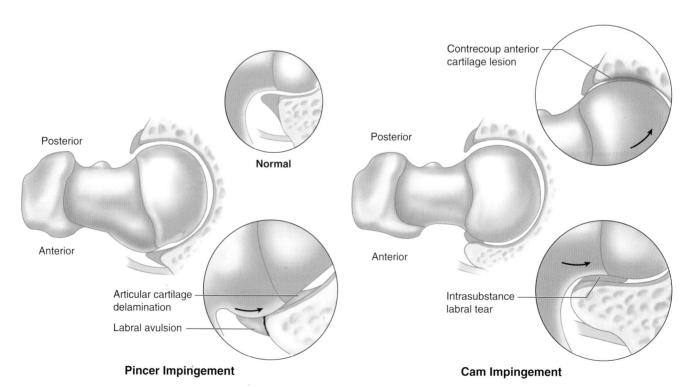

FIGURE 4-23 Femoroacetabular impingement pathophysiology.

■ Evaluation
- ▦ Groin or hip pain in association with limitation in ROM, especially flexion and internal rotation, can be a symptom.
- ▦ Patients generally have more passive external rotation than internal rotation.
- ▦ A positive result of an anterior impingement test is reproduction of symptoms with passive flexion, adduction, and internal rotation.

■ Imaging
- ▦ Plain radiographs should include anteroposterior pelvis and true lateral views with hip in 15 degrees of internal rotation (Figure 4-24).
  - A "**pistol-grip deformity**" demonstrating a nonspherical femoral head is seen in cam impingement.
  - A **crossover sign** is classically seen with acetabular retroversion causing pincer impingement.
    - Anterior wall crosses lateral to posterior wall
- ▦ Recent studies have demonstrated a high rate of false-positive radiographic findings.
  - Prevalence of coxa profunda has been demonstrated to be the same in asymptomatic patients as in those with diagnosed FAI.
  - More than 90% of asymptomatic adolescents have at least one radiographic parameter suggesting FAI, and 50% have two.
- ▦ A CT scan can give additional information about femoral-acetabular mismatch.
- ▦ MR arthrogram can be used to provide information about cartilage and labral injuries (Figure 4-25).

■ Treatment
- ▦ Treatment options include open or arthroscopic procedures to trim the femoral head and neck or acetabular rim, periacetabular osteotomy, femoral osteotomy, or combinations of these procedures with labral débridement or repair.
  - Grade III or IV arthritic change associated with poor outcomes

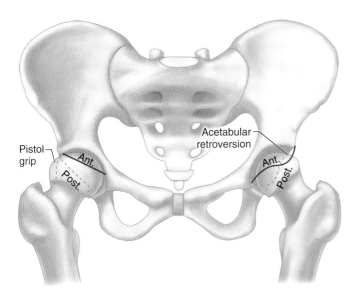

FIGURE 4-24 Radiographic abnormalities visualized in FAI. The right hip has a normal acetabulum (the *anterior line* does not cross the *posterior line*) but nonspherical femoral head. The left hip has a normal femoral head but retroverted acetabulum (the *anterior line* crosses the *posterior line*).

- ▦ Total hip arthroplasty is reserved for patients with significant arthritic changes.

OTHER HIP DISORDERS

■ Snapping hip (coxa saltans): two types—external and internal
- ▦ External
  - The iliotibial band abruptly catches on the greater trochanter or the iliopsoas impinges on the hip capsule.
  - More common in women with wide pelvises and prominent trochanters and can be exacerbated by running on banked surfaces.
  - Snapping may be reproduced with passive hip flexion from an adducted position.
  - Stretching and strengthening exercises, modalities such as ultrasonography, and occasionally surgical iliotibial lengthening may relieve the snapping.
- ▦ Internal
  - Iliopsoas tendon abruptly catches on underlying bony prominences
  - Diagnosed with extension and internal rotation of the hip from a flexed and externally rotated position
  - Dynamic ultrasonography, arthrography, and bursography may also be helpful in determining the diagnosis.

HIP ARTHROSCOPY

■ Indications
- ▦ As techniques improve, so do the indications. Hip arthroscopy is currently effective for the treatment of loose bodies, labral tears, chondral injuries, FAI, avascular necrosis, synovial disease, ruptured ligamentum teres, impinging osteophytes, and unexplained mechanical symptoms.

■ Setup
- ▦ Hip arthroscopy is typically performed with the patient in the supine or lateral position with approximately 50 lb (22.7 kg) of traction and a well-padded perineal post.

■ Portals
- ▦ Three portals are commonly used for instrumentation: one on each side of the greater trochanter and an additional anterior portal (Figure 4-26).

■ Compartments
- ▦ Three compartments are described:
  - The *central compartment* refers to the intraarticular portion of the hip joint between the cartilaginous portions of the proximal femur and acetabulum.
  - The *peripheral compartment* refers to the intraarticular portion of the hip joint along the neck of the femur and the edge of the acetabulum.
  - The *lateral compartment* refers to the extraarticular portion in the peritrochanteric region and trochanteric bursa.

■ Complications
- ▦ Complications, which are rare, are associated with traction injuries, iatrogenic chondral injuries, iatrogenic labral injury, and neurovascular injury caused by aberrant portal placement.
  - The sciatic and pudendal nerves are most frequently injured secondary to traction.

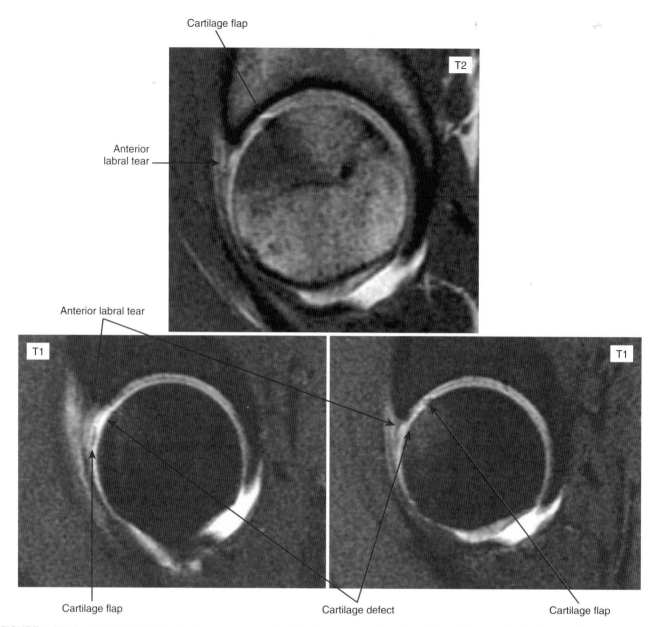

Cartilage flap

Anterior labral tear

T2

Anterior labral tear

T1

T1

Cartilage flap

Cartilage defect

Cartilage flap

FIGURE 4-25 Hip magnetic resonance arthrogram of anterior labral tear and cartilage flap. (From Morrison W: *Problem solving in musculoskeletal imaging*, Philadelphia, Mosby, 2008, Figure 11-56.)

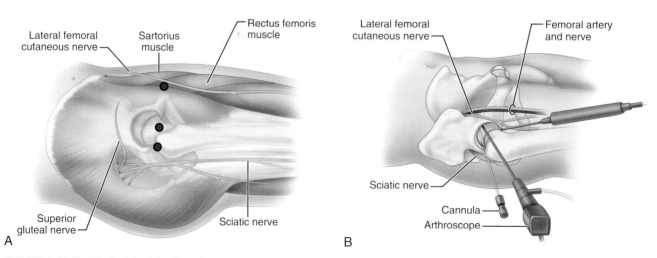

Lateral femoral cutaneous nerve

Sartorius muscle

Rectus femoris muscle

Lateral femoral cutaneous nerve

Femoral artery and nerve

Superior gluteal nerve

Sciatic nerve

Sciatic nerve

Cannula

Arthroscope

A

B

FIGURE 4-26 Portals *(red dots)* for hip arthroscopy are the anterior portal and two portals on either side of the greater trochanter. Superficial **(A)** and deep **(B)** structures. (From Canale ST, Beaty JH, editors: *Campbell's operative orthopaedics*, ed 12, Philadelphia, Mosby, 2013, Figure 51-59.)

- The maximum traction weight, not the length of traction time, has been associated with sciatic nerve injury.
- The anterior portal puts the lateral femoral cutaneous nerve at risk.
  - Also at risk are the ascending branch of the lateral femoral circumflex artery and the femoral neurovascular bundle.
- The anterolateral portal is associated with injury to the superior gluteal nerve.
- The posterolateral portal places the sciatic nerve at risk, particularly when the hip is externally rotated.
- Heterotopic ossification has been reported to occur following hip arthroscopy. Indomethacin has been shown to reduce the incidence.

SECTION 3 SHOULDER

ANATOMY (SEE CHAPTER 2, ANATOMY, FOR A THOROUGH DISCUSSION OF SHOULDER ANATOMY.)

- ■ **Osteology**
- Clavicle
  - An S-shaped bone, it is the last to ossify (the medial growth plate fuses in the early 20s).
- Scapula
  - Serves as the insertion site for 17 muscles
  - Three important prominences: glenoid, coracoid process, and acromion
  - Glenoid
    - The shoulder "socket," or glenoid cavity, is a lateral projection of the scapula.
    - Rim is surrounded by fibrocartilaginous thickening (the labrum), which serves to both deepen the socket (acting as a chock block) and anchor the inferior glenohumeral ligament complex.
    - Pear-shaped surface with an average upward tilt of 5 degrees and an average range of 7 degrees of retroversion to 10 degrees of anteversion
  - Coracoid process
    - Site of attachment of pectoralis minor, coracoacromial ligament, coracoclavicular ligaments and the conjoint tendon
    - On average, measures approximately 4.3 cm in length. The distance between the tip of the acromion and coracoclavicular ligaments is 2.6 to 2.8 cm. This is the available length for coracoid transfer.
  - Acromion
    - The result of fusion of four secondary ossification centers (from anterior to posterior): preacromion, mesoacromion, metacromion, basiacromion
    - Os acromiale, an unfused secondary ossification center, occurs with a 3% incidence; in 60% of affected patients, it is bilateral.
      - The most common location is at the junction of the mesoacromion and meta-acromion.
      - Persistent symptoms may be treated with open reduction and internal fixation.
- Humeral head
  - Is approximately spheroidal in 90% of individuals and has an average diameter of 43 mm
  - Normally retroverted an average of 30 degrees to the transepicondylar axis of the distal humerus
  - Articular surface inclined an average of 130 degrees superiorly in relation to the shaft.
  - **Vascular supply is derived primarily from posterior humeral circumflex artery**
- ■ **Articulations (four joints): glenohumeral, sternoclavicular, acromioclavicular, and scapulothoracic**

- Glenohumeral joint
  - Spheroidal (ball-and-socket) joint, it is the principal articulation of the shoulder and is stabilized by both static and dynamic restraints (see the following discussion on biomechanics).
  - Part of the static restraints, the glenohumeral ligaments are discrete capsular thickenings that act as a kind of rein to limit excessive rotation or translation of the humeral head; they are the superior glenohumeral ligament (SGHL), middle glenohumeral ligament (MGHL), and inferior glenohumeral ligament (IGHL) complex. The IGHL has both an anterior band (aIGHL) and posterior band (pIGHL) (Figure 4-27)
    - The aIGHL originates at the 3 o'clock position of the glenoid, and the pIGHL originates at the 8 o'clock position.
  - Additional capsular elements include the coracohumeral ligament, posterior capsule (thinnest portion [<1 mm] of shoulder capsule), and the rotator interval.
    - Contents of the rotator interval include the coracohumeral ligament, SGHL, biceps tendon, and glenohumeral capsule
    - Bounded medially by the lateral coracoid base, superiorly by the anterior edge of the supraspinatus, and inferiorly by the superior border of the subscapularis
      - Transverse humeral ligament forms its apex laterally
- Sternoclavicular joint
  - Gliding joint with a disc that serves to anchor the shoulder girdle to the chest wall
  - Elevation of the arm from 0 to 90 degrees produces clavicular rotation about its longitudinal axis and elevation at the sternoclavicular joint of 0 to 40 degrees. The posterior capsule is the primary restraint of excessive anterior and posterior translation.
- Acromioclavicular joint
  - The articulation of the scapula with the clavicle occurs through a diarthrodial joint containing an incomplete intraarticular disc.
  - Stabilized by the acromioclavicular ligaments, which primarily resist anteroposterior translation, and the coracoclavicular ligaments, which prevent inferior translation of the coracoid and acromion from the clavicle (Figure 4-28).
    - The conoid ligament provides superior restraint while the trapezoid ligament provides posterior restraint.

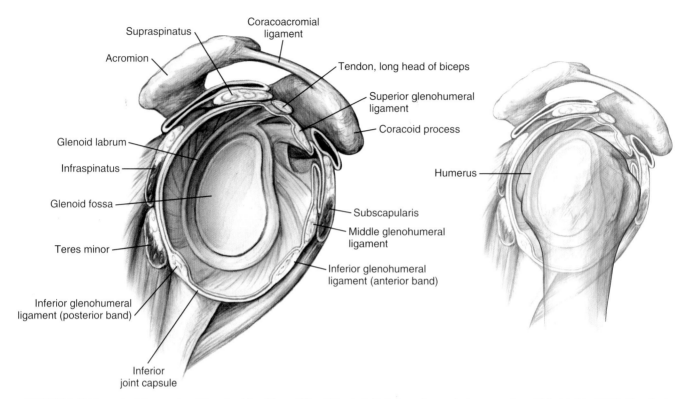

FIGURE 4-27 Important ligaments of the shoulder. (From Miller MD, et al: *Orthopaedic surgical approaches,* Philadelphia, 2008, Elsevier.)

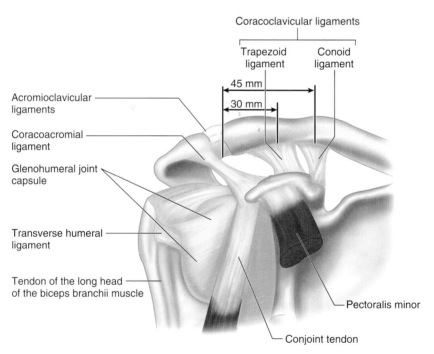

FIGURE 4-28 Anatomy of the superior shoulder suspensory complex and adjacent structures.

- The acromioclavicular joint is best evaluated in the Zanca view, in which the x-ray beam is directed 10 degrees cephalad at 50% of normal penetrance (see Table 4-7).
- Scapulothoracic joint
  - The medial border of the scapula articulates with the posterior aspect of the second to seventh ribs.
  - Angled 30 degrees anteriorly and has a 3-degree upward tilt
  - There are two major scapulothoracic bursae.
  - The ratio of glenohumeral to scapulothoracic motion during shoulder abduction is approximately 2 : 1.

BIOMECHANICS

- **The shoulder is stabilized by both static and dynamic restraints.**
- Static restraints (Table 4-5 and Figure 4-29)
  - Structures that provide unidirectional limitations to translation
  - Include the glenoid labrum, articular version, articular conformity, negative intraarticular pressure, capsule (posterior capsule and rotator interval), and glenohumeral ligaments
  - Glenoid labrum increases depth of glenoid concavity
    - Serves to anchor the glenohumeral ligaments
  - The SGHL and coracohumeral ligament are reinforcing structures of the rotator interval, limiting inferior translation and external rotation when the arm is adducted and posterior translation when the arm is flexed forward, adducted, and internally rotated.
    - Imbrication of the rotator interval decreases inferior and posterior translation, whereas its release produces increased forward flexion and external rotation.
  - The middle glenohumeral ligament limits external rotation of the adducted humerus, inferior translation of the adducted and externally rotated humerus, and anterior and posterior translation of the partly abducted (at 45 degrees) and externally rotated arm.
  - **The inferior glenohumeral ligament complex serves as the primary restraint to anterior, posterior, and inferior glenohumeral translation at 45 to 90 degrees of glenohumeral elevation. The aIGHL is important in external rotation and the pIGHL important in internal rotation.**

- **Dynamic restraints**
  - These include joint concavity compression produced by synchronized contraction of the rotator cuff, acting to stabilize the humeral head within the glenoid; increased capsular tension produced by direct attachments of the rotator cuff to the capsule; the scapular stabilizers that act to maintain a stable glenoid platform ("ball on a seal's nose"); and proprioception.
- **Throwing**
  - Significant forces are generated during throwing and can result in anatomic variation and injury.
  - Typically there is greater external rotation and a loss of internal rotation of the dominant shoulder in comparison with the nondominant shoulder; this condition is referred to as *glenohumeral internal rotation deficit* (GIRD).
  - The anterior capsule is selectively stretched, whereas the posterior capsule is tightened. These developments can predispose to both instability and internal impingement.
  - Bony changes have also been observed in the dominant shoulder, including increased humeral head retroversion and glenoid retroversion.
  - The five phases of throwing are shown in Figure 4-30.
  - Maximal torque is generated during two actions: maximal external rotation (late cocking) and just after ball release (deceleration).
    - The late cocking phase is associated with SLAP (superior labrum from anterior to posterior) tears and internal impingement.
    - **The deceleration phase is associated with tensile failure of the posterior aspect of the supraspinatus and anterior half of the infraspinatus.**
      - The rotator cuff must offset the high-energy forces during deceleration.
  - The scapula must rotate during throwing. It retracts during the late cocking phase and then protracts during the acceleration phase.
  - Scapular dyskinesis is extremely common in patients with a disabled throwing shoulder.
    - Control of scapular retraction and posterior tilt is lost.
    - Results in scapular protraction, anterior tilt, and excessive internal rotation
      - Anterior tilt results in external impingement.
      - Internal rotation results in internal impingement.
      - Loss of control causes decreased rotator cuff strength and increased anterior capsular strain.

Table 4-5	Static Shoulder Restraints	
STRUCTURE	**ARM POSITION**	**RESTRAINT**
Superior GHL	Adduction	Inferior translation External rotation
Middle GHL	Flexion, adduction, and internal rotation	Posterior translation
	Adduction	External rotation
	Adduction and external rotation	Inferior translation
	45 degrees abduction and external rotation	Anterior and posterior translation
Inferior GHL, anterior band	90 degrees abduction and external rotation	Anterior translation Inferior translation
Inferior GHL, posterior band	90 degrees abduction and internal rotation	Posterior translation Inferior translation
Rotator interval (superior GHL and coracohumeral ligament)	Adduction	Inferior translation
Posterior capsule	Flexion, adduction, and internal rotation	Posterior translation

GHL, Glenohumeral ligament.

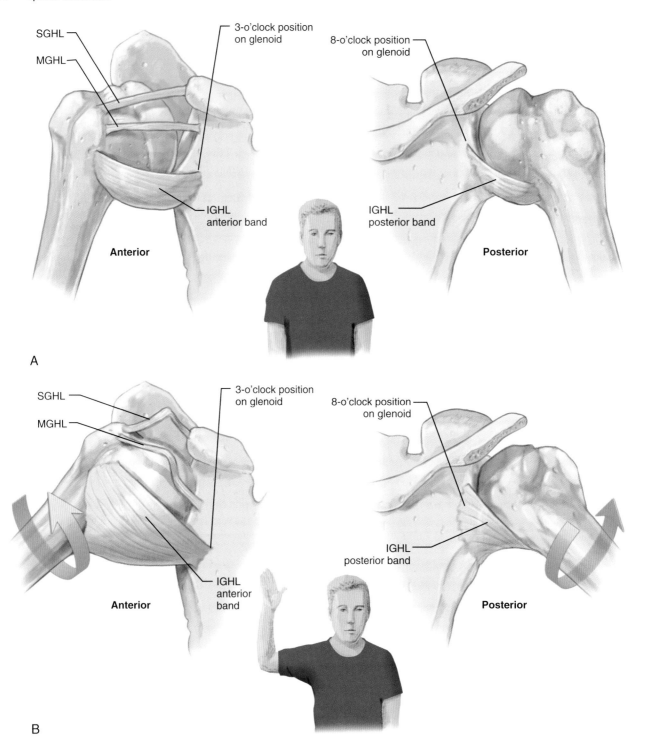

FIGURE 4-29 Dynamic relationship of the glenohumeral ligaments. **A,** In 0 degrees of abduction, the superior glenohumeral ligament (SGHL) is taut. **B,** As the arm is brought into the "apprehension position" of abduction and external rotation, the anterior band of the inferior glenohumeral ligament (IGHL) is pulled superiorly and anteriorly to span the midportion of the glenohumeral joint, thus providing anterior stability. *MGHL,* Middle glenohumeral ligament.

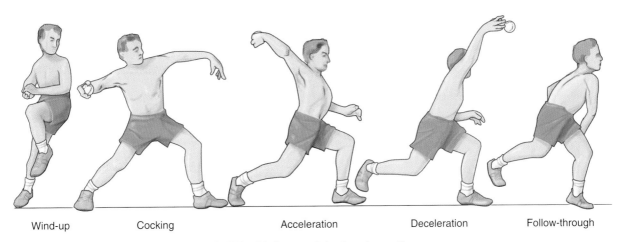

| Wind-up | Cocking | Acceleration | Deceleration | Follow-through |

FIGURE 4-30 Stages of the throwing motion.

Table 4-6 Shoulder: Key Examination Points

EXAMINATION	TECHNIQUE	SIGNIFICANCE
IMPINGEMENT/ROTATOR CUFF		
Impingement sign	Passive FF > 90 degrees	Pain indicates impingement syndrome
Impingement test	Passive FF > 90 degrees continues after subacromial injection	Relief of pain indicates impingement syndrome
Hawkins test	Passive FF of 90 degrees and IR	Pain indicates impingement syndrome
Jobe test	Resisted pronation/FF of 90 degrees	Pain indicates supraspinatus lesion
Drop-arm test	Maintaining FF in plane of scapula	Inability indicates supraspinatus lesion
Hornblower sign	Resisted maximal ER/abduction of 90 degrees	Pain indicates infraspinatus, supraspinatus, or post-supraspinatus lesion
Rubber band sign	Resisted maximal ER/slight abduction	Pain indicates infraspinatus lesion
Liftoff test	Arm in IR behind back	Inability to elevate from back indicates subscapularis lesion
Modified liftoff test	Resisted arm held off back	Inability to keep arm elevated when off back indicates subscapularis lesion
Belly-push test	Elbow held anterior with abduction pressure	Inability to hold elbow forward indicates subscapularis lesion
INSTABILITY		
Apprehension test	Supine abduction in 90 degrees and ER	Apprehension indicates anterior instability
Relocation test	Apprehension with posterior force	Relief of apprehension indicates anterior instability
Load-and-shift test	Anterior/posterior force on humeral head	Degree of translation reflects laxity or instability
Modified load-and-shift test	Supine load/shift with elbow bending	Degree of translation reflects laxity or instability
Jerk test	Post force with arm adduction and FF	A "clunk" sound indicates posterior subluxation
Sulcus sign	Inferior force with arm at side	Increased acromiohumeral interval reflects inferior laxity or instability (see Table 4-11 for sulcus grading)
LABRUM/BICEPS		
O'Brien (active compression) test	10 degrees adduction, 90 degrees FF, maximal pronation	Pain with resistance indicates SLAP lesion
Anterior slide test	Hand on hip, joint loading	Pain with resistance indicates SLAP lesion
Crank test	Full abduction, humeral loading, rotation	Pain indicates SLAP lesion
Speed test	Resisted FF in scapular plane	Pain indicates bicipital tendinitis
Yerguson test	Resisted supination	Pain indicates bicipital tendinitis
MISCELLANEOUS		
Spurling maneuver	Lateral flexion, rotation, cervical loading	Cervical spine disease or injury
Wright test	Extension-abduction-ER of arm with neck rotated away	Loss of pulse and reproduction of symptoms indicates thoracic outlet syndrome

ER, External rotation; *ext,* extension; *FF,* forward flexion; *IR,* internal rotation.

DIAGNOSTIC TECHNIQUES

■ History
- ▥ Age and chief complaint are two important considerations.
- ▥ Instability, acromioclavicular injuries, and distal clavicle osteolysis are more common in young patients.
- ▥ Rotator cuff tears, arthritis, and proximal humeral fractures are more common in older patients.

- ▥ Direct blows are usually responsible for acromioclavicular separations.
- ▥ Instability occurs with injury to the abducted externally rotated arm.
- ▥ Chronic overhead pain and night pain are associated with rotator cuff tears.

■ Physical examination
- ▥ Important physical examination points (Table 4-6)
- ▥ Note that to evaluate true ROM of the glenohumeral joint, scapula must be stabilized

- It is vital to use a combination of physical examination maneuvers to arrive at a diagnosis.
- **Imaging of the shoulder**
- Standard views:
  - Anteroposterior (AP) view
  - Glenohumeral "true" AP (Grashey) view
  - Axillary lateral view
    - Crucial view to evaluate glenohumeral dislocation
  - Scapular Y view
  - Acromioclavicular AP (Zanca) view
    - Taken with 10-degree cephalic tilt and 50% penetrance
- Additional views include rotational views, supine and prone views, and tilted views.
- Several findings and their significance are listed in Table 4-7.

SHOULDER ARTHROSCOPY

- **Portals**
- Standard portals
  - Posterior portal (2 cm distal and medial to the posterolateral border of the acromion, used primarily for viewing)
  - Anterior portal (just anterior to acromioclavicular joint)
  - Lateral portal (1-2 cm distal to lateral acromial edge)
- Additional portals
  - Supraspinatus (Neviaser) portal for anterior glenoid visualization (through supraspinatus fossa)
  - Anterolateral and posterolateral portals (port of Wilmington, just anterior to posterolateral corner of acromion) are useful for labral or SLAP tears and rotator cuff repair.
  - Anteroinferior (5 o'clock position) portal for Bankart repair and stabilization procedures
  - Posteroinferior (7 o'clock position) portal for stabilization procedures
- Hazards
  - Posterior portal: axillary nerve, suprascapular nerve, suprascapular artery
  - Anterior portals: cephalic vein, axillary artery, axillary nerve
  - Superior portals: suprascapular artery, suprascapular nerve

- **Technique**
- Intraarticular structures should be systematically evaluated.
- As the number and variety of arthroscopic procedures increase, so does the opportunity for iatrogenic injury.
- Maintaining adequate visualization through hemostasis, avoiding chondral abrasion, maintaining adequate flow with thermal devices, and preventing fluid extravasation by preserving muscle fascial layers help minimize the risk.
- **The axillary nerve is approximately 12 mm distal to the 6 o'clock position.**
- The axillary nerve has often branched into its four divisions at this position.
  - From proximal to distal: branch to teres minor, branch supplying lateral cutaneous innervation (superior lateral brachial cutaneous nerve), branch to posterior deltoid, branch to anterior deltoid
    - This explains why the majority of postoperative axillary neuropraxias are reported as typically isolated sensory abnormalities. The branch to teres minor is very difficult to evaluate clinically.

SHOULDER INSTABILITY

- **Instability is a pathologic condition manifesting as pain as a result of excessive translation of the humeral head on the glenoid during active shoulder motion; it represents a spectrum of injury to the shoulder stabilizers.**
- Can be divided along a spectrum between unidirectional and multidirectional. Matsen coined the acronyms TUBS and AMBRI as mnemonics.
  - TUBS: Traumatic unilateral dislocations with a Bankart lesion often necessitate surgery because they typically occur in young patients and have recurrence rates of up to 90% with nonoperative management. Anterior instability is much more common than posterior instability.
  - AMBRI: Atraumatic multidirectional bilateral shoulder dislocation/subluxation often responds to rehabilitation, and sometimes an inferior capsular shift or plication is required.

Table 4-7	Shoulder Injuries: Radiographic Findings	
VIEW/SIGN	**FINDINGS**	**SIGNIFICANCE**
View of supraspinatus outlet	Acromial structure (types I to III)	Type III acromion associated with impingement
View of 30-degree caudal tilt	Subacromial spurring	Area below level of clavicle is impingement area
Zanca 10-degree cephalic tilt	AC joint disease	AC DJD, distal clavicle osteolysis
West Point view	AI glenoid evaluation	Bony Bankart lesion seen with instability
Apical oblique (Garth) view	AI glenoid evaluation; humeral head evaluation	Bony Bankart lesion seen with instability; Hill-Sachs defect
Stryker notch	Humeral head evaluation	Hill-Sachs impression fracture
Anteroposterior internal rotation	Humeral head evaluation	Hill-Sachs defect
Hobbs view	SC injury	Anteroposterior dislocations
Serendipity view	SC injury	Anteroposterior dislocations
45-degree abduction, true anteroposterior view	Glenohumeral space	Subtle DJD
Arthrography	Rotator cuff injuries	Dye above cuff indicates tear
CT	Fractures	Classification is easier
MRI ± arthrography	Soft tissue evaluation	Labral, cuff, muscle tears

■ **Anterior instability**

■ Introduction
- Most common type of shoulder instability
- Typically the result of trauma to the arm when in the abducted and externally rotated position
- Fundamentally the pathoanatomy can be capsulolabral, osseous, or both.
- Capsulolabral pathoanatomy (Figure 4-31)
  - Bankart described the "essential lesion" of anterior shoulder instability to be an anteroinferior labral tear, so it bears the eponymous term *Bankart lesion.*
    - A Bankart lesion has been arbitrarily defined as an avulsion of the anterior-inferior capsulolabral complex with extension into the scapular periosteum and rupture of the periosteal tissue.
    - Found to occur in 90% of patients with recurrent anterior shoulder instability
  - A variety of other capsulolabral lesions have been described: Perthes lesion, anterior labroligamentous periosteal sleeve avulsion (ALPSA) lesion, and humeral avulsion of the glenohumeral ligaments (HAGL) lesion (Table 4-8).

- A HAGL lesion has an incidence between 1% and 9% and has typically necessitated open repair in the past because of its inferior location. However, newer arthroscopic techniques are being developed.
- Osseous pathoanatomy
  - A degree of bone injury either to the glenoid or humeral head is thought to occur in almost every patient with anterior shoulder instability.
  - Glenoid bone loss may occur either as an identifiable fragment with its attached capsulolabral structures (bony Bankart lesion) or as a result of impaction and erosion.
  - Some glenoid bone loss is present in 40% of first-time dislocators and 85% of recurrent dislocators.
    - Important to recognize glenoid bone loss preoperatively; significant bone loss has been associated with an increased rate of recurrence following Bankart repair. Significant bone loss has been defined as approximately 20% to 25% of the width of the glenoid at the level of the bare spot. This corresponds to approximately 6 to 8 mm of bone loss.

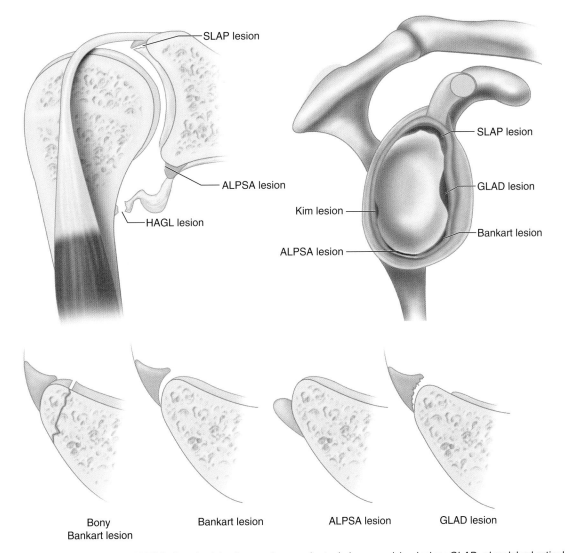

 FIGURE 4-31 Capsulolabral lesions. *ALPSA,* Anterior labroligamentous periosteal sleeve avulsion lesion; *GLAD,* glenolabral articular disruption; *HAGL,* humeral avulsion of the glenohumeral ligaments; *SLAP,* superior labrum anterior to posterior.

Table 4-8	Capsulolabral Lesions
LESION	**DESCRIPTION**
ASSOCIATED WITH ANTERIOR INSTABILITY	
Perthes	Avulsion of anterior-inferior glenolabral complex with preservation of medial scapular neck periosteum
Bankart	Complete avulsion of anterior-inferior glenolabral complex along with a piece of scapular neck periosteum
Bony Bankart	Osseous avulsion fracture of anterior-inferior glenolabral complex
ALPSA	Avulsion of anterior-inferior glenolabral complex with stripping of medial scapular neck periosteum but preservation of a medial hinge; loose fragment subsequently scars medially down scapular neck
HAGL	Avulsion of glenohumeral ligaments from their humeral-sided attachment
NOT ASSOCIATED WITH INSTABILITY	
Glenolabral articular disruption (GLAD)	Superficial tear of anterior-inferior labrum with associated cartilage injury but preservation of anterior-inferior glenolabral complex; presents with painful shoulder but not a cause of shoulder instability
SLAP	Disruption of superior labrum, originally described to stop at midglenoid notch*

ALPSA, Anterior labroligamentous periosteal sleeve avulsion lesion; *HAGL,* humeral avulsion of the glenohumeral ligaments lesion.
*Recent descriptions have associated SLAP (superior labrum anterior to posterior) tears with Bankart lesions, but SLAP lesions alone are not a cause of shoulder instability.

- The bone fragment in a bony Bankart lesion has been shown to undergo rapid absorption within 1 year of the primary injury.
- Humeral-sided bone injury typically occurs to the posterior superior humeral head and has been termed a *Hill-Sachs lesion* after the two radiologists who described it.
  - A Hill-Sachs lesion can be found in 40% of patients with recurrent subluxations but no dislocations, 90% of first-time dislocators, and almost 100% of recurrent dislocators.
  - An "engaging" Hill-Sachs lesion is oriented in such a manner that placing the shoulder in abduction and external rotation results in the humeral head losing contact with the glenoid and subsequent subluxation or dislocation of the glenohumeral joint.
- Age at first dislocation is the most important factor in predicting recurrence. Rate of redislocation:
  - Almost 100% in persons with open growth plates
  - 70% to 95% of persons younger than 20 years
  - 60% to 80% in persons aged 20 to 30 years
  - 15% to 20% in persons older than 40 years
- Associated injuries
  - Typically occur in older patients. Up to 40% of patients have an associated injury.
  - Dislocation with greater tuberosity fracture is the most common scenario, occurring in 15% of older patients. This has the best prognosis for risk of redislocation.
  - Rotator cuff tears, axillary nerve palsy, brachial plexus palsy, and axillary artery injury can also occur. The axillary nerve is susceptible to injury after anterior dislocation because of its relatively fixed position.
- History and physical examination
  - Typically present with a history of trauma
  - Note should be made of age at first dislocation, increasing ease of dislocation, frequency of recurrence, duration of symptoms, and ability to self-reduce.
  - Physical examination should focus on both diagnosis and identification of associated injuries.

- The apprehension-relocation test (Fowler test) is the most sensitive. The arm is placed into abduction and external rotation. As the arm is brought into this position, the patient experiences a sense of instability. The examiner then places a posterior force on the arm and the sense of instability is relieved.
- The load-and-shift test can be used to "classify" degrees of instability based on distance of humeral head translation: 1+: 0 to 1 cm of translation to before glenoid rim; 2+: 1 to 2 cm of translation to glenoid rim; 3+: more than 2 cm translation or over glenoid rim.
- An evaluation of generalized laxity should be performed.
- Imaging
  - Radiographs, CT, and MRI all have a role.
  - Standard radiographs, including an axillary view, are obtained to ensure the shoulder is located.
    - Specialized views are helpful for detecting glenoid and humeral head bone loss (see Table 4-7).
  - CT scan (Figure 4-32)
    - **Permits accurate identification of glenoid bone loss.** Recent studies suggest three-dimensional reconstructions are more reliable for measurement purposes.
  - MRI (Figure 4-33)
    - Typically an MR arthrogram is performed to increase sensitivity.
    - An *AB*duction-*E*xternal *R*otation (ABER) view further increases sensitivity
- Treatment
  - Reduction
    - Variety of techniques described. Traction-countertraction is most commonly employed. The Milch maneuver (slow abduction and external rotation) has some evidence suggesting increased success rates.
    - Recent Cochrane review suggests no difference between intraarticular injection of lidocaine and intravenous sedation with regard to the success rate of reduction, pain during reduction, or postprocedural pain

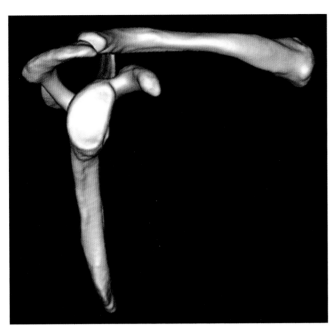

FIGURE 4-32 Three-dimensional reconstruction of computed tomography scan of the glenoid and scapula demonstrating approximately 20% anterior glenoid bone loss.

- An axillary view radiograph is mandatory to confirm reduction.
- Sling immobilization
  - Duration of immobilization has not been found to influence rates of redislocation.
  - Positioning the arm in external rotation has shown some success in the literature in reducing redislocation rates. However, the most recent studies have failed to confirm these early results, and meta-analyses suggest no difference between immobilization in internal or external immobilization.
- Surgical stabilization (see Table 4-9)
  - Management of the first-time shoulder dislocation remains controversial. There is support in the literature for stabilization of first-time dislocators, with reduced rates of redislocation and improved quality-of-life outcome measurements.
  - A multitude of surgical techniques have been described. Many are historical, but some of these are still important to be aware of because their long-term complications continue to be clinical concerns.
- Surgical techniques (Table 4-9 and Figure 4-34)
  - Debate continues on whether arthroscopic Bankart repair produces results equivalent to the current gold standard of open Bankart repair.
    - Several smaller randomized controlled trials have demonstrated similar outcomes.
    - Mohtadi and colleagues (2014) performed the largest randomized trial to date and have shown equivalent patient quality-of-life scores but significantly higher redislocation rates in the arthroscopic group. Specifically they have suggested that open repair be performed in males younger than 25 and in

patients with identifiable Hill-Sachs lesions on radiographs.
- In the setting of a bony Bankart repair, the bone fragment should be incorporated into the repair.
- A **Latarjet procedure should be considered when glenoid deficiency is greater than 20% to 25% of the glenoid width. It is also useful in a revision setting.**
  - The mechanism of stabilization of the Latarjet is threefold: (1) sling effect from subscapularis and conjoint tendon, (2) bone block effect from the transferred coracoid, (3) capsular repair effect of suturing coracoacromial ligament to the capsule.
- Chronic dislocations with humeral articular deficiency greater than 40% should be treated with allograft in younger patients and hemiarthroplasty in older patients.
- Rotator interval closure results in decreased external rotation in shoulder adduction and posteroinferior translation.
- *Remplissage* means "to fill" in French and involves tenodesis of the posterior capsule and infraspinatus into a Hill-Sachs lesion. Precise indications are not yet defined, but early evidence suggests medium to large or engaging Hill-Sachs lesions.
- Thermal capsular shrinkage is no longer recommended because of high rates of redislocation and the potential for capsular necrosis and subsequent capsular deficiency. **Postthermal capsular necrosis is treated with allograft anterior capsulolabral reconstruction.**
- Postoperative rehabilitation
  - Following Bankart repair, immobilization is typically performed for 3 to 6 weeks.
- Complications
  - Dependent on the procedure
  - Recurrent instability is the most common and occurs in upwards of 10% of patients
  - Infection and axillary nerve injury are other common complications of almost all instability procedures.
  - Dislocation arthropathy is a common late-occurring condition.
  - Latarjet complications include injury to the musculocutaneous nerve, fibrous union or nonunion of the coracoid, and screw breakage.

Posterior instability
- Much less common than anterior instability
- May be the result of traumatic or atraumatic causes
  - Trauma to the arm in flexion, adduction, and internal rotation is the most common cause.
  - Typically the result of higher-energy trauma
  - **Electric shocks and epileptic seizures are also a frequent cause. These result in posterior dislocation because the stronger shoulder internal rotators (latissimus dorsi, pectoralis major, subscapularis and teres major) overpower the weak external rotators (infraspinatus and teres minor).**
- Weightlifters, football linemen, swimmers, and gymnasts are the most frequently affected athletes.
- **Patients may exhibit positive results with load-and-shift and jerk testing.**
- Acute posterior dislocations are frequently missed.

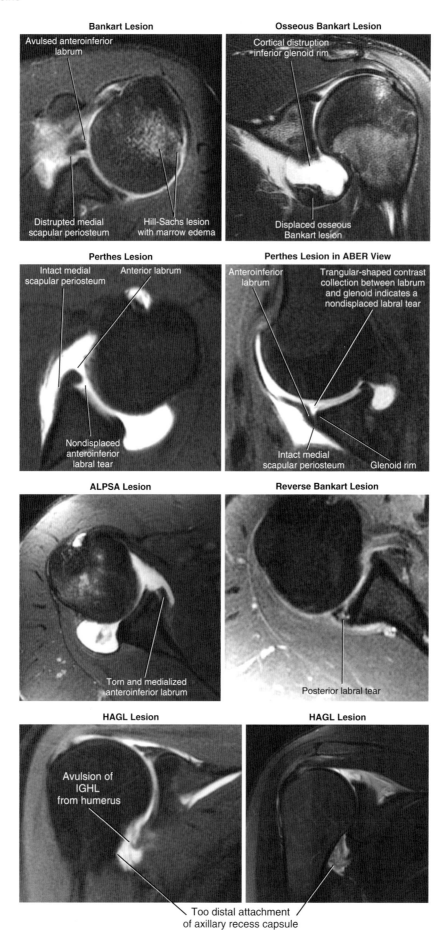

FIGURE 4-33 Magnetic resonance imaging appearance of the various soft tissue pathologies associated with shoulder instability. *ABER,* Abduction external rotation; *ALPSA,* anterior labroligamentous periosteal sleeve avulsion; *HAGL,* humeral avulsion of the glenohumeral ligaments.

Table 4-9 Surgical Options for Anterior Shoulder Instability

PROCEDURE	ESSENTIAL FEATURES	COMMENTS, KEY COMPLICATIONS
OPEN		
Bankart repair	Reattach labrum and IGHL to anterior glenoid; often combined with capsular shift	Gold standard; occasionally preferred in contact athletes
Latarjet coracoid transfer	Distal 2 cm of coracoid transferred to anterior glenoid neck with two-screw fixation and reattachment of CA ligament to anterior glenohumeral capsule	Primary procedure in patients with > 25% glenoid bone loss
Anterior capsulolabral reconstruction	Glenoid-based capsular shift	Designed for overhead athletes; may be performed as adjunct to Bankart
ARTHROSCOPIC		
Bankart repair	Reattach labrum and IGHL to anterior glenoid with use of suture anchors	Most common operation for anterior instability
Coracoid transfer (hybrid Bristow-Latarjet)	Distal 2 cm of coracoid transferred to anterior glenoid neck; CA ligament preserved	Investigational
SUPPLEMENTARY		
Remplissage	Arthroscopic infraspinatus and posterior capsule fixation into Hill-Sachs lesion using suture anchors	Investigational; performed in moderate to large Hill-Sachs lesions; medialized sutures limit external rotation
Humeral head allograft	Osteoarticular allograft inserted into Hill-Sachs lesion	Performed in large Hill-Sachs lesions
Partial humeral head resurfacing	Cobalt-chrome component inserted into Hill-Sachs lesions; typically performed with Latarjet	Alternative to humeral head allograft
Rotator interval closure	Open or arthroscopic superior capsular shift of MGHL to SGHL	Limits external rotation
REVISION		
Allograft bone grafting of glenoid	Iliac crest or distal tibia secured to anterior glenoid neck with screws	Performed in severe glenoid bone loss
Humeral hemiarthroplasty	Humeral component retroverted 50 degrees to achieve stability	Indicated in older patients with > 45% humeral head bone loss and glenohumeral arthritis
Rotational humeral osteotomy	Subcapital external rotational osteotomy to rotate Hill-Sachs lesion outside glenoid track	Performed in severe Hill-Sachs lesions
Allograft anterior capsulolabral reconstruction	Allograft tendon used to reconstruct anterior band of IGHL and MGHL	Performed in severe capsular deficiency due to systemic soft tissue disorders, electrothermal capsular necrosis, or repeated surgical procedures without bone loss
HISTORICAL		
Bristow coracoid transfer	Distal 1 cm of coracoid transferred and secured with 1 screw; CA ligament preserved	Higher rate of recurrence
Caspari technique	Arthroscopic transglenoid suture repair of glenoid labrum	Higher rate of recurrence; injury to suprascapular nerve
Staple capsulorrhaphy	Reattachment of capsule to glenoid neck with a staple	High rate of pain, higher rate of recurrence, reduced internal and external rotation, staple migration
Putti-Platt	Subscapularis advancement and shortening	Reduced external rotation, posterior glenoid arthritis
Magnusson-Stack	Subscapularis transfer to greater tuberosity	Reduced external rotation
Thermal capsular shrinkage	Use of thermal energy to reduce capsular volume	Higher rate of recurrence; can result in capsular deficiency and chondral damage

AGHL, Anterior glenohumeral ligament; *CA,* coracoacromial; *IGHL,* inferior glenohumeral ligament; *MGHL,* middle glenohumeral ligament.

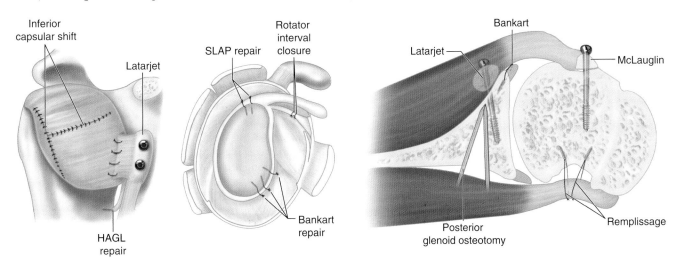

FIGURE 4-34 Various surgical procedures for treatment of shoulder instability.

- A fixed posterior shoulder dislocation is diagnosed by lack of external rotation.
- Patients may present with their arms internally rotated and with observable coracoid and posterior prominence.
- **Anteroposterior radiographs are unreliable but may demonstrate a "lightbulb" sign. An axillary lateral radiograph is critical in making the diagnosis.**
- When they are recognized, posterior dislocations respond well to acute reduction and immobilization.
- Rehabilitation focuses on rotator cuff and deltoid strengthening.
- Surgical intervention is typically performed only after rehabilitation has failed.
  - Patients with traumatic causes have been traditionally viewed as having a better prognosis following surgery.
  - The surgical procedure is dependent on the pathology. Posterior labral repair is most common.
  - Closure of the rotator interval may augment repairs.
  - Posterior glenoid version may be corrected with a posterior glenoid osteotomy.
- For chronic unrecognized posterior dislocations, several procedures may be performed, dependent on the degree of bone loss both in the humeral head and glenoid.
  - The Neer modification of the McLaughlin procedure involves transfer of the lesser tuberosity and associated subscapularis tendon into the reverse Hill-Sachs lesion.
  - Hemiarthroplasty or total shoulder arthroplasty is recommended when more than 35% to 40% of articular humeral-sided loss is present. Segmental reconstruction with allograft has initial promising results.
- A Kim lesion is an incomplete and concealed avulsion of the posteroinferior labrum (Figure 4-35).
  - May be associated with posterior and multidirectional instability
  - The jerk (posterior lesion) and Kim (posteroinferior lesion) tests have been shown to be highly sensitive and specific.
  - MR arthrography can be helpful in establishing the diagnosis, but findings may be subtle or falsely negative.
  - After failure of conservative treatment, arthroscopic labroplasty (with a posterior capsular shift in primary posterior instability) or posterior labroplasty (with an inferior capsular shift and rotator interval closure when associated with multidirectional instability) has been effective.
- Multidirectional instability (MDI)
- Represents the AMBRI spectrum of instability. Fundamentally thought to be the result of capsular laxity, but scapular muscular dysfunction is also a critical portion.
- Typically presents with an insidious onset of pain and sensation of looseness about the shoulder. Traumatic onset is rare. May affect both shoulders. Often associated with gymnasts, swimmers, and volleyball players.
- Physical examination reveals increased generalized laxity (Beighton criteria) and a positive sulcus sign. The sulcus sign should reproduce the patient's symptoms. Scapular dyskinesis is common.

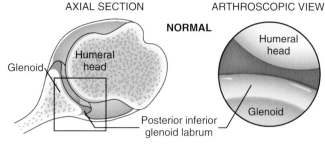
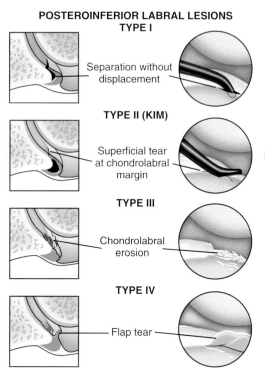

FIGURE 4-35 The Kim lesion is an incomplete and concealed avulsion of the posteroinferior labrum that may be associated with posterior and multidirectional instability.

- The focus of treatment is prolonged rehabilitation. This should focus on rotator cuff and deltoid strengthening, as well as correction of scapulothoracic mechanics.
- If 6 months to 1 year of rehabilitation has failed, inferior capsular shift or arthroscopic capsular plication is considered.
  - Five plication stitches are equivalent to an open capsular shift.

SUBACROMIAL IMPINGEMENT SYNDROME

- An extremely common cause of shoulder pain
- Debate exists as to the etiology, but likely represents a combination of extrinsic compression and intrinsic degeneration
- Extrinsic compression is from the anterior acromion, the coracoacromial ligament, and the acromioclavicular joint.
- Intrinsic degeneration occurs in the supraspinatus, and the resultant weakness causes narrowing of the subacromial space and abutment of the rotator cuff against the acromion.
  - Histologically, tendinopathy is characterized by disorganized collagen fibers and mucoid degeneration. Inflammatory cells are typically absent.

■ Patients present with an insidious onset of pain that is worse with overhead activity and at night. Neer and Hawkins signs are present. strength is normal.

■ Radiographs may demonstrate a hooked acromion.

■ Physical therapy, NSAID, and subacromial corticosteroid injections are the mainstay of treatment.

▦ The posterior approach for subacromial injection has been shown to be least accurate in women.

■ Symptoms that do not respond to a minimum of 4 to 6 months of nonoperative treatment may respond favorably to subacromial decompression and acromioplasty.

▦ Exceptions to decompression include massive irreparable rotator cuff tears that may benefit from débridement, with preservation of the coracoacromial arch to prevent anterosuperior humeral migration.

▦ Additional exceptions include the acute traumatic rotator cuff tear and injury in the overhead-movement athlete who may benefit from limited acromial smoothing and bursectomy, which is required for visualization and limiting postoperative irritation of the repair site.

■ Patients with workers' compensation claims have poor subjective outcomes after subacromial decompression.

ROTATOR CUFF DISEASE

■ **Overview**

▦ Rotator cuff disease is a continuum beginning with mild impingement and progressing toward partial tear, full-thickness tear, massive tear, and finally arthropathy of the rotator cuff.

▦ Tears associated with chronic impingement syndrome typically begin on the bursal surface or within the tendon substance, in contrast to those that occur on the articular surface because of tension failure in younger athletes participating in overhead activities.

▦ A variety of types of rotator cuff tears exist (Figure 4-36).
  • Full-thickness tears may take a crescent, U-shape, L-shape, or massive contracted pattern. The pattern often dictates repair technique.

▦ The majority of tears involve the supraspinatus and infraspinatus.
  • Subscapularis tears are discussed in the following section.

▦ DeOrio and Colfield classification based on tear size:
  • Small: less than 1 cm
  • Medium: 1 to 3 cm
  • Large: 3 to 5 cm
  • Massive: larger than 5 cm (two tendons)
    • Classification does not predict prognosis

▦ As tears increase in size or in chronicity, the muscle atrophies and a fatty infiltration occurs.

■ **Epidemiology**

▦ Some 28% of patients older than 60 years have a full-thickness tear, whereas 65% of those older than 70 have a full-thickness tear.

▦ Patients older than 60 with a tear have a 50% risk of having bilateral tears.

▦ In those with a unilateral painful full-thickness tear, there is a 56% chance of having an asymptomatic contralateral full- or partial-thickness tear.

▦ Of those with an asymptomatic tear, 50% will develop symptoms in 3 years, and of these patients, 40% may have progression of the tear.

■ **History and physical examination**

▦ Patients typically present with an insidious onset of pain exacerbated by overhead activities.

▦ Complaints of night discomfort, pain in the deltoid region, muscular weakness, and differences in active versus passive ROM are common; more significant weakness and loss of motion indicate a higher degree of cuff involvement.

▦ Acute pain and weakness may be seen after traumatic rotator cuff rupture.

▦ In young athletes, it is critical to confirm or exclude glenohumeral instability that causes a secondary impingement (nonoutlet impingement) from primary impingement syndrome (pathologic process within the subacromial space).

▦ For specific testing, refer to Table 4-6.

■ **Imaging**

▦ May demonstrate classic changes within the acromion or coracoacromial ligament (spurring and calcification) in addition to cystic changes within the greater tuberosity

▦ With chronic rotator cuff disease, superior migration of the humeral head with extensive degenerative change may be present.

▦ Ultrasonography: increasing in popularity as a tool both for diagnosis of rotator cuff disease and for confirmation of intraarticular or subacromial location of injections

▦ MRI is used to define the extent of tear, degree of tear retraction, and presence of muscular atrophy (Figure 4-37).
  • MRI is key for evaluating fatty infiltration. The *tangent sign* is defined as failure of the supraspinatus muscle belly to cross a line from the superior border of the coracoid to the superior border of the scapular spine (Figure 4-38).
    • It has been found to correlate with muscle atrophy and fatty infiltration of the supraspinatus. Patients with a positive tangent sign are more likely to have an irreparable rotator cuff tear.

■ **Treatment**

▦ Nonoperative treatment
  • Asymptomatic full-thickness tears should be treated nonoperatively.
  • Indicated for noncompliant patients, elderly patients (>65 years), medical contraindications to surgery, rotator cuff arthropathy, and athletes with a combined situation of instability and cuff tearing resulting from articular-side partial-thickness failure
  • Activity modification, avoiding repeated forward flexion beyond 90 degrees, and an aggressive program for strengthening the rotator cuff and stabilizing the scapula are initiated.
  • In addition, oral antiinflammatory medications, therapeutic modalities, and judicious use of subacromial steroid injections may be implemented.

▦ Operative treatment
  • Primary indication for surgical intervention is significant pain.
  • Chronic full-thickness tears that have failed to respond to nonoperative management may be treated surgically.
    • However, the evidence is weak for this.
  • Full-thickness acute tears should be repaired early because the disease process is accelerated in this setting.

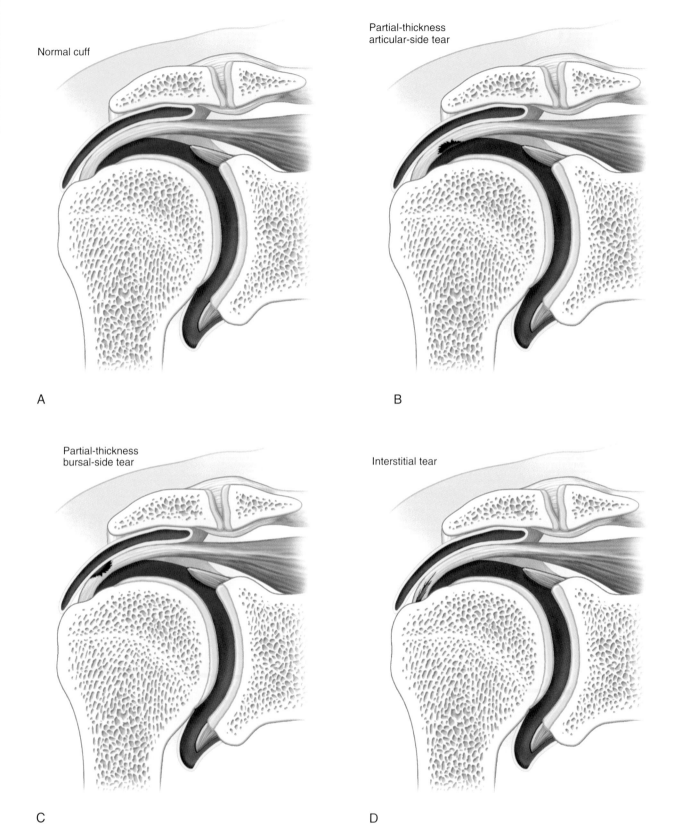

Normal cuff

Partial-thickness
articular-side tear

A

B

Partial-thickness
bursal-side tear

Interstitial tear

C

D

FIGURE 4-36 Patterns of rotator cuff tear. **A,** Normal rotator cuff. **B,** Partial-thickness articular sided tear. **C,** Partial-thickness bursal-side tear. **D,** Partial-thickness interstitial tear.

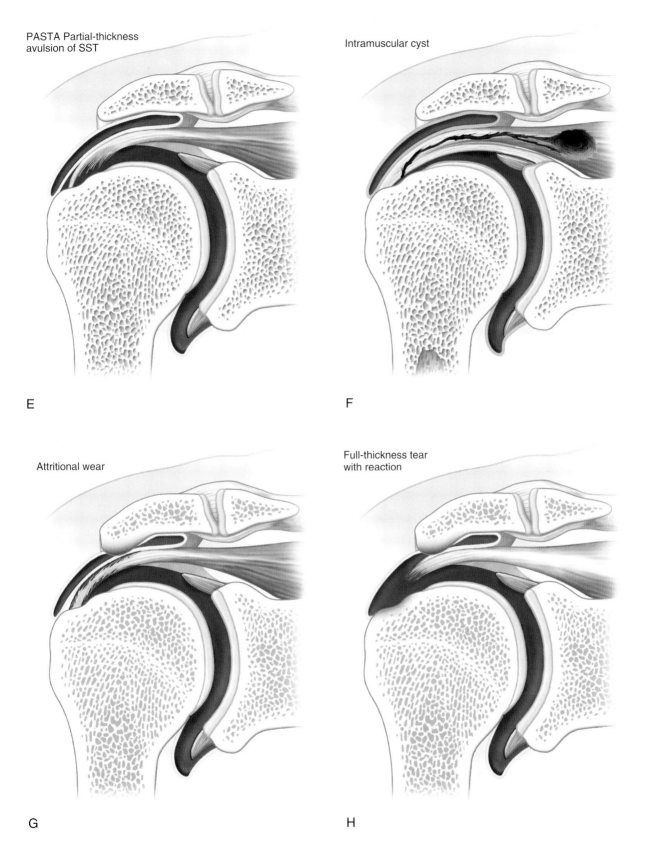

PASTA Partial-thickness
avulsion of SST

Intramuscular cyst

E

F

Attritional wear

Full-thickness tear
with reaction

G

H

FIGURE 4-36, cont'd E, Partial-thickness articular surface supraspinatus avulsion (PASTA lesion). **F,** Partial-thickness articular-side tear with intramuscular cyst. **G,** Attritional fraying of the tendon. **H,** Full-thickness tear.

Continued

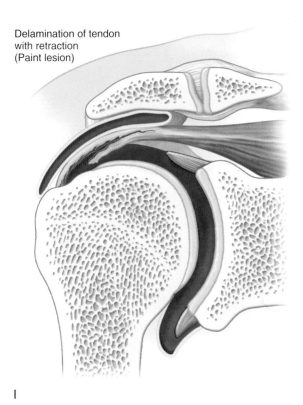

Delamination of tendon with retraction (Paint lesion)

I

FIGURE 4-36, cont'd I, Partial-thickness articular-sided tear with delamination and retraction of the deeper fibers.

- Surgery reliably decreases pain and improves motion and function.
- Surgical techniques
  - The operative approach has evolved from a classic open approach to a "mini-open" or deltoid-sparing approach and to an all-arthroscopic technique.
  - Regardless of the technique, the rate-limiting step for recovery is biologic healing of the rotator cuff tendon to the humerus, which is estimated to require a minimum of 8 to 12 weeks.
  - Routine acromioplasty is no longer recommended during rotator cuff repair.
  - Surgical techniques have evolved to include double-row and suture-bridge fixation techniques, which have improved biomechanical strength in vitro. Clinical correlation is still controversial.
  - **Blood flow to the repaired rotator cuff is achieved from the peribursal tissue and bone anchor site.** Vascularity has been shown to increase with exercise.
- **Special situations**
- Articular-side partial-thickness tears (e.g., partial articular supraspinatus tendon avulsion [PASTA]): Treatment with débridement versus repair remains controversial. Tears in which more than 7 mm of bone lateral to the articular margin is exposed should be considered significant and represent 50% of the tendon insertion.
  - Considerations include the depth of the tear, pattern of the tear (avulsion versus degeneration), amount of footprint uncovered, and activity level of the patient.
  - Patients with a preponderance of impingement findings and a tear of less than 50% thickness may

benefit from débridement and subacromial decompression.
- Large and massive tears
  - The failure rate is higher; tissue failure is most common.
  - Irreparable tears are more likely to occur when the acromiohumeral distance appears shorter (<7 mm) on anteroposterior radiograph.
  - Larger, more retracted tears (>40 mm length/width) are characterized by fatty atrophy, supraspinatus width of less than 5 mm at glenoid margin, high signal in infraspinatus
  - Regardless of healing, most patients report clinical improvement following repair.
- Irreparable tears
  - Combined tears of supraspinatus and infraspinatus may be treated with latissimus dorsi tendon transfer to the greater tuberosity in patients younger than age 65 who have no glenohumeral osteoarthritis.
  - **If pain is the major symptom and motion remains preserved, débridement with biceps tenotomy has been found to be useful**
  - If pseudoparalysis and glenohumeral arthritis is present, a reverse total shoulder arthroplasty may be performed.
  - Xenograft patches have not been found to be helpful.
- **Results**
- Although excellent results have been reported with rotator cuff repair, a high percentage of such tears either do not heal or recur.
  - The majority of failures occur within the first 3 to 6 months.
  - Failure typically occurs as a result of tissue pulling through the sutures.
- Despite this outcome, functional and subjective results remain excellent. A correlation appears to exist between younger age and repair success.
- **Failure rates have been reported to be higher in the following patient groups:**
  - Age 65 years or older
  - Massive tear
  - Moderate to severe muscle atrophy on T1-weighted oblique sagittal MRI
  - Over 50% fatty infiltration of the involved rotator cuff muscle belly
  - Tear retraction to the level of the glenoid
  - Diabetes
  - Smokers
  - Inability to participate in rehabilitation
- **Rehabilitation**
- Rehabilitation following rotator cuff repair is controversial.
- **Recent reports suggest no difference in clinical outcomes or healing rates with early motion versus delayed motion protocols.**
- **Complications**
- Approximately 6% to 8% of patients have continued pain and weakness following rotator cuff repair.
- Ultrasound is the imaging modality of choice for evaluation of a failed rotator cuff repair, but accuracy is highly technician dependent.
- Revision repair should be performed in the symptomatic patient who is younger than age 65 and has no significant fatty atrophy, no significant tendon retraction, no glenohumeral arthritis, and no pseudoparalysis.

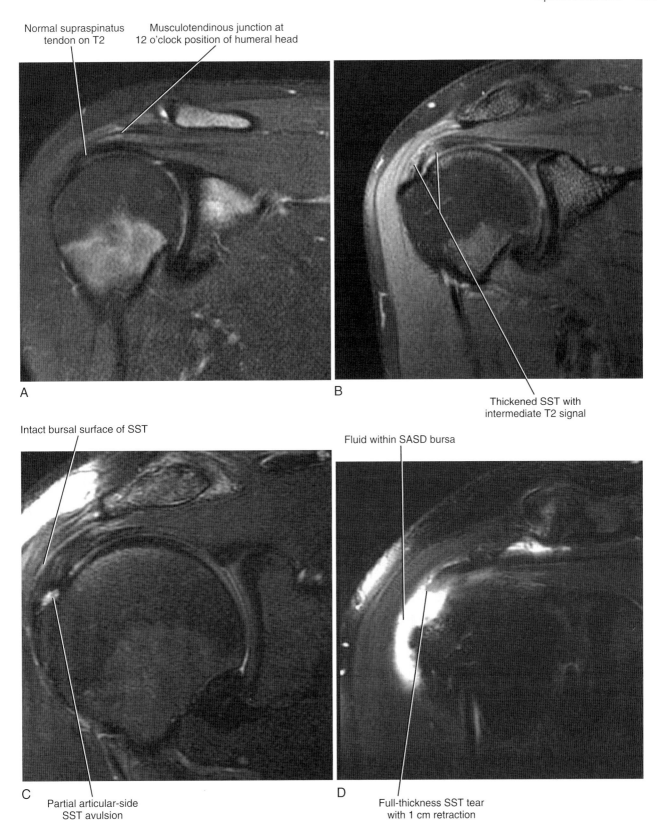

Normal supraspinatus
tendon on T2

Musculotendinous junction at
12 o'clock position of humeral head

A

B

Thickened SST with
intermediate T2 signal

Intact bursal surface of SST

Fluid within SASD bursa

C

Partial articular-side
SST avulsion

D

Full-thickness SST tear
with 1 cm retraction

FIGURE 4-37 Appearance of rotator cuff tears on MRI. **A,** Normal. **B,** Thickened supraspinatus tendon (SST). **C,** Partial SST avulsion. **D,** Full-thickness SST tear with fluid within subacromial-subdeltoid (SASD) space.

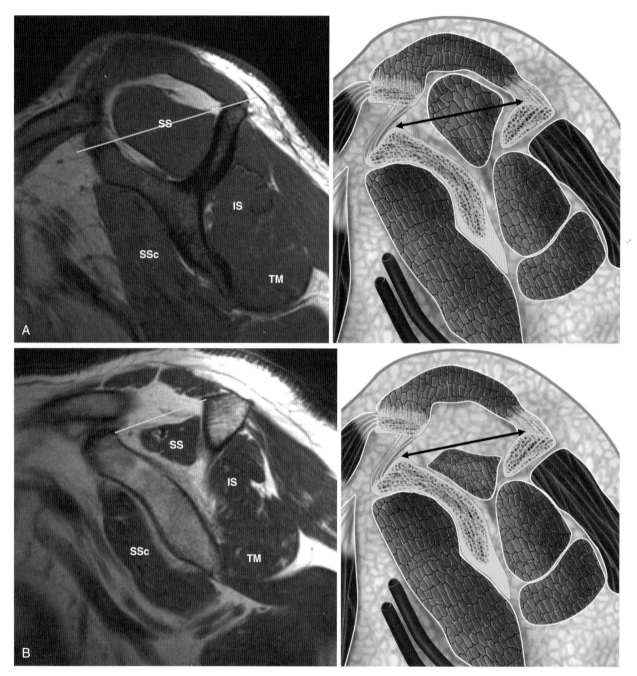

FIGURE 4-38 The tangent sign. This is defined as failure of the supraspinatus muscle belly to cross a line from the superior border of the coracoid to the superior border of the scapular spine. It correlates with muscular atrophy and fatty infiltration of the supraspinatus. **A,** Normal. **B,** Positive tangent sign. *IS,* Infraspinatus; *SS,* supraspinatus; *SSc,* subscapularis; *TM,* teres minor.

- A well-balanced partial repair is comparable to total repair.
- Latissimus dorsi tendon transfer may be considered in the younger patient with massive rotator cuff tear or significant fatty atrophy.
- A reverse total shoulder arthroplasty may be considered in an older patient with massive rotator cuff tear and other poor prognostic indicators.

SUBSCAPULARIS TEARS

- May occur after anterior dislocation and anterior shoulder surgery (e.g., shoulder arthroplasty)
- Symptoms include increased external rotation and the presence of a liftoff, modified liftoff, or belly-press sign.

- The appearance of an empty bicipital groove on axial MRI, with tear of the transverse humeral ligament, is often associated with subscapularis tear.
- At arthroscopy, a chronic subscapularis tear can be identified by the *comma sign,* which represents an avulsed sghl and chl (so-called comma tissue).
- Surgical treatment, either open or arthroscopic, is generally indicated; in chronic cases, a pectoralis transfer is occasionally required.
- Transfer of the pectoralis major places the musculocutaneous nerve at risk.

ROTATOR CUFF ARTHROPATHY

- Defined as a massive rotator cuff tear combined with fixed superior migration of the humeral head and severe

glenohumeral arthrosis, presumably caused by chronic loss of the concavity-compression effect
- Tendon transfer (latissimus/teres) for younger, active patients has been advocated.
- Inferior results have been reported for latissimus transfer in the presence of a subscapularis tear. This is due to a loss of the centering effect of the subscapularis on the humeral head during abduction and elevation.
- Hemiarthroplasty might be helpful if the anterior deltoid is preserved.
- This is a good option for patients whose predominant symptom is pain.
- Use of a reverse total shoulder arthroplasty (rtsa) has become increasingly popular for treatment of rotator cuff arthropathy.
  - It requires a competent deltoid and good glenoid bone stock.
  - It is recommended only for older patients (typically > 70 years) with low functional demands.
  - More predictable functional results are seen with the reverse prosthesis than with hemiarthroplasty, but a high rate of complications (40%) has been reported with its use.

SUBCORACOID IMPINGEMENT

- Patients with long or excessively laterally placed coracoid processes may have impingement of this process on the proximal humerus with forward flexion (120-130 degrees) and internal rotation of the arm.
- It may occur after surgery that causes posterior capsular tightness and loss of internal rotation.
- Local anesthetic injection should relieve these symptoms.
- CT performed with the arms crossed on the chest is helpful in evaluating this problem.
- A distance of less than 7 mm between the humerus and coracoid process is considered abnormal.
- Treatment of chronic symptoms involves resection of the lateral aspect of the coracoid process and reattachment of the conjoined tendon to the remaining coracoid.
- Arthroscopic coracoplasty has also been successful in treating this condition without detachment of the conjoined muscle group.

INTERNAL IMPINGEMENT

- Also termed *secondary impingement*
- Defined as contact between the articular side of the rotator cuff and the posterosuperior rim of the glenoid labrum when the arm is abducted and externally rotated
  - Occurs in the late cocking and early acceleration phases of throwing
- Etiology somewhat controversial
  - Alteration in glenohumeral kinematics leads to a posterosuperior shift of the humeral head; abduction and external rotation of the arm, in turn, lead to the internal impingement.
  - It is often associated with GIRD secondary to a tight posteroinferior capsule. (See Biomechanics; Throwing.)
  - This may cause pain associated with SLAP/biceps anchor disease, as well as undersurface rotator cuff tears of the posterior aspect of the supraspinatus and infraspinatus tendons.

- Presents with pain in the late cocking phase of throwing and associated loss of velocity and lack of command
- Bennett lesion (mineralization of the posterior inferior glenoid) is occasionally seen on radiographs or CT.
- Diagnosis can be aided with MR arthrography.
  - An abduction–external rotation (ABER) view may shows the internal impingement and associated lesions.
- Treatment
  - Primary treatment should include physical therapy and avoidance of aggravating activities.
  - Patients with GIRD may benefit from posterior and posteroinferior capsular stretching exercises such as the sleeper stretch, as well as stretching of the pectoralis minor tendon.
  - Operative treatment includes arthroscopic débridement or repair of the labrum, with débridement of the undersurface rotator cuff lesion.
    - A "peel-back" phenomenon of the superior labrum can be appreciated intraoperatively with abduction and external rotation of the arm.
  - Some authorities suggest repairing the rotator cuff if it is significantly thinned either by a transcuff technique or by taking down the remaining thinned cuff and advancing the unaffected normal tendon.
  - A posterior capsular release can be considered in patients who have GIRD and in whom nonoperative stretching has not caused improvement.

SUPERIOR LABRUM ANTERIOR TO POSTERIOR (SLAP) LESIONS

- Introduction
  - SLAP tears are uncommon injuries; comprise approximately 5% of all shoulder injuries
  - The superior labrum is more loosely adherent to the glenoid compared with the anterior-inferior labrum. Typically it attaches more medially, off the glenoid face.
  - Biceps tendon insertion into the superior labrum is complex:
    - 50% of tendon fibers insert to superior labrum
    - 50% insert to supraglenoid tubercle
      - 6.6 mm from the glenoid face at the 12 o'clock position
  - A variety of anatomic variants occur at the superior labrum and may be mistaken for pathology (Figure 4-39).
    - Three most common are a sublabral foramen, sublabral foramen with a thickened middle glenohumeral ligament (9% of shoulders), and the *Buford complex*, defined as an absent anterosuperior labrum with a thickened middle glenohumeral ligament (1.5% of shoulders).
    - Attempted repair with attachment of MGHL to the glenoid rim may result in limited shoulder external rotation
  - The original Snyder classification is most commonly used and has been expanded from four types to many more (Figure 4-40; see Table 4-10).
    - Type II is the most common (IIA is anterior, IIB is posterior, IIC is anterior and posterior).
- History and physical examination
  - May be traumatic or insidious onset of pain and mechanical symptoms

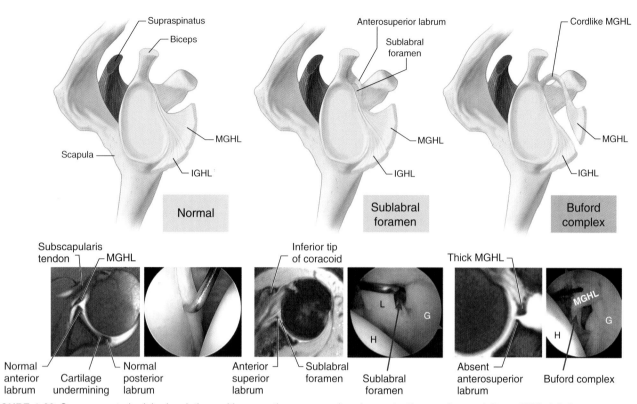

FIGURE 4-39 Common anterior labral variations with magnetic resonance imaging and arthroscopic correlations. *IGHL,* Inferior glenohumeral ligament; *MGHL,* middle glenohumeral ligament.

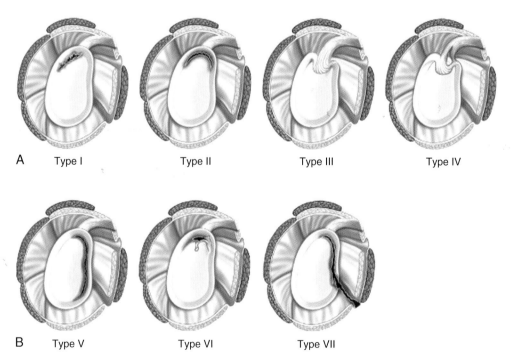

FIGURE 4-40 Expanded Snyder classification of SLAP (superior labrum from anterior to posterior) tears. **A,** Types I to IV. **B,** Types V to VII. (From Kepler CK, et al: Superior labral tear. In Reider B, Terry M, Provencher MT, editors: *Operative techniques: sports medicine surgery,* Philadelphia, Saunders Elsevier, 2009.)

TYPE	DESCRIPTION	TREATMENT
	Table 4-10	**Classification and Treatment of SLAP Tears**
I	Biceps fraying, intact anchor on superior labrum	Arthroscopic débridement
II	Detachment of biceps anchor	Repair versus tenotomy/tenodesis
III	Bucket-handle superior labral tear; biceps intact	Arthroscopic débridement
IV	Bucket-handle tear of superior labrum into biceps	<30% of tendon involvement: débridement >30%: repair or débridement and/or tenodesis of tendon
V	Labral tear + SLAP lesion	Stabilization of both
VI	Superior flap tear	Débridement
VII	Capsular injury + SLAP lesion	Repair and stabilization

- Traction, compression, or repetitive overhead throwing mechanism
- No single physical examination maneuver is specific for SLAP tear.
  - O'Brien test, compression-rotation test, Speed test, dynamic labral shear test, Kibler anterior slide test, crank test, and Kim biceps load test (see Table 4-6)

- **Imaging**
- MR arthrography is the modality of choice.
- Diagnosed either by abnormal morphology of the superior labrum or increased signal in the substance or under the superior labrum (Figure 4-41)
  - Signal that appears irregular and extends lateral to the glenoid or posterior to the biceps tendon is suggestive of a SLAP tear.
- **A paralabral cyst is indicative of a SLAP tear (or posterior labral tear).**
  - **Cyst may extend to spinoglenoid notch and compress the suprascapular nerve, leading to infraspinatus wasting**
- **Treatment (Table 4-10)**
- Highly controversial, particularly regarding type II lesions
- Nonoperative management
  - Should be attempted in virtually all patients
  - Rotator cuff strengthening and scapular stabilization
  - Throwers benefit from stretching of the posterior capsule.
  - Intraarticular injections
- Operative management
  - Arthroscopy may demonstrate a "peel-back" test where the posterosuperior labrum detaches in abduction and external rotation (the late cocking phase).
  - Surgical technique is dictated by the type of SLAP tear.
  - Controversy exists regarding repair versus tenotomy/tenodesis of type II lesions.
    - Some consensus that patients older than 40 years with obvious biceps pathology and degenerative labral changes are best treated with débridement and tenotomy/tenodesis

- If repair is chosen, there is conflicting biomechanical evidence to suggest one repair technique over another.
- If concomitant rotator cuff tear, recent studies have found no advantage to repairing SLAP at time of rotator cuff repair. May result in increased rate of stiffness if repaired.
  - Recent studies have suggested biceps tenotomy should be performed at the time of rotator cuff repair.
- **Postoperative rehabilitation**
- **Relatively high incidence of postoperative stiffness, so motion is begun early. Pendulums are initiated immediately.**
- **Passive and active assisted exercises are begun 7 to 10 days postoperatively.**
- Avoid resistive biceps exercises and external rotation with the arm in 90 degrees of abduction.
- **Complications**
- Stiffness is common after SLAP repair. One study demonstrated a 78% rate of stiffness.
  - Stiffness should be initially managed with physical therapy. If symptoms persist, arthroscopic capsular release may be performed.
- Persistent symptoms, articular cartilage injury, and loose or prominent hardware are other frequent complications following SLAP repair.

PROXIMAL BICEPS TENDON PATHOLOGY

- **Biceps tendinitis**
- Often associated with impingement, rotator cuff tears (subscapularis and leading-edge supraspinatus tears), and stenosis of the bicipital groove
- Like most other cases of "tendinitis," this is probably best considered to be a "tendinosis."
- Diagnosis is made by direct palpation with the arm externally rotated 10 degrees, and confirmed with Speed and Yergason tests.
- Initial management includes strengthening and local corticosteroid injection (around but not into the tendon).
- Surgical release (with or without tenodesis) is usually reserved for refractory cases.
- **Tenotomy without tenodesis is associated with subjective cramping and potential for cosmetic deformity ("Popeye deformity"). Weakness is not associated with tenotomy**
- Tenodesis may result in "groove pain" if the technique of the tenodesis retains portion of the tendon in the intertubercular groove. A subpectoral tenodesis technique reduces the risk of groove pain.
- **Biceps tendon subluxation**
- **Most commonly associated with a partial or complete subscapularis tear** (Figure 4-42)
  - Tear of the coracohumeral ligament or transverse humeral ligament may produce tendon subluxation as well.
- Arm abduction and external rotation may produce a palpable click as the tendon subluxates or dislocates outside the groove.
- Nonoperative treatment is similar to that for tendinitis, whereas operative treatment includes repair of the subscapularis and supporting structures of the bicipital groove but more often involves tenotomy or tenodesis with or without a subscapularis repair.

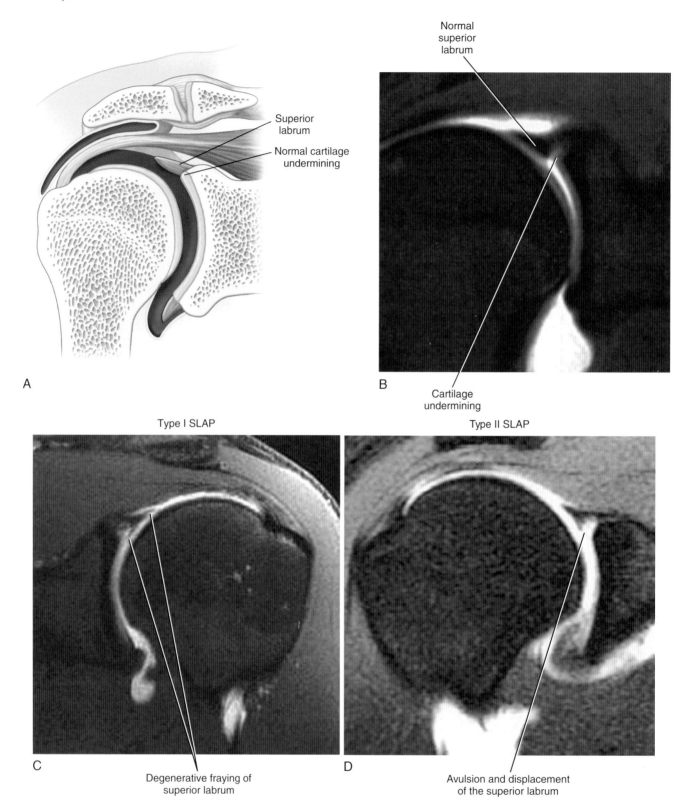

FIGURE 4-41 Appearance of SLAP tears on MRI. **A and B,** Normal anatomy. **C,** Type I SLAP. **D,** Type II SLAP.

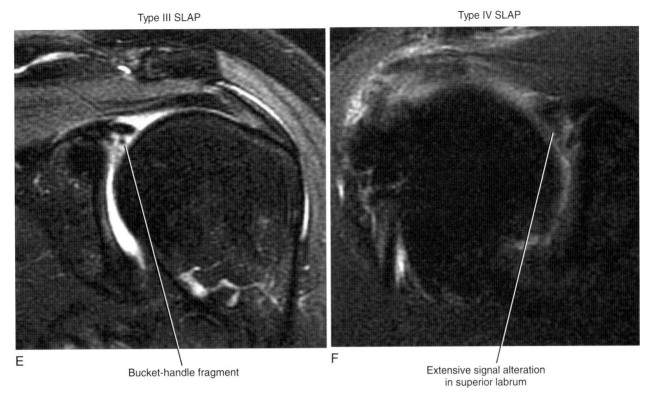

Type III SLAP

Type IV SLAP

E

Bucket-handle fragment

F

Extensive signal alteration
in superior labrum

FIGURE 4-41, cont'd E, Type III SLAP. **F,** Type IV SLAP.

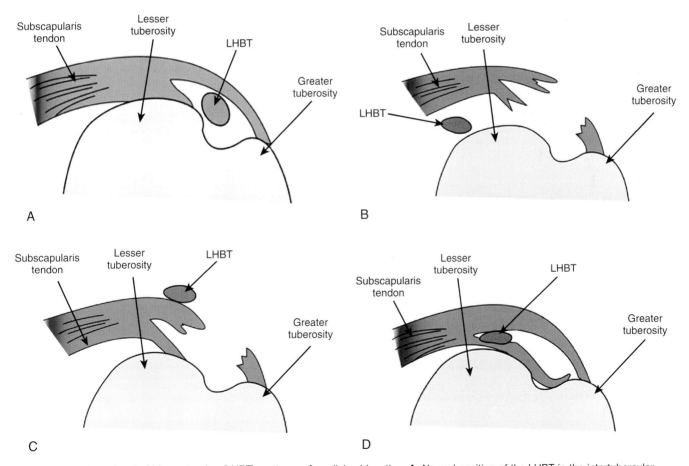

FIGURE 4-42 Long head of biceps tendon (LHBT), patterns of medial subluxation. **A,** Normal position of the LHBT in the intertubercular groove. **B,** Disruption or avulsion of the deep fibers of the subscapularis tendon off of the lesser tuberosity in conjunction with disruption of the coracohumeral ligament allows intraarticular subluxation of the LHBT. **C,** Disruption of the transverse humeral ligament along with disruption of the coracohumeral ligament allows extraarticular medial subluxation of the LHBT. **D,** Disruption of the coracohumeral ligament with an intact subscapularis tendon allows the LHBT to sublux medially into the substance of the subscapularis tendon, resulting in an interstitial tear of the subscapularis tendon and muscle.

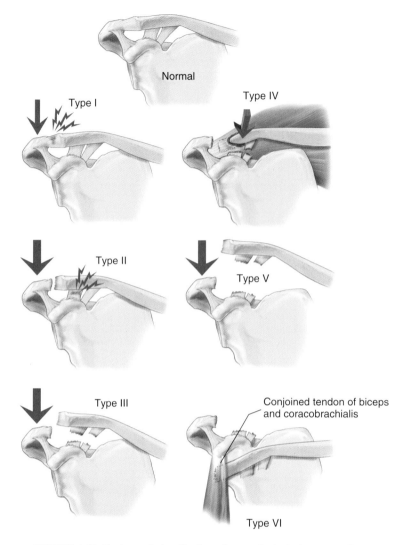

Normal

Type I

Type IV

Type II

Type V

Type III

Conjoined tendon of biceps and coracobrachialis

Type VI

FIGURE 4-43 Rockwood classification of acromioclavicular separations.

ACROMIOCLAVICULAR AND STERNOCLAVICULAR INJURIES

■ Acromioclavicular separation

▥ Overview
- These injuries are typically caused by a direct blow to the shoulder, are common athletic injuries, and can be classified into six types (Figure 4-43 and Table 4-11).
- A Zanca view is obtained to visualize the acromioclavicular joint. The x-ray beam is directed 10 degrees cephalad at 50% of normal penetrance (see Table 4-7).
- Type V injury is defined by a coracoclavicular distance that is greater than 100% that of the opposite side (bilateral acromioclavicular views are required).
- Type IV injury can be diagnosed on only an axillary lateral view.

▥ Conservative management
- **A brief period of immobilization followed by rehabilitation is appropriate for types I, II, and many III.**

▥ Treatment of type III injuries
- Management of type III injuries is somewhat controversial; most authorities advocate conservative treatment, especially in elderly patients, inactive patients, or patients who do not perform manual labor. Some authorities advocate surgical reduction and repair or reconstruction.
- The literature suggests that among patients treated immediately with surgery, the need for reoperation is higher than with primary surgery for those who are initially treated nonoperatively.

▥ Management of types IV through VI injuries
- These are typically treated surgically.

▥ Surgical treatment of failed conservatively treated injuries or acute treatment
- Reconstruction of the coracoclavicular ligament with a free soft tissue graft is becoming popular to allow for an anatomic reconstruction. Excessive medialization of the clavicular tunnels has been associated with a higher rate of failure.
- The coracoid tunnel technique is associated with a risk of coracoid fracture.
- The distal clavicle is often resected in the chronic situation, and the coracoacromial ligament may then be transferred to the distal clavicle (modified Weaver-Dunn procedure).
- Backup coracoclavicular stabilization is usually required for a successful outcome.

Table 4-11	Acromioclavicular Joint Injury Patterns and Management					
TYPE	**AC LIGAMENT INJURY**	**CC LIGAMENT INJURY**	**DELTOTRAPEZIAL FASCIA**	**CLINICAL FINDINGS**	**RADIOGRAPHIC FINDINGS**	**TREATMENT**
I	Intact	Intact	Intact	AC tenderness	Normal	Nonoperative
II	Ruptured	Intact	Intact	Pain with motion; clavicle is unstable in horizontal plane	Lateral end of clavicle is slightly elevated; stress views show < 100% separation	Nonoperative
III	Ruptured	Ruptured	Mild injury	Clavicle is unstable in both horizontal and vertical planes, extremity is adducted, and acromion is depressed relative to clavicle	Plain films and stress radiographs are abnormal—100% separation; in reality, acromion and upper extremity are displaced inferior to lateral clavicle	Nonoperative; consider operative if overhead athlete or heavy laborer
IV	Ruptured	Ruptured	Injured as clavicle is posteriorly displaced	Possible skin tenting and posterior fullness	Clavicle is displaced posteriorly on axillary view	Operative
V	Ruptured	Ruptured	Injured and stripped off clavicle	More severe type III injury; shoulder with severe droop; type III injury if shoulder shrug does not reduce it	100% to 300% increase in clavicle-to-acromion distance	Operative
VI	Ruptured	Ruptured	Possible injury	Rare inferior dislocation of distal clavicle; accompanied by other severe injuries; transient paresthesias	Clavicle is lodged behind intact conjoined tendon	Operative

From Miller MS, Thompson SR: *DeLee and Drez's orthopaedic sports medicine,* ed 4, Philadelphia, Saunders, 2014, Table 60-2.

■ **Acromioclavicular degenerative joint disease**

▨ As a result of the transmission of large loads through a small surface area, the acromioclavicular joint may begin to degenerate as early as the second decade of life.

▨ In addition, direct blows or low-grade acromioclavicular separation may cause posttraumatic arthritis.

▨ Diagnosed by direct palpation; other diagnostic features are pain elicited by crossed-chest adduction, radiographic evidence of osteophytes and joint-space narrowing, and pain relief with selective acromioclavicular joint injection.

▨ **Treatment includes both open and arthroscopic distal clavicle resections (Mumford procedure) with resection of less than 1 cm of the distal clavicle to preserve the posterior-superior capsule and avoid anterior and posterior instability and pain.**

▨ Arthroscopic excision has the advantage of allowing evaluation of the glenohumeral joint at time of surgery.

■ **Distal clavicle osteolysis**

▨ Common in weightlifters and in persons with a history of traumatic injury

▨ Radiographs of the distal clavicle reveal osteopenia, osteolysis, tapering, and cystic changes.

▨ After failure of selective corticosteroid injection, NSAIDs, and activity modification, this condition responds favorably to distal clavicle excision.

■ **Sternoclavicular subluxation and dislocation**

▨ Often caused by motor vehicle accidents or direct trauma but can be spontaneous and atraumatic during overhead elevation of the arm

▨ The posterior capsule is the most important anatomic restraint for anteroposterior translation.

▨ Plain imaging includes the Hobbs and Serendipity views; best diagnosed by CT.

▨ Closed reduction is often successful.

• Anterior dislocation should be first treated with acute closed reduction.

• **Posterior dislocation should be treated with closed reduction and open reduction if necessary, particularly with compression of the posterior structures.** Consultation with a cardiothoracic surgeon may be appropriate.

▨ Use of hardware should be avoided whenever possible.

▨ Failures of reductions and chronic dislocations are treated conservatively.

MUSCLE RUPTURES

■ **Pectoralis major**

▨ Injury to this muscle is caused by excessive tension on a maximally eccentrically contracted muscle, often found in weightlifters.

▨ Most commonly results in a tendinous avulsion

▨ Localized swelling and ecchymosis, a palpable defect (axillary webbing), and weakness with adduction and internal rotation are characteristic findings.

▨ Surgical repair to bone is performed in complete ruptures. Partial ruptures may be treated nonoperatively.

▨ Pectoralis major ruptures have not been reported in women.

■ **Deltoid**

▨ Complete rupture of this muscle is unusual; injuries are most often strains or partial tears.

▨ Repair to bone is required for complete ruptures.

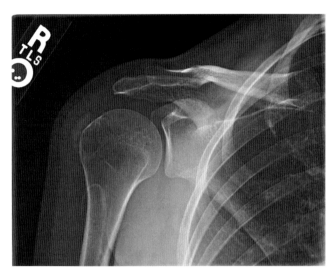

FIGURE 4-44 Radiographic appearance of calcific tendonitis.

- Iatrogenic injury occasionally occurs during open rotator cuff repair; some patients require deltoidplasty, which consists of mobilization and anterior transfer of the middle third of the deltoid. Unfortunately, this procedure is not always possible or successful.

■ Triceps
- Ruptures of the triceps are most often associated with systemic illness (e.g., renal osteodystrophy) or steroid use.
- Primary repair of avulsions is indicated.

■ Latissimus dorsi rupture
- This is a very rare condition manifesting with local tenderness and pain with shoulder adduction and internal rotation.
- Although nonoperative treatment may allow resumption of activities, operative repair has been described for high-demand athletes.

■ Calcific tendonitis
- A self-limiting condition of unknown origin that affects predominantly the supraspinatus tendon and occurs slightly more frequently in women.
  - Not related to a generalized disease process
- Calcium is deposited in the fibrocartilaginous matrix of the tendon as calcium carbonate apatite
- Three stages have been elucidated: precalcific, calcific, and postcalcific. Calcific stage is subdivided into formative and resorptive phases.
  - Resorptive phase associated with acute, sudden onset of extremely severe pain
- Radiographs demonstrate characteristic calcification within the tendon (Figure 4-44).
- Nonoperative treatment is the rule, consisting of physical therapy, modalities, and injections.
- "Needling" of the lesion under image guidance has been described and is often successful.
- Arthroscopic or open removal of the deposit is occasionally necessary.
- The rotator cuff should be repaired if it is significantly involved.

SHOULDER STIFFNESS

■ A stiff shoulder may be posttraumatic, postsurgical, or the result of "frozen shoulder."

- Posttraumatic or postsurgical stiffness results from excessive scar formation
- Motion loss is related to the area of surgery or trauma and may involve the humeroscapular motion interface between the proximal humerus and overlying deltoid and conjoined tendon, as well as contracture of the rotator cuff and capsule.
- Initial nonoperative management is the rule
- Prolonged posttraumatic shoulder stiffness is unlikely to respond to nonsurgical treatment, and a manipulation under anesthesia and open or arthroscopic lysis of adhesions may be performed.

■ Frozen shoulder
- This disorder (also known as *adhesive capsulitis*) is characterized by pain and restricted glenohumeral joint motion, especially external rotation.
- Typically affects individuals aged 40 to 70 years. The nondominant side is more frequently affected.
- The majority of cases are idiopathic. Patients with diabetes or thyroid disease are disproportionally affected. Other associations are trauma after chest or breast surgery and prolonged immobilization.
- The essential lesion involves the coracohumeral ligament and the rotator interval capsule.
- **Histologically there is evidence of inflammation and fibrosis. There is a dense matrix of type-III collagen containing fibroblasts and myofibroblasts that appear similar to Dupuytren disease**
- **Diagnosis is clinical, typically an insidious onset of pain followed by selective loss of external rotation. In later stages, global ROM loss occurs. Classically, active ROM and passive ROM are equivalent.**
  - Other two causes of selective loss of external rotation are glenohumeral osteoarthritis and a locked posterior shoulder dislocation. For this reason, radiographs must be obtained prior to making a diagnosis of frozen shoulder.
- Arthrography may demonstrate a loss of the normal axillary recess, revealing contracture of the joint capsule.
- MRI may demonstrate thickening of the glenohumeral joint capsule along the axillary pouch, thickening of the coracohumeral ligament, obliteration of the subcoracoid fat triangle and rotator interval synovitis. However, none of these are pathognomonic.
- Overwhelmingly the majority may be treated nonoperatively. Approximately 90% of patients respond to physical therapy, corticosteroid injection, and NSAIDs. Occasionally, distention arthrography is employed.
- Patients who fail 12 to 16 weeks of nonsurgical treatment are offered arthroscopic capsular release.
  - This procedure places the axillary nerve at risk.
  - Selective capsular release versus complete capsular release techniques are employed.

NERVE DISORDERS

■ Brachial plexus injury
- Minor traction and compression injuries, commonly known by football players as "burners" or "stingers," can be serious if they are recurrent or persist for more than a short time.
- Results from compression of the plexus between the shoulder pad and the superior medial scapula

when the pad is compressed into the Erb point (superior to the clavicle).

▤ Complete resolution of symptoms is required before the patient returns to play.

▤ If burners occur more than one time, the player should be removed from competition until cervical spine radiographs can be obtained.

▤ Brachial plexus injuries can also be seen following anterior glenohumeral dislocations and should not be confused with massive rotator cuff tears.

■ **Thoracic outlet syndrome**

▤ Results from compression of the nerves and vessels that pass through the scalene muscles and first rib

▤ This condition can be associated with cervical rib, scapular ptosis, or scalene muscle abnormalities.

▤ Patients may note pain and ulnar paresthesias.

▤ Positive findings with the Wright test (see Table 4-6) and on neurologic evaluation can be diagnostic.

▤ First-rib resection is occasionally required.

■ **Long thoracic nerve palsy**

▤ Injury to this nerve can result in medial scapular winging secondary to serratus anterior dysfunction (see Scapular winging later).

▤ This condition can be caused by a compression injury (e.g., in backpackers) or a traction injury (as seen in weightlifters).

▤ Simple observation is usually called for because many of these injuries spontaneously resolve within 18 months.

▤ Treatment with a modified thoracolumbar brace may be beneficial, and in rare cases, pectoralis major transfer may be required for chronic palsies that do not improve.

■ **Suprascapular nerve compression**

▤ This nerve may become compressed by various structures, including a ganglion in the spinoglenoid notch or suprascapular notch and a fracture callus in the area of the transverse scapular ligament (Figure 4-45).

▤ **Weakness and atrophy of the supraspinatus (proximal lesions) and infraspinatus are present along with pain over the dorsal aspect of the shoulder.**

  • Cysts within the spinoglenoid notch affect only the infraspinatus.

▤ Electrodiagnostic studies and MRI may confirm and elucidate the nature of the nerve compression.

▤ Compression caused by a cyst in association with a SLAP lesion may respond to arthroscopic decompression and labral repair (Figure 4-46).

▤ In the absence of a structural lesion, release of the transverse scapular ligament may provide relief.

■ **Quadrilateral space syndrome**

▤ This condition is defined as axillary nerve or posterior humeral circumflex artery compression within the quadrilateral space.

▤ Most commonly caused by a fibrous band between the teres major and the long head of the triceps

▤ Characterized by pain and paresthesias with overhead activity, as well as weakness or atrophy of the teres minor and deltoid

▤ Most often seen in athletes who participate in throwing activities; associated with late cocking and acceleration with the abducted, extended, and externally rotated arm. Diagnosis is confirmed by the arteriographic appearance of compression of the posterior humeral circumflex artery.

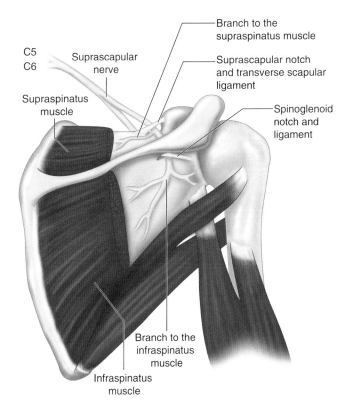

FIGURE 4-45 Anatomy of the suprascapular nerve and potential sites of compression.

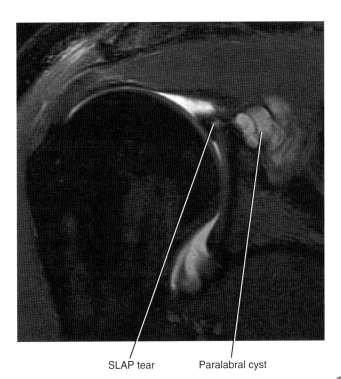

FIGURE 4-46 SLAP tear with adjacent paralabral cyst. Coronal T2-weighted image demonstrates abnormal signal within the superior labrum representing a SLAP tear and an adjacent paralabral cyst dissecting into the suprascapular notch.

■ **Other nerve injuries**

▤ Other injuries—including those of the axillary nerve, spinal accessory nerve (lateral scapular winging), and musculocutaneous nerve—are usually the result of surgical injury to these structures.

- Observation for several months is appropriate before exploration and repair of the affected nerve is considered.
- **Severe combined neurologic injury resulting in rotator cuff and deltoid paralysis that has failed neurolysis and tendon transfer may be treated with shoulder arthrodesis.**

OTHER SHOULDER DISORDERS

■ Glenohumeral degenerative joint disease

- Although it is more common in older patients, athletes who engage in throwing may develop arthritis at a younger age than usual.
- Osteoarthrosis typically results in posterior glenoid wear, whereas rheumatoid arthritis results in central glenoid wear.

- Arthritis may also be associated with other shoulder disorders, including instability and rotator cuff disease.
- Certain iatrogenic factors may also contribute to the development of osteoarthritis of the shoulder, including the use of hardware in and around the shoulder and overtightening of the shoulder capsule during shoulder reconstruction.
- Chondrolysis, possibly secondary to thermal ablation or intraarticular pain pumps, is another iatrogenic factor in degenerative joint disease.
- Radiographs, including a true anteroposterior view taken in abduction, can be helpful in characterizing the amount of arthritis.
- In some cases, arthroscopic débridement may be a temporizing measure before joint arthroplasty is considered.
- Progressive pain, decreased ROM, and inability to perform activities of daily living are reasonable

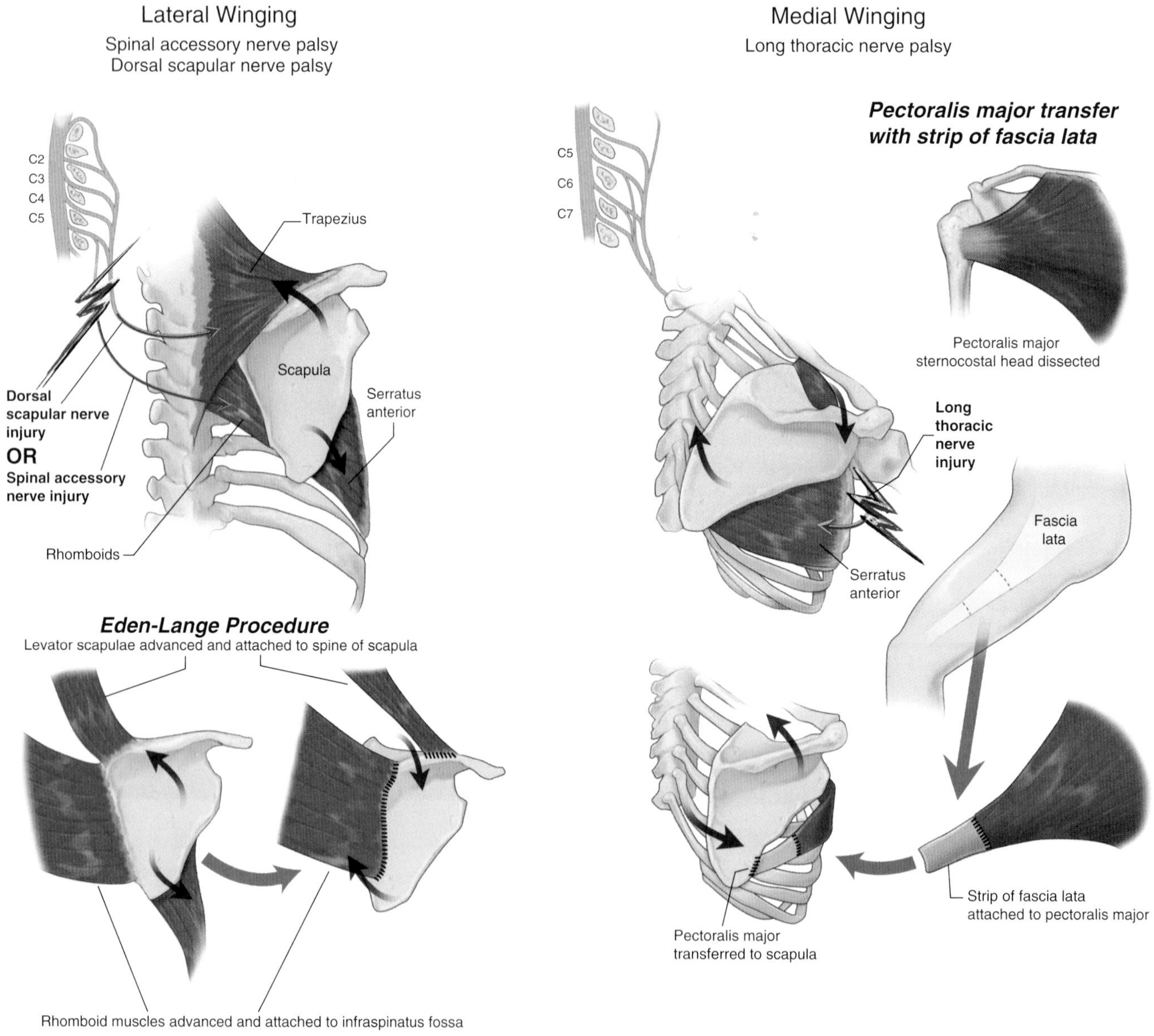

FIGURE 4-47 Lateral and medial scapular winging. Lateral winging may be treated with the Eden-Lange procedure in which the levator scapulae and rhomboid are transferred laterally on the scapula. Medial winging may be treated with pectoralis major transfer supplemented with a strip of fascia lata.

indications for considering prosthetic replacement or humeral head resurfacing.

- Complications of arthroplasty most commonly include glenoid loosening.
- **Scapulothoracic crepitus**
- Also known as *snapping scapula syndrome*
- Manifestation: painful scapulothoracic crepitus in association with elevation of the arm
- Scapulothoracic dyskinesis may be present, and pain is generally relieved with manual stabilization of the scapula.
- Many possible causes of symptomatic crepitus exist.
- The differential diagnosis includes osteochondroma and elastofibroma dorsi.
- Patients may respond to scapular strengthening exercises, local corticosteroid injections, or antiinflammatory medications.
- For more refractory cases, open or arthroscopic bursectomy and sometimes resection of the superomedial scapular border are necessary.
- **Scapular winging (Figure 4-47)**
- Can occur as a result of a nerve injury, bony abnormality, muscle contracture, intraarticular disease, or voluntarily
- The description of the direction of the winging is based on the movement of the inferior border of the scapula.
- **Nerve injuries include injury to the spinal accessory nerve (trapezius palsy, lateral winging), the long thoracic nerve (serratus anterior palsy, medial winging), and the dorsal scapular nerve (rhomboid palsy).**
- Osseous causes include osteochondromas and fracture malunions.
- Selective muscle strengthening may ameliorate winging.
- Surgical treatment includes lateral transfer of the levator scapulae and rhomboid muscles (Eden-Lange procedure) for lateral winging and pectoralis major transfer for medial winging.
- **Complex regional pain syndrome (formerly known as *reflex sympathetic dystrophy*)**
- As in the knee, this condition responds poorly to both conservative and surgical treatments.
- In a litigious medicolegal environment, it is often associated with malingering and issues of secondary gain.
- Diagnosis may be confirmed with a three-phase bone scan.
- Treatment options are numerous and may include sympathetic nerve block.

- **Little Leaguer shoulder**
- Commonly occurs in young baseball players and is actually a Salter-Harris type I fracture or stress reaction of the proximal humerus
- Overuse of the shoulder as a result of failure to limit pitch count and provide periods of adequate rest are the key factors implicated in the development of this condition.
- It has also been suggested that breaking pitches not be thrown until after skeletal maturity is reached.
- Radiographs may demonstrate widening of the proximal humeral physis in comparison with the contralateral proximal humerus (Figure 4-48).
- MRI can assist with the diagnosis if it is in question.
- The condition responds to rest and activity modification, with return to play allowed when symptoms have resolved completely.
- Recommendations regarding age and pitch counts have been made.

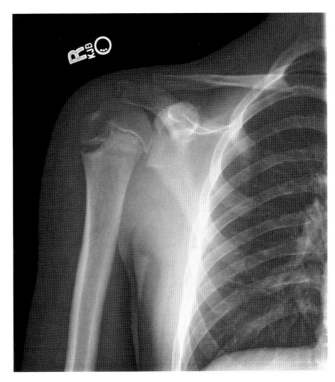

FIGURE 4-48 Radiographic appearance of Little Leaguer shoulder demonstrating widening of the proximal humeral physis.

SECTION 4 MEDICAL ASPECTS OF SPORTS MEDICINE

PREPARTICIPATION PHYSICAL EXAMINATION

- History and physical examination most helpful and cost-effective for identifying musculoskeletal and medical problems
- Family history of sudden cardiac death or any personal history of exertional chest pain or dyspnea necessitates further evaluation and cardiac workup.
- For National Collegiate Athletic Association (NCAA) purposes, final responsibility for medical disqualification rests with the team physician. life-threatening illnesses must be reported and are adequate grounds for disqualification

MUSCLE PHYSIOLOGY

- **Three types of muscle: I, IIA, and IIB**
- Type I muscle is slow twitching/aerobic and is helpful in endurance sports.
  - Training can increase the number of mitochondria and increase capillary density.

- Types IIA and IIB muscles are fast twitching/anaerobic and are helpful for sprinters.
- **These muscles have high contraction speeds, quick relaxation, and low triglyceride stores.**
- **The mode of energy utilization differentiates type iia from type iib muscle: iia has both aerobic and anaerobic capabilities, whereas iib is primarily anaerobic.**
- **Immobilization of muscle results in a shorter position with a decreased ability to generate tension.**

EXERCISE

- **Benefits**
- Done on a regular basis, exercise can decrease heart rate and blood pressure (hypertension), decrease insulin requirements in diabetic patients, decrease cardiovascular risk, and increase lean body mass.
- Also been shown to reduce risk of cancer, osteoporosis, and hypercholesterolemia
- **Aerobic threshold and conditioning**
- The aerobic threshold can be determined by measuring oxygen consumption and is useful for evaluating endurance athletes.
- Sports-specific conditioning involves aerobic and anaerobic conditioning in different proportions in accordance with the season and sport.
- In the off-season, long-distance runs can enable sprinters to increase aerobic recovery capability after sprints.
- Several exercise categories have been described. Stretching has also been shown to have a beneficial effect.
- **Delayed-onset muscle soreness**
- This condition often follows unaccustomed eccentric exercise, usually appearing 24 to 48 hours after the activity.
- Cause involves inflammation and edema of the connective tissue, with elevated creatine kinase levels

CARDIAC ABNORMALITIES IN ATHLETES

- **Sudden cardiac death**
- Usually related to an underlying heart condition
- Hypertrophic cardiomyopathy is the most common cause of sudden death in young athletes. Commotio cordis is second most common.
- Screening that includes electrocardiography (ECG) can identify this problem early.
  - Universal screening of athletes with an ECG is controversial and varies across the world.
- Diastolic murmurs found on routine examination warrant further cardiac evaluation.
- **Hypertrophic cardiomyopathy**
- Autosomal dominant with variable penetrance; thousands of mutations affect more than 10 genes
- May be asymptomatic or may present with exertional dyspnea or fatigue
- Murmurs that increase in intensity with Valsalva maneuvers are consistent with hypertrophic cardiomyopathy.
- Sports participation is contraindicated
- **Commotio cordis**
- Defined as sudden death from relatively mild chest wall impact
- Precise mechanism is unknown but may be due to onset of ventricular fibrillation from direct impact. The timing of impact during the cardiac cycle may be critical;

experimental evidence suggests the impact must occur 15 to 30 milliseconds before the T-wave peak.
  - This represents only 1% of the cardiac cycle and may help explain the rarity of the condition.
- Typically occurs in adolescents, and males account for 95% of victims
  - More compliant chest walls are thought to be the reason for young-age affliction.
- Management is immediate cardiopulmonary resuscitation and cardioversion.
- Previous reported survival rates were between 10% and 25%, but recent reports suggest improved rates owing to increased awareness and availability of defibrillators.

CONCUSSION

- **Defined as a brain injury due to an impulsive force transmitted to the head**
- Typically results in functional impartment with no structural injury
- **Symptoms and signs of concussion are highly variable.**
- 90% of concussions do NOT involve a loss of consciousness
- Can present with a headache, emotional lability, cognitive impairment, behavioral changes and sleep disturbance
- **Sideline evaluation**
- First priority is to exclude a cervical spine injury
  - Cannot exclude a cervical spine injury if the patient is unconscious
  - If cervical spine injury is suspected, the patient should have a cervical collar placed and be transported on a backboard to hospital for further evaluation.
- Concussion should be evaluated using a sideline assessment tool such as the Sport Concussion Assessment Tool 3 (SCAT3). This tool includes concentration and memory tasks, as well as the Balance Error Scoring System and Glasgow Coma Scale.
- The patient should be closely monitored.
- **Any player with diagnosed concussion is not allowed to return to play on the day of injury. The player must be cleared by a licensed healthcare professional prior to returning to play thereafter.**
- **Concussion investigations**
- Brain CT scan is not routinely obtained unless evaluation suggests an intracerebral or structural lesion.
  - Indications include loss of consciousness for more than 5 minutes, a focal neurologic lesion, Glasgow Coma Scale score less than 15, or worsening symptoms.
- Neuropsychological testing
  - Useful as an adjunct but should not be used as a sole determination of when to return to play
- **Management**
- **Same-day return to play is prohibited.**
- Physical and cognitive rest are the cornerstones of management.
- Approximately 90% of patients will recover within 10 days.
  - Persistent symptoms should be managed in a multidisciplinary fashion.
- A gradual return-to-play and return-to-school protocol should be followed (Table 4-12)
- **Second-impact syndrome**
- May occur with a second minor blow before initial symptoms have resolved

Table 4-12 Zurich Graduated Return-to-Play Protocol

REHABILITATION STAGE	FUNCTIONAL EXERCISE AT EACH STAGE OF REHABILITATION	OBJECTIVE OF EACH STAGE
1. No activity	Complete physical and cognitive rest	Recovery
2. Light aerobic exercise	Walking, swimming, or stationary cycling, keeping intensity <70% of maximum predicted heart rate No resistance training	Increase heart rate
3. Sport-specific exercise	Skating drills in ice hockey, running drills in soccer; no head impact activities	Add movement
4. Noncontact training drills	Progression to more complex training drills, such as passing drills in football and ice hockey May start progressive resistance training	Exercise, coordination, and cognitive load
5. Full contact practice	After medical clearance, participate in normal training activities	Restore confidence and assess functional skills by coaching staff
6. Return to play	Normal game play	

- Leads to loss of autoregulation of the brain's blood supply and potential herniation
- Second-impact syndrome is associated with a mortality rate of 50%.
- **Complications**
- Posttraumatic headaches
  - Recent research has demonstrated athletes who have headaches following concussion have a protracted recovery rate.
- Depression
- Chronic traumatic encephalitis (CTE)
  - Mean age of onset, age 42 years
  - Earliest signs are cognitive difficulty.
  - Mood disturbance and suicidal ideation may be present.
- Chronic neurobehavioral impairment

SICKLE CELL DISEASE

- **Sickle cell disease is a condition of red blood cells; due to defect in the β-globin chain of adult hemoglobin (Hba) that produces sickle hemoglobin (HbS)**
- Inheritance of two copies of HbS results in an HbSS phenotype and sickle cell disease.
- Inheritance of a single copy of HbS results in an HbAS phenotype and sickle cell trait.
- **Sickle cell trait is extremely common in African Americans, with a prevalence of 8% to 10%.**
- **Typically, sickle cell trait is an asymptomatic condition.**
- However, significant exertional activity, such as sports participation or military training, can result in exertional sickling.
- Intense heat or extreme altitude can lower the threshold for exertional sickling.

- Recent data have demonstrated that athletes with sickle cell trait have a 37 times greater relative risk of sudden death.
- Many sporting organizations, including the NCAA, requiring screening via blood tests
- Notably, all U.S. states perform neonatal screening for sickle cell trait.
- **Three major concerns with sickle cell trait:**
- Exertional rhabdomyolysis
  - Life threatening
  - Sickled red blood cells result in muscle ischemia and rhabdomyolysis.
- Splenic infarction
  - Often precipitated at higher altitudes
  - Presents as left upper quadrant abdominal pain
- Gross hematuria
  - Typically occurs from left kidney and should prompt medical evaluation
- **Sickle cell trait is not a contraindication to participation in any athletic activity.**
- **Important precautions must be taken.**
- **Maintain hydration.**
- **Permit adequate rest and recovery between intense exercise.**
- **Allow access to supplemental oxygen, particularly when at altitude.**

METABOLIC ISSUES IN ATHLETES

- **Dehydration**
- Fluid and electrolyte loss can lead to decreased cardiovascular function and work capacity.
- Absorption is increased with solutions of low osmolarity (<10%).
- Hyponatremia should be suspected in individuals who have participated in prolonged vigorous exercise and have been consuming free water.
- Rehydration with carbohydrate-containing fluids is recommended for exercise lasting longer than an hour.
- **Nutritional supplements**
- Continue to be a source of controversy
- Creatine, one of the more popular supplements, increases water retention in cells.
- In-season use can increase the incidence of dehydration and cramps.

ERGOGENIC DRUGS

- **Anabolic steroids**
- Derivatives of testosterone are abused by athletes attempting to increase muscle mass and strength and increase erythropoiesis.
- Adverse effects include liver dysfunction, hypercholesterolemia, cardiomyopathy, testicular atrophy, hypercoagulability, fluid and electrolyte imbalances, gynecomastia, acne, mood disturbances (particularly increased aggression), and irreversible alopecia.
  - Heart disease can result from increased plasma levels of low-density lipoprotein and decreased levels of high-density lipoprotein.
- Urine sampling has been the standard for evaluation by the International Olympic Committee.

- **Human growth hormone (HGH)**
  - Made from recombinant DNA; illegal use of this drug is common
  - Athletes attempting to increase muscle size and weight abuse this drug, which has side effects similar to those of steroids, as well as hypertension and gigantism.
  - Difficult to detect if suspected
  - Insulinlike growth factor (IGF)-1 has effects similar to those of HGH.
- **Prohormones**
  - Derivatives of testosterone, dehydroepiandrosterone (DHEA) and androstenedione have been used as anabolic agents; their effects are controversial.

FEMALE ATHLETE–RELATED ISSUES

- **Physiologic differences**
  - Women are typically smaller and lighter and have higher percentages of body fat.
  - Lower maximal oxygen consumption, cardiac output, hemoglobin, and muscular mass and strength are also important considerations.
  - Other differences contribute to the increased incidence of patellofemoral disorders, stress fractures, and knee ACL injuries in girls and women (especially in basketball, soccer, and rugby).
- **Female athlete triad**
  - Originally defined as disordered eating, amenorrhea, and osteoporosis
  - **Current definition is low energy availability (with or without an eating disorder), menstrual dysfunction, and altered bone mineral density**
  - Energy availability
    - Decreased energy intake may be facilitated by purging, fasting, laxatives, diuretics, and diet pills.
    - Anorexia and bulimia are the most common forms of eating disorders.
  - Menstrual dysfunction
    - *Amenorrhea* is defined as absence of menstrual cycles lasting longer than 3 months. *Oligomenorrhea* is a menstrual cycle longer than 35 days.
    - Oligomenorrhea is extremely common in female athletes. Prevalence may be as high as 20% to 40%.
    - Menstrual dysfunction is thought to be due to low energy availability.
      - Occurs when intake falls below 30 kcal/kg lean body mass per day
  - Bone mineral density (BMD)
    - Dual energy x-ray absorptiometry (DEXA) is the study of choice for evaluating BMD
    - Z-scores (age- and gender-matched controls) should be used instead of T-scores (30-year-old adult controls)
      - Osteopenia is defined as a Z-score between −1.0 and −2.0
      - Osteoporosis is defined as a Z-score below −2.0
    - Stress fractures are extremely common.
    - Long-distance female runners have been found to have the lowest average total BMD compared to other sports.
    - Low BMD is largely due to the hypoestrogenic state causing increased bone resorption.
      - Lack of suppressive effect of estrogen on osteoclasts
  - Treatment
    - Requires a multidisciplinary approach

- Nutritional counseling is critical. Psychotherapy, cognitive-behavioral therapy, and group therapy may be necessary if an eating disorder is present.
- Hormone replacement therapy and oral contraceptives may also be used.
  - If BMD fails to respond to nutritional counseling, an oral contraceptive should be initiated.
  - Bisphosphonates are approved only for postmenopausal osteoporosis. Off-label use should also be avoided owing to potential teratogenic effects.

INFECTIOUS DISEASE IN ATHLETES

- **The skin is the most common site of infection in athletes, representing over half of all infectious disease outbreaks.**
- **Person-to-person contact is the most common mode of transmission.**
- **Football, wrestling, and rugby are the most commonly involved sports.**
- **Herpes simplex virus (HSV) and *Staphylococcus* aureus infections are the most common pathogens.**
- **Bacterial skin infections**
  - Transmission occurs by means of direct person-to-person contact through disruptions in skin integrity.
  - Methicillin-resistant *S. aureus* (MRSA) prevalence has significantly increased in the community.
    - Must be considered in the differential diagnosis of any skin lesion
    - Often confused for a spider bite
  - *S. aureus* lesions are typically erythematous areas with a fluctuant mass, yellow or white center, and central head
  - Diffuse cellulitis suggests *Streptococcus* infection.
  - Simple abscesses may be treated with moist heat and topical mupirocin for 10 days. Incision and drainage may be performed if the infection persists.
  - Oral empirical antimicrobial therapy with coverage for MRSA should be started if the lesions are severe or extensive: 5 to 10 days of therapy with trimethoprim-sulfamethoxazole, doxycycline, clindamycin, linezolid, or minocycline.
  - Return-to-play criteria:
    - No new skin lesions for 48 hours
    - Oral antibiotic therapy for 48 to 72 hours (guidelines vary)
    - No actively weeping or draining lesions
  - Prevention is key.
    - Good personal hygiene, discourage body shaving, avoid sharing personal items, clean high-touch surfaces
    - Athletes with infections should avoid common-use water facilities.
- **Herpes simplex virus**
  - HSV-1 is the most common cause of herpes labialis (lips), and HSV-2 is the most common cause of urogenital herpes.
  - Transmitted by skin-to-skin contact or contact with bodily fluids
  - Highly infectious
    - 33% likelihood of contracting HSV if sparring with an infected partner
  - Lesions typically occur on the lips, head, extremities, and trunk.
  - Diagnosis is made by a cluster of vesicles on an erythematous base.
    - Lesions may crust or scab.

- Tissue culture is not necessary.
- Oral systemic antivirals are taken for 5 days. Acyclovir, valacyclovir, and famciclovir are options.
- Return-to-play criteria:
  - No systemic symptoms
  - No new lesions for 72 hours
  - No moist lesions; all lesions must be dried and surrounded by a firm adherent crust
  - Oral antiviral therapy for 120 hours
- **HIV**
- An athlete's HIV status is confidential; by itself, HIV infection is insufficient reason to restrict athletic participation.
- Wound care in this population is the same as that for all athletes, with the use of universal precautions, application of compressive dressings, and waiting until bleeding has stopped before a return to play.
- **Infectious mononucleosis**
- Caused by Epstein-Barr virus
- Classic triad is high fever, sore throat, and lymphadenopathy.
- Splenomegaly occurs in 50% to 100% of patients.
- Three complications with regard to athletes:
  - Splenic rupture
    - Usually occurs within first 3 weeks of illness
    - Due to lymphocytic infiltration
    - Very rare
  - Severe tonsillar enlargement
    - Upper respiratory tract blockage and acute respiratory compromise
  - Chronic fatigue
    - Can last for 3 months
- Treatment is symptomatic.
- Participation in contact sports should be restricted for 3 to 5 weeks, and splenomegaly must have resolved before a return to play.
- **Meningitis**
- A concern in athletes because of the ease of spread from the "close quarters" environment of the training room
- Symptoms include fever, headache, and nuchal rigidity.
- Evaluation of cerebrospinal fluid is important for identifying cases of bacterial meningitis.

MISCELLANEOUS SPORTS-RELATED INJURIES AND ISSUES

- **Blunt trauma**
- Can cause injury to solid organs
- These injuries may be subtle, and diagnosing them requires a high index of suspicion.
- The kidney is the most commonly injured organ (especially in boxing), followed by the spleen (injured in football).
- **Chest injuries**
- Can be serious and necessitate immediate on-field action
- Decreased breath sounds, deviated trachea, and hypotension may signify a tension pneumothorax.
  - Treatment entails placing a 14-gauge intravenous needle in the second intercostal space at the midclavicular line, followed by placement of a chest tube.
- Airway obstructions must also be anticipated and treated.
- Rib fractures may also occur in contact sports.
- The player usually has "had the air knocked out" of him or her, which can be related to a problem with the diaphragm.

- **Eye injuries**
- These injuries are best avoided with proper protection.
- A hyphema (blood in the eye) is associated with a vitreous or retinal injury in more than 50% of cases.
- **Ear injuries**
- Auricular hematomas ("cauliflower ear"), common in wrestlers, should be treated with aspiration and wrapping.
- **Tooth injuries**
- The tooth or teeth should be replaced immediately but may be temporarily placed in the buccal fold or in milk if necessary.
- Crown fracture is the most common maxillofacial injury in ice hockey.
- **Heat illness**
- **Heat stroke, common during the football preseason, is characterized by collapse, with neurologic deficits, tachycardia, tachypnea, hypotension, and anhidrosis.**
- **Treatment involves rapidly cooling the body's core temperature and hydration.**
- Heat stroke is the second leading cause of death in football players.
- **Cold injury**
- Treatment involves rewarming the patient in a warm-water bath (110°-112° F).
- **Exercise-induced bronchospasm**
- Involves transient airway obstruction that results from exertion
- Symptoms include the triad of coughing, shortness of breath, and wheezing.
- Commonly occurs in cold-weather sports, and the diagnosis is confirmed by a low forced expiratory volume.
- Provocative pulmonary testing is required for diagnosis.
- Treatment is with inhaled glucocorticoids.
- Inhaled β_2 agonists are used as rescue therapy.
- **Pneumothorax**
- A chest tube or large-bore angiocatheter must be inserted at the second intercostal space for tension pneumothorax.
- **Deep venous thrombosis (DVT) after knee arthroscopy**
- The incidence of DVT after knee arthroscopy is 10%; 2% of the cases are proximal without prophylaxis.
- For patients at high risk for DVT (older age, personal or family history of DVT, concomitant medical illness), it is prudent to treat with prophylaxis against DVT.
- **On-field bleeding**
- The affected player must be immediately removed from play and may not return until the bleeding has stopped and the wound has been covered with an occlusive dressing.
- **Special athletes**
- Special considerations may be necessary for patients with congenital heart disease and Down syndrome.
- Patients with Down syndrome may have congenital cervical instability, which should be assessed radiographically before sports participation.
- An atlanto-dens interval of more than 9 mm on flexion and extension views is an indication for surgical fusion.

SELECTED BIBLIOGRAPHY

The selected bibliography for this chapter can be found on https://expertconsult.inkling.com.

TESTABLE CONCEPTS

SECTION 1 KNEE

- The most common causes of an acute hemarthrosis: ACL tear (70%), isolated meniscus tear (15%), osteochondral fracture, patellar dislocation
- The vascular supply of the meniscus is a primary determinant of healing potential; tears in the peripheral third have the highest potential for healing.
- The gold standard for meniscal repair is the inside-out technique with vertical mattress sutures. The saphenous nerve is at risk in medial repairs; the peroneal nerve is at risk in lateral repairs.
- ACL anatomy: AM bundle is an anterior restraint, and PL bundle is a rotatory restraint.
- The sMCL origin is proximal and posterior to the medial epicondyle of the femur. Radiographically, originates slightly anterior to the junction of the posterior femoral cortex reference line and Blumensaat line.
- The posterior oblique ligament is the primary stabilizer against internal rotation and valgus between 0 and 30 degrees of knee flexion.
- The MPFL femoral attachment is anterior and distal to the adductor tubercle; or proximal to the attachment of the superficial medial collateral ligament; or proximal and posterior to the medial epicondyle. Radiographically, originates slightly anterior to the posterior femoral cortex reference line and immediately posterior to the most posterior aspect of the Blumensaat line (Schottle point).
- The LCL femoral origin is proximal and posterior to the lateral femoral epicondyle; or posterior and proximal to the insertion of the popliteus tendon.
- The popliteus femoral insertion is distal, anterior, and deep to the LCL. It internally rotates the tibia.
- The posterior horn of the medial meniscus is a major secondary stabilizer against anterior tibial translation in an ACL-deficient knee.
- Opening to varus or valgus stress testing at only 30 degrees of knee flexion indicates an isolated collateral injury. Opening in full extension indicates a combined cruciate and collateral injury.
- During knee arthroscopy, the posterolateral compartment can be best visualized by placing the arthroscope through the interval of the ACL and lateral femoral condyle or a posterolateral portal.
- Partial meniscectomy increases peak stresses in the affected compartment.
- The gold standard for meniscal repair is the inside-out technique with vertical mattress sutures. Regardless of the technique used, it is essential to protect the saphenous nerve branches (anterior to both the semitendinosis and gracilis muscles and posterior to the inferior border of the sartorius muscle) during medial repairs and to protect the peroneal nerve (posterior to the biceps femoris) during lateral repairs.
- Meniscal cysts occur primarily in conjunction with horizontal cleavage tears of the lateral meniscus.
- Discoid menisci should be observed if asymptomatic.
- If meniscal transplantation is considered, ligamentous deficiency and limb malalignment must be addressed. Contraindications include inflammatory arthritis or significant osteoarthritis.
- Following meniscal transplantation, allograft tissue often remains hypocellular or acellular. The most common complication is meniscal tear.
- The ACL injury rate is 2 to 8 times higher in female athletes than in male athletes because of smaller notches, smaller ligaments, increased generalized ligament laxity, increased knee laxity, and different landing biomechanics in women and girls.
- The Lachman test is the most sensitive examination for acute ACL injuries, whereas results of the pivot shift test are correlated most closely with outcome after ACL reconstruction. The pivot shift is a reduction of the subluxated lateral tibial plateau by the iliotibial band when moving from full extension to flexion.
- MRI evaluation of ACL injuries demonstrates characteristic "bone bruises" in more than half of cases; these bruises are typically located near the sulcus terminalis on the lateral femoral condyle and the posterolateral aspect of the tibia.
- Initial management consists of physical therapy for mobilization. Immobilization is avoided. Full range of motion and good quadriceps control should be achieved prior to surgery.
- A more horizontal graft position may reduce rotational instability.
- BPTB autografts demonstrate faster incorporation into the bone tunnels than do hamstring autografts and are often the graft of choice for patients desiring an early return to sports activity.
- The most common technical error in ACL surgery is placement of the femoral tunnel too far anteriorly, which results in limited flexion. Vertical graft placement results in decreased rotational stability.
- Arthrofibrosis is the most common complication following ACL reconstruction and is associated with a loss of patellar translation.
- No high-level evidence to suggest that ACL reconstruction reduces the risk of developing arthritis
- ACL rehabilitation should avoid open-chain quadriceps-activating exercises from 0 to 30 degrees of knee flexion.
- PCL injuries often result from a fall onto the ground with a plantar-flexed foot.
- PCL reconstruction should be reserved for functionally unstable knees or combined injuries. Single-bundle reconstructions should be tensioned in 90 degrees of flexion. Tibial inlay has biomechanical advantages such as avoiding the killer turn.
- PCL rehabilitation should avoid open-chain hamstring-activating exercises.
- Multiligament knee injuries require an immediate neurovascular examination. Vascular consultation should be obtained on any patient with absent pulses or an ankle-brachial index (ABI) less than 0.9.
- Chronic grade III posterolateral corner injuries often necessitate a valgus opening wedge osteotomy.
- Osteochondritis dissecans should be monitored in children with open physes. Adult lesions do not resolve and should be treated.
- Marrow-stimulating techniques, including microfracture, drilling, and abrasion arthroplasty, involve perforation of the subchondral bone after removal of the "tidemark" cartilage, with eventual clot formation and fibrocartilaginous repair tissue (type I collagen with inferior wear characteristics).
- No definitive research has demonstrated superiority of any cartilage restoration procedure. Current best available research suggests that for smaller lesions, microfracture, OATS, and ACI have similar recovery periods and functional results.
- Patellar tendonitis is associated with pain and tenderness near the inferior border of the patella (worse in extension than in flexion). Treatment is with NSAIDs and strengthening, including eccentric exercise and ultrasound.
- Iliotibial band friction syndrome presents with localized tenderness at the lateral femoral condyle, worse with the knee flexed 30 degrees.
- MRI evaluation of patellar dislocation demonstrates a classic bone bruise pattern involving the lateral femoral condyle and medial patella.
- Patellofemoral pain syndrome is most often due to muscular weakness, with weak quadriceps, hip abductors, and core musculature. Management is focused on prolonged rehabilitation.
- Conservative management is the mainstay of symptomatic bipartite patella.
- Lateral patellar facet compression syndrome should be treated with a lateral release only in the setting of objective evidence of lateral tilt

TESTABLE CONCEPTS

that has not responded to extensive nonoperative management. Lateral tilt is best evaluated by measurement of the lateral patellofemoral angle.

SECTION 2 PELVIS, HIP, AND THIGH

- Quadriceps contusions are acutely managed with overnight immobilization in hyperflexion.
- Athletic pubalgia (sports hernia) is the result of abdominal hyperextension and thigh hyperabduction, which result in injury to the muscles of the abdominal wall and adductor longus. Treatment is primarily nonoperative.
- MRI is the most specific test for detecting stress fractures. Treatment typically includes protected weight bearing, rest, cross-training, analgesics, and therapeutic modalities.
- Femoral neck stress fractures that occur on the inferior surface (compression side) can be treated nonoperatively.
- FAI presents with groin pain and limited ROM, especially in flexion and IR. A positive result of an anterior impingement test is reproduction of symptoms with passive flexion, adduction, and internal rotation.
- External snapping hip occurs when the iliotibial band abruptly catches on the greater trochanter, whereas internal snapping hip occurs when the iliopsoas impinges on the hip capsule.
- Complications of hip arthroscopy typically result from traction injuries or iatrogenic neurovascular injury from aberrant portal placement. Use of an anterior portal places the lateral femoral cutaneous nerve at risk. Use of an anterolateral portal places the superior gluteal nerve at risk. Use of a posterolateral portal places the sciatic nerve at risk, especially when the hip is externally rotated.

SECTION 3 SHOULDER

- The most common location for an os acromiale is at the junction of the mesoacromion and meta-acromion.
- Humeral head blood supply is primarily from the posterior humeral circumflex artery.
- The contents of the rotator interval include the coracohumeral ligament, SGHL, biceps tendon, and glenohumeral capsule. The SGHL and coracohumeral ligament limit inferior translation and external rotation when the arm is adducted and posterior translation when the arm is flexed forward, adducted, and internally rotated. Rotator interval closure results in decreased external rotation in shoulder adduction and posteroinferior translation.
- The inferior glenohumeral ligament complex serves as the primary restraint to anterior, posterior, and inferior glenohumeral translation at 45 to 90 degrees of glenohumeral elevation. The aIGHL is important in external rotation and the pIGHL important in internal rotation.
- In the throwing shoulder, the scapula must rotate during throwing. It retracts during the late cocking phase and then protracts during the acceleration phase. The deceleration phase is associated with tensile failure of the posterior aspect of the supraspinatus and anterior half of the infraspinatus.
- In shoulder arthroscopy, the posterior portal places the axillary nerve, suprascapular nerve, and suprascapular artery at risk.
- Traumatic anterior shoulder dislocations typically result when the arm is abducted and in external rotation. The axillary nerve is susceptible to injury.
- Instability is often associated with a Bankart lesion (anteroinferior labral tear) with disrupted medial scapular periosteum. A three-dimensional CT scan should be obtained if suspicion of glenoid bone loss exists.
- A HAGL lesion has an incidence between 1% and 9% and has typically necessitated open repair in the past because of its inferior

location. However, newer arthroscopic techniques are being developed.
- Age at time of initial dislocation is an important risk factor for recurrent shoulder instability.
- Several open and arthroscopic techniques have been developed to address instability. Glenoid deficiency greater than 25% of the humeral head is a specific indication for coracoid transfer (Latarjet procedure). Failure of rehabilitation for multidirectional instability is an indication for capsular shift. Chronic dislocation with greater than 40% of articular surface deficit is an indication for allograft in young patients and for prosthesis in older patients.
- Remplissage involves tenodesis of the posterior capsule and infraspinatus into a Hill-Sachs lesion. Precise indications are not yet defined, but early evidence suggests medium to large or engaging Hill-Sachs lesions.
- Postthermal capsular necrosis is treated with allograft anterior capsulolabral reconstruction.
- Physical examination for posterior instability includes load-and-shift and jerk testing.
- A fixed posterior shoulder dislocation is diagnosed by lack of external rotation. Anteroposterior radiographs are unreliable but may demonstrate a "lightbulb" sign. An axillary lateral radiograph is critical in making the diagnosis.
- For chronic unrecognized posterior dislocations, several procedures may be performed, dependent on the degree of bone loss both in the humeral head and glenoid. The Neer modification of the McLaughlin procedure involves transfer of the lesser tuberosity and associated subscapularis tendon into the reverse Hill-Sachs lesion.
- Multidirectional instability should be treated with extended rehabilitation that focuses on scapular stabilization before operative intervention is considered. Closed kinetic chain exercises should be emphasized.
- The prevalence of asymptomatic rotator cuff tears increases with age: 28% of those older than 60 years have a full-thickness tear, whereas 65% of those older than 70 years have a full-thickness tear.
- Asymptomatic full-thickness rotator cuff tears should be treated nonoperatively. The primary indication for surgical intervention is significant pain.
- Blood flow to the repaired rotator cuff is achieved from the peribursal tissue and bone anchor site.
- Acute rotator cuff tears should be repaired early because the disease process is accelerated in this setting.
- Rotator cuff repair rehabilitation protocols have no difference in clinical outcomes or healing rates with early motion compared to delayed motion.
- Irreparable combined tears of the supraspinatus and infraspinatus may be treated with latissimus dorsi tendon transfer to the greater tuberosity. If pain is the major symptom and motion remains preserved, débridement with biceps tenotomy has been found to be useful. Inferior results have been reported for latissimus transfer in the presence of a subscapularis tear.
- Signs of a subscapularis tear include increased external rotation and the presence of a liftoff, modified liftoff, or belly-press sign. The appearance of an empty bicipital groove on axial MRI with tear of the transverse humeral ligament is often associated with subscapularis tear. At arthroscopy, a chronic subscapularis tear can be identified by the comma sign, which represents an avulsed SGHL and CHL (so-called comma tissue).
- In athletes who participate in throwing activities, there is greater external rotation and a loss of internal rotation of the dominant shoulder than in the nondominant shoulder (GIRD). Initial treatment is

posterior and posteroinferior capsular stretching exercises, such as the sleeper stretch, as well as stretching of the pectoralis minor tendon.

- Internal impingement is defined as contact between the articular side of the rotator cuff and the posterosuperior rim of the glenoid labrum when the arm is abducted and externally rotated. Alteration of the glenohumeral kinematics leads to a posterosuperior shift of the humeral head; abduction and external rotation of the arm, in turn, lead to the internal impingement.

- SLAP tear management is controversial. If repair is undertaken, stiffness is a common complication, and motion should begin early.

- Biceps tenotomy without tenodesis is associated with subjective cramping and potential for cosmetic deformity ("Popeye deformity"). Weakness is not associated with tenotomy.

- For type III acromioclavicular separations, recommended management is conservative in elderly patients, inactive patients, and patients who do not perform manual labor.

- Distal clavicle resection for AC joint arthritis should entail resection of less than 1 cm of the distal clavicle to preserve the posterior-superior capsule and avoid anterior and posterior instability and pain.

- Sternoclavicular dislocation is best diagnosed by CT. Posterior dislocation should be treated with closed reduction and open reduction if necessary, particularly with compression of the posterior structures.

- Calcifying tendinitis is a self-limiting condition of unknown origin that affects predominantly the supraspinatus tendon. Radiographs demonstrate characteristic calcification within the tendon.

- Frozen shoulder histology demonstrates evidence of inflammation and evidence of fibrosis. There is a dense matrix of type-III collagen containing fibroblasts and myofibroblasts that appear similar to Dupuytren's disease. On examination, active ROM and passive ROM are equivalent.

- Suprascapular nerve compression by a ganglion in the spinoglenoid notch affects only the infraspinatus. Compression caused by a cyst in association with a SLAP lesion may respond to arthroscopic decompression and labral repair.

- Quadrilateral space syndrome is defined as axillary nerve or posterior humeral circumflex artery compression within the quadrilateral space, which results in pain and paresthesias with overhead activity,

as well as weakness or atrophy of the teres minor and deltoid. This is most often seen in athletes who participate in throwing activities and is associated with late cocking and acceleration with the abducted, extended, and externally rotated arm.

- Medial scapular winging is caused by damage to the long thoracic nerve. Lateral scapular winging is caused by damage to the spinal accessory nerve.

SECTION 4 MEDICAL ASPECTS OF SPORTS MEDICINE

- The history and physical examination is the most helpful and cost-effective for identifying musculoskeletal and medical problems.

- Hypertrophic cardiomyopathy is the most common cause of sudden death in young athletes. Sports participation is contraindicated.

- Any player with diagnosed concussion is not allowed to return to play on the day of injury. The player must be cleared by a licensed healthcare professional prior to returning to play thereafter.

- Sickle cell trait is not a contraindication to participation in any athletic activity. Important precautions must be taken: maintain hydration, permit adequate rest and recovery between intense exercise, allow access to supplemental oxygen (particularly when at altitude).

- Adverse effects of anabolic steroids include liver dysfunction, hypercholesterolemia, cardiomyopathy, testicular atrophy, gynecomastia, acne, mood disturbances (particularly increased aggression), and irreversible alopecia. Heart disease results from increased plasma levels of low-density lipoprotein and decreased levels of high-density lipoprotein.

- The "female athlete triad" consists of low energy availability (with or without an eating disorder), menstrual dysfunction, and altered bone mineral density. Insufficient caloric intake is the most common cause of secondary amenorrhea.

- MRSA transmission occurs by direct person-to-person contact through disruptions in skin integrity.

- Athletes with infectious mononucleosis should be restricted from contact sports participation for 3 to 5 weeks, and splenomegaly must have resolved before they return to play.

- Heat stroke is characterized by collapse, with neurologic deficits, tachycardia, tachypnea, hypotension, and anhidrosis. Treatment involves rapidly cooling the body's core temperature and hydration.

CHAPTER 5

ADULT RECONSTRUCTION

Edward J. McPherson, James A. Browne, and Stephen R. Thompson

CONTENTS

Continued

CONTENTS

SECTION 1 EVALUATION OF THE ADULT HIP PATIENT

Patient assessment of hip pain includes a physical examination and diagnostic radiographic modalities.

PHYSICAL EXAMINATION TESTS FOR HIP IRRITABILITY

- **Impingement test**
- Hip flexion to 90 degrees
- Hip adduction and internal rotation yield pain response.
- Hip internal rotation only yields pain response.
- Pain located in area of anterior hip with pain radiating to either posterior hip or lateral hip
- **Roll test**
- Patient is positioned supine. Finger rolling of leg (at calf level) into internal rotation and external rotation

- Leg will feel stiff or will occasionally grab.
- **Stinchfield test**
- Patient is positioned supine. Active straight leg raise of approximately 20 cm against mild resistance by examiner.
- Patient will feel pain in anterior hip against resistance.
- **Patrick test**
- Patient is positioned supine. Leg is positioned in figure-four position.
- Pain will be elicited in area of anterior hip region or posterior hip region.
- Be careful with interpretation of test. If pain is located over posterior pelvis, this indicates referred pain from L5-S1 facets or sacroiliac joint and not hip joint.

STUDIES

- ■ **Radiographs**
- ▥ Still the standard imaging modality for initial evaluation of hip pain
- ▥ See Section 2 for discussion of imaging studies in dysplasia and impingement.
- ■ **Computed tomographic (CT) scan**
- ▥ Three-dimensional CT with pelvic remodeling may be indicated for preoperative planning for reconstruction associated with dysplasia surgery, femoroacetabular impingement, and complex primary or revision total hip arthroplasty (THA).
- ■ **Magnetic resonance imaging (MRI)**
- ▥ Used when osteonecrosis suspected
- ▥ Gadolinium MRI arthrogram useful when labral pathology suspected, especially when associated with femoral acetabular impingement

SECTION 2 STRUCTURAL HIP DISORDERS IN THE ADULT

NATURAL HISTORY

- ■ **Many cases of mild dysplasia or femoroacetabular impingement (FAI) may be asymptomatic and go unrecognized on radiographs.**
- ■ **Hip pain in adults younger than 50 years often the result of an underlying structural problem**
- ■ **Initial presentation of symptoms may be soon followed by degeneration.**
- ▥ Increasing evidence suggests that FAI is an important contributing factor to the majority of adult hip arthritis.

SPECTRUM OF PRESENTATION

- ■ **Subtle**
- ▥ Patients may present with symptoms from associated labral pathology.
- ▥ Chondral surface delamination and chondral flap tears may also cause symptoms.
- ▥ Abductor muscle fatigue may be presenting symptom of dysplasia
- ■ **Advanced morphologic changes with significant arthritis**

CLASSIFICATION OF ADULT HIP DYSPLASIA

- ■ **Acetabulum (Box 5-1 and Figure 5-1)**
- ▥ Shallow acetabulum with lack of anterior and lateral coverage
- ▥ Decreased acetabular depth (socket < a hemisphere with upsloping acetabular index)
- ▥ Varying degrees of superolateral subluxation and lateralization of femoral head
- ▥ High articular contact stresses near superolateral rim
- ▥ Crowe classification
  - Grade 1: less than 50% femoral head subluxation and less than 10% proximal displacement of the femur (mild)
  - Grade 2: between 50% and 75% subluxation of the femoral head and 10 to 15% proximal displacement of the femur
  - Grade 3: between 75% and 100% subluxation of the femoral head and 15 to 20% proximal displacement of the femur
  - Grade 4: greater than 100% subluxation of the femoral head with greater than 20% proximal displacement of the femur with a deficient true acetabulum
- ■ **Proximal femur**
- ▥ High neck-shaft angle (coxa valga)
- ▥ Increased femoral anteversion

- ■ **Clinical syndrome**
- ▥ Increased contact stresses can lead to pain and degenerative changes of articular cartilage.

TREATMENT OF DYSPLASIA

- ■ **Treatment depends upon extent of deformity and location.**
- ■ **Surgical correction goals are to relieve pain and correct anatomic deformity. Long-term goal is to reduce occurrence of degenerative joint disease.**

Box 5-1	Acetabular Dysplasia Classical Definitions

Lateral CE angle < 20 degrees
- CE angle = head center to acetabular edge angle
- Measured on anteroposterior pelvis radiograph

Anterior CE angle < 20 degrees
- Measured on standing lateral (false profile) view

Acetabular index > 5 degrees
- Measured on anteroposterior pelvis radiograph

CE, Center edge.

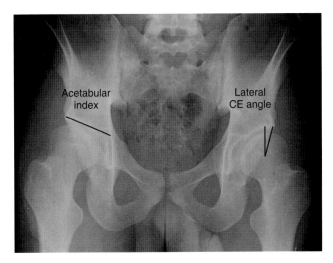

FIGURE 5-1 Anteroposterior pelvis radiograph displaying lateral center edge (CE) angle and acetabular index. Both hips in this case show a shallow socket dysplasia. The acetabular index should normally be horizontal, and the lateral CE angle should be 30 degrees.

- Surgical correction addresses main anatomic deformity: shallow socket or proximal femur abnormality.
- **Periacetabular osteotomy (Figure 5-2)**
- Most common technique used to correct tilt and version of socket
- Allows for large degree of correction
- Permits joint medicalization (i.e., center of hip rotation is positioned medial)
  - Lowers joint reactive forces
- Technical advantages
  - Does not violate the posterior column
  - Does not violate abductors
  - Allows early weight bearing
  - Relatively low complication rate and morbidity
- Goals of surgery
  - Acetabular roof index to zero
  - Head coverage: lateral center edge (CE) angle into normal range
  - Restore appropriate socket anteversion
    - Avoid overcorrection with subsequent retroversion and secondary FAI
- Conversion to THA
  - Previous hardware may be left in place if it does not interfere with placement of the acetabular component.
  - Previous osteotomy may have retroverted the socket, and internal landmarks may not be reliable to guide cup placement.
- **Proximal femur osteotomy**
- **THA**
- Reserved for patients with degenerative joint disease who are no longer candidates for hip preservation

FEMOROACETABULAR IMPINGEMENT

- **Acetabulum (Figure 5-3; see Figure 5-2)**
- Excessive bone present along rim of acetabulum results in overcoverage

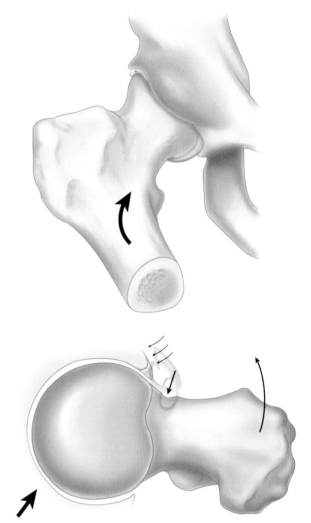

FIGURE 5-3 Pincer-type impingement: an acetabular side disorder where a prominent anterosuperior acetabular rim impinges on the femoral neck during flexion, leading to labral injury.

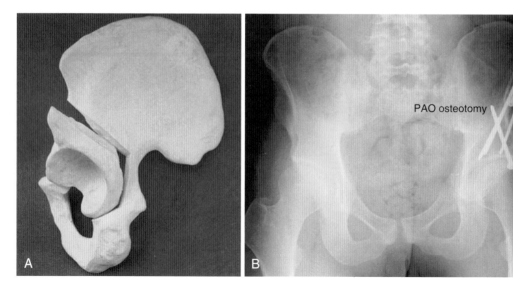

FIGURE 5-2 A, Model demonstrating periacetabular osteotomy (PAO). In the PAO technique, the posterior column is preserved. This maintains pelvic stability and allows for significant correction of acetabular tilt and version. **B,** Five-year postoperative radiograph of PAO. Notice acetabular index restored to horizontal and improved lateral center edge angle.

- Acetabular retroversion (crossover sign)
- Excessively deep socket
  - Coxa profunda occurs when acetabular fossa is medial to ilioischial line
  - Acetabular protrusio occurs when medial aspect of femoral head is medial to ilioischial line
- Acetabular index may be downsloping.
- **Proximal femur (Figures 5-4 through 5-6)**
- Offset between edge of femoral head and edge of femoral neck is reduced (i.e., reduced head-neck ratio).
- α-Angle may be used to measure head-neck offset.
  - Normally 40 degrees or less
- Typically due to excessive bone at junction of femoral head and neck
  - Aspherical head
  - Slipped capital femoral epiphysis deformity
- Pistol grip deformity may be present on radiographs.
- **Clinical syndrome**
- Abnormal impingement between femoral neck and anterosuperior acetabulum with flexion and internal rotation of the hip
  - Cam impingement is due to a femoral problem.
  - Pincer impingement is due to an acetabular problem.

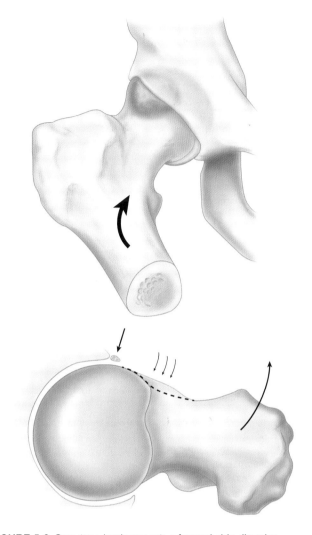

Proximal Femoral Dysplasia

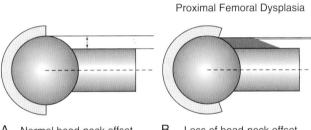

A Normal head-neck offset   B Loss of head-neck offset

FIGURE 5-4 A, Diagram demonstrating normal head-neck offset. Offset is measured using lines parallel to the line defining the femoral head center and neck midline. **B,** In femoral neck dysplasia, the offset between the femoral head and neck is significantly reduced. A reduced head-neck offset increases the risk for neck impingement upon the acetabular rim.

FIGURE 5-6 Cam-type impingement: a femoral side disorder where an aspherical femoral head causes impingement of the neck against the anterior edge of the acetabulum during flexion, resulting in labral injury and chondral delamination.

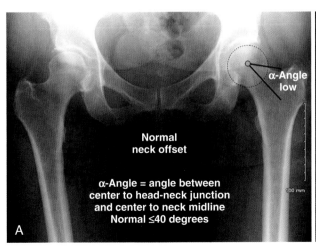

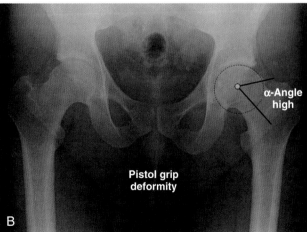

FIGURE 5-5 A, Anteroposterior radiograph measuring α-angle. The α-angle is a method to evaluate head-neck dysplasia. The α-angle is formed between the lines of femoral head center and neck midline, and femoral head center and head-neck junction. Normal α-angle is typically 40 degrees or less. **B,** Anteroposterior radiograph measuring α-angle in a dysplastic proximal femur. α-Angle is increased.

- The majority of cases have combined cam and pincer impingement.
- Activity-related groin pain exacerbated by hip flexion activities
- Impingement test is positive on clinical examination.
- Significant limitation of hip internal rotation tested at 90 degrees due to mechanical block
- Impingement can result in labral tears (pincer) and shearing delamination of the acetabular cartilage (cam).

TREATMENT OF FAI

- Surgical treatment varies according to patient anatomy.
- Labrum should be repaired when possible; results appear to be superior to labral débridement.

Labrum repair > Labrum DEBRIDEMENT

- **Surgical hip dislocation (Ganz trochanteric osteotomy)**
- Allows excellent exposure of proximal femur and acetabulum
- Permits treatment of severe deformities
- Preserves femoral head blood supply
- Allows for repair of soft tissues (labrum and chondral flap tears)
- Complications are rare (<5%) but include trochanteric nonunion and heterotopic bone formation.
- Anterior Z-capsulotomy preserves posterior vessels to femoral neck and minimizes risk for osteonecrosis.
- **Hip arthroscopy**
- See Chapter 4, Sports Medicine, for discussion.
- **Periacetabular osteotomy**
- Less common procedure for FAI
- May be used to address a retroverted socket

SECTION 3 OSTEONECROSIS OF THE HIP

OCCURRENCE

- Incidence not precisely known
- No comprehensive information on number of asymptomatic cases
- More common in males
- Typically affects patients in late 30s or early 40s

ETIOLOGY (SEE CHAPTER 1, BASIC SCIENCE)

- Hypercoagulable states may explain many *idiopathic* cases of osteonecrosis of the hip.
- In all cases, end-stage result is vascular occlusion in the juxtaarticular sinusoids adjacent to joint.

CLINICAL PRESENTATION

- Initial pain with sit to stand, stairs, inclines, and impact loading
- Pain location tends to be most noticeable in anterior hip.
- Can be acute in onset (acute infarct phenomenon), which can mimic an acute injury

IMAGING

- Start first with radiographs.
- Pelvis, anteroposterior (AP), and lateral radiographs
- If osteonecrosis detected, must image contralateral hip
  - Fifty percent of osteonecrosis cases have bilateral involvement.
- MRI is the standard imaging modality when radiographs are negative and osteonecrosis is suspected.

STAGING (TABLE 5-1)

- Modified Ficat system (incorporates MRI information)

TREATMENT

- **Nonsurgical**
- Bisphosphonate treatment will decrease risk for head collapse.
- Must start *before* crescent sign
- **Surgical treatment**
- Surgical treatment depends on these major variables:
  - Head collapse (i.e., crescent)
    - Yes or no
  - Age
    - 40 or younger
  - Irreversible etiology
    - Yes or no
  - Examples of irreversible etiology
    - Continued steroid use
    - Idiopathic
    - Hypercoagulable state
  - Extent of head involvement (by osteonecrosis)
    - Described as *volume* head involvement
    - Volume head involvement equals percent head involved on AP image multiplied by percent head involved on lateral image (e.g., 50% × 50% = 25% volume head involvement).
    - A—small lesion: less than 15% head involvement
    - B—medium lesion: 15% to 30% head involvement
    - C—large lesion: greater than 30% head involvement
- Younger age and crescent (or worse)
  - THA is recommended treatment.
    - Cementless cup and stem
    - Improved bearing technology
    - Good pain relief and function

Table 5-1	Modified Ficat Staging System for Osteonecrosis of the Hip			
STAGE	**MRI**	**BONE SCAN**	**RADIOGRAPHS**	**PATIENT STATUS**
0	Positive	Positive	Negative	Asymptomatic
1	Positive	Positive	Negative	Symptomatic
2	Positive	Positive	Positive—no crescent	Symptomatic
3	Positive	Positive	Positive—crescent	Symptomatic
4	Positive	Positive	Positive—head flattening, DJD	Symptomatic

DJD, Degenerative joint disease; MRI, magnetic resonance imaging.

- Younger age and no crescent
  - Common treatments
    - Core decompression
      - Treatment principles
        - Core decompression relieves pressure buildup within the femoral head by the inflammatory process.
        - Pressure relief translates to pain relief.
        - Stimulates a healing response
          - Bone and vascular neogenesis
      - Indications
        - No crescent
        - *Reversible etiology*
          - Patients on chronic steroids have poor results with core decompression.
        - Small head lesion (A lesion)
          - Patients with medium and large head lesions frequently collapse.
  - Vascularized fibular strut (Figure 5-7)
    - Treatment principles
      - Surgical removal of necrotic segment
      - Large core hole is needed.
      - Vascularized fibular strut is placed up against subchondral plate of femoral head to prevent collapse.
      - Particulate bone grafting of adjacent resected bone
    - Indications
      - Medium (B) and large (C) lesions
      - No crescent (preferred)
        - Reasonable success with crescent and minimal head collapse
      - Reversible etiology

- Less common treatments
  - Curettage of necrotic bone and bone grafting through femoral neck trap door
  - Rotational proximal femoral osteotomy
    - Must be able to rotate osteonecrotic segment out of weight-bearing zone and maintain good hip function
- Age 40 years or older and medium (B) or large (C) lesion
  - Best option is total hip replacement.
  - Medium to large lesions prone to collapse
- Older than 40 years and small (A) lesion
  - Best option is core decompression.
    - Patient must have reversible etiology.
    - Core decompression contraindicated if on chronic corticosteroid treatment
    - Result of vascularized fibular graft less predictable in older population.

TRANSIENT OSTEOPOROSIS OF THE HIP

- Uncommon cause of groin pain and inability to bear weight
- Commonly affects pregnant women or patients in their fifth decade of life
- Radiographs may appear normal or show only subtle osteopenia in the head and neck.
- MRI appearance is similar to bone marrow edema, with diffusely increased signal in the head and neck on T2-weighted images.
- Spontaneous recovery may take **several months** and often resolves in the pregnant patient early in the postpartum period.
- Protected weight bearing to protect against stress fracture
- Surgical intervention rarely indicated

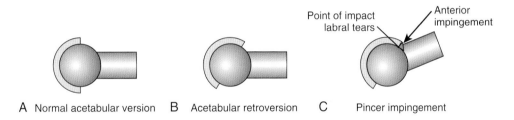

A Normal acetabular version   B Acetabular retroversion   C   Pincer impingement

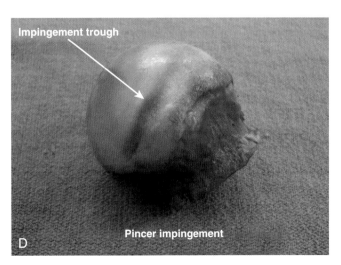

FIGURE 5-7 Pincer-type femoral acetabular impingement. **A,** Diagram showing normal acetabulum and proximal femur. **B,** Diagram depicting acetabular retroversion. Retroverted acetabulum will limit functional hip flexion. **C,** Mechanics of pincer impingement. In hip flexion, the femoral neck abuts acetabular rim. Typically this results in localized damage to the labrum. **D,** Ex vivo demonstration of pincer impingement. In this case, repetitive pincer impingement created a bony indentation trough on the femoral head at the site of flexion impingement.

SECTION 4 HIP ARTHRITIS TREATMENT

NONOPERATIVE

- **Activity modification**
- Reduce impact-loading exercises.
- Reduce weight.
- Avoid stairs, inclines, squatting.
- **Nonsteroidal antiinflammatory drugs (NSAIDs)**
- Cyclooxygenase (COX)-2 inhibition
- **Joint injections**
- Corticosteroid—antiinflammatory treatment
- Hyaluronate
  - Backbone of proteoglycan chain of articular cartilage
  - Improves joint rheology
- Approved by U.S. Food and Drug Administration (FDA) for knee use only in United States
- **Assist device (cane or crutch)**
- Opposite hand of affected hip

OPERATIVE

- **Arthroscopy**
- Best indication
  - Traumatic labral tear *not* associated with dysplasia
  - Hip joint shows mechanical signs of locking, catching, and clicking.
- Beware of labral resection in dysplasia.
  - Acetabular labrum provides stability in a shallow acetabular socket (labrum usually hypertrophic).
  - Isolated removal of labrum will typically result in rapid progression of joint degeneration and pain.
  - In cases of significant dysplasia, arthroscopic débridement is *not* recommended.
- Other indications
  - Loose body removal
  - Débridement of chondral flap tears
  - Synovitis
    - Diagnostic biopsy and therapeutic lavage
  - Diagnostic procedure
    - Undiagnosed mechanical hip pain
  - Degenerative arthritis
    - Therapeutic effect inversely related to severity of arthritis
    - Not helpful in moderate to advanced disease
    - Generally, will help only mechanical symptoms, not arthritic ache
- Arthroscopy technique
  - Traction required
  - Fluoroscopy required
  - Long cannulated trochars that are designed for hip joint
- Arthroscopy complications
  - Nerve injury—most frequent
    - Pudendal—due to traction post
    - Lateral femoral cutaneous—due to portal placement
    - Femoral—due to portal placement
  - Instrument breakage
  - Portal hematoma

- **Osteotomy (adult)**
- Salvage osteotomy
  - Abandoned in favor of THA for degenerative hip arthritis
- Reconstructive osteotomy
  - Periacetabular osteotomy—preferred procedure in the adult to correct early hip degeneration due to dysplasia
  - See the section Hip Dysplasia.
- **THA**
- See Section 5, Total Hip Arthroplasty.
- **Hip fusion**
- Less frequently used as THA technology advances
- Classical indication
  - Very young male laborer
  - *Unilateral* hip arthritis
- Energy expenditure
  - Approximately 30% increase in energy output during ambulation
- Collateral arthritis
  - Abnormal gait causes arthritis in these adjacent joints in 60% of patients.
    - Lumbar spine
    - Contralateral hip
    - Ipsilateral knee
  - Symptoms of pain typically start within 25 years of hip fusion.
- Hip fusion technique
  - Preserve abductor complex.
    - Many fusions are taken down for disabling pain in adjacent joints.
    - Select fusion technique that allows successful conversion to THA.
    - Greater trochanteric osteotomy with lateral plate fixation is preferred technique.
    - Be careful not to injure superior gluteal nerve, which innervates abductor complex.
- Fusion position
  - 20 to 25 degrees of flexion
  - *Neutral abduction*
    - Increased back and knee pain when fusion is in abduction
  - Neutral or slight external rotation of 10 degrees
- Fusion conversion to THA
  - Indications
    - Disabling back pain—most common
    - Disabling ipsilateral knee pain with instability
      - Excess knee stress will cause knee ligament stretch-out if fusion position is incorrect.
    - Disabling contralateral hip pain
- Function after conversion to THA
  - Hip function and clinical results directly related to integrity of abductor complex
    - Preoperative electromyogram of gluteus medius required
  - When hip abductor complex nonfunctional
    - Severe lurching gait will result.
    - THA will require *constrained* acetabular component.

■ **Resection arthroplasty**

▦ Usually last step before hip disarticulation in a frustrating downward clinical course

▦ Indications

- Incurable infection
  - Patients are most often immunocompromised.
  - Recurrent periprosthetic THA infection
  - Failed hip fusion with infection
  - Chronic destructive septic arthritis
- Noncompliant patient with recurrent THA dislocation
  - Usually multiply revised patient
  - Psychiatric condition
  - Profound dementia
  - Limb paresis or paralysis
  - Drug-seeking behavior
- Nonambulator
  - Intractable pain from arthritis
  - Hip fracture with open decubitus ulcers
  - Significant contracture interfering with hygiene and posture
- Failed hip fusion in patient with prior major trauma to hip and/or pelvis
  - Soft tissue loss to hip region precludes successful placement of THA.
  - Neurologic injury to extremity precludes successful function of THA.

■ **Hemiarthroplasty**

▦ Relegated to specific limited role

- Fracture treatment in low-demand elderly patient
  - Best indication—displaced subcapital hip fracture with little or no prior history of symptomatic hip arthritis
- Patient not able to comply with standard THA precautions
- Best indication for THA for hip fracture
  - High activity level
  - Subcapital or high neck fracture
  - Younger population (age ≤ 70 years)
  - Low risk for dislocation (no dementia or Parkinson disease)

▦ Hemiarthroplasty advantage

- Stability
  - Maximize head/neck ratio.
  - Large-diameter ball requires more distance to travel before dislocation.
  - Suction fit provided by labrum
- Enhanced stability negated if labrum and capsule resected

▦ Hemiarthroplasty disadvantage

- Groin pain in active individuals
- Increased osteolysis (compared to THA) in active individual
- Protrusio deformity if ball not sized well and osteoporosis present (Figure 5-8)

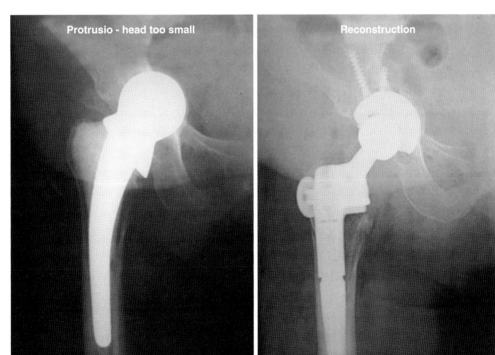

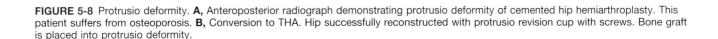

FIGURE 5-8 Protrusio deformity. **A,** Anteroposterior radiograph demonstrating protrusio deformity of cemented hip hemiarthroplasty. This patient suffers from osteoporosis. **B,** Conversion to THA. Hip successfully reconstructed with protrusio revision cup with screws. Bone graft is placed into protrusio deformity.

SECTION 5 TOTAL HIP ARTHROPLASTY

INDICATIONS

- Debilitating pain affecting activities of daily living
- Pain not well controlled by conservative measures
- Medically fit for surgery
- No active infection—anywhere

SURGICAL APPROACHES FOR THA

- The most common surgical approaches for THA are listed in Table 5-2.

TEMPLATING FOR THA

- Templating for THA can help achieve appropriate restoration of biomechanics.

- Standard radiograph with a known magnification should be used.
- Goal is to optimize limb length and femoral offset (Figure 5-9).

IMPLANT FIXATION

- Methods of fixation
- Cement
  - Polymethylmethacrylate (PMMA)
- Cementless
  - Biologic fixation—bone growth into the prosthesis secures implant
  - Two methods
    - Bone *ingrowth*—porous coating
    - Bone *ongrowth*—grit coating

Table 5-2	Most Common Surgical Approaches for THA				
APPROACH	**MUSCULAR INTERVAL**	**INTERNERVOUS INTERVAL**	**STRUCTURES AT RISK**	**PROS**	**CONS**
Anterior (Smith-Petersen)	Superficial: sartorius and tensor fascia latae Deep: rectus and gluteus medius	Femoral nerve and superior gluteal nerve	Lateral femoral cutaneous nerve Ascending branch of the lateral femoral circumflex artery	Stability Rapid recovery	Difficult femoral exposure Limits access to the posterior acetabulum A specialized table may be necessary.
Anterolateral approach (Watson-Jones)	Tensor fascia latae and gluteus medius	None	Branch of the superior gluteal nerve	Stability	Difficult femoral exposure Denervation or damage to the abductors
Lateral approach (Hardinge)	Splitting of the gluteus medius and sometimes vastus lateralis	None	Superior gluteal artery and nerve	Stability Improved exposure of femur compared to anterior and anterolateral	Damage to abductors (limp) Heterotopic ossification
Posterior or posterolateral (Southern)	Splitting of the gluteus maximus Tenotomies of the external rotators	None	Sciatic nerve	Extensile approach Quick recovery Low rate of complications	Slightly higher dislocation rate reported

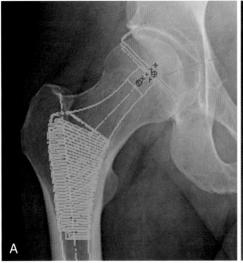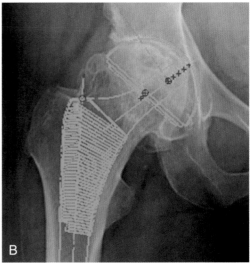

FIGURE 5-9 If the hip seen in **A** is inserted as templated, the expected outcome would be decreased leg length and offset compared to the native hip. Compare this to figure **B,** where the patient would have increased leg length and offset.

■ Cement fixation

▨ Microinterlock with endosteal bone

▨ Cement will fatigue with cyclic loading.

- Fatigue starts at stress points within the cement mantle.
- A *mantle defect* is an area where the prosthesis touches bone. This is an area of significant stress concentration (Figure 5-10).

▨ Cemented cups fail at a higher rate than cemented stems.

- Acetabular cup is positioned at an angle (i.e., theta [θ] angle) relative to longitudinal axis of leg. This creates shear and tension forces at cement-bone interface.
- Cement is strongest in *compression* and weaker in tension.
- Cemented stems fail at a lower rate than cups because stems see primarily a compression force.

■ Cemented stem failure

▨ Young, active patients are thought to have increased risk for failure over time.

▨ International registry data have demonstrated good survivorship with many cemented stem designs.

■ Cement technique—success

▨ Porosity reduction during mixing

- Decreased porosity reduces stress points in cement.
- Vacuum mixing—most common method to reduce cement porosity

▨ *Pressurization* of cement before component insertion

- Enhances cement interdigitation with bone

▨ *Pulsatile lavage* of bone before cementing

- Clean, dry bone allows better cement interdigitation.

▨ *Stem centralization* with distal stem centralizer

- Maintains uniform cement mantle (i.e., no mantle defects)

▨ *Stiff stem* lessens bending stress upon cement mantle.

- Cobalt chromium and stainless steel stems have performed better than titanium.

■ Biologic fixation

▨ Bone ingrowth (Figure 5-11)

- Prosthesis is fabricated with metal pores into metallic alloy. Bone grows into the porous structure, stabilizing the prosthesis to bone.
- Successful bone ingrowth is based upon the following factors:
  - Optimal pore size
    - Between 50 and 150 μm
  - Pore depth (i.e., deeper distance into metal) is directly related to increased fixation strength.
  - Optimal metal porosity
    - Porosity of 40% to 50% is best.
  - Minimize gap distance between prosthesis and bone.
    - Gaps between metal and bone must be less than 50 μm.
    - Bone will not grow across anything wider than this.
  - Minimal implant micromotion
    - Implant must have an *initial rigid fixation* for bone to grow into prosthesis.
      - Bone fixation less than 30 μm
      - Fibrous fixation greater than 150 μm
      - Fibrous encapsulation—gross macromotion
  - Cortical contact with bone
    - Cancellous bone is not weight bearing.
    - Implants must be placed upon cortical bone to allow physiologic load transfer to weight-bearing regions of bone.
    - Shear and torsional strength stronger when implant is adjacent to cortical bone as opposed to cancellous bone
  - Viable bone
    - Prior irradiation to pelvis and hip increases risk for aseptic loosening of bone ingrowth/ongrowth implants.

■ Initial rigid fixation for cementless hip implants

▨ Initial rigid implant fixation to host bone is required for long-term osteointegration. Two techniques are used: *press fit* technique and *line-to-line* technique.

▨ Press fit technique (Figure 5-12)

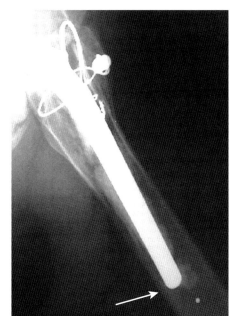

Cemented Stem

Mantle defect
- Prosthesis touches bone
- Area of stress concentration
- Higher stem loosening rate

FIGURE 5-10 Lateral radiograph of cemented femoral stem with mantle defect. Note distal stem tip that touches bone.

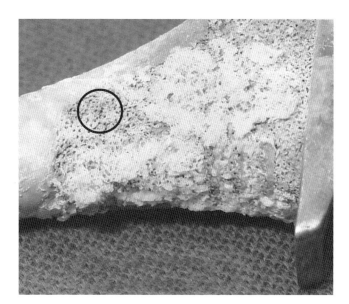

FIGURE 5-11 Ex vivo retrieval of bone ingrowth femoral stem. Note metallic pores *(circle)* that allow bone to grow into prosthesis and osteointegrate.

Press Fit Technique—Stem

Press Fit Technique—Cup

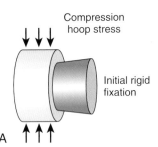

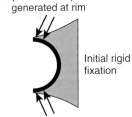

A

B

FIGURE 5-12 Diagram of press fit technique for cementless hip fixation. **A,** The canal of the femur is prepared with serial reaming and/or broaching to achieve desired implant size (remember that cortical contact is preferred). An implant of slightly larger size is impacted into position. The stem usually has a gradual wedge taper. The wedging effect generates compression hoop stresses that hold the implant still to allow bone to grow into implant interface. **B,** The acetabulum is prepared with serial hemispheric reamers to achieve desired implant size (ream to cortical margin of acetabular rim). An implant of slightly larger size is impacted into position. The wedge effect occurs at the rim of the acetabulum. The compression hoop stress generated at the rim holds the implant still to allow bone to grow into the implant interface.

- Bone is prepared such that a slightly oversized implant (relative to bone contour) is wedged into position.
  - Femoral stem typically has a gradual taper design to allow press fit into bone. Stem is typically 0.5 to 1 mm larger in size.
  - Acetabular cup is a hemispheric design. Cup is typically 1 mm larger in size. Press fit is against the acetabular rim. Screws are *not* required.
- Complication of press fit technique
  - Fracture is the most common complication.
    - The main reason for fracture is *underreaming*.
    - Acetabular fracture
      - If cup is stable, add screws.
      - If cup is unstable, remove cup and stabilize fracture. Reinsert cup with screws.
    - Femur fracture
      - Femur fractures are typically *proximal* in the calcar and due to wedge splitting of bone.
      - If crack is small and stem is stable, limit weight bearing and do not change stem.
      - If stem is unstable, remove stem and stabilize fracture typically with cerclage wires or cables. Reinsert stem. If remains unstable then insert revision stem.
- Line-to-line technique
  - Bone is prepared such that contour of bone is same size as implant.
    - Femoral stem has an *extensive porous coating* that provides an initial *frictional fit*. The rough surface provides enough resistance to motion that the implant is stable once impacted into final position. The frictional fit is also known as *scratch fit* or *interference fit*.
    - Acetabular cup is placed into position. Cup is a hemispheric design. Cup is secured with multiple screws placed into bone.
- Complication of line-to-line technique
  - Fracture is complication seen with femoral stem insertion; fracture typically occurs at distal stem tip.

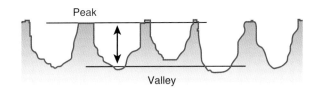

FIGURE 5-13 Surface roughness (R_a) of bone ongrowth prosthesis. R_a is defined as the average peak to valley on the surface of the implant. The value is typically in micrometers (μm).

- The force required to insert a straight stem into a bowed femur with a frictional fit can exceed the strength of the bone. The area of stress concentration is at the stem tip because of the modulus mismatch (bone/implant proximal vs. hollow bone distal).

BONE ONGROWTH FIXATION

■ Description
- Prosthetic surface is prepared by blasting surface with an abrasive grit material. Nickname is *grit blast fixation.*
- Implant material for grit blast fixation is always titanium alloy.
- Grit blasting process creates microdivots—no pores, just divots. Divot diameter approximately the same size as pore hole for a porous-coated implant.
- Bone grows *onto* rough surface, stabilizing prosthesis.

■ Surface roughness (R_a) (Figure 5-13)
- R_a is defined as average peak to valley on the surface of the implant.
- Implant roughness determines strength of biologic fixation.
  - Linear relation of R_a to fixation strength

■ Technique
- Initial rigid fixation of implant is always a *press fit* technique.
- Femoral stem design is typically a high-angle double-wedge taper (wedge in both coronal and sagittal planes) (Figure 5-14).
- Grit surface is extensile. Fixation strength with grit blast fixation is significantly lower than porous coating, and therefore the area of surface coating is greater.
- There are very few cups designed with bone ongrowth surface coating.

■ Complication of bone ongrowth
- Fracture
  - Bone ongrowth stem requires a very tight press fit to maintain initial rigid fixation. The double-wedge taper design is prone to proximal fracture.
- Aseptic loosening
  - Stem settling occurs when initial rigid fixation is not good enough to allow osteointegration.

HYDROXYAPATITE

- **Formula is $Ca_{10}(PO_4)_6 (OH)_2$.**
- ***Osteoconductive* only**
- **Effect—allows more rapid closure of gaps between bone and prosthesis**
- Bidirectional closure of space between prosthesis and bone

Bone Ongrowth

Technique
- Always press fit technique
- Design typically a high-angle wedge taper design
- Long-term fixation biologic

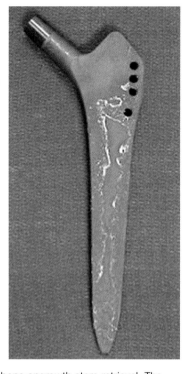

FIGURE 5-14 Photograph of bone ongrowth stem retrieval. The design of the stem has a sharp angle wedge design in two planes. The edges of the implant are sharp to provide rotational stability. Notice the rather scant amount of bone on the surface of this prosthesis. Implant was found biologically stable at the time of removal.

- Osteoblasts adhere to hydroxyapatite surface during implantation and then grow toward bone.
- Clinically shortens time to biological fixation
- **Success requires**
- High crystallinity—amorphous areas of hydroxyapatite will dissolve.
- Optimal thickness—a thick coating will crack and shear off.
  - Thickness under 50 to 70 μm preferred
- Surface roughness
  - Higher implant R_a provides increased metal-hydroxyapatite interface fracture toughness.

PRIMARY THA—FIXATION SELECTION

- **Cup**
- Porous-coated cementless cup is preferred choice.
- Porous-coated hemispheric cementless cups have reliable long-term results.
- **Stem**
- Both cementless and cemented fixation are acceptable techniques in primary THA.
- Cementless stem indications
  - High–activity-level patient (cement would cyclically fatigue over time)
  - Young male patient (higher loading stress would cause cement cracks at stress points)

FEMORAL STEM LOADING

- **Proximal porous coating (Figure 5-15)**
- Mechanical load is transferred to metaphysis and proximal diaphysis. This is termed *proximal bone loading*.

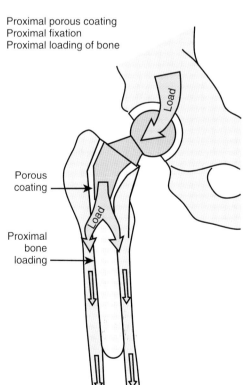

Proximal porous coating
Proximal fixation
Proximal loading of bone

Load

Porous coating

Load

Proximal bone loading

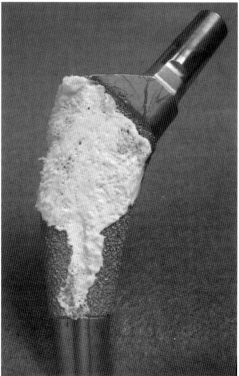

FIGURE 5-15 Diagram and retrieval photograph of proximal bone loading in a proximal porous-coated implant. With proximal porous coating, loading forces are transferred through the porous coating into the metaphysis and proximal diaphysis. This helps maintain proximal bone density.

- Proximal bone density is better maintained with proximal porous-coated implants.
- **Extensive porous coating (Figure 5-16)**
- More of the mechanical load bypasses the proximal femur because porous ingrowth is present throughout the diaphysis. This is termed *distal bone loading*.
- In a well-fixed extensively porous-coated femoral stem there will be endosteal consolidation of bone near the end of the stem. This is called a *spot weld* (Figure 5-17).
- **Cemented stem**
- In a well-fixed cemented stem, the mechanical load is distributed throughout the cement mantle. Similar to an extensively porous-coated stem, more of the load bypasses the proximal femur. A cemented femoral stem is considered *distal bone loading*.

FEMORAL STRESS SHIELDING

- **Description**
- Proximal femoral bone density loss observed over time in the presence of a solidly fixed implant; typically refers to cementless implants
- **Etiology**
- *Stem stiffness* is main factor.
  - Problem is modulus mismatch between stem and femoral cortex.
  - Hoek's law: when two springs are placed next to each other and loaded, more force is transmitted through the stiff spring and less through the flexible spring. Thus a cementless femoral stem that has a higher modulus than bone (i.e., stiff spring) sees much more loading stress than the surrounding proximal femur.
- Extent of porous coating is less important.
- **Factors affecting stem stiffness**
- Stem diameter is most important.
  - Stem stiffness approximates *radius*^{4} of stem.
  - Larger diameter stems are exponentially stiffer.
- Metallurgy
  - Co-Cr alloy is stiffer than titanium alloy.
- Stem geometry
  - More stiff
    - Solid and round stems
  - Less stiff
    - Hollow, slots, flutes, taper designs
- **Archetypical scenario creating stress shielding**
- Large-diameter stem of 16 mm or greater
- Co-Cr alloy stem
- Round, solid, cylindrical stem shaft
- Extensive porous coating
  - Distal bone loading

FEMORAL STEM BREAKAGE (FIGURE 5-18)

- Failure mode is *cantilever bending.*
- Seen with smaller-diameter stems (cemented or cementless)
- **Clinical scenario**
- Stem is fixed distally and loose on top.
- Loading of stem creates cyclic bending stress.
- Fracture occurs generally in middle portion where stems taper and become thin.

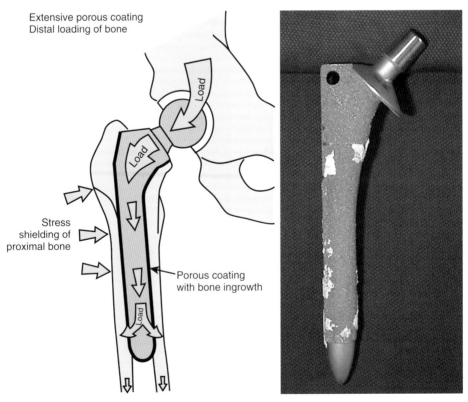

FIGURE 5-16 Diagram and retrieval photograph of distal bone loading in an extensively porous-coated prosthesis. With extensive porous coating, a majority of bone ingrowth occurs in the femoral diaphysis. Loading forces are transferred through the porous coating into the more distal diaphysis. As a result, bone density in the proximal femur is reduced because it does not see as much load.

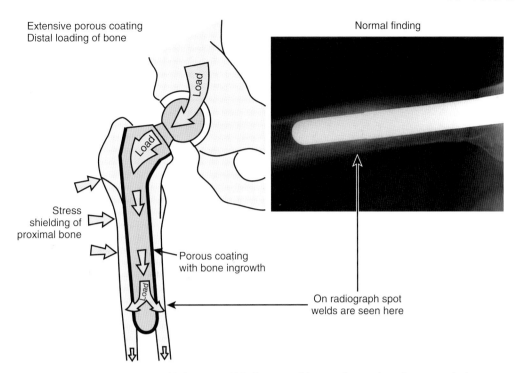

Extensive porous coating
Distal loading of bone

Normal finding

Stress
shielding of
proximal bone

Porous coating
with bone ingrowth

On radiograph spot
welds are seen here

FIGURE 5-17 Diagram and radiograph of spot weld. A spot weld indicates stable osteointegration of an extensively porous-coated implant. In contrast, a bony pedestal is bone accumulation within the medullary canal below the tip of a mechanically loose stem. The bony pedestal seeks to keep the stem from sinking further down the medullary canal.

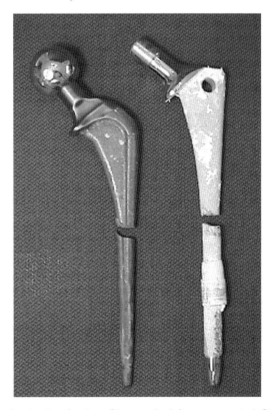

FIGURE 5-18 Photograph of stem retrievals due to stem fracture. Stem on the left was cemented. Stem on the right was cementless. Both stems have narrow-diameter stems, and both fractured in the typical region—the transition to the narrow part of the stem.

SECTION 6 REVISION THA

PRESENTATION

- *Start-up pain* is the most common initial presentation of loosening.
- Groin pain indicates a loose acetabular cup.
- Thigh pain indicates a loose femoral stem.
- Infection must always be ruled out as a cause of pain.
- Anterior iliopsoas impingement and tendinitis is poorly understood and may be the cause of a painful THA when a prominent or malpositioned cup is present and no other causes can be found.

ACETABULAR SIDE (FIGURE 5-19)

- Identify bone defects in acetabulum and pelvis.
- *Cavitary deficiency* is a loss of cancellous bone without compromise of main structural bone support.
- *Segmental deficiency* is loss of main bony support structures.
  - Acetabular rim
  - Acetabular column
  - Medial wall
- Combined deficiencies
- Well-fixed cementless implant with osteolytic defect
- Can be treated with débridement, bone grafting, and bearing component exchange
- Contraindications to this are a poorly positioned cup, poor implant design, an ongrowth fixation surface, or damaged locking mechanism.

- Significance of bone defects
- Major segmental bone deficiencies require a reconstruction cage, structural bone graft, or modular porous metal augments.
- A structure bone graft (a graft that reconstructs a segmental defect) alone without a cage has a high loosening rate.
- Fixation revision of acetabulum (Table 5-3)
- Cementless porous biologic fixation is preferred.
  - A cemented cup with impaction bone grafting is used more frequently outside of North America
- Hemispheric porous cup with screw is most common solution.
  - Must have at least two thirds of rim and a reasonable initial press fit to work
  - Requires at least 50% contact with host acetabular bone
  - Recommended cup replacement is to recreate the native center of rotation.
    - Cup placement should be inferior and medial (i.e., low and in).
      - Lowest joint reactive forces
    - Cup placement superior and lateral (i.e., up and out) is not recommended.
      - Highest joint reactive forces
      - Higher wear and component loosening
  - Fill cavitary deficiencies with particulate bone graft.
  - Acetabular porous metal wedge augmentation is an acceptable adjuvant to hemispheric cup to achieve stability and fixation when necessary

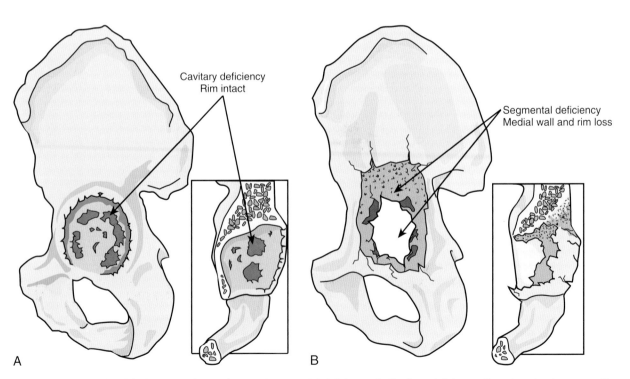

FIGURE 5-19 Diagrams of pelvis demonstrating cavitary and segmental deficiency. **A,** Cavitary deficiency. Bone loss involves cancellous bone. Main support structures are intact. **B,** Segmental deficiency. In this diagram there is structural loss of the medial wall and superior acetabular rim. Segmental defects are more difficult to reconstruct.

▦ Reconstruction cage (Figure 5-20)
  • Recommended when segmental bone deficiencies prevent initial rigid fixation of a hemispheric porous cup in desired position
  • Bone graft
    • Cage placement is against acetabulum and pelvis. Bone graft is placed behind cage.
      • Particulate graft preferred
      • Bulk support allograft when needed
  • Acetabular cup insertion
    • Acetabular cup is cemented into reconstruction cage.
▦ Modular porous metal construct (Figure 5-21)
  • Increasingly being used for cases of severe bone loss

• May allow achievement of mechanical stability an osseointegration when less than 50% host bone contact is available for a hemispherical implant
• Can help facilitate restoration of the hip center of rotation by filling superior defects
• Different highly porous metal options available including tantalum (75% porous by volume)
• Intraoperative flexibility to match defects
• May be combined with a cup in a so-called cup-cage construct
▦ Triflange cup (Figure 5-22)
  • Severe cases of bone loss where defect-matching techniques are limited
  • Decision to use made preoperatively as they are made custom for each patient based on a CT scan
▦ Acetabular screw placement (Figure 5-23)
  • *Posterior-superior* quadrant is the safe zone for acetabular screw placement. This is preferred zone for screw placement.
  • *Anterior-superior* quadrant is considered the zone of death. Screws and/or drill that penetrate too far risk laceration to the external iliac artery and veins.
    • Should a major vessel injury occur during screw placement, the hip wound should be immediately packed tight. Without closing the hip wound, an anterior pelvic incision is made to gain proximal control of the bleeding artery. Repair of the bleeding source is then addressed.
▦ Pelvic dissociation
  • Defined as separation of the superior aspect of the pelvis from the inferior aspect by fracture and/or osteolysis
    • Risk factors are female sex, massive pelvic bone loss (osteolysis), and rheumatoid arthritis.
    • Treatment/options
      • Multiflange reconstruction cage is preferred.
      • Posterior pelvic reconstruction plate to ilium and ischium followed by hemispheric cup, jumbo cup, or highly porous metal component with augmentation, as dictated by the remaining bone

Table 5-3	Reconstruction Options for Acetabular Revision
ACETABULAR REVISION OPTION	**CLINICAL PEARLS**
Hemispheric porous-coated cup	May be used in conjunction with adjunct techniques of bone grafting; screw fixation recommended
Highly porous metal cup	Appears to be effective in achieving biologic fixation in cases of severe bone defects; augments may be used for structural support; cup-cage construct can be used to offload cup.
Antiprotrusio cage	Useful in cases of severe bone defects or pelvic discontinuity; spans areas of healthy host bone and accommodates bone grafting deep to the cage; relies on mechanical fixation alone
Customized triflange implant	Requires several weeks or a month to obtain implant; serves as a good salvage option in cases of catastrophic bone loss and discontinuity; may achieve biologic fixation

Modified from Taylor ED, Browne JA: Reconstruction options for acetabular revision, *World J Orthop* 3:95–100, 2012, Figure 1.

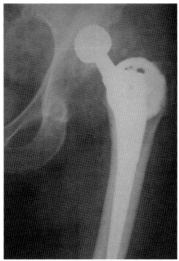 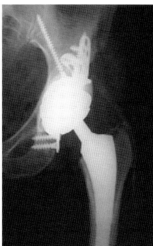 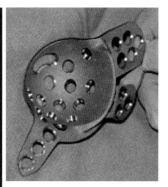

Acetabular cup is cemented into cage

FIGURE 5-20 Reconstruction cage for segmental acetabular deficiency. *Left,* Displaced acetabular cup. Note segmental bone loss of posterior acetabulum. *Center,* Pelvic reconstruction with a triflange cage. The cage is secured to bone with screws. Acetabular cup is cemented into the cage. *Right,* Triflange cage before insertion.

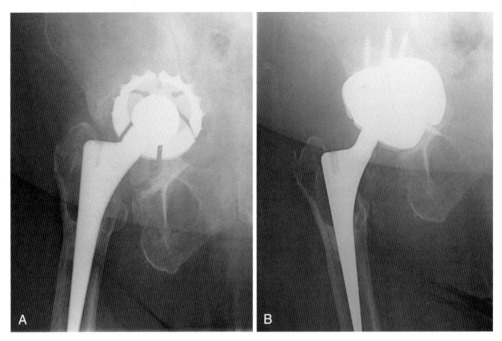

FIGURE 5-21 A, Preoperative radiograph showing failed acetabular component with large medial defect and intact rim. **B,** Postoperative radiography demonstrating the revision acetabular construct using tantalum augments as "footings" to support cup. (From Taylor ED, Browne JA: Reconstruction options for acetabular revision, *World J Orthop* 3:95–100, 2012, Figure 1.)

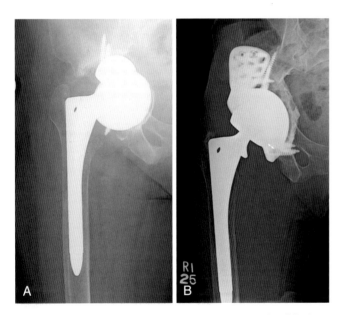

FIGURE 5-22 A, Preoperative radiography demonstrating failed revision acetabular component with massive bone loss and pelvic discontinuity. **B,** Postoperative radiographs showing custom triflange cup reconstruction. (From Taylor ED, Browne JA: Reconstruction options for acetabular revision, *World J Orthop* 3:95–100, 2012, Figure 1.)

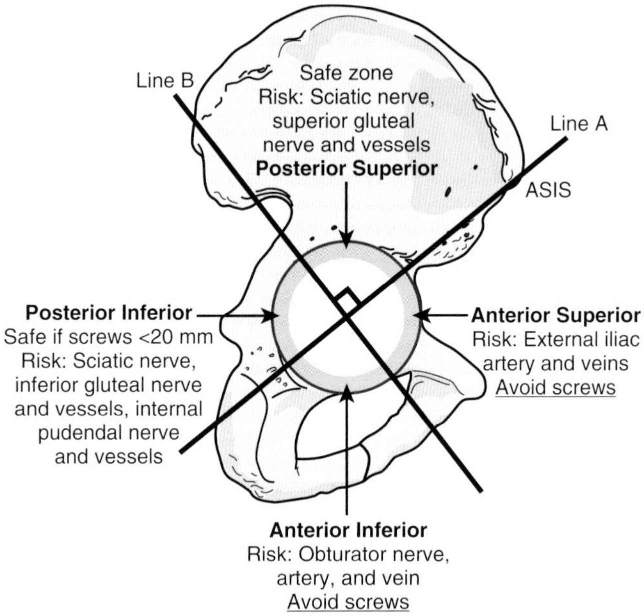

FIGURE 5-23 Diagram showing four quadrants for acetabular screw placement. *Line A* is formed by drawing a line from the anterior superior iliac spine (ASIS) to the center of the acetabular socket. *Line B* is then drawn perpendicular to line A, also passing through center of socket.

FEMORAL SIDE (FIGURE 5-24)

- **Identify bone defects in femur.**
- *Cavitary deficiency* is loss of endosteal bone. Cortical tube remains intact.
  - Endosteal ectasia is a form of cavitary deficiency in which the outer cortex has increased in diameter as a result of mechanical irritation by a loose femoral stem.
- Segmental bone deficiency is a loss of part of the cortical tube either in the form of holes or complete loss of a portion of the proximal femur.
- Combined deficiencies
- **Significance of bone defects**
- Revision femoral stem must bypass the most distal defect.
  - New implant must bypass most distal cortical defect by a minimum of *two cortical diameters*. Otherwise there is an increased risk for fracture at the tip of the stem.

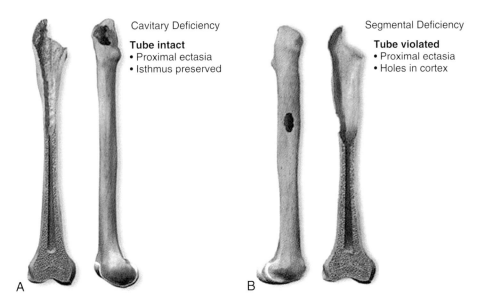

FIGURE 5-24 Diagrams of proximal femur demonstrating cavitary and segmental deficiencies. **A,** Cavitary deficiency. Bone loss involves cancellous bone and endosteal cortical bone within the femur. The outer cortical tube remains intact. The overall strength of the tube is diminished. **B,** Segmental deficiency. In this diagram the segmental defect is the hole in the diaphysis. A proximal cortical ectasia is also present (cavitary defect).

- The revision stem must prevent bending movements from passing through the region of the cortical hole, which is a weak point.
- Extensive metadiaphyseal bone loss and a nonsupportive diaphysis (Paprosky type IV classification) requires a femoral replacing endoprosthesis or an allograft-prosthetic composite
- **Fixation revision of femur**
- Cementless porous biologic fixation is preferred.
  - Cemented revision stems without impaction bone grafting have high failure rates at intermediate term and limited indications in the revision setting.
- Extensive porous-coated long-stem prosthesis is common solution.
  - An extensive grit-blasted stem with splines is also an accepted solution.
  - Typically made of Co-Cr
  - Achieve fixation in the diaphysis
  - Longer stems may be bowed, and engagement of the stem in the canal will dictate anteversion.
  - Stem should bypass defects and be long enough to achieve initial rigid fixation.
  - Extensively grit-blasted stem with splines also an accepted solution
- Tapered fluted implants
  - Made of more flexible titanium with a roughened surface
  - Achieve stability in the diaphysis
  - Taper design provides axial stability, whereas flutes provide rotational control.
  - Modular junctions allow for freedom in component anteversion but may increase the risk for breakage.
- Cemented revision stem
  - High failure rate at intermediate term
  - Recommended in patients with irradiated bone
  - Acceptable use in very elderly or very low-demand patient when immediate full weight bearing is needed

- Impaction grafting technique
  - Acceptable revision technique with greater popularity outside North America
  - Surgical technique
    - Place distal cement restrictor into diaphysis.
    - Impact particulate allograft bone (fresh frozen bone recommended) into endosteal canal. Bone is impacted around a femoral stem trial.
    - Cement polished tapered stem into impacted allograft bone.
    - Polished tapered stem is allowed to settle slightly within cement. Mechanical load forces are transmitted as compression forces upon allograft bone.
    - Allograft heals to endosteal bone.
    - Cement stays interdigitated with allograft.
    - Endosteal bone is restored.
  - Indication
    - Used to reconstitute cortical bone when there is significant cortical ectasia
    - Must have intact cortical tube. Small cortical defects can be covered with an external mesh or allograft strut.
      - Must not devascularize bone in process of covering hole
  - Complication of impaction grafting
    - **Most common complications are fracture and subsidence.**
    - Choice of allograft and morcellization technique are important factors affecting success.
- Segmental bone deficiency of femur
  - Cortical holes are reinforced with allograft cortical struts secured with cerclage cables (or wires).
  - Proximal cortical deficiencies may be restored with modular metallic endoprosthetic segments or with a bulk support allograft.
  - Proximal allograft technique

- Cement revision stem into proximal allograft.
- Connect allograft to host femur with a **step cut** or using an **intussusception** (telescoping) technique.
- Hold allograft to native femur with cables, plate, and/or allograft cortical strut.

■ **Modular bearing change**

▨ Indications
- Significant linear polyethylene (PE) wear associated with progressive radiographic osteolysis and/or mechanical symptoms of subluxation
- Implants must be well fixed to bone.

▨ Complications
- **Most common complication is dislocation.**
  - Patients generally feel well and fail to allow adequate soft tissue healing.

▨ Technique
- Must exchange both liner and head
- Bone graft osteolytic lesions behind cup with particulate graft through cup holes or small iliac trap door

▨ Cementing PE bearing into fixed porous cup
- Indicated when there is a damaged/worn locking mechanism or replacement PE bearing is not available
- Technique requirements
  - Optimize PE cup position to avoid neck impingement.
    - This reduces chance of hip instability.
  - Deep seating of PE liner into metal cup
    - This maximizes surface contact with cement and minimizes risk for PE cup debonding from cement.
  - Roughen back side of PE liner insert.
    - This increases surface area for bonding with cement.
  - Roughen inside surface of metal cup shell.
    - This also increases surface area for bonding with cement.
  - Close matching of PE liner to metal shell is *not important.*

SECTION 7 POLYETHYLENE WEAR AND OSTEOLYSIS IN THA

INTRODUCTION

■ **PE wear debris is the main culprit (when using traditional PE cup bearing). PE wear comes from two sources.**

▨ PE bearing wear—head-cup articulation

▨ *Backside wear*—occurs when the PE insert rubs against the metal shell, creating PE debris. This occurs because the PE locking mechanism does not completely inhibit PE micromotion against the metal shell. The more backside micromotion allowed, the more PE debris generated.

■ *Submicron*-sized particles shed by the PE bearing are responsible for eliciting the osteolysis reaction.

▨ Billions of particles are generated.
- Osteolysis more likely when the number of PE particles exceeds 10 billion particles per gram of tissue.

■ *Adhesive* bearing wear is the most important process that generates submicron-sized PE particles.

▨ Types of PE bearing wear
- **Adhesive wear** (Figures 5-25 and 5-26)—**most important mechanism in osteolysis process**
- Abrasive wear—rough femoral head surface causes mechanical scratching of PE surface with loss of PE material (*cheese grater* effect).

Primary articulation
PE beads being pulled off with each cycle

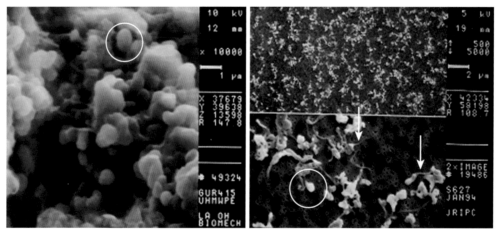

FIGURE 5-25 Scanning electron microscope photographs demonstrating adhesive wear in a polyethylene (PE) cup bearing. *Left,* Surface profile of a PE cup. Note submicron-sized beads that are melted together. *Top right,* PE particles collected after a bearing simulator test. *Bottom right,* Magnified view reveals that the particles collected *(circle)* are actually the beads pulled off the surface of the cup. *Arrows* point to the tails on the beads, indicating the beads are individually pulled off as the femoral head moves against the PE cup.

- Third-body particles—particles within joint space get between head and PE cup, causing abrasion. These particles cause PE to be removed from cup surface. Third-body particle sources include:
  - Cement debris
  - Metal debris shed from cup or stem
  - Metal debris from metal corrosion at modular metal-metal interfaces (i.e., modular junctions)
  - Hydroxyapatite debris shed from implant surfaces
  - Abrasive material introduced at time of prosthetic joint implantation (i.e., metal debris from drill bit)

OSTEOLYSIS PROCESS

- Phagocytes of submicron-sized PE particles by macrophage; macrophage becomes activated
- Additional macrophage recruitment via **cytokines released by** activated macrophage
- Release of osteolytic factors (cytokines) by the activated macrophage; these factors include:
- Tumor necrosis factor (TNF)-α—interleukin (IL)-1β
- Transforming growth factor (TGF)-β—IL-6
- Platelet-derived growth factor (PDGF)—receptor activator of nuclear factor κB ligand (RANKL)
- Bone resorption mediated **via RANKL**
- Mechanism of bone resorption mediated by osteoblast/RANKL (Figure 5-27)
- RANKL is produced by the osteoblast.
- RANKL attaches to RANK receptor on osteoclast, which activates bone resorption process.
- Osteoprotegerin, produced by many cell lines, blocks RANKL and mitigates bone resorption.
- The only cell that resorbs bone is the osteoclast.
- The RANKL/osteoprotegerin ratio in the bone microenvironment determines overall bone homeostasis.

OSTEOLYSIS AROUND THA PROSTHESIS—EFFECTIVE JOINT SPACE

- Intraarticular generation by PE particles elicits an inflammatory response that results in a **hydrostatic pressure buildup** within **the joint.**

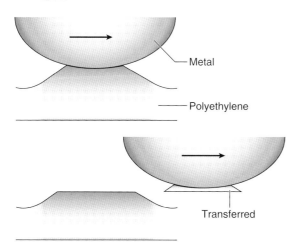

FIGURE 5-26 Adhesive wear occurs when the atomic forces occurring between the two opposing surfaces are stronger than the inherent strength of either material. In THA, adhesive wear results in small portions of the PE surface adhering and transferring to the opposing metal femoral head. This leads to wear particle generation and the creation of pits and voids in the PE.

- PE particles are then disseminated throughout the **effective joint space** (Figure 5-28).
- *Effective joint space* is defined as any contiguous area around the joint where the implant touches bone and includes the area around the cup, stem, and screws.
- Osteolysis can occur anywhere within the effective joint space (Figure 5-29).
- Fluid moves in the path of least resistance.
  - Areas well sealed by biologic integration will inhibit particle dissemination.

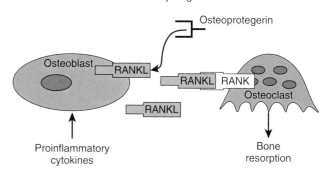

FIGURE 5-27 Diagrammatic representation of osteolysis-induced resorption of bone. Proinflammatory cytokines released by the activated macrophage reach the osteoblast, which in turn upregulates the production of receptor activator of nuclear factor κB ligand (RANKL). RANKL is produced on the surface of the osteoblast but is also released by the osteoblast in a soluble form. RANKL attaches to RANK receptor on the osteoclast surface. This induces osteoclastogenesis, resulting in bone resorption. RANKL is blocked by osteoprotegerin (expressed by osteoblasts and many other cell lines). The RANKL/osteoprotegerin ratio in the bone microenvironment determines overall bone homeostasis.

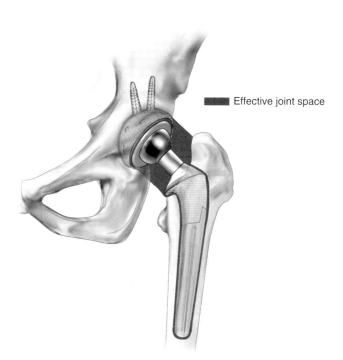

FIGURE 5-28 Effective joint space and osteolysis. Diagram of THA depicts area of effective joint space. The effective joint space includes any area where the prosthesis touches bone. PE particulate debris can be pumped anywhere within the effective joint space if there is a path for PE particles to be pumped.

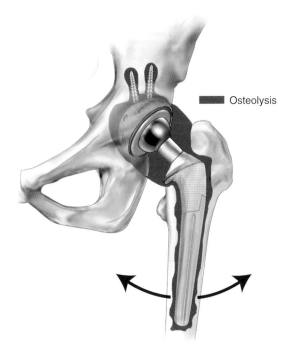

FIGURE 5-29 Diagram shows osteolysis around THA prosthesis. Remember that fluid (and PE particles) will move in path of least resistance. Prosthetic design, therefore, influences where osteolysis is likely to occur.

- Areas that are vulnerable to particulate debris dissemination include:
  - Smooth areas next to porous areas
  - Screw holes in cup
  - Surface area around screws
  - Debonded cement-bone interfaces
  - Cement mantle defects
- With an extensively porous-coated stem, most osteolysis is seen at the greater trochanter and proximal femur. This can lead to late insufficiency fracture of the greater trochanter.
- Proximal porous-coated femoral stems that do not have circumferential porous coating allow particles to be pumped toward distal stem region.
  - More osteolysis is seen at stem tip.

PARTICLE DEBRIS FORMATION—LINEAR VERSUS VOLUMETRIC WEAR

- **Volumetric wear** is main determinant of the number of PE particles generated.
- Volumetric wear is directly related to the square of the radius of the head (Figure 5-30).
- The wear track generated *approximates* a cylinder. The volume of a cylinder, and hence the amount of PE debris generated, is formulated as follows:

$$V = 3.14 \, r^2 w$$

where *V* is the volumetric wear of the PE cup, *r* is the radius of the femoral head, and *w* is the linear head wear (i.e., the distance the head has penetrated into the cup).
- **Head size** is most important factor in predicting the amount of PE particles generated.
- Linear wear rates in excess of 0.1 mm/yr are associated with osteolysis.

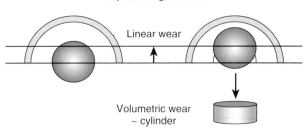

FIGURE 5-30 Diagram of PE wear in THA. As the head wears through the PE cup, a wear track is generated. Liner wear is measured where femoral head has penetrated into the PE cup. The wear track generated approximates a cylinder.

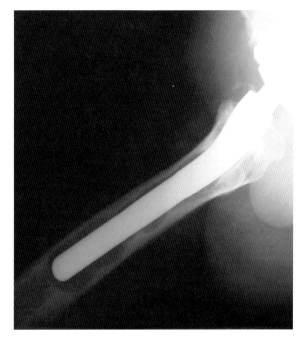

FIGURE 5-31 Lateral radiograph of femoral stem demonstrating osteolysis in THA. The classical finding is endosteal scalloping of femoral cortex.

- **Volumetric wear versus linear—the tradeoff**
- The following comparison is for *traditional* PE cup (i.e., does not include improved bearing technology).
- Small head—22 mm
  - Will have higher linear wear than 32-mm head
  - Will have lower volumetric wear than 32-mm head
  - Failure is more likely to result from wear through PE cup.
- Large head—32 mm
  - Will have lower linear wear than 22-mm head
  - Will have higher volumetric wear than 22-mm head
  - Failure is more likely to result from osteolysis.
- Compromise head—28 mm
  - Less volumetric wear than 32-mm head
  - Less linear wear than 22-mm head
  - Better stability than 22-mm head
  - Thus most hip systems use 28-mm head size.

OSTEOLYSIS—RADIOGRAPHIC FINDINGS IN THA

- **Endosteal scalloping** in femoral endosteal canal is hallmark finding (Figure 5-31).
- Round lytic lesions behind acetabular cup with screw holes is common finding.
- Round lytic lesion surrounding acetabular screw is also a typical finding.
- Osteolytic lesions develop later in prosthetic life cycle (usually starting after 10 years). Osteolytic lesions spotted within the first 2 to 3 years of the prosthetic life cycle are most likely a result of infection.

OSTEOLYSIS REDUCTION

- **Alternative bearing surfaces**
- Goal is to reduce macrophage-induced reaction.
  - Eliminate PE in hip system.
  - Less PE particles
  - Smaller PE particles that do not activate macrophage
- **Bisphosphonates**
- Inhibit osteoclast activity
- **Osteoprotegerin**
- Blocks RANKL activity, inhibiting osteoclastogenesis

SECTION 8 PERIPROSTHETIC THA FRACTURE

TIME OF FRACTURE

- **Intraoperative or early postoperative**
- Relates to surgical technique, implant design, and quality of host bone
- **Late**
- Associated with low-level trauma plus concomitant risk factors
  - Osteolysis
  - Stem loosening with bone abrasion
  - Segmental bone defect (i.e., hole in bone)
- **Most late fractures occur at stem tip.**
  - This is area of greatest modulus mismatch.
    - Bone and stem—stiff
    - Hollow bone distal—flexible

INTRAOPERATIVE FRACTURE

- **Highest risk is with cementless implants.**
- **Acetabular fracture**
- **Most common reason for fracture is underreaming.**
- Underreaming of 2 mm or more associated with higher fracture risk.
- Cup may be left in place if stable and additional screws used to enhance fixation.
- An unstable cup needs to be revised and may require a posterior column plate.
- **Femoral fracture**
- A longitudinal split in the calcar encountered when implanting a tapered proximally coated stem may be treated with stem removal, cabling, and reinsertion.
- If this does not result in a stable implant, a stem that bypasses the fracture and achieves diaphyseal fixation may be needed.

EARLY POSTOPERATIVE FRACTURE

- **Acetabular fracture**
- Overmedializing the cup can lead to fracture of the medial wall and intrapelvic migration of the acetabular component.
- **Femur fracture**
- Often a result of unrecognized intraoperative fracture
- **Wedge taper cementless stems**
  - Associated with **proximal** femur fractures
- **Cylindrical fully porous-coated stems**
  - Associated with **distal** femoral cracks

- **Treatment**
- If implant is loose and unstable
  - Open reduction with internal fixation (ORIF) and component revision
- If implant still maintains initial rigid fixation
  - Observation and limited weight bearing if just a crack
  - Prosthetic retention plus ORIF of fracture if there is significant fracture displacement or implant migration

LATE FRACTURE

- **Treatment guided by the Vancouver classification (Figure 5-32)**
- Fractures in the trochanteric area (Vancouver A)
  - Fractures involving the greater trochanter (Vancouver type A$_G$) can be treated nonoperatively if minimal displacement
    - ORIF considered for significant displacement or nonunion
    - ORIF *not* recommended in presence of massive osteolysis—inadequate bone for fixation and fracture healing
  - Fractures involving the lesser trochanter (Vancouver type A$_L$) treated nonoperatively with protected weight bearing even if displaced
- Fractures around or just distal to the stem (Vancouver B)
  - If the stem is well fixed (Vancouver B1), treatment is with ORIF.
    - Locking plate with unicortical screws and cables
    - Allograft struts with cables
  - If the stem is loose with good bone stock remaining (Vancouver B2), implant must be revised.
    - A broken cement mantle indicates a loose stem.
    - Diaphyseal engaging cementless revision stem preferred (fully porous coated cylindrical or tapered fluted modular implant may be used)
    - Fracture fragments typically secured proximally around revision femoral implant using wires or cables
  - If the stem is loose and poor bone stock is present in the proximal femur (Vancouver B3), implant must be revised and bone stock augmented.
    - Allograft-prosthetic composite (young patients)
    - Proximal femoral replacement (elderly or low-demand patients)
- Fractures well distal to femoral stem (Vancouver C)
  - Treated with ORIF using standard osteosynthesis techniques
  - Avoid creating stress riser, and overlap plate and femoral stem.

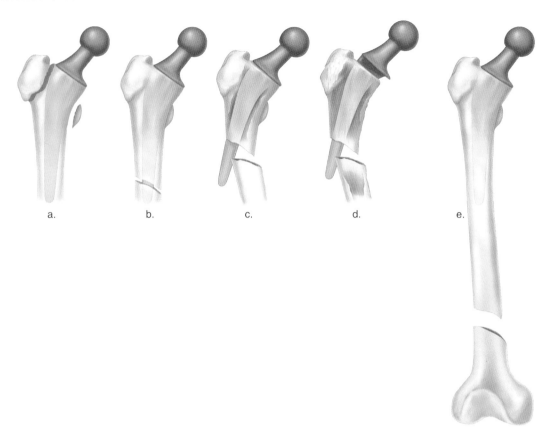

FIGURE 5-32 Vancouver classification of periprosthetic hip fractures. Type A fractures (a) include greater and lesser trochanteric fractures. Type B fractures occur around or just below the implant and include B1 fractures with a well-fixed stem (b), B2 fractures around a loose stem (c), and B3 fractures around a loose stem with poor remaining bone stock (d). Type C fractures (e) occur well distal to the femoral prosthesis.

SECTION 9 HIP RESURFACING ARTHROPLASTY

ADVANTAGES

- Preservation of proximal femur bone stock in young patients
- Improved stability compared to standard THA with small heads (22-32 mm)
- Theoretically easier to revise to THA

RELATIVE CONTRAINDICATIONS

- Coxa vara—increased risk for neck fracture
- Vertical shear force on neck
- Female of childbearing age
- Metal ions cross into the placenta.
- Renal failure
- Functioning of kidneys required to excrete metal ions

- Loss of bone stock, small anatomy, poor hip mechanics
- Metal hypersensitivity

COMPLICATIONS

- **Most common early complication (within first 3 years) is femoral neck fracture (1% to 4%)**
- Risk factors: notching of the neck, female, poor bone quality, varus implant position, small components, disruption of blood flow to femoral head
- Increased incidence of groin pain has been reported compared to THA.
- Abnormal soft tissue reactions secondary to metal-on-metal bearing

SECTION 10 THA—MISCELLANEOUS

THA—NERVE INJURY

- Involved nerves: 80% sciatic nerve, 20% femoral nerve
- **Compression is most common pathologic mechanism of injury.**
- In patients who have a nerve injury after primary THA, only 35% to 40% will recover to normal strength.

- **Sciatic nerve travels closest to acetabulum at the level of ischium.**
- During surgery, the most common reason for sciatic nerve injury is errant retractor placement causing excess compression to nerve.
- Peroneal nerve division is most often involved because this part of nerve is closest to acetabulum.

- Risk factors for nerve injury
- Female
- Posttraumatic arthritis
- Revision surgery
- Developmental dysplasia of the hip
- Developmental dysplasia of the hip
- Risk for nerve palsy increases with lengthening of leg over 3.5 cm.
- Postoperative functional footdrop
- Clinical scenario—patient sits in chair after surgery and develops footdrop.
  - With hip flexed 90 degrees in chair, there is too much tension on sciatic nerve.
  - Treatment—place patient back into bed.
    - Hip placed in extension (bed flat)
    - Knee flexed on one to two pillows
    - This position provides least tension on sciatic nerve.
- Postoperative hematoma
- A hip hematoma from anticoagulation can cause sciatic nerve palsy.
  - Compression is mechanism of injury.
  - Treatment is immediate evacuation of hematoma.

THA—ANATOMY

- Medial femoral circumflex artery
- Located underneath quadratus femoris muscle or gluteus maximus tendon
- Cutting deep to this area risks laceration to vessel.
  - Treatment is ligation/cauterization.
- Ascending branch of the lateral femoral circumflex artery
- At risk during direct anterior approach to THA and should be ligated
- Passes upward beneath tensor fasciae latae and is encountered in the space between tensor fasciae latae and sartorius
- Transverse acetabular ligament and obturator vessels
- Transverse acetabular ligament extends between the two cotyloid pads at the inferior aspect of the acetabulum.
- Errant retractor placement inferior to the ligament can cause damage to **obturator artery** and vein.
  - Treatment is ligation/cauterization.

THA—SPECIFIC COMPLICATIONS AND HOST RISK FACTORS

- Sickle cell disease
- Associated with early prosthetic loosening
  - Mechanism is extended bone infarct disease.
- Psoriatic arthritis
- Associated with higher periprosthetic infection rate
- Ankylosing spondylitis
- Associated with higher risk for heterotopic ossification
- Hip hyperextension due to fixed pelvic deformity can lead to a higher anterior dislocation rate.
- Parkinson disease
- Higher dislocation rate
- Higher perioperative mortality
- Higher perioperative medical complications
- Higher reoperation rate
- Paget disease
- Increased blood loss

- Good results may be still obtained with cementless fixation.
- Dialysis
- Higher risk of infection and loosening
- Fat emboli syndrome
- Occurs with femoral stem insertion
- Fat and bone marrow emboli are pressurized into bloodstream.
- Intraoperative hypotension, hypoxia, mental status changes, and petechial rash are hallmark findings.
- Treatment is volume and respiratory support.

VENOUS THROMBOSIS IN THA

- Activation of clotting cascade begins during surgery.
- Greatest risk for activation occurs during insertion of femoral component. Applies to both cemented and cementless implants.
- Mechanism for thrombogenesis
  - Femoral venous **occlusion** during preparation and insertion of femoral component
  - Typically, leg is twisted and mechanically levered during femoral stem preparation and insertion.

HETEROTOPIC OSSIFICATION

- Small amounts of clinically insignificant heterotopic ossification (HO) are common and likely present in a majority of THA.
- Risk factors: male, ankylosing spondylitis, those with hypertrophic subtype of arthritis, posttraumatic arthritis, head injury, and history of HO
- Prevention
- Careful handling of soft tissues
- Prophylaxis with oral indomethacin or radiation therapy (700-800 Gy) within 24 hours prior to surgery or 72 hours after surgery
- Treatment
- No effective treatment in early postoperative period once the process has started
- Indication for surgical resection is significant loss of motion.
- Process should be mature and stable on serial radiographs before proceeding with resection.
- Heterotopic bone may recur after operative resection.

ILIOPSOAS IMPINGEMENT

- Underrecognized cause of groin pain after THA
- Discomfort with resisted hip flexion and straight leg raise
- Cross-table lateral radiograph or CT may show a **retroverted cup or anterior overhang of the acetabular component**.
- An injection may be used to confirm the diagnosis.
- Treatment is with release or resection of the iliopsoas tendon, alone or in combination with acetabular revision for an anterior overhanging component.

THA—IMPLANT FACTS

- THA biomaterials—Young's modulus relative values (Table 5-4)
- THA bearing friction—relative values (Table 5-5)

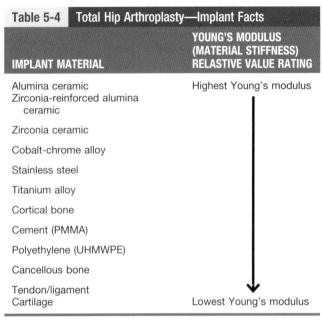

Table 5-4	Total Hip Arthroplasty—Implant Facts
IMPLANT MATERIAL	**YOUNG'S MODULUS (MATERIAL STIFFNESS) RELATIVE VALUE RATING**
Alumina ceramic	Highest Young's modulus
Zirconia-reinforced alumina ceramic	
Zirconia ceramic	
Cobalt-chrome alloy	
Stainless steel	
Titanium alloy	
Cortical bone	
Cement (PMMA)	
Polyethylene (UHMWPE)	
Cancellous bone	
Tendon/ligament Cartilage	Lowest Young's modulus

PMMA, Polymethylmethacrylate; *UHMWPE*, ultra-high-molecular-weight polyethylene.

Table 5-5	Bearing Friction
BEARING MATERIAL	**COEFFICIENT OF FRICTION RELATIVE VALUE RATING**
Articular cartilage	Highest Young's modulus
Al_2O_3 on Al_2O_3 (alumina on alumina)	
Co-Cr alloy on Co-Cr alloy	
Metal on PE	
Ice on ice	
Steel on steel	Lowest Young's modulus

Co-Cr, Cobalt-chrome; *PE*, polyethylene.

SECTION 11 THA—JOINT STABILITY

Dislocation in THA frequently is a multifactorial issue. Treatment is patient specific, and the solution depends on the problem.

INCIDENCE OF THA DISLOCATION

- **Primary THA—typically 1% to 2%**
- **Revision THA—typically 5% to 7%**
- **Highest incidence of dislocation**
- THA in the elderly patient (age > 80 years) for failed ORIF of femoral neck fracture—reasons:
  - Muscular weakness
  - Mental compromise
  - Loss of balance and coordination

RISK FACTORS FOR DISLOCATION

- **Female**
- **THA for osteonecrosis**
- **Posterolateral approach**
- **Smaller head size**
- **Greater trochanteric nonunion**
- **Revision THA**
- **Obesity**
- **Alcoholism**
- **Neuromuscular conditions**

DISLOCATING THA—ASSESSMENT

- **Component design**
- **Component alignment**
- **Soft tissue tension**
- **Soft tissue function**

COMPONENT DESIGN

- **Prosthetic range of motion (ROM) consists of two parts:**
- Primary arc range (Figure 5-33)
- Lever range (Figure 5-34)
  - Range allowed as hip starts to lever out of socket

PRIMARY ARC RANGE

- **Primary arc range is controlled by the head/neck ratio (Figure 5-35).**
- Head diameter/neck diameter is head/neck ratio.
- **Best stability is achieved by maximizing head/neck ratio (Figure 5-36).**
- **Additions to acetabulum and/or femoral neck decrease primary arc range.**
- Neck skirt (also known as *femoral head collar on femoral stem*)
  - Decreases head/neck ratio
- Acetabular hoods
  - Decrease primary arc range (Figure 5-37)
- **Acetabular constrained cups**
  - **Markedly decrease primary arc range (Figure 5-38)**
  - Rule—constrained cups should be avoided as much as possible.

LEVER RANGE

- **Lever range is controlled by head radius (Figure 5-39).**
- A large head has higher excursion distance and is more stable.
- **Most stable construct is a bipolar hemiarthroplasty (two pivot points).**

COMPONENT DESIGN—BEST RANGE IN THA

- ■ **High primary arc range**
- ▨ Maximize head/neck ratio
- ▨ No additions to cup or neck
- ■ **High excursion distance**
- ▨ Large diameter head

COMPONENT ALIGNMENT

- ■ **Primary arc range must be centered within patient's functional hip range (Figure 5-40).**
- ■ **Component malalignment does not decrease primary arc range.**
- ■ **Placement of components in a malaligned position results in a stable side and unstable side of the functional hip range.**
- ■ Implant positioning in THA
- ▨ Cup anteversion—20 to 30 degrees (Figure 5-41)
- ▨ Cup theta (θ)-angle (also known as *coronal tilt*)—35 to 40 degrees (Figure 5-42)
- ▨ Stem anteversion—10 to 15 degrees (Figure 5-43)
- ■ **Cup malposition**
- ▨ Retroversion—risk is posterior dislocation.
- ▨ Excess anteversion—risk is anterior dislocation.
- ▨ High θ-angle (vertical cup)—risk is posterior-superior dislocation.
- ▨ Low θ-angle (horizontal cup)—risk is inferior dislocation.
- ■ **Stem malposition**
- ▨ Retroversion—risk is posterior dislocation.
- ▨ Excess anteversion—risk is anterior dislocation.

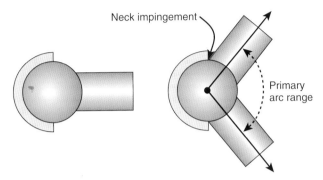

FIGURE 5-33 Diagram demonstrating primary arc range in THA. At the end of hip range, neck impingement occurs, limiting motion. Primary arc range is the arc of motion allowed between the two ends of impingement.

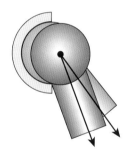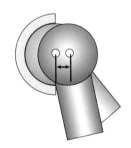

FIGURE 5-34 Diagram demonstrating lever range and excursion distance. *Left,* lever range. When the femoral neck impinges on the acetabular cup, it begins to lever out of socket. The range of motion allowed before the hip dislocates is termed the lever range. *Right,* Excursion distance. As the hip begins to lever, the femoral head is lifted out of socket. The excursion distance is the distance the head must travel to dislocate. The excursion distance is equal to the radius of the femoral head

Primary arc range controlled by

Head/neck ratio

$$\frac{\text{Head diameter}}{\text{Neck diameter}} \propto \text{Primary arc range}$$

Increased   Decreased

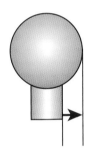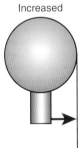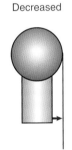

FIGURE 5-35 Diagram demonstrating head/neck ratio. Diagram on *left* defines head diameter/neck diameter as head/neck ratio. *Center* diagram shows an increased head/neck ratio when, in this example, the femoral neck diameter is decreased. Diagram on *right* shows a decreased head/neck ratio when, in this example, the femoral head diameter is decreased.

Increasing head/neck ratio
Same neck taper

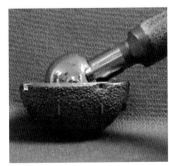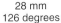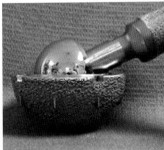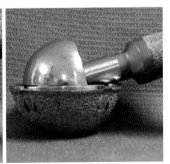

| 28 mm | 32 mm | 38 mm |
| 126 degrees | 131 degrees | 154 degrees |

FIGURE 5-36 Photographs showing how increasing head/neck ratio increases primary arc range. In this demonstration, the neck diameter remains constant. As the head diameter increases, the head/neck ratio increases, and primary arc range increases as well.

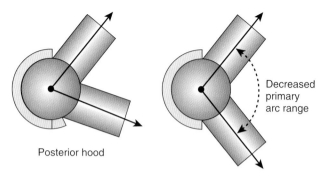

FIGURE 5-37 Diagram showing the addition of an acetabular posterior hood. The addition of an acetabular hood significantly reduces primary arc range.

SOFT TISSUE TENSION

- ■ **Abductor complex is key to hip stability.**
  - ▨ Consists primarily of gluteus medius muscle and gluteus minimus muscle
  - ▨ Prosthetic implant design and positioning must maintain/restore proper abductor hip tension.
- ■ **Restoration of abductor tension achieved by the following (Figure 5-44):**
  - ▨ Restored normal hip center of rotation
  - ▨ Restored head offset

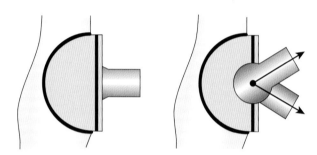

FIGURE 5-38 Diagram of constrained acetabular cup. A constrained liner covers the femoral head past its equator. This keeps the ball from coming out of socket. This has the adverse effect of severely restricting primary arc range.

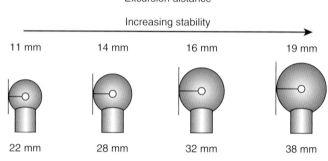

FIGURE 5-39 Diagram demonstrating excursion distance and effect on hip stability. Excursion distance is equal to the radius of the femoral head. By increasing femoral head diameter, excursion distance is increased. This increases hip stability.

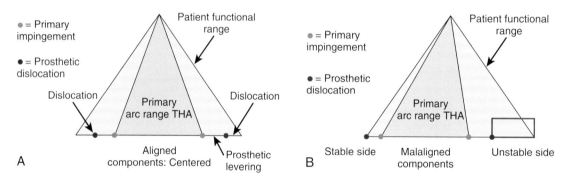

FIGURE 5-40 Diagrammatic representation of component malposition showing its effect on hip stability. **A,** Primary THA arc range centered within patient's functional hip range. Generally, THA arc range is less than patient's hip range because of smaller head size. **B,** Component malalignment. Note that THA arc range has not changed. Instead, malposition allows the patient to exceed primary arc range and lever range. This in effect creates a stable side and an unstable side.

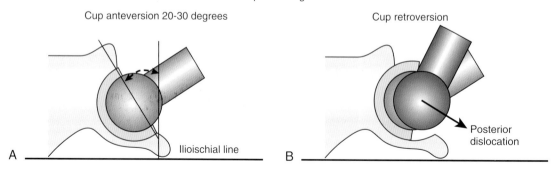

FIGURE 5-41 Diagram of acetabular cup version. **A,** In this figure, cup anteversion is referenced relative to the ilioischial line. The cup should be placed at 20 to 30 degrees of anteversion. **B,** With a retroverted cup, the femur impinges and levers in flexion, which can result in posterior hip dislocation.

- ▦ Restored femoral neck length
- ■ **Reduced hip offset—problems:**
- ▦ Weakened abductor complex
- ▦ Increased joint reaction force (decreased abductor lever arm)
- ▦ Positive Trendelenburg sign
- ▦ Gluteus medius lurch with walking
- ▦ Increased risk for dislocation
- ■ **Short neck length—problems:**
- ▦ Short neck length occurs by making a low neck cut or using a short prosthetic neck length (or both).
- ▦ Shortens abductor muscle length, resulting in abductor weakness
- ▦ Decreases hip offset, which also weakens abductor complex
- ▦ Results in bony impingement of greater trochanter against pelvis during hip range (Figure 5-45)
  - • Causes pain
  - • Allows hip levering and increases risk for dislocation

Preoperative Templating

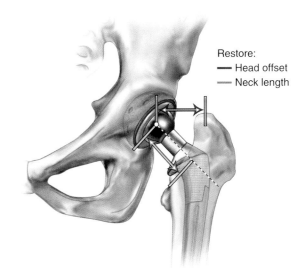

FIGURE 5-44 Diagram demonstrating head offset and femoral neck length. Head offset is the distance from the hip head center to the lateral femur (either the greater trochanteric tip or a line that is centered within the femoral medullary canal). Femoral neck length is the distance from femoral head center to the base of the femoral neck (usually the top of the lesser trochanter is used as the reference mark). Preoperative hip templating is used to make sure that the appropriate implant design and femoral neck osteotomy level are chosen to restore preoperative values.

Component alignment
(acetabular tilt—θ-angle)

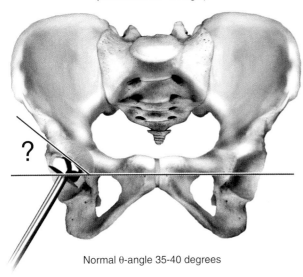

Normal θ-angle 35-40 degrees

FIGURE 5-42 Diagram of theta (θ)-angle. In the coronal plane, the cup should be placed at a θ-angle of 35 to 40 degrees. A low θ-angle cup is a risk for abduction impingement. A high θ-angle cup increases risk for posterior-superior dislocation.

Component Alignment

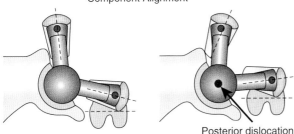

A Stem anteversion 10-15 degrees   B   Stem retroversion

FIGURE 5-43 Diagram of stem anteversion. **A,** Normal stem anteversion of 10 to 15 degrees. This allows functional hip flexion without impingement. **B,** Stem retroversion. With a retroverted stem, the proximal femur impinges early against pelvis. This can result in levering and posterior dislocation.

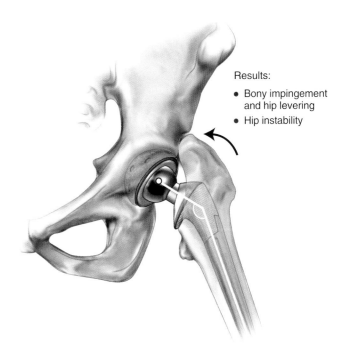

FIGURE 5-45 Diagram showing effect of decreased neck length. A decreased neck length brings the proximal femur closer to the pelvis. As the hip is ranged, the greater trochanter is more likely to abut the pelvis. This causes hip levering and increases risk for hip instability.

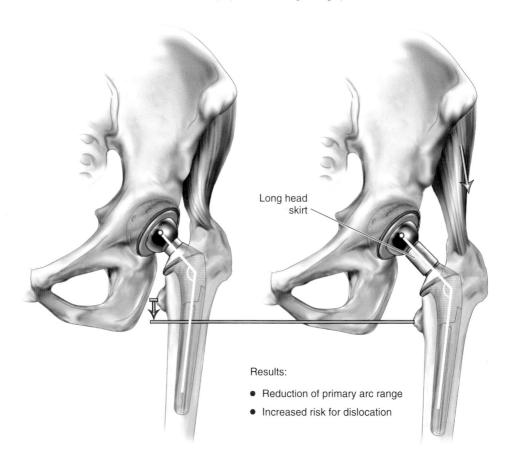

Long Femoral Neck with Skirt
(improved bending strength)

Long head
skirt

Results:

● Reduction of primary arc range

● Increased risk for dislocation

FIGURE 5-46 Diagram demonstrating the problem of using a long femoral head. A low neck cut is compensated by employing a long femoral neck (typically 9 mm or longer). When using a long head, a metal skirt is added to improve bending strength (to prevent metal fatigue and failure). The thick metal skirt can significantly reduce primary arc range, resulting in an increased risk for dislocation.

▦ Shortens leg length

■ **Restored neck length using long head—problems:**

▦ A short femoral neck cut can be compensated with an extra-long prosthetic neck length. However, **a long neck length requires a skirt** (Figure 5-46).
  • A skirt decreases primary arc range.
  • Increases risk for dislocation
  • **If the prosthetic neck-shaft angle is lower than the native hip, the addition of neck length will excessively increase neck offset.**
    • This can cause trochanteric bursitis and chronic lateral hip pain (Figure 5-47).

■ **Narrow-offset femoral stem design**

▦ A femoral stem with an offset designed with more narrow angle than the native hip will reduce hip offset. This reduces abductor tension and increases risk for hip dislocation.

▦ A narrow-offset stem can be compensated by employing a longer femoral head length (i.e., neck length). This creates two potential problems.
  • Addition of neck length to restore offset will excessively lengthen the leg.
  • Addition of a long neck requires a skirt, which decreases primary arc range and increases risk for dislocation.

■ **Greater trochanteric escape (Figure 5-48)**

▦ Greater trochanteric escape occurs when the greater trochanter pulls away from the proximal femur.
  • Usually a result of failed trochanter fixation after revision THA
    • Can also occur from trauma (usually associated with osteolysis in greater trochanter)
    • Successful reattachment is difficult and often fails.
  • Problems
    • Because the hip abductor complex attaches to the greater trochanter, trochanteric escape results in a loss of hip compression and increases risk for hip dislocation.
    • There is increased external and internal hip rotation because the greater trochanter no longer restricts rotation range. This also increases the risk for dislocation because the hip can more easily approach and exceed lever range.
    • The greater trochanter fragment can impinge between the hip and pelvis, causing hip levering.

▦ Treatment
  • Maximize head/neck ratio.
    • No neck skirts and no acetabular hoods
  • Resect greater trochanter fragment to prevent impingement levering.
  • Constrained acetabular cup is last resort.

Low Neck-Shaft Angle
(more varus)

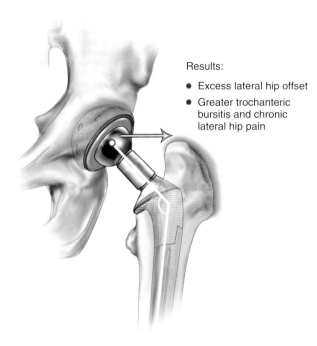

Results:

- Excess lateral hip offset
- Greater trochanteric bursitis and chronic lateral hip pain

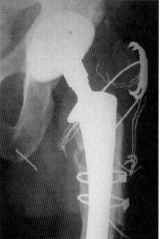

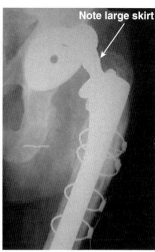

Trochanteric escape

Dislocation after débridement
Revised to constrained
polyethylene insert

FIGURE 5-47 Diagram demonstrating the problem of excess lateral hip offset. A low neck cut is compensated by employing a longer femoral head length (i.e., neck length). However, when the neck-shaft angle of the prosthesis is lower (i.e., more varus) than the native femoral neck, the addition of neck length excessively increases hip offset. This causes excess tension of the iliotibial band over the greater trochanter, which causes chronic pain and bursitis.

FIGURE 5-48 Radiographs showing trochanteric escape after revision THA. The radiograph on *left* shows greater trochanter pulled away from the proximal femur. The greater trochanter was damaged from osteolysis, leaving little surface area for healing. Cyclic fatigue eventually resulted in cable breakage and detachment of the greater trochanter from the femur. When the greater trochanter is not attached to the vastus lateralis, it will be pulled cephalad toward the joint region. In this region, the greater trochanteric fragment is an impingement source. Radiograph on *right* shows subsequent dislocation. When the greater trochanter is not attached to the femur, prosthetic rotation range is increased and the hip is more likely to lever out of socket. Also note head skirt *(arrow)*, which diminishes primary arc range.

SOFT TISSUE FUNCTION

- The soft tissues about the hip are controlled by several body systems. All are integrated together to provide hip stability. The three main factors controlling soft tissue function include
  - Central nervous system (CNS)
  - Peripheral nervous system
  - Local soft tissue integrity (surrounding hip region)
- CNS mechanisms causing disruption to hip function and increasing risk for dislocation
  - Muscle dysfunction
  - Sensory impairment
  - Impaired coordination
  - Impaired balance
  - Cognitive loss of restraint (i.e., compliance/memory)
- CNS conditions affecting hip function
  - Cerebral dysfunction
    - Stroke, seizure, CNS disease
  - Cerebellar dysfunction
    - Balance/coordination
  - Delirium
    - Medications, withdrawal phenomenon
  - Dementia
  - Psychiatric
    - Psychosis, addiction
- Peripheral nervous system mechanisms causing disruption to hip function, increasing risk for dislocation
  - Muscle dysfunction
  - Sensory impairment
  - Pain

- Peripheral nervous system conditions affecting hip
  - Spinal stenosis
  - Radiculopathy
  - Neuropathy
  - Paralysis/paresis
- Local soft tissue integrity mechanisms causing disruption to hip function and increasing risk for dislocation
  - Muscle dysfunction
  - Soft tissue dysfunction (other than muscle)
  - Soft tissue loss
  - Skeletal deformity
    - **Example: patients with ankylosing spondylitis have increased risk for anterior dislocation.**
- Local soft tissue conditions affecting hip function
  - Trauma
    - Soft tissue loss
    - Myoligamentous disruption
  - Deconditioning
    - Poor health
    - Aging process
  - Irradiation
    - Radiation fibrosis with soft tissue contraction
  - Dysplasia
    - Musculoskeletal hypoplasia
  - Osteolysis
    - Bone loss
    - Myotendinous disruption
  - Collagen abnormalities
    - Clinical hyperelasticity
  - Myopathy
  - Malignancy
  - Infection

DISLOCATING THA—TREATMENT

- ■ **Each case of hip dislocation is unique. There is not one common treatment.**
- ■ **In each case assess:**
- ▦ Component design
- ▦ Component alignment
- ▦ Soft tissue tension
- ▦ Soft tissue function
- ■ **Clinical review of dislocating event important**
- ▦ Was dislocation at extreme end range or within usual activities of daily living?
- ▦ Patient's cognition—impaired versus normal
- ▦ Clinical examination
  - • Determine where THA starts to lever and sublux.
- ■ **Radiographic review**
- ▦ Scrutinize implant design and position.
- ■ **Initial treatment for dislocated THA**
- ▦ **Two thirds of patients with a first-time THA dislocation can be successfully treated with closed measures.**
- ▦ Closed reduction
  - • Sedation or anesthesia preferred to minimize soft tissue trauma
  - • During closed reduction, take hip through full range and assess position of dislocation.
    - • Determine if subluxation is within patient's activities of daily living or at extreme end range.
  - • Posterior hip dislocation
    - • In supine position, the leg will lie in **internal rotation, adduction,** and shortened position.
    - • Reduction maneuver for posterior hip dislocation
      - • Flexion to 80 to 90 degrees
      - • Internal rotation
      - • Adduction
      - • Distraction
  - • Anterior hip dislocation
    - • In supine position, the leg will lie in **external rotation, slight abduction,** and slightly shortened position.
    - • Reduction maneuver for anterior hip dislocation
      - • Extension
      - • External rotation
      - • Slight abduction
      - • Distraction
  - • Postreduction treatment
    - • Education—hip precautions
    - • Immobilization of joint—(usually 6 weeks)
      - • Spica brace/cast
      - • Knee immobilizer—this will keep patient from putting hip in a compromised position.
    - • Physical therapy
      - • Focus on strength, balance, agility, coordination
    - • Optimization of medical conditions
- ■ **Surgical treatment**
- ▦ Surgical options
  - • Implant revision
  - • Greater trochanteric advancement
  - • Constrained acetabular socket
  - • Conversion to bipolar hemiarthroplasty
  - • Resection arthroplasty
- ▦ Rule 1—surgical treatment

- • If any implant component is malaligned, it needs to be changed.
  - • May require complete hip revision
- ▦ Component revision—goals
  - • Maximize head/neck ratio to increase primary arc range.
    - • No neck skirts or acetabular hoods
  - • Accurate component alignment
  - • Recreate center of hip rotation and head offset.
  - • Stabilize greater trochanter (if possible) if it is detached.
- ▦ Greater trochanter advancement (also known as *Charnley tensioning*) (Figure 5-49)
  - • Technique is to perform trochanteric osteotomy, advance greater trochanter distally on lateral femur, and resecure with claw, cables, and/or wires.
  - • By advancing greater trochanter distally, the abductor complex is tensioned tighter, which increases hip compression forces.
  - • Requirements
    - • No component malalignment
    - • Adequate distal bone surface for bony fixation and bone healing
    - • Intact superior gluteal nerve
- ■ **Constrained PE socket**
  - • A constrained PE socket encloses the femoral head and *mechanically* prevents hip from distracting out of socket.
  - • **Reserved for the multiple dislocator with soft tissue dysfunction**
  - • Best indications:
    - • Elderly patient (i.e., low demand) with **normal component alignment**
    - • Abductor deficiency/dysfunction
    - • Central neurologic decline
    - • Revision THA with reconstruction cage (Figure 5-50)
      - • Significant soft tissue dissection and potential muscle dysfunction with cage placement
  - • Contraindication
    - • Cup malposition
  - • Constrained cup—failure mechanisms
    - • Because a constrained cup significantly reduces primary arc range (as low as 60- to 70-degree arc range), the cup is exposed to more frequent and more intense lever range forces. With repetitive loading, the constrained cup will fail via two different mechanisms.
      - • The PE deforms at the edges of the socket and the hip dislocates.
      - • The PE does not deform. In this case the levering forces are then transmitted to the acetabular prosthetic-bone interface, resulting in mechanical cup loosening.
- ▦ Bipolar hemiarthroplasty conversion
  - • Technique—remove acetabular component. Ream remaining bone to a hemisphere. Press fit bipolar ball to rim of acetabulum (minimizes risk for medial migration of head).
  - • Requirements
    - • Fully intact acetabular bone
      - • No segmental rim deficiencies, otherwise the bipolar ball will dislocate
    - • Good bone density

Trochanter Advancement
(adductors are retensioned)

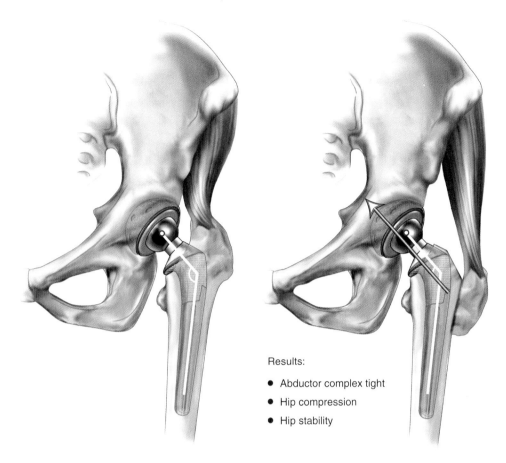

Results:

- Abductor complex tight
- Hip compression
- Hip stability

FIGURE 5-49 Example of greater trochanteric advancement. Diagram on the *left* shows implants in good alignment, but the abductor sleeve is lax in tension. When the greater trochanter is distally advanced *(right)*, the abductor tension is improved, resulting in increased hip compression forces. This improves hip stability.

- Rim fit technique
- Advantage
  - Maximize fully head/neck ratio.
  - Bipolar construct has a little more inherent stability than monopolar ball.
- Disadvantages
  - Groin pain—metal articulating on bone (Figure 5-51)
  - Medial migration of head developing into protrusio deformity
  - Accelerated PE wear
    - Larger overall PE wear surface area
- Resection arthroplasty
  - Indications
    - Nonambulator
    - Neurologic deficits where stability cannot be achieved
    - Recurrent/ongoing periprosthetic infection
    - Drug-seeking behavior with purposeful voluntary dislocations

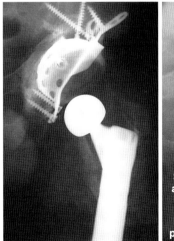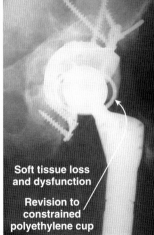

Soft tissue loss and dysfunction

Revision to constrained polyethylene cup

FIGURE 5-50 Radiographs showing dislocation in a multiply revised THA. In this example the patient had multiple risk factors for dislocation: cage revision, greater trochanteric escape, spinal stenosis, and peripheral neuropathy. Note the loss of soft tissue tension as the hip has literally dropped out of socket *(left)*. Stability was achieved with placement of a constrained PE socket *(right)*.

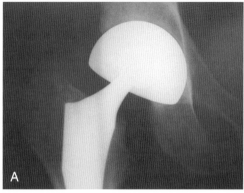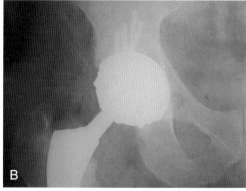

FIGURE 5-51 Example of hemiarthroplasty for recurrent THA dislocation. This 66-year-old man was revised for recurrent THA dislocation. **A,** Bipolar ball articulating on bone. Although hip was stable, this active patient experienced significant groin pain. **B,** The acetabular socket was revised to a fixed acetabular socket with revision of femoral component to provide proper acetabular and femoral component alignment. This patient remains stable with current construct.

SECTION 12 THA—ARTICULAR BEARING TECHNOLOGY

BEARING TYPES

- **Hard on soft (traditional)**
- Metal on PE
- Ceramic on PE
- **Hard on hard (alternative)**
- Metal on metal
- Ceramic on ceramic
- Metal-ceramic

HARD-ON-SOFT BEARING

- **Lubrication mechanism**
- Boundary lubrication
  - Asperities (surface rough points) on each surface make contact with each other—always.
  - Boundary lubricant (i.e., synovial fluid) separates surfaces just enough to prevent severe wear.
- **Bearing couples**
- Alumina ceramic on PE—good
- Co-Cr alloy on PE—good
- Zirconia ceramic on PE—not good
- Stainless steel on PE—fair
- Titanium alloy on PE—bad
- **Zirconia ceramic on PE—problem**
- Zirconia ceramic in vivo undergoes **phase transformation.** This means surface architecture changes over time, making the surface more rough.
  - **Yttrium-stabilized tetragonal crystal phase changes to monoclinic crystal phase.**
  - Monoclinic phase has increased surface roughness—increased PE wear.
- **Titanium alloy on PE—avoid**
- Titanium alloy head is easily scratched (Figure 5-52).
  - **Results in increased abrasive wear**
  - Causes rapid PE wear
- **Factors affecting wear**
- Surface roughness of head
- Sphericity of head
- PE manufacturing process
- PE sterilization process
- PE irradiation modification

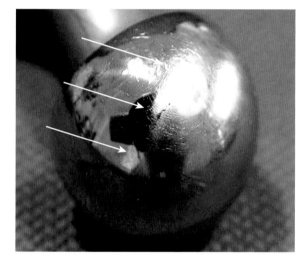

FIGURE 5-52 Femoral head retrieval of cemented femoral stem with nonmodular titanium femoral head. *Arrows* point to hemisphere of abrasive wear. This area articulates with the PE cup. It has become scratched by third-body particles that have entered the joint-bearing region. This roughened surface greatly increases PE wear.

- PE shelf life
- **Surface roughness of head**
- Co-Cr head (Figure 5-53)
  - Carbide asperities stick up and cause scratching.
- Ceramic head (Figure 5-54)
  - Residual pits on surface create roughness.
- Metal smearing—ceramic heads (Figure 5-55)
  - Metal smearing—transfer of metal to surface of ceramic head (ceramic head is not scratched)
  - Source of metal smear is hip subluxation with subsequent metal transfer from acetabular cup.
  - There is increased surface roughness in metal smear region.
  - Increased roughness causes increased wear.
- **Sphericity of head**
- Areas out of round are high stress points. These areas increase PE wear.

Hard on Soft

Surface roughness of head

- Co-Cr head
  - Carbide asperities stick up and cause scratching

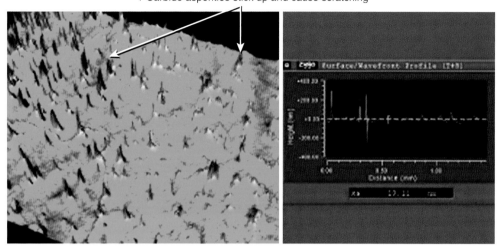

FIGURE 5-53 Scanning photomicrograph of cobalt chrome (Co-Cr) alloy head. The sharp peaks emanating from the surface are carbide asperities that protrude from the surface. (Courtesy Ian Clarke, PhD, and Donaldson Arthritis Research Foundation.)

- ■ **PE manufacturing process—four methods:**
- ▨ Ram bar extrusion—machine component
- ▨ Sheet molding—machine component
- ▨ Compression molding—machine component
- ▨ **Direct compression molding—no machining—best wear**
- ■ **Ram bar extrusion process—problem (Figure 5-56)**
- ▨ With ram bar extrusion process, calcium stearate is added to keep PE from binding up during extrusion process.
- ▨ **Addition of calcium stearate to PE adversely affects PE wear rates.**
- ▨ Calcium stearate in PE causes the following problems:
  - Inconsistent PE consolidation
  - **Results in unfused PE resin particles**
  - Increased PE oxidation potential
  - Reduced mechanical properties of PE
- ▨ Calcium stearate *should not* be added to PE.
- ■ **Direct compression molding**
- ▨ Implant is made directly from the mold. There is no secondary machining of the bearing surface.
- ▨ Bearing surface is less rough.
- ▨ **Best wear of the four manufacturing techniques**
- ■ **PE sterilization process—three methods:**
- ▨ Ethylene oxide gas
- ▨ Gas plasma spray (peroxide)
- ▨ Low-dose irradiation (generally between 2.5 and 4.5 Mrad)
- ■ **Irradiation of PE (Figure 5-57)**
- ▨ Major key point—irradiation of PE in air is bad.
- ▨ Irradiation of PE—sequence of events
  - **Irradiation of PE ruptures PE bond, creating free radicals.**
  - Free radicals can rebond via two different pathways.
    - In presence of oxygen (i.e., air), the free radical can bond with oxygen, resulting in PE **chain scission.** This is termed *oxidized PE.*
    - In absence of oxygen, the free radical will bond with an adjacent chain to create a **cross-link.** This is termed *cross-linked PE.*

Hard on Soft

Surface roughness of head

- Ceramic head
  - Residual pits on surface create roughness

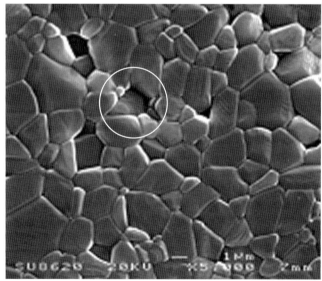

FIGURE 5-54 Scanning micrograph of surface of a ceramic head. Note residual pits *(circle)* on surface. These small areas create the roughness of a ceramic surface.

- ▨ Oxidized PE—main problem
  - **Oxidation of PE results in greatly reduced mechanical properties.**
  - Reduced mechanical properties cause accelerated PE wear and can also lead to catastrophic PE wear.
- ▨ Cross-linked PE—advantage
  - Improved resistance to adhesive and abrasive wear
  - Improved wear compared to non–cross-linked PE
  - Irradiation of PE in an oxygen-free environment is the preferred process.

- Methods to maintain the PE implant in an oxygen-free environment
  - Vacuum packaging
  - Oxygen-free gas packaging: argon or nitrogen
- **PE sterilization methods—comparison**
- Ethylene oxide and gas plasma
  - No cross-linking of PE
  - **Generally higher wear rate for same product compared to oxygen-free irradiation cross-linking process**
- Low-dose irradiation in oxygen-free environment
  - Cross-linking of PE
- **PE irradiation modification**
- This is not a sterilization process.

- Involves high-dose irradiation
  - 5 to 15 Mrad (10 Mrad = 100 kGy)
- **Product produced is highly cross-linked PE (HCLPE)**
- **HCLPE**
- Advantages compared to standard PE
  - Better wear resistance
  - PE wear particles tend to be **smaller** in size.
    - Potentially less osteolysis reaction
  - Generally, decreased number of particles generated (this is process dependent)
- Disadvantages compared to standard PE
  - Decreased tensile strength
    - Pulling force to break
  - Decreased fatigue strength
    - Maximum cyclic stress the material can withstand
  - Decreased fracture toughness
    - Force to propagate a crack

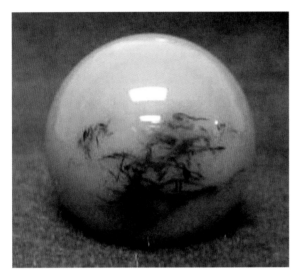

FIGURE 5-55 Photograph of a ceramic head retrieval demonstrating metal smear. With repetitive hip subluxation, metal from the acetabular cup is transferred to the ceramic head. The greater the smear area, the higher the rate of PE wear.

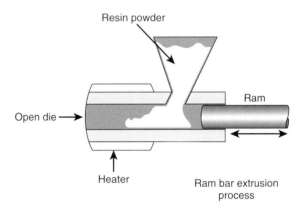

FIGURE 5-56 Diagram of ram bar extrusion process. PE powder is poured into chamber. The chamber is heated, and the bar of melted PE is pushed out the end of the die. Calcium stearate is added to the PE power to prevent it from sticking to surfaces of the die.

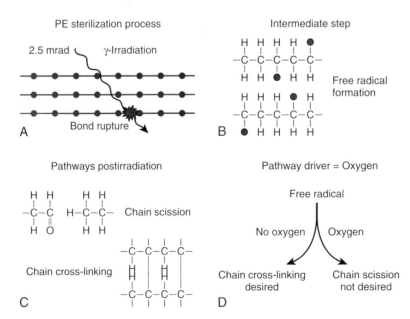

FIGURE 5-57 Diagram depicting irradiation process of PE. Irradiation of PE causes bond rupture **(A)**, which creates free radicals **(B)**. Free radicals can combine with oxygen to create an oxidized form of PE, which results in chair scission, or, in the absence of oxygen, the PE chains can form cross-links **(C)**. The presence or absence of oxygen determines the pathway the PE free radicals will take **(D)**. Cross-linking is the desired pathway.

- Decreased ductility
  - Elongation without fracture
- **HCLPE manufacturing process**
- Several different methods to produce HCLPE
  - Processes produce HCLPE products that are *not equivalent.*
- First-generation HCLPE process consists of:
  - High-dose irradiation
  - Heating of PE
  - Sterile packaging
- The major factors important to HCLPE production include:
  - High-dose irradiation
  - PE microstructure
  - PE crystallinity
  - PE heating process
- High-dose irradiation
  - The higher the dose of irradiation, the greater amount of free radicals generated.
  - **Problem—residual free radicals after cross-linking do remain.**
    - This is an oxidation risk.
- PE (officially ultra-high–molecular-weight PE [UHMWPE]) microstructure
  - PE in a manufactured implant exists in two forms (i.e., phases; Figure 5-58).
    - Crystalline phase
      - Provides mechanical strength to PE
    - Amorphous phase
      - Only amorphous regions of PE cross-link.
- PE properties—crystallinity
  - Optimum crystallinity 45% to 65%
  - Decreased crystallinity less than 45%
    - Decreases mechanical properties
    - PE more prone to macroscopic failure (i.e., cracks)
  - Increased crystallinity greater than 65%
    - The large crystalline phase leaves a very small amorphous phase.

- The greatly reduced amorphous region is more susceptible to chain scission oxidation.
- Creates significant increase in particulate debris
- PE heating during HCLPE process
  - **Two techniques of heating PE:**
    - **Annealing—heat PE to a level below melting point.**
    - **Melting—heat above PE melting point.**
      - UHMWPE melting point—140°C (284°F)
  - Reason for PE heating:
    - Postirradiation heating eliminates free radicals.
    - **Melting terminates all free radicals.**
    - Annealing eliminates some but not all free radicals.
      - Risk—potential for in vivo oxidation of PE, resulting in PE debris formation
  - Melting of HCLPE—problem
    - **Melting of PE reduces mechanical properties.**
    - Reason: cross-linking of free radicals occurs during melting, which prevents recrystallization.
    - Result—lowered crystallinity with lowered mechanical properties
    - Clinical relevance
      - **Cracking of PE cup may occur at edges of plastic with neck impingement.**
      - In the knee—edge loading or excess PE post loading may cause macroscopic cracks.
  - Annealing of HCLPE—problem
    - Annealing of PE increases oxidation potential.
    - Reason: crystalline areas maintain free radicals.
      - During annealing, crystalline areas do not unravel and eliminate free radicals.
      - Crystalline areas do not cross-link, so free radicals remain, leading to oxidation risk.
  - Melted versus annealed HCLPE properties (Table 5-6)
    - Several different methods to produce HCLPE.
      - Processes that produce HCLPE are *not equivalent.*
    - Each process attempts to:
      - Decrease the amount of free radicals
      - Improve oxidation resistance
      - Minimize adverse mechanical properties
- Second-generation HCLPE processing
  - Similar to first generation, but with additional PE processing to further reduce free radicals
  - Second-generation process
    - High-dose irradiation
    - Processing of PE—combination of:
      - Heating
      - PE treatment
    - Sterile packaging
  - Second-generation PE treatments
    - Mechanical compression
    - Vitamin E impregnation
    - Sequential processing

HCLPE Processing

UHMWPE - Two phases

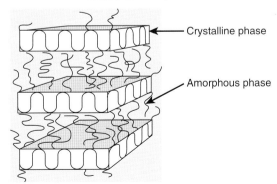

Crystalline phase

Amorphous phase

Only amorphous areas cross-link

FIGURE 5-58 Diagram of ultra-high-molecular-weight polyethylene (UHMWPE) phases. The UHMWPE in an implant exists in two forms (phases): the crystalline phase and the amorphous phase. The crystalline phase provides the mechanical properties to the PE. When the PE is irradiated, only the amorphous areas cross-link. *HCLPE,* Highly cross-linked polyethylene.

Table 5-6	Comparison of Melted versus Annealed HCLPE First-Generation Properties	
IRRADIATED AND MELTED		**IRRADIATED AND ANNEALED**
Low crystallinity (<50%)		Good crystallinity (>55%)
Low strength (<40 MPa)		Good strength (>45 MPa)
No oxidation potential		Potential for oxidation
Potential for macroscopic failure		Potential for osteolysis

HCLPE, Highly cross-linked polyethylene.

- Mechanical compression technique
  - Heat anneal, then compress rod of plastic down to a smaller-diameter rod.
  - Mechanical compression allows PE chains to be closer aligned.
  - Free radicals are more likely to be recombined.
  - Mechanical compression creates **anisotropic properties** on surface of bearing.
    - This means the PE wear properties vary according to the main orientation of the PE chains.
- Vitamin E enrichment of PE
  - Heat anneal PE
  - PE is soaked in vitamin E bath.
  - Vitamin E serves as a free-radical scavenger.
    - Vitamin E donates a hydrogen ion to the PE chain.
- Sequential processing
  - Irradiation and low-heat anneal
  - Repeat sequence several times.
  - More reduction of free radicals
- HCLPE—clinical performance
  - Clinical studies demonstrate reduction in wear rates and the incidence of osteolysis compared to standard UHMWPE implants at 10 years' follow-up.
    - Low wear rate of HCLPE appears to be independent of head diameter, with significant reductions in wear seen even with large head size.

- **PE shelf life**
- Irradiated PE packed in oxygen-free environment minimizes oxidation.
- However, any remaining free radicals stay in the PE indefinitely.
  - Any remaining free radicals are an oxidation risk.
  - When PE is oxidized, chain scission occurs, which results in increased PE particle debris.
- Remaining free radicals in PE—relative rank
  - Ethylene oxide and gas plasma—low
  - Irradiation (gamma irradiation) plus heat treatment—some
  - Irradiation alone—a lot
- PE product storage
  - Depending on packaging technique, oxygen can diffuse back into PE product.
  - Result—**on-the-shelf oxidation**
- PE packaging
  - Amount of oxygen that diffuses back into the package depends on two main variables:
    - **Packaging material—most important factor**
      - Defined as diffusion capability
    - Time on shelf
- On-shelf oxidation—worst-case scenario
  - Gamma irradiation
  - Product packaging in air (i.e., oxygen)
  - Long shelf life of 5 years or more
  - Result is rapid PE wear.
- On-shelf oxidation—worrisome scenario
  - High-dose γ-irradiation—HCLPE
  - Heat anneal
  - Permeable oxygen packing
  - Long shelf life of 5 years or more
- On-shelf oxidation—worry about these products:
  - Jumbo or extra small implants that are rarely used
  - Less frequent procedures—examples:
    - Unicompartmental replacement
    - Elbow/ankle replacement

HARD-ON-HARD BEARING

- **Lubrication mechanism**
- **Boundary lubrication** when hip at rest or slow motion
- **Hydrodynamic (also known as *fluid film*) lubrication** while walking
- **Hydrodynamic lubrication**
- Asperities on each surface are small (i.e., highly polished surfaces) and do not make contact.
- Fluid film lubrication *always* requires angular velocity.
  - Ball must be moving at significant speed.
- Factors affecting fluid film state:
  - Radial clearance
  - R_a (surface roughness)
  - Bearing size
  - Sphericity
  - Bearing material
- Radial clearance (Figure 5-59)
  - Radial clearance is defined as:
    - Radius of cup minus radius of head
  - Radial clearance defines **contact area** of bearing.
    - Best radial clearance (value depends on biomaterial used) provides **polar contact** with **high conformity.** This value will provide best bearing wear rate.
- R_a
  - The smoother the bearing surfaces, the better the chance for fluid film lubrication.
  - Supersmooth surfaces are used for hard-on-hard THA alternative bearings.
  - Hard-on-hard bearings—surface roughness
    - Metal (Co-Cr)—R_a 0.01 μm
    - Ceramics—R_a 0.006 μm
  - Comparison
    - Red blood cell diameter—R_a 100 μm
    - Machined PE—R_a 7.0 μm
- Bearing size
  - The greater the head radius, the better the chance for fluid film lubrication.
    - **Head radius is directly related to the lambda (λ)-ratio** (a formula defining fluid film mechanics).

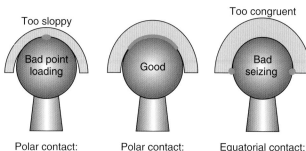

Contact area changes by changing radius between cup and ball

Too sloppy | Too congruent

Bad point loading | Good | Bad seizing

Polar contact: Low conformity | Polar contact: High conformity | Equatorial contact: Fluid "lockout"

FIGURE 5-59 Diagram showing effect of radial clearance and surface contact area of alternative hard-on-hard THA bearing. *Left,* A relatively high radial clearance. With a high radial clearance, hip loading is concentrated in a small polar contact region. This is disadvantageous and causes higher wear rates. *Right,* A relatively low radial clearance. With a low radial clearance, fluid is not able to effectively ingress and egress the bearing region. This creates a fluid lockout state, which causes high friction and wear. *Center,* Ideal radial clearance, which allows adequate fluid flow within the bearing but also provides optimum surface contact area for best wear.

The higher the λ-ratio, the better the chance for fluid film mechanics.

▦ Sphericity
- Desired goal is perfectly round.
  - Sphericity depends on manufacturing technique and good quality assurance.
  - Goal is to keep sphericity less than 7 µm.
  - High points cause localized stress points that increase friction.

▦ Bearing material
- Metal (Co-Cr alloy)—high carbide (i.e., high carbon content alloy) content is better. A high carbide content creates a harder bearing surface, which provides better bearing wear.
- Ceramics—generally smoother than superpolished Co-Cr alloy

■ **Stripe line**

▦ Primarily described on ceramic-ceramic bearings, but similar effect can occur on metal-metal bearings

▦ **Defined as an area of roughness created on the head and cup as a result of repetitive subclinical subluxation; hip is in lever range** (Figure 5-60)
- Subluxation with sit to stand
- Repetitive end-range activities
- Subluxation as head distracts out of socket during end swing phase
- Stripe line is detected microscopically. It is not caused by metal smear effect.

▦ Stripe line indicates abnormal bearing wear mechanics.
- Technical goals surgically are to reduce lever range subluxation with better component design, positioning, and offset.

■ **Metal-metal wear**

▦ Very small particles generated
- 0.015- to 0.12-µm particles (i.e., nanometer-sized particles)

▦ Very low linear wear

▦ Very low volumetric wear

▦ However, **absolute number of particles generated is significantly greater than comparable PE bearing.**

▦ Run-in wear
- Described mainly for metal-metal bearing
- Run-in wear is the higher wear rate seen within the first 1 million cycles (≈1 year of high activity).

- Etiology—in vivo polishing of the two new round bearing surfaces
  - **Polish out high points**
    - Areas out of round
    - Areas of prominent carbide asperities
  - Very small changes occur in diameters with polishing.
- **After run-in wear, the wear rate reduces to a lower steady state rate.**

■ **Metal-metal debris response**

▦ Very small nanometer particles can dissolve to generate cobalt and low-valence (Cr^{3+}) chromium ions.

▦ **With normal bearing wear, there will be detectable cobalt and chromium levels in urine and blood.**

▦ **Serum and urine levels correlate to bearing wear rate.**
- High blood levels of cobalt and chromium (after run-in phrase) correlate to abnormal bearing wear.
  - Usually a result of repetitive subclinical subluxation and poor prosthetic mating

▦ Biologic response to wear debris
- Metal debris from metal-metal bearing processed by the **T-cell lymphocyte**
- Two distinct responses:
  - Hypersensitivity reaction
    - Seen immediately after implantation
  - Particulate-induced T-cell response (PITR) or adverse local soft tissue reaction (ALTR)
    - Seen later (3-5 years)

▦ Hypersensitivity response
- Generally rare
- Almost always associated with nickel (Ni^{2+}) ion
- Reaction starts after placement of implant in vivo
  - Pain and ache start soon after postoperative recovery.
- Persistent dull ache (24/7 characteristic)
- Fluid aspiration—low white blood cell (WBC) count
- Treatment is replacement with nickel-free implant (i.e., remove Co-Cr alloy metal).

▦ Adverse local soft tissue response (ALTR)
- Likely related to continued debris formation at a **high rate in susceptible patients** with a predisposition
  - Patients with malpositioned implants (particularly a cup abduction angle > 55 degrees) often have increased wear.
  - Edge wear (maximum area of wear crosses over edge of cup) leads to large increase in local contact

Area of Pathologic Wear

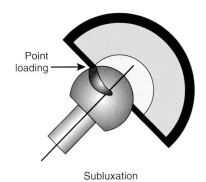

Point loading

Subluxation

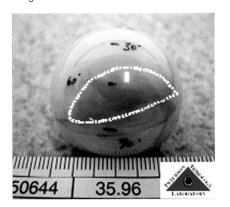

FIGURE 5-60 *Left,* Diagram depicting stripe line. With repetitive subclinical subluxation, the prosthetic head rotates upon the edge of cup bearing. This is a high-contact-stress scenario that roughens the articular surface of the femoral head. *Right,* Slide attempts to show stripe line, which is highlighted on the ball. Stripe line detection requires microscopic review.

pressures and breakdown of boundary lubrication (Figure 5-61).
  • Cup position does not explain all failures.
• Ultimate response may be **pseudotumor formation** (mass or cystic fluid collection).
  • May be more common in patients with high serum cobalt and chromium levels, but correlation is weak.
  • No cut-off values for ion levels have been identified.
• Involves a highly activated RANKL system
• The activated T-cell response has many associated cytokines, including:
  • IL-2, IL-6
  • Interferon (IFN)-γ
  • RANKL (which stimulates osteoclastogenesis)
▧ ALTR/pseudotumor response—clinical presentation
  • Pain and ache in hip common, although may be clinically silent
    • Detectable with cross-sectional imaging (typically MRI with metal artifact reduction sequence or ultrasound) (Figure 5-62)
  • Osteolysis may be seen around implants.
  • Tissues show inflammatory mass, primarily of lymphocytes.
    • Pathologic finding known as *aseptic lymphocyte-dominated vasculitis-associated lesion* (ALVAL)

• Grading systems have been developed to determine the severity of ALVAL.
• Regional tissues around the hip show necrosis thought to be secondary to cobalt and chrome toxicity.
• Major concern is for destruction of abductors.
  • Revision surgery often recommended to avoid progressive soft tissue damage
  • Abductor loss is very difficult to treat, so avoidance is paramount.
▧ ALTR/pseudotumor treatment
  • Remove Co-Cr bearing.
  • Revise loose implants.
    • Use titanium alloy implants for revision.
  • Radical soft tissue débridement
    • Debulk toxic tissues.
  • Use ceramic-PE bearing or ceramic-ceramic bearing (no Co-Cr heads).
■ **Metal-metal—specific conditions**
▧ Avoid metal-metal bearing in a woman of childbearing age.
  • Metal ions do cross placenta.
▧ Avoid in renal failure.
  • Metal ions no longer eliminated.
■ **Metal-metal—cancer risk**

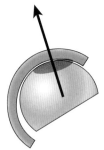 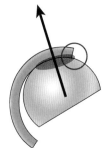 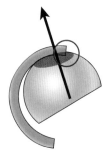 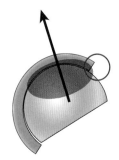

Well functioning   Reduced coverage   Steep inclination   Reduced clearance

FIGURE 5-61 Edge wear occurs when the maximum area of wear crosses over the edge of the cup and has been associated with increased wear rates in metal-on-metal bearings. Potential causes of edge wear are shown and include reduced coverage of the head from a cup that is less than a hemisphere, a cup that is excessively vertical, or reduced clearance between the head and the cup.

PITR (ALVAL)
Atypical Lymphocytic and Vasculitic
Associated Lesion

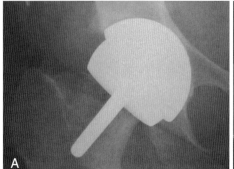 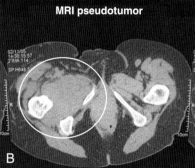 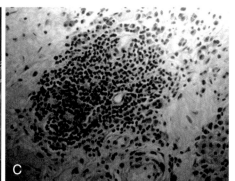

FIGURE 5-62 Case example of pseudotumor following metal-metal resurfacing arthroplasty. **A,** Radiograph of total articular resurfacing (TAR) implant with osteolysis in superior cup region and around superior femoral neck region. **B,** MRI of local hip region showing large mass that extends into pelvis *(circle).* **C,** At surgery, the large inflammatory mass shows aggregates of T cells surrounding vascular structures. Special staining will also reveal metal debris particles in these regions. *PITR,* Particulate-induced T-cell response.

- To date, with metal-metal bearing use, there has been **no increased risk for cancer** compared with standardized populations.
- However, with high-bearing-wear scenarios, the local tissues are subject to potential metaplasia/dysplasia from metal ions.

■ **Ceramic-ceramic bearing**
- First-generation alumina—high head fracture rate (up to 13.4%)—reasons:
  - More related to neck impingement (Figure 5-63)
    - Adverse head/neck ratio
    - Ceramic heads with thick skirts
  - Poor manufacturing technique
  - Low ceramic density
  - Coarse microstructure
- Third-generation alumina results in lower fracture rate.
  - Improved manufacturing technique
  - Hot isostatic pressed technique
  - High ceramic density
  - Finer microstructure
  - Skirt elimination results in better head/neck ratio.
- Advantage
  - Lowest wear
    - Generally less wear (both linear and volumetric) than metal-metal
    - Fewer particles generated than with metal-metal
  - Bioinert debris
    - No ionization of particles
    - No cancer risk
    - No dysplasia/metaplasia effects on local soft tissues
- Disadvantage
  - Head size limitation
    - Ceramic socket must be placed within a metal acetabular shell. Also, ceramic socket must have a minimum thickness to limit fracture. These factors limit ultimate ceramic head size.
    - Stability is less than large-diameter metal-metal bearing.
    - Fluid film mechanics less optimal with smaller head radius.

- Head length limitation
  - No skirts allowed
  - Can potentially limit hip offset, leading to hip impingement and instability
- Hip squeak
  - Psychologically affects patients with daily audible squeak
  - Etiology—perfect storm consisting of:
    - Implant malpositioning
    - Lever range wear
    - Stripe line formation, which creates an arcuate rough area on head and disrupts lubrication
    - Implant resonance—vibratory resonance created by lever range over rough region is amplified by prosthetic construct, which may be audible in ear frequency range.
  - Disruption in lubrication will lead to squeaking in all hard-on-hard bearings.
  - Treatment is revision of the cup to PE bearing with head change (head is damaged by squeak).
- Fracture
  - The Achilles' heel of this material when used for hip bearing
  - **Fracture is due to low toughness of material.**
  - Fracture treatment
    - Must replace with another ceramic-ceramic bearing
    - **After fracture, microscopic shards of ceramic remain and are severely abrasive.**
    - If a PE bearing is placed after ceramic bearing fracture, there will be rapid PE wear.

■ Head change
- Any ceramic head placed on a used femoral neck must have an internal titanium jacket (Figure 5-64).
- A used femoral neck is roughened by wear and corrosion.
- A new ceramic head (without a metal jacket) placed on a roughened neck can fracture with repetitive hip loading. High points on roughened neck cause a *burst fracture*.

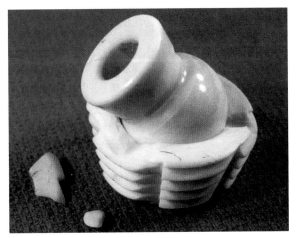

FIGURE 5-63 Photograph of retrieved first-generation ceramic-ceramic THA. Note very thick neck, which was required for strength in first-generation systems. The enlarged neck adversely reduced head/neck ratio. Also note acetabular fracture resulting from neck impingement.

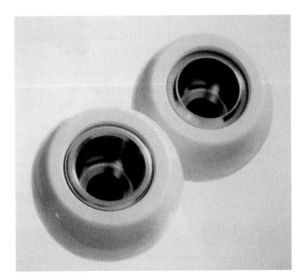

FIGURE 5-64 Photograph of internal metal jacket in ceramic head. This internal metal sleeve protects the head from burst fracture when placed onto a used femoral neck that has been roughened by use.

TRUNNION CORROSION

- There has been increasing attention on the potential for metal ion release from the modular junction between the head and stem
  - Mechanically-assisted crevice corrosion seen on majority of retrievals for failed metal-on-metal hips
  - Large diameter femoral heads, larger femoral component offsets, and varus stems increase the mechanical stress on trunnion (toggle effect)
  - Process has been associated with ALTR and pseudotumor formation
  - Has been reported in metal on PE bearings

SECTION 13 KNEE ARTHRITIS ASSESSMENT

Patient assessment of knee pain includes a physical examination and diagnostic radiographic modalities.

CLINICAL PRESENTATION

- **Pain with weight bearing**
  - Aggravated by stairs, hills, sit to stand
- **Bowing deformity and instability**
  - Seen later in presentation

IMAGING STUDIES

- **Radiographs are still the standard for initial evaluation. Images should include:**
  - Weight-bearing AP and lateral
  - **Weight-bearing 45-degree bent knee,** imaged posterior to anterior
    - X-ray plate is positioned parallel to tibia.
  - Sunrise view (i.e., merchant view)
  - Extension and flexion lateral
- **MRI**
  - Grossly overused in the arthritic patient population
  - If the joint space is significantly narrowed on radiograph, then MRI is *not* indicated.
  - Used when osteonecrosis is suspected
- **CT scan**
  - Three-dimensional CT with remodeling used for preoperative planning for reconstruction associated with dysplasia planning, posttrauma planning, and complex total knee arthroplasty (TKA) planning

SECTION 14 KNEE ARTHRITIS TREATMENT

NONOPERATIVE

- **Activity modification**
  - Reduce impact-loading exercises
- **Reduce weight**
  - Avoid stairs, inclines, squatting
- **NSAIDs**
  - COX-2 inhibition
- **Acetaminophen**
- **Patellar taping**
  - Used when there is patellar maltracking
- **Physical therapy**
  - Focus is on quadriceps strengthening
- **Joint injections**
  - Corticosteroid–antiinflammatory treatment
  - Hyaluronate
    - Backbone of proteoglycan chain of articular cartilage
    - Improves joint rheology
- **Unloading brace**
  - Helpful, but compliance low
  - Best suited for exercise activity
- **Assist device (cane or crutch)**
  - Opposite hand of affected knee
  - **Up to 50% reduction** of joint reactive force of affected knee

OPERATIVE

- **Arthroscopy**
- **Palliative treatment only**
  - Use selectively.
    - Overaggressive articular shaving accelerates natural course of degeneration.
  - **Success directly related to degree of mechanical symptoms noted preoperatively**
    - Meniscal tears with catching and locking
    - Loose bodies
    - Unstable cartilaginous flaps
  - **Success inversely related to severity of arthritis**
    - Not helpful in moderate to advanced disease
    - Will not take away toothache pain caused by reactive bone edema from mechanical overload
  - Palliative results less effective in the presence of knee malalignment (varus or excess valgus)
    - Malalignment causes mechanical overload and bone pain.
- **Osteotomy**
  - Best indication
    - Young active patient generally younger than age 50
  - **Most likely to succeed when disease affects predominantly one compartment**
  - **For varus knee malalignment:**
    - Treatment is valgus-producing proximal tibial osteotomy.
    - Reason: problem is usually due to **proximal tibial varus**.
      - Goal of surgery: correct the deforming problem.
    - **Osteotomy goal: maintain joint line of knee perpendicular to mechanical axis of leg.**
      - Mechanical axis of leg defined as center of hip through center of knee to center of ankle
  - **For valgus knee malalignment:**
    - Treatment is varus-producing supracondylar femoral osteotomy.
    - Reason: problem typically is result of **lateral femoral condylar hypoplasia.**

- Goal of surgery: correct the deforming problem.
- **Osteotomy goal: maintain joint line of knee perpendicular to the mechanical axis of leg.**
- Valgus-producing tibial osteotomy (for varus knee deformity)
  - Selection criteria
    - Clinical examination and radiographs show other two compartments are free of arthritis.
    - Patient is **physiologically young** and has an occupation or activity level that makes arthroplasty less appropriate.
  - Contraindications
    - Inflammatory arthritis
    - Lack of flexion—minimum of 90 degrees needed
    - Flexion contracture over 10 degrees
    - Ligament instability
      - Especially varus thrust gait (this indicates lateral compartment ligament/capsular stretch-out)
      - Femoral-tibial subluxation greater than 1 cm (viewed on AP radiograph)
      - Note: ACL deficiency acceptable
    - Medial compartment bone loss
    - Lateral compartment joint narrowing
      - Detected by valgus stress radiograph
  - Osteotomy less successful when
    - Smoking
    - Age 60 years or older
    - Varus deformity of 10 degrees or more
      - There is just not enough bone to remove to correct deformity.
    - Concomitant arthritis in other compartments
  - Main problems
    - Closed-wedge technique
      - Patella baja deformity
      - Loss of tibial posterior slope
    - Open-wedge technique
      - Patella baja deformity
      - Nonunion
      - Loss of valgus correction (i.e., collapse of open wedge)
- Varus-producing femoral osteotomy (for valgus knee deformity)
  - Selection criteria
    - Valgus deformity of 12 degrees or greater
      - Clinical pain isolated to lateral knee compartment
    - Clinical examination and radiographs show medial knee compartment free of arthritis.
    - Patellofemoral joint should also be free of arthritis, but minimally symptomatic patellofemoral disease is acceptable (reduction of Q angle improves patellofemoral mechanics and reduces pain).
    - Patient is physiologically young and has an occupation or activity level that makes arthroplasty less appropriate.
  - Contraindications
    - Inflammatory arthritis
    - **Prior medial meniscectomy**
    - Lack of flexion—minimum of 90 degrees needed
    - Flexion contracture over 10 degrees
    - Ligament instability
      - Especially valgus thrust gait (this indicates medial compartment ligament/capsular stretch-out)
      - Femoral-tibial subluxation seen on AP radiograph
    - Medial compartment joint narrowing

- Detected by **varus stress** radiograph
- Age older than 65—relative contraindication
- Osteoporosis—relative contraindication
- Main problems
  - Nonunion
  - Loss of varus correction
    - Seen more in patients with osteopenia/osteoporosis
  - Residual patellofemoral maltracking may require a lateral retinacular release.

- **Unicompartmental arthroplasty**
- Used for patients in whom arthritis predominantly affects one compartment
  - Most common is medial compartment replacement.
- Advantage
  - Quicker recovery compared to TKA and osteotomy
  - Fewer short-term complications
  - Better knee function
    - ACL is not sacrificed as it is in TKA.
  - Smaller incision
    - Shorter hospital stay with less postoperative pain
- Results
  - High rate of short-term to midterm satisfaction
  - However, **long-term survivorship is not comparable** to TKA when measured by revision rates.
- Contraindications
  - Inflammatory arthritis
  - **Significant fixed deformity**
    - Must be able to correct deformity on clinical examination (e.g., must correct resting varus attitude to normal valgus)
  - Previous meniscectomy in opposite compartment
  - ACL deficiency—key
    - ACL deficiency is an *absolute* contraindication for a mobile-bearing unicompartmental replacement.
  - Flexion contracture greater than 10 degrees
  - Tricompartmental arthritis
- Selection criteria—important
  - Pain must be localized to the compartment being replaced.
  - Anterior knee pain means significant patellofemoral disease.
  - Diffuse or global pain means tricompartmental disease.
- Technique
  - Do not overcorrect.
    - Overcorrection places increased load to unresurfaced compartment.
    - Can cause early failure due to arthritis
  - For varus deformity
    - Correct to 1 to 5 degrees of clinical valgus
- Complication
  - Stress fracture
    - Always involves **tibial side**
    - Associated with heavy weight and high activity level
    - Clinically, pain-free interval, then spontaneous onset of pain with activity
    - Aspiration of knee shows **blood.**
- Failure mechanisms
  - Overcorrection at time of surgery
    - Risk is disease progression in opposite compartment.
  - Undercorrection at time of surgery
    - Risk is implant overload with subsequent failure.
  - Fixed-bearing implants
    - More likely to fail from mechanical loosening
  - Mobile-bearing implants

- More likely to fail from disease progression
- Patellar impingement upon femoral implant
  - Patellar pain requiring revision to TKA
- **Isolated patellofemoral arthritis**
- TKA (not patellofemoral arthroplasty) is recommended choice in older patients.
  - Superior functional results compared to patellectomy or patellofemoral arthroplasty.
- Lateral retinacular release commonly seen with isolated patellofemoral arthritis.

- Maltracking is usually the cause of isolated patellofemoral arthritis.
- Patellofemoral replacement procedure
  - Precise soft tissue balancing required for successful result
    - Residual maltracking causes pain.
    - Must restore a patellofemoral alignment to a normal Q angle
- **TKA: see next section.**

SECTION 15 TOTAL KNEE ARTHROPLASTY

INDICATIONS

- **Debilitating pain affecting activities of daily living**
- **Pain not well controlled by conservative measures**
- **Medically fit for surgery**
- **No active infection—anywhere**

TKA SURVIVAL

- **Best survival**
- Well-balanced knee
- **Neutral mechanical alignment**
- **Decreased survivorship**
- Young age—55 years or less
- Osteoarthritis
- Reason: high activity level
- **Increased survivorship**
- Old age—70 years or older
- Rheumatoid arthritis
- Reason: low activity level
- Cemented fixation (all components)

TECHNICAL GOALS OF TKA

- **Restore neutral mechanical alignment of limb**
- **Restore joint line**
- **Balanced ligaments**
- **Normal Q angle**

PREOPERATIVE PLANNING FOR TKA

- **Preoperative radiographs should include:**
- *Standing* bilateral AP knees
- Extension and flexion lateral
- Sunrise (merchant view)
- Standing *full-length* AP hip to ankle when:
  - Bony angular deformity present
  - Very short stature
    - Below 60 inches (152 cm)
  - Very tall stature
    - Above 75 inches (190 cm)
- **Radiographic analysis**
- Determine end cuts—femur and tibia.
- Determine position of femoral canal entry site at the knee.
- Identify bone defects.
- Identify joint subluxation.
- Identify ligament stretch-out.
  - If varus thrust gait is evident, then standing single-leg AP radiographs are recommended (Figure 5-65).
- Determine anticipated ligament releases.

- Anticipate extent of constraint needed from preoperative review of radiographs.
- **End cuts—distal femur and proximal tibia**
- **Goal with end cuts is to restore neutral mechanical alignment of the limb.**
  - *Neutral mechanical alignment* is defined as a line from hip head center, through knee center, to ankle center.
- Preoperative analysis of femur (review of full-length radiographs) is used to determine the following (Figure 5-66):
  - Anatomic axis of femur (AAF)
    - A line that bisects the medullary canal of the femur
    - The AAF, drawn to the distal end of the femur, **determines *entry point* for the femoral medullary guide rod** for the cutting jigs.
  - Mechanical axis of femur (MAF)
    - A line from center of distal femur to center of femoral head
    - **Significance—distal femur is cut *perpendicular* to MAF.**
      - This allows even mechanical loading to knee implant.
  - Valgus cut angle
    - Defined as angle between AAF and MAF
    - Intramedullary guide rod is placed into femur (this defines AAF).

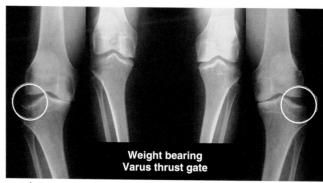

**Weight bearing
Varus thrust gate**

Lateral ligament stretch-out
Standing single-leg study

FIGURE 5-65 Preoperative review of patient in preparation of TKA. Standing anteroposterior *(middle radiograph)* shows varus attitude of knees. Patient clinically had significant varus thrust bilaterally. Standing single-leg-stance radiographs *(left and right radiographs)* demonstrate severity of lateral ligament stretch-out. In this case, a revision knee system was ordered to accommodate potential instability problems that may be encountered during balancing and trialing.

- Distal femoral cut jig is assembled to intramedullary guide rod.
- Surgeon selects valgus cut angle (typically between 4 and 7 degrees).
- Distal femur should end up being *perpendicular* to MAF.
- Always measure valgus cut angle in tall and short patients (Figure 5-67).
  - Hip offset remains relatively constant.
  - Femur length, therefore, has more influence upon valgus cut angle.
- Preoperative analysis tibia (review of full-length radiograph) is used to determine the following (Figure 5-68):
  - Anatomic axis of tibia (AAT)
    - A line that bisects the medullary canal of the tibia
    - The AAT, drawn through the proximal tibia, **determines the entry point for the tibial medullary guide.**
      - Both intramedullary and extramedullary cutting jigs for the proximal tibial end cut are acceptable techniques.
  - Mechanical axis of tibia (MAT)
    - A line from center of proximal tibia to the center of ankle
    - **Significance—proximal tibia is cut *perpendicular* to MAT.**
      - This allows even mechanical loading to knee implant.
  - Tibial cut angle
    - Defined as angle between AAT and MAT
    - Intramedullary guide technique
      - Intramedullary guide is placed into tibia.
      - Proximal tibia cut jig is assembled onto intramedullary guide.
      - Surgeon selects tibial cut angle (usually 0 degrees).

- Proximal tibia should end up being cut *perpendicular* to MAT.
- Extramedullary guide technique
  - The extramedullary guide technique is placed over the anterior tibia. A jig distally holds guide centered over ankle. A proximal jig holds guide centered over proximal tibia (landmark is **medial one-third region of tibial tubercle**).
- Surgeon selects tibial cut angle.
- In most cases the AAT and MAT are coincident. Therefore tibial cut angle is zero.
- When there is a tibial deformity (e.g., fracture or bowing deformity), the AAT and MAT are divergent. The tibial cut angle is then carefully measured and selected to provide a proximal tibial end cut perpendicular to MAT.

BONE CUTS IN TKA—GOALS

- Measured resection—replace bone and cartilage with implants that are of the same thickness.
- Maintains joint line, which is important for proper ligament function
- Maintains ligament tension
- Accurate bone cuts are accomplished with cutting jigs.

CORONAL PLANE LIGAMENT BALANCING IN TKA

- Correction of varus or valgus deformity
- Balancing goals
- Equal ligament tension in medial and lateral compartments tested in extension and in flexion
- Principle (Figure 5-69)
- Release concave side—tight side
- Retension convex side—loose side
- Varus deformity
- Convex side is lateral—loose

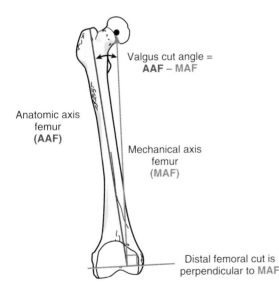

FIGURE 5-66 Diagram showing preoperative measurements of femur to make distal femoral end cut. The distal femur is cut perpendicular to the mechanical axis of the femur. The anatomic axis of the femur (AAF) is defined clinically by the intramedullary guide that is placed into the canal. A cutting jig is placed onto the medullary guide rod. The distal valgus cut angle is the value set into the cutting jig to make the distal femoral cut perpendicular to the mechanical axis. Also note the location where the AAF exits the distal femur. This is the position to open the distal femur to insert the medullary guide rod.

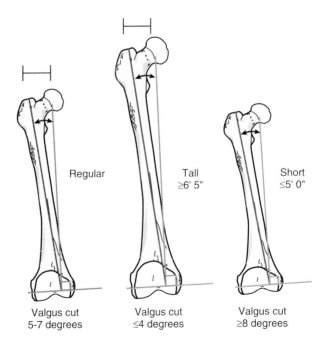

FIGURE 5-67 Effect of femoral length on valgus cut angle. Hip offset does not vary widely. Therefore valgus cut angle is more influenced by femoral length. Tall patients will have a lower valgus cut angle, whereas short patients will have a higher valgus cut angle.

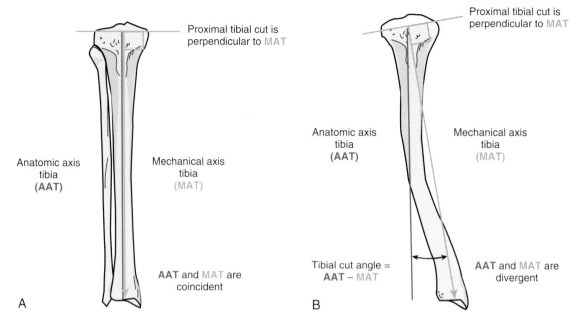

 FIGURE 5-68 Diagrams showing preoperative measurements of tibia to make proximal tibial end cut. The proximal tibia is cut perpendicular to the mechanical axis of the tibia (MAT). **A,** Usually the anatomic axis of the tibia (AAT) and MAT are coincident. In this situation the tibial end cut is zero. **B,** In the situation where a tibial angular deformity is present, the AAT and MAT are divergent. The tibial cut angle is carefully measured to make a tibia end cut perpendicular to the MAT.

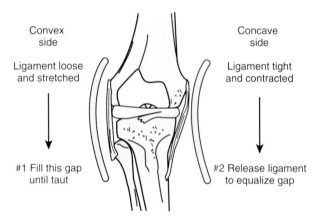

 FIGURE 5-69 Diagram demonstrating principle of coronal plane balance in TKA. The knee in this example has a varus deformity. The lateral side of the knee is the convex side where the ligaments have been stretched from the deformity. On this side, the lateral joint space is filled with the prosthesis until the ligament is once again under normal tension. The concave side is the medial side where the ligament is tight and contracted. The medial ligament complex is released until there is equal tension between the medial and lateral compartments.

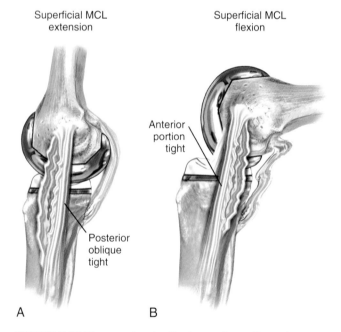

FIGURE 5-70 Diagram showing the two major portions of superficial medial collateral ligament (MCL). **A,** In extension, the posterior oblique portion of the ligament is taut. The posterior oblique portion is released for medial extension ligament contracture. **B,** In flexion, the anterior portion is tight. The anterior portion is released for medial flexion ligament contracture. (Courtesy Leo Whiteside, MD.)

- Concave side is medial—medial compartment release needed
- Medial compartment release in sequence
  - Osteophytes
  - Deep medial collateral ligament (MCL; also known as *meniscal tibial ligament*)
    - Includes medial knee capsule
  - Posterior medial corner
    - Capsule
    - Semimembranosus
  - **Superficial MCL—key structure** (Figure 5-70)
    - Posterior oblique portion tight in extension
      - Release for medial extension tightness
    - Anterior portion tight in flexion
      - Release for medial flexion tightness
- **Valgus deformity**
- Convex side is medial side—loose
- Concave side is lateral side—lateral compartment release needed

LCL Release

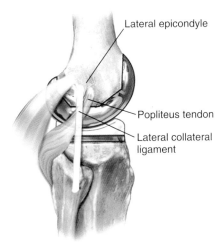

Lateral epicondyle

Popliteus tendon

Lateral collateral ligament

FIGURE 5-71 Anatomic relationship of popliteus tendon to lateral collateral ligament (LCL). The popliteal tendon inserts onto lateral epicondyle just in front of (distal and anterior to) lateral collateral ligament.

- ▨ Lateral compartment release in sequence
  - Osteophytes
  - Lateral capsule
  - Iliotibial band—key structure
    - **Tight in extension**
      - Release for lateral extension tightness
  - Popliteus—key structure
    - **Tight in flexion**
      - Release for lateral flexion tightness
    - Release popliteus off anterior portion of lateral epicondyle (Figure 5-71).
  - Lateral collateral ligament—last
- ■ **Extraarticular coronal bone deformity and TKA**
- ▨ General rules
  - The closer the extraarticular coronal bone deformity is to the knee joint, the greater the mechanical malalignment at the joint line.
    - For any given magnitude, a deformity farther away from the knee, the smaller the intraarticular bone cut needed to correct the mechanical alignment.
  - An extraarticular deformity within the distal one-fourth of the femur or proximal one fourth of the tibia are the most difficult to correct if making bone cuts only at the knee joint. Reasons:
    - Large bone resections required may compromise ligament attachment sites.
    - Large bone resections adversely affect implant sizing, fitting, and rotational alignment.
    - Extreme releases required to balance the knee often render the ligament incompetent.
  - **McPherson one-fourth rule:** when coronal deformity is within the distal one fourth of the femur or proximal one fourth of the tibia and deformity is 20 degrees or more, the recommended treatment is:
    - Concomitant osteotomy and TKA
      - Closing wedge osteotomy preferred
      - Diaphyseal press fit stem with splines recommended
        - Provides rotation stability and obviates the need for additional fixation at osteotomy site

Flexion Gap

Controlled by
- **Posterior** cut of femur
- Tibial cut
- PCL

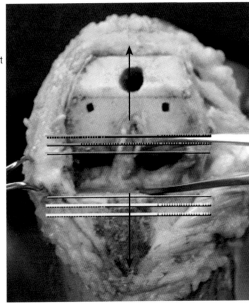

FIGURE 5-72 Intraoperative photo of knee showing structures that control flexion gap space. Knee is at 90 degrees of flexion. The gap between the green and yellow lines is the flexion gap, created after making bone cuts in the "posterior" femoral condyles and the proximal tibia. The flexion gap can be increased by cutting more posterior femur, cutting more proximal tibia, or removing (recessing) the PCL.

FLEXION DEFORMITY (I.E., FLEXION CONTRACTURE)

- ■ Concave side is posterior—posterior knee release required
- ■ Posterior knee release—in sequence
- ▨ Osteophytes
- ▨ Posterior capsule
- ▨ Gastrocnemius muscle origin
- ■ **Posterior releases are performed with the knee flexed (generally at 90 degrees of flexion).**
- ▨ Less danger to popliteal artery

SAGITTAL PLANE BALANCING IN TKA

- ■ Also known as *balancing the gaps*
- ■ Balancing goal
- ▨ Full extension and full flexion
- ■ Importance
- ▨ Full functional knee range
- ▨ Stability
- ▨ Pain relief
  - Unbalanced gaps cause pain from tightness or pain from instability.
- ■ Flexion gap—controlled by (Figure 5-72)
- ▨ **Posterior** cut of femur
- ▨ Tibial cut
- ▨ **Posterior** cruciate ligament (PCL)
- ■ Extension gap—controlled by (Figure 5-73)
- ▨ **Distal** cut of femur
- ▨ Tibial cut
- ▨ Posterior capsule
- ■ Balancing the gaps
- ▨ McPherson rule
  - **Symmetric** gap problem—adjust **tibia first.**
  - **Asymmetric** gap problem—adjust **femur first.**

- Table 5-7 and Figure 5-74 review **all sagittal plane gap scenarios.** Follow above rule, and this will guide you to a solution.
  - For some gap imbalance scenarios, there is more than one possible solution.

Extension Gap

Controlled by
- **_Distal_** cut of femur
- Tibial cut
- Posterior capsule

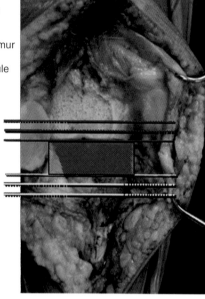

FIGURE 5-73 Intraoperative photo of knee showing structures that control extension gap space. The extension gap is controlled by the distal cut of the femur, the tibial cut, and the posterior capsule. Knee is in extension. The rectangle is the extension gap created after making bone cuts in the "distal" femur and the proximal tibia. The extension gap can be increased by cutting more "distal" femur, cutting more proximal tibia, or recessing the posterior capsule.

TKA—COMPLICATIONS

- **Femoral notch**
- Occurs when making anterior femoral bone cut and saw cuts into femoral cortex
  - This happens when cutting jig is placed a little too low on distal femur.
- An anterior femoral notch
  - Lessens load needed to cause fracture
  - In torsional load, there is no change in fracture location.
  - In **bending,** fracture starts at notch, creating a short oblique fracture.
  - **Caution—do not manipulate a TKA with a notch.**
- **Peroneal nerve palsy**
- **Deformity most likely to cause nerve palsy with TKA is valgus flexion deformity.**
  - Valgus deformity plus
  - Flexion contracture
- **When peroneal palsy is identified postoperatively, the first treatment is:**
  - **Remove compressive wraps and flex the knee.**
- If the nerve is not cut, most palsies will resolve within 3 months.
- If nerve palsy does not resolve after 3 months and nerve has not been cut (test by electromyogram/nerve conduction velocity):
  - Recommendation is to explore and decompress the peroneal nerve.
- **Lateral retinacular release**
- The artery at risk for transection is the **lateral superior genicular artery.**
  - Transection of this artery increases risk for **osteonecrosis** of the patella.

Table 5-7	**Review of Sagittal Plane TKA Gap Scenarios Sagittal Plane Balancing—Total Knee Replacement**	
SCENARIO	**PROBLEM**	**SOLUTIONS**
Tight in extension (contracture) Tight in flexion (will not bend fully)	Symmetric gap • Did not cut enough tibial bone	1. Cut more proximal tibia
Loose in extension (recurvatum) Loose in flexion (large drawer test)	Symmetric gap • Cut too much tibial bone	1. Use thicker polyethylene insert 2. Metallic tibial augmentation
Extension good Loose in flexion (large drawer test)	Asymmetric gap • Cut too much posterior femur	1. Increase size of femoral component from anterior to posterior (i.e., go up to next size). Fill posterior gap with either cement or metal augmentation. 2. Translate femoral component posteriorly (femur size unchanged). Fill posterior gap with either cement or metal augmentation. 3. Use thicker polyethylene insert and readdress as tight extension gap.
Tight in extension (contracture) Flexion good	Asymmetric gap • Did not release enough posterior capsule or • Did not cut enough distal femur	1. Release posterior capsule. 2. Take off more distal femur bone (1-2 mm at a time).
Extension good Tight in flexion (will not bend fully)	Asymmetric gap • Did not cut enough posterior bone or • PCL scarred and too tight (assuming use of a PCL-retaining knee system) • No posterior slope in tibial bone cut (i.e., anterior slope)	1. Decrease size of femoral component from anterior to posterior (i.e., recut to next smaller size). 2. Recess PCL. 3. Check posterior slope of tibia, and recut if anterior slope is present.
Loose in extension (recurvatum) Flexion good	Asymmetric gap • Cut too much distal femur or • Anteroposterior size too big	1. Distal femoral augmentation 2. Use thicker tibial polyethylene inset, and readdress as tight flexion gap. 3. Decrease size of femoral component from anterior to posterior (i.e., recut to next smaller size), and readdress as symmetric gap problem.

PCL, Posterior cruciate ligament; _TKA,_ total knee arthroplasty.

Flexion Gap is Loose

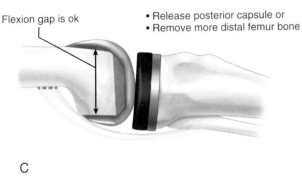

Larger femoral component

Fill gap with metal aug or cement

A

Flexion Gap is Loose

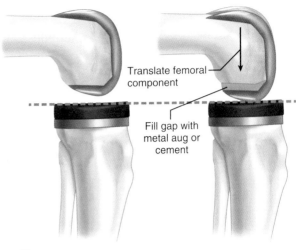

Translate femoral component

Fill gap with metal aug or cement

B

Extension Gap is Tight

Flexion gap is ok

• Release posterior capsule or
• Remove more distal femur bone

C

Flexion Gap is Tight

Flexion gap is too full

• Remove more posterior femur bone
• Use smaller femoral component

D

Flexion Gap is Tight - CR Knee Design

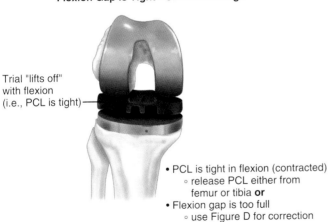

Trial "lifts off" with flexion (i.e., PCL is tight)

• PCL is tight in flexion (contracted)
  ◦ release PCL either from femur or tibia **or**
• Flexion gap is too full
  ◦ use Figure D for correction

E

Extension Gap is Loose

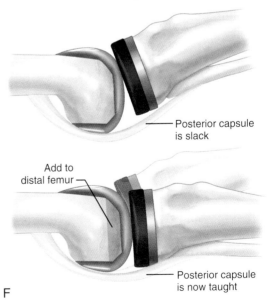

Posterior capsule is slack

Add to distal femur

Posterior capsule is now taught

F

FIGURE 5-74 Illustrations of scenarios presented in Table 5-7.

- **Patella fracture**
- Causes
  - Overresection of patella bone
    - **Minimum thickness is 13 mm.**
  - Compromised circulation
    - Big lateral retinacular release (transection of lateral superior geniculate)
    - Osteonecrosis with fracture and fragmentation
  - Patellofemoral maltracking
  - Direct trauma
- Treatment
  - Patella component solid and minimal lag
    - Controlled motion brace is initially locked in extension. Slowly increase flexion in increments.
  - Loose patella component
    - Component revision if there is enough remaining bone; remove smaller fragments.
    - Component resection if there is not enough remaining bone to support resurfacing
  - Significant extensor lag
    - Extensor reconstruction
- **Intraoperative MCL injury**
- Recommended treatment is to convert to revision prosthesis with high post for varus/valgus support (i.e., constrained post, not a posterior stabilized post).
- Primary repair of MCL is acceptable.
  - Postoperative brace with full knee range for 6 weeks
- **Extensor disruption**
- Almost always occurs at patellar tendon attachment to tibial tubercle
- Direct repair and nonsurgical treatment **do not work.**
- Extensor allograft reconstruction provides best chance for successful salvage.
  - **Fresh frozen allograft preferred**
    - Better healing compared to irradiated allografts
  - When allograft is used, the allograft is tensioned as tight as possible with the knee in **full extension.**
    - This gives best chance to minimize residual knee lag.
- **Arthrofibrosis**
- Manipulation of postoperative knee should be between **4 and 8 weeks.**
  - Late manipulation has high rate of fracture.

- Late stiffness—a big problem
  - Arthrotomy with scar resection and reduction of modular PE thickness is not recommended.
    - Very high failure rate with recurrent pain and stiffness
  - Revision TKA is recommended if preoperatively a problem with alignment, sizing, or component positioning can be identified.
- **Postoperative flexion contracture**
- In a well-balanced TKA (with full intraoperative ROM) a postoperative flexion contracture is due to **hamstring tightness and spasm.**
  - Treatment is therapy.
  - Keep knee straight at rest.
    - No pillows under knee
- **Postoperative TKA range**
- The most important predictor of postoperative knee range is *preoperative* knee range.
- **Osteolysis**
- Presentation in TKA
  - Starts later in life of implant—8 to 12 years
  - Gradual increase in effusion and weight-bearing pain
  - Mild warmth in knee
    - Not hot
    - No erythema
  - Normal infection laboratory results
    - Normal quantitative C-reactive protein (CRP)
  - Aspiration negative
    - Normal WBC count
      - A WBC count greater than 2500 cells/µL is suspicious for infection.
    - No crystals
    - Cultures are negative.
  - Radiographs show round lytic lesions behind implant (Figure 5-75).
    - **Most common site is behind posterior femoral condyle.**
- Treatment
  - If implants are mechanically loose, then revision TKA
    - Radical débridement of osteolytic bone lesions
    - Fill segmental defects with bone graft or metal augmentation

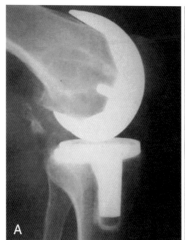 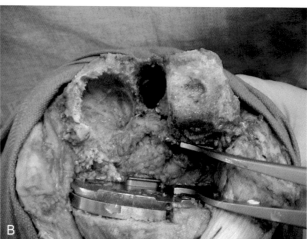

FIGURE 5-75 Osteolysis in TKA. **A,** Classical radiographic appearance of osteolysis in a TKA that is 10 years old. Note large round lytic lesions behind the posterior femoral condyle. **B,** Intraoperative photograph of same knee. Note severe bone loss in medial femoral condyle. This lesion required structural bone allograft. Knee was revised using a constrained revision knee system because the medial collateral ligament attachment onto the medial femoral condyle was compromised from osteolytic bone loss.

- If implants are mechanically stable, then retain implants and change modular tibial PE bearing
  - Radical débridement of osteolytic bone lesions
  - Fill segmental defects with bone graft and/or cement

- **Heterotopic ossification**
- Overview
  - HO forms in periarticular tissues after surgery without a well-defined precipitating event.
  - Transformation of primitive mesenchymal cells into osteoblastic tissues occurs **within 16 hours of surgical procedures,** with maximum stimulus for HO formation occurring within 32 hours.
    - Optimal prophylaxis should be instituted preoperatively or within the first 24 to 48 hours postoperatively.
  - HO in TKA is relatively frequent (small islands of bone seen in periarticular tissues), but **symptomatic HO is rare (≤1%)**; problems include:
    - Loss of motion (extension and/or flexion)
    - Pain
    - Clicks, crunch, snaps
- Risk factors
  - Hypertrophic osteoarthritis
  - DISH—diffuse idiopathic skeletal hyperostosis
    - Increased bone density (secondary to hypertrophic bone) correlates with increased risk of HO.
  - Patient with prior history of HO after surgery
  - Ankylosing spondylitis
  - Surgical technique
    - Periosteal stripping/damage, especially of the femur
    - Femoral notch
    - Tearing/trauma to quadriceps mechanism
  - Postoperative conditions
    - Knee hematoma and/or effusion
    - Forced manipulation for stiffness
    - Limited knee motion due to pain and inadequate compliance with therapy
- Diagnosis
  - Standing AP and lateral radiographs
    - Most common site is anterior femoral cortex superior to femoral prosthesis
    - Also frequent: islands of bone within tissue of suprapatellar soft tissue
- Treatment
  - Remember, spontaneous resolution of pain and restricted knee range does occur as the inflammatory process abates and the HO process matures; **first step is to wait and continue with therapy.**
  - Surgical removal of HO masses is indicated when pain and limited motion persist.
    - Excision procedure should be performed when HO process has matured.
      - Preferred timing of surgery is 12 to 18 months after index TKA.
      - HO process is considered mature when bone scan of HO region is "quiet" (i.e., scintigraphy of HO site is of similar intensity to adjacent bone).
      - Serum alkaline phosphate level (indicator of bone remodeling) must also return to normal levels.
- Prophylaxis
  - Two effective treatments; treatment should be applied to those patients with known risk factors:
    - Single-dose external beam radiation (600-800 Gy) given preoperatively or postoperatively by

postoperative day 5 (all data are for THA; no data for TKA).
  - NSAIDs
    - Treatment regimen of 7 to 14 days is considered effective (most data are from THA literature).
    - Documented NSAIDs inhibiting formation of HO include indomethacin, aspirin, naproxen, ibuprofen, diclofenac, ketorolac, and tromethamine.

- **Periprosthetic femur fracture**
- Rule 1: If implants are mechanically loose
  - Treatment is revision TKA and ORIF of fracture.
    - Usually use spline diaphyseal stem, which provides rotational stability to TKA implant
  - Treatment with fracture resection and endoprosthetic hinge TKA is an acceptable alternative when:
    - Highly comminuted fracture and
    - Patient is elderly and/or
    - Bone is significantly osteoporotic
- Rule 2: If implants are mechanically stable
  - Treatment options
    - ORIF with premolded supracondylar plate (first choice)
      - Submuscular plating lowers nonunion rate compared with extensile approach.
    - Revision TKA and ORIF of femur fracture is acceptable.
      - Usually used when TKA is symptomatically painful prior to injury
    - Fracture resection and endoprosthetic hinge TKA is an acceptable alternative when:
      - Highly comminuted fracture and
      - Patient is elderly and/or
      - Bone is significantly osteoporotic
    - Retrograde nailing is best suited for distal **diaphyseal** fracture.
      - A small knee arthrotomy is recommended to visualize knee and make sure that the nail does not impinge upon polyethylene bearing causing damage/breakage to bearing.

- **Periprosthetic joint infection (PJI)**
- Principles also apply to THA and TSA.
- Risk factors
  - Diabetes
  - Smoking
  - Autoimmune inflammatory disease states including:
    - Rheumatoid arthritis
    - Psoriatic arthritis
    - Systemic lupus erythematosus
    - Ankylosing spondylitis
  - Immune suppression medications:
    - TNF-α inhibitors including:
      - Infliximab (Remicade)
      - Adalimumab (Humira)
      - Certolizumab pegol (Cimzia)
      - Golimumab (Simponi)
      - Etanercept (Enbrel)
    - TNF-α inhibitors increase the risk for opportunistic infections including:
      - Mycobacteria, fungus, *Legionella,* and *Listeria*
      - Reason: TNF-α stabilizes old granulomas. Using TNF inhibitors leads to granuloma dissociation

Bacterial Adherence   Biofilm Formation   Mature Biofilm

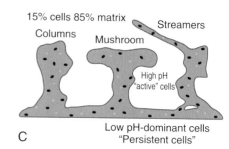

FIGURE 5-76 Diagram depicting biofilm formation on a prosthetic implant. **A,** Bacteria within the joint space adhere to implant (via adhesins) and multiply. Once the population of bacteria reaches a predetermined concentration (defined as a quorum), the colony expresses the biofilm. **B,** The biofilm under ideal conditions can rapidly proliferate and develop into mature biofilm. **C,** Mature biofilm state, in which bacteria interact with each other with signaling molecules and nanowires.

and release of the organisms; thus the infection is reactivated.
- Antimetabolites including:
  - Methotrexate
  - Leflunomide (Arava)
  - Azathioprine
  - Cyclophosphamide (Cytoxan)
- Glucocorticoids
- Obesity
◼ Biofilm (Figure 5-76)
- The most important factor influencing periprosthetic infection treatment
- All bacteria make biofilm.
- Biofilm consists of approximately 15% cells and 85% **polysaccharide** matrix.
- Biofilm forms on:
  - All foreign materials
  - Devitalized tissues
    - Soft tissue and bone
- Biofilm, once established, matures into sophisticated microenvironment.
  - Bacteria communicate with signaling molecules and nanowires.
    - **Nanowires** are very small cell-to-cell connections that allow bacteria in a biofilm to communicate with each other.
- Clinical importance of biofilm state
  - Bacteria become 1000 to 1500 times more resistant to antibiotics.
- Essentially, bacteria within a biofilm state cannot be killed with standard dosing regimens of antibiotics.
  - In vivo, biofilm can colonize, grow, and cover a surface within 4 to 8 days.
  - Effective treatment for established biofilm infection requires:
    - Implant and foreign body removal
    - Removal of all devitalized bone and soft tissue
  - **Inadequate débridement of biofilm material is the reason for treatment failure and infection recurrence.**
    - This includes retained cement and metal left in the medullary canals adjacent to the affected prosthetic joint.
◼ Diagnosis
- Most current based upon International Consensus Meeting of Musculoskeletal Infection Societies.
- A definite diagnosis of PJI can be made when the following clinical conditions are met:

- A **sinus tract** communicates with the affected prosthetic joint; _OR_
- A **pathogen is isolated by culture from two separate fluid or tissue samples** obtained from the affected prosthetic joint; _OR_
- **Four of the following six criteria exist:**
  - Elevated serum erythrocyte sedimentation rate (ESR) or elevated serum C-reactive protein (CRP) concentration
  - Elevated synovial WBC count
    - Acute PJI (early postoperative or from hematogenous seeding event to prosthetic joint): 20,000 WBCs/mL or more
    - Chronic PJI: 2500 WBCs/mL or more
  - Elevated synovial neutrophil percentage (neutrophils are commonly referred to in laboratory tests as PMNs [polymorphonuclear leukocytes])
    - Acute PJI: 89% neutrophils (PMNs) or more
    - Chronic PJI: 70% neutrophils (PMNs) or more
  - Isolation of a pathogen in one culture from fluid or tissue obtained from the affected prosthetic joint
  - Presence of purulence in the affected prosthetic joint
  - Greater than five neutrophils per high power field in five high-power fields observed from histologic review of periprosthetic tissue at 400 times magnification
◼ Treatment algorithm
- Classification
  - Acute infection (<3 weeks **known duration**)
    - Nonbiofilm state
    - Implants are salvageable.
    - Treatment is surgical.
  - Chronic infection
    - Biofilm state
    - Implants are not salvageable
    - Treatment is surgical and implants are removed.
- Acute periprosthetic infection
  - Currently, acute infection is defined as known infection of less than 3 weeks' duration.
    - Reason: no method to identify a biofilm with routine laboratory tests; 3 weeks has been selected as a reasonable time frame to treat as acute.
  - Treatment
    - Radical débridement surgery, including synovectomy and lavage

- Modular bearings are exchanged.
  - Must access all prosthetic spaces and flush bacteria
  - Intravenous antibiotic therapy for 4 to 6 weeks
  - **Arthroscopic lavage of an acutely infected joint replacement is *not* acceptable treatment.**
- Failure
  - If infection recurs, treat as a chronic infection. Do not attempt second débridement surgery.
- Chronic periprosthetic infection
  - Currently, chronic infection is defined as known infection for more than 3 weeks' duration.
  - Treatment
    - Implant removal
    - Radical débridement, including synovectomy, removal of necrotic bone and all devitalized soft tissue, and copious lavage
    - Stabilization of joint with high-dose-antibiotic–loaded methylmethacrylate spacer
      - Static spacer is used if joint stability is compromised by soft tissue and/or bone loss.
      - Articulated spacer is used if joint stability preserved.
    - Types of spacers:
      - Antibiotic-loaded acrylic cement (ALAC)
        - Construct consists primarily of high-dose-antibiotic–loaded methylmethacrylate cement
      - Prostalac (prosthesis and ALAC)
        - Construct that contains temporary metal and plastic prosthesis along with ALAC
      - Both constructs are acceptable for treatment. There is no proven superiority of ALAC versus Prostalac.
    - Intravenous antibiotic therapy for 4 to 6 weeks
    - Second-stage reconstruction
  - Second-stage reconstruction—options:
    - Reimplant joint arthroplasty
      - Most common treatment
      - Requires revision/salvage system to accommodate bone and soft tissue loss from infection débridement surgery
    - Arthrodesis
      - Used when there is significant loss of functional tissues
      - Must have adequate bone stock for fusion
    - Prosthetic endofusion device

- Bone defects are spanned by modular rods connected at the knee.
- Device maintains functional leg length compared with classic arthrodesis.
- Amputation—indications:
  - Neuropathy and chronic pain are too debilitating to consider reimplantation.
  - Recurrent infection after resection arthroplasty
    - Patient is too medically compromised to help combat infection
- Permanent resection
  - Patient is unfit for surgery.
- Infection prevention—total joint replacement
  - Infection prevention—proven
    - Prophylactic antibiotics
      - Administer **30 minutes before** skin incision.
      - Continue for 24 hours after surgery.
    - **Vertical** laminar air flow
      - **Vertical flow systems are superior to horizontal flow systems.**
      - Reason: horizontal flow systems create large vortex currents that circulate unfiltered air into the surgical wound.
    - Antibiotic-impregnated cement
      - No more than 1 g of antibiotic per 40-g packet of cement (do not want to reduce mechanical properties of cement)
      - Indicated for higher-risk patients
      - Use may be associated with increased rates of aseptic loosening.
      - Reason: even 1 g of antibiotic powder may reduce mechanical properties of the cement enough to cause premature cement fatigue in high-load situations.
- Wound coverage
  - Medial gastrocnemius rotational flap
    - The *workhorse* for deficiencies about the knee
    - Blood supply—medial sural artery
    - Used to cover medial and anterior deficiencies
    - Good excursion
  - Lateral gastrocnemius rotational flap
    - Blood supply—lateral sural artery
    - Used to cover lateral soft tissue deficiencies
    - Little excursion
    - **Risk—peroneal nerve palsy** from traction of the flap as it is pulled anteriorly to lateral side of knee

SECTION 16 TKA DESIGN

DESIGN CATEGORIES

- **Designs are categorized based upon an increasing level of mechanical constraint in knee system.**
- Least constrained
  - Cruciate-retaining TKA—**remove ACL and keep PCL**
  - Cruciate-sacrificing TKA—**remove ACL and PCL**
  - Both used for straightforward primary TKA
- Constrained
  - Constrained nonhinge TKA
  - Used for complex primary or revision TKA
- Highly constrained
  - Hinge TKA
  - Used for complex revision TKA

CRUCIATE-RETAINING PRIMARY TKA DESIGN

- **Description (Figure 5-77)**
- PCL helps regulate flexion stability.
- PCL tension influences femoral rollback.
  - Rollback is defined as the progressive posterior change in femoral-tibial contact point as the knee moves into flexion.
- Generally, cruciate-retaining implants have more flat PE inserts to accommodate for flexion rollback.
- **PCL retention—advantages**
- Bone conserving
- More consistent joint line restoration
  - Keeping PCL keeps flexion gap smaller.

- More proprioceptive feedback by keeping PCL
- **PCL retention—disadvantages**
- Harder to balance with severe deformities
  - **Avoid cruciate-retaining implants when:**
    - **Varus greater than 10 degrees**
    - **Valgus greater than 15 degrees**
- PCL balance is critical for long-term bearing wear.
  - **A tight PCL in flexion causes increased PE wear.**
    - Must balance PCL in flexion
    - Avoid lift-off (Figure 5-78).
    - PCL can be released off femur or tibia.
    - PCL balance is sometimes hard to assess intraoperatively.
  - Excess recession (i.e., release) can result in late failure caused by flexion instability and repetitive subluxation.
    - Flexion instability is characterized by:
      - Knee effusion
      - Chronic pain
      - Inability to reciprocate stairs
      - Inability to arise from low chair
      - Knee buckling
- Late rupture of PCL with resultant instability
  - PE particle debris can cause osteolysis and result in disruption of PCL from bony attachments.
  - Traumatic fall onto flexed knee can cause rupture.
- Paradoxical forward sliding as knee flexes
  - With ACL removed, knee kinematics are **drastically** altered.

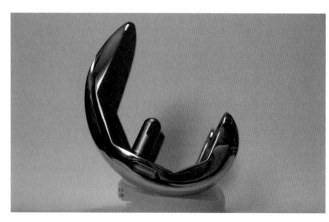

FIGURE 5-77 Lateral view of cruciate-retaining (CR) TKA implant. This is the typical profile of the femoral component. In this design the posterior cruciate ligament is retained. The PE insert is generally more flat to allow the femur to roll back onto the posterior part of bearing.

- As knee flexes, there is paradoxical forward-sliding movement, which causes sliding wear on PE insert.
  - Sliding wear causes significant PE wear.

CRUCIATE-SACRIFICING PRIMARY TKA DESIGN

- **Two options:**
- Spine and cam mechanism in the posterior aspect of the knee
  - Also called **posterior stabilized knee**
- An extended anterior PE lip
  - Also called **anterior stabilized knee**

POSTERIOR STABILIZED PRIMARY TKA DESIGN

- **Description (Figure 5-79)**
- A cam connects between the two posterior femoral condyles.
- The cam engages a tibial PE post during flexion.
- The cam and post control rollback.
- Generally, posterior stabilized implants have more dished (i.e., congruent) PE inserts.
- **Posterior stabilized knee—advantages:**
- Easier balancing in severe coronal deformities (i.e., varus/valgus) because both ACL and PCL are removed
- Controlled flexion kinematics with spine and cam, less sliding wear
- **Posterior stabilized knee—disadvantages:**
- Femoral cam jump (Figure 5-80)
  - Occurs when flexion gap is left too loose
  - Mechanism of cam jump
    - Varus or valgus stress when knee is flexed
    - Patient usually lying in bed or sitting on floor
    - Flexion gap opens up, and femoral cam then rotates in front of post and then comes to rest in front of tibial post.
  - Closed reduction maneuver
    - Knee is positioned at 90 degrees of flexion off the table (dependent dangle) under anesthesia.
    - An anterior drawer maneuver is performed.
      - Will feel clunk as knee is reduced
  - Ultimate solution requires knee revision to address loose flexion gap.
  - **Causes of loose flexion gap:**
    - Overrelease of popliteus
      - Inadvertently occurs also with saw blade
    - Overrelease of *anterior portion* of superficial MCL
    - Anterior translation of femoral component

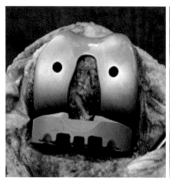
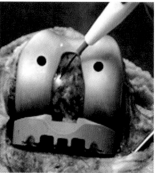
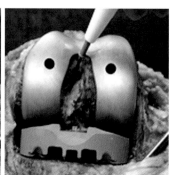

FIGURE 5-78 Intraoperative demonstration of posterior cruciate ligament (PCL) recession. PCL release off intercondylar notch allows flexion gap to increase in increments. Photograph on left shows classical presentation of tight PCL. With the knee in flexion, the tight PCL levers the anterior portion of the tibial insert upward creating lift-off. Sequential photographs show release of PCL just enough to allow tibial insert to lie back onto tibial. This sequence is termed *balancing the PCL*.

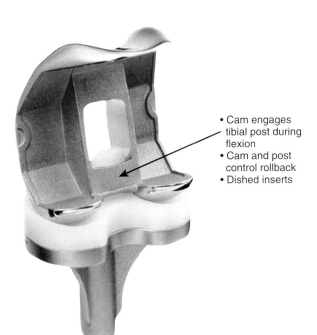

• Cam engages tibial post during flexion
• Cam and post control rollback
• Dished inserts

FIGURE 5-79 Posterior-lateral view of posterior stabilized (PS) implant. This is the typical profile of the femoral and tibial component. The cam on the femur engages a tibial post when the knee moves into flexion. This prevents anterior translation of the femur on the tibia, which stabilizes the knee in flexion in the absence of a posterior cruciate ligament.

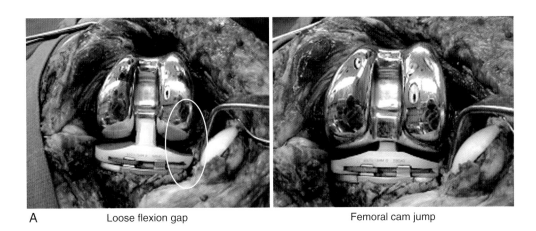

A   Loose flexion gap   Femoral cam jump

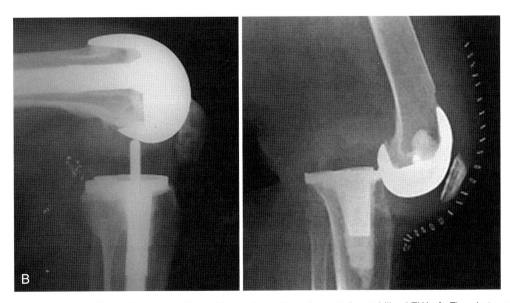

FIGURE 5-80 Intraoperative and radiographic presentation of femoral cam jump in posterior stabilized TKA. **A,** The photograph on *left* shows loose flexion gap. The *circled area* highlights loose lateral flexion gap caused by popliteal tendon deficiency. As the knee is stressed into varus, the tibia then rotates out in front of the tibial post. The cam then comes to rest in front of the tibial post. **B,** Two different presentations of femoral cam jump. Radiograph on *left* shows femur perched in front of tibial post (reinforced in this case with a metal post). Radiograph on *right* shows femur completely dislocated anteriorly when knee is brought into extension after cam jump.

▥ Patella clunk syndrome
- Scar tissue (descriptively, a nodule of scar) superior to patella gets caught in box as knee moves from flexion into extension.
- Scar catches in box, then releases with a clunk.
- Clunk occurs in range between 30 and 45 degrees.
- Treatment is removal of suprapatellar scar nodule (Figure 5-81).
  - Arthroscopic removal is acceptable.
  - Miniarthrotomy is also acceptable.
- Preventive treatment (Figure 5-82)
  - Synovectomy and débridement of all scar from quadriceps tendon at time of TKA

▥ Tibial post wear and breakage
- Tibial post is an additional PE surface that can cause wear and enhance risk for osteolysis.
- Aseptic loosening and osteolysis **are correlated with tibial post wear** and damage.
- **If the knee hyperextends, the edge of the femoral box can impinge on the anterior tibial post** (Figure 5-83).
  - Causes anterior post damage and fatigue
  - Causes increased PE wear and osteolysis
- Anterior tibial post wear occurs when TKA components are in **net hyperextension.** This includes:
  - Flexion of femoral component on distal femur
  - Excess tibial posterior slope
  - Knee hyperextension (i.e., loose extension gap)
  - Anterior translation of tibial component on tibia (i.e., placing tibial implant toward front of tibia rather than placing on posterior tibial rim)
  - **Anterior translation of femoral component has** *no effect* **on anterior tibial post impingement.**

▥ Additional bone is removed from middle of distal femur.
- Bone removed can be substantial in a small knee.

▥ Flexion gap is bigger.
- Flexion gap opens up when PCL is removed.
- **To balance the extension gap, additional distal femur bone is removed in a posterior stabilized TKA.**
  - Consequence of additional distal femoral bone removal
    - Joint line elevation with possible baja deformity
  - The maximum joint line elevation allowed in primary TKA is 8 mm.
    - This ensures proper kinematic function and stability of collateral ligaments.

■ Posterior stabilized TKA—indications:
▥ Patellectomy
- Cruciate-retaining knee with a flat PE is prone to anterior subluxation when patella is absent.
▥ Inflammatory arthritis
- PCL is at risk for rupture with erosive disease process.
▥ Trauma with PCL rupture or attenuation

ANTERIOR STABILIZED PRIMARY TKA DESIGN

■ Description (Figure 5-84)
▥ A cruciate-retaining femoral component is used.
▥ The PCL is removed (or highly recessed).
▥ Tibial insert is a highly congruent bearing with a raised anterior PE lip.
▥ No mechanism for rollback
▥ Anterior lip resists anterior translation.

■ Anterior stabilized knee—advantages:
▥ Easier balancing in severe deformities (i.e., varus/valgus)
▥ Bone conserving
▥ Operative versatility
- Do not have to switch to posterior stabilized system when PCL is lost or overreleased
▥ Regulated flexion kinematics
- High congruency limits sliding wear.
- Knee flexion is achieved by:
  - Placing tibial knee flexion center posteriorly. This is called posterior offset center of rotation.
  - Placing tibial component with native posterior slope. By doing so, femur is less likely to impinge upon posterior tibia in flexion.

■ Anterior stabilized knee—disadvantages:
▥ Increased PE surface area
- This increases risk for increased PE wear debris and osteolysis.
▥ Minimal rollback
- Must adjust surgical technique to attain high flexion
  - Posterior translation of tibial component on tibia, when possible
  - Recreate native tibial posterior slope
▥ Flexion gap laxity causes rotational instability and pain.
- Similar to posterior stabilized design, a loose flexion gap will cause instability usually in midflexion.
- Mechanism of **midflexion instability**
  - Varus or valgus stress when knee is flexed (between 50 and 90 degrees)

Treatment — Arthroscopy

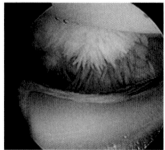 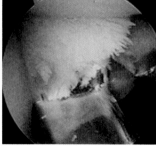 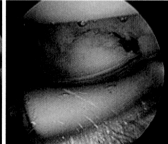

| Nodule superior to patella | Incarceration of nodule in box with flexion | Scar débridement with scope |

FIGURE 5-81 Arthroscopic photographs demonstrating patella clunk syndrome. Classical appearance of fibrotic scar nodule in suprapatellar region *(left)*. Incarceration of scar in posterior stabilized box as knee is brought from flexion into extension *(center)*. Arthroscopic removal of nodule *(right)*.

Preventative treatment

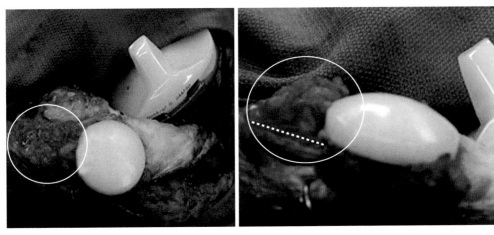

Remove tissue down to quadriceps tendon

FIGURE 5-82 Inflammatory tissue *(circle)* around arthritic patella at time of primary TKA *(left)*. This tissue, if not removed, will cause patellar clunk syndrome. This tissue should be aggressively débrided to level of quadriceps tendon *(dotted line, right)*.

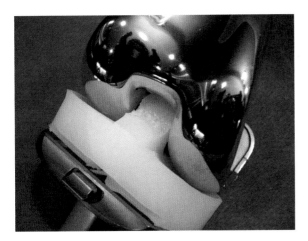

FIGURE 5-83 Photograph of posterior stabilized implant with anterior tibial post wear. Note indentation on anterior post where the edge of femoral box impinges upon anterior tibial post. This occurs when the knee moves into hyperextension.

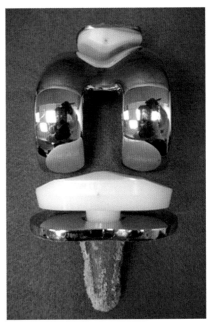

FIGURE 5-85 Retrieval of a primary TKA with a tibial rotating platform. Tibial PE component has a yoke that inserts into tibial baseplate. The tibial PE bearing rotates on a polished tibial baseplate.

- Patient usually lying in bed or sitting on floor
- Flexion gap opens up, and tibia rotates anteriorly. This creates a subluxing event, but knee usually does not lock up.
- Pain is experienced when reciprocating stairs, arising from a chair, or negotiating uneven surfaces; it is usually associated with a knee effusion.
- Treatment requires revision to address loose flexion gap.

TIBIAL ROTATING PLATFORM IN PRIMARY TKA

▪ Description (Figure 5-85)

▦ The tibial PE bearing rotates on a polished metal tibial baseplate.

▦ The rotating platform can be used with both anterior stabilized (high congruent) and posterior stabilized TKA designs.

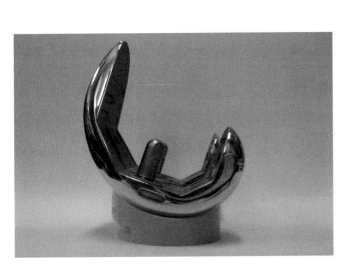

FIGURE 5-84 Lateral view of anterior stabilized (AS) TKA design. This is the typical profile of the femoral and tibial component. The tibial PE bearing is highly congruent and also has a raised anterior PE lip to resist anterior translation. In this design there is minimal rollback.

- The PCL is removed when using a tibial rotating platform.
- **Rotating platform knee—advantages:**
- Better articular conformity through entire knee range
  - Theoretically less PE wear
- **Equivalent survivorship to fixed-bearing knee, but not superior**
  - Wear and osteolysis still seen
- **Rotating platform knee—disadvantages:**
- **Bearing spinout** (Figure 5-86)
  - **Occurs when flexion gap is left too loose**
  - Mechanism of spinout:
    - Varus or valgus stress when knee is flexed
    - Patient usually lying in bed or sitting on floor
    - Flexion gap opens up, and tibia rotates behind femur.
    - Femur then comes to rest in front of tibial PE bearing and locks into spinout position.
  - Closed reduction maneuver
    - Knee is positioned at 90 degrees of flexion off the side of the table (dependent dangle) under anesthesia.
    - Tibial bearing is manipulated by digital palpation and pressure into reduced position.
  - Ultimate solution requires knee revision to address loose flexion gap.

MODULARITY IN PRIMARY TKA

- **Modular tibial component is now standard.**
- Metal baseplate
- Modular PE insert
- Stems can be attached to tibia and/or femur.
- **Modularity—advantages**
- Greater intraoperative flexibility
- Modular bearing change for worn PE in well-fixed implants—thus major revision is avoided
- **Modularity—disadvantages:**
- **Backside PE wear**
  - Backside wear occurs when the tibial locking mechanism allows micromotion to occur between tibial baseplate and **backside surface of tibial PE bearing**.
  - More osteolysis with modular designs
  - Locking mechanisms for tibial PE inserts do not completely eliminate micromotion.

- Backside wear is **_not_ a problem with a monoblock design**.
  - With monoblock design, the tibial PE bearing is pressed onto metal baseplate at the factory.
  - There is no backside wear with monoblock designs.
- Backside wear—reduction
  - Polished tibial baseplate
  - Tighter locking mechanisms

CONSTRAINT IN TKA

- **Reason:**
- Soft tissues about knee will not support prosthesis.
  - Loss of key vital support structures
- Prosthesis must then accommodate for loss of soft tissue support.
- **Constraint options**
- High tibial post nonhinged
- Hinge with rotating tibial platform
- Hinge with no rotating tibial platform
  - Rarely used
- **Constrained nonhinged TKA**
- Definition (Figure 5-87)
  - High central post that **substitutes for MCL** and lateral collateral ligament function
  - A standard **posterior stabilized** post is **not constrained.**
- Indications:
  - Residual flexion gap laxity—most common reason
    - Owing to soft tissue weakness, the extension and flexion gaps cannot be completely balanced.
  - MCL attenuation
  - Lateral collateral ligament attenuation and deficiency
  - MCL complete deficiency
    - Relative (still debatable)
  - Charcot arthropathy
    - Relative (still debatable)
- Disadvantages:
  - More constraint upon implant places more forces through implant and implant-bone interface. This causes:
    - Higher rate of aseptic loosening
    - More PE wear/damage to PE post
  - Constrained high-post knee system **requires medullary stem support** in femur and tibia to help distribute increased load forces (i.e., load shares) through the implant and into host diaphyseal bone.

Rotating Platform

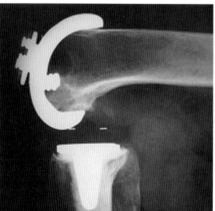
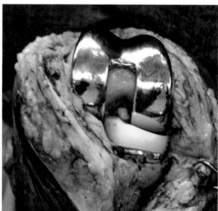

FIGURE 5-86 Demonstration of bearing spinout. Radiograph on *left* shows classical appearance of bearing spinout. Note that femur profile has no central box. Therefore this radiograph is not of a posterior stabilized knee with cam jump. Photograph on *right* is intraoperative appearance of same patient. Note that the lateral tibial PE component is completely posterior to the lateral femoral condyle.

■ Hinge TKA

- ▨ Definition (Figure 5-88)
  - Femoral and tibial components are linked with a connecting bar and bearings.
  - There is a fixed extension stop.
  - Most designs incorporate a tibial rotating platform.
    - This reduces torque stress to implant bone interface.
- ▨ Indications
  - Global instability
    - Due to trauma or infection
  - Hyperextension instability (Figure 5-89)
    - This is *absolute* **indication** for hinge.
    - Hyperextension conditions include:
      - Postpolio knee
        - Increased knee extension forces to lock and hold knee in extension during gait, eventually causing posterior capsule to stretch out
      - Erosion of posterior capsular attachments to bone as a result of:
        - Advanced bony osteolysis
        - Autoimmune disease states (particularly rheumatoid arthritis)
    - Native knee removal
      - Tumor
      - High-energy fracture with communication
      - Massive infection

A posterior stabilized knee
is *not* constrained

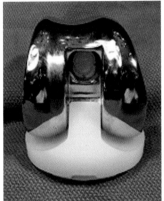 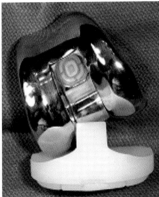 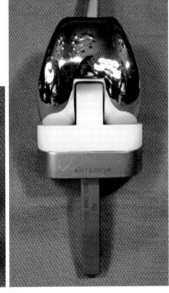

Posterior stabilized knee
No varus/valgus support

Constrained
high post

FIGURE 5-87 Diagram showing high-post constrained TKA. Photographs on *left* show a typical posterior stabilized TKA. If medial collateral ligament or lateral collateral ligament function is lost, the posterior stabilized post will not resist varus or valgus forces and the knee will be unstable. The photograph on the *right* shows a constrained high-post design. This PE post is very tall and will not allow varus or valgus opening of the knee.

Hinge Basics

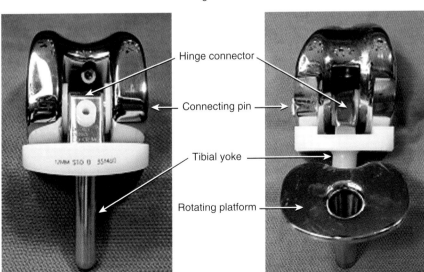

FIGURE 5-88 Diagram showing basic components of hinge TKA. In all hinge systems, the femur is connected to the tibia via a connecting post placed into the middle of the knee. A connecting pin of metal is placed through femur and tibial post. A locking pin keeps connecting pin in position. A tibial yoke rests in the tibial component. This allows rotation of the tibia.

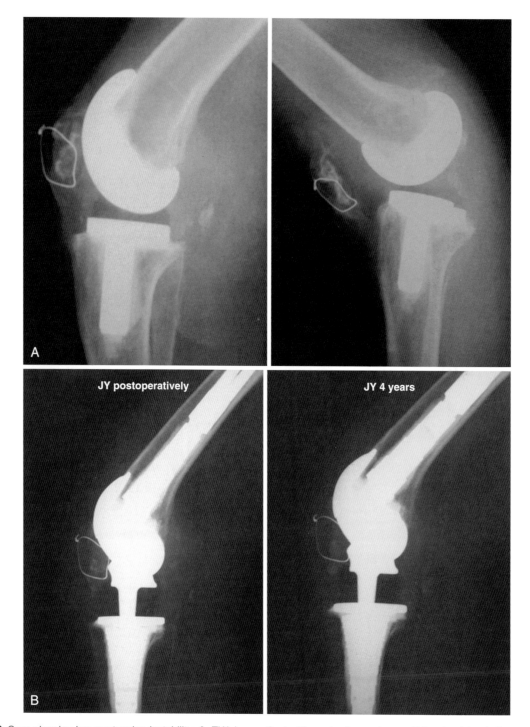

FIGURE 5-89 Case showing hyperextension instability. **A,** TKA in a patient with postpolio syndrome. Extension lateral shows severe hyperextension, which on presentation was only mildly painful. However, the patient had significant difficulty with walking. **B,** Revision to a hinge TKA.

SECTION 17 REVISION TKA

PREOPERATIVE EVALUATION

- Revision of a painful TKA without an identified specific cause for pain is likely to have a poor outcome.
- Must first identify intrinsic intraarticular source of pain versus extrinsic source of pain
- Extrinsic sources of knee pain
- Referred pain from the hip
  - Most common missed diagnosis
  - Hip pain typically refers to anterior-medial knee region (distal branch of obturator nerve)
- Referred pain from the spine
  - Typically L3 nerve root
- Extraarticular at the knee
  - Allodynia—chronic regional pain syndrome
  - Local superficial neuroma
- Intrinsic sources of knee pain
- Mechanical loosening

- Osteolysis with PE debris synovitis
- Malposition and/or malalignment of implants
- Instability
- Infection
  - Typically, **constant global pain** with abnormal infection laboratory results and positive aspiration studies
- Hypersensitivity
  - Typically, constant global pain with normal infection laboratory results and negative aspiration studies
  - Most common metal ion involved in knee hypersensitivity is **nickel.**
  - Diagnosis made by serum lymphocyte T-cell proliferation test (LTT), *not* **skin patch test**
- **Intraarticular aspiration**
- WBC count greater than 2500/μL raises suspicion for low-grade infection.
- **Intraarticular lidocaine challenge**
- Administer at least 15 mL of lidocaine or 50/50 mixture of lidocaine/Marcaine.
- A positive test should take away over 90% of pain.
  - This indicates that pain eminates primarily from within the knee joint.
- **CT scan**
- Evaluation for rotational malalignment of implants
  - Compare posterior condylar axis of metallic condyles with epicondylar axis.
    - Posterior condylar axis should be parallel or slightly externally rotated to epicondylar axis.
  - Tibial implant axis should lie over medial third of tibial tubercle.
    - A tibial implant axis that lies medial tibial tubercle indicates malalignment.

SURGICAL APPROACH

- **Use prior incisions.**
- **Avoid making skin bridges with a new incision.**
- **Lifting a subcutaneous soft tissue flap is much safer than a second incision with a skin bridge.**
- **Difficult exposure sequence**
- Extended proximal arthrotomy
  - To most proximal end of tendon
- Externally rotate tibial bone from soft tissue envelope
  - Subperiosteal dissection of soft tissues from medial tibial tubercle all the way around to posterior-medial corner of knee
  - Release posterior-medial corner structures and, if needed, posterior tibial capsule
- Lateral knee débridement
  - Remove scar from patella, tendon, and lateral gutter
- Lateral retinacular release
  - Gradually avert patella
- Quadriceps tendon snip (usually 2 cm)
  - Transverse snip at most proximal region

- **Tibial tubercle osteotomy**
- Use as last resort
- Best indication is stiff TKA (<90 degree flexion) with patella baja deformity

IMPLANT SYSTEM

- **Have comprehensive revision system available.**
- Revision surgery is often unpredictable.
- Constrained tibial insert option is a must.
- Stems and metallic augmentations

MODULAR BEARING CHANGE FOR *PREMATURE* EXCESSIVE WEAR

- **Most current tibial PE bearings should last at least 13 to 15 years with an average patient wear scenario in a well balanced knee.**
- **Failure rate of isolated modular bearing change for excessive premature PE failure is 30% to 40%.**
- **Reasons for premature failure:**
- Unappreciated malalignment
- Poor knee balancing in either coronal or sagittal plane
- **Isolated modular bearing change in this scenario is not recommended.**

REVISION TKA—TECHNIQUE

- **Implant removal**
- **Joint line restoration with tibia first**
- Joint line is generally 1.5 cm superior to top of fibular head.
- Failure to restore joint line will result in decreased flexion.
- **Femur restoration**
- Gap balancing
- Adjust for patellar positioning.
  - Avoid baja impingement.

REVISION TKA—PATELLA

- **Isolated patella component failure usually indicates subtle malalignment in patellar tracking.**
- Higher failure rate for isolated patellar revision
- Consider full revision.
- **A mechanically loose patellar component can cause significant patellar bone loss.**
- **For revision to another patellar component, bone thickness must be at least 12 mm, and there must be enough bone to support PE pegs within bone.**
- If bone is inadequate for revision resurfacing:
  - Débridement of patella with bone retention is acceptable.
  - Patellectomy is recommended for bony fragmentation.

SECTION 18 PATELLAR TRACKING IN TKA

INTRODUCTION

- **The most common complications in TKA involve abnormalities in patellar tracking.**
- **Preoperative maltracking** is the only predictor of postoperative maltracking.

- **Most important factors for successful patellar tracking:**
- Maintaining normal Q angle
- Proper component rotation
- Maintaining normal patellofemoral tension

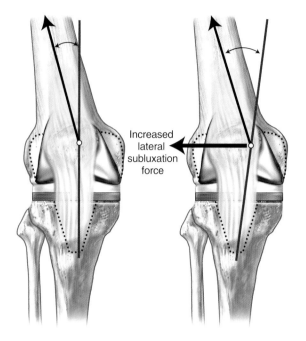

FIGURE 5-90 Diagram depicting effect of an increased Q angle in TKA. As the Q angle increases, so does the resultant lateral subluxation force. Because the shape of the resurfaced patella is a dome, this design is less able to resist the lateral pull effect. The result is an increased risk for patellar subluxation.

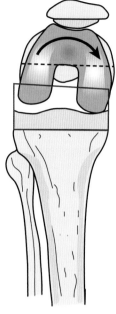

FIGURE 5-91 Diagram showing adverse effect of internal rotation of femoral component. Diagram depicts TKA at 90 degrees of flexion. With internal rotation of femur, the patellar groove faces inward and the flexion gap becomes asymmetric. Patellar tracking and flexion kinematics are both adversely affected.

Q ANGLE IN TKA

- Q angle **definition—the angle between a line defining the axial pull of the quadriceps tendon and a line bisecting the patellar tendon**
- Reasons an increased Q angle in TKA is bad (Figure 5-90):
- An increased Q angle increases the resultant lateral subluxation force (i.e., lateral pull effect).
- Prosthetic patellar replacements (by design) are less restrained than native patella.
- Prosthetic patellar replacements are therefore more likely to sublux with increased Q angle forces.
- Q angle goal in TKA
- Restore proper Q angle with techniques that do not compromise mechanical alignment or stability of the knee.

TKA TECHNIQUES TO OPTIMIZE PATELLAR TRACKING

- Reduce excess valgus.
- Valgus deformity must be corrected to a neutral mechanical alignment—*always.*
- Severe valgus deformities that require radical ligamentous releases can be adequately managed with sophisticated revision-style prosthetic systems.
- Component positioning
- Patellar maltracking—causes:
  - Internal rotation of:
    - Femoral component
    - Tibial component
  - Medialization of:
    - Femoral component
    - Tibial component
- Femoral component rotation
- Do not internally rotate femoral component.
- Internal rotation of femur—resultant problems (Figure 5-91)

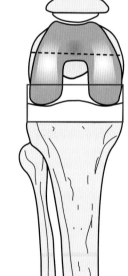

FIGURE 5-92 Diagram showing proper positioning of femoral component in slight external rotation. With slight external rotation, the patellar groove is centered under the patella and the flexion gap is balanced, which optimizes flexion kinematics.

- Relative lateral tilt of patella
  - Patellar groove faces inward.
- Trapezoidal flexion gap
  - Unbalanced flexion gap
- Technique goal is slight external rotation of femur (Figure 5-92).
  - Patellar groove is centered under patella.
  - Rectangular flexion gap
    - Balanced flexion gap

Slight External Rotation of Femoral Component

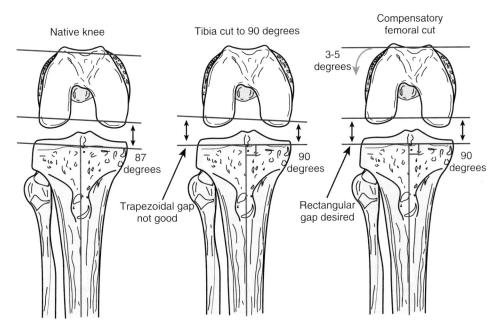

FIGURE 5-93 Diagrams demonstrating proper component rotation during TKA. *Left,* Native knee in flexion. In many instances, the native proximal tibia is actually in slight varus (average is 3 degrees). *Center,* In TKA procedure, the proximal tibia is cut perpendicular to mechanical axis. This leaves the flexion gap asymmetric and unbalanced. *Right,* Compensatory cut on femur, which is externally rotated to create a rectangular (i.e., balanced) flexion gap and to optimize patellar tracking.

- External rotation of femoral component (Figure 5-93)—Why?
  - Commonly the native proximal tibia is actually in slight varus.
    - Average is 3 degrees varus.
  - During TKA, the proximal tibia is cut perpendicular to mechanical axis.
  - This results in trapezoidal flexion gap (i.e., unbalanced flexion gap).
  - To compensate, the femoral component is externally rotated a similar amount to obtain a rectangular flexion gap (i.e., balanced flexion gap) and also optimize patellar tracking.
- External rotation of femoral component—techniques
  - There are five established techniques to determine proper femoral component rotation. All methods are acceptable (Figure 5-94).
    - Anteroposterior axis method
      - *Anteroposterior axis* is defined as line from intercondylar notch (specifically the most lateral border of PCL) to center of trochlear groove.
      - A line drawn perpendicular to anteroposterior axis is used to set femoral rotation.
    - Epicondylar axis method
      - The epicondylar axis is a line drawn from the center of the medial epicondyle to the center of the lateral epicondyle.
      - Femoral rotation is set along this line.
    - Posterior condylar axis method
      - The posterior condylar axis is a line connecting the apex of the medial femoral condyle and lateral femoral condyle measured at 90 degrees of flexion.
      - The femoral rotation line is mechanically chosen along a line that is 3 degrees externally rotated to this line (acceptable range is 3-5 degrees of external rotation).

- Tibial alignment axis method
  - The proximal tibial cut is with a cutting jig set 90 degrees to the mechanical axis of the tibia.
  - With the knee at 90 degrees of flexion, the same guide is used to set femoral component rotation by drawing rotation line on the femur.
- Gap balance axis method
  - The proximal tibia is cut first.
  - With the knee at 90 degrees of flexion, tension devices are placed under the medial and lateral femoral condyles. A set tension is then applied to the flexion gap.
  - **The femoral rotation line is drawn to create a *rectangular* flexion gap.**
- **Beware of lateral femoral condylar hypoplasia.**
  - In this condition the lateral femoral condyle is small due to hypoplastic development.
    - Clinically, a knee with lateral femoral condylar hypoplasia presents with a prominent valgus deformity. With the knee viewed in flexion, the lateral femoral condyle looks small relative to the medial femoral condyle.
  - **In lateral femoral condylar hypoplasia the posterior axis *cannot* be used.**
    - If the posterior condylar axis is used as the rotation reference, the femur will be placed in internal rotation and the flexion gap will be unbalanced.
- **Tibial component rotation**
- Do not internally rotate tibial component.
- Internal rotation of tibia—resultant problem (Figure 5-95)
  - Increases Q angle
  - Increases lateral subluxation force
- Tibial component positioning should lie over medial half of tibial tubercle.

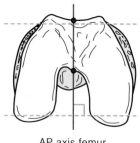

A AP axis femur (Leo Whiteside)

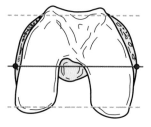

B Epicondylar axis (John Insall)

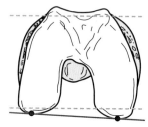

C Posterior condylar axis (set 3 degrees of external rotation into jig)

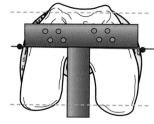

D Tibial alignment axis (Richard Scott)

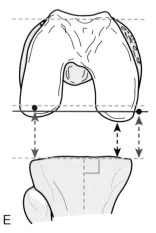

- Tensiometers placed under LFC and MFC
- External rotation set to create a *rectangular gap*

Gap balance (Michael Freeman)

E

 FIGURE 5-94 Diagrams showing methods to determine femoral component rotation. **A,** In the anteroposterior (AP) axis method, the AP line is drawn from the center of the intercondylar notch to the center of the trochlear groove. The femoral rotation is set along a line perpendicular to the AP axis. **B,** The epicondylar axis is a line drawn from the center of the medial and lateral epicondyles. Femoral rotation is set parallel to this line. **C,** Posterior condylar axis. The posterior condylar line is drawn between the two femoral condyles (at 90 degrees of flexion). Femoral rotation is set at 3 degrees of external rotation relative to this line. **D,** Tibial alignment axis. The tibial jig, used to cut the tibia at 90 degrees to the tibial mechanical axis, is also used to set femoral rotation. Either the jig is raised or a block is placed upon the jig to draw the femoral rotation line. **E,** Gap balance axis method. Tensiometers are placed into the flexion gap, and tension is applied to the flexion gap. The femoral rotation line is drawn to create a rectangular flexion gap with the knee ligaments under tension. *LFC,* Lateral femoral condyle; *MFC,* medial femoral condyle.

■ Implant medialization
- Do not medialize femoral component.
  - Reason: medialization of femur moves patellar groove medial relative to tibial tubercle. Result is **net increase in Q angle.**
  - Lateralization is acceptable.

Internal rotation tibial component = External rotation of tibial tubercle

Tibial implant should line up over medial half of tibial tubercle

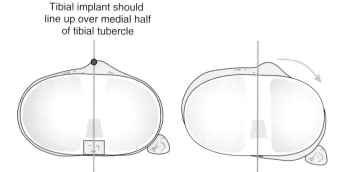

FIGURE 5-95 Diagram showing tibial component rotation in TKA. For optimal patellar tracking, the tibial component should be rotated over the medial half of the tibial tubercle *(left).* Avoid internally rotating tibia *(right).* When tibial component is internally rotated, the tibial tubercle is positioned in external rotation relative to the knee flexion plane. This increases the Q angle, which increases lateral subluxation forces.

Result
- Net decrease in Q angle
  - Center of patellar dome is medial to center of patellar tendon

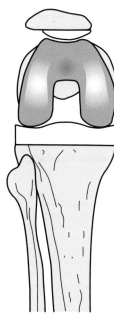

FIGURE 5-96 Diagram showing medialized patellar component. In this technique, a small patellar dome is used. It is placed in a medialized position. The center of the patellar dome, being medial to the center of the patellar tendon, reduces net Q angle.

- Do not medialize tibial component.
  - Reason: medialization moves knee articulation medial relative to tibial tubercle. Result is **net increase in Q angle.**
  - Lateralization is acceptable.
- Patellar component medialization is acceptable (Figure 5-96).
  - Reason: center of the patellar component is placed medial to the center of the patellar tendon. Result is net decrease in Q angle.
  - Avoid lateralization of patellar component.

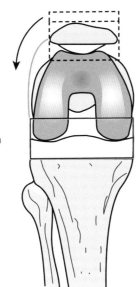

 FIGURE 5-97 Diagram showing patellar height. Measuring patellar height before and after patellofemoral resurfacing is important in maintaining normal retinacular tension. Increasing patellar height *(upper box, arrow)* increases retinacular tension. This increases lateral pulling forces on patella.

■ **Patellofemoral tensioning (also called *third-gap balancing*)**
▨ Restoring normal patellar height maintains normal retinacular tension (Figure 5-97).
  • **Increasing net patellar height increases retinacular tension.**
  • **Increased retinacular tension will increase lateral pull forces upon patella, causing maltracking.**
▨ Patellofemoral height (i.e., patellofemoral gap) is controlled by sum of total of:
  • Patella bone thickness
  • Patella implant thickness
  • Trochlea bone thickness
  • Trochlea implant thickness
▨ Increased patellofemoral gap—worst case
  • Thin bone cut on patella
    • Remaining patellar bone is too thick.
  • Thick PE implant (by design)
  • Thin bone cut on trochlea
    • Remaining trochlear bone is too thick.
  • Thick femoral trochlear implant (by design)

INTRAOPERATIVE ASSESSMENT OF MALTRACKING

■ If maltracking is seen with TKA implants in place, ***first* release tourniquet,** then reevaluate before making any changes.
■ The tourniquet can alter extensor tension and falsely create increased lateral pull forces.

POSTOPERATIVE ASSESSMENT OF MALTRACKING

■ If physical examination and plain radiographs do not reveal the cause of postoperative patellar maltracking, a CT scan can be used to determine rotational alignment of femoral and tibial components.

PATELLA BAJA

■ **Frequently seen after**
▨ Proximal tibial osteotomy (both closed and open wedge techniques)

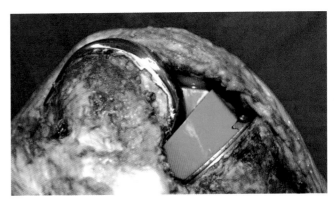

FIGURE 5-98 Intraoperative photograph of TKA with patella baja. With baja deformity, the patella component impinges upon the tibial component, limiting flexion and causing pain.

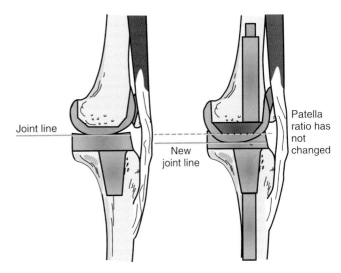

FIGURE 5-99 Technique to reduce patella baja impingement in TKA. *Left,* Patella baja and starting joint line. *Right,* Lowered joint line achieved by cutting more tibial bone and adding distal femoral augmentation.

▨ Tibial tubercle transfer/slide
▨ Trauma
■ **Baja in TKA will cause (Figure 5-98):**
▨ Loss of knee flexion
▨ Impingement pain in flexion
■ **Operative solutions to reduce baja in TKA**
▨ Superior placement of patellar component
  • Use smaller patellar dome placed superiorly on patella.
  • Trim/taper inferior bone to reduce flexion impingement.
  • Useful for mild baja deformity
▨ Lower joint line—sophisticated technique (Figures 5-99 and 5-100)
  • Make a lower tibial bone cut.
  • Add distal femoral metallic augmentation.
  • Requires revision knee system
▨ Cephalad transfer of tibial tubercle/anterior tibia
  • Procedure is risky.
    • Bone healing not always predictable (especially around a cemented tibial component)
    • Clinically, patient may have residual functional extensor lag.

Painful TKA

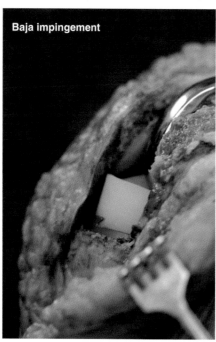
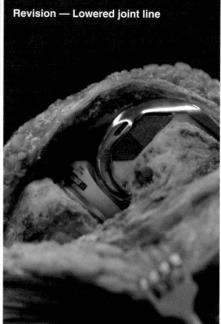

FIGURE 5-100 Intraoperative demonstration of lowering joint line to correct patella baja. *Left,* Baja impingement in flexion. *Right,* Same knee after revision TKA. The joint line was lowered by making a lower tibial bone cut and reducing tibial component thickness. Notice distal femoral augmentation used to bring femur more distal.

- Patellectomy for extreme cases
  - Patellectomy alters anterior knee tension.
    - Need to use cruciate substituting (or constrained) knee system

PATELLAR RESURFACING VERSUS NONRESURFACING

- Between the two techniques, there is not an established superior method.
- Patellar resurfacing—problems
- Patella component loosening
  - Due to maltracking
  - Due to osteolysis
- Patella *clunk* and *crunch*
  - Clunk occurs when suprapatellar scar tissue gets entrapped within the posterior stabilized box as the knee comes from flexion into extension.
  - Clunk is unique to posterior stabilized design.
  - Patellar crunch occurs when scar accumulates around patellar component, creating a crunching noise as the knee comes from flexion to extension.
- Patella fracture
  - Reason: bone cut too thin
  - Minimum thickness for patella is 13 mm.

- Avascular necrosis of patella with fragmentation
  - Reason: peripatellar devascularization due to lateral retinacular release
    - Disruption of lateral superior geniculate artery
- Unresurfaced patella problems
- Anterior knee pain
  - Incidence increases over time.
    - Articular cartilage wears away, and there is point loading upon patellar bone.
  - Results of secondary resurfacing are variable.
    - Pain relief not predictable
- Patella nonresurfacing—criteria
- Noninflammatory arthritis
- Lower activity level
- No dysplasia or maltracking
- No baja
- Patella nonresurfacing—requirements
- Need anatomic femoral component
  - V-shape trochlea groove to match native patella
  - Deep trochlear groove to prevent overstuffing of patellar gap
- Circumferential denervation of patella with electrocautery

SECTION 19 CATASTROPHIC WEAR IN TKA

PREMATURE FAILURE OF TKA IMPLANT

- Etiology is macroscopic PE failure.
- Problem is not a microscopic PE wear problem.
- Clinically, patient presents with a large knee effusion that may or may not be painful.
- Osteolysis is present but is a secondary problem.

- Multiple factors are involved to create the *perfect storm* of catastrophic wear.

FACTORS INVOLVED IN CATASTROPHIC WEAR

- PE thickness
- Articular geometry

Articular Geometry

Low contact area

High contact load

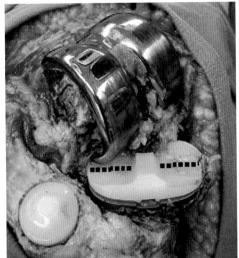
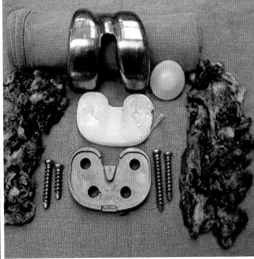

FIGURE 5-101 Intraoperative photograph of TKA with catastrophic wear after 9 years. *Left,* Flat PE bearing articulating with a flat style femoral component. This allows for only a thin line of contact *(dotted line)* during knee load. The stresses generated upon the PE are excessive and the PE fails macroscopically. *Right,* Inflammatory debris removed at the time of revision.

- Knee kinematics
- Surgical technique
- PE processing

POLYETHYLENE THICKNESS

- Thin PE breaks.
- To keep knee bearing contact stress below the yield strength of UHMWPE (12 to 20 mPA), the PE must be **at least 8 mm.**
- This applies to "traditional" PE that is not highly cross-linked.
- Many second-generation knee systems had PE knee inserts that had a PE thickness of 4 to 5 mm in the thinnest region.
- Current designs ensure that PE thickness in the thinnest areas of the insert is at least 8 mm.

ARTICULAR GEOMETRY (FIGURE 5-101)

- Avoid flat PE.
- Knee loads will exceed yield strength of UHMWPE.
- Thin line of joint contact during loading in flat PE insert
- Results in high contact loads to PE
- Goals of articulation
  - **Maximize contact area.**
  - Minimize contact loads (i.e., force/area).
  - Best design is biplanar congruency (Figure 5-102).
    - Congruent design in coronal plane and
    - Congruent design in sagittal plane

KNEE KINEMATICS

- **Sliding wear is bad for PE.**
- Sliding wear occurs when the ACL is sacrificed.
- When the ACL is removed and the PCL remains, the femur slides across the tibial PE during flexion and extension.
- Sliding movements are most pronounced in a cruciate-retaining knee with a flat PE insert.

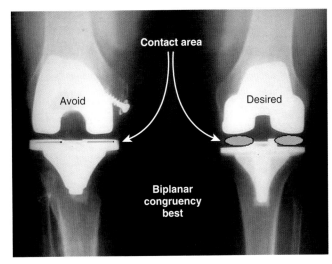

FIGURE 5-102 Radiograph showing two different articular bearing designs in TKA. Left knee has a flat bearing design in the coronal plane. The contact area is a line, and contact loads are high. Right knee has a congruent design in the coronal plane. The contact area of this design is an ellipse, and the contact loads are low.

- Sliding movements are least pronounced in a posterior stabilized or anterior stabilized knee with a **congruent PE insert.**
- Sliding wear across the tibia in laboratory testing creates severe surface and subsurface cracking with high wear.
- Current knee prosthetic systems are designed to minimize tibial sliding wear.

SURGICAL TECHNIQUE

- A tight flexion gap hastens sliding-wear effect.
- Stress is amplified with:
  - Tight PCL
  - Anterior tibial slope (Figure 5-103)

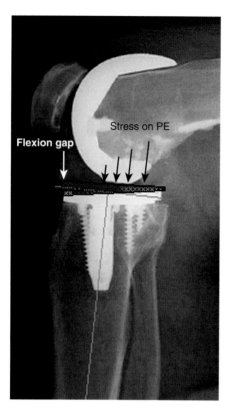

FIGURE 5-103 Radiograph demonstrating effect of anterior slope on PE stress loads. In this radiograph, the *gold lines* define a neutral tibial slope. Compared to the neutral slope line, the tibial component is positioned with an anterior slope. As the knee flexes, the flexion gap *(triangle)* becomes smaller. Consequently, at end flexion the contact stresses on the PE become excessively high *(arrows)*.

POLYETHYLENE PROCESSING (REVIEW SECTION 12)

- ■ **Fabrication**
- ▥ Ram bar extruded PE is not good.
  - • Variation in PE quality within the bar
- ▥ Calcium stearate additive is bad.
  - • Causes fusion defects in PE
- ▥ **Best PE fabrication process: direct compression molding**
  - • PE powder is placed into a mold, heated, and compressed. This creates an implant directly from the mold.
- ■ **Sterilization**
- ▥ Irradiated PE in air is bad.
  - • Oxidized PE chains
  - • **Reduced *mechanical strength* of PE**
- ■ **Machining (cutting-tool effect)**
- ▥ The cutting tool used to machine PE microscopically **stretches PE chains** (Figure 5-104).
  - • Amorphous areas are stretched.
- ▥ **The cutting-tool stretch effect is most pronounced 1 to 2 mm *below* the cut surface of the PE.**
- ▥ The stretched PE chains are more susceptible to radiation, resulting in greater oxidation in this region.
- ▥ **The clinical finding of the PE stretch/oxidation effect is the classical white band of oxidation in the subsurface of the PE** (Figure 5-105).

PERFECT STORM SCENARIO FOR CATASTROPHIC WEAR (FIGURE 5-106)

- ■ **Metal-backed tibial baseplate with bone-conserving tibial bone cut**
- ▥ Thin PE of 5 mm

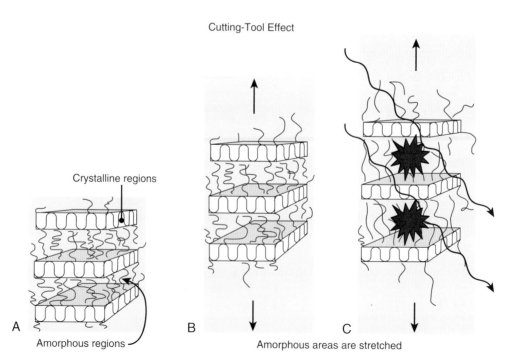

Cutting-Tool Effect

FIGURE 5-104 Diagram depicting the effect of machining upon PE. As the high-speed cutting tool removes the PE, the remaining nearby PE has stretched. Stretching occurs in the amorphous areas. The stretch effect is most pronounced in the PE 1 to 2 mm below the surface of the cut PE. The stretched PE chains are more susceptible to radiation, resulting in greater oxidation in this region.

- Flat bearing design in coronal plane
- Low contact area (a line)
- High contact load
- PCL retention with flat PE insert
- High sliding wear
- Ram bar PE with calcium stearate additive
- Fusion defects in PE
- γ-Irradiation sterilization in air (i.e., oxygen)
- Weakened mechanical properties of PE
- Machined PE surface
- Cutting-tool stretch effect upon PE

MEASURES TO MITIGATE CATASTROPHIC PE WEAR

- PE thickness at least 8 mm (for traditional PE)

- Congruent bearing design
- High contact area
- Low contact load
- Sliding wear on tibia minimized
- PCL substitution or
- PCL *accepting* prosthesis
  - PCL is used as a static stabilizer only (seen with anterior stabilized knee).
- Direct compression molded PE bearing
- No machining of articular surface
- Inert PE irradiation
- γ-Irradiation sterilization in **oxygen-free** environment
- Quality packaging to minimize on-the-shelf oxidation
  - Must keep oxygen from diffusing back into PE through packaging

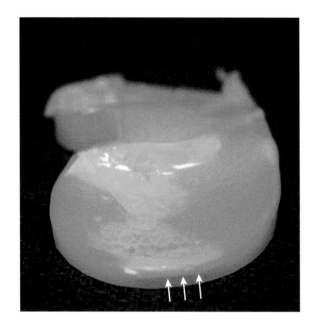

FIGURE 5-105 Retrieval PE knee insert after 9 years in vivo. Note classical white band of oxidation located 1 to 2 mm below machined surface of PE *(arrows)*. The knee was revised for catastrophic wear.

Catastrophic PE Failure

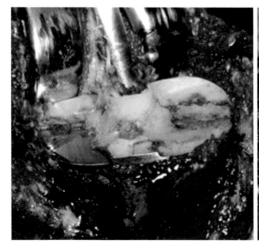 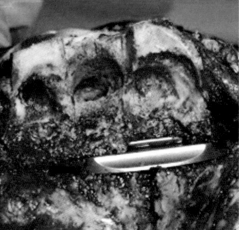

FIGURE 5-106 Intraoperative photographs of 8-year-old TKA in 58-year-old man. Patient presented with painless effusion. *Left,* Complete macroscopic failure of PE bearing. *Right,* Effect of osteolysis in femur. Reconstruction required extensive bone allografts and complex revision knee system.

SECTION 20 GLENOHUMERAL ARTHRITIS

INTRODUCTION

- **Etiology**
- Primary osteoarthritis (OA)
- Post-dislocation ("dislocation arthropathy")
- Posttraumatic
- Postsurgical (typically "capsulorrhaphy arthropathy")
- Rotator cuff deficiency ("cuff tear arthropathy")
- Chondrolysis
- Rheumatoid disease
- Osteonecrosis
- Neuropathic arthritis ("Charcot arthropathy")
- Septic arthritis
- **Primary OA**
- More common in women and patients older than 60 years
- Classic features of joint space narrowing and inferior humeral head osteophyte
- First radiographic sign may be fixed posterior humeral head subluxation, owing to tight anterior capsule.
- **Results in classic posterior glenoid wear**
- **Dislocation arthropathy**
- Due to articular cartilage damage from shear and impaction
- Increased age, posterior dislocation, and associated glenoid fractures associated with higher incidence
  - Number of dislocations and surgical stabilization have not been found to be associated.
- The 25-year follow-up data of primary anterior dislocations have shown an incidence of 56% of radiographically evidence arthrosis at final follow up.
- **Capsulorrhaphy arthropathy**
- Due to overtightening of capsule and resultant abnormal translation of the humeral head on the glenoid away from the capsulorrhaphy side
- Subscapularis transfer or imbrication is also a cause, but these procedures are rarely performed.
- Often associated with severe posterior glenoid erosion
- **Cuff tear arthropathy (CTA)**
- Incidence of arthropathy in patients with significant rotator cuff tears is approximately 4% to 20%.
- Due to a complex series of events that culminate in a loss of the concavity-compression effect of the glenohumeral joint. This results in nutritional and biomechanical alterations, causing articular cartilage loss and loss of humeral head bone density. Superior migration of the humeral head occurs, resulting in abutment against the coracoacromial arch and further degenerative changes.
- **Chondrolysis**
- Recently characterized entity that typically occurs after shoulder arthroscopy
- Etiology is uncertain.
  - Associated with use of radiofrequency energy, continuous postoperative anesthetic infusion, low-grade infection, bioabsorbable suture anchors, and contrast medium
- Presents with worsening pain and gradual reduction in ROM.

- Almost complete dissolution of articular cartilage on humeral head and glenoid
  - Classically differentiated from primary OA by an absence of osteophyte formation until late in the process
- **Rheumatoid disease**
- Shoulder affected in 90% of patients with rheumatoid disease
- Erosive nature of rheumatoid disease results in central glenoid wear (compared to posterior glenoid wear in OA) and subsequent medialization of the humeral head.
- **Osteonecrosis**
- May be traumatic or nontraumatic
  - Traumatic causes most frequently due to 3- or 4-part humeral head fractures
  - 35% incidence of osteonecrosis for 3-part fracture and 90% for 4-part fracture
  - Nontraumatic causes are the same as for other anatomic areas and include steroid use, alcohol use, metabolic causes, and hemoglobinopathies.
- Staging of humeral head osteonecrosis is similar to that of femoral head.
- **Neuropathic arthropathy**
- Loss of trophic and protective effects of the shoulder nerve supply
- Most commonly due to syringomyelia (syrinx), followed by leprosy. Other causes include CNS disorders and diabetes.
- Results in severe destructive arthropathy

HISTORY AND PHYSICAL EXAMINATION

- **Progressively worsening shoulder pain**
- **Loss of ROM, particularly loss of external rotation due to anterior and inferior capsular ligament contraction**
- **Important to examine for strength of rotator cuff musculature**
- Subscapularis integrity should be very carefully evaluated.
- **Significant clinical overlap with other shoulder conditions; radiographs are essential for diagnosis.**

IMAGING

- **The etiology of glenohumeral arthritis can often be determined from radiographs (Figure 5-107).**
- **True AP and axillary views are the most important.**
- **Primary OA**
- Posterior glenoid wear
- Central humeral head wear ("Friar Tuck" pattern)
- Inferior humeral head osteophyte ("goat's beard")
- Posterior humeral head subluxation
- **Rheumatoid disease**
- Central glenoid wear
- Medialization of humeral head with loss of humeral head offset
- Significant osteopenia within the humeral head and glenoid
- Osteophytes are infrequent.
- Periarticular erosions
- **Cuff tear arthropathy**
- Proximal migration of the humeral head
  - Decreased acromiohumeral distance

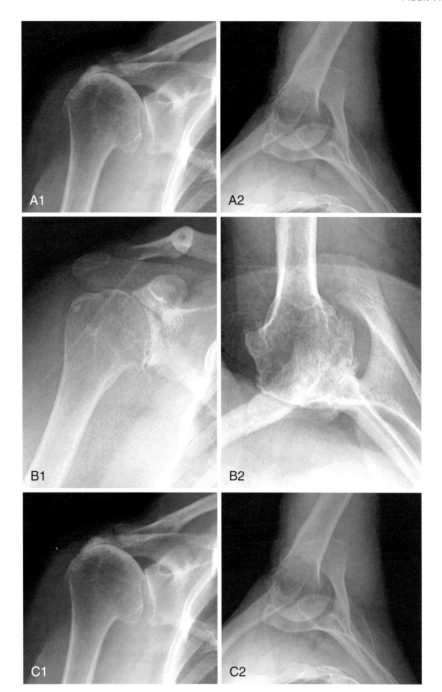

FIGURE 5-107 Radiographic features of glenohumeral arthritis based on etiology **(A-C).** (From Gartsman GM, Edwards TB: *Shoulder arthroplasty,* Philadelphia, 2008, Saunders, Figures 6-1 and 24-5; Miller MD, Thompson SR: *DeLee & Drez's orthopaedic sports medicine,* ed 4, Philadelphia, 2015, Saunders, Figure 56-4; and Brower AC, Flemming DJ: *Arthritis in black and white,* ed 3, Philadelphia, 2012, Saunders, Figures 6-1 and 6-3.)

- Femoralization of proximal humerus
  - Humeral head becomes more rounded as the tuberosities erode from chronic abrasion against the coracoacromial arch.
- Acetabularization of coracoacromial arch
  - Acromion undersurface becomes sclerotic and concave from the humeral head abrasion.
- **CT scan is an important investigation, particularly to determine glenoid morphology and remaining glenoid bone stock (Figure 5-108).**
- Normally the glenoid is 3 degrees retroverted and the humerus is approximately 20 to 30 degrees retroverted.
- Walch classification used for primary OA (Figure 5-109)
- **MRI is used particularly to determine rotator cuff integrity.**

- 5% to 10% incidence of full thickness rotator cuff tears in primary OA; 25% to 40% in rheumatoid disease

TREATMENT

- **Treatment for shoulder arthritis is similar to treatment of arthritis in the knee and hip. Nonoperative modalities include activity modification, NSAIDs, physical therapy focusing on capsular stretching, and corticosteroid injections.**
- **In broad terms, surgical treatment options can be separated based on whether there is an intact rotator cuff.**
- Intact rotator cuff: shoulder hemiarthroplasty, hemiarthroplasty with biologic glenoid resurfacing, total shoulder arthroplasty (TSA)

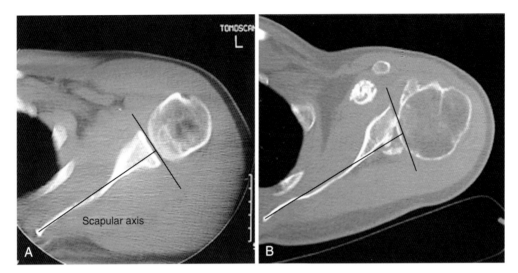

FIGURE 5-108 CT scans demonstrating glenoid version. **A,** Neutral glenoid version. Version is determined by drawing a line along the scapular axis and a line from anterior glenoid to posterior glenoid. Normal version is neutral to slight anteversion. **B,** Glenoid retroversion in a patient with osteoarthritis. Note the significant amount of posterior glenoid wear and posterior displacement of humeral head.

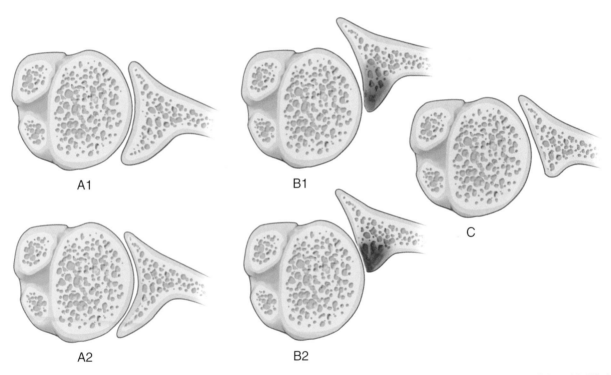

FIGURE 5-109 Walch classification of glenoid morphology (From Miller MD, Thompson SR: *DeLee & Drez's orthopaedic sports medicine,* ed 4, Philadelphia, 2015, Saunders, Figure 56-6.)

- ▨ **Deficient rotator cuff: hemiarthroplasty, reverse shoulder arthroplasty (RSA)**
- ■ **Contraindications to shoulder arthroplasty**
- ▨ Nonfunctioning deltoid and rotator cuff
- ▨ Intractable instability
- ▨ Active infection
- ▨ Charcot arthropathy
- ▨ Poor patient compliance
- ■ **Nonarthroplasty surgical interventions for shoulder arthritis are generally reserved for relatively young patients.**

- ▨ Comprehensive arthroscopic management ("CAM procedure") includes glenohumeral débridement, capsular release, and removal of humeral osteophytes.
- ■ **Shoulder arthrodesis remains an alternative for failed prosthetic reconstructions, combined rotator cuff and deltoid deficiency, paralytic disorders, infection, and intractable instability.**

SECTION 21 SHOULDER HEMIARTHROPLASTY

Shoulder hemiarthroplasty involves replacement of the humeral head only.

INDICATIONS

- Best indication: young patient with early-stage osteonecrosis before degenerative changes occur on glenoid side
- Indications are decreasing because of improved long-term results of total shoulder arthroplasty compared to hemiarthroplasty, as well as the advent of reverse shoulder arthroplasty for cuff tear arthropathy.

REQUIREMENTS

- Normal glenoid bone stock and anatomy
- Normal or near-normal glenoid articular cartilage

COMPLICATIONS

- Late glenoid pain
- As glenoid surface wears, pain increases.
- Eccentric glenoid bone loss complicating revision surgery

CONVERSION FROM HEMIARTHROPLASTY TO TSA

- Can be difficult, and pain relief is not always predictable.

HEMIARTHROPLASTY FOR CUFF TEAR ARTHROPATHY (CTA)

- In general, a reverse total shoulder arthroplasty is now preferred over shoulder hemiarthroplasty for CTA.
- However, if a hemiarthroplasty is selected, the following technical issues apply:
- Use of anatomic head sizing and avoidance of "overstuffing" with a large head. Overstuffing is associated with increased pain.
- Preservation of the coracoacromial ligament
  - If the coracoacromial ligament is removed, the anterior acromial arch is disrupted.
  - The humeral head can escape and dislocate anterosuperiorly.

SECTION 22 TOTAL SHOULDER ARTHROPLASTY

INTRODUCTION

- Involves glenoid resurfacing and humeral head replacement (Figure 5-110)
- Indicated for shoulder arthritis with intact and functional rotator cuff

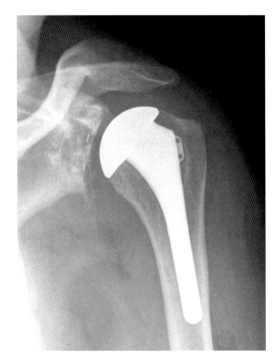

FIGURE 5-110 An anteroposterior radiograph of total shoulder arthroplasty for primary osteoarthritis. (From Miller MD, Thompson SR: *DeLee & Drez's orthopaedic sports medicine,* ed 4, Philadelphia, 2015, Saunders, Figure 56-10.)

- Preferred procedure for shoulder OA and inflammatory arthritis
- Superior pain relief compared to hemiarthroplasty
- Results of hemiarthroplasty conversion to TSA show variable satisfaction
- Problems with hemiarthroplasty conversion to TSA:
  - Severe glenoid bone loss. Results in compromised or difficult glenoid component fixation
  - Unpredictable pain relief
  - Unpredictable final shoulder ROM

REQUIREMENTS

- Rotator cuff must be intact and functional.
- Isolated reparable supraspinatus tear without retraction is acceptable condition to proceed with TSA.
- Incidence of full-thickness rotator cuff tears in patients undergoing TSA is 5% to 10%.

COMPONENT POSITIONING

- Humeral stem is positioned in retroversion.
- Accepted range: 25 to 45 degrees retroversion
- Excessive humeral bone removal during humeral neck osteotomy places the rotator cuff tendons at risk of injury.
- Glenoid is positioned in neutral.
- Avoid glenoid retroversion.
- Eccentric posterior glenoid wear management
  - From 0 to 15 degrees of retroversion can be managed with eccentric glenoid reaming.
  - Over 15 degrees may require posterior glenoid bone grafting or augmented glenoid component. Alternatively, a reverse shoulder arthroplasty may be used.

REHABILITATION

- Avoid excessive passive external rotation exercises.
- Classically caused by patient pushing self up from a low chair
- Excessive passive external rotation results in tear and pull-off of subscapularis tendon from lesser tuberosity.
- Presents as weakness in belly-press test, inability to perform lift-off test, and increased amount of passive external rotation compared to the uninvolved shoulder
- Results in anterior shoulder instability, the most common instability pattern after TSA
- Diagnosis is with ultrasound.

- Treatment of subscapularis pull-off is early surgical exploration and repair of the detached subscapularis tendon. In some cases, repair must be augmented with transfer of pectoralis major tendon.

COMPLICATIONS

- Implant loosening
- Primarily due to glenoid-sided failure
- Infection
- Associated with males and young patient age
- *Propionibacterium acnes* and *Staphylococcus* spp. are the most common pathogens.

SECTION 23 REVERSE TOTAL SHOULDER ARTHROPLASTY (RTSA)

INTRODUCTION

- Involves insertion of following implants (Figure 5-111)
- A porous-coated baseplate is secured to the glenoid with a central screw and multiple peripheral screws. Fixation is cementless.
- A glenosphere (i.e., ball) is assembled to baseplate.
- A humeral stem is inserted into canal (cemented or cementless technique).
- A humeral PE socket is assembled to the humeral stem.

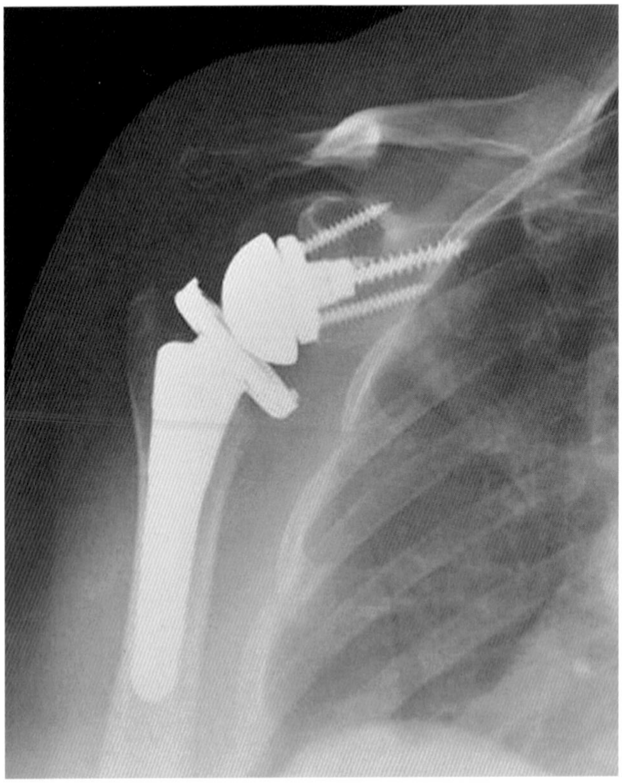

FIGURE 5-111 Radiograph of a reverse total shoulder arthroplasty (rTSA). In the rTSA system, a porous-coated glenoid baseplate is inserted into the glenoid and secured with a central screw and peripheral screws. A glenosphere (i.e., ball) is attached to the baseplate. A humeral stem is placed into the humerus. A PE cup is then assembled to the proximal humeral stem via a Morse taper junction. Note inferior tilt of glenoid component, which aids in deltoid tensioning.

- Resolves problem of superior migration of humeral head with CTA
- As deltoid contracts, the humerus rotates around glenosphere. Elevation power is provided by the deltoid.
  - Translational force of the deltoid is converted to rotational motion.
- Deltoid power and efficiency are improved by increasing humeral offset via medialization of the center of rotation.
- **A reverse TSA (when indicated) is best treatment for CTA.**
- Better functional ROM compared to hemiarthroplasty
- Better pain relief compared to hemiarthroplasty

REQUIREMENTS

- Intact axillary nerve
- Full function of deltoid
- Adequate glenoid bone stock
- Soft tissue tension is adjusted by varying the length of the glenosphere and humeral socket.
- Stability is provided by:
  - Deltoid tensioning
    - Adjust humeral offset.
    - Glenoid tilt
  - Head diameter
    - Larger diameter is more stable.
  - Component positioning

COMPONENT POSITIONING

- Glenosphere must be positioned as low as possible on the glenoid.
- This minimizes risk for scapular notching by humeral socket.
- Glenoid baseplate (and glenosphere) should be tilted inferiorly 10 to 15 degrees.
- This is key to enhancing deltoid tensioning and thus providing implant stability.
- Humeral stem is positioned in retroversion.
- 25 to 40 degrees retroversion preferred

COMPLICATIONS

- Dislocation of a reverse TSA most commonly is anterior.
- **Mechanism of dislocation is shoulder hyperextension and external rotation. In this position, the humeral socket levers posteriorly and dislocates.**
- Classically results from pushing up on chair armrest
- Occurs in approximately 9% of patients

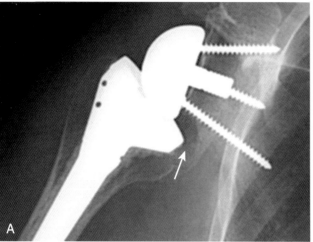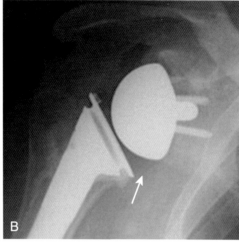

 FIGURE 5-112 Scapular notching in reverse shoulder arthroplasty. **A,** A typical varus implant without scapular notching *(arrow).* **B,** A typical valgus implant showing scapular notching *(arrow).* (From Jarrett CD et al: Reverse shoulder arthroplasty, *Orthop Clin North Am* 44:389–408, 2013, Figure 8.)

- Most important risk factor is an irreparable subscapularis at the time of surgery
- Lesser risk factors include proximal humeral nonunion, prior failed arthroplasty and preoperative fixed glenohumeral dislocation
- Scapular notching (Figure 5-112)
- Extremely common
  - Incidence between 50% and 90% of rTSA
- Results from repeated contact between inferior scapular neck and humeral component (or humerus)
- Clinical presentation is variable.
  - Notching may cause pain.
  - Notching may lead to fracture.
  - Notching may cause levering and dislocation.

- Minimize notching by:
  - Positioning glenoid baseplate (and glenosphere) as low as possible on glenoid bone
  - Optimize glenosphere head length; this pushes humeral socket away from scapula.
  - Increase glenosphere size.
- Infection
- Associated with prior failed arthroplasty and age younger than 65
- To date, diabetes, smoking, obesity, and inflammatory arthropathy have *not* been associated with increased rates of infection.

SECTION 24 INFECTION IN SHOULDER ARTHROPLASTY

INTRODUCTION

- Periprosthetic shoulder infections are unlike infections in hip and knee arthroplasty.
- Clinical presentation and diagnostic evaluation are different.

COMMON ORGANISMS

- *Propionibacterium acnes* and coagulase-negative *Staphylococcus* are increasingly recognized and common causes of shoulder arthroplasty infection.
- Incision of dermal sebaceous glands may be a source of *P. acnes.*

HISTORY AND PHYSICAL EXAMINATION

- **Pain is the most common complaint.**
- **A persistent draining sinus is second most common.**
- Stiffness, erythema, effusion, fever, chills, and night sweats are other common presentations.
- Risk factors for infection are *unlike* those for THA or TKA.
- Postoperative hematoma, young age, male sex, arthroplasty for trauma, and revision surgery have been the only identified risk factors.

INVESTIGATIONS

- Radiographs are essential to exclude other causes.
- Signs of infection include effusion, endosteal scalloping, periprosthetic radiolucent lines, and bony resorption.
- Bone scans should not be routinely obtained; their efficacy has not been demonstrated.
- Serology
- ESR and CRP have not demonstrated sufficient sensitivity or specificity to suggest periprosthetic shoulder infection.
- Joint aspiration
- No universal guidelines on when to aspirate a suspected infected shoulder arthroplasty
- Synovial leukocyte counts above 500 cells/μL have been found to be suggestive, but this is not universally accepted.
- Recent investigations have suggested a role for synovial α-defensin levels, but this is investigational.
- Synovial fluid culture is critical.

MICROBIOLOGY

- Synovial fluid and tissue cultures are the gold standard for diagnosis of infection.

- Cultures should be held anywhere from 14 to 28 days to detect *P. acnes*. Cultures should be on aerobic, anaerobic, and broth media.
- At surgery, it has been recommended that at least four different specimens be obtained.
- No current association between intraoperative frozen-section findings (e.g., >5 neutrophils per high power field) and diagnosis of periprosthetic shoulder infection

MANAGEMENT

- Surgical options:
- Antibiotic suppression, irrigation and débridement with component retention, resection arthroplasty, one-stage revision, two-stage revision, fusion, and amputation
- Acute infections may respond to incision and drainage.
- Chronic infections are optimally treated with two-stage (component extraction, antibiotic spacer placement, and delayed reimplantation) revision surgery. Some recent studies demonstrate efficacy with single-stage revision.
- Antibiotics
- Generally guided by culture results and consultation with infectious disease physicians

SELECTED BIBLIOGRAPHY

The selected bibliography for this chapter can be found on https://expertconsult.inkling.com.

TESTABLE CONCEPTS

- Osteonecrosis of the femoral head
  - Alcohol, steroids, trauma, sickle cell
  - Medial femoral circumflex artery
  - Total hip for collapse
  - Size and location of the lesion predict progression in asymptomatic patients
- Femoroacetabular impingement
  - Cam and pincer
  - Radiographic identification (crossover, ischial spine prominence, head-neck offset)
  - Exam: flexion adduction internal rotation (FADIR)
  - Hip preservation for symptomatic young patients with defined structural lesions
  - Address structural problems on both sides of joint and preserve labrum.
  - Arthroplasty for advanced arthritis
- Hip dysplasia
  - Anteversion of acetabulum and femur
  - Lateral center-edge angle (Wiberg) and sourcil (Tonnis) angle
  - Address all pathology (both sides of joint).
  - Do not scope the dysplastic hip.
  - Repair the labrum (do not débride if given the option).
  - PAO for the acetabulum (preserves posterior column)
  - THA for arthritis or subluxation (limb lengthening a concern—sciatic nerve)
- Total hip approaches (Table 5-8)
  - Know intervals and nervous innervation.
  - Safe zone 5 cm above tip of trochanter (superior gluteal artery and nerve)
  - If doing MIS and something goes wrong, convert to traditional approach.
- THA materials
  - Young's modulus (stiffness): ceramic, Co-Cr-Mo, stainless steel, titanium
  - Titanium—self-passivation (oxide layer)
  - Femoral stem breakage—cantilever bending
  - Irradiation/cross-linking of PE: wear resistance increases, mechanical strength decreases.
  - Oxidation—decreases mechanical properties (strength) and increases stiffness (elastic modulus)
  - PE manufacturing—direct compression (good), calcium stearate (bad), gamma in air (bad)
- THA fixation
  - Cemented cups fail at higher rate than cemented stems (cementless preferred for cup)
  - Survivorship approximately 1% per year
  - Cemented femur—no sharp edges, avoid flexible materials (Ti) and precoat/roughened implant
  - Cementless femur—circumferential coating, flexible material may reduce stress shielding.
  - Stress shielding—large, stiff, distally fixed stem (look for spot welds and proximal osteopenia).
  - Hydroxyapatite—$Ca_{10}(PO_4)_6(OH)_2$—delamination can occur.
  - Ingrowth—live host bone, appropriate ingrowth material, no motion (<150 μm)
- THA implant position/technique
  - Acetabulum inclination: 40 degrees (30-50)
  - Acetabulum anteversion: 20 degrees (10-40)
  - Femur anteversion: 15 degrees (5-20)
  - Combined anteversion: 35-40 degrees
  - Direction of dislocation is direction of excess.

Table 5-8	Surgical Approaches for Total Hip Arthroplasty			
APPROACH	**MUSCULAR INTERVAL**	**NERVOUS INTERVAL**	**PROS**	**CONS**
Direct anterior	Sartorius-TFL Rectus-Glut Med	Femoral-SGN	Stability Rapid recovery?	Femoral exposure Specialized table?
Lateral	Medius and vastus lateralis splitting	NA	Stability	Abductor recovery Extend distal only
Anterolateral	Medius-TFL	NA	Stability	Femoral exposure TFL denervation
Posterior	Maximus split ER tenotomies	NA	Extensile Muscle recovery	Instability

TESTABLE CONCEPTS

- Intraoperative calcar crack with cementless stem—expose, remove stem, wire/cable, reinsert (if stable)
- Hip stability
  - Head-to-neck diameter ratio—increase ROM to impingement.
  - Large diameter heads—jump distance
  - ROM to impingement decreased by lipped/hooded liners, skirts/collars, constrained liners
- Osteolysis
  - Associated with PE wear
  - Adhesive wear more important than abrasive wear
  - Phagocytosis of submicron PE particles by *macrophage*; bone resorption by osteoclasts
  - Key radiographic features—eccentric head position, endosteal scalloping
- Bearings
  - Lubrication (fluid-film > mixed > boundary)
  - Metal-on-metal—contraindications include female of child-bearing age, renal failure
  - Theoretical benefits—large head/stability, low wear, no fracture risk
  - Sensitive to implant position, clearance, implant size, coverage arc
  - Edge wear—impingement, microseparation, edge loading
  - ALTR/ALVAL—*lymphocyte*, similar features to delayed type IV hypersensitivity reaction
  - Hip resurfacing—preservation of bone stock, femoral neck fractures (1%)
  - COC—lowest wear couple
  - Disadvantages—fracture risk, squeaking
- Hip arthrodesis
  - Young, male laborer
  - Adjacent joint degeneration most common cause for conversion to THA
  - Position: 20 to 25 degrees of flexion, 0 degrees abduction, 0-10 degrees external rotation
  - Walking function depends on abductors.
- Patient-specific considerations for THA
  - Sickle cell: early loosening
  - Psoriatic arthritis: infection
  - Ankylosing spondylitis: HO
  - Parkinson disease: dislocation, mortality
  - Dialysis: infection, loosening
  - Irradiation: cement versus highly porous metals
- Treatment of PE wear
  - Revise if symptomatic or massive lytic defect
  - May leave cup if well-positioned and well fixed
  - Dislocation is most common complication (use large head).
  - Bone grafting controversial
- Dislocation (Figure 5-113)
  - Constrained liners only for abductor deficiency with well-positioned implants
- Revision THA
  - Femur—diaphyseal engaging cementless stem typical answer (need diaphysis)
  - Acetabulum—cementless hemispherical cup is solution 95% of the time
  - Pelvic discontinuity requires plan B.
  - Screw placement—zone of death is anterior-superior (external iliac).
- Periprosthetic fracture
  - Calcar crack can be treated with stem removal, cabling, and stem reinsertion.

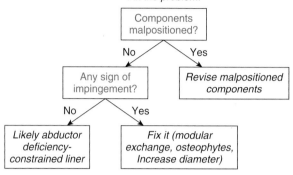

Treatment of Dislocation
Why did it dislocate? Patient, surgeon, implant
Fix the problem.

FIGURE 5-113 Surgical approach to recurrent THA dislocation.

- Type B—if stem is loose, revise the implant; if stem well-fixed, ORIF.

SECTION 14 KNEE ARTHRITIS TREATMENT

- Knee osteotomy is typically indicated in the active patient younger than age 50.
  - Varus knee—valgus-producing high tibial osteotomy
  - Valgus knee—varus-producing supracondylar femoral osteotomy
  - Contraindications: inflammatory arthritis, less than 90 degrees of knee flexion, collateral ligament insufficiency
- Unicompartmental arthroplasty
  - Advantages: quicker recovery, smaller incision, better knee function
  - Disadvantages: long-term survivorship not as good as TKA
  - Contraindications: inflammatory arthritis, greater than 10 degrees of flexion contracture, fixed varus/valgus deformity, ACL deficiency, tricompartmental arthritis
  - Complications: stress fracture of tibia, patellar impingement

SECTION 15 TOTAL KNEE ARTHROPLASTY

- Varus knee balancing
  - Medial compartment release needed
  - Osteophytes, deep medial collateral ligament (MCL), posteromedial corner (capsule and semimembranosus), superficial MCL (posterior oblique tight in extension, anterior tight in flexion)
- Valgus knee balancing
  - Lateral compartment release needed
  - Osteophytes, lateral capsule, iliotibial band (tight in extension), popliteus (tight in flexion), lateral collateral ligament
- Flexion deformity balancing
  - Osteophytes, posterior capsule, gastrocnemius muscle origin
- Sagittal plane balancing
  - Flexion gap—*posterior* cut of femur, tibial cut, and posterior cruciate ligament (PCL)
  - Extension gap—*distal* cut of femur, tibial cut, posterior capsule
  - For some gap imbalance scenarios, there is more than one possible solution.
  - McPherson's rule
    - Symmetrical gap problem—adjust tibia first.
    - Asymmetrical gap problem—adjust femur first.
- TKA complications
  - Femoral notching—lessens load needed to cause fracture with knee bending; avoid knee manipulation with femoral notch

TESTABLE CONCEPTS

- Peroneal nerve palsy—valgus knee with flexion contracture most at risk. Initial treatment is remove compressive dressing and flex knee.
  - Most recover within 3 months if nerve is not cut. If nerve palsy does not resolve, explore and decompress peroneal nerve.
- Patella osteonecrosis—lateral retinacular release transects the lateral superior genicular artery.
- Extensor disruption—*cannot repair;* must use allograft reconstruction
- HO—optimal prophylaxis (pre- or postoperatively within first 24-48 hours): single-dose external beam radiation (600-800 Gy), NSAIDs
- Periprosthetic joint infection—definite diagnosis can be made when a sinus tract communicates with affected joint <u>or</u> a pathogen is isolated by culture from two separate fluid or tissue samples <u>or</u> four of the following six exist:
  - (1) Elevated ESR or CRP concentration, (2) elevated synovial WBC count, (3) elevated synovial neutrophil percentage, (4) isolation of a pathogen by culture from one fluid or tissue sample, (5) presence of purulence, or (6) greater than five neutrophils per high power field observed from histologic review
- Biofilm:
  - Made by all bacteria
  - Once established cannot be eradicated with any current treatment regimen
  - Effective treatment requires prosthetic removal and radical soft tissue débridement.
- Infection treatment:
  - Acute (known infection <3 weeks)—irrigation and débridement, exchange of modular bearings, component retention, and intravenous antibiotics
  - Chronic (biofilm state)—implant removal, irrigation and débridement, joint stabilization with antibiotic-loaded cement spacer, intravenous antibiotics, and second-stage reconstruction

SECTION 16 TKA DESIGN

- PCL tension influences femoral rollback. Femoral rollback is defined as progressive posterior change in femoral-tibial contact point as knee moves into flexion.
- PCL retention
  - Advantages: bone conserving, consistent joint line restoration, improved proprioception
  - Disadvantages: harder to balance, excess recession can result in late failure caused by flexion instability
- Posterior stabilized TKA must be used if patellectomy, inflammatory arthritis, or PCL previously ruptured.
- Maximum joint line elevation is 8 mm to avoid patella baja deformity and decreased knee flexion.
- Modular tibial components can have backside PE wear from micromotion between tibial baseplate and tibial PE bearing.
- A constrained TKA must be used if the soft tissues will not support a standard prosthesis.
  - Indicated for residual flexion gap laxity, MCL or lateral collateral ligament deficiency, and Charcot arthropathy.

SECTION 18 PATELLAR TRACKING IN TKA

- Femoral and tibial components—do not internally rotate or medialize.

- In a valgus knee, the lateral condyle is frequently hypoplastic and the posterior condylar axis cannot be used as a guide for rotation.
- Patellar component medialization is acceptable because it decreases the Q angle.
- Maltracking
  - Intraoperatively—first release the tourniquet and reassess.
  - Postoperatively—if examination and radiographs are acceptable, a CT scan can be used to determine rotational alignment of components.
- Patella baja results in loss of knee flexion and impingement pain. Seen after proximal tibial closed- or open-wedge osteotomy, tibial tubercle osteotomy, and trauma.

SECTION 19 CATASTROPHIC WEAR IN TKA

- Five key factors to avoid catastrophic PE wear:
  - PE thickness—greater than 8 mm
  - Articular geometry—avoid flat PE.
  - Knee kinematics—minimize tibial sliding wear.
  - Surgical technique—avoid tight flexion gap.
  - PE processing—use direct compression molding and inert PE irradiation (i.e., irradiate PE in an oxygen-free environment).

SECTION 20 GLENOHUMERAL ARTHRITIS

- Primary glenohumeral OA results in classic posterior glenoid wear. Inflammatory arthropathies typically cause centralized glenoid wear.
- The etiology of glenohumeral OA can often be determined from radiographs.

SECTION 21 SHOULDER HEMIARTHROPLASTY

- In broad terms, surgical treatment options can be separated based on whether there is an intact rotator cuff.
  - Intact rotator cuff: shoulder hemiarthroplasty, hemiarthroplasty with biologic glenoid resurfacing, total shoulder arthroplasty (TSA)
  - Deficient rotator cuff: hemiarthroplasty, reverse shoulder arthroplasty (RSA)

SECTION 22 TOTAL SHOULDER ARTHROPLASTY

- TSA is the preferred procedure for shoulder OA and inflammatory arthritis. It has superior pain relief compared to hemiarthroplasty.
  - The rotator cuff must be intact and functional.
  - An isolated reparable supraspinatus tear without retraction is an acceptable condition to proceed with TSA. Approximately 5% to 10% of patients undergoing TSA have a full-thickness tear.
  - Excessive humeral bone removal during humeral neck osteotomy places the rotator cuff tendons at risk of injury.
  - An eccentric posteriorly worn glenoid should be managed based on the degree of retroversion.
    - 0 to 15 degrees: eccentric glenoid reaming
    - More than 15 degrees: posterior glenoid grafting, augmented glenoid component, or conversion to RSA
  - The most common instability pattern after TSA is anterior instability. Diagnosis is via ultrasound.

SECTION 23 REVERSE TOTAL SHOULDER ARTHROPLASTY (RTSA)

- A reverse TSA is the best treatment for cuff tear arthropathy (CTA)
  - Mechanism of dislocation is shoulder hyperextension and external rotation. In this position, the humeral socket levers posteriorly and dislocates. Classically results from pushing up on chair armrest.
  - Most important risk factor is an irreparable subscapularis at the time of surgery. Lesser risk factors include proximal humeral

TESTABLE CONCEPTS

nonunion, prior failed arthroplasty, and preoperative fixed glenohumeral dislocation.
- Scapular notching is extremely common. The clinical presentation is variable but often may present with pain. Notching is minimized by positioning the glenoid baseplate (and glenosphere) as low as possible on glenoid bone.

SECTION 24 INFECTION IN SHOULDER ARTHROPLASTY

- Infection following shoulder arthroplasty most commonly presents with pain. A persistent sinus is the second most common presentation.

- Risk factors are unlike those for THA or TKA.
- Synovial fluid and tissue cultures are the gold standard for diagnosis of infection.
- Cultures should be held anywhere from 14 to 28 days to detect *P. acnes.* Cultures should be on aerobic, anaerobic, and broth media.

CHAPTER 6

DISORDERS OF THE FOOT AND ANKLE

Anish R. Kadakia and Jeffrey D. Seybold

CONTENTS

SECTION 1 BIOMECHANICS OF THE FOOT AND ANKLE

- ◼ Primary functions of foot and ankle: to provide weight bearing support and forward ambulation
- ◼ Anatomy
- ▦ Ankle
  - Ankle mortise formed by tibial plafond, medial malleolus, and lateral malleolus (Figure 6-1)
  - Mortise articulates with dome of talar body
  - Mortise widens and ankle becomes more stable in dorsiflexion owing to shape of talar dome (wider anteriorly)
    - Mortise widens 1 to 1.5 mm during motion from plantar flexion to dorsiflexion
  - A simplified model of the ankle joint has a horizontal axis from anteromedial to posterolateral and a coronal axis from superomedial directed distally and laterally to the tip of the fibula (between the malleoli) (Figure 6-2).

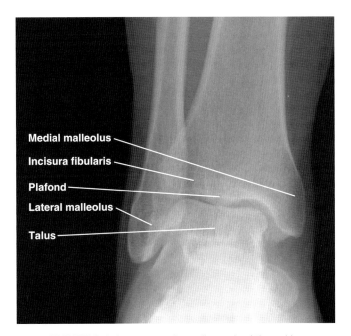

FIGURE 6-1 Anteroposterior radiograph of the ankle.

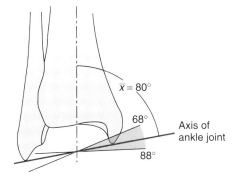

FIGURE 6-2 Angle between the axis of the ankle joint and the long axis of the tibia. (From Hsu J et al: *AAOS atlas of orthoses and assistive devices*, Philadelphia, 2008, Elsevier.)

- Responsible for most sagittal plane motion of foot and ankle
  - 23 to 48 degrees plantar flexion
  - 10 to 23 degrees dorsiflexion
- Also contributes to inversion/eversion and rotation
- ▦ Distal tibiofibular joint
  - Distal fibula—convex medial surface
  - Incisura fibularis—concave surface of distal lateral tibia
  - Fibula rotates (≈2 degrees) within incisura during ankle motion and ambulation. Ankle dorsiflexion results in external rotation and proximal translation of fibula.
- ▦ Ligamentous anatomy (Figure 6-3)
  - Lateral ankle ligaments function as a restraint to varus/inversion forces at ankle.
    - Anterior talofibular ligament (ATFL) originates from anteroinferior aspect of lateral malleolus (1 cm proximal to its tip) and extends to lateral aspect of talar neck.
    - Calcaneofibular ligament (CFL) extends from tip of lateral malleolus to lateral aspect of calcaneus.
    - Posterior talofibular ligament (PTFL) extends from posterior lateral malleolus to posterolateral talus.
    - ATFL is the weakest ankle ligament; PTFL is the strongest.
  - Distal tibiofibular joint (ankle syndesmosis) and fibula provide stability against lateral talar translation.
  - **Deltoid ligament complex—main ankle stabilizer during stance**
    - Deep deltoid ligament extends from apex of medial malleolus to medial talar body and functions primarily to resist lateral talar translation.
    - Superficial deltoid ligament extends from distal medial malleolus to navicular bone, sustentaculum tali of calcaneus, medial talus, and spring ligament. Functions primarily to resist valgus/eversion ankle forces (i.e., talar tilt).
- ▦ Hindfoot and midfoot
  - Hindfoot includes talus, calcaneus, and cuboid; subtalar, calcaneocuboid (CC), and talonavicular (TN) joints are included (Figure 6-4). Hindfoot functions primarily in inversion and eversion.
    - Inversion motion is normally greater than eversion.
    - Limited eversion accommodation contributes to stiffness and disability derived from even a mild cavovarus foot deformity.
    - **Spring ligament connects calcaneus to navicular along the medial hindfoot.**
      - Supports the talar head and is incompetent in adult acquired flatfoot deformity
    - **Subtalar joint motion is interrelated to tibial rotation.**
      - Internal tibial rotation results in subtalar eversion.
        - Late heel strike and foot flat
      - External tibial rotation results in subtalar inversion.
        - Initial heel strike and toe-off
  - Midfoot begins at articulation between navicular and cuneiforms, along with cuboid and fourth and fifth metatarsals. Midfoot also includes tarsometatarsal (TMT) joints.

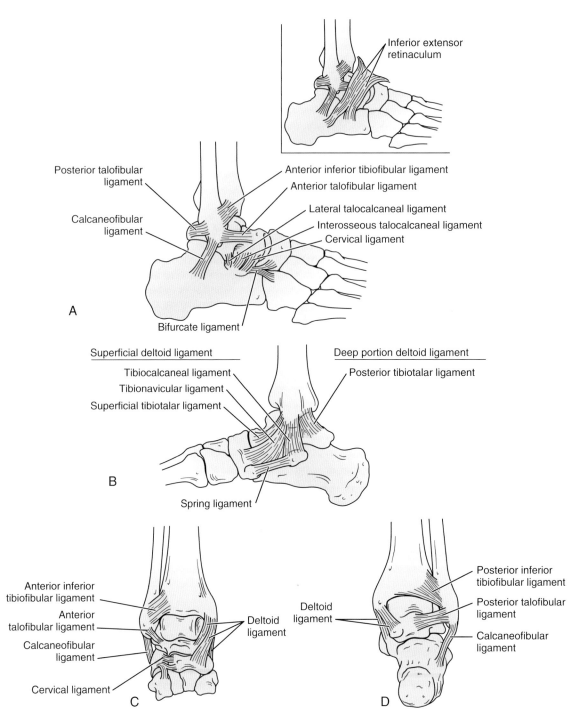

FIGURE 6-3 Ligaments of the ankle and subtalar joint. **A,** Lateral view. **B,** Medial view. **C,** Anterior view. **D,** Posterior view. (From Miller MD: *Core knowledge in orthopaedics—sports medicine,* Philadelphia, 2006, Elsevier.)

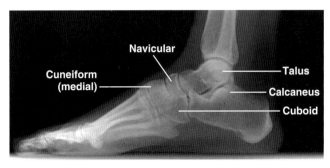

FIGURE 6-4 Lateral radiograph of the foot.

- Midfoot functions in adduction and abduction.
- CC and TN joints are collectively referred to as the *midtarsal, transverse tarsal,* or *Chopart joint.*
  - This joint is important for providing hindfoot and midfoot stability to produce a rigid lever at heel rise.
  - During foot flat (hindfoot valgus, forefoot abduction, and dorsiflexion of ankle), the transverse tarsal joints are parallel and supple, adapting to uneven ground.
  - During toe-off (hindfoot varus, forefoot adduction, and plantar flexion of ankle), these joints become

EVERSION INVERSION

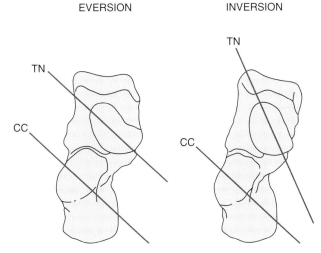

FIGURE 6-5 Function of the transverse tarsal joint. When the heel is everted, the transverse tarsal joints are parallel and unlocked, allowing the foot to be supple and pronate and accommodate to the floor. When the heel is inverted (varus), the transverse tarsal joint is divergent and locked, allowing for a stable hindfoot/midfoot complex for toe-off. *CC,* Calcaneocuboid; *TN,* talonavicular.

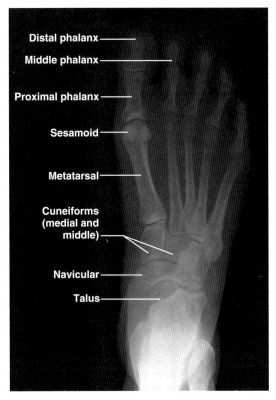

FIGURE 6-6 Anteroposterior radiograph of the foot.

divergent and lock, providing stiffness to the foot for forward propulsion (Figure 6-5).
- Failure of posterior tibial tendon (PTT) to lock transverse tarsal joints is the biomechanical etiology for lack of a heel rise in patients with PTT dysfunction (PTTD).
- Midfoot provides an important bridge between hindfoot and forefoot, giving both flexibility and stability necessary for normal gait and other activities.
- Ligamentous stability to midfoot is provided through longitudinal and transverse ligaments on plantar and dorsal aspects of each joint.
  - Plantar ligaments are thicker and stronger than their dorsal counterparts.
  - **Primary stabilizer of longitudinal arch is the interosseous ligaments, NOT the plantar fascia**; plantar fascia is a secondary stabilizer.
- Lisfranc joint complex has a specialized bony and ligamentous structure, providing stability to this joint.
  - The second metatarsal extends more proximally than surrounding metatarsals. This "keystone" effect imparts inherent bony stability.
  - Dorsal and plantar ligaments extend from the second metatarsal to each of the three cuneiforms.
  - **Largest and strongest of these ligaments is the Lisfranc ligament, traveling from medial cuneiform to base of second metatarsal.**
- The foot is also divided into three columns.
  - **Medial column** includes the first metatarsal, the medial cuneiform, and the navicular.
  - **Middle column** includes the second and third metatarsals, the middle cuneiform, and the lateral cuneiform.
    - Rigidity of the middle column allows for a rigid lever arm during push-off.

- **Lateral column** includes the fourth and fifth metatarsals and the cuboid.
  - Sagittal mobility of the lateral column imparts flexibility necessary for walking on uneven ground.
  - Lateral column has the most sagittal mobility (≈10 degrees in dorsiflexion and plantar flexion), and middle column has the least (≈2 degrees in dorsiflexion and plantar flexion).
- Foot has longitudinal and transverse arches, with arch stability provided by a combination of the bony architecture, ligamentous attachments, and muscle forces.
  - Stability of the midfoot allows for push-off during gait and other activities.
- Forefoot
  - Forefoot includes all structures distal to the TMT joints (Figure 6-6).
  - First metatarsal is the widest and shortest and bears 50% of the weight during gait.
  - Second metatarsal is usually the longest and experiences more stress than the other lesser metatarsals.
    - Second metatarsal is more commonly involved in stress fractures.
  - Lesser toes are controlled by a delicate muscle balance:
    - Extrinsic muscles
      - Extensor digitorum longus [EDL]
      - Flexor digitorum longus [FDL]
    - Intrinsic muscles—metatarsophalangeal (MTP) flexion and proximal interphalangeal (PIP) extension
      - Interossei
      - Lumbricals

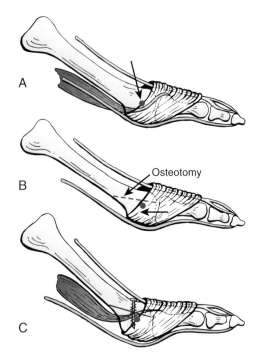

FIGURE 6-7 Axis of the metatarsophalangeal joint before and after Weil osteotomy. **A,** Lesser metatarsal before osteotomy; note intrinsics are plantar to the axis. **B,** Osteotomy is above the center of the metatarsal head. **C,** Following the osteotomy and proximal translation of the capital fragment, the intrinsics course dorsal to the axis of rotation. This can lead to metatarsophalangeal joint dorsiflexion. (From Coughlin MJ et al: *Surgery of the foot and ankle,* ed 8, Philadelphia, 2006, Mosby.)

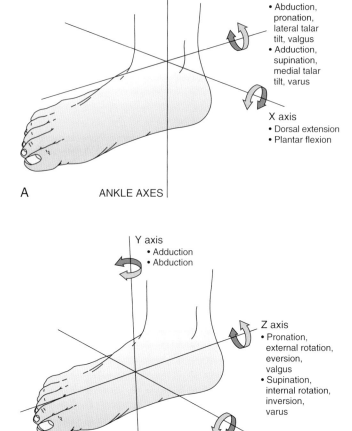

FIGURE 6-8 Axes of rotation of the ankle **(A)** and foot **(B).** (From Myerson MS: *Foot and ankle disorders,* Philadelphia, 2000, Elsevier.)

- Passive restraints
  - Plantar plate—disrupted in a hammertoe and crossover toe
  - Extensor hood—primary distal insertion point of the long extensors, which function to extend MTP joint but NOT PIP joint
  - Joint capsule
  - Collateral ligaments

- **Intrinsic tendons** pass plantar (providing a flexion force) to MTP joint axis proximally and pass dorsal to the axis distally (providing an extension force).
  - **Plantar migration of this axis after a Weil (oblique shortening) osteotomy of the metatarsal leads to a "floating" toe. The tendons are now relatively dorsal to the MTP axis of rotation** (Figure 6-7).
  - Loss of intrinsic function as seen in hereditary motor sensory neuropathy or diabetic neuropathy predictably leads to claw toes.

Foot positions versus foot motions

- Foot positions are defined differently than foot motions.
- Foot positions are:
  - Varus/valgus—hindfoot
  - Abduction/adduction—midfoot
  - Equinus/calcaneus—ankle
- Foot motions in the three axes of rotation are illustrated in Figure 6-8 and summarized in Table 6-1.
  - The critical assessment is to determine the relationship of the forefoot to the hindfoot.

Table 6-1	Motions of the Foot and Ankle
PLANE OF MOTION	**MOTION**
Sagittal (X-axis)	Dorsiflexion
	Plantar flexion
Frontal (coronal) (Z-axis)	Inversion
	Eversion
Transverse (Y-axis)	Forefoot/midfoot
	Adduction
	Abduction
	Ankle/hindfoot
	Internal rotation
	External rotation
Triplanar motion	Supination
	Adduction
	Inversion
	Plantar flexion
	Pronation
	Abduction
	Eversion
	Dorsiflexion

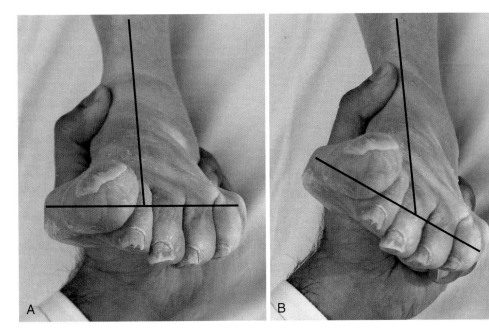

FIGURE 6-9 A patient with long-standing pes planovalgus deformity. **A,** With the hindfoot in valgus, the foot is plantigrade to the ground. **B,** With the hindfoot corrected to neutral, the forefoot supination becomes evident with the elevated first ray. Failure to correct this deformity will cause any surgical correction to fail because the hindfoot will go back into valgus as the first ray must contact the ground.

- If the heel is in a neutral position (subtalar neutral), the forefoot should be parallel with the floor to meet the ground flush (plantigrade).
  - If the first ray is elevated, the forefoot is in varus position. If the first ray is flexed, the forefoot is in valgus position (see Figure 6-3). This should not be confused with hindfoot varus or valgus.
  - Example: in a long-standing flatfoot deformity the heel is valgus and the forefoot has compensated by going into varus or supinating to keep the foot flat to the ground.
    - Once the heel has been corrected, the elevated first ray can be easily seen (Figure 6-9).

■ **Gait cycle**
▥ One full gait cycle from heel strike to heel strike is termed a *stride.*
- Each stride is composed of a stance phase (heel strike to toe-off; 62% of cycle) and a swing phase (toe-off to heel strike; 38% of cycle) (Figure 6-10).
- *Walking* is defined by a period of double limb support in addition to always having one foot in contact with the ground throughout the gait cycle.
- Ground reaction forces are approximately 1.5 times body weight during walking and 3 to 4 times body weight during running.
  - This difference is due to the increased load after the float phase of running, in which there is no foot in contact with the ground.
- As the speed of gait increases, the stance phase decreases.
▥ Soft-tissue contributions to gait mechanics
- Swing phase
  - Anterior tibialis—contracts concentrically
    - Loss of function results in a foot drop and steppage gait.

- **Heel strike**
  - **Anterior tibialis—contracts eccentrically**
    - Controls the rate at which foot strikes the ground. In patients with foot drop, the rapid strike of the foot can result in a loud "slap" during heel strike.
  - Hindfoot—locked/inverted at initial strike; passively everts during transition from heel strike to foot flat
    - Allows for energy absorption. Failure to evert in patients with cavovarus deformity increases forces to lateral foot, resulting in stress fractures (fifth metatarsal), callus formation, and ankle instability.
- Foot flat
  - Gastrocnemius-soleus complex—eccentric contraction
    - Controls forward progression of body over the foot
    - **Loss of function results in a calcaneus gait with heel pain**
  - Hindfoot—unlocked/everted for ground accommodation
- Toe-off
  - Gastrocnemius-soleus complex—concentric contraction
  - In addition, as foot progresses from heel strike to toe-off, the following changes allow foot to convert from a flexible shock absorber to a rigid propellant:
    - Plantar fascia, which attaches to plantar medial heel and runs the length of the arch to the bases of each proximal phalanx, is tightened as MTP joints extend. The longitudinal arch is accentuated.
      - This is called the *windlass mechanism* (Figure 6-11).
    - Hindfoot supinates, with firing of the PTT.
    - Transverse tarsal joint locks and provides a rigid lever arm for toe-off.

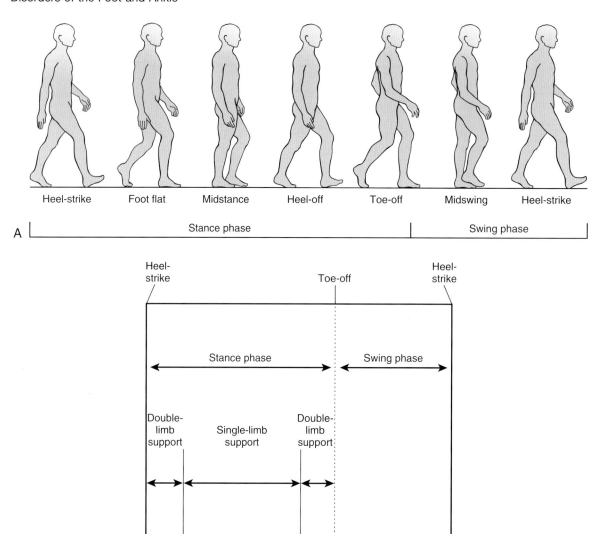

FIGURE 6-10 The gait cycle. **A,** The normal phases of gait. **B,** Time dimensions of normal gait cycle. (From Miller MD: *Core knowledge in orthopaedics—sports medicine,* Philadelphia, 2006, Elsevier.)

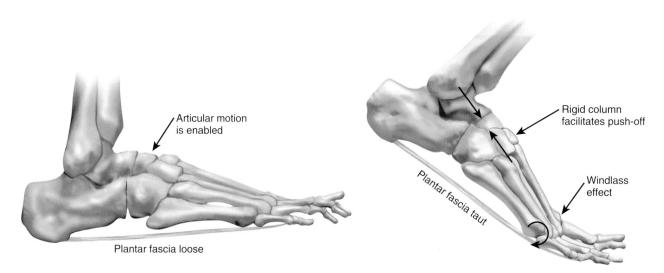

FIGURE 6-11 Windlass mechanism and function of the plantar fascia. When the foot is at rest, there is some mobility between the bones of the midfoot, allowing flexibility. During the push-off phase of gait, this flexibility would be detrimental. The plantar fascia, which inserts distal to the metatarsophalangeal joints, tightens as the toes are dorsiflexed, which pulls the tarsal bones together and "locks" them into a rigid column. This effect has been likened to a windlass, which is a rope or chain extending over a drum used to raise and lower sails and anchors on a ship. (From Morrison W, Sanders T: *Problem solving in musculoskeletal imaging,* St. Louis, 2008, Mosby.)

SECTION 2 PHYSICAL EXAMINATION OF THE FOOT AND ANKLE

■ Inspection

▨ Foot and ankle should be inspected for:
- Symmetry
- Callouses—areas of abnormally increased pressure
- Signs of peripheral vascular disease—lack of hair, increased skin pigmentation (hemosiderin deposition)
- Swelling—symmetric (likely systemic etiology) versus asymmetric (trauma, venous thrombosis, cellulitis, osteomyelitis, focal musculoskeletal etiology) (Figure 6-12)
- Ecchymosis—plantar ecchymosis associated with TMT injury (Lisfranc injury) (Figure 6-13)
- Alignment
  - Neutral
  - Cavovarus—elevated longitudinal arch with hindfoot varus and plantar-flexed first ray (Figure 6-14)
- Pes planus—flat longitudinal arch with hindfoot valgus (Figure 6-15)
  - Must differentiate hindfoot-driven versus midfoot-driven etiology
    - Midfoot driven secondary to degenerative joint disease (DJD) or chronic Lisfranc injury
      - Treatment—midfoot fusion with realignment
    - Hindfoot driven (adult) secondary to PTTD (most common)
      - Treatment—FDL tendon transfer with medial slide calcaneal osteotomy or triple arthrodesis

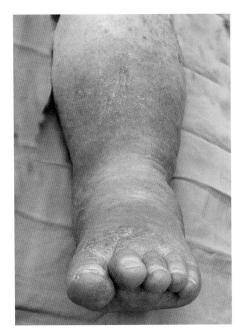

FIGURE 6-12 This patient presented with chronic osteomyelitis of the leg, with a past medical history significant for diabetes mellitus and peripheral vascular disease. Note no hair growth in distal half of leg, along with significant swelling of the limb.

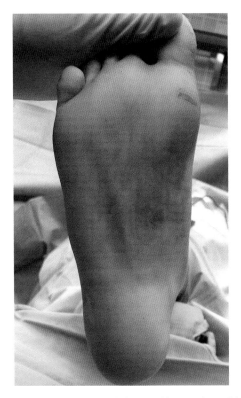

FIGURE 6-13 Plantar ecchymosis is noted in a patient with a Lisfranc (tarsometatarsal) injury.

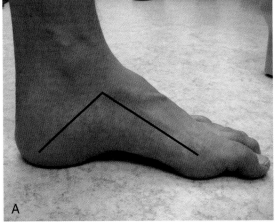
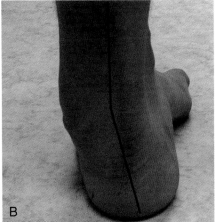

FIGURE 6-14 Note the plantar-flexed first ray **(A)** and varus position of the hindfoot **(B)** in a patient with a cavovarus deformity.

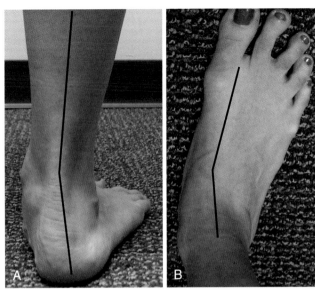

FIGURE 6-15 Valgus position of the hindfoot **(A)** with forefoot abduction **(B)** in a patient with a pes planovalgus deformity.

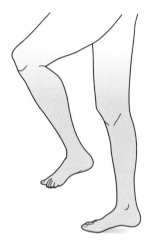

FIGURE 6-16 Steppage gait consists of each knee being excessively raised when walking. This maneuver compensates for a loss of position sense by elevating the feet to ensure they will clear the ground, stairs, and other obstacles. It is a classical sign of posterior column spinal cord damage from tabes dorsalis. However, peripheral neuropathies more commonly impair position sense and lead to this gait abnormality. (From Kaufman D: *Clinical neurology for psychiatrists*, ed 6, Philadelphia, 2006, Elsevier.)

- Hindfoot driven (pediatric) secondary to abnormal skeletal development
  - Treatment—lateral column lengthening
- Gait evaluation
  - Steppage gait—increased knee and hip flexion during swing phase to ensure toes clear the floor (Figure 6-16)
    - Secondary to foot drop (peroneal nerve palsy or neuropathy)
  - **Calcaneus gait—increased ankle dorsiflexion during heel strike**
    - **Secondary to triceps surae (gastrocnemius-soleus) weakness**
  - Antalgic gait—shortened stance phase on the affected side
    - Secondary to pain, most commonly DJD

- Short stance phase minimizes amount of time pressure is placed to affected limb, decreasing pain.
- **Vascular examination**
- Palpate dorsalis pedis and posterior tibial pulses; if not present, consider noninvasive studies.
  - Predictive for healing
    - Doppler ultrasonography
      - Triphasic waveforms are normal.
    - Ankle-brachial index (ABI)
      - Greater than 0.5, with normal ranging from 0.9 to 1.3
      - Greater than 1.3 indicates inelastic vessels (calcified—common in diabetics); NOT indicative of good flow.
    - Toe pressures
      - Greater than 40 mm Hg
    - Transcutaneous oxygen pressures (TcPO$_2$)
      - Greater than 30 mm Hg
- **Neurologic examination**
- Sensory examination should assess the following five cutaneous nerves that supply the feet (Figure 6-17):
  - Superficial peroneal (Figure 6-18)
    - Medial dorsal cutaneous—dorsomedial foot
    - Intermediate dorsal cutaneous—dorsolateral foot
  - Deep peroneal—first dorsal web space
  - Sural—posterolateral border of the leg and the lateral border of the foot (Figure 6-19)
  - Tibial—plantar foot (Figure 6-20)
    - Medial calcaneal
    - Medial plantar
    - Lateral plantar
- Inability to sense a Semmes-Weinstein 5.07 monofilament is consistent with neuropathy.
  - **Most predictive sign for development of a foot ulceration**
- **Motor examination**
- When assessing strength, keep in mind the relation the tendon has to the axis of the ankle. For example, if it passes medially and posteriorly, the function of that structure will be to provide plantar flexion and inversion (tibialis posterior).
- When assessing motor function of the foot and ankle, the following muscles should be tested:
  - Tibialis anterior—ankle dorsiflexion, L3-4
  - Extensor hallucis longus—great-toe extension, L4-5
  - Peroneus longus and brevis—hindfoot eversion, L5-S1
  - Posterior tibialis—hindfoot inversion, L4-5
  - Gastrocnemius complex—ankle plantar flexion, S1
- It is important to remember that neurologic deficits can be secondary to more proximal pathology (e.g., central nervous system, spinal cord, nerve root).
- **Palpation and stability**
- Palpation of the tendinous and bony anatomy of the foot and ankle is facilitated by its subcutaneous nature. A detailed examination can typically reproduce the patient's source of pain, allowing examiner to identify the cause without the need for supplementary studies.
- The courses of all tendons are checked both at rest and during contraction for swelling, nodules, and subluxation.
- Tinel sign should be sought for:
  - Tibial nerve at the tarsal tunnel
  - Superficial peroneal nerve as it exits the fascia of the lateral compartment (anterolateral leg)

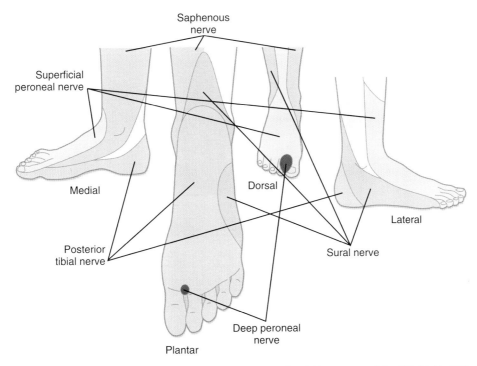

FIGURE 6-17 Sensory nerve distribution of the ankle. (From Adams J et al: *Emergency medicine,* Philadelphia, 2008, Elsevier.)

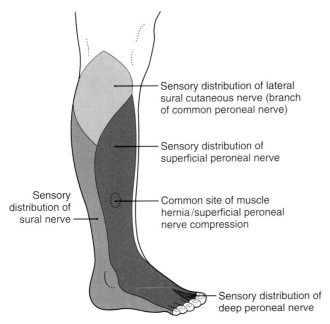

FIGURE 6-18 Sensory distribution of superficial peroneal nerve. Note typical location of muscle hernia/superficial peroneal nerve compression. (From Frontera W et al: *Clinical sports medicine: medical management and rehabilitation,* Philadelphia, 2006, Elsevier.)

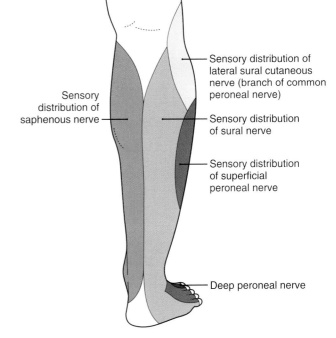

FIGURE 6-19 Sensory distribution of sural nerve. (From Frontera W et al: *Clinical sports medicine: medical management and rehabilitation,* Philadelphia, 2006, Elsevier.)

- Deep peroneal nerve (anterior tarsal tunnel syndrome) at anterior ankle and hindfoot; may be compressed at inferior extensor retinaculum
- Web spaces can be palpated for evidence of interdigital neuromas with an associated **Mulder sign.**
  - With dorsal pressure applied to the web space, the metatarsal heads are compressed with the contralateral hand. An audible click along with radiating pain into the affected toes is a positive sign.
- Stability of the lateral ankle ligaments can be assessed with the anterior drawer and varus talar tilt tests (Figure 6-21).
  - Anterior drawer test
    - Anterior pressure on the hindfoot with ankle in plantar flexion evaluates ATFL.

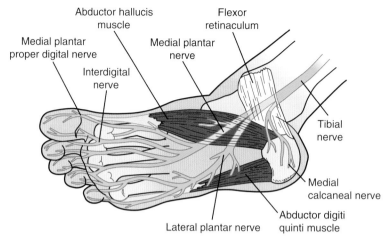

FIGURE 6-20 The tarsal tunnel and its neural contents—the terminal portion of the tibial nerve, the medial plantar nerve, the lateral plantar nerve, and the medial calcaneal nerve—are illustrated, as are the digital nerves. (From Dyck P, Thomas PK: *Peripheral neuropathy,* ed 4, Philadelphia, 2005, Saunders.)

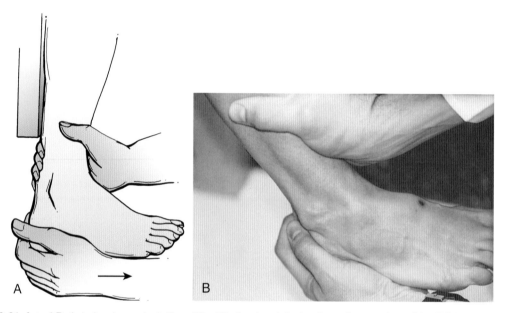

FIGURE 6-21 A and **B,** Anterior drawer test. (From Miller MD: *Core knowledge in orthopaedics—sports medicine,* Philadelphia, 2006, Elsevier.)

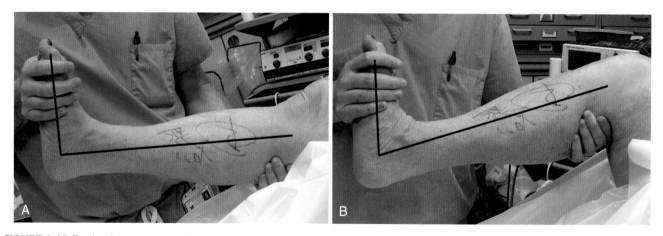

FIGURE 6-22 Testing for a gastrocnemius contracture. **A,** With the knee extended, equinus of the ankle is noted, with an inability to dorsiflex past neutral. **B,** With knee flexion, the soleus muscle is isolated, and in this case an increase of 5 degrees of dorsiflexion is noted. This is consistent with an isolated contracture of the gastrocnemius. If no change in dorsiflexion occurred, both the soleus and gastrocnemius are contracted and Achilles lengthening is required.

- Varus stress test
  - **Inversion of the ankle in plantarflexion evaluates the ATFL.**
  - Inversion of ankle in dorsiflexion evaluates CFL.
- Range of motion (ROM)
- Both passive and active ROM should be compared with contralateral side.
- There is a high rate of variability of normal motion of the joints of the foot and ankle, with no defined absolute normal.

- ROM that is limited to the contralateral side or painful is abnormal.
- Increased ROM, specifically ankle dorsiflexion, is critical to identify and may be associated with an Achilles rupture.
- **Silverskiöld test (difference in ankle dorsiflexion with knee flexed vs. extended while hindfoot is in neutral position) can help differentiate between gastrocnemius and Achilles contractures** (Figure 6-22).
  - Increased ankle dorsiflexion with knee flexed is indicative of an isolated gastrocnemius contracture.

SECTION 3 RADIOGRAPHIC EVALUATION OF THE FOOT AND ANKLE

- Weight-bearing views should be obtained when possible.
- Standard views of the ankle are:
  - Anteroposterior (AP)
  - Lateral
  - Mortise (view of 15 degrees of internal rotation along transmalleolar axis)
  - Gravity or manual external rotation stress is critical in the evaluation of suspected deltoid ligament (SER IV) and syndesmotic injuries (Figure 6-23).
  - Anterior drawer and talar tilt views are helpful in cases of suspected ankle instability (Figures 6-24 and 6-25).
- Standard views of the foot should include:
  - AP—medial and middle column visualized
  - Lateral
    - Sagittal alignment of the foot visualized (pes planus, cavus)
    - Dorsal osteophytes are easily identified at the hindfoot/midfoot and signify early DJD.
  - Oblique—middle and lateral column visualized
- Special views are provided as the clinical presentation warrants (Table 6-2).
- Comparison views of the contralateral foot or ankle are not routinely ordered but can be helpful.
  - Used primarily in the setting of a suspected ligamentous injury (syndesmotic, Lisfranc, or plantar plate of the first MTP)

- Imaging procedures
- Computed tomography (CT) of the foot and ankle is especially useful for complex fractures (pilon, calcaneus, talus, midfoot, Lisfranc) and tarsal coalition.
- Magnetic resonance imaging (MRI) aids evaluation of osteochondral defects, osteonecrosis, neoplasm, and other soft tissue pathologies or tendon injuries.
- Bone scans are sensitive for identification of stress fractures.
- Indium-tagged white blood cell (WBC) scan is both sensitive and specific in detection of osteomyelitis.

Table 6-2	Special Radiographic Views of the Foot and Ankle
VIEW	**SPECIFIC PURPOSE**
Canale view—15 degree internal rotation for foot	Talar neck view for fracture
Harris view—axial heel view	Calcaneus fractures
Sesamoid view—axial sesamoid view	Sesamoid fracture or arthritis
Broden view—talocalcaneal (subtalar) medial oblique views at 10-degree variations	Posterior, medial, and anterior facets of subtalar joint for fracture or arthritis

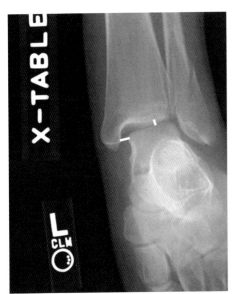

FIGURE 6-23 Gravity stress ankle radiograph demonstrating increased medial clear space (>4 mm) and greater than the superior clear space with associated fibular fracture displacement.

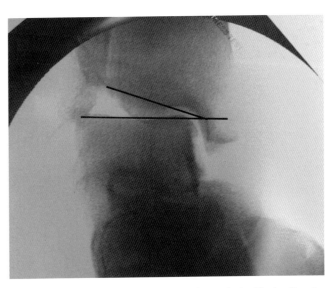

FIGURE 6-24 Varus stress radiograph of a patient with significant talar tilt of more than 15 degrees. (From Miller MD, Sanders T: *Presentation, imaging and treatment of common musculoskeletal conditions,* Philadelphia, 2011, Elsevier.)

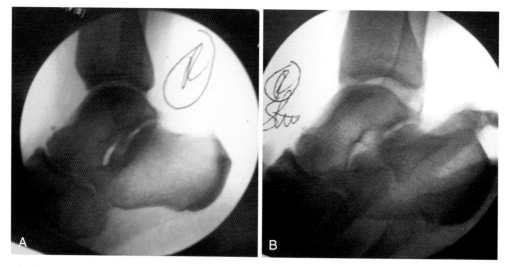

FIGURE 6-25 Anterior drawer stress radiograph demonstrating the anterior translation of the talus **(B)** relative to the normal position of the talus in the unstressed radiograph **(A).** (From Miller MD, Sanders T: *Presentation, imaging and treatment of common musculoskeletal conditions*, Philadelphia, 2011, Elsevier.)

SECTION 4 ADULT HALLUX VALGUS

- ■ **Overview**
- ▨ *Hallux valgus* is defined as lateral deviation of the great toe, with medial deviation of first metatarsal.
- ▨ Pathophysiology: likely multifactorial
  - • Intrinsic factors such as genetic predisposition, ligamentous laxity, and predisposing anatomy (convex metatarsal head, pes planus) are contributory.
  - • Extrinsic factors such as certain types of shoewear (narrow toe box, high heels) also play a role.
- ■ **Pathoanatomy (Figure 6-26)**
- ▨ Medial capsular attenuation

- ▨ Proximal phalanx drifts laterally, leading to the following conditions:
  - • Plantar-lateral migration of abductor hallucis; change in position causes the muscle to plantar flex and pronate the hallux.
  - • Stretching of the extensor hood of the extensor hallucis longus
  - • Lateral deviation of the extensor hallucis longus and flexor hallucis longus (FHL), causing a muscular imbalance and deforming force for valgus progression and pronation of the great toe (Figure 6-27)

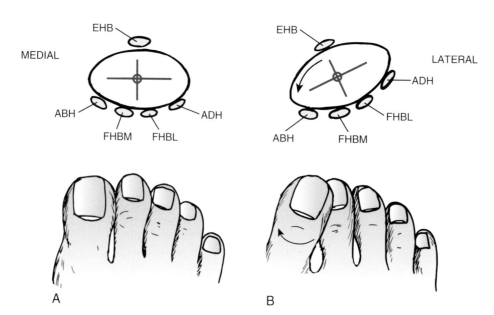

FIGURE 6-26 Schematic representation of tendons around the first metatarsal head. **A,** Normal articulation in a balanced state. **B,** Relationship of the tendons in hallux valgus deformity. *ABH,* Abductor hallucis; *ADH,* adductor hallucis; *EHB,* extensor hallucis brevis; *FHBL,* flexor hallucis brevis lateral head; *FHBM,* flexor hallucis brevis medial head. (From Coughlin MJ et al: *Surgery of the foot and ankle*, ed 8, Philadelphia, 2006, Mosby.)

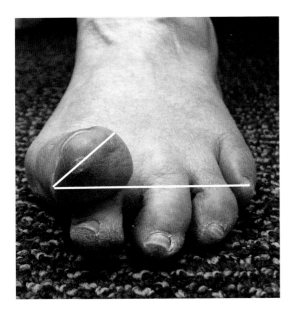

FIGURE 6-27 Pronation of the great toe is easily noted by comparing the angulation of the nail of the great toe relative to the floor. (From Miller MD, Sanders T: *Presentation, imaging and treatment of common musculoskeletal conditions,* Philadelphia, 2011, Elsevier.)

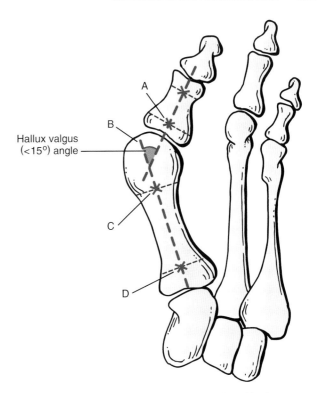

Hallux valgus (<15°) angle

FIGURE 6-28 Hallux valgus angle. Marks are placed in the mid-diaphyseal region of the proximal phalanx and the first metatarsal at an equal distance from the medial and lateral cortices. The longitudinal axis of the proximal phalanx is determined by an axis drawn though points A and B, and the longitudinal axis of the first metatarsal is determined by a line drawn through points C and D. The hallux valgus angle is formed by the intersection of the diaphyseal axes of the first metatarsal (line CD) and the proximal phalanx (line AB). (From Coughlin MJ et al: *Surgery of the foot and ankle,* ed 8, Philadelphia, 2006, Mosby.)

- First metatarsal head moves medially off the sesamoids, increasing the intermetatarsal angle (IMA).
- Secondary contracture of the lateral capsule, adductor hallucis, lateral metatarsal-sesamoid ligament, and intermetatarsal ligament
- Radiographs
  - Multiple measurements can be obtained from standard radiographs that guide treatment options.
    - Hallux valgus angle (HVA): angle formed by line along first metatarsal shaft and line along shaft of proximal phalanx (Figure 6-28)
      - Normal: less than 15 degrees
    - First-second intermetatarsal angle (IMA): angle formed by line along first metatarsal shaft and line along second metatarsal shaft (Figure 6-29)
      - Normal: less than 9 degrees
    - Hallux valgus interphalangeus (HVI) angle: angle formed by line along shaft of proximal phalanx and line along shaft of distal phalanx (Figure 6-30)
      - Normal: less than 10 degrees
      - Associated with a congruent deformity
    - Distal metatarsal articular angle (DMAA): angle formed by line along articular surface of first metatarsal and line perpendicular to axis of first metatarsal (Figure 6-31)
      - Normal: less than 10 degrees
      - Increased angle associated with a congruent deformity
  - Congruency of first MTP joint must be determined (Figure 6-32).
    - Congruency is determined by comparing the line connecting the medial and lateral edge of the first metatarsal head articular surface with the similar line for the proximal phalanx.
      - When these lines are parallel, the joint is congruent.
        - Increased DMAA
          - Distal redirectional osteotomy of the metatarsal head (medial closing wedge)

- Increased HVI
  - Akin osteotomy—medial closing wedge osteotomy of the phalanx
- Both of these operations may be required in addition to an osteotomy of the metatarsal to correct the increased IMA. Performing these osteotomies does NOT exclude additional distal or proximal metatarsal correction.
      - When these lines are divergent, the joint is incongruent.
        - Patients may present with both an incongruent joint and increased DMAA or HVI in severe deformities.
  - Position of sesamoids should be noted; in more severe or chronic deformities, the sesamoids are frequently displaced laterally.
  - Presence of first MTP joint and first TMT joint degenerative changes should be noted.
    - A stiff or arthritic MTP joint requires a first MTP arthrodesis.

■ **Nonoperative treatment**

■ Adjusting shoewear and increasing the size of the toe box may limit pain with pressure along the prominent dorsomedial eminence.

■ There is no role for "corrective" braces or splints.

■ **Operative treatment**

■ The best indication for operative intervention is pain that has not responded to adjusting shoewear or activity.

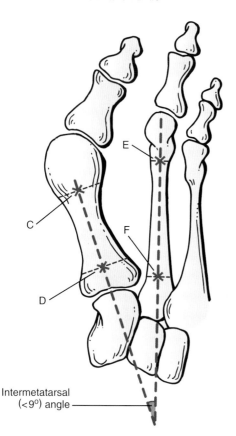

FIGURE 6-29 First-second intermetatarsal angle. Mid-diaphyseal reference points are placed equidistant from the medial and lateral cortices of the first and second metatarsals in both the proximal and distal mid-diaphyseal region. The longitudinal axis is drawn for both the first metatarsal (line CD) and the second metatarsal (line EF). The first-second intermetatarsal angle is formed by the intersection of these two axes (line CD and line EF). (From Coughlin MJ et al: *Surgery of the foot and ankle,* ed 8, Philadelphia, 2006, Mosby.)

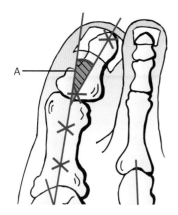

FIGURE 6-30 Hallux valgus interphalangeal angle. Mid-diaphyseal reference points are drawn on the proximal phalanx, and on the distal phalanx a reference point is placed at the distal tip of the phalanx and at the midpoint of the articular surface of the distal phalanx. A line is drawn to connect the reference points for the axes of each phalanx. Point A shows the proximal phalanx axis. The intersection of the axis of the distal phalanx with the longitudinal axis of the proximal phalanx forms the hallux valgus interphalangeal axis. (From Coughlin MJ et al: *Surgery of the foot and ankle,* ed 8, Philadelphia, 2006, Mosby.)

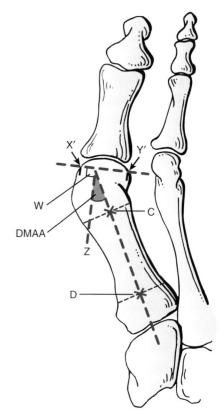

FIGURE 6-31 Distal metatarsal articular angle (DMAA). The DMAA defines the relationship of the articular surface of the distal first metatarsal with the longitudinal axis of the first metatarsal. Points are placed on the most medial and lateral extent of the distal metatarsal articular surface (X′, Y′). A line drawn to connect these two points defines the "slope laterally of the articular surface." Another line through points W and Z is drawn perpendicular to the first line X′Y′. A third line through points C and D defines the longitudinal axis of the first metatarsal. The angle subtended by the perpendicular line (W, Z) and the longitudinal axis of the first metatarsal (C, D) defines the DMAA. (From Coughlin MJ et al: *Surgery of the foot and ankle*, ed 8, Philadelphia, 2006, Mosby.)

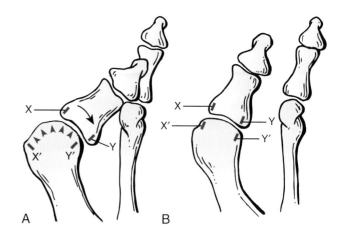

FIGURE 6-32 Congruency versus subluxation. **A,** Hallux valgus deformity with subluxation (noncongruent joint) is characterized by lateral deviation of the articular surface of the proximal phalanx in relation to the articular surface of the distal first metatarsal. **B,** Hallux valgus deformity with a nonsubluxated (congruent) metatarsophalangeal joint is caused most often by lateral inclination of the distal metatarsal articular surface. Points X and Y determine the medial and lateral extent of the articular surface of the proximal phalanx; points X′ and Y′ determine the medial and lateral extent of the metatarsal articular surface. Note the lateral slope of the distal metatarsal articular surface. (From Coughlin MJ et al: *Surgery of the foot and ankle,* ed 8, Philadelphia, 2006, Mosby.)

Surgical correction of a hallux valgus deformity is NOT a cosmetic procedure.

- The appropriate surgical procedure is dictated by the abnormal radiographic angular measurements in concordance with underlying clinical abnormalities.
  - The patient's physical examination and associated pathology dictates the appropriate surgical procedure regardless of the angular measurements.
    - First MTP fusion required: IMA will correct with realignment of first MTP; concomitant metatarsal osteotomy NOT required (Figure 6-33)
      - Rheumatoid arthritis (RA)
      - Osteoarthritis
        - Painful or stiff first MTP—deformity cannot be passively corrected
      - Spasticity
        - Stroke
        - Cerebral palsy
    - Lapidus (first TMT realignment arthrodesis) required:
      - Ligamentous laxity
      - First TMT DJD
  - Procedures never appropriate in isolation (high recurrence rate):
    - Distal soft tissue release (modified McBride)
      - Modification—retention of the lateral (fibular) sesamoid
    - Medial eminence resection
    - Medial capsular imbrication
    - Isolated osteotomy without associated soft tissue correction

- Algorithmic approach to identifying the appropriate surgical intervention (Box 6-1):
  - All patients should undergo a soft tissue release with all associated osteotomies and first TMT arthrodesis (Lapidus).
  - IMA 13 degrees or less and HVA 40 degrees or less
    - Distal metatarsal osteotomy (chevron)
    - Distal soft tissue release
    - Medial eminence resection and capsular repair
  - IMA greater than 13 degrees or HVA greater than 40 degrees
    - Proximal metatarsal osteotomy/scarf
    - Distal soft tissue release

Box 6-1	**Algorithm for Surgical Correction of Hallux Valgus**

IMA ≤ 13 degrees AND HVA ≤ 40 degrees
  Distal metatarsal osteotomy (chevron)
IMA > 13 degrees OR HVA > 40 degrees
  Proximal metatarsal osteotomy
Instability of the first TMT/joint laxity
  Lapidus (fusion of first TMT joint)
Arthritis or spasticity
  First MTP fusion
Increased DMMA
  Distal metatarsal redirectional osteotomy in addition to metatarsal translational osteotomy
HVI
  Akin osteotomy

DMMA, Distal metatarsal articular angle; *HVA*, hallux valgus angle; *HVI*, hallux valgus interphalangeus; *IMA*, intermetatarsal angle; *MTP*, metatarsophalangeal; *TMT*, tarsometatarsal.

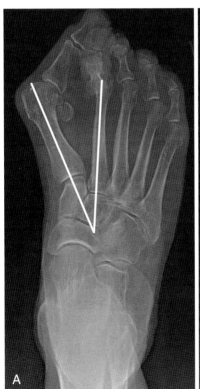
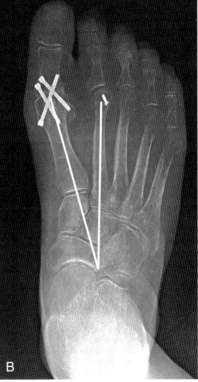

FIGURE 6-33 A, Preoperative anteroposterior radiograph of a patient with a hallux valgus deformity with associated stiffness and pain within the joint. **B,** Postoperative radiograph demonstrates correction of both the hallux valgus deformity and the intermetatarsal angle without the need for an additional metatarsal osteotomy.

- Medial eminence resection and capsular repair
- Instability of first TMT/joint hyperlaxity
  - Lapidus (fusion of first TMT joint) (Figure 6-34)
  - Soft tissue release
  - Medial eminence resection and capsular repair
- **Increased DMAA (>10 degrees)**
  - **Distal medial closing wedge metatarsal osteotomy in addition to what is required based on angular measurements** (Figure 6-35)
    - **IMA 13 degrees or less and HVA 40 degrees or less**
      - **Distal biplanar closing wedge metatarsal osteotomy**
        - Translate and redirect the metatarsal head simultaneously.
    - **IMA greater than 13 degrees or HVA greater than 40 degrees**
      - **Proximal metatarsal osteotomy AND distal medial closing wedge metatarsal osteotomy**
  - Instability of first TMT/joint hyperlaxity
    - Lapidus AND distal medial closing wedge metatarsal osteotomy
- Hallux valgus interphalangeus
  - Akin osteotomy
    - Can be done in isolation if no other deformity present

- Commonly performed in addition to procedures required to correct HVA and IMA (Figure 6-36)
- **■ Operative complications**
- ▦ Avascular necrosis (AVN)
  - Distal metatarsal osteotomy and lateral soft tissue release may be performed simultaneously without increased risk of AVN.
    - Intraoperative laser Doppler studied demonstrated medial capsulotomy primary insult to metatarsal head blood flow.
- ▦ Recurrence
  - Can occur with any procedure—highly associated with:
    - **Undercorrection of IMA**
    - Isolated soft tissue reconstruction (modified McBride)
    - Isolated resection of the medial eminence
- ▦ Dorsal malunion
  - Results in transfer metatarsalgia—highly associated with:
    - Lapidus (first TMT fusion)
    - Proximal crescentic osteotomy
- ▦ Hallux varus
  - Resection of the fibular sesamoid (original McBride)
  - Overresection of the medial eminence
  - Excessive lateral release
  - Overcorrection of IMA
- ▦ Nonunion
  - Highest risk associated with a Lapidus procedure

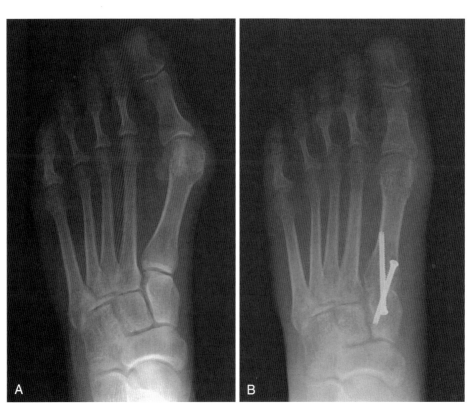

FIGURE 6-34 A, Preoperative radiograph of a patient with hallux valgus and first tarsometatarsal instability. B, Correction was successfully achieved with a Lapidus procedure using two crossed screws for fixation. (From Miller MD, Sanders T: *Presentation, imaging and treatment of common musculoskeletal conditions,* Philadelphia, 2011, Elsevier.)

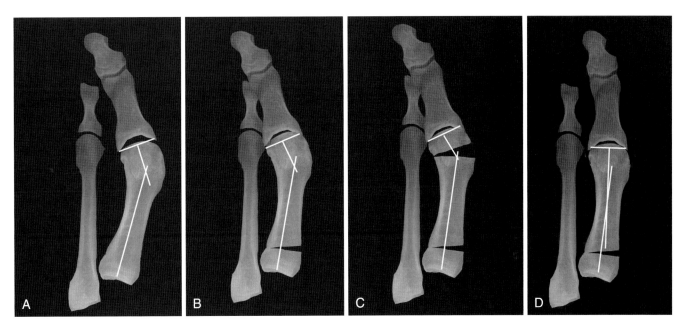

FIGURE 6-35 A, Hallux valgus deformity secondary to an increased intermetatarsal angle (IMA) and distal metatarsal articular angle (DMAA). **B,** Correction of the IMA with a proximal osteotomy causes the proximal phalanx to override the second toe secondary to the DMAA. **C,** A distal closed-wedge osteotomy is performed. **D,** With closure of the osteotomy, the phalanx is now directed parallel to the metatarsal shaft, correcting the overall deformity.

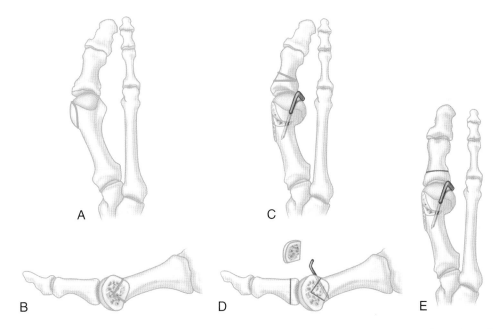

FIGURE 6-36 A, Resection of medial eminence parallel to medial border of foot. **B,** Chevron osteotomy cut is made, and metatarsal head is shifted laterally 2.5 to 3 mm. **C,** Osteotomy is fixed with 0.045-inch smooth pin, and protruding medial border of metatarsal is osteotomized flush with metatarsal head. **D,** Akin cut parallels concavity at base of proximal phalanx, and 1-mm wedge of bone is removed. **E,** Suture closure of Akin osteotomy corrects residual valgus of hallux. (From Canale ST, Beaty J: *Campbell's operative orthopaedics,* ed 11, Philadelphia, 2007, Elsevier.)

SECTION 5 JUVENILE AND ADOLESCENT HALLUX VALGUS

■ Factors

- Several critical factors separate these patients from adult patients with hallux valgus deformity.
- Recurrence of the deformity after surgical correction is the most common complication (Figure 6-37).
- Proximal osteotomy is performed through the medial cuneiform in patients with an open first metatarsal physis.
  - If arthrodesis of the first TMT is required for laxity, surgical intervention is delayed until physeal closure.
- The deformity is secondary to underlying bony and ligamentous anatomy, which must be addressed to prevent recurrence.
  - Varus of the first metatarsal with a large IMA is commonly present.
  - DMAA is typically increased.
  - Hallux valgus interphalangeus (HVI) may be present.
  - Ligamentous laxity may be present, and a history of Ehlers-Danlos or Marfan syndrome should be elicited.
    - Examine for generalized hyperlaxity to determine if a first TMT arthrodesis is required.
  - Family history is frequently positive for hallux valgus.
- Operative correction
  - Single, double, or triple osteotomies are required to correct the deformity, applying the same principles as described for evaluation of adult hallux valgus.

- In cases of ligamentous laxity, a first TMT arthrodesis substitutes for a proximal osteotomy to correct the IMA. The first metatarsal physeal plate must be closed.
  - Single osteotomy
    - HVI
      - Akin osteotomy
    - Increased DMAA, IMA 13 degrees or less
      - Biplanar distal chevron osteotomy for DMAA and IMA
  - Double osteotomy
    - HVI with increased DMAA, IMA 13 degrees or less
      - Akin osteotomy for HVI
      - Biplanar distal chevron osteotomy for DMAA and IMA
    - IMA greater than 13 degrees, with increased DMAA
      - Biplanar distal chevron osteotomy for DMAA
      - Opening wedge medial cuneiform osteotomy
  - Triple osteotomy
    - HVI with increased DMAA, IMA greater than 13 degrees
      - Akin osteotomy for HVI
      - Biplanar distal chevron osteotomy for DMAA
      - Opening wedge medial cuneiform osteotomy

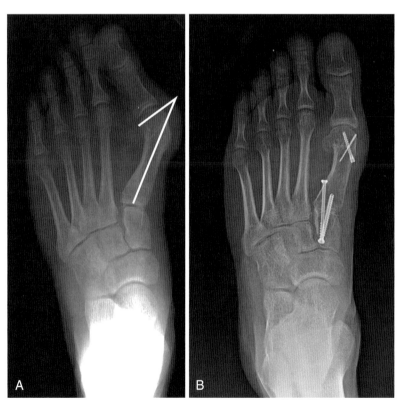

FIGURE 6-37 A, Juvenile hallux valgus recurrence in a patient who underwent a prior isolated proximal osteotomy. The deformity is associated with a large intermetatarsal angle and increased distal metatarsal articular angle. In addition, on examination the patient was noted to have hyperlaxity. **B,** A Lapidus procedure with a medial closed-wedge osteotomy of the distal metatarsal is required to achieve a long-lasting correction.

SECTION 6 HALLUX VARUS

- **Etiology**
- Medial deviation of the great toe is most often an iatrogenic deformity secondary to overcorrection of hallux valgus.
  - Overresection of the medial eminence
  - Excessive lateral release
  - 0-degree or negative IMA (Figure 6-38)
- **Nonoperative treatment**
- Limited to accommodation of the deformity with shoe modifications and shoe stretching
- **Operative treatment**
- Dependent upon whether deformity is flexible (reducible) or rigid (irreducible)

- Flexible deformity can be corrected with a soft tissue procedure.
  - **Release of abductor hallucis muscle and fascia**
  - **Transfer of a portion of extensor hallucis longus (EHL) or brevis (EHB) tendon under the transverse intermetatarsal (IM) ligament to the distal metatarsal neck (taken from lateral to medial)** (Figure 6-39)
    - The distal portion of the tendon is left intact, creating a static stabilizer to correct the deformity.
- Fixed deformity, deformity with limited first MTP motion, or presence of first MTP DJD is treated with a first MTP arthrodesis.

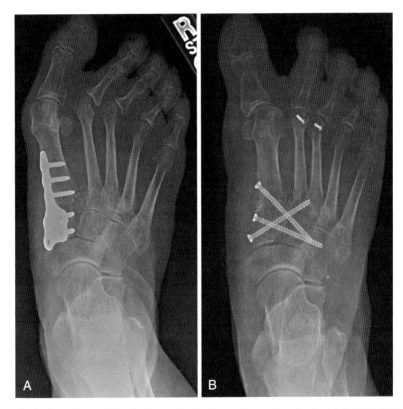

FIGURE 6-38 A, Recurrence of a hallux valgus deformity in a patient who underwent a prior Lapidus procedure. The increased intermetatarsal angle (IMA) occurred secondary to disruption of the intercuneiform. **B,** A revision procedure with arthrodesis of the intercuneiform joint resulted in an overcorrection of the IMA, resulting in hallux varus. The patient had a flexible deformity and was able to wear shoes without pain.

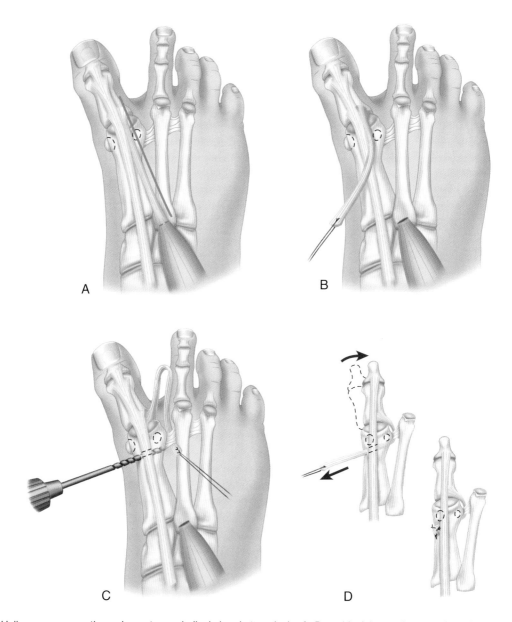

A

B

C

D

FIGURE 6-39 Hallux varus correction using extensor hallucis brevis tenodesis. **A,** Dorsal incision and transection of extensor hallucis brevis tendon. **B,** Transected tendon is passed deep to transverse metatarsal ligament from distal to proximal. **C,** Hole is drilled in dorsomedial first metatarsal. **D,** Extensor hallucis brevis tendon is pulled through drill hole and secured with sutures to periosteum or bone. (From Canale ST, Beaty J: *Campbell's operative orthopaedics,* ed 11, Philadelphia, 2007, Elsevier. Redrawn from Juliano PJ et al: Biomechanical assessment of a new tenodesis for correction of hallux varus, *Foot Ankle Int* 17:17, 1996.)

SECTION 7 LESSER-TOE DEFORMITIES

■ **Anatomy and function**

■ Static stability of the lesser toes is provided by the congruency of the MTP and interphalangeal joints.
  • Plantar plate—plantar aponeurosis and capsule—provides a soft tissue block to metatarsal head depression and prevents hyperextension of the MTP joint.
  • Persistent hyperextension at MTP joint may lead to attenuation and weakening of plantar structures.

■ Dynamic stability is provided by the various tendons that insert on lesser toes (Figure 6-40).
  • Extensor digitorum longus (EDL): primary extensor of MTP joint
    • Runs through a sling over dorsal surface of MTP joint before splitting into a central slip that inserts on the middle phalanx and two dorsolateral slips that reconverge to insert at the base of the distal phalanx.

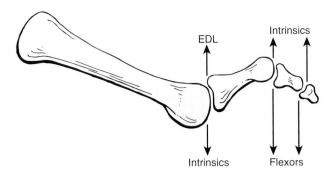

FIGURE 6-40 Diagram demonstrates the relationship of the intrinsic and extrinsic muscles about a lesser toe. The smaller intrinsic muscles are overpowered by the extrinsic muscles, leading to a hammer-toe deformity. *EDL,* Extensor digitorum longus. (From Coughlin MJ et al: *Surgery of the foot and ankle,* ed 8, Philadelphia, 2006, Mosby.)

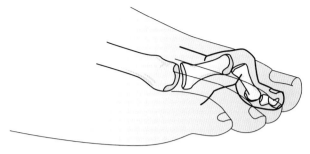

FIGURE 6-41 Hammer-toe deformity. (From DiGiovanni C: *Core knowledge in orthopaedics—foot and ankle,* Philadelphia, 2007, Elsevier.)

- Distal extensor effect of the EDL is neutralized when the proximal phalanx is dorsiflexed, as in hammer toe or claw toe deformities.
- Extensor digitorum brevis (EDB) extends PIP joints and inserts on lateral aspect of EDL tendon on all but the fifth toe.
- Flexor digitorum longus (FDL): primary plantar flexor of distal interphalangeal (DIP) joints as it inserts on plantar aspect of distal phalanges; also weakly plantar flexes MTP joints.
- Flexor digitorum brevis (FDB) splits at the level of the MTP joint and inserts on plantar lateral aspects of middle phalanges. The FDB is the primary plantar flexor of the PIP joints.
- Intrinsic muscles of the foot include the lumbricals, which originate from the FDL tendon and insert on the extensor sheath over the MTP joints, and four dorsal and three plantar interossei muscles, which insert on the medial aspect of the proximal phalanges.
  - These muscles act similarly to the intrinsic muscles of the hand, flexing the MTP joints and extending the PIP and DIP joints.
  - Pull of the intrinsics is plantar to the rotational axis of the MTP joints.
  - Plantar translation of the metatarsal head after a distal osteotomy of the metatarsal places the intrinsics dorsal to the axis of rotation of the MTP joint, creating the "floating toe."
- Extrinsic muscles (EDL and FDL) overpower intrinsic muscles in positioning the lesser toes in hammer- and claw-toe deformities, with the EDL driving MTP joint extension and the FDL driving PIP and DIP joint flexion.
  - EDL is also a weak antagonist to flexion at interphalangeal joints, and likewise the FDL is a weak antagonist to extension at MTP joint.
  - Dorsiflexion of the proximal phalanx at MTP joint neutralizes these weak antagonist effects and accentuates the developing deformity.
- Lesser-toe deformities occur much more commonly in women (up to a 5 : 1 ratio), thought to be secondary to high-fashion shoewear that constricts the forefoot and maintains the MTP joints in hyperextension.
  - A hammer deformity most commonly involves the second toe, owing to its relative length compared to the remainder of the lesser toes. A short toe box will cause the second toe to buckle and extend at the MTP joint.
  - Chronic positioning of the MTP joint in hyperextension will attenuate the static plantar structures, allowing depression of the metatarsal head, migration of the fat pad distally, and imbalance of the dynamic forces on the toe as described earlier.

■ Hammer-toe deformity

- The characteristic hammer-toe deformity is flexion of the PIP joint. With weight bearing, the MTP joint will appear dorsiflexed; this should correct with elevation of the foot off the ground (Figure 6-41).
- The term *complex hammer toe* refers to concomitant dorsiflexion of the MTP joint that does not correct and is more appropriately termed (and treated as) a *claw toe*.
- Treatment is dependent upon the flexibility of the deformity (Table 6-3).
  - Flexible deformity
    - Nonoperative—protective padding, tall toe-box shoes, corrective hammer-toe splints are effective.
    - Operative—flexor tenotomy or flexor to extensor tendon transfer
  - Fixed deformity
    - Nonoperative—accommodative shoes and protective padding can minimize callous formation. A corrective splint should NOT be used.
    - **Operative—PIP arthroplasty (resection of distal neck and head of proximal phalanx) or PIP arthrodesis** (Figure 6-42)

■ Claw-toe deformity (intrinsic minus toe)

- Characterized by flexion of the PIP and DIP joints in the setting of fixed hyperextension of the MTP joint (Figure 6-43)
  - Clawing typically involves multiple toes and is often bilateral.
  - Cavus deformity, neuromuscular diseases that affect the balance of the extrinsic and intrinsic musculature, inflammatory arthropathies that lead to attenuation of soft tissue structures and instability of the MTP joint, and trauma have all been implicated in the etiology of claw toes.
  - Claw toes are a noted complication of compartment syndrome involving the deep compartments of the foot.

Table 6-3	Surgical Treatment of Lesser-Toe Deformities	
DEFORMITY	SURGICAL OPTIONS	COMMENTS
HAMMER TOE		
Flexible	Girdlestone-Taylor FDL flexor-to-extensor tendon transfer	Add EDL lengthening or tenotomy if active flexion <10-15 degrees
Fixed	PIP arthroplasty or arthrodesis	
MALLET TOE		
Flexible	FDL tenotomy	
Fixed	Excisional arthroplasty or arthrodesis of the DIP joint	
CLAW TOE		
Flexible	FDL flexor-to-extensor tendon transfer with EDB tenotomy and EDL lengthening	Look for underlying neuromuscular etiology when >2 toes are involved
Fixed	Weil osteotomy (oblique shortening osteotomy of the metatarsal) with MTP capsulotomy Extensor lengthening PIP arthroplasty or arthrodesis	
Crossover 2nd toe	Extensor digitorum brevis tendon transfer with medial capsular release Flexor-to-extensor tendon transfer	Weil osteotomy should be performed if the MTP is dislocated

DIP, Distal interphalangeal; *EDB,* extensor digitorum brevis; *EDL,* extensor digitorum longus; *FDL,* flexor digitorum longus; *MTP,* metatarsophalangeal; *PIP,* proximal interphalangeal.

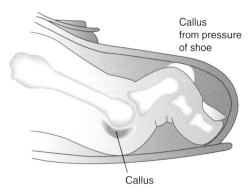

FIGURE 6-42 Dorsal aspect of the proximal interphalangeal joint strikes the toe box, leading to callus formation. An intractable plantar keratosis may develop beneath the metatarsal head. (From DeLee J: *DeLee and Drez's orthopaedic sports medicine,* ed 3, Philadelphia, 2011, Saunders.)

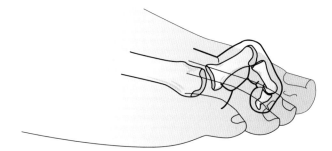

FIGURE 6-43 Claw-toe deformity with fixed hyperextension of the MTP joint with PIP and DIP joint flexion. (From DiGiovanni C: *Core knowledge in orthopaedics—foot and ankle,* Philadelphia, 2007, Elsevier.)

- Treatment is dependent upon the flexibility of the deformity (see Table 6-3).
  - Flexible deformity
    - Nonoperative—shoe modification, padding over any prominent or painful callosities, and use of orthotics to offload and support a potentially painful, plantarly subluxed metatarsal head
    - Operative
      - Flexor-to-extensor tendon transfer of the FDL alters the function of the FDL to function as an intrinsic and maintain correction (Figure 6-44).
      - Lengthening of the EDL and EDB is typically required.
  - Fixed deformity
    - Nonoperative—shoe modification, padding over any prominent or painful callosities, and use of orthotics to offload and support a potentially painful, plantarly subluxed metatarsal head
    - Operative

- PIP arthroplasty or arthrodesis, along with MTP joint capsulotomy and extensor lengthening
- **Dislocated MTP joint requires use of a Weil or distal metatarsal shortening osteotomy to reduce MTP joint** (Figure 6-45).

■ **Mallet-toe deformity**
■ A mallet toe consists of an isolated flexion deformity at the DIP joint (Figure 6-46).
■ Treatment (see Table 6-3)
  - Nonoperative—similar methods to those used in treating patients with hammer-toe and claw-toe deformities
  - Operative
    - Flexible
      - Flexor tenotomy
    - Fixed
      - DIP arthroplasty (excision of the distal neck and head of the middle phalanx) or DIP fusion
      - Extensor repair can be performed to minimize recurrence.

■ **Crossover-toe deformity (see Table 6-3)**
■ Multiplanar instability of the second toe may cause the toe to lie dorsomedially relative to the hallux (Figure 6-47).

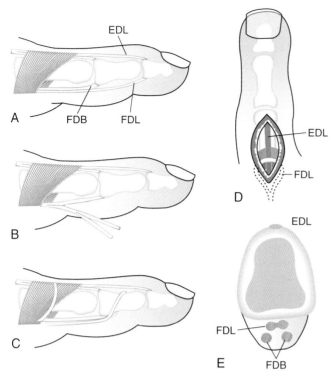

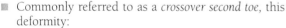

FIGURE 6-44 Technique of flexor tendon transfer. **A,** Lateral view shows flexor digitorum longus (FDL), flexor digitorum brevis (FDB), and extensor digitorum longus (EDL). **B,** The flexor digitorum longus is detached through a distal puncture wound and is delivered through a transverse incision at the plantar metatarsophalangeal joint flexion crease. **C,** The tendon is split longitudinally, and each half is delivered on either side of the proximal phalanx and is sutured into either the extensor expansion or the corresponding limb of the flexor tendon. **D,** Dorsal view shows transferred flexor digitorum longus tendon. **E,** Cross-sectional view shows the characteristic position of the flexor digitorum longus tendon. It is deep to the flexor digitorum brevis and is characterized by a midline raphe. (From DeLee J: *DeLee and Drez's orthopaedic sports medicine,* ed 3, Philadelphia, 2011, Saunders.)

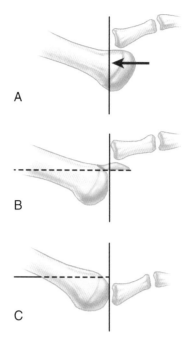

FIGURE 6-45 Weil osteotomy. **A,** Before surgery. **B,** After proximal displacement of metatarsal head. **C,** After resection of distal tip of dorsal fragment. (From Canale ST, Beaty J: *Campbell's operative orthopaedics,* ed 11, Philadelphia, 2007, Elsevier. Redrawn from Vandeputte G et al: The Weil osteotomy of the lesser metatarsals: a clinical and pedobarographic follow-up study, *Foot Ankle* 21:370, 2000.)

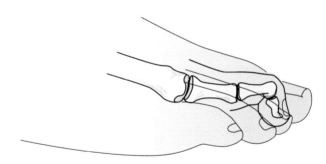

FIGURE 6-46 Mallet-toe deformity. (From DiGiovanni C: *Core knowledge in orthopaedics—foot and ankle,* Philadelphia, 2007, Elsevier.)

- Commonly referred to as a *crossover second toe,* this deformity:
  - **Requires disruption of the plantar plate—KEY component**
  - Requires attenuation of the lateral collateral ligament
  - **May be iatrogenic, caused by steroid injection within the MTP joint, resulting in plantar plate attenuation**
- Treatment
  - Nonoperative—toe taping and corrective splints can minimize the discomfort but will not permanently correct the deformity.
  - Operative
    - For complete tears of the plantar plate, plantar plate repair has been advocated, with promising results. Plantar plate repair typically requires a shortening osteotomy of the distal metatarsal to aid in visualization and tissue repair.
    - Flexor-to-extensor tendon transfer with release of the medial collateral ligament
    - EDB tendon transfer with rerouting plantar to the intermetatarsal ligament

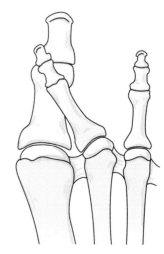

FIGURE 6-47 A crossover-toe deformity resulting from a rupture of the lateral collateral ligament and plantar plate and contracture of the medial collateral ligament. (From DiGiovanni C: *Core knowledge in orthopaedics—foot and ankle,* Philadelphia, 2007, Elsevier.)

- Distal metatarsal osteotomy (Weil) required if severe subluxation or dislocation of the MTP joint

■ **MTP joint instability**

▧ Mild subluxation of the MTP joint that presents with pain and swelling without any deformity

- Drawer test results in pain within the joint (Figure 6-48).
  - Most sensitive physical examination test to evaluate for plantar plate injury

▧ More commonly seen in athletes (runners, tennis)

▧ If the diagnosis is in question, an MR arthrogram of the involved joint will identify any injuries to the plantar plate or collateral ligaments.

▧ Treatment
- Nonoperative
  - Toe taping and stabilizing lesser-toe orthotics
  - **Steroid injections are contraindicated and may result in iatrogenic creation of a crossover-toe deformity.**
- Operative
  - MTP synovectomy with reconstruction of the MTP joint capsule for isolated synovitis
  - If severe instability or deformity, a flexor-to-extensor tendon transfer is traditionally performed to stabilize MTP joint.
  - For complete tears of the plantar plate, plantar plate repair has been advocated with promising results. Plantar plate repair typically requires a shortening osteotomy of the distal metatarsal to aid in visualization and tissue repair.

■ **Freiberg disease/infraction**

▧ Osteochondrosis of one of the lesser metatarsals, most commonly involving the second metatarsal

▧ Patients have pain localized over the affected metatarsal head.
- The second metatarsal is affected in over two thirds of cases. The third metatarsal accounts for most of the

remaining cases. The fourth is affected in less than 5% of cases. The first and fifth metatarsals are rarely affected.
- Pain is worse with ambulation and activities; relieved with rest.

▧ Common radiographic findings in Freiberg disease include:
- Resorption of the central metatarsal bone adjacent to the articular surface, with flattening of the metatarsal head (Figure 6-49)
- Osteochondral loose bodies
- Joint space narrowing in late-stage disease, with associated osteophyte formation along with collapse of the articular surface (Figure 6-50)

▧ Nonoperative treatment
- Common strategies consist of activity modification, shoewear modification (hard sole), orthotics (metatarsal bar), and a period of protected weight bearing.

▧ Operative treatment
- For early-stage disease, joint débridement should be considered.
  - All synovitis, osteophytes, and loose bodies are débrided through a dorsal incision.
  - This should be considered for patients with relatively good articular surface congruity and minimal metatarsal deformity.

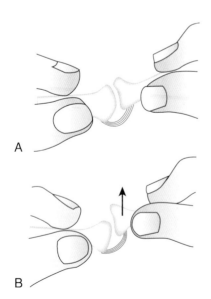

FIGURE 6-48 A dorsal plantar drawer test is administered by thrusting the toe in a dorsal plantar direction. With capsulitis or metatarsophalangeal (MTP) joint instability, pain is elicited. When a patient complains of presumable MTP pain but no deformity is present, eliciting pain with a drawer test assists in making the correct diagnosis. (From DeLee J: *DeLee and Drez's orthopaedic sports medicine*, ed 3, Philadelphia, 2011, Saunders.)

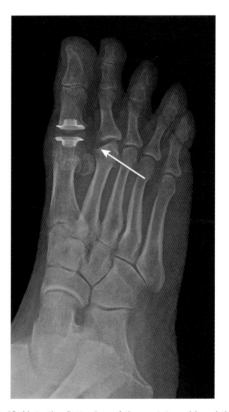

FIGURE 6-49 Note the flattening of the metatarsal head that is commonly seen with Freiberg disease *(arrow)*. This patient had a prior silicone arthroplasty of the great toe and developed Freiberg disease secondary to overload. (From Miller MD, Sanders T: *Presentation, imaging and treatment of common musculoskeletal conditions*, Philadelphia, 2011, Elsevier.)

- Many studies have reported good results with dorsal closing wedge metaphyseal osteotomy of the affected metatarsal (Figure 6-51).
  - This is done in conjunction with a thorough débridement of synovitis, abnormal cartilage, osteophytes, and necrotic bone.
  - This osteotomy serves to rotate the plantar aspect of the articular surface, which is typically well-preserved, to a more superior position, where it then articulates with the phalanx.

■ Fifth-toe deformities

- Several types of deformity exist, including underlapping, overlapping, rotatory, and cock-up toes.
- Subluxation at the fifth MTP results in weakened push-off during ambulation, a loss of coverage of the fifth metatarsal head, and subsequent callus formation under the dorsolateral aspect of the fifth toe.
- Nonoperative treatment
  - For an overlapping fifth toe, stretching or taping may be helpful, along with shoes with a wide toe box.
- Operative treatment
  - Cock-up fifth toe
    - EDL transfer into the abductor digiti minimi, with rerouting inferior to the phalanx
    - Release of the dorsomedial capsule and Z-plasty of the skin may be required.
  - Congenital curly toe (underlapping)
    - Tenotomy of FDL and FDB has been recommended in children with flexible deformities.
  - Syndactylization is reserved for salvage after failed operative intervention.

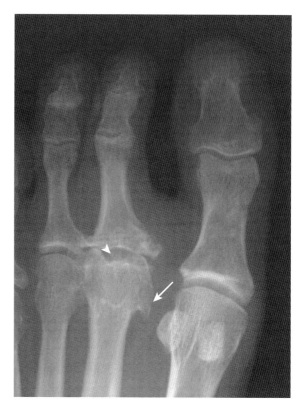

FIGURE 6-50 Coned-down anteroposterior view of the forefoot demonstrating the natural history and long-term sequela of untreated Freiberg disease. Note the significant subchondral cysts *(arrowhead)* and osteophyte formation *(arrow)* indicating osteoarthritis. (From Miller MD, Sanders T: *Presentation, imaging and treatment of common musculoskeletal conditions,* Philadelphia, 2011, Elsevier.)

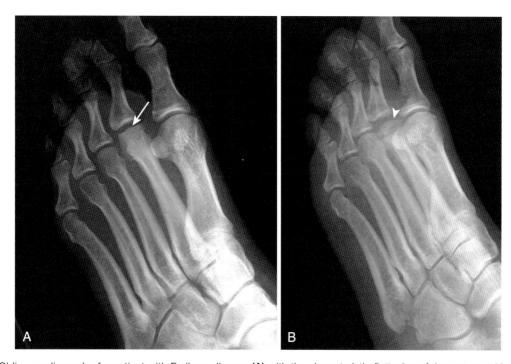

FIGURE 6-51 Oblique radiograph of a patient with Freiberg disease **(A)** with the characteristic flattening of the metatarsal head *(arrow)* treated with a dorsal closed-wedge osteotomy **(B).** Note how the contour of the metatarsal head has been recreated *(arrowhead).* (From Miller MD, Sanders T: *Presentation, imaging and treatment of common musculoskeletal conditions,* Philadelphia, 2011, Elsevier.)

SECTION 8 HYPERKERATOTIC PATHOLOGIES

HARD CORNS (HELOMATA DURUM)

■ Diagnosis

■ Commonly occur over the metaphyseal aspect of the phalanges at MTP or interphalangeal joints, especially of the fifth toe
  - Secondary to extrinsic pressure (on the border of the foot)
■ Secondary to frictional irritation or from pressure over bony prominences (Figure 6-52)
■ Examination reveals epidermal hyperplasia with a conical central area.

■ Nonoperative treatment

■ Shaving or paring the corn with a pumice stone, followed by removal of the central inverted "seed" of the corn
■ Modification of shoewear and protective padding reduces extrinsic pressure.

■ Operative treatment

■ Reserved for refractory cases that fail conservative management
■ Excision of bony prominences at the interphalangeal joint
■ Partial cheilectomy of the metatarsal head and hemiphalangectomy of the proximal phalanx can also be effective.

SOFT CORNS (HELOMATA MOLLE)

■ Diagnosis

■ Hyperkeratoses that develop as the result of moisture in web space and pressure from neighboring phalangeal condyles (Figure 6-53)
■ Two main types:
  - Prominent medial condyle of the fifth proximal phalanx contacts the lateral base of the fourth proximal phalanx or metatarsal head.
  - Distal phalangeal exostosis abuts its neighboring toe at various locations.
■ Macerated and friable skin with thickened callus, usually deep in the web space
■ Mediolateral squeezing of toes causes significant pain.

■ Nonoperative treatment

■ Absorptive padding in web space and accommodative shoewear
  - Decreases contact pressure between toes and wicks excess moisture

■ Operative treatment

■ Excision of offending bony prominences and adjacent skin lesions
  - Avoid web space incisions to minimize risk of infection.
■ Proximal lesions
  - Basilar hemiphalangectomy with lateral condyle excision of the metatarsal head
  - Web space syndactylization also effective

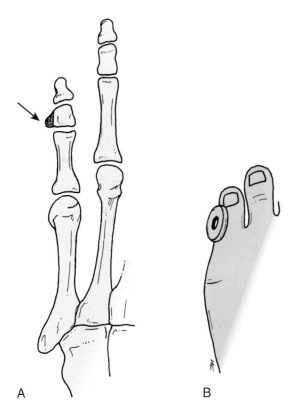

FIGURE 6-52 **A,** An underlying exostosis *(arrow)* combined with restrictive footwear leads to a hard corn. **B,** A pad may be used to relieve pressure. (From Porter D, Schon L: *Baxter's the foot and ankle in sport,* ed 2, Philadelphia, 2007, Elsevier.)

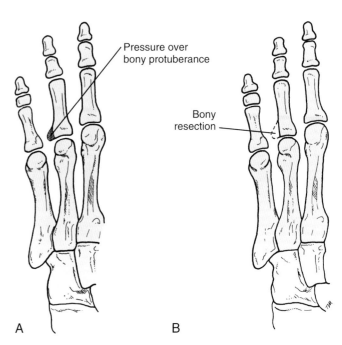

FIGURE 6-53 **A,** A soft corn may develop over the base of the proximal phalanx. **B,** Resection of the bony prominence. (From Porter D, Schon L: *Baxter's the foot and ankle in sport,* ed 2, Philadelphia, 2007, Elsevier.)

INTRACTABLE PLANTAR KERATOSIS (IPK)

- Plantar callus secondary to excess pressure from metatarsal head
- Predisposing factors: fat pad atrophy, plantar-flexed first ray, equinus contracture, intrinsic-minus toe contracture, and hypertrophy of the sesamoid
- Two main types: (Figure 6-54)
- Discrete form
  - Localized callus with a hyperkeratotic core, usually caused by prominence of fibular condyle
  - Commonly associated with a prominent tibial sesamoid
  - Nonoperative treatment
    - Callus trimming and soft metatarsal pads
    - Consider total contact orthosis or extended steel shank for patients with significant fat pad atrophy.
  - Operative treatment
    - Shaving of the plantar surface of the tibial sesamoid or fibular metatarsal condylectomy
    - Consider complete excision of the tibial sesamoid in more advanced cases.
    - Consider dorsiflexion osteotomy in patients with a plantar-flexed first ray.
  - Diffuse form
  - Secondary to pressure phenomenon from the entire metatarsal head
  - Commonly associated with an elongated metatarsal, an excessively plantar-flexed metatarsal, or transfer lesion
  - Nonoperative treatment—similar to the discrete form of IPK
  - Operative treatment
    - Shortening or dorsiflexion metatarsal osteotomy is the surgical treatment of choice.
    - Complete plantar condylectomy is also effective and favored over the original Duvries arthroplasty (which included resection of the metatarsal head that occasionally led to transfer metatarsalgia).

BUNIONETTE DEFORMITY (TAILOR'S BUNION)

- Diagnosis
- Prominence over distal aspect of fifth metatarsal head

- Causes pain over lateral or plantar aspect of MTP joint, particularly with compressive shoewear
- Bunionette deformity in conjunction with ipsilateral hallux valgus and metatarsus primus varus is termed *splayfoot.*
- Three distinct types have been described, based on the anatomic location of the deformity along the fifth metatarsal.
  - Type I deformity—distinguished by presence of an enlarged fifth metatarsal head (Figure 6-55)
  - Type II deformity—demonstrates lateral bowing of fifth metatarsal diaphysis (Figure 6-56)
  - Type III deformity—demonstrates an abnormally widened fourth-fifth metatarsal angle (normal, <8 degrees) (Figure 6-57)

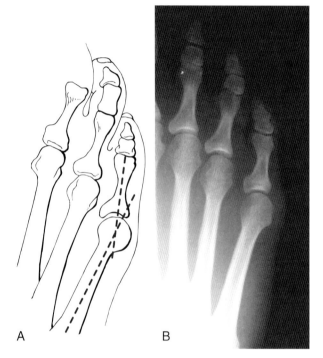

FIGURE 6-55 A and **B,** Type I bunionette deformity is characterized by an enlarged fifth metatarsal head. (From Coughlin MJ et al: *Surgery of the foot and ankle,* ed 8, Philadelphia, 2006, Mosby.)

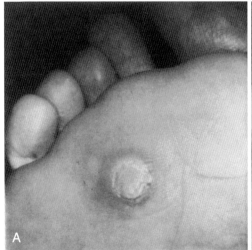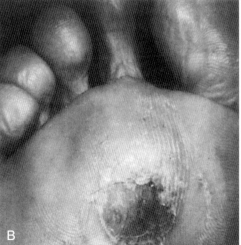

FIGURE 6-54 A, Discrete callus in a tennis player with an enlarged fibular condyle. **B,** Diffuse callus in a runner. (From Porter D, Schon L: *Baxter's the foot and ankle in sport,* ed 2, Philadelphia, 2007, Elsevier.)

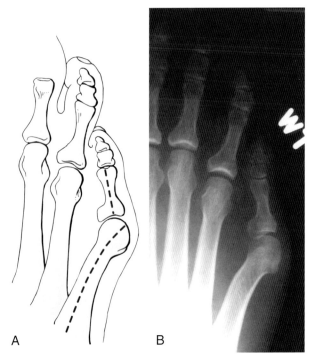

FIGURE 6-56 A and **B,** Type II bunionette deformity is characterized by lateral bowing of the fifth metatarsal head. (From Coughlin MJ et al: *Surgery of the foot and ankle,* ed 8, Philadelphia, 2006, Mosby.)

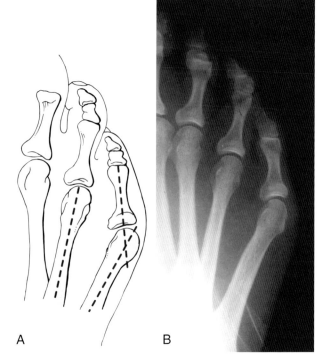

FIGURE 6-57 A and **B,** Type III bunionette deformity is characterized by an abnormally wide fourth-fifth intermetatarsal angle. (From Coughlin MJ et al: *Surgery of the foot and ankle,* ed 8, Philadelphia, 2006, Mosby.)

■ Conservative treatment
  • Shoewear modification, strategic padding, and shaving the symptomatic callus is usually effective.
  • With plantar callus or associated pes planus, consider a metatarsal pad or custom orthotic device.
■ Surgical treatment
  • **Lateral metatarsal head condylectomy (type I)**

• **Distal fifth metatarsal osteotomy (i.e., chevron; type II)**
• **Oblique diaphyseal osteotomy (type III)**
• Consider metatarsal head resection for salvage.
• Proximal osteotomy should be avoided owing to the tenuous blood supply at the proximal metadiaphyseal junction of the fifth metatarsal.

SECTION 9 SESAMOIDS

ANATOMY

■ Medial (tibial) and lateral (fibular) hallucal sesamoids are part of a strong sesamoid capsuloligamentous complex.
■ Enveloped within the two heads of the flexor hallucis brevis (FHB) tendon, separated by an intersesamoid ridge called the *crista*
■ Attached to proximal phalanx via the plantar plate
■ Suspended by the collateral ligaments of MTP joint, metatarsosesamoid ligaments, intersesamoid ligament, abductor hallucis tendon, and adductor hallucis tendon
■ Analogous to the patella, they provide a mechanism to increase the mechanical advantage of the pulley function of the intrinsics (FHB).
■ Protect the FHL and disperse the forces beneath the first metatarsal head

DEFORMITIES

■ Sesamoid disorders can include acute injury (fracture, dislocation, sprain/"turf toe"), sesamoiditis, stress fracture, arthrosis, AVN, and IPK.
■ Diagnosis
■ Chief complaint is pain under the first metatarsal head, especially with toe-off.
■ Physical examination—tenderness with direct palpation of the involved sesamoid, pain with first-MTP ROM
■ Radiographs—in addition to AP and lateral views, lateral oblique (fibular sesamoid) and medial oblique (tibial sesamoid) views isolate each bone, and axial view shows the articulation with metatarsal head (Figure 6-58).

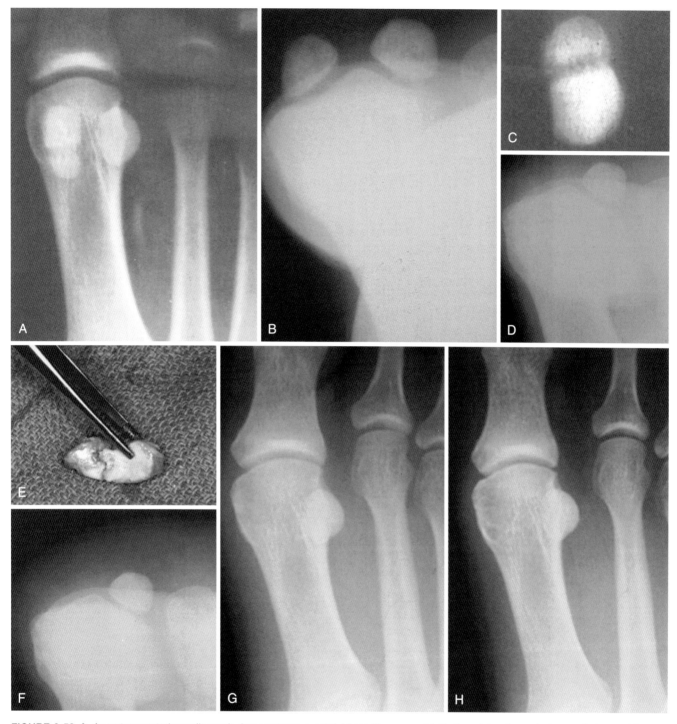

FIGURE 6-58 A, An anteroposterior radiograph demonstrates a painful bipartite sesamoid. **B,** An axial radiograph does not show evidence of a fracture or bipartite sesamoid. **C,** Radiograph of a pathology specimen showing rounded edges pathognomonic of a bipartite sesamoid. **D,** Axial view following excision of medial sesamoid. **E,** Gross pathology of a specimen. **F** and **G,** Immediately following surgery. **H,** At 19-year follow-up after medial sesamoid excision. Alignment of the first metatarsophalangeal joint is well maintained. (From Coughlin MJ et al: *Surgery of the foot and ankle,* ed 8, Philadelphia, 2006, Mosby.)

- Mechanism of injury—forced dorsiflexion of the first MTP joint, repetitive loading
  - Turf toe—forced dorsiflexion can result in avulsion of the plantar plate off the base of the phalanx and subsequent proximal migration of the sesamoids.
  - Tibial sesamoid is more frequently involved in trauma but also more likely to be bipartite or multipartite.

- **Conservative treatment**
- Turf toe
  - Grade 1—capsular strain
    - Signs—normal ROM, weight bearing without difficulty, normal radiographs
    - Treatment—stiff insole, taping, with immediate return to play

- Grade 2—partial capsular tear
  - Signs—painful ROM, limited weight bearing, normal radiographs
  - Treatment—no athletic activity for 2 weeks, stiff insole, return to play if painless 60-degree dorsiflexion present
- Grade 3—complete tear of the plantar plate
  - Signs—severe pain with palpation, limited and painful ROM, abnormal radiographs (fracture, proximal sesamoid migration)
  - Treatment—superior results demonstrated with operative repair of the plantar plate over conservative care
- Sesamoid fracture
  - Initial treatment with a fracture boot to limit the stress across the sesamoid
  - Transition to sesamoid relief pad (dancer's pad) with gradual resumption of activity
- Sesamoiditis
  - Treated with antiinflammatory medications, rest, ice, and activity and shoewear modification
- **Operative treatment**
- Symptomatic nonunions or cases that prove refractory to conservative care can be treated surgically with bone grafting or with partial or complete sesamoidectomy.
- Results of sesamoidectomy are the most predictable.
- Excision of the proximal or distal pole achieves the best results and should be performed if the fracture pattern allows.
- **Complications of medial and lateral sesamoidectomy are hallux valgus and varus, respectively.**

- Repairing the defect with capsule (or a slip of abductor hallucis for the tibial sesamoid) helps prevent this complication.
- **Cock-up deformity (or claw toe) will occur if both sesamoids are excised** (Figure 6-59).
- Care should be taken to avoid injury to the FHL and loss of flexor function, especially in the high-performance athlete.

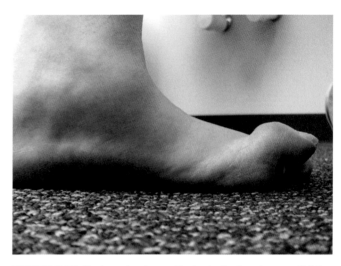

FIGURE 6-59 Cock-up toe in a patient who had undergone tibial and fibular sesamoidectomies. Both sesamoids should never be resected to prevent this complication. A first metatarsophalangeal joint fusion can be done concomitantly to prevent this from occurring.

SECTION 10 ACCESSORY BONES (Figure 6-60)

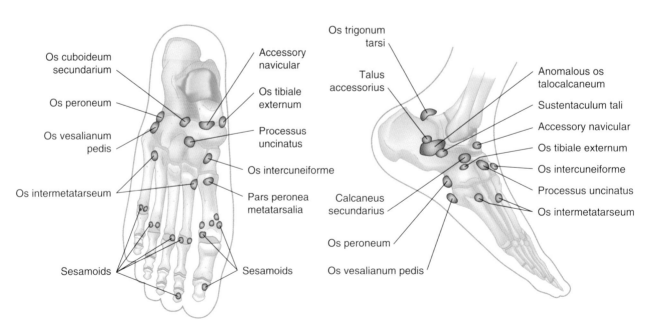

FIGURE 6-60 Accessory ossicles of the foot. (From Berquist TH, editor: *Radiology of the foot and ankle,* New York, 1989, Raven Press. In Mark J et al: *Rosen's emergency medicine,* ed 7, Philadelphia, 2009, Elsevier.)

SECTION 11 NEUROLOGIC DISORDERS

INTERDIGITAL NEURITIS (MORTON NEUROMA)

■ Definition

▨ Compressive neuropathy of the interdigital nerve, usually between the third and fourth metatarsals (Figure 6-61)

▨ The pathophysiology of this condition is still poorly understood.
- Theories include compression/tension around the intermetatarsal ligament, repetitive microtrauma, vascular changes, excessive bursal tissue, endoneural edema, and eventual neural fibrosis.

■ Diagnosis

▨ Patients will frequently report pain and burning on the plantar aspect of the web space, with over 60% of patients noting pain radiating into the toe distally. Numbness is reported in only 40% of patients.

▨ Exacerbated by footwear with narrow toe boxes and high heels

▨ Physical examination
- Palpation between and just distal to the metatarsal heads elicits plantar tenderness.
- Compressing the medial and lateral aspect of the forefoot while palpating the web space structures can provoke symptoms and occasionally a bursal "click" (Mulder click).
- Metatarsalgia and MTP synovitis often present similarly and should be ruled out.

▨ Radiographs
- Plain films should be performed to rule out bony masses or deformity.

- MRI can be used to identify other pathologies, but not required for diagnosis.

■ Nonoperative treatment

▨ Shoewear modification (avoiding high heels and narrow toe boxes) is the most important and effective intervention.

▨ Metatarsal pads placed proximal to the focus of pain can prevent direct pressure and widen the intermetatarsal space during weight bearing, thereby indirectly decompressing the nerve.

▨ Corticosteroid injections can have moderate effectiveness (≈50% of patients report positive response).

■ Operative treatment

▨ Excision of neuroma
- Dorsal approach most common
  - Incise the transverse intermetatarsal ligament.
  - Identify the common digital nerve and its branches, and resect the nerve 2 to 3 cm proximal to the intermetatarsal ligament (proximal to the small plantar branches), which allows the proximal stump to retract (Figure 6-62).
  - Minimizes formation of stump neuroma, the most common complication
  - Difficult visualization results in a 4% rate of failure to excise the neuroma.
  - Overall success rates approach 80%.
- Plantar approach
  - Decreases the rate of missed neuroma excision
  - Does not require incision of the transverse intermetatarsal ligament

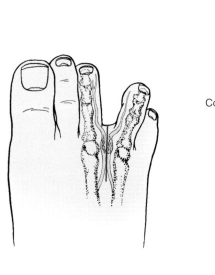
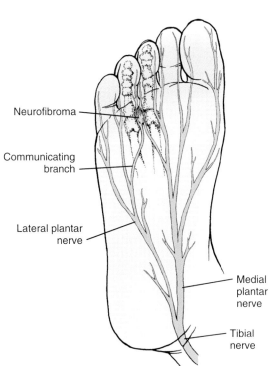

Neurofibroma

Communicating branch

Lateral plantar nerve

Medial plantar nerve

Tibial nerve

FIGURE 6-61 Most common anatomic location of interdigital neuroma; plantar and dorsal views. (From Canale ST, Beaty J: *Campbell's operative orthopedics,* ed 11, Philadelphia, 2007, Elsevier. Modified from McElvenny RT: The etiology and surgical treatment of intractable pain about the fourth metatarsophalangeal joint (Morton's toe), *J Bone Joint Surg* 25:675, 1943.)

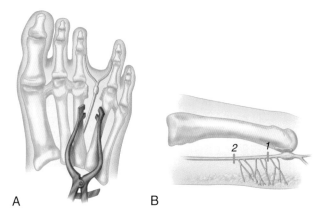

FIGURE 6-62 A, Lamina spreader used to expose neuroma. **B,** Lateral view of plantar branches of digital nerve. *1,* Previously recommended level of neurectomy; *2,* currently recommended level of neurectomy (3 cm proximal to ligament) to avoid plantarly directed nerve branches. (From Canale ST, Beaty J: *Campbell's operative orthopaedics,* ed 11, Philadelphia, 2007, Elsevier. Modified from Weinfeld SB, Myerson MS: Interdigital neuritis: diagnosis and treatment, *J Am Acad Orthop Surg* 4:328, 1996.)

- Increased risk (5%) of painful plantar scar
- Typically used for revision neuroma resection

RECURRENT NEUROMA

- **Definition**
- Bulbous enlargement of the neural stump (or secondary glioma)
- Usually caused by inadequate proximal resection or failure of the nerve to retract
- Neural stump adheres to adjacent bone and soft tissue, causing a traction neuritis.
- **Diagnosis**
- Localized pain and tenderness to palpation (Tinel sign) in web space of previous neuroma resection, at or proximal to metatarsal heads
- Must rule out "irritable" tibial nerve
  - Palpate along tibial nerve and branches distal to flexor retinaculum.
- Recurrent neuroma is likely if symptoms are localized and reproducible.
- **Nonoperative treatment—similar to primary neuroma (see earlier)**
- **Operative treatment**
- Excision of the stump neuroma can be performed through another dorsal incision or through a plantar incision.
- Plantar incision allows access to a very proximal location in which to place the resected neuroma stump.
  - Preferred approach for revision neuroma excision
- The new stump should be transposed into muscle tissue if possible.
- Success rate after excision of a recurrent or stump neuroma is 65% to 75%.

TARSAL TUNNEL SYNDROME

- **Definition**
- Compressive neuropathy of the tibial nerve within the fibroosseous tunnel posterior and inferior to the medial malleolus

- Bounded by the flexor retinaculum (laciniate ligament) superficially; the medial talus, medial calcaneus, and sustentaculum tali deep; and the abductor hallucis inferiorly
- The tarsal tunnel also contains the tibialis posterior, FHL and FDL tendons, the posterior tibial artery, the venae comitantes, and the numerous septa that subdivide the tunnel.
- Reported causes of tarsal tunnel syndrome include tenosynovitis, engorged or varicose vessels, synovial or ganglion cysts, pigmented villonodular synovitis, nerve sheath tumors, lipomas, fracture of the sustentaculum tali or medial tubercle of the posterior process of the talus, middle facet tarsal coalition, and accessory muscles.
- Systemic diseases such as diabetes mellitus, RA, and ankylosing spondylitis may have an indirect effect by causing inflammatory edema.
- **Diagnosis**
- Symptoms of tarsal tunnel syndrome may be vague and misleading.
  - Include a burning sensation on the plantar surface of the foot and medial ankle and occasional sharp pains or paresthesias
  - Prolonged standing, walking, or running can exacerbate the symptoms.
- Physical examination
  - Percussion of the entire course of the distal tibial nerve and its branches should be performed.
    - Tinel sign, radiating pain or discomfort with continuous deep compression over the nerve, or diminished two-point discrimination may be elicited.
  - Sensory examination is usually unpredictable.
  - Assess hindfoot alignment—pes planus may cause increased tension on the nerve.
  - Wasting of the abductor hallucis or abductor digiti quinti may be seen if the medial or lateral plantar nerve are involved, respectively.
- **Diagnostic tests**
- Electrodiagnostic studies should be performed to help make the diagnosis or determine a different level of compression.
  - Sensory nerve conduction studies are more commonly abnormal than motor nerve conduction studies.
  - Electromyography (EMG) abnormalities are less sensitive.
- MRI may identify the presence of a mass occupying lesion, which if present must be excised (Figure 6-63).
  - Surgical decompression with mass excision results in more predictable symptomatic improvement compared to patients who do not have a mass occupying lesion.
- Correlation with history and physical examination findings is essential.
- **Nonoperative treatment**
- Management should begin with conservative measures unless there is a suspicious mass or suspected malignancy.
- Medications such as NSAIDs, vitamin B₆, and tricyclic antidepressants are most commonly prescribed.
  - Selective serotonin reuptake inhibitors (SSRIs), and antiseizure medications (gabapentin, pregabalin) are also used.
- Physical therapy may include stretching, massage, desensitization, and iontophoresis.

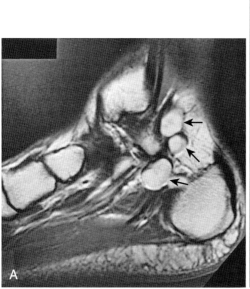
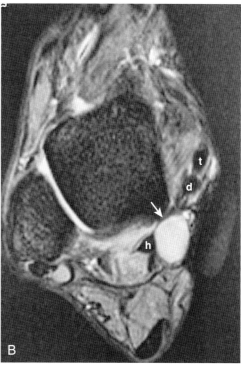

FIGURE 6-63 Tarsal tunnel syndrome from schwannomas. **A,** T1-weighted contrast-enhanced sagittal image of the hindfoot. Three round masses *(arrows)* that show enhancement are running through the tarsal tunnel. **B,** T2-weighted axial image of the hindfoot. One of the schwannomas is shown as a high-signal mass *(arrow)* in the space normally occupied by the posterior tibial nerve, artery, and vein. *d,* Flexor digitorum tendon; *h,* flexor hallucis tendon; *t,* tibialis posterior tendon. (From Helms C et al: *Musculoskeletal MRI,* ed 2, Philadelphia, 2009, Saunders.)

- Orthoses to correct hindfoot valgus (medial heel wedge) play an important role as well.
- In cases of acute inflammation or severe limitation because of pain, a brief course of a CAM walker boot or short leg cast may be helpful.
- **Operative treatment**
- Space-occupying lesion should be excised, with concomitant nerve release.
- If appropriate conservative management for 3 to 6 months is unsuccessful, surgical intervention is warranted.
- Longitudinal incision made over the course of the tibial nerve; curves distally behind medial malleolus to the abductor musculature (Figure 6-64)
- The nerve is identified proximally, and the proximal investing fascia and flexor retinaculum are released.
  - Care must be taken to release the superficial and deep fascia of the abductor hallucis muscle.
- Endoscopic tarsal tunnel release is not recommended.
- Recurrence of tarsal tunnel syndrome is a challenging problem.
  - Incomplete release is the most common etiology, though intrinsic nerve damage may play a role in recurrent symptoms.
  - Revision release may be of benefit if incomplete release is suspected, though results are often poor.
- **Lateral plantar nerve**
- Provides sensation to the plantar lateral aspect of the foot
- **May be injured during surgical approaches that require a plantar incision, such as a tibiotalocalcaneal (TTC) arthrodesis with an intramedullary nail**

- **First branch of the lateral plantar nerve (Baxter nerve) may be a source of chronic plantar medial heel pain.**
  - **Associated with long-distance runners/marathon runners**
- **Medial plantar nerve**
- Provides sensation to the plantar medial aspect of the foot
- Entrapment occurs at the knot of Henry (junction of FDL and FHL tendons).
- Most common etiology is external compression from orthotic devices.
- Also called *jogger's foot,* conservative treatment is often successful and includes avoidance of orthotics or pressure along the plantar medial hindfoot.

ANTERIOR TARSAL TUNNEL SYNDROME

- **Definition**
- Compressive neuropathy of the deep peroneal nerve in the fibroosseous tunnel formed by the Y-shaped inferior extensor retinaculum (Figure 6-65)
- The nerve divides into the lateral motor and the medial sensory branches within the tunnel and is accompanied by the dorsalis pedis artery.
- Common causes of compression include tightly laced shoes, anterior osteophytes at the tibiotalar and TN articulations, a bony prominence associated with pes cavus deformity or fracture, ganglion cysts, and tendinitis of the EDL, EHL, or tibialis anterior (Figure 6-66).

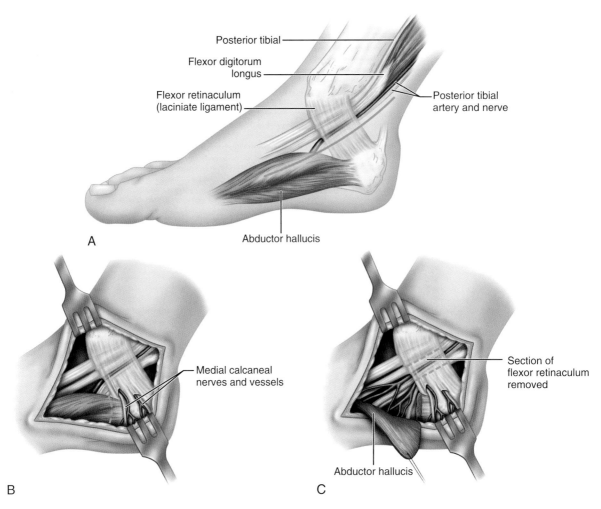

Posterior tibial

Flexor digitorum longus

Flexor retinaculum (laciniate ligament)

Posterior tibial artery and nerve

Abductor hallucis

A

Medial calcaneal nerves and vessels

Section of flexor retinaculum removed

Abductor hallucis

B   C

FIGURE 6-64 Tarsal tunnel release. **A,** Skin incision. **B,** Note branches of medial calcaneal nerve and artery penetrating retinaculum. Broken line indicates incision for reflecting abductor hallucis muscle. **C,** Abductor hallucis is reflected plantarward, and section of flexor retinaculum to be removed is outlined. (From Canale ST, Beaty J: *Campbell's operative orthopaedics,* ed 11, Philadelphia, 2007, Elsevier.)

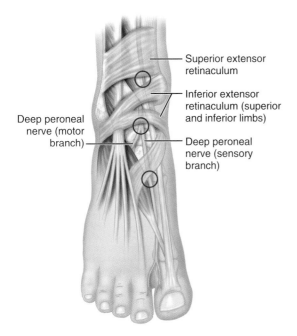

Superior extensor retinaculum

Inferior extensor retinaculum (superior and inferior limbs)

Deep peroneal nerve (motor branch)

Deep peroneal nerve (sensory branch)

FIGURE 6-65 Deep peroneal nerve entrapment. Circles denote areas of impingement. (From Mann RA, Baxter DE: Diseases of the nerves. In Mann RA, Coughlin MJ, editors: *Surgery of the foot and ankle,* ed 6, St Louis, 1993, Mosby.)

■ **Diagnosis**
▪ Patients present with burning pain and paresthesias along the medial second toe, lateral hallux, and first web space, or even vague dorsal foot pain.
▪ Symptoms are often worse at night as the ankle assumes a plantar-flexed posture, and with shallow, laced shoes.
▪ Physical examination
  • Decreased two-point discrimination, positive Tinel sign along course of the deep peroneal nerve
  • Pain may be worse with plantar flexion of ankle as the nerve is stretched.

■ **Nonoperative treatment**
▪ Night splints, NSAIDs, diagnostic/therapeutic injections, shoe tongue padding, and footwear with loose lacing or alternative lacing techniques are the conservative approaches.

■ **Operative treatment**
▪ Surgical release involves incising the inferior extensor retinaculum, releasing both branches of the nerve, excising bone spurs, and carefully repairing the bony capsule to avoid exposing the nerve to bleeding bone while protecting the dorsalis pedis artery.
▪ Patients should understand that relief of the paresthesias and dysesthesias may take weeks or months.

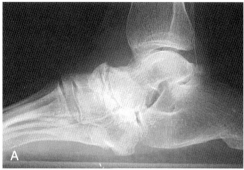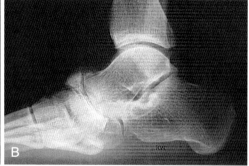

FIGURE 6-66 Arthritis of the talonavicular joint **(A)** or nonunion of a navicular fracture **(B)** can compress the deep peroneal nerve. (From Myerson MS: *Foot and ankle disorders,* Philadelphia, 2000, Elsevier.)

SUPERFICIAL PERONEAL NERVE ENTRAPMENT

■ **Definition**

▨ Compressive neuropathy of the superficial peroneal nerve as it exits from the lateral compartment into the anterior ankle

▨ The opening in the fascia is approximately 12 cm proximal to the tip of the lateral malleolus.

▨ Neuritis may occur after an inversion injury or with fascial defects.

▨ **The nerve can also be damaged or entrapped in scar tissue at the anterolateral portal following ankle arthroscopic procedures.**

■ **Diagnosis**

▨ Symptoms include burning pain and tingling over the dorsum of the foot.

▨ Symptoms exacerbate with plantar flexion and inversion.

▨ Tinel sign is frequently present over the nerve as it exits the lateral compartment.

■ **Nonoperative treatment includes NSAIDs, diagnostic/ therapeutic injections, and other nerve modalities with physical therapy. Surgical release of the nerve with fasciotomy is indicated if nonoperative treatment fails.**

SURAL OR SAPHENOUS NERVE ENTRAPMENT

■ Entrapment of the sural or saphenous nerves is rare, typically occurring only after surgical procedures as the nerves become entrapped in scar tissue.

■ Conservative treatments may be successful, but neurolysis or resection of neuroma with burial of the nerve end is indicated for refractory cases.

■ The sural nerve is prone to injury with lateral hindfoot procedures that use a sinus tarsi approach. The traditional extensile lateral calcaneus approach places the sural nerve at risk at both the proximal and distal ends of the incision.

SEQUELAE OF UPPER MOTOR NEURON DISORDERS

■ **Definition**

▨ Most commonly secondary to traumatic brain injury, stroke, and spinal cord injury

▨ Disruption of the upper motor neuron pathways can lead to paralysis, muscular imbalance, and acquired spasticity, which ultimately may cause deformity of the foot and ankle.

▨ Secondary problems include fixed contractures, calluses, pressure sores, hygiene issues, joint subluxation, shoewear difficulties, and dissatisfaction with physical appearance.

▨ **The most common deformity of the foot and ankle is equinovarus.**

   • The equinus component is caused by overactivity of the gastrocnemius-soleus complex.

   • The varus is due to relative overactivity of the tibialis anterior, with lesser contributions from the FHL, FDL, and tibialis posterior.

■ **Nonoperative treatment**

▨ Early intervention with physical therapy, stretching and strengthening, and maintenance of joint ROM.

▨ Other modalities include splinting, serial casting, oral muscle relaxants, phenol and lidocaine nerve blocks, and botulinum type A toxin injections.

   • Phenol blocks have a proven history, will often have longer-lasting effects, and are less expensive than botulinum toxin.

   • Advantage of botulinum is ease of delivery—requires only an injection into the muscle belly, rather than a precise injection around the motor nerve.

■ **Operative treatment**

▨ Surgery for acquired spasticity should be delayed at least 6 months after onset to allow for maximum recovery.

▨ Equinus deformity is addressed with either an open Z-lengthening of the Achilles tendon or a percutaneous triple hemisection technique (Figure 6-67).

▨ Varus deformity is addressed with a split anterior tibialis tendon transfer (SPLATT) to the lateral cuneiform or cuboid or total anterior tibial tendon transfer to the lateral cuneiform.

   • If the varus deformity is fixed, lateral closing wedge calcaneal osteotomy or subtalar fusion may be necessary.

▨ Release of the toe flexors is often required secondary to a tenodesis effect as the ankle is brought into a plantigrade position.

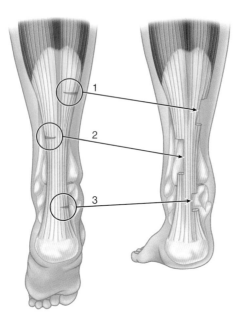

FIGURE 6-67 Incisions for percutaneous Achilles tendon lengthening. Cut ends slide on themselves with forceful dorsiflexion of foot. (From Canale ST, Beaty J: *Campbell's operative orthopaedics,* ed 11, Philadelphia, 2007, Elsevier. Modified from Hsu JD, Hsu CL: Motor unit disease. In Jahss MH, editor: *Disorders of the foot,* Philadelphia, 1982, Saunders.)

CHARCOT-MARIE-TOOTH DISEASE (CMT)

■ Definition
- CMT is the most common inherited progressive peripheral neuropathy, affecting approximately 1 in every 2500 people.
- Many genetic variants of CMT disease; as a group are referred to as *hereditary motor-sensory neuropathies* (HMSNs)
- Type 1 HMSN is the most common presentation of CMT.
  - Usually autosomal dominant with a duplication of chromosome 17
- An abnormal myelin sheath protein is the basis of CMT degenerative neuropathy.
- The earlier the onset, the more severe the neurologic findings

■ Diagnosis
- Deformity and awkward gait are common initial complaints, with weakness, lateral ankle instability, and lateral foot pain presenting later.
- Physical examination
  - Bilateral symmetric pes cavovarus deformity is caused by motor imbalance.
    - **Tibialis anterior (TA) and peroneus brevis (PB) weakness seen early**
    - **First ray is plantar flexed because of relative unopposed pull of peroneus longus (PL > TA)** (Figure 6-68).
      - This creates forefoot cavus and compensatory hindfoot varus (tripod effect).
    - **Hindfoot pulled farther into varus because of relative unopposed pull of posterior tibial (PT) muscle (PT > PB)**
      - Plantar-flexed first ray and hindfoot varus leads to external rotation of distal tibia and fibula.

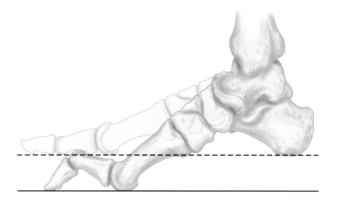

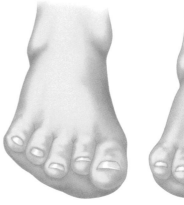
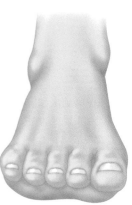

FIGURE 6-68 Lateral and frontal view of plantar-flexed first ray as seen in Charcot-Marie-Tooth disease. (From Canale ST, Beaty J: *Campbell's operative orthopaedics,* ed 11, Philadelphia, 2007, Elsevier.)

- Intrinsic (EDB, EHB, interossei) wasting leads to overpull of extrinsics (EHL, EDL, FHL, FDL), which causes claw-toe deformity.
  - Weak TA leads to recruitment of EHL and EDL during swing phase of gait, worsening claw-toe deformity.
  - Prominent and tender calluses may be present beneath the metatarsal heads.
- Coleman block test (Figure 6-69) **should be used to determine if a hindfoot varus deformity is secondary to the plantar-flexed first ray or an independent component.**
  - **Deformity corrects with Coleman block— forefoot-driven hindfoot varus.**
    - **Surgical correction involves dorsiflexion osteotomy of the first metatarsal.**
  - **Deformity does not correct with Coleman block— hindfoot varus independent of the forefoot.**
    - **Surgical correction involves:**
      - **Dorsiflexion osteotomy of the first metatarsal (forefoot) AND**
      - **Lateral closing calcaneal osteotomy (hindfoot)**
- Sensory deficit is variable.
  - Proprioception, vibration, and two-point discrimination affected first
  - Severe sensory loss may lead to recurrent ulceration, deep infection, and even neuropathic arthropathy.

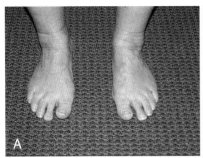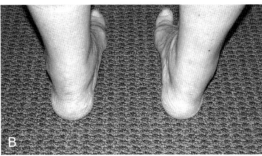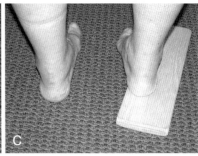

FIGURE 6-69 A, Unilateral cavus foot on left (patient's right foot). Note the appearance of the medial heel on the left, while on the opposite side the medial heel is not visible. **B,** Right varus heel alignment on the same patient viewed from behind. Note the normal heel alignment of the left foot. **C,** Correction of heel alignment on Coleman block testing on the same patient. Note the same alignment of both feet while right foot is on the block, implying forefoot-driven cavus. (From DiGiovanni C: *Core knowledge in orthopaedics—foot and ankle,* Philadelphia, 2007, Elsevier.)

■ **Treatment**
▓ Flexible deformity (hindfoot can be passively manipulated)
  • In an adolescent with closed physes and a supple deformity, surgical treatment rather than brace management is currently recommended because of the progressive pattern of this disease.
  • Operative treatment involves:
    • Release of the plantar fascia
    • Closing wedge dorsiflexion osteotomy of first metatarsal
      • Always required; if deformity corrects with Coleman block test, no other bony correction is required.
      • Lateral calcaneal slide and/or closing wedge osteotomy if deformity does NOT correct with the Coleman block (Figure 6-70)
    • Transfer of peroneus longus into peroneus brevis at the level of the distal fibula
    • Frequently an Achilles tendon lengthening (TAL) is required.
    • Forefoot correction is performed according to the guidelines outlined previously.
    • A flexible clawed hallux can be surgically treated with a Jones procedure (arthrodesis of interphalangeal joint and transfer of EHL to first metatarsal).
▓ Fixed deformity (hindfoot cannot be passively manipulated)
  • Nonoperative management can be attempted with a brace.
    • Locked-ankle, short-leg ankle-foot orthosis (AFO) with an outside (varus-correcting or lateral) T-strap is recommended.
    • Rocker sole can improve gait and decrease energy expenditure.
  • Operative treatment includes:
    • Triple arthrodesis usually required for hindfoot correction
    • PTT transfer through the interosseous membrane, and TAL can correct equinus contracture and dorsiflexion weakness.
    • Plantar fascia release and dorsiflexion osteotomy of the first metatarsal
    • Forefoot correction is performed according to the guidelines outlined previously.

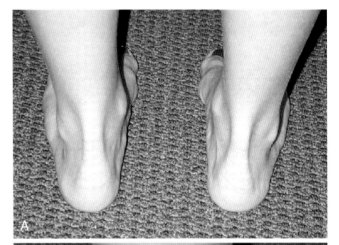
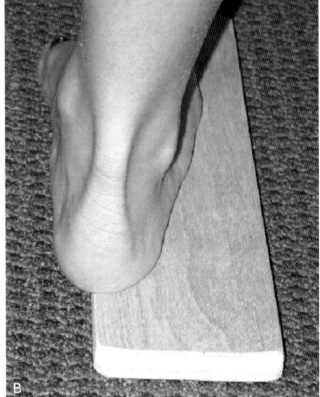

FIGURE 6-70 A, Unilateral right heel varus. **B,** Same patient on a Coleman block with no change in heel position, indicating hindfoot-driven cavus.

PERIPHERAL NERVE INJURY AND TENDON TRANSFERS

- Traumatic injuries to the lower extremity can result in injury to the nerves and/or musculature, resulting in a paralytic deformity.
- **Use of AFO can be a successful nonoperative treatment; however, many patients desire to become brace free.**
- Principles of tendon transfers
- Deformity must be flexible (passive ROM must be present). A rigid deformity requires an arthrodesis.
- Preoperative physical examination is critical to determine which tendons should be transferred.
  - Assess which muscles are still active—must have at least four-fifths strength to transfer.
  - Redirect a deforming force to create a restoring force.
- Peroneal nerve palsy
- Loss of the anterior and lateral compartments—loss of active dorsiflexion and eversion

- Deformity—equinovarus
- Transfer PTT (deforming force) through the interosseous membrane anteriorly to the dorsal midfoot (restores dorsiflexion) with an Achilles tendon lengthening.
- Compartment syndrome—loss of the anterior and deep posterior compartments
- Deformity—cavovarus (PL) with equinus (Achilles)
- Treatment—Achilles tendon lengthening with transfer of the PL (deforming force) to the dorsolateral midfoot (restores dorsiflexion).
- Unique cases such as compartment syndrome or traumatic injury can create variable patterns of motor loss. Correction of the deformity is unique to each case, dependent upon the remnant motor function.

SECTION 12 ARTHRITIC DISEASE

CRYSTALLINE DISEASE

- **Gout**
- Pathology
  - Abnormal purine metabolism results in precipitation and deposition of monosodium urate crystals into synovium-lined joints.
  - Induces a severe inflammatory response
  - Induced by certain medications that increase serum uric acid, localized trauma, alcohol, or purine-rich foods, as well as by the postsurgical state
  - Men are more commonly affected than women.
- Diagnosis
  - Patients complain of sudden joint pain, with a characteristic history ("not even a sheet could touch it").
  - Physical examination—intense signs of inflammation (redness, swelling, warmth, tenderness) and pain with ROM
  - The great-toe MTP joint is most often involved (50%-75% of initial attacks).
    - 90% of patients with chronic gouty attacks will have one or more episodes involving the hallux MTP joint **(podagra).**
  - Characteristic radiographic signs:
    - Inordinate soft tissue enlargement about the MTP joint
    - Bony erosions both at a distance from and within the joint articular surface
      - Extensive articular and periarticular destruction can occur in chronic conditions (Figure 6-71).
      - Secondary to large deposits of gouty residue **(tophi)**
- **Definitive diagnosis—needle aspiration of the joint**
  - Indicated in the presence of an acute swollen painful joint; fluid sent for crystals and Gram stain with culture
  - Pathognomonic signs: needle-shaped monosodium urate crystals, which under polarized light are strongly negatively birefringent

- Critical to rule out an acute septic joint, which will be determined from the aspiration
- Serum uric acid may or may not be elevated and should be not used to confirm or refute the diagnosis.
- Treatment
- **Acute attacks treated with indomethacin or colchicine**
- **Chronic attacks treated with allopurinol**
- Joint destruction or deposition of large quantities of tophi may require arthrodesis and/or débridement of tophaceous debris.

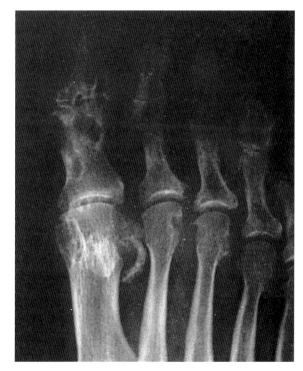

FIGURE 6-71 Gouty arthritis. Multiple punched-out lesions are present. (From Mercier L: *Practical orthopaedics*, ed 6, Philadelphia, 2008, Elsevier.)

■ Pseudogout (chondrocalcinosis)
- Pathology
  - Deposition of calcium pyrophosphate dihydrate (CPPD) crystals in or about a joint may lead to severe initial inflammatory response.
  - Usually articular, with less periarticular soft tissue involvement than gout
  - Commonly affects the knee but may present in articulations of the foot or ankle
- Diagnosis
  - Joint aspiration reveals weakly positive birefringent crystals with varied shapes under polarized light microscopy.
  - Lesser MTP, TN, and subtalar joints can be affected.
  - Characteristic radiographic signs:
    - Intraarticular calcifications commonly seen (unlike gout) (Figure 6-72)
    - Joint destruction can occur with recurrent attacks over a long period, but this is rare.
- Treatment—rest, oral NSAIDs for acute synovitis, protected weight bearing, and corticosteroid injections

SERONEGATIVE SPONDYLOARTHROPATHY (SNSA)

■ Definition
- Inflammatory arthritides that are negative for rheumatoid factor
- Distinguished from RA clinically by a higher incidence of involvement of entheses (i.e., the interface between collagen and bone where ligament, tendon, and capsular tissue insert into bone)
- Involvement of this transitional tissue is found in psoriatic arthritis, ankylosing spondylitis, Reiter syndrome, and inflammatory bowel disease.
- May destroy articular cartilage but characteristically are more destructive toward collagen and fibrocartilage

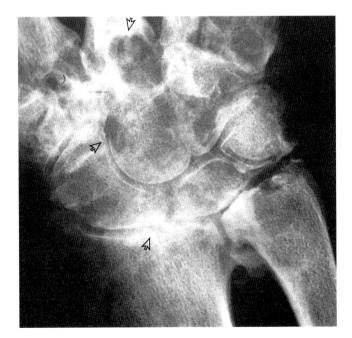

FIGURE 6-72 Wrist abnormalities in gout. Diffuse disease of all compartments of the wrist is evident. Erosions *(arrows)* are most prominent at the common carpometacarpal compartment *(upper arrow)*. (From Resnick D: The radiographic manifestations of gouty arthritis. *CRC Crit Rev Diagn Imaging* 9:265, 1977.)

■ Diagnosis
- Often presents in the foot as plantar fasciitis, Achilles tendinitis, or posterior tibial tendinopathy
- **Psoriatic arthritis can present with swollen and inflamed distal joints or, more classically, as dactylitis ("sausage digit").**
- **Periarticular bony erosion may occur, causing a classic "pencil-in-cup" sign typical of psoriatic arthritis** (Figure 6-73).
- **Additional findings may include nail pitting, onycholysis, and keratosis.**

■ Treatment
- Pharmacologic agents such as NSAIDs, or occasionally salicylates or cytotoxic drugs under the direction and observation of a rheumatologist, are the mainstays of treatment.
- Intraarticular corticosteroid injections may improve symptoms, especially for acute flares.
- Surgical intervention is sometimes required for small joint erosions, recalcitrant Achilles tendinopathy, and plantar fasciitis.

RHEUMATOID ARTHRITIS

■ Definition
- Chronic symmetric polyarthropathy that most commonly presents in the third and fourth decades and is more prevalent in women.
- Synovitis causes ligament and capsular laxity and cartilage and bony erosion.
- Vasculitis and soft tissue fragility is common, requiring diligent care of the soft tissues during nonoperative and operative management.
- Use of immune-mediating pharmacologic therapies in the perioperative period should be discussed with a rheumatologist because complications can result.
  - Most can be continued (prednisone, methotrexate, hydroxychloroquine), but the newer biologic agents (e.g., TNF antagonists) should be discontinued.
  - **Most significant risk factor for development of a postoperative wound infection: history of previous wound infection**

■ Diagnosis
- Foot involvement very common in rheumatoid patients
  - Forefoot more commonly involved than midfoot or hindfoot
- Patients complain of forefoot swelling, poorly defined pain, and eventually deformity.
- MTP joint pathophysiology:
  - Chronic synovitis leads to incompetence of the joint capsules and collateral ligaments.
  - Toes sublux or dislocate dorsally, deviate laterally into valgus, and develop hammering (Figure 6-74).
  - Intrinsic muscles worsen the claw-toe deformity.
  - Plantar fat pad migrates distally and atrophies, causing metatarsalgia and painful keratoses.
  - As lesser toes deviate laterally, hallux valgus occurs and transfer metatarsalgia worsens.
- Midfoot and hindfoot are less commonly and less severely involved in RA.
  - Significant midfoot/hindfoot arthrosis (TN joint characteristic)
  - Often results in a pes planovalgus deformity

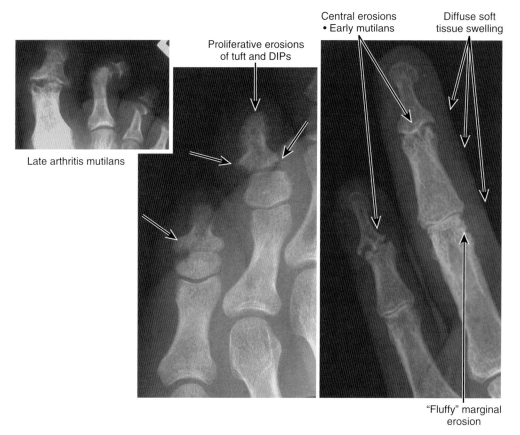

Central erosions
• Early mutilans

Diffuse soft
tissue swelling

Proliferative erosions
of tuft and DIPs

Late arthritis mutilans

"Fluffy" marginal
erosion

FIGURE 6-73 Psoriatic arthritis. Erosions classically have a proliferative appearance, with a fluffy or whiskered quality. Central erosions can lead to joint destruction with a "pencil-in-cup" pattern. *DIPs,* Distal interphalangeal joints. (From Morrison W, Sanders T: *Problem solving in musculoskeletal imaging,* Philadelphia, 2008, Elsevier.)

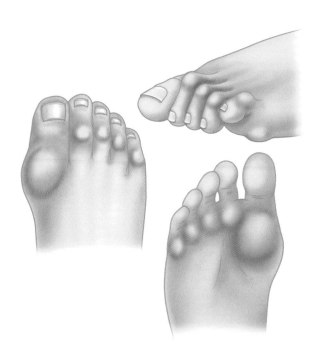

FIGURE 6-74 Rheumatoid foot. Note multiple deformities of rheumatoid arthritis of forefoot with hallux valgus, subluxed and dislocated metatarsophalangeal joints, claw toes, hammer toes, and bursal formation. (From Canale ST, Beaty J: *Campbell's operative orthopaedics,* ed 11, Philadelphia, 2007, Elsevier.)

- Underlying cause of flatfoot deformity must be carefully assessed to determine whether it is midfoot driven or hindfoot driven.
- Midfoot etiology—TMT joints subluxated, with a congruent hindfoot (Figure 6-75)
  - Treatment—realignment midfoot arthrodesis
- Hindfoot etiology—transverse tarsal and subtalar joints are subluxated, with a normal midfoot.
  - Treatment—triple arthrodesis
- ▪ Tibiotalar joint also commonly involved—easily differentiated from osteoarthritis by lack of osteophyte formation, osteopenia, and symmetric joint space narrowing (Figure 6-76)
  - Ankle arthrodesis is currently the treatment of choice, with ankle replacement emerging as a more reliable technique.
    - A tibiotalar and subtalar (TTC) arthrodesis performed with an intramedullary nail risks a tibial stress fracture in these patients.
      - This complication is best treated conservatively with a cast.
  - Risks of wound complications after total ankle arthroplasty have been shown to increase in patients with RA.
- ▪ **Treatment**
- ▪ Nonoperative treatment
  - Rest, NSAIDs, immune-modulating drugs under the direction of rheumatologists, toe taping, orthoses, and careful use of corticosteroid injections may help symptoms related to synovitis.

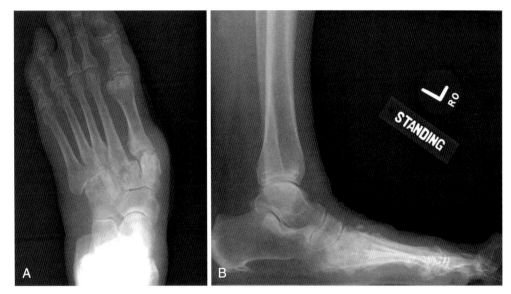

FIGURE 6-75 A, Anteroposterior radiograph of a patient with rheumatoid arthritis with a flatfoot deformity that is secondary to midfoot arthritis. Note how the first and second metatarsals are subluxated laterally relative to the cuneiforms. **B,** The lateral radiograph demonstrates loss of the longitudinal arch centered at the tarsometatarsal joints, with obvious degenerative changes. Surgical treatment is a realignment midfoot arthrodesis. Care must be taken in differentiating this from a hindfoot-driven flatfoot, where the deformity is centered at the talonavicular joint.

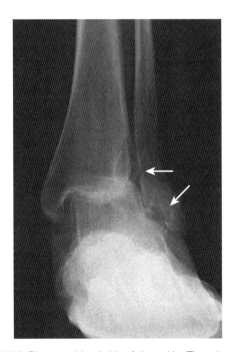

FIGURE 6-76 Rheumatoid arthritis of the ankle. There is diffuse loss of cartilage space with erosions of the fibula *(arrows)*. The scalloping along the medial border of the distal fibula is designated the *fibular notch sign* and is a characteristic finding in rheumatoid arthritis. The hindfoot is in valgus alignment. (From Firestein G et al: *Kelley's textbook of rheumatology,* ed 8, Philadelphia, 2008, Elsevier.)

- ▨ Operative treatment
  - • Late (in presence of deformity)—"rheumatoid forefoot reconstruction" (Hoffman procedure) (Figure 6-77)
    - • First MTP arthrodesis, lesser metatarsal head resection with pinning of the lesser MTP joints, and closed osteoclasis of the interphalangeal joints versus PIP arthroplasty
      - • Silicone arthroplasty not recommended; complications are cock-up deformity, silicone synovitis, and osteolysis.

- • Accomplished through three well-placed longitudinal dorsal incisions (Figure 6-78)
- • Extensor brevis tenotomy and Z-lengthening of the extensor longus tendons may be necessary.
- • Most common complication of forefoot arthroplasty is intractable plantar keratoses.
- • Midfoot, hindfoot, or ankle arthrodesis indicated as above

OSTEOARTHRITIS

▨ Definition

- ▨ Osteoarthritis and posttraumatic arthritis share similarities in the mechanical nature of the problem, clinical presentation, and treatment algorithm.
- ▨ Posttraumatic arthritis is most common in the hindfoot, tibiotalar, and TMT articulations.
- ▨ Osteoarthritis commonly affects the first MTP joint and the midfoot joints (TMT, intercuneiform, naviculocuneiform (NC), and TN joints).
- ▨ Lateral ankle instability, PTT insufficiency, and neuromuscular deformities also commonly contribute to degenerative arthritis.
- ▨ Diagnosis
- ▨ Patients complain of dull, achy pain at the involved joint, usually worse with activity.
- ▨ Physical examination—tenderness to palpation at the joint surface, with loss of ROM, and pain with passive ROM
- ▨ Radiographs—loss of joint space, subchondral sclerosis and cysts, osteophyte formation (Figure 6-79)
- ▨ First MTP joint
  - • Tenderness over the dorsum of the joint, limited dorsiflexion secondary to large dorsal osteophyte, and pain with grind test
  - • Graded clinically and radiographically:
    - • Grade 0—normal radiographs, stiff on examination
    - • Grade I—mild dorsal osteophyte, joint space preserved, mild pain at extremes of ROM

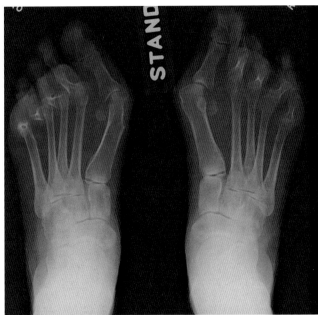

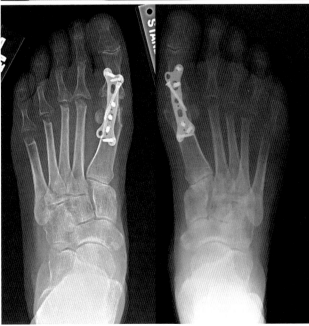

FIGURE 6-77 Preoperative **(A)** and postoperative **(B)** radiographs for rheumatoid forefoot reconstruction.

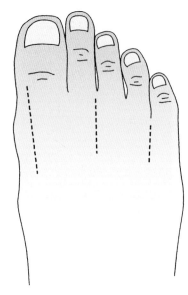

FIGURE 6-78 Incisions for first metatarsophalangeal (MTP) joint arthrodesis and lesser MTP joint resection arthroplasty for rheumatoid arthritis.

- Rigid flatfoot without arthritis is also common presentation but is not amenable to joint preservation surgery and should be treated with a triple arthrodesis.
- Tibiotalar joint
- Tenderness in anterior ankle joint line
- Limited ROM with pain, especially in extreme dorsiflexion
- May have associated varus or valgus deformity, either at ankle or more proximally especially with history of prior fracture or injury
- Radiographs show joint space narrowing, sclerosis and cysts, osteophytes, and possibly varus or valgus deformity.
  - Standing radiographs essential; may need long-leg alignment view with history of leg trauma
- May be associated with cavovarus deformity, rigid flatfoot (valgus), or chronic lateral ankle instability (varus)

■ **Nonoperative treatment**
▦ Initial treatment should include antiinflammatory medications, activity modification, orthotic support or bracing, and corticosteroid injections.
▦ **Hallux rigidus—stiff foot plate with an extension under the great toe (Morton extension)**
▦ **Midfoot (TMT) arthritis—stiff-soled or steel shank modified shoe with a rocker bottom in addition to a cushioned heel. Use of a full-length rigid foot orthotic can also be beneficial.**
▦ Hindfoot (ST, TN, CC) arthritis—AFO or rigid lace-up leather brace (Arizona type)
▦ **Tibiotalar arthritis—AFO or rigid lace-up leather brace (Arizona type). Shoe modification consists of a single hindfoot rocker-sole shoe.**
■ **Operative treatment**
▦ **Hallux rigidus:**
  - **Grades I and II (pain at extreme ROM only)— usually treated with dorsal cheilectomy (removal of all osteophytes including portion of dorsal metatarsal head with loss of cartilage (Figure 6-80)**

- Grade II—moderate osteophyte formation, joint space narrowing (<50%), moderate pain with ROM that may be more constant
- Grade III—severe osteophyte formation, substantial joint space narrowing (>50%), significant stiffness with pain at extreme ROM but not at midrange
- Grade IV—same as III but with pain at midrange of passive motion
- Subtalar, TN, CC joints
- Tenderness at the sinus tarsi (subtalar joint), dorsal TN joint, and/or lateral column
- Pain with passive hindfoot inversion/eversion (subtalar), midfoot ROM (TN, CC)
- Radiographs show varying severity of joint space narrowing and osteophyte formation.

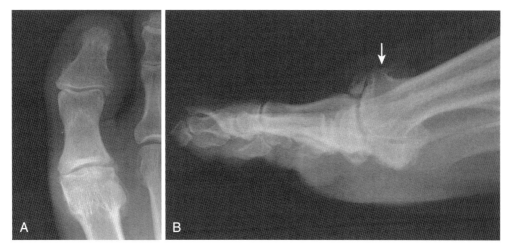

FIGURE 6-79 Hallux rigidus. **A,** Posteroanterior radiograph of the great toe shows cartilage space narrowing and hypertrophic lipping. **B,** The lateral radiograph shows a prominent dorsal osteophyte (arrow). (From Weissman B: *Imaging of arthritis and metabolic bone disease,* Philadelphia, 2009, Elsevier.)

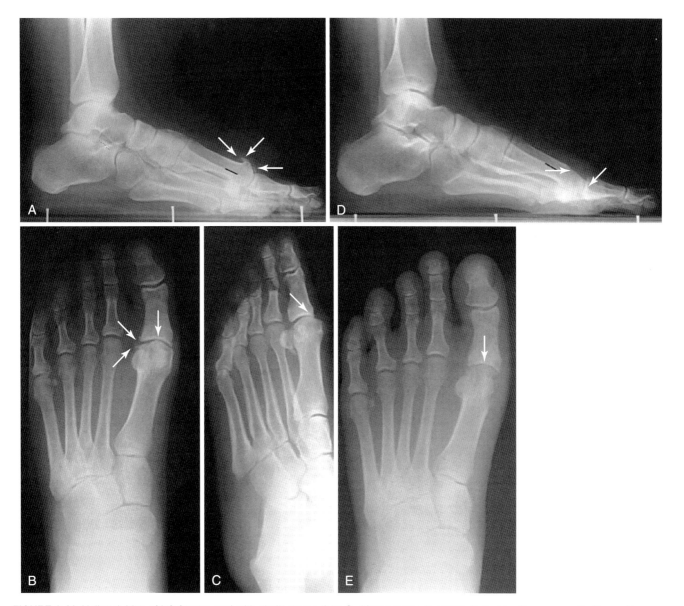

FIGURE 6-80 Hallux rigidus of left foot treated with cheilectomy. **A** to **C,** After surgery. **D** and **E,** One year after surgery. Radiographic hallmarks of hallux rigidus denoted by white arrows (dorsal osteophyte **[A]** and joint space narrowing **[B** and **C]**). Postoperative radiograph after cheilectomy (*white arrow;* **D**) with diminished but preserved joint space (*white arrow;* **E**). (From Canale ST, Beaty J: *Campbell's operative orthopaedics,* ed 11, Philadelphia, 2007, Elsevier.)

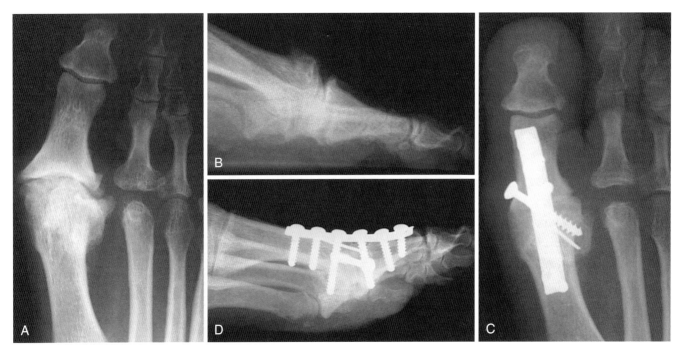

FIGURE 6-81 Fusion for severe hallux rigidus. **A** and **B,** Preoperative radiographs. **C** and **D,** Postoperative radiographs. (From Coughlin MJ et al: *Surgery of the foot and ankle,* ed 8, Philadelphia, 2006, Mosby.)

- **Grades III and IV (pain throughout ROM with positive grind)—best treated with arthrodesis** (Figure 6-81)
  - Position—neutral rotation, 10 to 15 degrees of dorsiflexion, and 5 degrees valgus
- Interposition arthroplasty with varying results— reserved for younger patients who require preserved hallux ROM
- Implant arthroplasty not recommended owing to poor results
  - **Silicone arthroplasty can result in a heavy synovitis with destruction of the joint.**
    - Isolated pain within the great toe
      - Removal of implant with synovectomy only is successful in providing pain relief.
    - Great toe pain with lesser metatarsalgia
      - Implant removal with bone grafting and arthrodesis to restore function of the great toe
- Midfoot joints
  - Midfoot arthrodesis is the treatment of choice.
    - In the setting of deformity (flatfoot) the joints must be reduced into an anatomic position to achieve a satisfactory result (realignment arthrodesis) (Figure 6-82).
    - *Medial column arthrodesis* **refers to fusion of both the NC and first TMT joints, occasionally required for a flatfoot deformity to stabilize the collapsed midfoot and restore the lateral–first TMT angle.**
      - In situ fusion in the setting of a deformity will predictably lead to a poor result.
- Hindfoot (ST, TN, CC) joints
  - **Arthrodesis of single joints leads to significant limitation in hindfoot inversion/eversion (TN > ST > CC).**

- Isolated TN fusion has a high rate of nonunion, and given the significant restriction of hindfoot motion from a TN fusion, an ST fusion is commonly performed in addition to ensure a union without causing any incremental functional deficit.
- Triple arthrodesis is also an appropriate option. If the CC joint is unaffected, it is more common to *not* include the CC joint in the arthrodesis ("medial double"). This is also an appropriate option for patients with compromise of the lateral soft tissues, which may increase the risk of wound complications or infection, because the approach can be performed through a single medial incision.
- Triple arthrodesis is usually performed to correct arthritis secondary to deformity (Figure 6-83).
  - Position—0 to 5 degrees of hindfoot valgus, neutral abduction/adduction, plantigrade (both the first and fifth metatarsal evenly strike the ground)
  - **Revision of a malunited triple arthrodesis requires:**
    - **Calcaneal osteotomy (corrects varus or valgus)**
    - **Transverse tarsal osteotomy (allows rotation of the foot into a plantigrade position)**
    - **Wedge resection can correct abduction (medial wedge) or adduction (lateral wedge).**
- Subtalar arthrodesis
  - Indications:
    - Subtalar DJD
    - Calcaneus fracture (Sanders IV) or late sequelae
    - Posttraumatic DJD secondary talus fracture (no deformity) (Figure 6-84)
    - Talocalcaneal coalition
    - Subtalar DJD
  - Increased nonunion rate with history of ankle arthrodesis or smoking; nonunion rate higher with prior ankle arthrodesis than with nicotine use

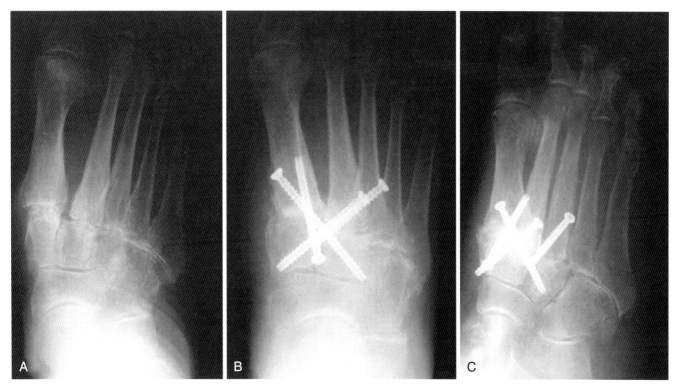

FIGURE 6-82 **A,** This posttraumatic deformity involved the entire midfoot, with all three columns seemingly affected. Despite the severity of the deformity, only the medial and middle columns were clinically symptomatic. **B** and **C,** Arthrodesis was performed with realignment and screw fixation. (From Myerson MS: *Reconstructive foot and ankle surgery: management of complications,* ed 2, Philadelphia, 2010, Elsevier.)

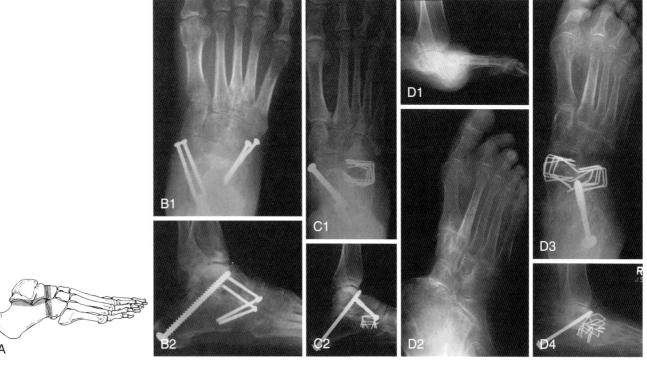

FIGURE 6-83 Triple arthrodesis, methods of internal fixation. **A,** Diagram of triple arthrodesis. **B,** Postoperative radiograph demonstrating triple arthrodesis with anatomic restoration of foot posture. **C,** Triple arthrodesis using 7.0-mm cannulated screws for the subtalar and talonavicular joints and multiple power staples for the calcaneocuboid joint. **D,** Correction of severe hindfoot deformity secondary to long-standing posterior tibial tendon dysfunction with restoration of the longitudinal arch using a 7.0-mm cannulated screw for the subtalar joint and power staples for the talonavicular and calcaneocuboid joints. Note that the height of the longitudinal arch has been restored and severe abduction of the foot is corrected. (From Coughlin MJ et al: *Surgery of the foot and ankle,* ed 8, Philadelphia, 2006, Mosby.)

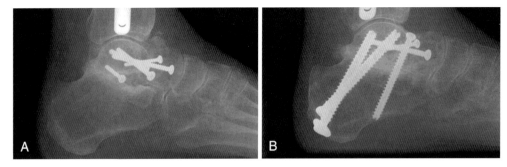

FIGURE 6-84 A, Preoperative radiograph of a patient with subtalar arthritis, the most common complication following a talus fracture. Importantly, the patient did not have a varus deformity with shortening of the medial column. **B,** Postoperative radiograph demonstrates a subtalar fusion that eliminated the patient's pain. If the patient had had a varus deformity, a triple arthrodesis would have been required.

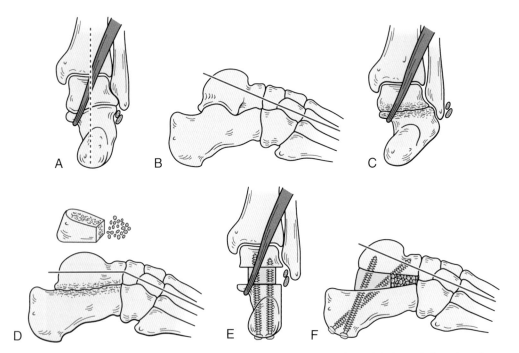

FIGURE 6-85 Subtalar fusion with distraction. **A,** The dashed line shows the alignment of the tibia through the tuber, the area where the flexor hallucis longus crosses at the back of the joint, and the location of the peroneal tendons under the fibular tip. **B,** Normal alignment of the subtalar joint and inclination of the talus are depicted. Notice that the all-important midaxial line of the talus continues directly through the midfoot and the apex of the first metatarsal in the medial column. **C,** After a typical high-energy calcaneal crush injury, the tuber is angled into varus while the lateral wall is angled and has exploded laterally toward valgus and impinges on the distal fibula, pushing the peroneal tendons out of their normal position. The subtalar joint is crushed and the hindfoot has lost height. **D,** The inclination of the talus is out of line with the medial column and markedly limits the range of dorsiflexion in the anterior dome of the talus. A wedge of posterior iliac crest tricortical bone will be used to open the talocalcaneal joint and restore height. **E,** Two large 6.5-mm bolts or fully threaded screws are positioned much as they would be for subtalar arthrodesis in situ. In this case, however, they serve as positioning screws rather than lag screws and maintain distraction of the talus from the calcaneus instead of compressing the graft. The exploded lateral wall is excised and the tuber repositioned with less varus tilt and in slight valgus alignment to the weight-bearing line of the tibia. **F,** Reconstruction restores ideal talar inclination and talar–naviculocuneiform–first metatarsal axial alignment. An anteroposterior radiographic view of the foot should be taken intraoperatively to ensure that the talocalcaneal alignment is correct in the transverse plane and that the foot is not significantly pronated or supinated. (From Browner B et al: *Skeletal trauma,* ed 4, Philadelphia, 2008, Elsevier. Adapted and redrawn from Hansen ST Jr: *Functional reconstruction of the foot and ankle,* Philadelphia, 2000, Lippincott Williams & Wilkins.)

- Subtalar bone-block arthrodesis (Figure 6-85)
  - Prior calcaneal fracture with loss of height
    - Results in anterior impingement, complaints of anterior ankle pain with ambulation in addition to hindfoot pain
  - Autograft or allograft bone block arthrodesis restores the height of the calcaneus.
    - Less successful at correcting residual hindfoot varus

- Tibiotalar joint
  - Arthrodesis provides excellent pain relief but also results in some restricted function (Figure 6-86).
    - Position—neutral dorsiflexion (90 degrees), 0 to 5 degrees hindfoot valgus, 5 to 10 degrees external rotation
      - Valgus and external rotation keep the hindfoot unlocked to allow for accommodative hindfoot motion.

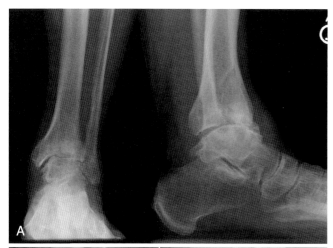

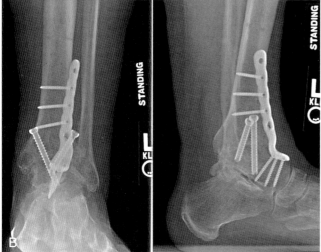

FIGURE 6-86 Preoperative anteroposterior and lateral radiographs of a patient with end-stage ankle arthritis **(A).** An ankle fusion was performed with an anterior plate and cross screws **(B).** The method of fixation is not as critical as ensuring a neutral clinical position of the ankle.

- Leads to radiographic arthritis in surrounding foot joints
  - Subtalar joint is the most common location of adjacent joint arthritis.
  - No evidence to show causation or progress of knee or hip arthritis
- Total ankle arthroplasty outcomes improving and are no longer considered experimental.
  - Pain relief equivalent to arthrodesis, function and gait slightly improved, higher risk of revision surgery
  - **Ankle replacement has shown the best outcome in patients with osteoarthritis.**
    - Superior to that shown in patients with rheumatoid or posttraumatic etiology
  - Syndesmotic fusion associated with decreased rate of failure with the Agility Ankle Replacement
    - Current generation of implants preserve the syndesmosis and distal fibula.
  - Newer-generation implants retain ligamentous and bony stabilizers and require careful anatomic balancing.
  - Salvage of failed implants is difficult given the amount of bone loss and current lack of available revision components. The most reliable current technique is a bone-block ankle arthrodesis (femoral head) with or without additional subtalar fusion.
  - Contraindications include severe coronal plane deformity, AVN, Charcot arthropathy, young age, history of infection.
- Distraction arthroplasty using thin-wire external fixation—limited role; may be option in younger patients with preserved ankle ROM
- Bipolar osteochondral allograft transplantation—limited data and high failure rates in most series

SECTION 13 POSTURAL DISORDERS

PES PLANUS (FLATFOOT DEFORMITY)

- ■ May be congenital (see Chapter 3, Pediatric Orthopaedics) or acquired (also called *adult-acquired flatfoot deformity* [AAFD])
- ■ Important to determine whether the deformity is flexible or fixed
- ▥ Fixed or rigid deformity requires a triple arthrodesis.
- ■ Pathology
- ▥ Most common cause of AAFD is PTTD.
  - PTT is the primary dynamic support for the arch.
  - PTT fires after the foot is flat to generate heel rise and lock the transverse tarsal joint for a rigid, stable foot during push-off.
  - Etiology of PTTD is multifactorial and includes:
    - Zone of hypovascularity 2 to 6 cm proximal to the PTT insertion on the navicular.

- Overload of the arch from activity or obesity
- Inflammatory disorders such as RA
- ▥ The spring (calcaneonavicular) ligament is the primary static stabilizer of the TN joint.
  - Incompetence of the spring ligament is associated with increased flatfoot deformity.
  - Isolated acute rupture of the spring ligament has been reported to cause an acute deformity without disease of the PTT.
  - Reconstruction of the spring ligament with allograft or autograft as an adjunct to standard flatfoot reconstruction has shown success in early series.
- ▥ Diagnosis
- ▥ **Patients complain of medial ankle/foot pain early, progressive loss of arch, and lateral ankle pain late (subfibular impingement).**

- Physical examination
  - Standing examination demonstrates asymmetric hindfoot valgus, depressed arch, and an abducted forefoot.
    - "Too many toes" when the foot is viewed posteriorly (Figure 6-87)
    - **Pain or inability to perform single-limb heel rise indicates insufficient PTT.**
  - Determine whether deformity is flexible (passively correctable to a plantigrade foot) or fixed (rigid deformity that is not passively correctable).
- Radiographs (Figure 6-88)
  - Pes planus indicated by negative lateral talo–first metatarsal angle (Meary angle)
  - Forefoot abduction indicated by TN uncoverage
- **Treatment—based upon stage of the deformity**
- Stage I—synovitis without deformity
  - Nonoperative
    - Immobilization (cast or boot)
    - Orthotic after acute swelling and pain subsided
      - Arch support with medial heel wedge
  - Operative
    - Synovectomy of PTT

- Stage II—flexible deformity is the critical feature; PTT is degenerated and functionally incompetent.
  - **Nonoperative**
    - **AFO in conjunction with physical therapy has demonstrated the highest success rate.**
    - Use of a full-length orthotic with an arch support, medial heel wedge, and medial forefoot support (if supination/forefoot varus present) is used after acute pain has resolved.
    - A lace-up ankle brace may also be used.
  - Operative
    - **Correction of all stage II deformities includes a tendon transfer (FDL or FHL) into the navicular to reconstruct the PTT.**
    - Presence of a gastrocnemius contracture should be assessed for and corrected with a gastrocnemius recession if present.
    - Stage IIA—defined by hindfoot valgus without significant forefoot abduction (<40% uncovering of the talus)
      - **Medial slide calcaneal osteotomy** (Figure 6-89)
    - Stage IIB—defined by forefoot abduction (>40% talar uncovering) in addition to hindfoot valgus
      - Lateral column lengthening (Figure 6-90)
      - Additional medial slide calcaneal osteotomy may be required.
    - Stage IIC—defined by fixed forefoot supination/varus (first ray is elevated after correction of the hindfoot

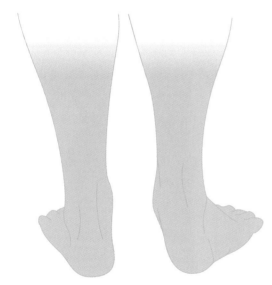

FIGURE 6-87 Patients with tendon ruptures have either a unilateral flatfoot or, in those who had previous flat feet, a relatively flatter foot on the involved side. Excessive forefoot abduction also can be suspected from posterior observation when more toes are visible lateral to the patient's heel on the involved side. This finding is called the *too-many-toes sign*. (From DeLee J: *DeLee and Drez's orthopaedic sports medicine,* ed 3, Philadelphia, 2011, Saunders.)

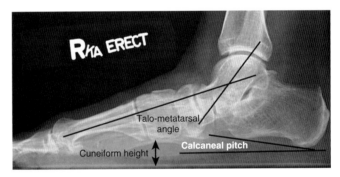

FIGURE 6-88 The lateral foot radiograph images the loss of alignment between the first metatarsal and midfoot. A talo–first metatarsal angle greater than 4 degrees signifies pes planus (as shown, 32 degrees). The calcaneal pitch angle is also determined on the lateral radiograph; a normal angle is between 17 and 32 degrees (12 degrees in this patient). Arch height loss is documented by a decrease in this angle. A loss of medial cuneiform–floor height is also indicative of loss of arch height. This is shown by the black arrow. (From DiGiovanni C: *Core knowledge in orthopaedics—foot and ankle,* Philadelphia, 2007, Elsevier.)

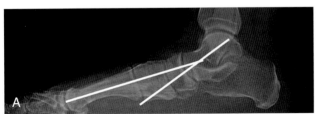
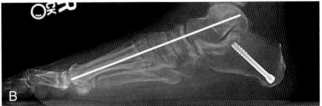

FIGURE 6-89 A, Preoperative radiograph of a patient with stage II posterior tibial tendon dysfunction. Note the break in the lateral talo–first metatarsal angle centered at the talonavicular joint. **B,** Excellent correction is noted on the postoperative radiograph, with restoration of the lateral talo–first metatarsal angle with colinearity of the first metatarsal and the talus.

to neutral) in addition to hindfoot valgus (Figure 6-91). Forefoot abduction may also be present.

- Stable medial column—navicular is colinear with first metatarsal.
  - **Cotton osteotomy (dorsal opening wedge osteotomy of the cuneiform) to plantar flex the first ray**
- Unstable medial column—plantar sag at NC or first TMT joint
  - Medial column fusion (based upon point of collapse)
    - Isolated first TMT fusion
    - Isolated NC fusion
    - Combined NC and TMT fusion (both joints are involved radiographically)
- Hindfoot treated based upon talar uncovering
  - Less than 40%—medial slide calcaneal osteotomy
  - More than 40%—lateral column lengthening and possible medial slide calcaneal osteotomy if residual hindfoot valgus
- **Stage II surgical summary**
  - **FDL or FHL tendon transfer for ALL patients**
  - **Gastrocnemius recession if contracture present**
  - **Hindfoot valgus—medial slide calcaneal osteotomy**
  - **Forefoot abduction—lateral column lengthening**

- Forefoot supination
  - **Stable medial column—Cotton osteotomy**
  - Unstable medial column—first TMT arthrodesis
- Stage III—defined by a fixed/rigid pes planovalgus deformity
  - Nonoperative
    - Accommodative rigid AFO or Arizona brace. Do *not* attempt to correct the deformity—increased risk of pain and pressure points, leading to ulceration.
  - Operative
    - Triple arthrodesis
    - Additional medial column stabilization is occasionally required for severe deformities (Figure 6-92)
    - TAL if equinus contracture present
- Stage IV—defined by incompetence of the deltoid ligament; standing AP ankle radiograph demonstrates lateral talar tilt (valgus) or ankle arthritis.
  - If the ankle valgus is passively correctable with minimal degenerative changes, an attempt can be made at deltoid ligament reconstruction with hindfoot reconstruction.
  - Rigid deformity or progressive arthritis requires TTC arthrodesis (Figure 6-93).
  - The most reliable operation for a stage IV deformity is a TTC fusion.

PES CAVUS DEFORMITY

- **Defined by a high-arched foot, often with associated heel varus (cavovarus)**
- **Pathology**
- Neuromuscular
  - Unilateral—rule out tethering of the spinal cord or spinal cord tumors.
  - Bilateral—most commonly Charcot-Marie-Tooth (see the section Neurologic Disorders)

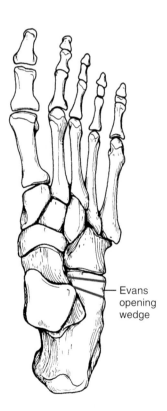

FIGURE 6-90 Evans anterior calcaneal osteotomy helps restore and stabilize longitudinal arch by elongating lateral column of foot. (From Coughlin M et al: *Surgery of the foot and ankle,* ed 8, Philadelphia, 2006, Elsevier. Modified from Pedowitz WJ, Kovatis P: Flatfoot in the adult, *J Am Acad Orthop Surg* 3:293, 1995.)

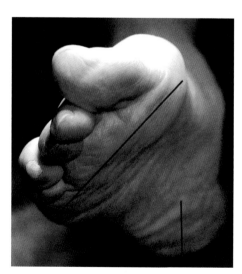

FIGURE 6-91 Demonstration of forefoot varus. The degree of forefoot varus is determined by placing the heel in neutral position, covering the head of the talus with the navicular, and then observing the relationship of the metatarsal heads to the neutral hindfoot. In fixed forefoot varus, the lateral border of the foot is more plantar flexed than the medial border. (From Coughlin MJ et al: *Surgery of the foot and ankle,* ed 8, Philadelphia, 2006, Mosby.)

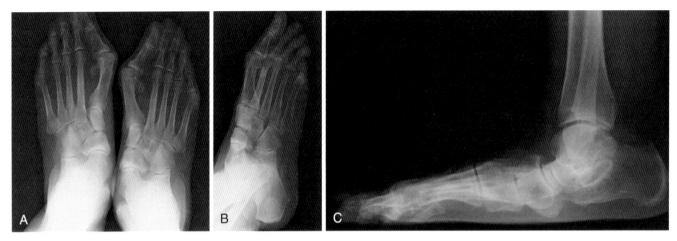

FIGURE 6-92 A to **C,** Rigid flatfoot deformity before treatment with a triple arthrodesis. (From Myerson MS: *Reconstructive foot and ankle surgery: management of complications,* ed 2, Philadelphia, 2010, Elsevier. [Photos courtesy John Campbell, MD, Baltimore, Md.])

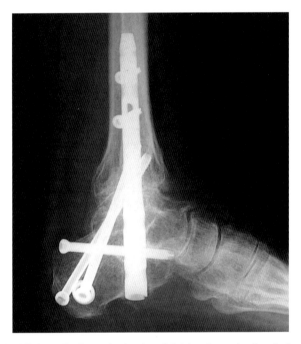

FIGURE 6-93 Radiograph showing tibiotalocalcaneal arthrodesis for involvement of the ankle and subtalar joints performed with an intramedullary device and augmented with screw fixation. (From DiGiovanni C: *Core knowledge in orthopaedics—foot and ankle,* Philadelphia, 2007, Elsevier.)

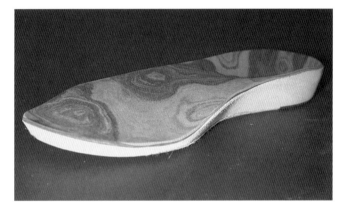

FIGURE 6-94 Cavus foot orthotic. Note the hollowed-out recess under the first metatarsal head and the laterally based forefoot wedge and lowered medial arch. (From DiGiovanni C: *Core knowledge in orthopaedics—foot and ankle,* Philadelphia, 2007, Elsevier.)

- Idiopathic—usually subtle, bilateral
- Traumatic—secondary to talus fracture malunion, compartment syndrome, crush injury
- ■ **Diagnosis**
- Patients complain of painful calluses under the first metatarsal, fifth metatarsal, and medial heel.
  - Secondary to the plantar-flexed first ray and varus hindfoot
- Often associated with lateral ankle ligament instability, peroneal tendon pathology
- ■ **Coleman block test used to assess flexibility of the hindfoot (out of varus) when the first**

metatarsal plantar flexion (forefoot valgus) is eliminated.
- Wooden block placed just lateral to the first ray; first metatarsal head then lies off the block, with remainder of block on the weight-bearing foot.
- If the hindfoot passively corrects into valgus, the deformity is forefoot driven (due to plantar-flexed first ray).
- ■ **Treatment**
- Nonoperative—orthotics with lateral heel wedge, decreased arch, and depressed first ray may be effective (Figure 6-94).
- Operative
  - **Forefoot-driven deformity—first metatarsal dorsiflexion osteotomy is indicated.**
  - With no or incomplete correction of the hindfoot with the Coleman block test, a lateral calcaneal closing wedge osteotomy (Figure 6-95) is indicated in addition to a dorsiflexion osteotomy of the first metatarsal (Figure 6-96).
    - A subtalar fusion or triple arthrodesis may be needed if arthritic symptoms are present.

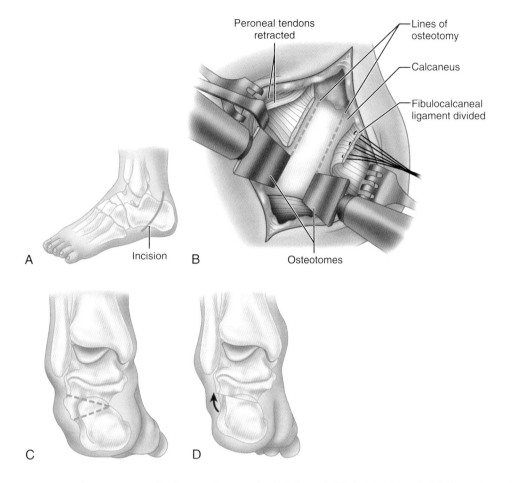

FIGURE 6-95 Dwyer closed-wedge osteotomy of calcaneus for varus heel. **A,** Lateral skin incision is made inferior and parallel to peroneal tendons. **B,** Wedge of bone is resected with its base laterally. **C,** Wedge of bone is tapered medially. **D,** Calcaneus is closed after bone has been removed, and varus deformity is corrected to slight valgus. (From Canale ST, Beaty J: *Campbell's operative orthopaedics,* ed 11, Philadelphia, 2007, Elsevier.)

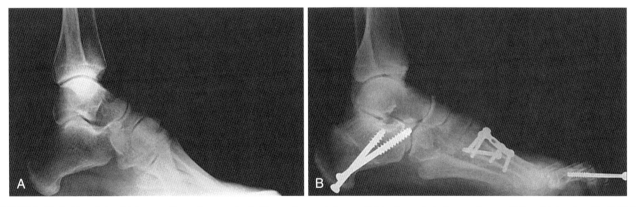

FIGURE 6-96 A, True lateral talar position of cavus foot. The radiograph is parallel to the axis between the medial and lateral malleoli. This view clearly shows the relationship of the talus to the calcaneus and the relative amount of dorsiflexion of the talus to the tibia. This view, however, distorts the forefoot, making the first metatarsal appear vertical. **B,** Postoperative radiograph demonstrates corrections of the foot. Hindfoot was repaired with a calcaneal slide transfixed with two screws. Note the slight cephalad positioning of the posterior fragment of the calcaneus. A majority of the correction was achieved by sliding this fragment laterally (out of varus). Midfoot was corrected with internal fixation with a dorsal closed-wedge osteotomy of the first metatarsal. In the forefoot correction, a single screw transfixes the interphalangeal joint of the hallux. The lesser toes were not corrected in this case. (From Coughlin MJ et al: *Surgery of the foot and ankle,* ed 8, Philadelphia, 2006, Mosby.)

SECTION 14 TENDON DISORDERS

ACHILLES TENDON

- The Achilles tendon is addressed in the section on heel pain.

PERONEAL TENDONS

- Most common disorders include tendinitis/tenosynovitis and tendon subluxation/dislocation, which often causes peroneus brevis degenerative tears.
- Diagnosis
- Acute or chronic localized swelling and tenderness over peroneal tendons
- **Common cause for chronic pain following an ankle sprain or chronic instability**
- Associated with cavovarus foot deformity
- Peroneal subluxation or dislocation
  - **Caused by forced eversion and dorsiflexion, leading to disruption of superior peroneal retinaculum (SPR)**
  - Pain and/or sensation of snapping in the retrofibular groove
  - Often causes peroneus brevis degenerative tears
  - Sudden dorsiflexion while downhill skiing is a common report.
  - Plain radiographs may demonstrate a rim fracture of the lateral aspect of the distal fibula.
- Acute rupture of the peroneus longus tendon at or through a fracture of the os peroneum can occur.
  - Radiographs show a retraction or fracture of the os peroneum.
- Treatment
- Nonoperative treatment
  - Chronic peroneal tendinosis or tenosynovitis is initially treated with activity modification, NSAIDs, lace-up ankle brace, and physical therapy.
  - Ultrasound or MRI can be used to aid diagnosis (Figure 6-97).
    - Ultrasound useful as dynamic tool to evaluate subluxation/dislocation.
    - False-positive results showing longitudinal tears common with MRI
- Operative treatment—based on the pathology
  - Tenosynovectomy, débridement, and repair of degenerative tears (usually peroneus brevis)
    - Synovitis or less than 50% diseased tendon
    - Groove deepening if shallow fibular groove
  - Excision and tenodesis
    - Required when there is a complete rupture or severely degenerative tendon (>50%) that prohibits repair
  - Hindfoot varus
    - Dwyer osteotomy (lateral closing wedge osteotomy of the calcaneus)
      - Limits risk of recurrent tears and continued pain
  - Peroneal subluxation or dislocation
    - Chronic
      - Requires repair/reconstruction of the SPR and fibular groove deepening
    - Acute
      - SPR repair/reconstruction

- Tendon transfer to fifth metatarsal
  - Over 50% degeneration of both peroneus longus and brevis requires excision of both tendons.
  - Good results reported with both lateral transfer of the FHL or FDL and allograft
  - Allograft may be used if peroneal muscles demonstrate adequate excursion at the time of surgery.

POSTERIOR TIBIAL TENDON

- The posterior tibial tendon is addressed in the section on pes planus deformity.

ANTERIOR TIBIAL TENDON

- Tenosynovitis uncommon but can be observed in patients with inflammatory arthritis
- NSAIDs and walking cast or boot recommended
- Corticosteroid injections may provide relief but increase the risk of tendon rupture.
- Complete ruptures rare—mainly occur in older patients
- Commonly missed diagnosis
- **Presents as painless anterior ankle mass**
- Foot drop may be subtle because of recruitment of toe extensors.
- **Primary repair generally improves functional results regardless of age.**
- **Interpositional graft may be required in delayed cases.**

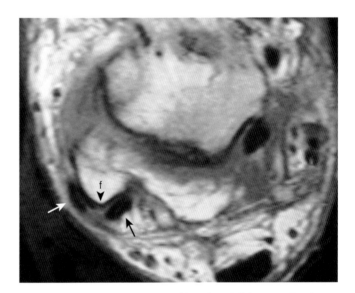

FIGURE 6-97 Peroneal tendon subluxation. Axial proton density MRI shows longitudinally torn peroneus brevis *(white arrow)* subluxed laterally and anteriorly from its normal position adjacent to the peroneus longus *(black arrow).* Note that the distal fibula has a rounded contour *(small black arrowhead),* a finding that can be associated with peroneal subluxation. *f,* Fibula. (From Manaster BJ et al: *Musculoskeletal imaging—the requisites,* ed 3, Philadelphia, 2006, Elsevier.)

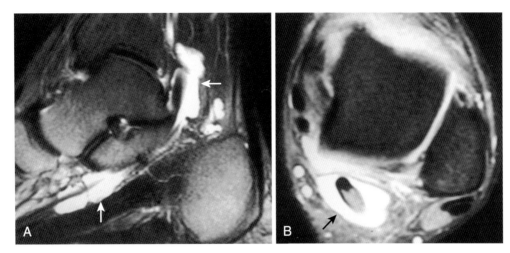

FIGURE 6-98 Abnormalities of the flexor hallucis longus tendon: tenosynovitis. Sagittal (TR/TE, 3400/98) **(A)** and transverse (TR/TE, 4000/14) **(B)** fast spin-echo MRIs reveal considerable fluid within the sheath *(arrows)* about the flexor hallucis longus tendon. The amount of fluid is out of proportion to that present in the ankle joint. (From Resnick D: *Internal derangements of joints*, ed 2, Philadelphia, 2006, Saunders.)

FLEXOR HALLUCIS LONGUS

- **Stenosing FHL tenosynovitis**
- Usually seen in dancers on pointe and gymnasts
- Posterior ankle pain, triggering of the hallux interphalangeal joint, and pain with resisted hallux plantar flexion
- Stenosis occurs along course of FHL between the posterolateral and posteromedial tubercles of the talus.

- MRI is the diagnostic modality of choice.
  - Fluid (high signal intensity) will be noted surrounding the FHL at the level of the ankle joint (Figure 6-98).
- **Nonoperative treatment—activity modification, consider boot immobilization for short period of rest, NSAIDs.**
- **Operative treatment—open (posteromedial approach) or arthroscopic FHL tenosynovectomy and release of the fascia**

SECTION 15 HEEL PAIN

PLANTAR HEEL PAIN

- **Plantar fasciitis**
- Definition
  - Painful heel condition that can affect both sedentary and active individuals and is most often seen in the adult population
  - Associated with a contracture of the gastrocnemius-soleus complex
- Pathology
  - Likely involves microtears at the origin of the plantar fascia, which initiates inflammation and an injury-repair process that leads to a traction osteophyte
  - 90% to 95% of patients will improve within a year regardless of the specific treatment offered.
- Diagnosis
  - Exquisite pain and tenderness over the plantar medial tuberosity of the calcaneus at the proximal insertion of the plantar fascia
  - Classic symptoms include pain with the first step in the morning and after prolonged sitting.
  - Bilateral symptoms are common.
  - Small subset of patients may experience pain and tenderness at the origin of the abductor hallucis, which may indicate entrapment or inflammation of the first branch of the lateral plantar nerve.

- Nonoperative treatment
  - **Plantar fascia–specific stretching protocols and Achilles tendon (heel cord) stretching are the key to effective nonoperative management.**
  - **Also includes cushioned heel inserts, night splints, physical therapy, walking casts, and antiinflammatory medications**
  - Cortisone injections may relieve pain but are associated with attenuation or rupture of the plantar fascia, fat atrophy.
  - Platelet rich plasma injections and low-intensity extracorporeal shock wave therapy (ESWT) have demonstrated success in limited studies.
- Operative treatment
  - Limited release of the plantar fascia (medial half) may be necessary in refractory cases.
    - Complete release can place the longitudinal arch of the foot at risk, overload the lateral column, and lead to dorsolateral foot pain and metatarsal stress fractures.
    - Concomitant release of the deep fascia of the abductor hallucis may relieve entrapment of the lateral plantar nerve and improve the surgical result (Figure 6-99).
    - Gastrocnemius recession has been advocated, with varied results.

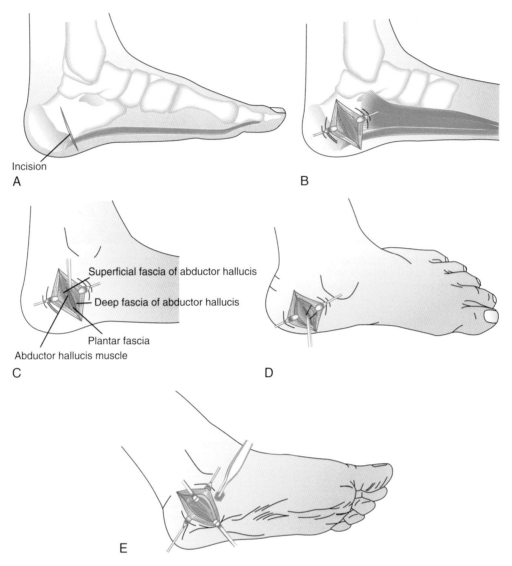

FIGURE 6-99 Plantar fascia and nerve release. **A,** Incision. **B,** Release of the abductor hallucis muscle. **C,** Abductor hallucis muscle is reflected proximally. **D,** Abductor hallucis is retracted distally. **E,** Resection of small medial portion of the plantar fascia. (From DeLee J: *DeLee and Drez's orthopaedic sports medicine,* ed 3, Philadelphia, 2011, Saunders.)

■ **Baxter neuritis (compression of first branch of lateral plantar nerve)**
■ Definition
  • Baxter neuritis presents as plantar medial heel pain that can be difficult to differentiate from plantar fasciitis.
  • Associated with athletes involved in running sports
  • Diagnosis
  • **Pain more medial over abductor hallucis (as compared to the more plantar pain seen with plantar fasciitis)**
  • Compression over Baxter nerve will reproduce the pain and may cause radiation into the plantar lateral foot.
  • Diagnostic tests
    • EMG/nerve conduction velocity (NCV) may demonstrate increased motor latency within the abductor digiti quinti.
    • MRI may demonstrate fatty infiltration of the abductor digiti quinti, best seen on the coronal views.

  ▨ Nonoperative treatment
    • Heel cord stretching and cushioned heel inserts
  ▨ Operative treatment
    • **Open release of Baxter nerve must include release of the deep fascia of the abductor hallucis.**
■ **Bony causes**
▨ **Calcaneal stress fractures**
    • **Most common in the active individual or military recruit**
    • **MRI typically used to aid diagnosis.**
    • **Treat with rest, protected weight bearing (cast, CAM walker).**
▨ Periostitis
    • Pain and tenderness in the central portion of the heel pad
    • Represents traumatic periosteal or bursal inflammation secondary to a known injury or atrophic heel pad
    • Treat with cushioned shoe inserts or a short course in a well-padded cast.
    • The examiner should be vigilant for other signs or symptoms suggesting inflammatory arthritis.

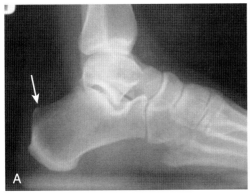
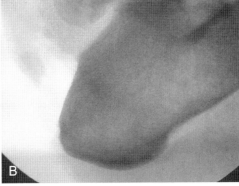

FIGURE 6-100 Preoperative **(A)** and intraoperative **(B)** radiographs of Haglund deformity *(arrow)*. (From Porter D, Schon L: *Baxter's the foot and ankle in sport,* ed 2, Philadelphia, 2007, Elsevier.)

▦ Sever disease
  • Also referred to as *calcaneal apophysitis*
  • More common in boys; typically appears between age 10 and 14 years, prior to closure of calcaneal apophysis and just before or during a growth spurt
  • Treatment includes activity modification, gastrocnemius stretching, and cushioned heel orthotics.
  • No correlation with symptoms and fragmentation of apophysis

ACHILLES DISORDERS

▦ Definition
▦ The Achilles tendon (comprising the gastrocnemius and soleus tendons) rotates 90 degrees laterally to insert on the posterior aspect of the calcaneal tuberosity.
▦ The retrocalcaneal bursa lies between the anterior surface of the Achilles tendon and the posterosuperior aspect of the calcaneus.
▦ *Haglund deformity* refers to an enlarged prominence of the posterosuperior calcaneal tuberosity.
▦ The Achilles accepts 2000 to 7000 N of stress, depending on the applied load, and transfers forces of 6 to 10 times body weight during a running stride.

▦ Physical examination
▦ Bony prominence, tendon thickening, and area of tenderness should be evaluated.
▦ The Silfverskiöld test evaluates for contracture.
  • Test ankle dorsiflexion with the knee extended and flexed and the hindfoot in neutral position.
  • Tightness in both knee flexion and extension indicates Achilles contracture.
  • Improvement in ankle dorsiflexion with knee flexion (relaxing the gastrocnemius origin proximal to the knee) indicates isolated gastrocnemius contracture.

▦ Retrocalcaneal bursitis/Haglund deformity
▦ Inflammation of the retrocalcaneal bursa that often occurs along with insertional tendinopathy and Haglund deformity
▦ Diagnosis
  • Patients present with deep posterior heel pain, fullness and tenderness with palpation medial and lateral to the tendon, and increased pain with ankle dorsiflexion.
  • Symptoms often seen in conjunction with insertional Achilles tendinopathy

  • Lateral foot radiographs will demonstrate Haglund deformity.
  • MRI is rarely necessary to make the diagnosis.
▦ Nonoperative treatment
  • NSAIDs, external padding, ice, heel-lift orthotics, and shoewear modification
  • Steroid injection should be avoided owing to inherent risk of Achilles rupture.
▦ Operative treatment—includes débridement of inflamed retrocalcaneal bursa along with excision of Haglund deformity when present (Figure 6-100)

▦ Insertional Achilles tendinopathy
▦ Degenerative process showing disorganized collagen and mucoid degeneration with minimal inflammatory cells
  • *Tendinopathy* is preferred description
▦ Comprises approximately one fourth of Achilles tendinopathy cases
▦ Diagnosis
  • Patients complain of pain, swelling, burning, and stiffness in the posterior heel.
  • Progressive enlargement of the bony prominence of the heel, along with pain caused by direct pressure from shoewear is common.
  • Tenderness localized to the Achilles tendon insertion on the posterior calcaneus, most often midline
  • Radiographic evaluation
    • Bone spur and intratendinous calcification seen on lateral foot radiograph (Figure 6-101)
    • MRI and ultrasound can be helpful to determine extent of Achilles tendon degeneration.
▦ Nonoperative treatment
  • **Activity and shoewear modification, heel lifts, stretching, physical therapy with eccentric training,** and silicone heel sleeves/pads to decrease pain from direct pressure are mainstays of conservative treatment.
  • Although it has been used, extracorporeal shockwave therapy lacks definitive data to support its use.
  • Steroid injections should be avoided.
  • Nonoperative treatment beneficial in approximately 50% to 70% of cases
▦ Operative treatment
  • Includes excision of retrocalcaneal bursa, resection of prominent superior calcaneal tuberosity, and débridement of degenerative tendon including calcification

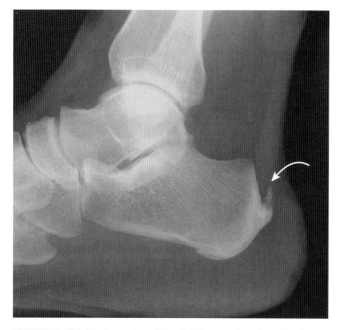

FIGURE 6-101 Radiography of the Achilles tendon. Insertional tendinosis. The distal tendon is thickened at its site of insertion onto the calcaneus, and an insertional enthesophyte has formed *(curved arrow)*. (From Weissman B: *Imaging of arthritis and metabolic bone disease,* Philadelphia, 2009, Elsevier.)

- If tendon detachment (>50%) is required for thorough débridement, reattachment with suture anchors is indicated.
- Lateral, midline, and medial J-shaped incisions have all been described.
- **FHL tendon transfer is indicated if more than 50% of the Achilles tendon requires excision** (Figure 6-102).

■ **Noninsertional Achilles tendinopathy**

▦ Includes inflammation of the paratenon alone, peritendinitis with a component of tendon thickening (commonly referred to as *tendinosis*), or tendinosis alone

▦ Multifactorial etiology includes overuse, mechanical imbalance, poor tissue vascularity and genetic predisposition, and fluoroquinolone antibiotics.

▦ Thought to involve the response to microscopic tearing of the tendon
  - Abnormal vascularization of the ventral mesotenal vessels 2 to 6 cm proximal to the insertion limits blood flow to diseased tissue and decreases capacity for healing.

▦ Accounts for nearly half of all Achilles tendinopathy cases

 ▦ Diagnosis
  - Patients often present with pain, swelling, and impaired performance, especially with running.
  - Tender area of fusiform thickening localized approximately 2 to 6 cm proximal to the insertion of the tendon
  - MRI will demonstrate thickening of the tendon, with intrasubstance intermediate signal intensity consistent with the disorganized tissue. In the setting of a chronic rupture, a large gap will be present between the hypoechoic (dark) tendon ends (Figure 6-103).

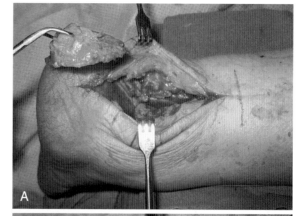

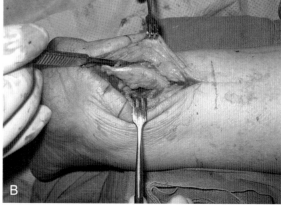

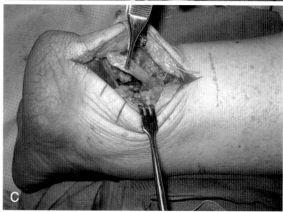

FIGURE 6-102 When the Achilles is degenerative at the insertion and proximally or when more than 50% of the tendon is involved, a flexor hallucis longus (FHL) graft should be considered **(A)**. The central approach is used to detach the Achilles posteriorly, and the prominent bone is resected **(B)**. The degenerative tendon is débrided **(C)**. The FHL tendon is harvested from behind the ankle and will be reattached through a tunnel or into a trough before repairing the Achilles tendon. (From Porter D, Schon L: *Baxter's the foot and ankle in sport,* ed 2, Philadelphia, 2007, Elsevier.)

▦ Nonoperative treatment
  - **Eccentric strengthening has demonstrated the highest success rate.**
  - Includes rest, activity modification, heel lifts, physical therapy with emphasis on modalities and eccentric strengthening exercises, and ESWT.
  - Other treatments with evolving evidence include glyceryl trinitrate patches, prolotherapy, and aprotinin injections.
  - Nonoperative treatment effective in approximately 50% to 70% of cases

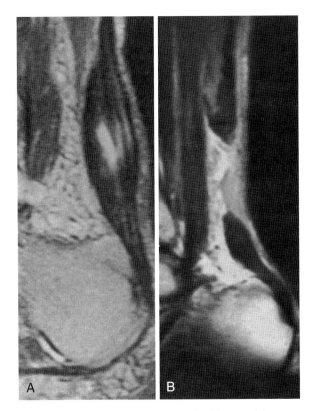

FIGURE 6-103 Chronic Achilles tendinosis with a partial or complete tear. **A,** Partial tear. Sagittal T2-weighted (TR/TE, 2000/70) spin-echo MRI shows an enlarged Achilles tendon containing irregular regions of high signal intensity. **B,** Complete tear. Sagittal intermediate-weighted (TR/TE, 3000/30) spin-echo MRI shows complete disruption of the Achilles tendon and a proximal segment that is inhomogeneous in signal intensity. Note the edema and hemorrhage of high signal intensity about the acutely torn tendon. (From Resnick D, Kransdorf M: *Bone and joint imaging,* ed 3, Philadelphia, 2004, Saunders.)

▣ Operative treatment
  ● Less invasive options include percutaneous longitudinal tenotomies in the area of degeneration, as well as stripping the anterior aspect of the tendon with large suture to free adhesions.
  ● For moderate to severe disease, open excision of the degenerated tendon tissue with tubularization has shown good results.
  ● **For more than 50% degenerative involvement of the Achilles, débridement with an FHL tendon transfer is recommended.**
    ● MRI evidence of significant involvement (diffuse thickening of the tendon without a focal area of disease) indicates the need for FHL transfer.
▇ **Acute Achilles tendon rupture**
▣ Most common tendon rupture in the lower extremity
▣ Complete rupture associated with sudden or violent dorsiflexion of ankle or lunge
▣ **Increased risk with prior intratendinous degeneration, fluoroquinolones, steroid injections, inflammatory arthritis**

▣ Frequently misdiagnosed (up to 20%) as ankle sprain or DVT, because active plantar flexion may be intact with activation of toe flexors and plantaris.
▣ Prodromal symptoms present in only 10% of patients
▣ Peak incidence in third to fifth decade of life
▣ Palpable gap in the tendon not always appreciated
▣ **Thompson test**
  ● Squeezing the calf with the ankle and foot at rest should result in passive plantar flexion of the foot.
  ● A positive (abnormal) test is strongly associated with Achilles rupture.
▣ The affected ankle demonstrates decreased plantar flexion tone with the patient in a prone position and the knees flexed.
▣ Imaging studies are often unnecessary; MRI or ultrasound may be helpful if the diagnosis is in question.
▣ Treatment
  ● Controversial because both nonoperative and operative treatments have shown good functional results and patient satisfaction in multiple studies.
  ● Nonoperative treatment has been historically associated with higher risk of rerupture (approaching 20%).
    ● However, current data has definitively demonstrated that the rate of rerupture with functional rehabilitation is equivalent to surgical repair.
    ● Cast immobilization longer than the initial 2 weeks after injury is *not* appropriate nonoperative management.
      ● Prolonged cast treatment is associated with a higher rerupture rate compared to surgical treatment and nonoperative functional rehabilitation.
    ● Surgical treatment has demonstrated superior power compared to nonoperative treatment.
      ● Neither course of treatment results in normal function compared to the normal extremity.
  ● **Operative treatment associated with increased risk of wound complications and infection**
    ● **Treated with aggressive débridement and culture-specific antibiotics**
  ● **Percutaneous techniques popular but traditionally increased risk of sural nerve injury**
  ● Early protected mobilization after 2 weeks of non–weight bearing and splint immobilization, generally with improved functional results compared to prolonged non–weight bearing and delayed rehabilitation
  ● Operative intervention cautioned in patients with diabetes mellitus, neuropathy, immunocompromised states, age older than 65 years, tobacco use, sedentary lifestyle, BMI above 30 kg/m^2, peripheral vascular disease, or local/systemic dermatologic disorders
▇ **Chronic Achilles tendon rupture**
▣ Nonoperative treatment—AFO
▣ **Operative treatment—in the setting of a chronic rupture, FHL transfer is the treatment of choice.** Allograft remains an option if excursion of the gastrocnemius-soleus muscle complex is retained.

SECTION 16 ANKLE PAIN AND SPORTS INJURIES

■ Ankle sprains
▦ Common in athletes, most frequently involves ATFL (weakest lateral ankle ligament)
▦ CFL is less commonly involved.
▦ The strong PTFL is rarely implicated.
▦ Ottawa ankle rules (Stiell et al., 1995) dictate radiographs appropriate only if tenderness at distal tibia or fibula, tenderness at base of fifth metatarsal or navicular, or inability to bear weight.
▦ Diagnosis
  • Patients often recall twisting mechanism, typically inversion.
  • Swelling, ecchymosis, pain with weight bearing all common.
  • Must assess for recurrent instability and ask for signs of loose body or osteochondral injury (mechanical symptoms such as locking or catching).
  • Radiographic evaluation
    • AP, mortise, and lateral x-rays of the ankle obtained; weight-bearing x-ray preferable if patient can tolerate
    • Foot x-rays should be obtained if any pain on examination—especially at base of fifth metatarsal or anterior process of calcaneus—to rule out fracture.
    • Assess for avulsion fractures, osteochondral defects, mortise or syndesmosis instability.
    • MRI typically reserved for patients with continued pain despite weeks of conservative treatment (immobilization, elevation, ice, NSAIDs) or concern for loose body or osteochondral defect
      • MRI may demonstrate attenuation or tear of the lateral ligamentous structures.
      • Bone bruising common in severe sprains and may result in longer time to pain-free activity and return to sports

▦ Nonoperative treatment
  • All patients initiated on RICE protocol (rest, ice, compression, elevation) with limited weight bearing if marked ankle joint-line tenderness or pain with weight-bearing activity
  • Progressive and protected weight bearing initiated as symptoms allow
  • **Physical therapy important for balance and proprioception, peroneal strengthening, and associated with a decreased rate of reinjury**
▦ Operative treatment
  • Reserved for patients with recurrent and symptomatic instability with excessive and asymmetric talar tilt and positive anterior drawer test, symptomatic osteochondral defects
  • Multiple procedures described; anatomic procedures typically first-line treatment and successful in 85% to 90% of cases
    • Modified Bröstrom procedure—anatomic reconstruction of ATFL supplemented with extensor retinaculum
    • Nonanatomic—peroneal tendon procedures (Evans procedure, Chrisman-Snook) or allograft procedures reserved for recurrent instability after initial operative treatment

▦ High ankle sprains
  • Sprains involving the syndesmosis ligaments require nearly twice as long to return to activity as "low" ankle sprains.
  • Pain in the anterior syndesmosis with syndesmosis squeeze or external rotation stress tests suggestive of injury
  • Stable injuries may be treated with RICE (see earlier).
  • Unstable injuries treated with operative intervention, especially in athletic population
  • Tibiofibular synostosis common complication. May be addressed with excision of synostosis or syndesmosis fusion if failed conservative treatment.
■ Anterior ankle impingement
▦ Soft tissue or bony condition leading to increased pain, decreased ROM, and occasionally a sense of instability
▦ Common in athletic population, especially if history of ankle sprains
▦ Pain with dorsiflexion and pivoting activities common
▦ Reproducible tenderness over anterior ankle joint line key to diagnosis
▦ Lateral radiographs may demonstrate osteophyte formation at anterior tibial plafond or dorsal talar neck. Best visualized with anteromedial oblique view.
▦ Ice, NSAIDs, brace immobilization, corticosteroid injections may provide relief.
▦ Operative intervention reserved for failure of conservative management; typically includes arthroscopic débridement of synovitis and bone spurs
■ Posterior ankle impingement
▦ Common in ballet dancers, gymnasts, soccer players, and downhill runners
▦ May be associated with os trigonum (present in 7% of adults), prominent posterolateral process of talus (Stieda process), or loose bodies
▦ Pain exacerbated and reproducible with maximum plantar flexion of ankle and push-off maneuvers
▦ May lead to synovitis of FHL tendon
▦ Nonoperative treatment as in anterior impingement
▦ **Operative intervention includes arthroscopic or open débridement of posterior synovitis and impinging bone.**
■ Osteochondral lesions
▦ **Most commonly due to trauma or repetitive microtrauma**
▦ Seen in up to 70% of ankle sprains, 75% of ankle fractures
▦ Location
  • Medial talar dome
    • Most common
    • Typically more posterior
    • Unreliable history of trauma; if provided, inversion sprain with plantar flexion
    • Larger and deeper than lateral lesions
  • Lateral talar dome
    • Less common
    • Central or anterior location
    • Usually history of acute trauma, inversion sprain with dorsiflexion
    • More often unstable, displaced, or symptomatic

- Patients often present with history of ankle injury, continued pain, and mechanical symptoms such as locking or catching with activity.
- Physical examination demonstrates deep pain over ankle joint line; palpation often does not reproduce described symptoms; ankle effusion common.
- Radiographic evaluation
  - AP, mortise, and lateral weight-bearing ankle x-ray obtained. May not demonstrate subtle lesions.
  - CT scan helpful for bony lesions, determining integrity of subchondral bone, identifying cysts, preoperative planning
  - MRI scan sensitive for all lesions, but edema pattern frequently overestimates severity of injury
    - Linear fluid signal deep to subchondral bone indicates unstable injury.
    - Sensitivity 92% for predicting stable versus unstable lesions
- Treatment
  - Acute stable defects may heal with rest, protected weight bearing.
  - Overall 45% excellent to good results with nonoperative treatment
  - Operative intervention reserved for unstable defects or patients with mechanical symptoms, symptoms not responding to conservative measures
  - Arthroscopic intervention most common
  - 80% to 85% success rate reported for nearly all interventions for defects smaller than 1.5 cm^2

- Débridement of defect to stable border with microfracture is first-line treatment.
- Large (>1 cm^2), cystic, or shoulder lesions; recurrent pain or refractory cases may be more effectively addressed with graft procedures, osteochondral autograft transplantation surgery, autologous chondrocyte implantation, and bulk allograft.
- Smaller than 1-cm-diameter lesions with stable cartilage cap amenable to retrograde drilling techniques
- Open intervention with medial malleolar osteotomy required for posterior defects
- Tibial defects with decreased success rates compared with talar lesions

■ Chronic exertional compartment syndrome
- Condition that may present in athletes (especially runners and cyclists) with pain that increases gradually with activity and eventually restricts performance. In severe cases, paresthesias may be noted secondary to compression of the superficial peroneal nerve.
  - Relief of pain and swelling quickly after rest is consistent with the disease process.
    - In contrast to stress fracture
- Compartment pressures should be measured before, during, and after exercise.
  - Pressures higher than 30 mm Hg 1 minute after exercise, 20 mm Hg 5 minutes after exercise, or

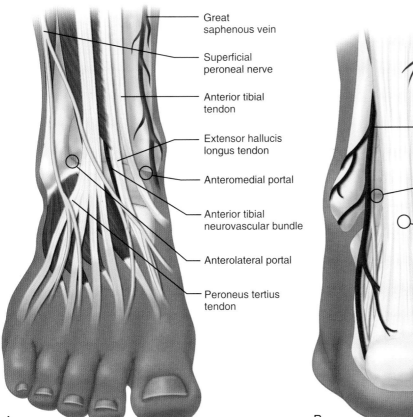

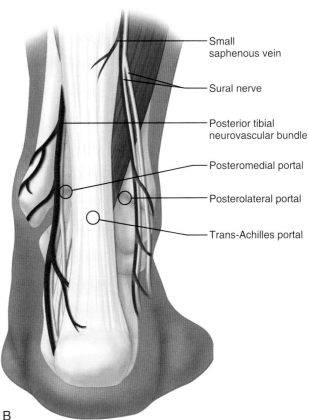

FIGURE 6-104 A, Anterior anatomy of ankle with diagram of standard portal placement. **B,** Posterior anatomy of ankle with diagram of standard portal placement. (Adapted from Miller MD, Chhabra A, Safran M: *Primer of arthroscopy,* Philadelphia, 2010, Saunders.)

absolute values higher than 15 mm Hg during rest can help establish the diagnosis.

- The anterior compartment is the more commonly involved and has the best prognosis for recovery.
- Fasciotomy is indicated for refractory cases.
- Popliteal artery entrapment syndrome is often confused with chronic posterior compartment syndrome.
  - Patients with popliteal artery entrapment syndrome present with intermittent claudication, including calf pain, cramping, coolness, and at times paresthesias into the foot.
  - Provocative tests include obliteration of pedal pulses with active plantar flexion or passive dorsiflexion of the ankle with Doppler recordings.
  - Treatment is release and recession of the medial head of the gastrocnemius.

- **Ankle arthroscopy pearls** (Figure 6-104)
- Position patients supine with a bump under the ipsilateral thigh to allow for traction on the ankle.

- Noninvasive traction devices or a sterile Ace wrap are commonly used to distract the ankle joint and allow for visualization of the joint.
- Distraction is often unnecessary for débridement of anterior spurs or synovitis.
- **The most common complication after ankle arthroscopy is nerve injury.**
  - **The superficial peroneal nerve is the most commonly injured as the anterolateral portal is established. The nerve can often be palpated and identified with plantar flexion of the ankle and fourth toe.**
  - The saphenous nerve may be injured with a wayward anteromedial portal.
  - Posteromedial and anterocentral portals are typically avoided to limit injury to the tibial nerve/posterior tibial artery and deep peroneal nerve/dorsalis pedis artery, respectively.
  - A "nick-and-spread" technique is advocated to avoid nerve injury.

SECTION 17 THE DIABETIC FOOT

PATHOPHYSIOLOGY

- **Diabetic neuropathy**
- The diagnosis of foot ulcerations results in the greatest rate of hospital admissions in diabetics, as well as lower extremity amputations.
- The combination of neuropathy and excess pressure on the plantar foot leads to ulceration.
- Sensation
  - Polyneuropathic loss of sensation begins in a stocking distribution of the feet and progresses proximally.
  - Diagnosed by the inability to perceive the 5.07 Semmes-Weinstein monofilament
  - Most patients (90%) who cannot feel the 5.07 monofilament have lost protective sensation to their feet and are at risk for ulceration.
  - With the Therapeutic Shoe Bill, money is allocated for neuropathic patients to purchase extra-depth shoes and total contact inserts (three per year) for ulcer prevention.
- Autonomic neuropathy
  - An abnormal sweating mechanism leads to a dry foot.
  - Vulnerable to fissuring cracks, which then become portals for infection
- Motor neuropathy
  - Most commonly involves the common peroneal nerve
  - Resultant loss of tibialis anterior motor function and a foot drop
  - Small intrinsic musculature of the foot also commonly affected, resulting in claw toes and subsequent toe-tip ulcerations due to excessive pressure
- **Hypomobility syndrome**
- Result of excessive glycosylation of the soft tissues of the extremities
- Leads to decreased joint ROM

- **Peripheral vascular disease**
- Occurs in 60% to 70% of patients who have had diabetes for over 10 years, involving both large and small vessels
- Noninvasive vascular examination should be performed when pulses not palpable.
  - Waveforms (normal is triphasic)
  - Ankle-brachial indices (minimum for healing, 0.45; normal, 1.0)
    - Calcifications in the artery can falsely elevate the ankle-brachial index. Greater than 1.3 is nonphysiologic and consistent with calcification of the vessels.
  - **Absolute toe pressures (minimum for healing, 40 mm Hg; normal, 100 mm Hg)**
- Transcutaneous oxygen measurements (PO_2) of the toes greater than 40 mm Hg have been found to be predictive of healing.
- **Immune system impairment**
- Poor cellular defenses, such as abnormal phagocytosis, altered chemotaxis of WBCs, and a poor cytotoxic environment (due to hyperglycemia) to fight off bacteria, lead to difficulty in fighting off infection once it has developed.
- **Metabolic deficiency**
- **Reduced total protein less than 6.0, WBC count less than 1500, and albumin levels less than 2.5 result in poor healing potential.**
  - **These parameters must be normalized with nutritional support prior to surgical intervention.**

CLINICAL PROBLEMS

- **Ulcers**
- Classification and treatment
  - Ulcer location (forefoot, midfoot, and heel) and the presence or absence of arterial disease influence healing rates.

- Depth-ischemia classification (modification of Wagner-Meggitt classification)
  - Depth
    - Grade 0
      - Skin intact with bony deformity—at risk
      - Treatment
        - Extra-depth shoe and pressure-relief insoles
    - **Grade 1**
      - **Localized superficial ulcer without tendon or bone involvement**
      - **Treatment**
        - **In-office ulcer débridement**
        - **Total contact cast**
    - Grade 2
      - Deep ulcer with exposed tendon or joint capsule
      - Treatment
        - Formal operative débridement of all exposed tendon and nonviable tissue
        - Followed by dressing changes and total contact casting once wound bed is healthy
    - **Grade 3**
      - **Extensive ulcer with exposed bone/ osteomyelitis or abscess**
      - **Treatment**
        - **Surgical débridement of exposed bone/ osteomyelitis and nonviable tissue**
        - Followed by dressing changes and total contact casting once wound bed is healthy
  - Ischemia
    - Grade A—normal vascularity
    - Grade B—ischemia without gangrene
      - Noninvasive vascular studies and surgical revascularization if indicated
    - Grade C—partial (forefoot) gangrene
      - Noninvasive vascular studies and surgical revascularization if indicated
      - Metabolic assessment

- Delay surgery if albumin below 2.5 or total protein below 6, and improve patient's nutritional status.
  - Operative intervention—partial foot amputation
- Grade D—complete foot gangrene
  - Same as with grade C
  - Operative intervention—below-knee or above-knee amputation
- Additional treatment
  - **Midfoot collapse may require ostectomy of bony prominence if stable deformity, or midfoot fusion if midfoot instability is present.**
  - **Equinus contracture is very common, and Achilles lengthening will offload the midfoot/forefoot.**
    - **Achilles lengthening required:**
      - **Recurrent forefoot/midfoot ulceration**
      - **Ulceration with equinus deformity**
  - Toe deformities often require joint resection or amputation.
- The ultimate goal is an ulcer-free, functional, plantigrade foot that can fit within a brace or shoe.
- **Charcot arthropathy**
- Chronic, progressive, destructive process affecting bone architecture and joint alignment in people lacking protective sensation (Figures 6-105 and 6-106)
- Occurs in approximately 1% to 1.5% of patients with diabetes; 7.5% of patients with diabetes and neuropathy
- Two theories regarding pathophysiology are neurotraumatic and neurovascular destruction.
- Classification: Eichenholtz stages of Charcot arthropathy (Table 6-4)
  - Related to the degree of warmth, swelling, and erythema
  - Continuum from bone resorption and fragmentation to bone formation and consolidation that takes 6 to 18 months

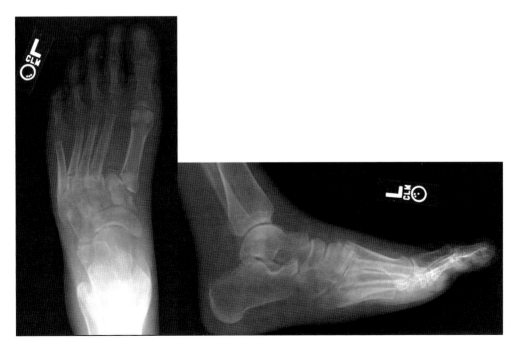

FIGURE 6-105 Patient with midfoot neuroarthropathy with bony and ligamentous components to the deformity. The patient had no prior antecedent trauma. The radiographic appearance is more suggestive of a high-energy injury, and in cases where no prior trauma or minor trauma was noted, one should consider the presence of neuroarthropathy.

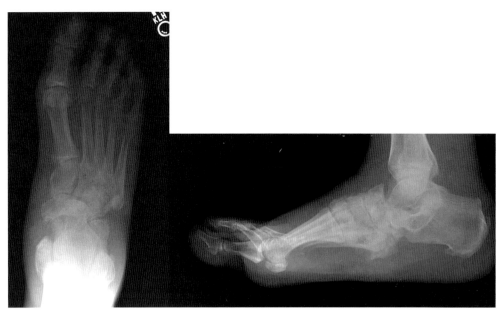

FIGURE 6-106 Patient with neuroarthropathy of the hindfoot.

Table 6-4	Stages of Charcot Arthropathy (Eichenholtz)*	
STAGE	**SIGNS AND SYMPTOMS**	**RADIOGRAPHS**
0: Clinical (prefragmentation)	Acute inflammation; confused with infection	Regional bone demineralization
1: Dissolution (fragmentation)	Acute inflammation, swelling, erythema, warmth; confused with infection	Regional bone demineralization, periarticular fragmentation, joint dislocation
2: Coalescence	Less inflammation, less swelling, less erythema	Absorption of bone debris; early bone healing and periosteal new bone formation
3: Resolution	Resolved erythema, swelling, and warmth; consolidation of healing	Smoothed bone edges, bony/fibrous ankylosis

*Based on the signs, symptoms, and radiographic changes that occur with the neuropathic joint/fracture over time.

- Also classified by location (Brodsky):
  - Type 1: midfoot (most common)—60%
  - Type 2: hindfoot (subtalar, TN, CC joints)—10%
  - Type 3A: tibiotalar joint—20%
  - Type 3B: fracture of calcaneal tuberosity—less than 10%
  - Type 4: combination of areas—less than 10%
  - Type 5: forefoot—less than 10%

▥ Patients complain of swelling, warmth, redness and deformity.
  - Pain may be present in up to 50% of patients.
  - Swelling and redness is typically resolved in morning.
  - Often confused with osteomyelitis clinically
  - Up to 35% present with bilateral disease.
▥ Treatment
  - Goal is to achieve stage 3 (resolution) while maintaining alignment, ambulatory status, and minimizing soft tissue breakdown.
  - **Initial treatment is immobilization and non–weight bearing.**
    - **Best with total contact cast**
    - Can transition to custom brace (AFO, or Charcot restraint orthosis walker [CROW] boot) once swelling and warmth subsides
    - Medication management includes bisphosphonates, neuroleptic medications, antidepressants, and topical anesthetics.

- Successful in up to 75% of cases
- Operative treatment
  - Stable deformity with recurrent ulcers secondary to prominence—exostectomy
  - **Unstable/unbraceable deformity—arthrodesis**
    - **Ankle and hindfoot Charcot best treated with arthrodesis, given the high likelihood of failure of nonoperative management**
    - **Midfoot Charcot treatment with plantar closing wedge osteotomy to correct deformity**
  - **TAL almost universally required**
  - Amputation as salvage
  - High complication rates—nearly 70%

■ Diabetic foot infections
▥ Occur contiguous to open skin wounds (ulceration, skin fissure, cut)
  - Hematogenous spread of infection into the foot or ankle is rare.
▥ Infections in the diabetic foot or ankle are either isolated soft tissue infections (cellulitis or abscess) or osteomyelitis.
  - If abscess suspected, perform needle aspirate or MRI.
    - MRI has high false-positive rate in the diagnosis of osteomyelitis, particularly with concurrent Charcot arthropathy.

- WBC-labeled scan or dual-image technetium/indium (Tc/In) scan is more sensitive and specific for osteomyelitis than isolated Tc scan.
- Contiguous osteomyelitis present in 67% percent of foot ulcerations that probe to bone
▨ Diabetic foot infections are polymicrobial.
  - Superficial wound culture does not identify the organism responsible for the infection and should not be performed.
  - Deep surgical cultures (or bone biopsy if exposed bone) provide most accurate result.
▨ Treat with initial broad-spectrum antibiotic coverage once surgical cultures obtained, and adjust once sensitivity returns.
▨ **Abscesses require surgical drainage and antibiotics.**
▨ Osteomyelitis is treated with antibiotics and surgical débridement.
  - **Culture-specific antibiotics from a bone biopsy have proven to be an effective tool in treating osteomyelitis, without the need for bone resection. Resection of all nonviable or infected soft tissue should also be performed.**
  - If culture-specific antibiotic therapy fails, surgical resection of infected bone and débridement of surrounding tissue is required in addition to antibiotic therapy.
  - Often results in more extensive débridement, including ray resection, partial calcanectomy

(calcaneal involvement), and partial or complete foot amputation
▨ **Amputation level**
▨ Transmetatarsal
  - Lowest energy expenditure
  - No tendon transfer needed
▨ Lisfranc
  - Must transfer peroneal tendons to the cuboid to prevent varus
  - TAL to prevent equinus
▨ Chopart
  - **Transfer anterior tibialis to talus to prevent equinus.**
  - **Achilles lengthening to prevent equinus**
▨ Syme
  - **Amputation level with the next lowest energy expenditure after a transmetatarsal amputation. Superior to both a Lisfranc and Chopart amputation with regard to the amount of energy required to ambulate.**
  - Contraindicated if history of heel ulcers
▨ Transtibial
  - **Superior results with postoperative casting for 3 to 5 days, with conversion to rigid removal dressing**
  - Critical to maintain full knee extension during healing
  - Typically transition to weight bearing in a temporary prosthesis by 6 weeks postoperatively

SECTION 18 TRAUMA

PHALANGEAL FRACTURES

▪ **Most common injuries to the forefoot**
▪ **Mechanism of injury**
▨ Usually caused by stubbing mechanism (axial loading with varus or valgus force) or by crush mechanism (heavy load dropped on the foot)
▪ **Diagnosis**
▨ Patients present with pain, ecchymosis, and swelling.
▨ AP, lateral, and oblique radiographs are usually suitable to detect fractures.
▪ **Treatment**
▨ Nondisplaced fractures with or without articular involvement
  - Stiff-soled shoes and protected weight bearing, "buddy taping"
▨ Displaced fractures
  - Closed reduction can be attempted, with gravity traction or pencil reduction followed by stiff-soled shoe and "buddy taping."
▨ Hallux fractures carry greater functional significance than those of the lesser toes.
  - Distal phalanx fractures often the result of a crush mechanism
    - If concomitant nail bed injury is present, considered an open fracture
    - Irrigation and débridement, nail bed repair, and antibiotic coverage

- Operative treatment—indicated for gross instability or intraarticular discontinuity greater than 2 mm
  - Fixation achieved with crossed K-wires or mini–fragment screws.
  - Most common complication is stiffness.

METATARSAL FRACTURES

▪ **Stability achieved by the bony architecture of the midfoot and the ligamentous attachments at the metatarsal bases and necks (intermetatarsal ligaments)**
▪ **Severe displacement of shaft fractures is uncommon unless multiple metatarsals are fractured.**
▪ **First and fifth metatarsals are more mobile and susceptible to injury.**
▪ **Mechanism of injury**
▨ Crush-type injury (which can result in severe soft tissue trauma), twisting forces
▨ When multiple metatarsals are fractured, a Lisfranc injury must be ruled out.
▪ **Diagnosis**
▨ Patients present with pain, ecchymosis, and swelling.
▨ Weight bearing is often painful and difficult.
▨ AP, lateral, and oblique radiographs are usually suitable to detect fractures.
▨ Plantar ecchymosis may signify a more significant injury involving the Lisfranc joint complex.

■ **First metatarsal fractures**

■ First metatarsal bears approximately one third of body weight.

  • Maintenance of alignment is very important.

■ Nondisplaced fractures—boot or hard-soled shoe, weight bearing as tolerated

■ Displaced fractures—surgical fixation; open reduction and internal fixation (ORIF) with lag screws or plate fixation

■ **Second, third, and fourth metatarsal fractures**

■ Majority are minimally displaced.

  • Treat with a low-tide walking boot or hard-soled shoe with arch support.

  • Isolated fractures are stable secondary to the intermetatarsal ligaments that are present both at the base and neck that help to prevent displacement.

■ Surgical fixation indicated in fractures with significant sagittal plane deformity (>10 degrees) or if the three central metatarsals are fractured. With multiple fractures, the intermetatarsal ligaments cannot provide stability, and therefore these are inherently unstable.

  • ORIF with plate-and-screw fixation or intramedullary antegrade-retrograde pinning technique

  • Care should be taken to maintain proper metatarsal length to minimize the risk of transfer metatarsalgia or plantar keratosis.

■ Metatarsal neck fractures

  • Most treated conservatively in boot or shoe

  • With multiple (central 3) and/or complete displacement, treat with open reduction and antegrade-retrograde pinning or plate-and-screw fixation.

■ Metatarsal base fractures

  • Primarily through metaphyseal bone, heal rapidly if stable

  • High suspicion for a Lisfranc injury should be present when these fractures are seen.

■ Metatarsal stress fractures

  • Common, often secondary to repetitive stress or cavovarus foot posture

  • MRI or bone scan will aid in the diagnosis.

  • Second metatarsal stress fracture is the most common and is classically described in amenorrheal dancers.

  • Treat in weight-bearing boot or hard-soled shoe.

  • Evaluate for metabolic bone disease in these patients (especially if insidious onset) or if there is no distinct causal event (increase in training, initiation of new activity).

  • Recurrent stress fracture in the presence of a cavovarus foot may require reconstruction of the cavovarus alignment to prevent recurrence.

■ **Fifth metatarsal fracture**

■ Represent a unique subset of forefoot injuries

■ Classification involves anatomic description of the fracture (Figure 6-107).

  • Zone 1—avulsion fracture of the proximal fifth metatarsal tuberosity

    • Occurs secondary to an inversion mechanism and subsequent pull of the lateral band of the plantar fascia and/or peroneus brevis tendon

    • Sometimes extends into the cubometatarsal joint

    • Most treated with protected weight bearing in shoe or boot

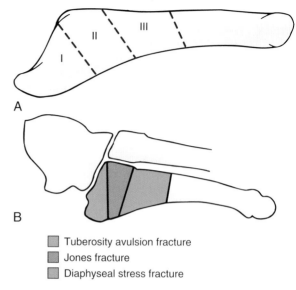

FIGURE 6-107 A and **B,** Three-part classification scheme as described by Botte. (From Coughlin MJ et al: *Surgery of the foot and ankle,* ed 8, Philadelphia, 2006, Mosby. [Courtesy M. Botte.])

  • Open reduction required if fifth metatarsal–cuboid articular surface is displaced or if fracture is rotated with the fractured surface of the proximal fragment no longer facing the distal fragment

  • Tenting of the skin is also an indication for fixation.

  • A lag screw placed obliquely from the base of the fifth metatarsal into the medial cortex of fifth metatarsal is the surgical treatment of choice.

  • Chronic pain from a previous avulsion fracture may be addressed with excision of the fragment and reattachment of the peroneus brevis.

• Zone 2—fractures of the metaphyseal-diaphyseal junction that extend into the fourth-fifth intermetatarsal articulation

  • Also known as a *Jones fracture* (Figure 6-108)

  • Acute zone 2 fractures can be treated with non–weight-bearing immobilization for 6 to 8 weeks.

    • Recurrent fracture after nonoperative intervention should be treated with intramedullary screw fixation.

  • **Elite athletes should be treated with intramedullary screw fixation.**

    • Minimum screw diameter of 4 mm

    • Returning to sports activity prior to radiographic union increases risk of nonunion.

• Zone 3—fractures of the proximal diaphysis usually secondary to stress

  • Mostly in athletes secondary to repetitive microtrauma

  • Occur in the vascular watershed region of the proximal fifth metatarsal

    • Slow healing time and greater risk of nonunion

  • High risk of refracture with nonoperative treatment when fracture is stress-related (33%)

  • Intramedullary screw fixation is surgical treatment of choice.

    • Bone grafting may be required in case of nonunion, significant resorption.

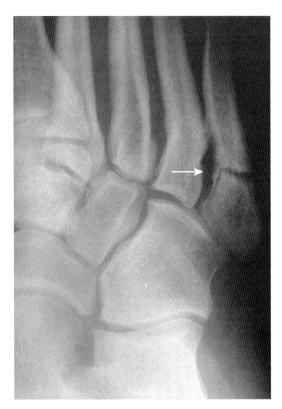

FIGURE 6-108 Jones fracture of the fifth metatarsal *(arrow).* (From Coughlin MJ et al: *Surgery of the foot and ankle,* ed 8, Philadelphia, 2006, Mosby.)

- Presence of a varus foot deformity is not uncommon in these patients, and concomitant lateral closing wedge calcaneal osteotomy should be considered to prevent recurrence (Figure 6-109).

FIRST MTP JOINT INJURIES

- ▓ Hallux MTP sprain ("turf toe")—see the section Sesamoids.
- ▓ Hallux MTP dislocation
- ▓ Usually a dorsal dislocation secondary to hyperextension
- ▓ Results in volar plate rupture at its insertion on the metatarsal neck
- ▓ The classification indicates which structures are injured as well as likelihood of achieving closed reduction.
  - Type I—intersesamoid ligament intact, likely plantar incarceration of the metatarsal head. Sesamoids may be intraarticular. No fracture present.
  - Irreducible by closed methods
  - Type IIA—intersesamoid ligament ruptured
  - Type IIB—associated sesamoid fracture (usually tibial sesamoid) (Figure 6-110)
  - High possibility of closed reduction
  - Type IIC—combination of type IIA and IIB
  - Treatment
  - Type I injuries require open reduction with dorsal longitudinal approach.
  - Type II injuries are possible to reduce closed.
    - They may have associated intraarticular fracture fragments that require excision.
  - If joint is unstable after reduction, pinning the joint for 3 to 4 weeks is indicated.

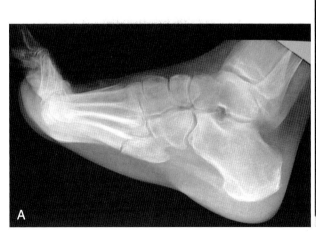
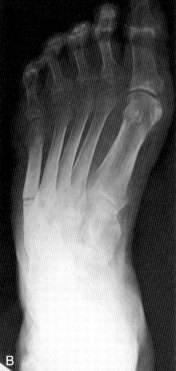

FIGURE 6-109 Watch for the Jones fracture in the varus foot. **A,** This patient had a cavovarus foot deformity secondary to a stroke. Chronic lateral foot overload resulted in a fifth metatarsal fracture and subsequent nonunion. **B,** The fracture appears incompletely healed after 6 months of symptoms. The patient underwent surgery, including intramedullary screw placement and hindfoot osteotomy with muscle transfers, to balance the deformity. (From DiGiovanni C: *Core knowledge in orthopaedics—foot and ankle,* Philadelphia, 2007, Elsevier.)

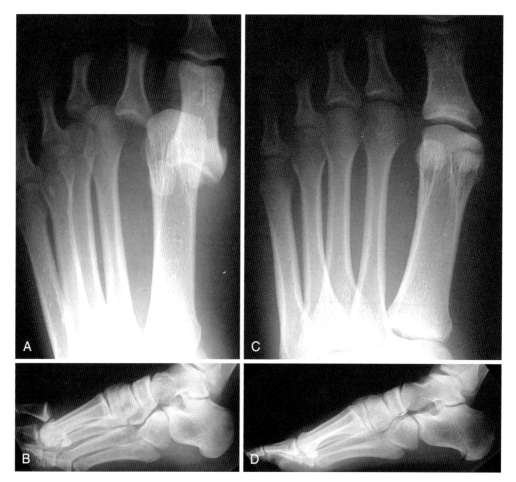

FIGURE 6-110 Type IIB dorsal dislocation of the first metatarsophalangeal joint, as seen on anteroposterior **(A)** and lateral **(B)** radiographs. Fracture through the medial sesamoid is best seen on the lateral view. Closed reduction was performed, also reducing the sesamoid fracture **(C** and **D)**. (From Coughlin MJ et al: *Surgery of the foot and ankle,* ed 8, Philadelphia, 2006, Mosby.)

 TARSOMETATARSAL FRACTURES AND DISLOCATIONS (LISFRANC INJURY)

- The Lisfranc articulation is a stable construct because of its bony architecture and strong ligaments.
- The base of the second metatarsal fits into a mortise formed by the proximally recessed middle cuneiform ("keystone configuration").
- In the coronal plane, the second metatarsal base serves as the cornerstone in a "Roman arch" configuration (Figure 6-111).
- Ligamentous anatomy of the TMT joints (Figure 6-112)
- Intermetatarsal ligaments between the second and fifth metatarsal bases
  - No direct ligamentous attachment from the first to second metatarsal
- Lisfranc ligament—critical to stabilizing second metatarsal and maintenance of midfoot arch
  - Between medial cuneiform and base of second metatarsal
  - Interosseous ligament is stiffest and strongest, dorsal is the weakest.
  - Plantar ligament inserts on base of second and third metatarsal.

- Mechanism of injury:
- Indirect
  - Axial loading of a plantar-flexed foot
  - Athletic injury (most common), fall from height
  - Subtle and have a higher likelihood of being misdiagnosed
- Direct
  - Motor vehicle accidents, crush injuries
  - Significant soft tissue injury, often open
- Diagnosis
- Injuries range from nondisplaced purely ligamentous disruptions to severe fracture-dislocations (Figure 6-113).
- More common in men
- Severe pain, inability to bear weight, marked swelling, and tenderness
- Plantar ecchymosis should raise suspicion for a TMT/Lisfranc injury.
- Radiographic evaluation
  - AP, lateral, and oblique radiographs should be obtained (Figure 6-114).
    - Lateral translation of the second metatarsal relative to the middle cuneiform is diagnostic of a Lisfranc injury.

Second cuneiform

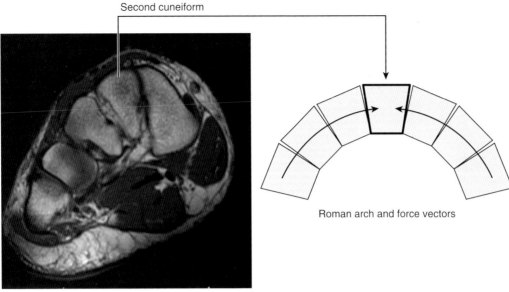

Transverse arch of the midfoot

Roman arch and force vectors

FIGURE 6-111 The second cuneiform and second metatarsal base are shaped like a keystone in the coronal plane. The Lisfranc joint is shaped like a Roman arch. This anatomy and stabilization by the Lisfranc ligament are important for support of the arch of the foot. (From Morrison W, Sanders T: *Problem solving in musculoskeletal imaging,* Philadelphia, 2008, Elsevier.)

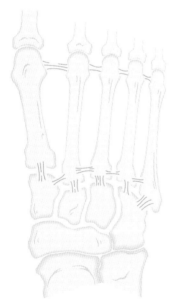

FIGURE 6-112 The Lisfranc articulation with its ligamentous attachments. Note the recessed second tarsometatarsal joint and the Lisfranc ligament in place of the first-second intermetatarsal ligament. (From DeLee J: *DeLee and Drez's orthopaedic sports medicine,* ed 3, Philadelphia, 2011, Saunders.)

- Weight-bearing radiographs with contralateral comparison view, abduction stress views, and single-limb weight-bearing views may be necessary to confirm diagnosis when clinical suspicion is high (Figure 6-115).
  - "Fleck sign" (Figure 6-116)
    - Small, bony avulsion from the base of the second metatarsal seen in the first intermetatarsal space
    - Diagnostic of a Lisfranc injury

- Proximal variant—forces transmit through the intercuneiform joint and out the NC joint; may be subtle (Figure 6-117)
- CT and MRI may be valuable in detecting occult fractures or ligamentous injury, aid in preoperative planning.

■ **Classification**

▨ Differentiating between purely ligamentous injuries and fracture-dislocations may have treatment implications.
- Primary arthrodesis of the TMT joints is an alternative to ORIF in a purely ligamentous injury.
- Multiple described classification schemes are not useful for determining treatment and prognosis.

■ **Treatment**

▨ Anatomic reduction is most predictive of good clinical results.

▨ Nonsurgical management is only indicated in cases with no displacement on weight bearing and stress radiographs and no evidence of bony injury on CT (usually dorsal sprains).

▨ Operative treatment—any displacement on radiographs or evidence of a bony injury is treated with ORIF.
- Should be delayed until soft tissue swelling has resolved
- **Anatomic reduction is mandatory and open reduction is often required as opposed to closed reduction with percutaneous fixation.**
- Fixation should proceed from proximal to distal and medial to lateral.
  - Medial and middle column (first, second, and third TMT joints; intercuneiform joints)
    - Typically stabilized with screw fixation across the involved joints (Figure 6-118)
    - Dorsal plating is gaining in popularity—less iatrogenic articular damage.
    - Fixation is commonly removed after 4 months to minimize the risk of hardware failure and restore the normal joint mechanics.

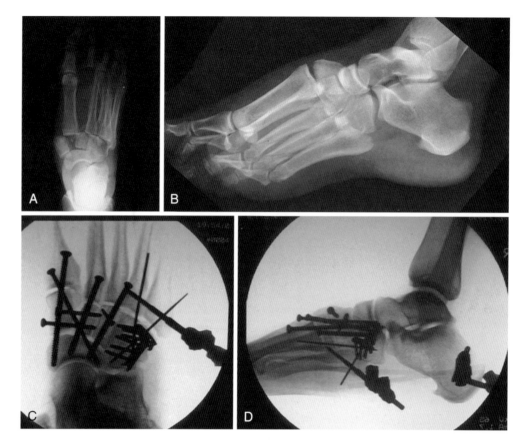

FIGURE 6-113 Commonly, intertarsal instability accompanies a Lisfranc (tarsometatarsal) injury. Sometimes it is occult, so a high index of suspicion should always be maintained intraoperatively and both clinical and radiographic stress examinations performed. Usually, however, it is overt (as in this case—**A, B**), and treatment is the same and demands rigid anatomic open reduction with internal fixation (ORIF) **(C, D)**. The intertarsal instability can often be initially aligned with a medial or lateral column external fixator, as was used for this patient, after which fixation is made easier for the surgeon and should begin proximally and proceed distally so that abnormal anatomy can be realigned to normal anatomy in a sequential manner. Note that this technique helped with disimpaction of the lateral cuboid nutcracker injury, which also required ORIF with bone grafting to restore integrity to the lateral column. (From Browner B et al: *Skeletal trauma,* ed 4, Philadelphia, 2008, Elsevier.)

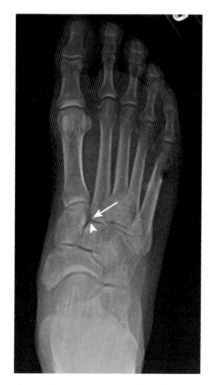

FIGURE 6-114 Normal anteroposterior weight-bearing radiograph demonstrating the alignment relationship between the base of the second metatarsal *(arrow)* and middle cuneiform *(arrowhead)*. Any lateral deviation of the second metatarsal relative to the middle cuneiform is consistent with a Lisfranc disruption and must be operatively treated. (From Miller MD, Sanders T: *Presentation, imaging and treatment of common musculoskeletal conditions,* Philadelphia, 2011, Elsevier.)

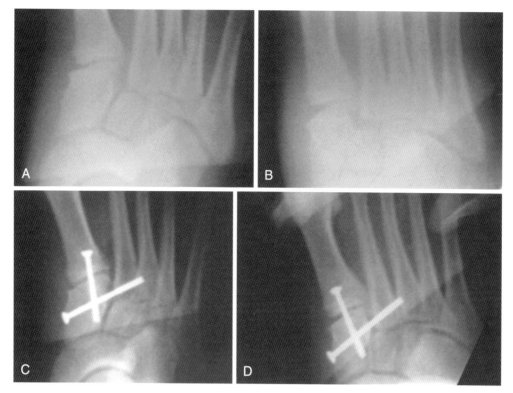

FIGURE 6-115 Anteroposterior and stress radiographs of foot with subtle Lisfranc dislocation. **A,** Radiograph appears normal. **B,** With stress into everted position, metatarsals sublux laterally. **C,** Postreduction radiograph reveals satisfactory reduction and internal fixation. **D,** Reduction maintained on eversion stress radiograph. (From Canale ST, Beaty J: *Campbell's operative orthopaedics,* ed 11, Philadelphia, 2007, Elsevier.)

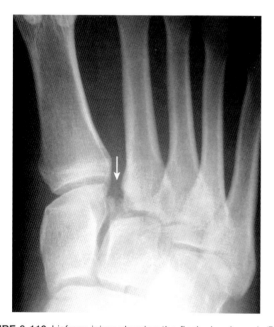

FIGURE 6-116 Lisfranc injury showing the fleck sign *(arrow).* (From Mercier L: *Practical orthopaedics,* ed 6, Philadelphia, 2008, Elsevier.)

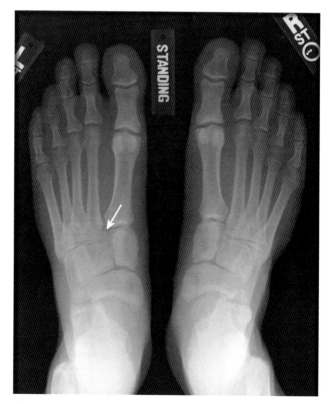

FIGURE 6-117 Patient with a Lisfranc injury identified by the fleck sign *(arrow).* In this case, the ligament itself remained intact and the injury occurred by avulsion of the ligament from the base of the second metatarsal. The function of the ligament is compromised, and operative intervention is indicated. (From Miller MD, Sanders T: *Presentation, imaging and treatment of common musculoskeletal conditions,* Philadelphia, 2011, Elsevier.)

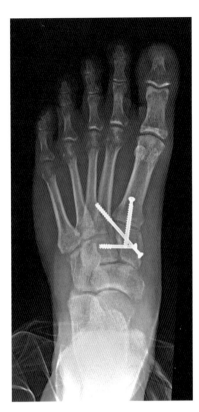

FIGURE 6-118 Postoperative radiograph of patient who was treated with screw fixation. In addition to a screw transfixing the first tarsometatarsal joint, the "Lisfranc" screw was used to hold the second metatarsal reduced. In this case instability of the intercuneiform joint was noted and required fixation. (From Miller MD, Sanders T: *Presentation, imaging and treatment of common musculoskeletal conditions*, Philadelphia, 2011, Elsevier.)

- Lateral column (fourth and fifth TMT joints)
  - Temporary fixation with K-wires, owing to mobile segment
  - Removed at 6 weeks
- Primary arthrodesis is an alternative treatment option, with some benefit seen in patients with purely ligamentous high-energy injury (dorsal subluxation or dislocation) or significant intraarticular comminution (Figure 6-119).
- Complications
  - Missed diagnosis or improper treatment may lead to traumatic planovalgus deformity or posttraumatic arthritis.
  - Midfoot realignment and arthrodesis is the appropriate salvage procedure (Figure 6-120).
  - Uncommon to require fourth or fifth TMT arthrodesis as part of fusion construct

MIDFOOT INJURIES (EXCLUDING LISFRANC INJURIES)

- **Midfoot consists of the navicular, the three cuneiforms, the cuboid, and their corresponding articulations.**
- **Acts as a stout connection between the forefoot and hindfoot**
- Relatively immobile, with strong plantar ligaments
- Serves an important shock-absorbing function
- Chopart and Lisfranc joints are therefore of greater functional importance than the articulations among the midfoot bones.

- Cuboid is critical to the integrity of the lateral column.
- **Cuboid injuries**
- Often associated with other midfoot or Lisfranc fractures/dislocations
- Radiographic evaluation
  - AP, lateral, and oblique (30-degree medial oblique is ideal) views
  - Weight-bearing/stress views can help ascertain midfoot stability if there is clinical concern.
  - CT may be required to define fracture fragments and articular congruity.
- Cuboid avulsion from the CC articulation
  - Most common; due to an inversion force (lateral ankle sprain)
  - Treat conservatively, with weight bearing as tolerated in boot or brace.
- Cuboid fractures
  - Results from forced plantar flexion and abduction of the forefoot resulting in an axial load
  - Often causes comminuted impacted fracture, or "nutcracker" fracture (Figure 6-121)
  - Treatment
    - Nondisplaced, minimal articular involvement—conservative treatment in boot
    - ORIF required when comminution or displacement compromises the length and alignment of the lateral column
    - Lateral column external fixation can be used as an aid to obtain length or for definitive fixation in severely comminuted cases (Figure 6-122).
- Cuboid syndrome
  - Painful subluxation seen in athletes, especially ballet dancers
  - The patient may have pain or a palpable "click" as the foot is brought from plantar flexion and inversion to dorsiflexion and eversion.
- Complete dislocation of the cuboid
  - Extremely rare, often due to higher-energy mechanisms
  - Usually displaced in a plantar and medial direction
- **Cuneiform injuries**
- Most occur in association with other midfoot injuries, in particular Lisfranc injuries.
- The medial cuneiform is the most commonly injured.
  - Displaced or unstable medial cuneiform injuries require anatomic reduction and stable fixation.
- **Navicular fractures**
- The navicular articulates with the talar head on its concave proximal surface and with the three cuneiforms distally.
- Rigidly fixed in the midfoot by dense ligamentous attachments
- Blood supply—dorsalis pedis supplies the dorsum, medial plantar branch of the posterior tibial artery supplies the plantar surface, and branches of these arteries create a plexus to supply the tuberosity.
  - The central portion of the bone is relatively less vascular and therefore at risk for stress injuries and nonunions.
- Classification and treatment
  - Navicular fractures classified as avulsion, tuberosity, body, and stress injuries

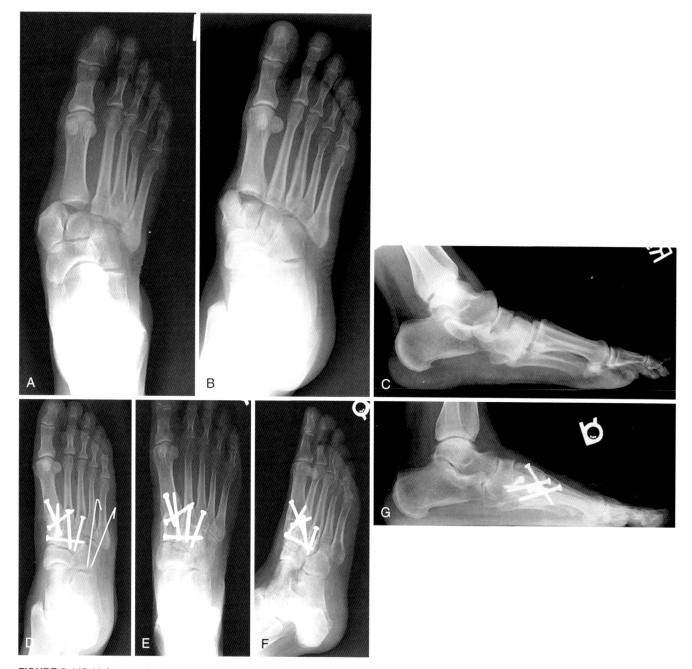

FIGURE 6-119 Lisfranc and midtarsal injury treated with primary arthrodesis of the first through third tarsometatarsal (TMT) joints. Anteroposterior **(A),** oblique **(B),** and lateral **(C)** radiographs of a Lisfranc injury with dorsolateral dislocation of all metatarsal bases without associated fracture. The lateral radiographs also show associated injury to the midtarsal joint with plantar fracture-dislocation of the navicular, which required open reduction and internal fixation to stabilize this articulation. Primary arthrodesis may be indicated in true TMT dislocations because the long-term stability of these joints depends on ligamentous healing, which is less reliable than bony healing. **D,** Oblique postoperative radiograph showing arthrodesis of the medial three TMT joints and provisional Kirschner-wire fixation of the fourth and fifth TMT joints. Weight-bearing anteroposterior **(E),** oblique **(F),** and lateral **(G)** radiographs 1 year postoperatively. (From Coughlin MJ et al: *Surgery of the foot and ankle,* ed 8, Philadelphia, 2006, Mosby.)

- Avulsion fractures
  - Ligamentous attachments (usually from dorsal TN joint) avulse a fragment of bone during inversion, twisting, and hyper–plantar flexion injuries.
  - Most common, treated symptomatically
- Navicular tuberosity fractures
  - Secondary to acute eversion of the foot with simultaneous contraction of the tibialis posterior

- Displacement usually minimal owing to broad attachment of the posterior tibial tendon
- Concomitant lateral injury is common (anterior process of the calcaneus, cuboid fracture).
- Treatment
  - Nondisplaced or minimally displaced fractures treated in cast or boot with protected weight bearing.

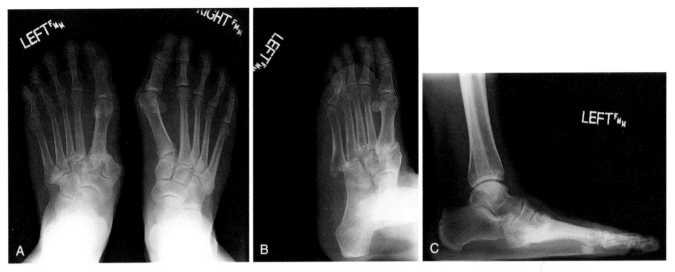

FIGURE 6-120 A to **C,** This severe posttraumatic deformity was symptomatic in each of the three midfoot columns. Note the severe abduction of the entire tarsometatarsal joint complex. (From Myerson MS: *Reconstructive foot and ankle surgery: management of complications,* ed 2, Philadelphia, 2010, Elsevier.)

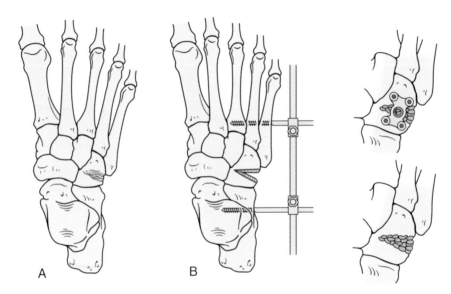

FIGURE 6-121 A, "Nutcracker impaction" injury of the cuboid shortens the lateral column of the foot, thereby causing a pes planus deformity because of a relative mismatch with the medial column. **B,** External fixation to distract the fracture corrects the deformity but leaves a void. Stable healing requires bone grafting, often augmented with a small buttress plate. (From Browner B et al: *Skeletal trauma,* ed 4, Philadelphia, 2008, Elsevier.)

- Fractures displaced more than 5 mm have a high chance of nonunion—surgical fixation recommended.
  - Small avulsions or symptomatic nonunions can be treated with excision.
- Navicular body fractures
  - Axial load to a plantar-flexed foot with either abduction or adduction through the midtarsal joints
  - Type I fracture—transverse in the coronal plane, dorsal fragment less than 50% of body
  - Type II fracture—dorsolateral to plantar medial, with resultant medialization (adduction) of the fragment and forefoot
  - Type III fracture—central or lateral comminution with possible lateral displacement of the foot

- Treatment
  - ORIF of even minimally displaced fractures is recommended.
  - Goal is to preserve TN and therefore hindfoot motion.
  - May require external fixation to preserve medial column length or as aid in fracture reduction
  - Primary or delayed arthrodesis of involved joints may be required with extensive comminution.
- Navicular stress fractures
  - Secondary to repetitive trauma, especially in running and jumping athletes
  - Cavus feet a predisposing factor
  - Typically occur in the central third of the navicular
  - Patients complain of vague dorsal midfoot or ankle pain.

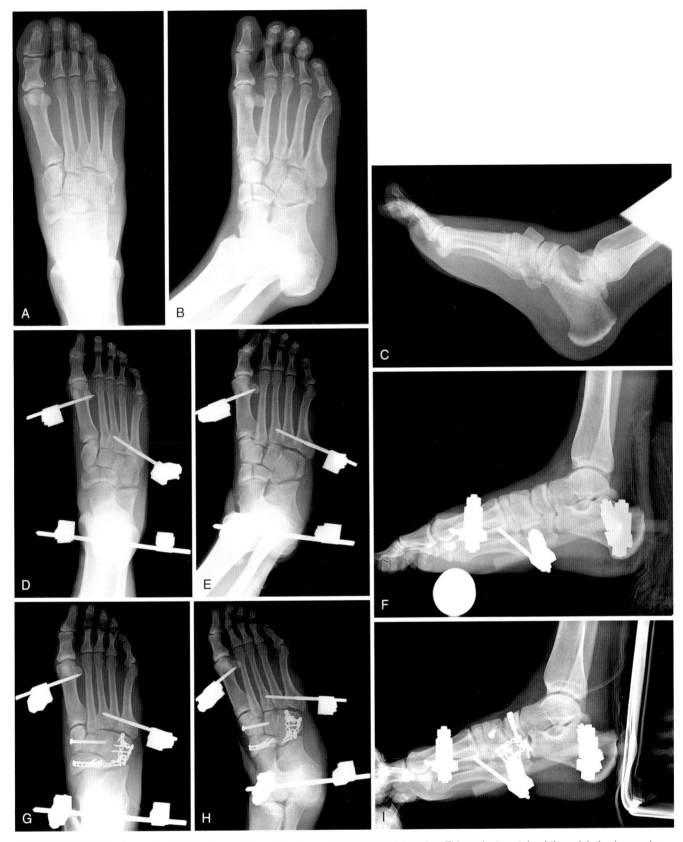

FIGURE 6-122 Navicular and cuboid fractures with middle (second) cuneiform dislocation. This patient sustained these injuries in a motor vehicle crash. **A** and **B,** Anteroposterior and oblique injury radiographs. **C,** Lateral injury radiograph. **D** to **F,** Definitive open reduction with internal fixation (ORIF) of this patient's injuries could not be accomplished acutely owing to profuse edema. Closed reduction of middle (second) cuneiform dislocation and of foot alignment was accomplished and held using a through-and-through calcaneal tuberosity pin, attached via carbon fiber rods to a distal first metatarsal pin medially and a proximal fourth and fifth metatarsal pin laterally. **G** to **I,** Definitive ORIF was accomplished after foot edema was controlled. A single intercuneiform screw holds the middle (second) cuneiform reduced. Plate fixation is noted on the navicular and cuboid, maintaining anatomic reduction. The medial and lateral external fixator was left in place for 6 weeks to supplement fixation support. (From DiGiovanni C: *Core knowledge in orthopaedics—foot and ankle,* Philadelphia, 2007, Elsevier.)

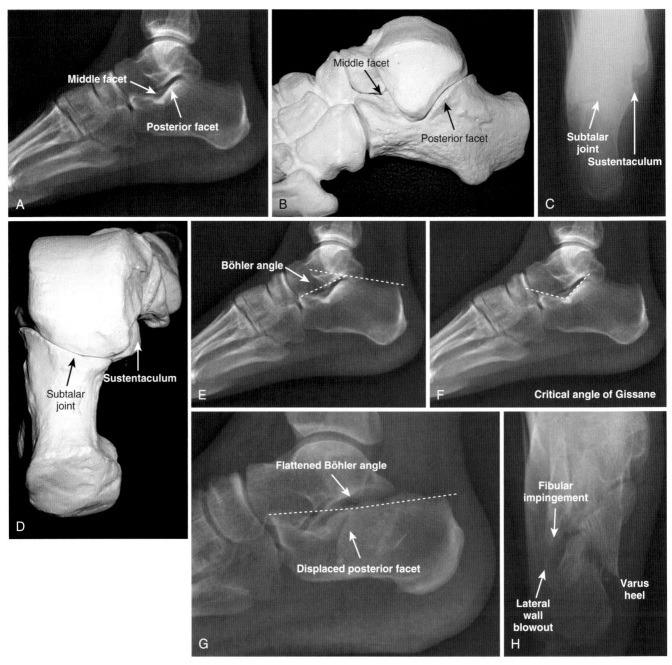

FIGURE 6-132 The normal **(A, C)** and pathologic **(G, H)** radiographic anatomy of the calcaneus. The lateral **(A, E, G)** and Harris axial **(C, H)** views of the calcaneus are useful in assessing the shape and alignment of the calcaneus. The lateral view **(A, E)** allows for the assessment of the posterior and middle facet positions as well as an assessment of calcaneal height (Böhler angle, **E**). The Böhler angle is formed by drawing two lines. The first is drawn from the highest point on the anterior process to the highest point on the posterior facet. The second line is tangential to the superior edge of the tuberosity. The normal value of the Böhler angle is 25 to 40 degrees. In the injured calcaneus **(G)**, the Böhler angle diminishes, corresponding to the loss of height ("flattening"). The critical angle of Gissane **(F)** is the angle formed by the intersection of a line drawn along the dorsal aspect of the anterior process of the calcaneus and a line drawn along the dorsal slope of the posterior facet. The normal value of the Gissane angle is 120 to 145 degrees. The axial view **(C, H)** is useful for determining displacement of the tuberosity, varus angulation, fibular abutment, and displacement of the lateral wall. (From Browner B et al: *Skeletal trauma,* ed 4, Philadelphia, 2008, Elsevier.)

- Prognosis
  - Worse outcomes correlate to higher fracture types.
  - Patients with significant intraarticular displacement, flattened Böhler angle, women, age younger than 29, and not involved in worker's compensation have improved clinical outcomes with operative compared to nonoperative management.

- Posttraumatic subtalar arthritis is common; may require arthrodesis.
  - 50% decreased ROM of subtalar joint expected after injury, regardless of treatment
  - Patients complain of pain over the sinus tarsi with limited inversion/eversion.
  - Superior outcomes demonstrated with arthrodesis after primary ORIF compared to patients who

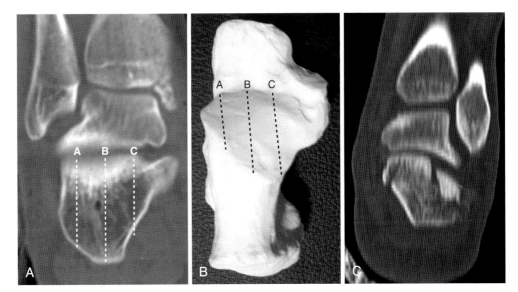

FIGURE 6-133 The Sanders classification is based on the fracture pattern through the posterior facet as seen on coronal CT scan. Type 1 fractures are nondisplaced. Type 2 fractures are two-part fractures of the posterior facet. Type 3 fractures are three-part fractures of the posterior facet. Type 4 fractures are highly comminuted, with four or more fragments to the posterior facet. **A** and **B,** Type 2 and type 3 fractures are further classified based on the location of the fracture lines (A, B, and C), as shown. **C,** Based on this classification system, this fracture would be a Sanders type 3AC. The prognosis for calcaneus fractures worsens as the comminution of the posterior facet worsens. (From DiGiovanni C: *Core knowledge in orthopaedics—foot and ankle,* Philadelphia, 2007, Elsevier.)

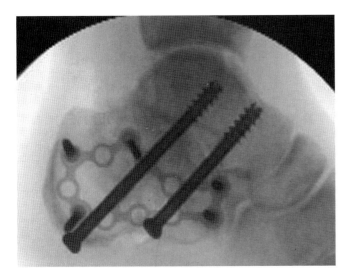

FIGURE 6-134 Primary subtalar fusion may be indicated in cases of severe comminution or destruction of the articular cartilage. Once reduction and fixation of the calcaneus is complete, the subtalar joint is denuded of cartilage. Compressive fixation is then applied across the subtalar joint. (From Browner B et al: *Skeletal trauma,* ed 4, Philadelphia, 2008, Elsevier.)

were treated initially with nonoperative management
  • Secondary to restoration of height and width of the hindfoot in operatively treated patients
• In cases with significant loss of calcaneal height, horizontal talus, and resultant anterior ankle pain, bone-block distraction arthrodesis of the subtalar joint is required.

PERITALAR (SUBTALAR) DISLOCATIONS

■ **Associated tarsal fractures in 90%**
▦ Medial—dorsomedial talar head, posterior tubercles of talus, lateral navicular

▦ Lateral—cuboid, anterior process of calcaneus, lateral process of talus and lateral malleolus
■ **Medial dislocation (Figure 6-135)**
▦ More common than lateral dislocations—85%
▦ Result from forceful inversion of the hindfoot, resulting in medial displacement of the calcaneus
▦ Reduction can usually be accomplished under sedation or general anesthesia.
▦ Most common obstacles to reduction are the EDB, the extensor retinaculum, the peroneal tendons, and the TN capsule.
■ **Lateral dislocation (Figure 6-136)**
▦ Less common than medial dislocations—15%
▦ Occurs with forceful eversion of the hindfoot, resulting in lateral displacement of the calcaneus
▦ Most common obstacles to reduction are an interposed posterior tibial tendon and FHL tendon.
■ **CT scan recommended in all cases to rule out small intraarticular fragments.**
■ **Treatment**
▦ Immobilization in boot or cast for 6 to 12 weeks if stable reduction
▦ Unstable reduction requires temporary stabilization with either K-wire fixation or external fixation.
▦ Intraarticular fragments should be removed surgically.

COMPARTMENT SYNDROME

■ **Leg compartment syndrome (see Chapter 11, Trauma)**
■ **Foot compartment syndrome**
▦ Anatomy (controversial)
  • Medial compartment—abductor hallucis, FHB
  • Central (calcaneal) compartments (three)
    • Superficial—FDB
    • Central—quadratus plantae
    • Deep—adductor hallucis and tibial neurovascular bundle

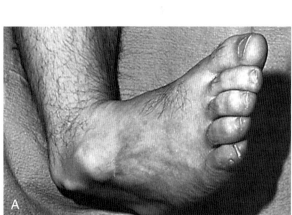 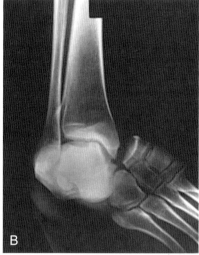

FIGURE 6-135 Medial subtalar dislocation. **A,** Posture of foot. Note prominence of head of talus. **B,** Radiographic appearance of dislocation. (From Canale ST, Beaty J: *Campbell's operative orthopaedics,* ed 11, Philadelphia, 2007, Elsevier; and DeLee JC, Curtis R: Subtalar dislocation of the foot, *J Bone Joint Surg* 64A:433, 1982.)

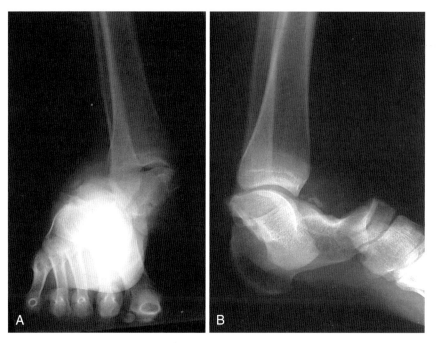

FIGURE 6-136 Anteroposterior **(A)** and lateral **(B)** radiographs of lateral subtalar dislocation. (From Coughlin MJ et al: *Surgery of the foot and ankle,* ed 8, Philadelphia, 2006, Mosby.)

- Lateral compartment—flexors, abductors, and opponens to the fifth toe
- Interosseous compartments (four)—interossei muscles
- The dorsalis pedis artery forms an anastomosis with the plantar arch by passing between the first and second metatarsal bases.
- Mechanism of injury
- When the intracompartmental fluid pressure meets or exceeds the capillary filling pressure (perfusion pressure), irreversible muscle and nerve damage can occur.

- In the foot, crush injuries are the most common cause.
- Calcaneus fractures carry a up to a 17% incidence of compartment syndrome.
- Diagnosis
- Diagnosis is made by constellation of clinical findings and high index of suspicion.
- Clinical findings include massive swelling, pain out of proportion to the injury that is not relieved by immobilization or appropriate analgesics, severe pain with passive motion of the toes (stretching the intrinsic muscles), and paresthesias and/or loss of light-touch perception and two-point discrimination.

- Presence of normal capillary refill and palpable and/or Doppler positive pulses do not rule out compartment syndrome.
- Compartment pressures can be measured to aid in the diagnosis.
  - Values greater than 30 mm Hg or those within 20 mm Hg of the diastolic pressure should raise suspicion of a compartment syndrome.
- Treatment
  - Fasciotomies can be performed through three incisions (see Figure 6-68).
    - Dorsomedial incision
      - Medial to second metatarsal
      - Releases first and second interosseous, medial, and deep central compartments
    - Dorsolateral incision
      - Lateral to fourth metatarsal
      - Releases third and fourth interosseous, lateral, superficial and middle central compartments
    - Medial incision
      - Plantar medial border of hindfoot
      - Releases calcaneal compartment
  - The wounds should be left open initially, with delayed closure or skin grafting performed as swelling improves.
  - Definitive treatment is compartment release.
    - The result of unrecognized and untreated compartment syndrome is NOT simply isolated claw toes.
    - Damage is not isolated to the musculature but also affects peripheral nerves. This commonly results in chronic pain with hypersensitivity that can be difficult or impossible to treat.
    - Benign neglect of a foot compartment syndrome is not appropriate management.

ANKLE FRACTURES

- **Typically a low-energy mechanism of injury, <u>rotational as opposed to axial load</u>**
- **Must always evaluate for deltoid or syndesmosis injury**
- **Diagnosis**
- Varied presentations depending on severity of injury
- Radiographic evaluation
  - AP, mortise, and lateral radiographs often sufficient to identify fracture pattern
  - **External rotation stress or gravity stress radiographs assess for deltoid integrity (Figure 6-137).**
    - <u>**Medial clear space widening with stress indicates deep deltoid disruption and implies unstable fracture pattern.**</u>
  - <u>CT scan</u> obtained for complex fracture patterns, posterior malleolar fractures (Figure 6-138)
  - Radiographic measurements helpful, but wide range of normal—comparison contralateral ankle radiographs may identify subtle instability of deltoid or syndesmosis.
    - Medial clear space less than 4 mm
    - Talocrural angle 83 (±4) degrees
    - Talar tilt less than 2 mm
    - Syndesmosis-tibial clear space less than 5 mm
    - Tibiofibular overlap less than 10 mm or 42% width of fibula

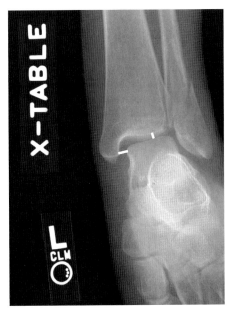

FIGURE 6-137 Gravity stress ankle radiograph showing increased medial clear space and fibular fracture displacement. Medial clear space widening with stress indicates deep deltoid disruption and implies unstable fracture pattern.

- Continuous curve along lateral talus and tip of distal fibula (Shenton line or "dime sign")
- **Classification**
- Lauge-Hansen
  - Describes position of foot (first word) and injury motion of the foot relative to the leg. Increasing stages include additional injuries to stage I.
  - **Supination-adduction (vertical medial malleolar fracture with low transverse fibular fracture) (Figure 6-139)**
    - Stage I—transverse distal fibula fracture at or below level of ATFL or lateral ligament injury
    - Stage II—oblique or vertical fracture of medial malleolus
      - Medial tibial plafond impaction occurs in up to 50% of cases and must be addressed.
  - **Supination–external rotation (oblique distal fibula at level of syndesmosis with or without transverse medial malleolar fracture) (Figure 6-140)**
    - Most common fracture pattern
    - Stage I—rupture of anterior inferior tibiofibular ligament (AITFL)
    - Stage II—oblique or spiral fracture of distal fibula
    - Stage III—rupture of posterior inferior tibiofibular ligament PITFL or avulsion fracture of posterior malleolus
    - Stage IV—transverse or oblique fracture of medial malleolus or deltoid disruption
    - Stress test typically performed to identify stable (SER-II) versus unstable (SER-IV) fracture patterns
  - **Pronation-abduction (comminuted fibular fracture above the level of the syndesmosis, obvious disruption of the syndesmosis, with or without medial malleolar fracture) (Figure 6-141)**
    - Stage I—rupture of deltoid ligament or transverse fracture of medial malleolus
    - Stage II—rupture of the AITFL or avulsion of anterolateral tibia

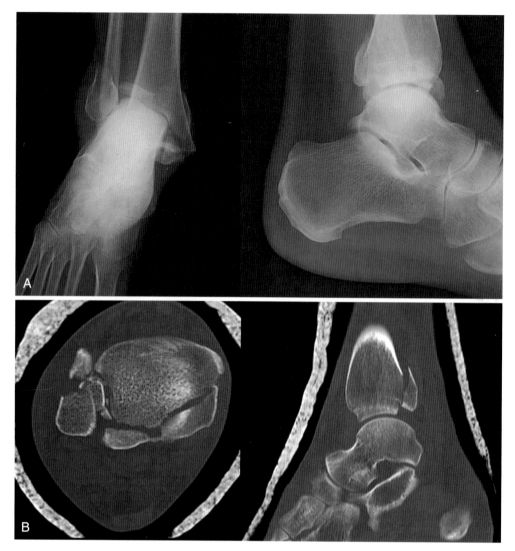

FIGURE 6-138 Fractures with a posterior malleolar component or fracture/dislocations are best evaluated with a CT scan to assess for the presence and displacement of articular fragments. The severity of this fracture on plain radiographs **(A)** can be underestimated when compared to the CT scan **(B).** Following review of the CT scan for these types of fractures, the operative approach is frequently altered.

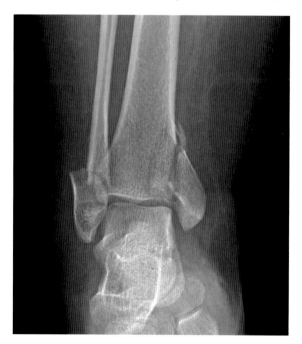

FIGURE 6-139 Supination adduction injury with a vertical fracture line through the medial malleolus. Use of an antiglide plate is critical in these injuries to prevent malunion.

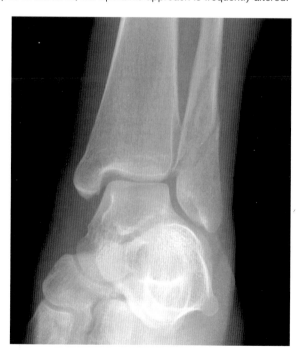

FIGURE 6-140 Oblique fibula fracture at level of syndesmosis seen on mortise radiograph, consistent with a supination–external rotation fracture pattern.

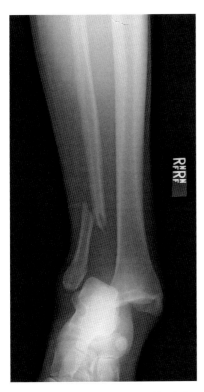

FIGURE 6-141 Transverse fibular fracture with obvious disruption of the syndesmosis and nearly complete subluxation of the talus. This injury pattern (or a comminuted fibula) is consistent with a pronation-abduction injury that consists of a large lateral translator force to the foot.

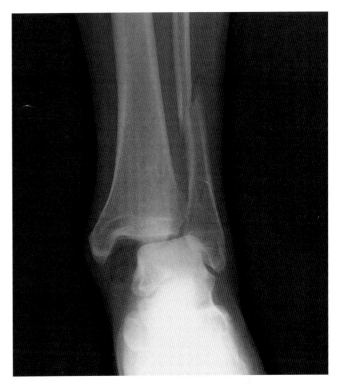

FIGURE 6-142 Suprasyndesmotic oblique fibula fracture with associated lateral talar translation that is consistent with a pronation–external rotation (PER) fracture pattern. Ankle dislocation is less common in a PER injury than in a pronation abduction (PAB) pattern.

- Stage III—oblique or spiral fracture of fibula above level of syndesmosis
- Stage IV—rupture of PITFL or avulsion fracture of posterior malleolus
- **Pronation–external rotation (oblique fracture of the fibula above the level of syndesmosis, with slight widening of the syndesmosis, with or without medial malleolar fracture)** (Figure 6-142)
  - Stage I—medial malleolus fracture
  - Stage II—anterior lip of tibial plafond fracture
  - Stage III—fracture of fibula above level of malleolus
  - Stage IV—rupture of PITFL or avulsion fracture of posterior malleolus
- Danis-Weber/OTA
  - Based on location of fibula fracture
  - 44-A—infrasyndesmotic
    - Stable, rarely require operative intervention
  - 44-B—trans-syndesmotic
    - Variably unstable, test with external rotation or gravity stress radiographs.
  - 44-C—suprasyndesmotic
    - Inherently unstable, require operative intervention
- Posterior malleolar fractures/posterior pilon
  - Significant attention has been placed on the role of the posterior malleolus when considering ankle fractures.
    - Greater than 2-mm displacement of the articular surface is associated with worse functional outcomes 1 year after injury.
      - Regardless of size of the posterior malleolar fragment
    - Stabilization of the posterior malleolus restores 70% of the stability of the syndesmosis.

- **Associated with spiral fractures of distal third of the tibia**
- Indications for ORIF are controversial because the historical criteria based on size may not be sufficient.
  - Displacement of the fracture greater than 2 mm or size greater than 25% of the articular surface is ideally treated with ORIF.
- Posterior pilon
  - Recently described fracture pattern with comminution of posterior malleolus
  - Indicative of more severe articular injury but commonly rotational mechanism of injury
  - Includes fracture of distal fibula and avulsion fracture of posterolateral portion of posterior malleolus (PITFL), variable patterns of posteromedial plafond and medial malleolus fractures (Figure 6-143)
  - Inherently unstable owing to syndesmosis instability
- Most commonly addressed with posterolateral approach with or without a posteromedial approach with direct fixation of posterior malleolar fractures and articular impaction
- Bosworth fracture-dislocation
  - Distal fibula entrapped behind incisura of distal tibia
  - Irreducible with closed methods, because interosseous membrane is intact

Treatment
- Must obtain stable reduction of ankle mortise
- One millimeter of lateral talar shift is associated with a 42% decrease in tibiotalar contact area.
- Syndesmosis instability must be addressed after fixation of fractures.

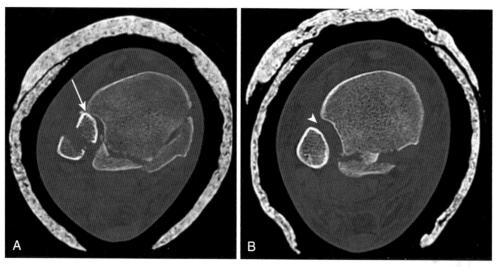

FIGURE 6-143 A, Axial CT scan of a patient with a posteromedial and posterolateral fragment with preserved integrity of the AITFL, as noted through lack of diastasis *(arrow)*. In this case, with fixation of the posterolateral fragment, the stability of the syndesmosis should be restored. **B,** The obvious widening of the anterior aspect of the syndesmosis is consistent with injury to the AITFL that will not be restored with reduction of the posterolateral fragment. In this case, supplemental fixation of the syndesmosis is required in addition to reduction and fixation of the posterior malleolus. Also note that given the interposed fragment between the posterolateral fragment and tibia, an indirect reduction of that piece is impossible.

 ■ **Braking response time for driving returns (on average) 9 weeks after operative fixation of ankle fractures.**
■ Nonoperative treatment
  • Indications
    • Systemic conditions precluding anesthesia, poor protoplasm for healing (severe diabetes, vascular disease), limited baseline weight-bearing activity
    • Isolated stable distal fibula fractures without deltoid insufficiency (Danis-Weber A or B)
    • Isolated avulsion fractures of tip of medial malleolus
    • Nondisplaced bimalleolar fractures in selected high-risk patients
  • Weight-bearing CAM boot for 6 weeks
  • Frequent radiographic follow-up indicated
■ Operative treatment
  • Indications
    • Displaced bimalleolar or trimalleolar fractures
    • Displaced distal fibula fractures with deltoid insufficiency (so-called bimalleolar equivalent fractures)
    • Displaced isolated medial malleolus fractures
    • Fracture patterns with syndesmosis disruption
    • Posterior malleolar fractures with greater than 25% articular involvement or more than 2 mm step-off (controversial)
    • Bosworth fracture-dislocations
    • Open fractures
  • Techniques for ORIF
    • Fibula
      • AP lag screw with lateral neutralization plate—spiral or oblique fracture patterns (Figure 6-144)
      • Posterolateral antiglide plate—biomechanically superior to lateral plate, increased risk of peroneal irritation
      • Anatomic locking plate—helpful for very distal fractures, osteoporotic bone, or comminution
        • This type of plate is not routinely required.

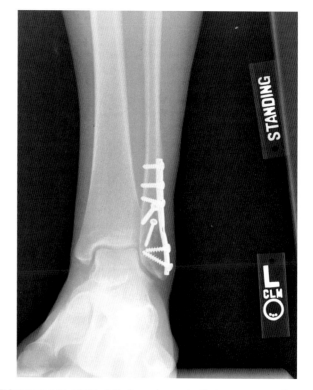

FIGURE 6-144 ORIF of fibula performed with lag screws and a lateral neutralization plate. A 2.7-mm or 3.5-mm screw may be used.

  • Medial malleolus
    • Partially threaded 4-mm screws most common technique
      • Bicortical 3.5-mm screws demonstrated superior biomechanical strength compared to unicortical 4.0-mm partially threaded cancellous screws. No

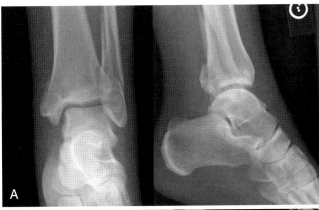

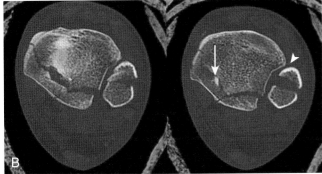

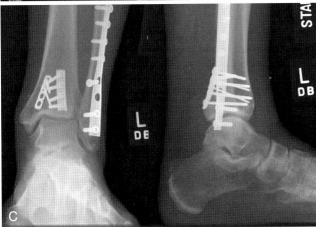

FIGURE 6-145 Anteroposterior and lateral views of a patient with a "posterior pilon" fracture. **A,** On the preoperative x-rays, a positive double-contour sign can be appreciated, indicating involvement of the whole posterior tibial metaphysis. **B,** This is confirmed on axial CT scans, where additional posteromedial comminution can be seen *(white arrow)* with syndesmotic gapping *(white arrowhead)* excluded. **C,** Postoperative x-rays demonstrate double plating of the posterior malleolar fragment.

proven clinical superiority has been demonstrated.
- **Medial buttress plate/screws parallel to joint—vertical fracture patterns (supination-adduction)**
- Posterior malleolus (Figure 6-145)
  - AP lag screws have been described; best indicated in nondisplaced fractures.
  - Posterior buttress plate—displaced fractures, posterior pilon fractures

- Syndesmosis (Figure 6-146)
  - Anatomic reduction of syndesmosis is critical. May directly visualize with dissection over anterior tibiofibular ligaments.
    - When using a clamp, it should be externally rotated 15 degrees relative to the foot in line with the axis of the syndesmosis.
      - Dorsiflexion of the ankle is not critical during reduction.
    - **The fibula is most unstable in the sagittal plane, and therefore a sagittal as well as coronal stress test should be performed.**
    - Obtaining a contralateral true lateral of the unaffected limb will allow comparison to verify fibular reduction of the affected limb.
      - This technique has been compared to intraoperative CT scan and has demonstrated high reproducibility in ensuring accurate syndesmotic reduction.
  - Controversies regarding fixation techniques
    - One versus two screws
    - Three versus four cortices
    - 3.5-mm versus 4.5-mm screws
    - Screws versus suture devices
    - Hardware removal versus retention of screws
  - If removing screws, leave in position for at least 12 to 16 weeks.
  - No proven benefit to screw removal; retained screw or broken screws have not been proven detrimental to function.
    - Radiographic improvement in tibiofibular alignment has been demonstrated after syndesmotic screw removal, however.
- Complications
  - **Malunion**
    - **Associated with insufficient fibular length (short fibula), medial clear space widening, and malreduction of the syndesmosis**
    - **Treatment**
      - **Fibular osteotomy to restore length, medial gutter débridement, and reconstruction of the syndesmosis**
  - Wound complications—5%
  - Deep infection—1% to 2% (up to 20% in diabetics)
  - Posttraumatic arthritis
    - Associated with malreduction or persistent mortise instability
    - Increased risk with higher-stage fracture patterns or involvement of tibial plafond (trimalleolar fractures worse than bimalleolar fractures)
- Special circumstances
  - Diabetic patients
    - **Non–weight-bearing period must be doubled relative to nondiabetic patients.**
      - 3 months
    - High rate of complications with both nonoperative and operative treatment
    - Biggest risk factor for complications is presence of neuropathy.
    - Skin complications, loss of reduction, and nonunion noted with cast treatment

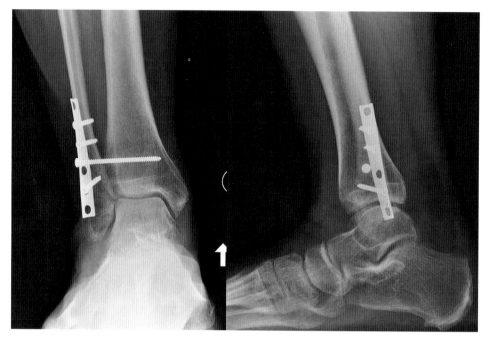

FIGURE 6-146 Single 3.5-mm tricortical screw for stabilization of the syndesmosis following ORIF of the fibula.

- Wound complications, deep infection, loss of reduction, and hardware failure noted with operative treatment
  - Up to 30% amputation rate
- Open fractures
  - Emergent irrigation and débridement indicated
  - Immediate ORIF if limited contamination

PILON (TIBIAL PLAFOND) FRACTURES

- Frequently comminuted intraarticular fractures of distal tibial plafond
- High-energy mechanism of injury, often associated with falls from height or motor vehicle collisions (axial loads)
- Most common in fourth decade of life, more common in men
- Poor outcomes more common in patients with lower income or education levels, preexisting medical comorbidities, males, workers compensation claims
- May note continued clinical improvement for up to 2 years
- Diagnosis
- Significant swelling, fracture blisters, and open injuries may be present.
- Radiographic evaluation
  - AP, mortise, and lateral x-rays of the ankle typically sufficient to evaluate fracture; tibia-fibula and foot x-rays may be required if concern for more extensive injury.
  - CT valuable to determine extent of intraarticular involvement and fracture planes for preoperative planning
    - Obtain after reduction of fracture; fragments frequently shift position after manipulation (Figure 6-147).
  - Three common fragments identified; are due to ligamentous attachments
    - Medial—deltoid ligament
    - Volkmann—posterior tibiofibular ligament
    - Chaput—anterior tibiofibular ligament

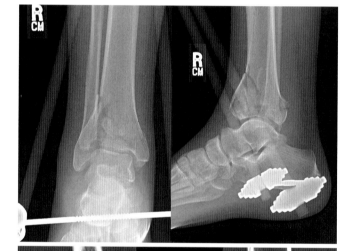

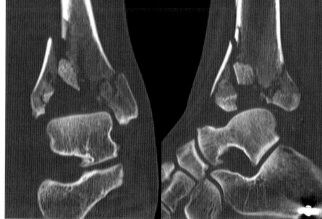

FIGURE 6-147 Given the severity of the injury, obtaining radiographs following placement of an external fixator is valuable in better understanding the fracture pattern. A CT scan is critical and should only performed after external fixator placement to evaluate the position of the intraarticular fragments that require reduction.

- Classification—common classifications include Ruedi-Allgower and AO/OTA and describe degree of comminution but generally not helpful to determine operative plan.
- Nonoperative treatment
- Indicated for patients unable to tolerate anesthesia or severe soft tissue or vascular compromise
- Stable fracture patterns without articular displacement may be amenable to nonoperative treatment.
- Operative treatment
- Limited internal fixation with external fixation is not the most effective treatment method for these injuries. If external fixation is performed, thin wire frames are ideal because they can be used to stabilize the articular surface and provide rigid fixation.
- **Primary temporary external fixation, delayed ORIF is the most commonly used method. Fixation of the fibula is not required at the index operation.**
  - Immediate ORIF is associated with an unacceptable rate of wound complications and therefore is not advocated.
  - **ORIF of tibia and fibula is delayed until soft tissue swelling resolves and any hemorrhagic blisters have epithelialized.**
  - Principles of ORIF (Figure 6-148):
    - Anatomic reduction and absolute rigid fixation of articular surface
    - Preserve tibial length.
    - Reconstruction of metaphyseal shell
    - Bone grafting of metaphyseal defects
    - Reattachment of metaphysis to diaphysis
      - Bridge plating technique is appropriate, without requirement to achieve anatomic reduction. Restoration of length, alignment, and rotation are critical.
- Complications
  - Wound dehiscence reported in 9% to 30%—decreased risk if soft tissue swelling allowed to resolve prior to tibial fixation
  - Infection—5% to 15%
  - Malunion or nonunion—increased risk with hybrid fixation, nicotine use, diabetes, poor bone quality
  - Nonunion most common at metaphyseal junction
  - Posttraumatic arthritis—may appear as early as 1 to 2 years following injury
  - Although primary arthrodesis has been described, ORIF is the most commonly performed method at this time.

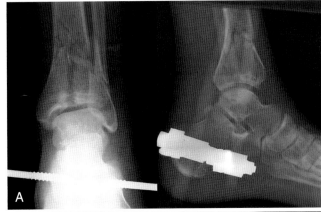
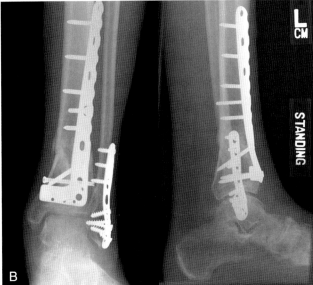

FIGURE 6-148 A, Preoperative radiographs of a pilon fracture that underwent initial spanning external fixation without ORIF of the fibula. **B,** Final fixation is noted 1 year postoperatively with ORIF of the tibia and fibula and restoration of the articular surface.

- **Normal return to braking time**
  - 6 weeks following initiation of weight bearing

SELECTED BIBLIOGRAPHY

The selected bibliography for this chapter can be found on https://expertconsult.inkling.com.

TESTABLE CONCEPTS

SECTION 1 BIOMECHANICS OF THE FOOT AND ANKLE

- At the distal tibiofibular joint, the fibula externally rotates and proximally translates with ankle dorsiflexion.
- In the toe-off phase of gait, the plantar fascia is tightened as the metatarsophalangeal (MTP) joints extend. The longitudinal arch is accentuated. This is termed the *windlass mechanism.* The hindfoot supinates and locks with firing of the posterior tibial tendon.
- Plantar migration of the metatarsal head after a Weil osteotomy may lead to cock-up toe deformity as the axis of pull of the intrinsics moves dorsal to the center of rotation.

SECTION 2 PHYSICAL EXAMINATION OF THE FOOT AND ANKLE

- Cavovarus alignment demonstrates an elevated longitudinal arch with hindfoot varus and a plantar-flexed first ray. Pes planus is noted with a flat longitudinal arch with hindfoot valgus.
- Vascular examination findings that are predictive for healing include toe pressure greater than 40 mm Hg and transcutaneous oxygen pressure greater than 30 mm Hg.
- Neurologic examination should include use of a Semmes-Weinstein 5.07 monofilament. Inability to sense this is consistent with neuropathy and the most predictive sign for the development of a foot ulceration.
- Stability of the lateral ankle ligaments can be assessed with the anterior drawer and varus talar tilt tests.
  - Anterior drawer test—anterior pressure on the hindfoot with the ankle in plantar flexion evaluates the anterior talofibular ligament.
  - Varus stress test—inversion of the ankle in dorsiflexion evaluates the calcaneofibular ligament.
- The Silfverskiöld test evaluates for contracture.
  - Test ankle dorsiflexion with the knee extended and flexed with the hindfoot in neutral alignment.
  - Tightness in both knee flexion and extension indicates Achilles contracture.
  - Improvement in ankle dorsiflexion with knee flexion (relaxing the gastrocnemius origin proximal to the knee) indicates isolated gastrocnemius contracture.

SECTIONS 4 AND 5 ADULT AND JUVENILE HALLUX VALGUS

- A key feature in the pathoanatomy of hallux valgus is lateral drift of the proximal phalanx, leading to plantar lateral migration of abductor hallucis, which results in plantar flexion and pronation.
- There are four key radiographic angular measurements in hallux valgus.
  - Hallux valgus angle (HVA), first-second intermetatarsal angle (IMA), hallux valgus interphalangeus (HVI) angle, and the distal metatarsal articular angle (DMAA)
- Congruency of the first MTP must also be determined by comparing the line connecting the medial and lateral edge of the first metatarsal head articular surface with the similar line for the proximal phalanx. When these lines are parallel, the joint is congruent.
- Appropriate surgical procedures are determined by two factors.
  - Angular measurements
  - Clinical scenario
  - Regardless of angular measurements, the following clinical abnormalities dictate surgical procedure.
  - Spasticity (stroke or cerebral palsy)—first MTP fusion
  - Osteoarthritis or rheumatoid arthritis—first MTP fusion
  - Ligamentous laxity—Lapidus (first tarsometatarsal [TMT] realignment arthrodesis)
  - First TMT degenerative joint disease (DJD)—Lapidus

- A distal soft tissue release (modified McBride) is never appropriate in isolation.
- In general, all patients should undergo a soft tissue release with all associated osteotomies and first TMT arthrodesis.
- Angular measurement guides for surgical procedure
  - IMA 13 degrees or less AND HVA 40 degrees or less—distal chevron
  - IMA greater than 13 degrees OR HVA greater than 40 degrees—proximal metatarsal osteotomy
- Complications
  - Recurrence—undercorrection of IMA or isolated soft tissue reconstruction. Recurrence of the deformity after surgical correction is the most common complication in juvenile and adolescent hallux valgus.
  - Dorsal malunion—Lapidus or proximal crescentic osteotomy; results in transfer metatarsalgia
  - Hallux varus—overresection of the medial eminence

SECTION 7 LESSER-TOE DEFORMITIES

- Hammer toe—proximal interphalangeal (PIP) flexion (MTP dorsiflexed but should correct with elevation). Fixed deformity is treated with PIP arthroplasty (resection of distal neck and head of proximal phalanx) or PIP arthrodesis.
- Claw toe—PIP and distal interphalangeal (DIP) flexion with fixed MTP hyperextension
  - Flexible—flexor-to-extensor tendon transfer of flexor digitorum longus (FDL)
  - Fixed—PIP arthroplasty/arthrodesis with MTP capsulotomy and extensor lengthening. A dislocated MTP joint requires use of a distal metatarsal osteotomy (e.g., Weil) to reduce MTP joint.
- Mallet toe—DIP flexion; flexible deformity treated with flexor tenotomy; fixed deformity with DIP arthroplasty or fusion
- Crossover toe—sagittal and axial plane deformities. Key component is disruption of the plantar plate. May be iatrogenic from steroid injection within MTP joint. Address with EDB transfer.
- Freiberg disease—osteochondrosis of metatarsal head. Early-stage disease is treated with joint débridement. A dorsal closed-wedge metaphyseal osteotomy may also be performed.
- Congenital curly toe—perform tenotomy of FDL and flexor digitorum brevis in children with flexible deformities.

SECTION 8 HYPERKERATOTIC PATHOLOGIES

- Bunionette deformity is treated based on the anatomic location of deformity.
  - Enlarged fifth metatarsal head—lateral condylectomy
  - Lateral bowing of fifth metatarsal diaphysis—distal metatarsal osteotomy
  - Widened fourth-fifth metatarsal angle—oblique diaphyseal osteotomy

SECTION 9 SESAMOIDS

- Turf toe mechanism of injury is forced dorsiflexion resulting in avulsion of the plantar plate off the base of the phalanx and subsequent proximal migration of the sesamoids.
  - Complete tears of the plantar plate treated with operative repair have demonstrated superior results compared to conservative care.
- Complications of medial and lateral sesamoidectomy are hallux valgus and varus, respectively.
- Cock-up deformity (or claw toe) will occur if both sesamoids are excised.

TESTABLE CONCEPTS

SECTION 11 NEUROLOGIC DISORDERS

- Interdigital neuritis (Morton neuroma) is a compressive neuropathy of the interdigital nerve, usually between the third and fourth metatarsals. Surgical treatment is via a dorsal approach, incision of the transverse intermetatarsal ligament and resection of the nerve 2 to 3 cm proximal to the intermetatarsal ligament.
- The lateral plantar nerve may be injured during surgical approaches that require a plantar incision, such as a tibiotalocalcaneal arthrodesis with an intramedullary nail.
- Upper motor neuron disorders most commonly result in an equinovarus foot deformity.
  - Equinus—overactivity of gastrocnemius-soleus complex
  - Equinus deformity is addressed with either an open Z-lengthening of the Achilles tendon or a percutaneous triple-hemisection technique.
  - Varus—overactivity of tibialis anterior (lesser contributions from flexor hallucis longus [FHL], FDL, and tibialis posterior)
  - Varus deformity is addressed with a split anterior tibialis tendon transfer (SPLATT) to the lateral cuneiform or cuboid or total anterior tibial tendon transfer to the lateral cuneiform.
- Type I hereditary motor-sensory neuropathy is the most common presentation of Charcot-Marie-Tooth disease (CMT).
  - Usually autosomal dominant with a duplication of chromosome 17
- Treatment of a flexible cavus deformity involves:
  - Release of the plantar fascia
  - Transfer of the peroneus longus into the peroneus brevis at the level of the distal fibula
  - A closed-wedge dorsiflexion osteotomy of the first metatarsal is always required.
  - If the deformity does not correct with Coleman block, perform a lateral calcaneal slide and/or closed-wedge osteotomy.
- Nonoperative treatment of a fixed deformity
  - Locked-ankle, short-leg ankle-foot orthosis (AFO) with an outside (varus-correcting or lateral) T-strap is recommended.
    - Rocker sole can improve gait and decrease energy expenditure.
- Peroneal nerve palsy results in loss of the anterior and lateral compartments with loss of active dorsiflexion and eversion. This results in equinovarus.
  - Transfer posterior tibial tendon (PTT) through the interosseous membrane anteriorly to the dorsal midfoot to restore dorsiflexion. Achilles tendon should be lengthened.

SECTION 12 ARTHRITIC DISEASE

- Foot involvement very common in rheumatoid patients with the forefoot more commonly involved than the midfoot or hindfoot
  - The toes sublux or dislocate dorsally, deviate laterally into valgus, and develop hammering.
  - "Rheumatoid forefoot reconstruction"—first MTP arthrodesis, lesser metatarsal head resection with pinning of the lesser MTP joints, and closed osteoclasis of the interphalangeal joints versus PIP arthroplasty
  - The most common complication of forefoot arthroplasty is intractable plantar keratoses.
- Osteoarthritis etiology is typically posttraumatic in the hindfoot and tibiotalar articulations, while idiopathic in the first MTP and midfoot joints.
- First MTP (hallux rigidus)—tenderness over dorsum of joint, limited dorsiflexion due to large dorsal osteophyte and pain with grind test
  - Initial treatment is a stiff foot plate with extension under great toe (Morton extension).

- Surgical treatment in those with pain at extremes of range of motion (ROM)—dorsal cheilectomy.
  - Pain throughout ROM with positive grind—arthrodesis (neutral rotation, 10 to 15 degrees of dorsiflexion, and slight valgus)
- Hindfoot arthritis—triple arthrodesis to correct arthritis secondary to deformity (0 to 5 degrees of hindfoot valgus, neutral abduction/adduction, plantigrade)
  - Revision of malunited triple arthrodesis requires calcaneal osteotomy and/or transverse tarsal osteotomy.
- Subtalar arthritis—Subtalar fusion nonunion risk is increased with history of ankle arthrodesis and smoking.
- Prior calcaneal fracture with loss of height results in anterior impingement, anterior ankle pain, and hindfoot pain and is treated with subtalar bone-block arthrodesis.
- Tibiotalar arthritis—Arthrodesis provides excellent pain relief with some restricted function.
  - The ideal position for fusion is neutral dorsiflexion, 0 to 5 degrees of hindfoot valgus, and 5 to 10 degrees of external rotation.
  - Leads to eventual arthritis in surrounding foot, most commonly the subtalar joint
  - Total ankle arthroplasty has shown the best outcome in patients with osteoarthritis. Syndesmotic fusion is associated with a decreased rate of failure for the Agility Ankle Replacement.

SECTION 13 POSTURAL DISORDERS

- Pes planus (flatfoot) deformity is most commonly caused by posterior tibial tendon dysfunction in the adult. There is a zone of hypovascularity 2 to 6 cm from the PTT attachment on the navicular.
  - Standing examination demonstrates asymmetric hindfoot valgus, depressed arch, and an abducted forefoot.
  - "Too many toes" when the foot is viewed posteriorly
  - Pain or an inability to perform a single-limb heel-rise indicates an insufficient PTT.
  - Radiographs demonstrate a negative lateral talo–first metatarsal angle (Meary angle) and talonavicular uncoverage
  - Treatment is based on whether the deformity is flexible or fixed.
  - Stage II surgical summary
    - FDL or FHL tendon transfer for ALL patients, gastrocnemius recession if contracture present, hindfoot valgus—medial slide calcaneal osteotomy
    - Forefoot abduction—lateral column lengthening
    - Forefoot supination
      - Stable medial column—Cotton osteotomy
      - Unstable medial column—first TMT arthrodesis
  - Stage III or fixed deformity is treated with a triple arthrodesis.
- Pes cavus etiology is neuromuscular, idiopathic, or traumatic (talus fracture malunion).
  - The Coleman block test is used to assess the flexibility of the hindfoot (out of varus) when the first metatarsal plantar flexion (forefoot valgus) is eliminated.
    - If the hindfoot passively corrects into valgus, the deformity is forefoot driven (due to plantar-flexed first ray).
  - Conservative treatment includes orthotics with a lateral heel wedge, decreased arch, and depressed first ray.
  - Surgical treatment for forefoot-driven deformity—first metatarsal dorsiflexion osteotomy
  - Surgical treatment for flexible hindfoot deformity—lateral calcaneal closed-wedge osteotomy and first metatarsal dorsiflexion osteotomy

TESTABLE CONCEPTS

SECTION 14 TENDON DISORDERS

- Peroneal tendon subluxation is caused by forced eversion and dorsiflexion, leading to disruption of superior peroneal retinaculum. This requires repair/reconstruction of the superior peroneal retinaculum and fibular groove deepening.
- FHL tenosynovitis is classically seen in dancers.
  - Posteromedial ankle pain, triggering of first interphalangeal joint, and pain with resisted hallux plantar flexion
  - Operative treatment is FHL tenosynovectomy and release of the fascia.

SECTION 15 HEEL PAIN

- Plantar fasciitis classically presents with exquisite pain and tenderness over the plantar medial tuberosity of the calcaneus at the proximal insertion of the plantar fascia. There is pain with the first step in the morning and after prolonged sitting. It is frequently associated with an Achilles or gastrocnemius contracture.
  - Nonoperative management includes both plantar fascia–specific stretching and Achilles stretching. Management also includes cushioned heel inserts, night splints, physical therapy, walking casts, cortisone injections, and antiinflammatory medications.
  - Operative management includes limited (medial half) release of the plantar fascia. Complete release can place the longitudinal arch of the foot at risk, overload the lateral column, and lead to dorsolateral foot pain and metatarsal stress fractures.
  - Other invasive options with evolving evidence include gastrocnemius recession and extracorporeal shock wave therapy.
- Baxter neuritis is compression of the first branch of the lateral plantar nerve. It presents as plantar medial heel pain and can be difficult to differentiate from plantar fasciitis.
- Insertional Achilles tendinopathy treatment includes excision of the retrocalcaneal bursa, resection of a prominent superior calcaneal tuberosity, and débridement of the degenerative tendon.
  - If more than 50% tendon detachment is required, reattachment with suture anchors is indicated. FHL tendon transfer is indicated if more than 50% of tendon requires excision.
- In noninsertional Achilles tendinopathy, MRI evidence of significant diffuse involvement without a focal area of disease indicates need for an FHL transfer.
- The treatment of acute Achilles tendon ruptures remains controversial. Most studies noted that nonoperative treatment results in an elevated rerupture rate while operative treatment increases wound complication and infection risks.
- Chronic rupture of the Achilles tendon requires FHL transfer.

SECTION 16 ANKLE PAIN AND SPORTS INJURIES

- High ankle sprains are injuries to the syndesmosis ligaments. Pain is elicited with external rotation stress at the ankle. Synostosis is a common sequelae and may be treated by débridement or syndesmosis fusion.
- Chronic exertional compartment syndrome is an uncommon cause of leg pain in the athlete. The standard pressures for diagnosis include intracompartmental pressures greater than 30 mm Hg after 1 minute of exercise, greater than 20 mm Hg after 5 minutes of exercise, or absolute pressures greater than 15 mm Hg.
- Popliteal artery entrapment may be confused with chronic exertional compartment syndrome. Dorsal pedal pulses may be obliterated with active ankle plantar flexion or passive dorsiflexion.

SECTION 17 THE DIABETIC FOOT

- Ninety percent of patients who cannot feel the 5.07 monofilament have lost protective sensation to their feet and are at risk for ulceration.
- Motor neuropathy most commonly involves the common peroneal nerve with resultant loss of tibialis anterior motor function with a footdrop. The small intrinsic musculature is also commonly affected, resulting in claw toes and subsequent toe-tip ulcerations.
- Peripheral vascular disease occurs in 60% to 70% of diabetic patients, and noninvasive vascular examination should be performed when pulses are not palpable. Absolute toe pressures are normally 100 mm Hg, and the minimum for healing is 40 mm Hg.
- Transcutaneous oxygen measurements (TcP_{O_2}) of the toes greater than 40 mm Hg have been found to be predictive of healing.
- Metabolic deficiency also impairs wound healing. Total protein less than 6.0 g/dL, WBC count less than 1500, and albumin level less than 2.5 g/dL all predict poor healing potential.
- Diabetic ulcers
  - Diabetic ulcer management is based on the depth-ischemia classification
  - Equinus contracture is very common, and Achilles lengthening will offload the midfoot/forefoot; required in recurrent forefoot/midfoot ulceration or ulceration with equinus deformity
- Charcot arthropathy
  - Charcot arthropathy is a chronic, progressive, destructive process affecting bone architecture and joint alignment in people lacking protective sensation.
  - Eichenholtz classification
    - I—Fragmentation: hyperemia, hot, swollen, erythematous
    - II—Coalescence: beginning of reparative process
    - III—Consolidation: smoothed bone edges with bony/fibrous ankylosis
  - Midfoot most common location (60%)
  - Swelling and redness is classically diminished with elevation. It is often confused with osteomyelitis clinically.
  - Initial treatment is immobilization and non–weight bearing; best with a total-contact cast; transition to AFO or Charcot restraint orthosis walker boot once swelling/erythema subsides
- Diabetic foot infections
  - Diabetic foot infections are polymicrobial. Deep surgical cultures provide the most accurate result.
  - Treatment with initial broad-spectrum antibiotic coverage once surgical cultures obtained. Adjust once sensitivity returns.
  - Surgical resection of infected bone is indicated if culture-specific antibiotic therapy fails. Ray resection, partial calcanectomy or partial/complete foot amputation may be required.
  - Amputation level
    - Lisfranc—tarsometatarsal disarticulation; must transfer peroneal tendons to cuboid to prevent varus and perform Achilles lengthening to prevent equinus
    - Chopart—talonavicular and calcaneocuboid joint combined disarticulation; must transfer anterior tibialis to talus to prevent equinus and perform Achilles lengthening to prevent equinus
    - Syme—ankle disarticulation; second lowest energy expenditure after a transmetatarsal amputation. Heel ulcers are absolute contraindication.

TESTABLE CONCEPTS

SECTION 18 TRAUMA

- Metatarsal fractures
  - Second metatarsal stress fracture is the most common and is classically described in amenorrheal dancers.
    - Treat in weight-bearing boot or hard-soled shoe.
    - Evaluate for metabolic bone disease in these patients, especially if insidious onset or if there is no distinct causal event (increase in training, initiation of new activity).
  - Fifth metatarsal fractures can be divided anatomically into avulsion fractures, fractures of the metaphyseal-diaphyseal junction, and fractures of the proximal diaphysis.
    - Avulsion fractures—protected weight bearing
    - Metaphyseal-diaphyseal fractures—non–weight bearing; elite athletes or delayed healing treated with intramedullary screw fixation
    - Proximal diaphysis—intramedullary fixation
- Lisfranc ligament is between the medial cuneiform and base of second metatarsal.
  - Nonsurgical management of Lisfranc injuries is indicated in nondisplaced injuries.
  - Primary arthrodesis is an alternative treatment option, with some benefit seen in patients with purely ligamentous injury or significant intraarticular comminution.
  - Missed diagnosis or improper treatment may lead to traumatic planovalgus deformity or posttraumatic arthritis.
  - Midfoot realignment and arthrodesis is the appropriate salvage procedure.
- Navicular stress fractures are secondary to repetitive trauma, especially running and jumping. They typically occur in the central one third, and patients complain of vague dorsal midfoot or ankle pain.
  - Computed tomography (CT) is the gold standard for diagnosis.
  - Nondisplaced fractures should be treated with non–weight bearing.
- The talus blood supply is provided by the posterior tibial artery, dorsalis pedis artery, and perforating peroneal artery. The artery of the tarsal canal carries the main supply to the talar body.
- Talar neck fractures are commonly associated with medial neck comminution, leading to a varus deformity.
  - Varus malunion is highly associated with use of medial compression screws. This leads to a cavovarus deformity, limiting hindfoot eversion that results in lateral border foot pain.
  - Avascular necrosis (AVN) increases with the severity of the injury. Hawkins sign is a subchondral linear lucency of the talar dome that is indicative of talar revascularization. Sclerosis of the talar dome does not guarantee that AVN has occurred, but it is suggestive.
- Lateral process talus fractures are highly associated with snowboarding. They are also a source of continued pain after an ankle sprain.
- Extraarticular calcaneal fractures may endanger posterior skin if there is significant displacement. Urgent operative reduction and fixation is required.

- Intraarticular calcaneal fractures result in lateral wall blowout, resulting in subfibular impingement and peroneal tendon encroachment.
  - Indications for open reduction with internal fixation (ORIF)— posterior facet fracture displacement greater than 2 to 3 mm, flattening of Böhler angle, varus malalignment of tuberosity
  - Disruption of the medial soft tissue does not increase the complication rate for ORIF as opposed to lateral soft tissue trauma.
  - Delayed wound healing can occur in 25% of patients from an extensile approach. Risk for a deep infection is much lower at 1% to 4%.
  - FHL at risk during placement of screws from lateral to medial— specifically at the level of the sustentaculum (constant fragment)
  - Worse outcomes correlate to higher fracture types.
  - Patients with significant intraarticular displacement, flatter Böhler angle, age younger than 29 years, women, and those not involved in workers' compensation have improved clinical outcomes with surgical compared to nonoperative management.
  - Posttraumatic subtalar arthritis is common and may require arthrodesis. Patients complain of pain over the sinus tarsi, with limited inversion/eversion.
  - In cases with significant loss of calcaneal height, horizontal talus, and resultant anterior ankle pain, bone-block distraction arthrodesis of the subtalar joint is required.
- Subtalar dislocations are most commonly medial.
  - Associated tarsal bone fractures in 90% of dislocations
  - The most common obstacles to reduction of a medial dislocation are the extensor digitorum brevis, the extensor retinaculum, and the peroneal tendons.
  - Most common obstacles to reduction of a lateral dislocation are an interposed posterior tibial tendon and FHL tendon.
- Ankle fractures
  - Deltoid or syndesmosis stability must be assessed and treated operatively if unstable.
  - X-ray parameters of stability may be helpful, but a wide range of normal exists.
  - Lauge-Hansen classification system notes the position of the ankle first, and the injury motion of the ankle relative to the leg second.
  - Bosworth fracture-dislocations—posterior dislocation of the fibula relative to the tibial incisura; require operative reduction
  - Posterolateral fibular antiglide plates are biomechanically superior to lateral plates but cause increased peroneal irritation.
  - Medial buttress plate required for fixation of a vertical medial malleolus fracture
- Pilon fractures are severe injuries and may take up to 2 years for complete recovery.
  - Primary external fixation with delayed ORIF is advocated by many; allows for anatomic reduction of the fracture but increases risk of infection and wound complications.
  - Nonunion (most common at metaphysis) and posttraumatic DJD are common complications.

CHAPTER **7**

HAND, UPPER EXTREMITY, AND MICROVASCULAR SURGERY

Lance M. Brunton and A. Bobby Chhabra

CONTENTS

ANATOMY

- **Extensor anatomy (Figures 7-1 and 7-2)**
  - Extensor (dorsal) compartments of the wrist (Table 7-1)
  - **Extensor retinaculum—prevents tendon bowstringing at wrist**
  - **Juncturae tendinum—extensor tendon interconnections in hand that may mask proximal tendon lacerations**
  - **Sagittal bands—centralize the extensor mechanism and attach to the volar plate**
  - Central slip—terminal extensor digitorum communis tendon, inserts on base of middle phalanx (P2), aids in proximal interphalangeal (PIP) joint extension
  - Extensor mechanism receives contributions from the intrinsic muscles—interossei and lumbricals
  - Lateral bands—receive contributions from common extensor and intrinsics, converge to form terminal extensor tendon, which inserts on base of distal phalanx (P3)
  - **Transverse retinacular ligament—prevents dorsal subluxation of lateral bands**
  - **Triangular ligament—prevents volar subluxation of lateral bands**
  - Oblique retinacular ligament (ligament of Landsmeer)—helps link PIP and distal interphalangeal (DIP) joint extension
  - **Grayson/Cleland ligaments—fibrous investments lying volar and dorsal to digital neurovascular bundles, respectively (Grayson is ground; Cleland is ceiling)**
- **Flexor anatomy (Figures 7-3 through 7-5)**
  - Flexor digitorum profundus (FDP)—inserts at metadiaphyseal P3, flexes DIP joint, aids in PIP and MCP flexion

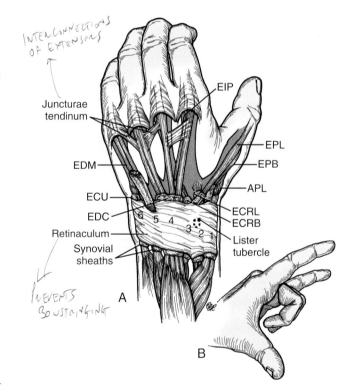

FIGURE 7-1 A, Extensor (dorsal) compartments of the wrist. The first compartment contains the abductor pollicis longus (APL) and extensor pollicis brevis (EPB); the second contains the radial wrist extensors, extensor carpi radialis longus (ECRL), and extensor carpi radialis brevis (ECRB); the third contains the extensor pollicis longus (EPL); the fourth contains the extensor digitorum communis (EDC) and extensor indicis proprius (EIP); the fifth contains the extensor digiti minimi (EDM); and the sixth contains the extensor carpi ulnaris (ECU). **B,** Depiction of independent index and small digit extension from EIP and EDM. (From Doyle JR: Extensor tendons—acute injuries. In Green DP et al, editors: *Green's operative hand surgery,* ed 5, New York, 2005, Churchill Livingstone, p 1881.)

Table 7-1	Extensor (Dorsal) Compartments of the Wrist		
COMPARTMENT	**TENDONS**	**ASSOCIATED PATHOLOGY**	**OTHER POINTS**
1	APL/EPB	de Quervain tenosynovitis	APL may have multiple slips, and EPB may have a separate compartment
2	ECRL/ECRB	Intersection syndrome	Radial to Lister tubercle
3	EPL	Late rupture after closed treatment of distal radius fracture	Ulnar to Lister tubercle; test by placing palm flat on table and lifting thumb
4	EDC/EIP	Extensor tenosynovitis	EIP ulnar to index EDC
			Small EDC present in only 25%
5	EDM	Vaughn-Jackson syndrome (initial)	EDM ulnar to small EDC
6	ECU	ECU instability	ECU subsheath part of TFCC

APL, Abductor pollicis longus; *ECRB,* extensor carpi radialis brevis; *ECRL,* extensor carpi radialis longus; *ECU,* extensor carpi ulnaris; *EDC,* extensor digitorum communis; *EDM,* extensor digiti minimi; *EIP,* extensor indicis proprius; *EPB,* extensor pollicis brevis; *EPL,* extensor pollicis longus; *TFCC,* triangular fibrocartilage complex.

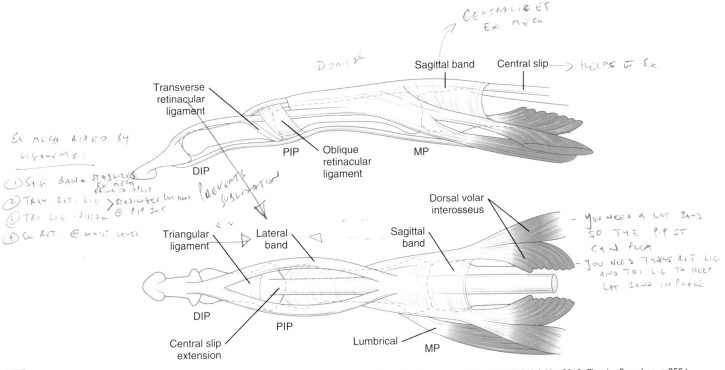

FIGURE 7-2 Depiction of the digital extensor mechanism. (From Tang JB, editor: *Tendon surgery of the hand,* Philadelphia, 2012, Elsevier Saunders, p 356.)

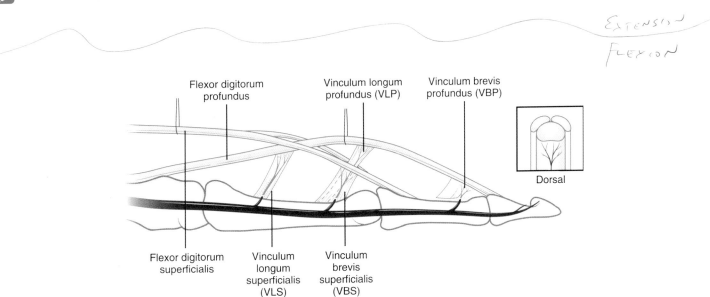

FIGURE 7-3 The blood vessels enter the flexor tendons through the vincular system. (From Tang JB, editor: *Tendon surgery of the hand,* Philadelphia, 2012, Elsevier Saunders, p 7.)

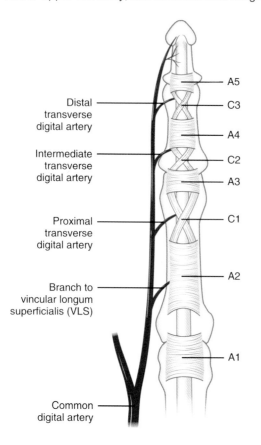

Distal transverse digital artery — A5

— C3

— A4

Intermediate transverse digital artery — C2

— A3

Proximal transverse digital artery — C1

Branch to vincular longum superficialis (VLS) — A2

— A1

Common digital artery

FIGURE 7-4 The tendon sheath contains the annular pulleys A1 to A5 and the cruciate pulleys C1 to C3. (From Tang JB, editor: *Tendon surgery of the hand,* Philadelphia, 2012, Elsevier Saunders, p 7.)

- **Middle, ring, and small FDP share common muscle belly in the forearm**
  - Index FDP often distinct muscle belly
- Flexor digitorum superficialis (FDS)—inserts at metadiaphyseal P2, flexes the PIP joint, aids in MCP flexion
  - Three to four individual muscle bellies in the forearm
  - **Small FDS—absent approximately 20% of the time**
- FDP tendon splits FDS at Campers chiasm at level of proximal phalanx (P1)
- Flexor tendon sheath—tunnel encompasses tendons distal to MCP joint
- Vascular supply to flexor tendons is both *intrinsic* (direct feeding vessels) and *extrinsic* (diffusion via synovial sheath)
- Each digital flexor tendon sheath has five annular pulleys (A1-A5) and three cruciate pulleys (C1-C3)
  - A2 and A4 pulleys—prevent flexor tendon bowstringing
- Thumb has at least two annular pulleys and an oblique pulley in between that prevents flexor pollicis longus (FPL) tendon bowstringing, although significant variation may exist
- Carpal tunnel contains the median nerve and nine flexor tendons (FPL, four FDS, and four FDP tendons)
  - FPL tendon—most radial structure in carpal tunnel
  - **Long and ring FDS tendons are volar to index and small FDS.**
  - Transverse carpal ligament (TCL)—roof of carpal tunnel

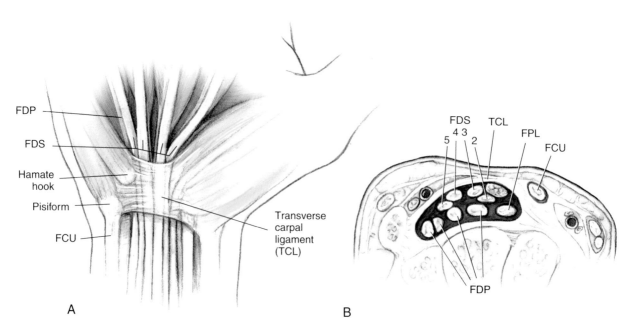

FDP
FDS
Hamate hook
Pisiform
FCU

Transverse carpal ligament (TCL)

A

FDS
5 4 3 2   TCL   FPL   FCU

FDP

B

FIGURE 7-5 Components of the carpal tunnel. **A,** Palmar view. **B,** Cross-sectional view. The roof of the carpal tunnel is the flexor retinaculum, which is composed of the deep forearm fascia, the transverse carpal ligament (TCL), and the distal aponeurosis between the thenar and hypothenar muscles. The carpal tunnel contains the median nerve and nine tendons: one flexor pollicis longus (FPL) and four each of the flexor digitorum superficialis (FDS) and flexor digitorum profundus (FDP) tendons. The FPL is dorsal to the flexor carpi radialis and is the most radial tendon within the carpal tunnel. *FCU,* Flexor carpi ulnaris. (From Miller MD et al, editors: *Orthopaedic surgical approaches,* Philadelphia, 2008, Saunders.)

- Ulnar tunnel (Guyon canal) contains ulnar nerve and artery
  - Volar carpal ligament—roof of Guyon canal (TCL is floor)
- Linburg sign—interconnections between FPL and index FDP in forearm; unilateral in up to 30%, bilateral in up to 15%

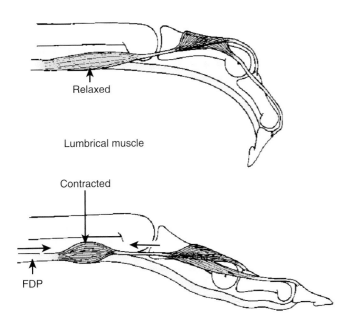

FIGURE 7-6 The lumbrical muscles flex the metacarpophalangeal joint and extend the proximal interphalangeal joint. *FDP,* Flexor digitorum profundus. (From Trumble TE, editor: *Principles of hand surgery and therapy,* Philadelphia, 2000, WB Saunders.)

- Palmaris longus (PL) tendon—present up to 85% of the time, common source of autograft for upper extremity reconstructive procedures
- Flexor carpi radialis (FCR) and flexor carpi ulnaris (FCU)—primary wrist flexors, insert on base of second metacarpal and pisiform, respectively
- **Intrinsic anatomy (Figure 7-6)**
- Includes four dorsal interosseous (digit abductors) and three palmar interosseous (digit adductor) muscles
  - Contribute to MCP flexion and interphalangeal (IP) extension—innervated by ulnar nerve
- **Lumbrical muscles originate on radial aspect of FDP tendons and pass volar to transverse metacarpal ligaments to insert on the radial lateral bands**
  - Contribute to interphalangeal joint extension, relax extrinsic flexor system
  - Radial two lumbricals—innervated by median nerve
  - Ulnar two lumbricals—innervated by ulnar nerve
- **Intrinsic tightness—PIP flexion less with MCP joints held in extension (intrinsics on stretch, extrinsics relaxed)**
- **Extrinsic tightness—PIP flexion less with MCP joints held in flexion (extrinsics on stretch, intrinsics relaxed)**
- **Neurovascular anatomy**
- Entire hand supplied by branches of the median, radial, and ulnar nerves
- Sensory innervation of the hand is depicted in Figure 7-7.
- Median nerve—innervates pronator teres, FDS, FCR, PL, radial two lumbricals
  - **Anterior interosseous branch of median nerve (AIN)—innervates FPL, index and long FDP (50% of time), pronator quadratus**

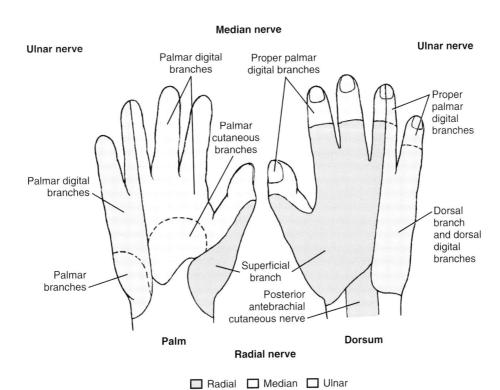

FIGURE 7-7 Sensory patterns of the median, ulnar, and radial nerves for the volar *(left)* and dorsal *(right)* aspects of the hand. (From Trumble TE, editor: *Principles of hand surgery and therapy,* Philadelphia, 2000, WB Saunders.)

- Palmar cutaneous branch of median nerve—usually lies between PL and FCR at distal wrist flexion crease
- Recurrent motor branch of median nerve—innervates abductor pollicis brevis, opponens pollicis, and superficial head of flexor pollicis brevis
- Ulnar nerve—innervates FCU, ring/small FDP, long FDP (50% of time), ulnar two lumbricals
  - Deep motor branch of ulnar nerve—innervates dorsal and volar interossei, abductor digiti minimi, flexor digitorum minimi, palmaris brevis, deep head of flexor pollicis brevis
- Martin-Gruber anastomoses
  - **Interconnections between motor fibers of the median and ulnar nerve in the forearm**
  - Occurs in approximately 17% of people
  - Four variations recognized
  - Motor branches from the median nerve connecting with the ulnar nerve to innervate "median" intrinsic muscles is most common (type 1)
- Riche-Cannieu anastomoses
  - Interconnections between motor fibers of the median and ulnar nerve in the hand
- Radial nerve proper—innervates lateral portion of brachialis (also musculocutaneous), triceps, anconeus, brachioradialis, extensor carpi radialis longus (ECRL)
  - Divides into superficial sensory branch and posterior interosseous nerve (PIN), which innervates all remaining extensor muscles
  - Extensor carpi radialis brevis (ECRB) has variable innervation from either radial nerve proper or PIN
  - Terminal branch of PIN lies at floor of fourth extensor compartment
- **Proper digital nerves lie volar to proper digital arteries**

DISTAL RADIUS FRACTURES

- **Introduction**
- Most common fracture of the upper extremity (>300,000 per year) in the United States, with bimodal distribution
- High-energy trauma in young (e.g., motor vehicle accident, fall from height)
- Low-energy falls in elderly persons with osteoporotic bone
- Most prevalent group—white women older than age 50 years
- **Anatomy**
- Distal radius articular surface—biconcave, scaphoid, and lunate facets
- Distal radioulnar joint (DRUJ)—articulation with ulna at sigmoid notch
- Lister tubercle—small dorsal prominence, landmark for dorsal approach to wrist
- Metaphysis—thin cortex, vulnerable to bending forces
- Brachioradialis insertion—major deforming force
- Normal wrist—distal radius bears 80% of axial load
- **Clinical evaluation**
- Pain, swelling, and deformity at the wrist after trauma
- Open injuries more common in young patients
- Examine for concurrent anatomic snuffbox and ulnar-sided wrist tenderness
- Evaluate shoulder and elbow
- Assess median and ulnar nerve function

- Acute carpal tunnel syndrome—characterized by progressive, evolving paresthesias and disproportionate pain; requires emergency median nerve decompression (carpal tunnel release)
- Mild, vague, and nonprogressive sensory dysfunction is not indicative of acute carpal tunnel syndrome.
- Ulnar nerve palsy after high-energy displaced distal radius fracture has also been described.
- **Radiographic evaluation (posteroanterior, lateral, and oblique views)**
- Intraarticular involvement
  - Evaluate fracture pattern, gap, and step-off
- Distal fragment angulation
  - Apex dorsal—Smith
  - Apex volar—Colles
- Radial height
  - Average 11 mm
- Radial inclination
  - Average 22 degrees (Figure 7-8)

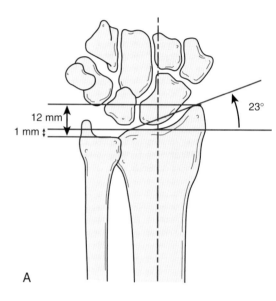

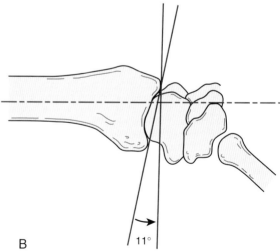

FIGURE 7-8 Schematic drawings of the average radial inclination **(A)** and volar tilt of the distal radius **(B).** (From Trumble TE et al, editors: *Core knowledge in orthopaedics: hand, elbow, and shoulder,* Philadelphia, 2006, Mosby, p 89.)

- Volar tilt (lunate fossa inclination)
  - Average 11 degrees
- Ulnar variance—neutral (normal), positive, or negative
  - Assessed with forearm in neutral rotation
  - Compare to contralateral side (Figure 7-9)
- DRUJ involvement
  - Assess true lateral radiograph for DRUJ alignment
- Associated fractures—ulnar styloid, distal ulna, carpus
  - **Isolated fracture of radial styloid (chauffeur fracture)—may be associated with scapholunate ligament disruption**
  - Radiocarpal dislocation may be purely ligamentous or associated with styloid fractures (radial and/or ulnar)
    - Beware of extremely distal fracture patterns
    - Highly unstable and difficult to reduce by closed means
    - Also termed "inferior arc" injury
- Other imaging studies—computed tomography (CT) for detail of complex intraarticular patterns; magnetic resonance imaging (MRI) for occult fracture, bone contusion, associated soft tissue injury

Classification

- Mostly descriptive
- Common eponyms (Colles, Smith, Barton, Hutchinson) predate radiography
- Over 10 other schemes exist (e.g., AO, Frykman, Fernandez, Melone, Mayo) but largely fail to help predict treatment or prognosis.

Treatment

- General goals—maintain reduction until union, restore function, prevent symptomatic posttraumatic radiocarpal osteoarthrosis
- Factors considered—age, medical condition, activity demands, bone quality, fracture stability, associated injuries
- Closed treatment
  - Definitive cast immobilization (favored over removable splints) sufficient in minimally displaced low-energy injuries, especially in functionally low-demand patients
    - Minimal initial displacement likely to remain stable
  - Closed reduction indicated in displaced fractures with abnormal radiographic parameters, especially in functionally high-demand patients
    - Dorsal hematoma block with local anesthetic
    - Finger traps, upper arm counterweight for ligamentotaxis

- Recreate deformity, manipulate distal fragment.
- Sugar tong plaster splint with three-point mold
- Keep MCP and IP joints free for motion.
- Radiographs obtained weekly for first 3 weeks
- **Loss of reduction correlates with increasing age.**
- Postreduction benchmarks (American Academy of Orthopaedic Surgeons guideline):
  - Radial shortening less than 3 mm
  - Dorsal articular tilt less than 10 degrees
  - Intraarticular step-off less than 2 mm
- Immobilization for 6 to 8 weeks (no evidence to support any particular type)
- Wrist and digit stiffness, muscle atrophy, and disuse osteopenia may result from prolonged immobilization.
- Operative treatment
  - Closed reduction and percutaneous pinning (CRPP)
    - Kapandji intrafocal pinning used rarely
  - External fixation
    - Bridging and nonbridging techniques described
    - Role in fractures with open contaminated wounds
    - Difficult to restore articular alignment and volar tilt
    - **Overdistraction may lead to increased risk of complex regional pain syndrome (CRPS)**
  - Distraction plating
    - Also termed *bridge plating* or "internal ex fix"
    - Secured second or third metacarpal and radial shaft (Figure 7-10)
    - Alternative to external fixation in highly comminuted fractures or in elderly patients with severe osteoporosis

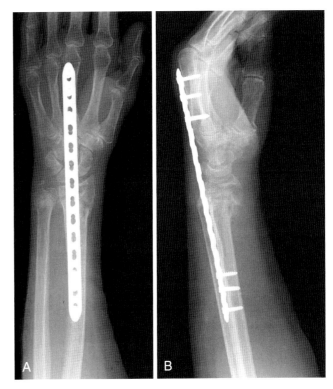

FIGURE 7-10 Immediate postoperative posteroanterior and lateral radiographs that demonstrate placement of a 14-hole distraction plate. Note that three bicortical screws were placed in the radial diaphysis and three bicortical screws were placed into the third metacarpal. (From Richard MJ et al: Distraction plating for the treatment of highly comminuted distal radius fractures in elderly patients, *J Hand Surg Am* 37:948–956, 2012.)

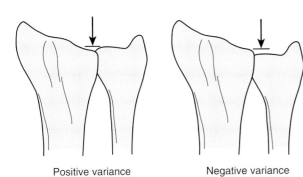

Positive variance   Negative variance

FIGURE 7-9 Ulnar variance of the distal radius. (From Trumble TE et al, editors: *Core knowledge in orthopaedics: hand, elbow, and shoulder,* Philadelphia, 2006, Mosby, p 89.)

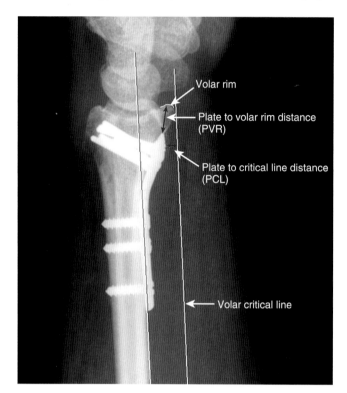

FIGURE 7-11 Measurements of plate position and prominence are demonstrated on this facet lateral radiograph. The plate-to–critical line distance (PCL) is measured with negative values for plates dorsal to the critical line and positive values for prominent plates volar to the critical line. The plate-to–volar rim (PVR) distance is measured with positive numbers for plates proximal to the volar rim and negative values for plates distal to the volar rim. This plate is appropriately positioned. (From Kitay A et al: Volar plate position and flexor tendon rupture following distal radius fracture fixation, *J Hand Surg Am* 38:1091–1096, 2013.)

- Disadvantage is second surgery to remove plate at 8 to 12 weeks
- Open reduction with internal fixation (ORIF)
  - Dorsal plating
    - Approach between third and fourth extensor compartments
    - Articular reduction directly visualized
    - Best for dorsally displaced fractures with dorsal bony defects
    - Historical disadvantage—extensor tendon irritation or rupture from prominent hardware
  - Volar plating
    - Henry approach between FCR and radial artery or through floor of FCR tendon sheath
    - Articular reduction not directly visualized, relies on fluoroscopic guidance
    - Fixed-angle and variable-angle plates available
    - Placed at or proximal to watershed line (Figure 7-11)
    - Best for Smith and Barton fracture patterns but often method of choice for dorsally displaced injuries as well
    - **Repair of the pronator quadratus following implant placement—no obvious benefit with respect to range of motion (ROM), grip strength, or avoidance of flexor tendon injury**

- Fragment-specific
  - Low-profile constructs, technically challenging
  - May be best suited for certain intraarticular fracture patterns including those with volar-ulnar ("critical corner") fragment
  - Hook plate may capture volar-ulnar fragment with less chance of flexor tendon irritation as compared to standard volar plate implant
- Intramedullary nailing
  - May have role in stable extraarticular patterns
  - Minimal long-term data to support use
- Arthroscopic assistance
  - Aids in articular reduction
  - Ensures that screws do not penetrate joint
- Injectable bone graft substitutes
  - Calcium phosphate
  - Coralline hydroxyapatite
- Evidence does not support any advantage of early versus delayed motion recovery after surgical fixation of distal radius.
- **Concurrent treatment of ulnar styloid fracture is not routinely necessary.**
  - No difference in multiple outcome measures when comparing patients undergoing ORIF of distal radius with and without ulnar styloid fixation
  - **Painful nonunion/DRUJ instability in small number of cases after radial fracture reduction (<10%)**
- Complications
  - Median nerve dysfunction (acute or delayed onset) is the most common complication following a distal radius fracture.
  - Extensor pollicis longus (EPL) tendon rupture
    - Most commonly occurs as a late complication following closed treatment because of sheath hematoma, attritional wear and/or vascular insufficiency near the Lister tubercle
    - Typically presents as a painless, acute loss of thumb extension
    - Treat with PL intercalary autograft or extensor indicis proprius (EIP)-to-EPL tendon transfer.
  - Distal radius nonunion is uncommon.
  - Asymptomatic malunion in a functionally low-demand patient does not require treatment
  - **Low-demand patients with pain from ulnocarpal impaction may benefit from distal ulna resection (Darrach procedure).**
  - **Corrective radius osteotomy with ORIF and bone grafting may be indicated for high-demand patients to prevent adaptive carpal instability and possible midcarpal arthritis** (Figure 7-12).
  - Presence of radiocarpal osteoarthrosis following intraarticular distal radius fracture with residual step-off is prevalent but does not necessarily correlate with patient-reported symptoms.
  - **Multiple case reports of flexor tendon pathology after volar plating**
    - FPL—most common rupture after volar plating; potentially due to improper plate placement distal to watershed zone
    - EPL—most common extensor tendon injured; potentially due to drill-bit penetration or dorsally prominent screws

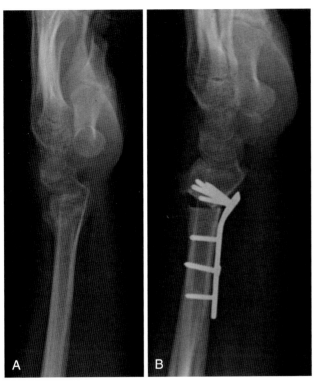

FIGURE 7-12 Lateral radiographs before and after corrective osteotomy of a dorsally angulated distal radius malunion with volar plate fixation. (From Ozer K et al: The role of bone allografts in the treatment of angular malunion for the distal radius, *J Hand Surg Am* 36:1804–1809, 2011.)

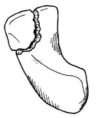 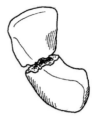 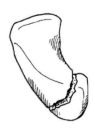

| Scaphoid tubercle fracture | Scaphoid waist fracture | Proximal pole fracture |

FIGURE 7-13 Scaphoid fractures can be simply described as involving the distal pole or tubercle, waist, or proximal pole. (From Trumble TE, editor: *Principles of hand surgery and therapy,* Philadelphia, 2000, WB Saunders.)

- Vitamin C in doses of at least 500 mg/day for 50 days may decrease the incidence of CRPS in women older than age 50 treated for a distal radius fracture, although previous supportive evidence has been recently disputed.

CARPAL FRACTURES AND INSTABILITY

▣ Anatomy
- Eight carpal bones aligned in two rows
- Proximal row—scaphoid, lunate, and triquetrum
  - Flexes with radial deviation, extends with ulnar deviation
- Distal row—trapezium, trapezoid, capitate, and hamate
- Pisiform is a sesamoid within the FCU tendon

- Functional "dart-thrower's motion" describes combined wrist extension–radial deviation to wrist flexion–ulnar deviation.
  - Occurs through midcarpal joint
  - Proximal row remains relatively immobile
- Carpus has a rich vascular supply with multiple anastomoses
- Scaphoid, lunate, and capitate may each have a large area supplied by a single interosseous vessel, making them more susceptible to osteonecrosis after trauma.
- Some evidence suggests a **proprioceptive role for the terminal branch of the PIN**, which may be compromised when this branch is sacrificed during dorsal approaches to the wrist that purposely denervate for a presumed analgesic effect in patients with chronic wrist pain.

▣ Scaphoid fractures
- **Most common carpal fracture, accounting for up to 15% of acute wrist injuries**
  - Anatomy
    - Approximately 75% covered by articular cartilage
    - Main blood supply comes from a dorsal branch of the radial artery, enters at dorsal ridge just distal to waist, and flows in retrograde fashion toward proximal pole
    - Additional branches off superficial volar branch of radial artery enter at distal tubercle and perfuse distal third
    - **Tenuous vascular anatomy renders waist and proximal pole fractures at risk for nonunion and posttraumatic osteonecrosis.**
  - Diagnosis
    - Suspect when chief complaint is radial-sided wrist pain after forced hyperextension and radial deviation of the wrist
    - Swelling, anatomic snuffbox/volar tubercle tenderness, limited wrist and/or thumb motion
    - Standard wrist radiographs and additional "scaphoid view"—approximately 30 degrees of wrist extension and 20 degrees of ulnar deviation displays scaphoid in best profile
    - Radiographs initially nondiagnostic in more than 30% of cases
    - With negative radiographs and high clinical suspicion, immobilize and repeat examination and radiographs in 2 weeks
    - **Bone scan, ultrasonography, CT, and MRI have all been used for earlier diagnosis.**
    - All of these are better for "ruling out" rather than "ruling in" a scaphoid fracture.
    - **MRI has highest sensitivity, specificity, and accuracy (all > 95%) with high positive and negative predictive values**
    - Neglect of injury for more than 4 weeks increases nonunion rate almost 10-fold.
  - Classification
    - Location (Figure 7-13)
      - Tubercle, distal pole, waist (most common), proximal pole

- Stability
  - Stable fractures characterized by transverse pattern, minimal comminution, and limited displacement
  - Unstable fractures often demonstrate more vertical or oblique patterns, significant comminution, and wide displacement.
  - **CT probably best modality for determining displacement and stability**
- Treatment
  - Nonoperative
    - Cast immobilization for nondisplaced fractures
    - No evidence to suggest that the type of cast affects outcome (e.g., long-arm vs. short-arm, standard vs. additional thumb spica component)
    - Expected time to union increases and overall union rate decreases as the fracture location becomes more proximal.
    - Consequently, length of cast immobilization should be greater for more proximal fractures.
  - Operative
    - **Indications include greater than 1 mm displacement, intrascaphoid angle greater than 35 degrees (humpback deformity), and trans-scaphoid perilunate dislocation**
    - Proximal pole fracture is also a relative indication.
    - Minimally displaced fractures may be treated with percutaneous internal fixation using a headless compression screw.
    - Formal ORIF for displaced injuries

- Regardless of incision size, guide-pin placement should be within the central axis of both the proximal and distal fragments.
- Approach dictated by fracture location and surgeon preference
- **Volar approach potentially avoids disruption to the main blood supply of the scaphoid.**
- Union rates of over 90% expected
- Aggressive physical therapy typically delayed until radiographic union achieved (average, 8-12 weeks)
- CT may be necessary to confirm union (bridging trabeculae)
- Complications
  - Include nonunion, malunion, osteonecrosis, and posttraumatic osteoarthrosis
  - Symptomatic early-stage scaphoid nonunion may be treated with ORIF and bone grafting (Figure 7-14).
  - Inlay (Russe) technique best used in cases with minimal deformity and a vascularized proximal pole
  - Scaphoid nonunion with accompanying humpback deformity requires open-wedge interposition (Fisk) graft to restore scaphoid length and carpal alignment.
  - Graft may be obtained from distal radius or iliac crest.
  - Presence of intraoperative punctate bleeding is the most reliable sign of a viable proximal pole.

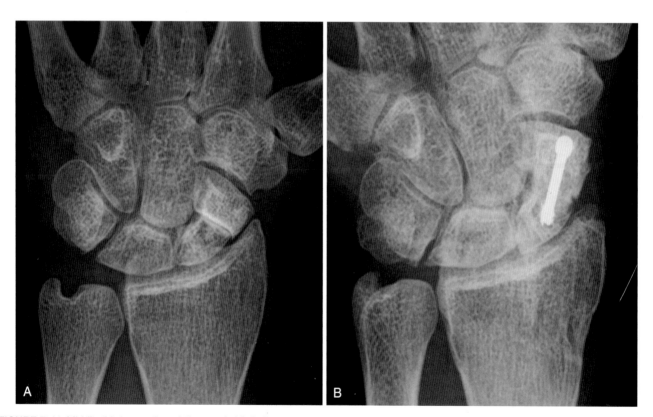

FIGURE 7-14 Middle-third nonunion of the scaphoid. **A,** Posteroanterior view obtained before surgery, showing sclerotic borders at the nonunion site and slight sharpening of the radial styloid. **B,** At 1 year after surgery, the scaphoid has healed and the donor site appears fully remodeled. (From Aguilela L, Garcia-Elias M: The anterolateral corner of the radial metaphysis as a source of bone graft for the treatment of scaphoid nonunion, *J Hand Surg Am* 37:1258–1262, 2013.)

- Vascularized bone grafting has a role in nonunions with avascular proximal pole
  - Most commonly harvested from dorsal aspect of distal radius, based on 1,2 intercompartmental supraretinacular artery (1,2 ICSRA)
  - May also be treated by free transfer of medial femoral condyle bone graft, supplied by descending medial genicular, and connected end-to-side to radial artery
- Untreated, chronic scaphoid nonunion may lead to characteristic progression of posttraumatic osteoarthrosis called *scaphoid nonunion advanced collapse* (SNAC) wrist:
  - Stage I—radioscaphoid arthritis
  - Stage II—involvement of scaphocapitate joint
  - Stage III—lunocapitate joint
  - Options for treatment of SNAC wrist include radial styloidectomy, distal scaphoid resection (Malerich procedure), proximal row carpectomy, scaphoid excision and four-corner (bone) fusion, and total wrist fusion, depending on stage of presentation and surgeon preference (Figures 7-15 and 7-16).

■ **Other carpal bone fractures—small fraction of wrist injuries**
▦ Lunate—may be seen with perilunate dislocation; treat with ORIF if displaced
▦ **Capitate neck—may occur in combination with scaphoid fracture or perilunate dislocation, treat with ORIF or intercarpal fusion**
▦ Triquetrum—majority are dorsal capsular avulsion fractures (wrist sprain) and require only a brief period of immobilization
▦ **Hook of hamate—often from blunt trauma to palm, frequently associated with sports (e.g., golf, baseball, hockey, racquet sports)**
  - **Imaging—carpal tunnel view, CT scan** (Figures 7-17 and 7-18)

- Symptomatic patients who fail trial of cast immobilization or those that present in delayed fashion are treated with fracture fragment excision.
- Flexor tendon rupture of the ring/small may be seen with chronic nonunion.
- Be aware of the bipartite hamate, which may be differentiated from a fracture by its smooth cortical surfaces.

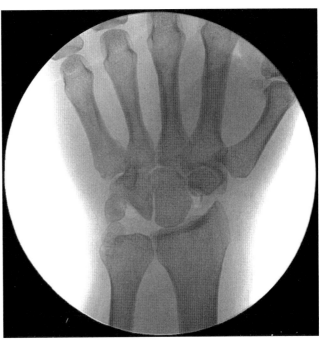

FIGURE 7-15 Fluoroscopic posteroanterior image immediately following proximal row carpectomy. (From Weiss ND et al: Arthroscopic proximal row carpectomy, *J Hand Surg Am* 36:577–582, 2012.)

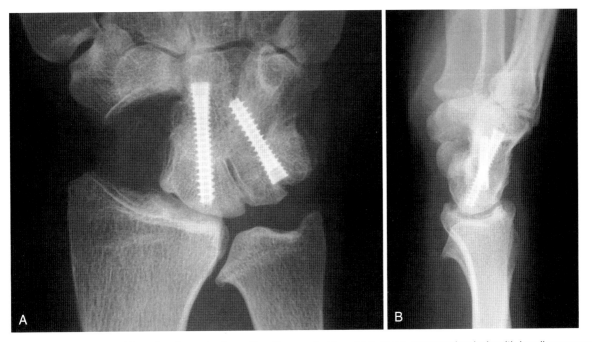

FIGURE 7-16 Posteroanterior and lateral radiographs 2 months after scaphoid excision and 4-corner arthrodesis with headless compression screws. (From Ozyurekoglu T, Turker T: Results of a method of 4-corner arthrodesis using headless compression screws, *J Hand Surg Am* 37:486–492, 2012.)

- Fractures of trapezoid or pisiform—extremely rare
  - Pisiform fractures are treated with cast immobilization.
  - If symptomatic nonunion occurs, pisiform excision can be performed.
- **Carpal instability**
- Disruption of normal kinematics of wrist
- Characterized by wrist pain, loss of motion, weakness
- If untreated, may lead to degenerative arthritis and disability
- Spectrum of injury from occult (predynamic) to dynamic to static

- Static instability detected on standard radiographs, whereas dynamic instability requires either stress radiographs or live fluoroscopy
- *Carpal instability dissociative* (CID) describes instability between individual carpal bones of single carpal row, such as dorsal intercalated segmental instability (DISI) and volar intercalated segmental instability (VISI) (Figures 7-19 and 7-20).
- *Carpal instability nondissociative* (CIND) describes instability between carpal rows, such as midcarpal or radiocarpal instability.
- Carpal instability resulting from a malunited distal radius fracture is an example of *carpal instability adaptive.*
- Perilunate dislocations combine CID and CIND and are classified as *carpal instability complex.*
- Specific injuries
  - DISI—most common form of carpal instability
    - Scapholunate ligament disruption
    - Dorsal fibers are stronger than volar fibers.

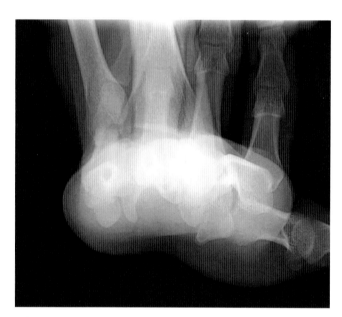

FIGURE 7-17 The carpal tunnel view demonstrates the hook of the hamate. (From Miller MD, Thompson SR, editors: *DeLee & Drez's orthopaedic sports medicine: principles and practice,* ed 4, Philadelphia, 2015, Elsevier Saunders, p 860.)

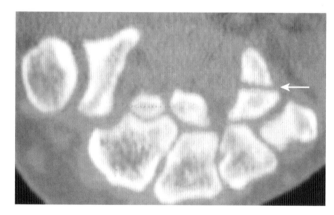

FIGURE 7-18 Sagittal computed tomographic scan view of a hook of hamate fracture *(arrow).* (From Trumble TE, editor: *Principles of hand surgery and therapy,* Philadelphia, 2000, WB Saunders.)

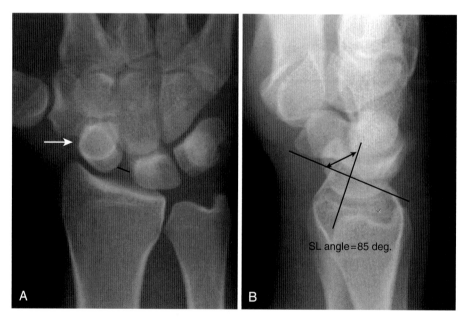

SL angle=85 deg.

FIGURE 7-19 A scapholunate (SL) ligament injury. **A,** Anteroposterior radiograph depicting SL injury. Notice the foreshortened scaphoid, with a cortical ring sign *(arrow),* as well as the widened SL interval *(black line).* **B,** Lateral radiograph of the wrist showing SL ligament disruption. Notice the dorsiflexed posture of the lunate and the increased SL angle. (From Miller MD, Thompson SR, editors: *DeLee & Drez's orthopaedic sports medicine: principles and practice,* ed 4, Philadelphia, 2015, Elsevier Saunders, p 830.)

- Secondary injury to stabilizing dorsal and/or volar extrinsic ligaments, volar scaphotrapeziotrapezoid (STT) ligaments
- Scaphoid hyperflexion and lunate hyperextension
- May be traumatic or result from inflammatory or crystalline arthropathy
- Physical examination findings
  - Dorsal wrist pain, often with loading
  - Diminished grip strength
  - Reproduction of pain/palpable clunk with scaphoid shift test (dorsally directed pressure over volar scaphoid tubercle while wrist brought from ulnar to radial deviation subluxates or dislocates scaphoid over dorsal ridge of distal radius that when released causes scaphoid to reduce with painful clunk)
  - A bilateral nonpainful clunk is a negative test result.
- Standard radiographs may reveal cortical ring sign, increased scapholunate angle (>70 degrees), or widened scapholunate interval (>3 mm).
- Bilateral clenched-fist (anteroposterior grip) comparison views may reveal a dynamic DISI with relatively widened scapholunate interval on affected side (stress radiographs)
- MRI best—but not perfect—for detection of scapholunate ligament injury
- **Gold standard: wrist arthroscopy**
  - Geissler classification (Table 7-2)
- Treatment depends on stage of instability
  - Partial ligament injuries (predynamic or dynamic instability) may improve with nonoperative treatment or arthroscopic débridement.
  - Acute scapholunate ligament rupture rarely amenable to primary repair alone
  - Delayed treatment may require open reduction of scapholunate interval and K-wire pinning with or without some form of dorsal capsulodesis or tendon autograft reconstruction.

- Various tendon (e.g., Brunelli) and bone-retinaculum-bone grafts have also been attempted for scapholunate reconstruction.
- Limited clinical data on reduction-association of scaphoid and lunate (RASL) procedure or other forms of implants to span scapholunate joint
- Cases of chronic untreated static instability may result in scapholunate advanced collapse (SLAC wrist)
- Three stages are described (Figure 7-21).
- Radioscaphoid and scaphocapitolunate joints are affected first.
- Radiolunate joint is spared until late stages.
- Treatment depends on condition of articular surfaces and competency of the radioscaphocapitate ligament.
- Options include radial styloidectomy, proximal row carpectomy, scaphoid excision and four-corner

GRADE	DESCRIPTION
Table 7-2	**Geissler Classification of Arthroscopic Scapholunate Ligament Disruption**
I	Attenuation or hemorrhage of interosseous ligament as seen from radiocarpal space. No incongruity of carpal alignment in midcarpal space.
II	Attenuation or hemorrhage of interosseous ligament as seen from radiocarpal space. There may be a slight gap (less than width of probe) between carpal bones in midcarpal space.
III	Incongruity or step-off of carpal alignment as seen from both radiocarpal and midcarpal space. Probe may be passed through gap between carpal bones.
IV	Incongruity or step-off of carpal alignment as seen from both radiocarpal and midcarpal space. There is gross instability with manipulation. A 2.7-mm arthroscope may be passed through the gap between carpal bones ("drive-through sign").

From Miller MD, Thompson SR, editors: *DeLee & Drez's orthopaedic sports medicine: principles and practice,* ed 4, Philadelphia, 2015, Elsevier Saunders, p 839.

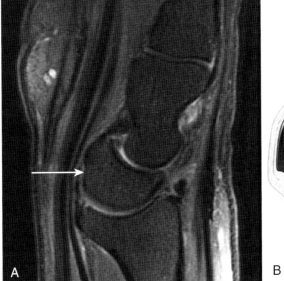
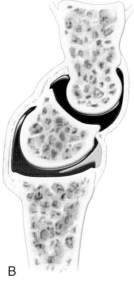

FIGURE 7-20 Dorsal intercalary segmental instability (DISI). **A,** The DISI posture of the lunate as seen on sagittal plane magnetic resonance imaging in a patient with scapholunate dissociation. Arrow points to the abnormally extended lunate. **B,** Artist's rendition of the DISI pattern. (From Miller MD, Thompson SR, editors: *DeLee & Drez's orthopaedic sports medicine: principles and practice,* ed 4, Philadelphia, 2015, Elsevier Saunders, p 831.)

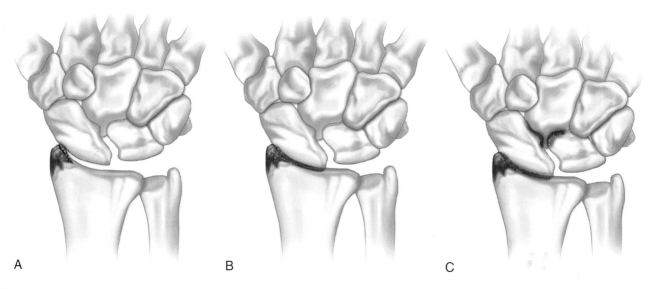

A   B   C

FIGURE 7-21 Progression of scapholunate advanced collapse. **A** and **B** depict progressive degenerative changes at the radioscaphoid joint. With advancing carpal collapse, the capitate may migrate proximally, resulting in midcarpal arthritis **(C)** and disruption of the Gilula lines radiographically. (© Mayo Clinic. Reproduced with permission of the Mayo Foundation.)

arthrodesis, isolated capitolunate arthrodesis, or total wrist arthrodesis.
- Denervation of the terminal branch of the PIN ± AIN is often done in conjunction with these procedures, although some dispute its benefit because of resulting reduction of proprioceptive wrist control.
- VISI—second most common form of carpal instability
  - Disruption of lunotriquetral interosseous ligament
  - Volar fibers are stronger than dorsal fibers.
  - Accompanying injury of the dorsal extrinsic ligaments (dorsal radiocarpal and intercarpal ligaments) may result in static instability.
  - Both the scaphoid and lunate tilt volarly.
  - Ulnar-sided wrist pain
  - Physical examination
    - Positive lunotriquetral shear test
  - Radiographs may show break in Gilula arc on posteroanterior view and decreased scapholunate angle to less than 30 degrees on lateral view.
  - MRI may show pathology of lunotriquetral ligament.
  - **Gold standard: wrist arthroscopy**
  - Treatment
    - Direct volar lunotriquetral ligament repair
    - FCU tendon augmentation
    - Lunotriquetral arthrodesis
    - Ulnar-shortening osteotomy for patients with concurrent ulnocarpal impaction syndrome
- Midcarpal CIND
  - Clunking wrist that may or may not be painful
  - Many patients have generalized ligamentous laxity.
  - History of trauma often absent
  - Sudden shift of proximal carpal row with active radial or ulnar deviation
  - Maximize nonoperative management
  - Midcarpal fusion preferred over attempt at soft tissue reconstruction
- Radiocarpal dislocation (CIND)
  - Rare, high-energy injuries
  - "Inferior arc" injury

- May be associated with intracarpal injury, acute carpal tunnel syndrome, possible compartment syndrome, other major musculoskeletal and/or organ injuries
- May be purely ligamentous or include radial and/or ulnar styloid fractures
- Ulnar translocation of the carpus signifies global ligamentous disruption.
  - Volar extrinsic ligaments
    - Radioscaphocapitate
    - Long radiolunate
    - Short radiolunate
    - Radioscapholunate, also termed *ligament of Testut*—vestigial neurovascular contents
- Moneim proposed two types based on accompanying intracarpal fracture or interosseous ligament injury.
- Dumontier and Graham stressed the distinction between injuries with small versus large radial styloid fractures.
- ORIF of styloid fractures may be enough to restore stability.
- May also require direct ligamentous repair and/or external fixation to neutralize forces
- Associated intracarpal injuries treated simultaneously
- **Carpal instability adaptive from distal radius malunion**
  - May result from deformities with more than 30 degrees of sagittal malalignment
  - Concern for midcarpal pain/arthritis
  - Treat with corrective osteotomy of the distal radius.
- Perilunate dislocations (carpal instability complex)
  - Potentially devastating injuries resulting from forced dorsiflexion, ulnar deviation, and supination of wrist
  - Approximately 25% of cases may be missed in the emergency department.
  - Mayfield described four stages of perilunar disruption of ligamentous constraints, proceeding in counterclockwise direction:
    - Stage I—scapholunate disruption
    - Stage II—scaphocapitate disruption

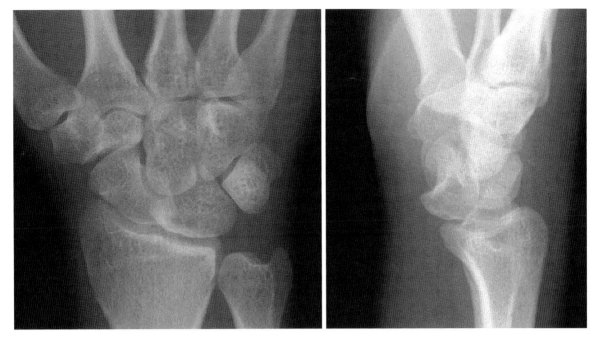

FIGURE 7-22 Posteroanterior *(left)* and lateral *(right)* radiographs of a perilunate dislocation. Notice the difficulty of assessing the dislocation on the posteroanterior view alone. On the lateral radiograph, the lunate is seen to be completely dislocated. (From Miller MD, Thompson SR, editors: *DeLee & Drez's orthopaedic sports medicine: principles and practice,* ed 4, Philadelphia, 2015, Elsevier Saunders, p 829.)

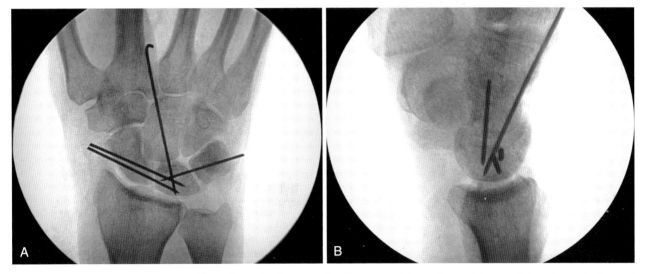

FIGURE 7-23 Posteroanterior and lateral plain radiographs demonstrating the appropriate position of intercarpal pins after reduction and ligamentous stabilization of a perilunate dislocation. (From Miller MD, Thompson SR, editors: *DeLee & Drez's orthopaedic sports medicine: principles and practice,* ed 4, Philadelphia, 2015, Elsevier Saunders, p 855.)

- Stage III—lunotriquetral disruption
  - Dorsal midcarpal dislocation
  - Capitate dorsal to lunate on lateral view
- Stage IV—circumferential disruption
  - Volar lunate dislocation—osteonecrosis of the lunate avoided because of attached volar extrinsic ligaments that sustain blood supply (Figure 7-22)
- Lesser-arc injuries—purely ligamentous
- Greater-arc injuries—carpal fracture (trans-scaphoid most common)
- Prompt attempt at closed reduction, especially in setting of acute carpal tunnel syndrome

- Stable closed reduction may allow for delayed definitive surgical management, but there is no role for closed treatment alone.
- Irreducible injuries necessitate urgent operative intervention.
  - ORIF may require dorsal and/or volar approach.
  - Combination of ligamentous repair, fracture fixation, dorsal capsulodesis, K-wire pinning of proximal row and midcarpal joint (Figure 7-23)
  - Carpal tunnel release for associated acute carpal tunnel syndrome
  - Cast immobilization for 2 to 3 months

- Late diagnosis leads to consistently poor outcomes
  - Methods of treating delayed and chronic perilunate dislocations are controversial.

METACARPAL AND PHALANGEAL INJURIES

■ Introduction
- ▦ Most frequently encountered injuries of skeletal system
- ▦ Vast majority treated nonoperatively
  - Many initially splinted with hand in intrinsic-plus or "safe" position
    - Wrist in 15 to 30 degrees of extension
    - MCP joints in 70 to 90 degrees of flexion
    - Interphalangeal joints in neutral
  - Immobilization for 3 to 4 weeks at most
- ▦ Surgical intervention may be indicated in open injuries, intraarticular fractures, irreducible fractures, digit malrotation (scissoring), and multiple fractures
- ▦ **Digit rotation assessed statically with wrist tenodesis and dynamically as patient initiates making a fist**
  - All fingertips should point toward volar scaphoid tubercle; compare to contralateral side.
- ▦ Goals of treatment are stable reduction, edema control, and early ROM.

■ Fractures and dislocations
- ▦ Metacarpal head   *HEAD*
  - Most commonly occurs in the index or middle finger
  - Some condylar injuries represent ligamentous avulsions.
  - Greater than 1 mm of articular step-off may warrant ORIF.   *>1mm = Sx*
  - Joint stiffness is common with both nonoperative and operative treatment.
  - **Associated open "fight bites" require urgent surgical débridement and assessment of extensor mechanism injury.**
  - Severe open or comminuted fractures (e.g., gunshot wounds) may be treated with spanning external fixation.
  - Arthroplasty or arthrodesis (especially index MCP) are other possible treatments.
- ▦ Metacarpal neck   *NECK*
  - Weakest portion of metacarpal
  - Most frequently involves the ring and small finger
  - "Boxer's fracture"— metacarpal neck fracture of the small finger, paradoxically from poor punching technique
  - Intrinsic muscles are major deforming force leading to apex dorsal angulation
  - Check for malrotation, pseudoclawing, and MCP joint extensor lag.
  - Many treated with closed reduction (Jahss maneuver) and 3 to 4 weeks of immobilization
  - Suggested acceptable angulation of each metacarpal neck:
    - Index and long fingers less than 15 to 20 degrees
    - Ring finger less than 30 to 40 degrees
    - Small finger less than 70 degrees (controversial)
  - Greater compensation from more mobile fourth and fifth carpometacarpal (CMC) joints
  - CRPP for irreducible fractures (antegrade, retrograde or transverse)

- ▦ Metacarpal shaft   *SHAFT — 5mm is max*
  - May be transverse, oblique, or spiral
  - May be associated with higher risk of malrotation
    - Just 5 degrees of malrotation results in 1.5 cm of digital overlap.
  - Suggested acceptable angulation of each metacarpal shaft:
    - Index and long fingers less than 10 degrees
    - Ring and small fingers less than 30 degrees
  - **Every 2 mm of metacarpal shortening leads to 7 degrees of extensor lag.**
  - **Up to 5 mm is acceptable without significant functional deficit.**
  - Irreducible displaced fractures are treated with CRPP or ORIF.
    - Intramedullary pinning may be performed antegrade or retrograde.
    - Lag screw fixation for fracture length twice the bone diameter
    - Prominent dorsal plates may interfere with extensor tendon function and necessitate later removal after union.
  - Multiple metacarpal shaft fractures are unstable injuries that often necessitate surgical intervention regardless of deformity.
- ▦ Metacarpal base fracture and CMC joint dislocation   *BASE*
  - Stable minimally displaced fractures of metacarpal base are treated nonoperatively. — *NON OP - STABLE/MIN DISPLACEMENT*
  - Ring and small CMC joint fracture-dislocations often result from higher-energy mechanisms
    - **Pronated 30-degree oblique radiograph provides best view**
    - CT scan for better detail of complex injuries
  - Small-finger CMC joint fracture-dislocation is termed a "reverse" or "baby" Bennett fracture.   *LIKE "BURMETTE"*
    - Extensor carpi ulnaris (ECU) tendon—major deforming force
  - Accompanying distal row carpal fractures may be seen.
  - Attempt at closed reduction is warranted, but these unstable injuries often require additional surgical stabilization.
    - CRPP or ORIF
  - Delayed treatment, painful malunion, or posttraumatic osteoarthrosis may require arthrodesis.
- ▦ Thumb metacarpal   *THUMB*
  - Most common pattern is extraarticular epibasal fracture
    - Up to 30 degrees of angulation acceptable secondary to compensatory CMC joint motion
    - Excessive angulation may lead to MCP joint hyperextension and requires CRPP or ORIF.
  - Bennett fracture—an intraarticular fracture-dislocation (Figure 7-24)
    - **Abductor pollicis longus (APL) and thumb extensors cause proximal, dorsal, and radial displacement of the metacarpal shaft.**
    - Adductor pollicis causes supination and adduction of the metacarpal shaft.
    - Anterior oblique or "beak" ligament keeps the volar-ulnar base fragment reduced to trapezium.
    - CRPP or ORIF is chosen based on the size of fragment.
    - Reduction with traction, palmar abduction, and pronation
    - Goal: less than 1 to 2 mm of articular step-off

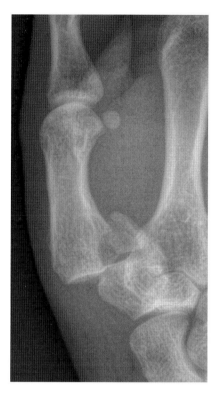

FIGURE 7-24 Lateral radiograph showing a Bennett fracture-subluxation. (From Zhang X et al: Treatment of a Bennett fracture using tension band wiring, *J Hand Surg Am* 37:427–433, 2012.)

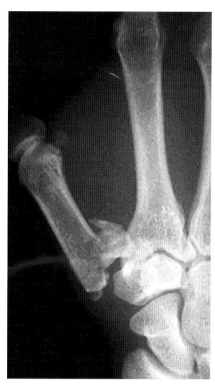

FIGURE 7-25 Radiograph of a Rolando fracture, which is a comminuted first metacarpal base injury. (From Trumble TE et al, editors: *Core knowledge in orthopaedics: hand, elbow, and shoulder*, Philadelphia, 2006, Mosby, p 66.)

- Rolando fracture—a comminuted intraarticular fracture that may be in shape of Y or T (Figure 7-25)
  - Degree of comminution and surgeon experience guides treatment, because CRPP, ORIF, and external fixation are all viable options.
- Thumb MCP ligamentous injuries
  - **Acute (skier) or chronic (gamekeeper) injury to the thumb MCP joint ulnar collateral ligament (UCL)**
  - Competent UCL critical for strong, effective pinch
  - Mechanism of injury is usually forceful thumb hyperextension and/or hyperabduction.
  - Dorsal-to-volar spectrum of injury potentially involving proper UCL, accessory UCL, and volar plate
  - Radiographs should be obtained before stress examination to rule out bony avulsion injury.
  - In the absence of fracture, stress MCP joint with radial deviation both at neutral and 30 degrees of flexion
    - Instability in 30 degrees of flexion indicates injury to proper UCL.
    - Instability in neutral indicates additional injury to accessory UCL and/or volar plate.
    - Threshold is greater than 35 degrees of opening or greater than 20 degrees difference compared to uninjured thumb.
  - Differentiation between complete and partial tears is difficult to determine by physical examination alone.
    - Stress radiographs and/or MRI may aid in the diagnosis.
  - Partial injuries may be initially treated with thumb spica cast immobilization for 4 to 6 weeks.
  - **In over 85% of cases, a complete injury is accompanied by a Stener lesion, in which the adductor pollicis aponeurosis is interposed between**

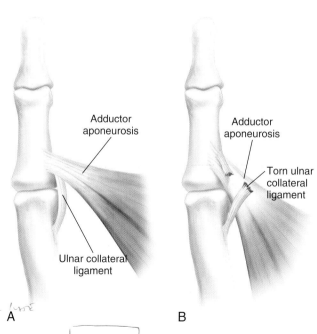

FIGURE 7-26 Stener lesion. The adductor aponeurosis separates the two ends of the ulnar collateral ligament, and the aponeurosis must be incised to repair the ligament. (From Morrison WB, Sanders TG: *Problem solving in musculoskeletal imaging*, Philadelphia, 2008, Elsevier.)

Labels in figure: Adductor aponeurosis; Ulnar collateral ligament; Adductor aponeurosis; Torn ulnar collateral ligament; A; B

the avulsed UCL and its insertion site on the base of the proximal phalanx (Figure 7-26).

- Presence of a Stener lesion may be palpable on examination, prevents proper healing, and requires surgical intervention to properly reattach the

ligament through drill holes, suture anchor, or interference screw.
- A displaced avulsion fracture of the base of the proximal phalanx may occasionally require ORIF if the fragment is large enough.
- Chronic UCL injuries require ligament reconstruction with either adjacent joint capsule or tendon graft, with or without pinning of joint.
  - Associated posttraumatic osteoarthrosis best treated by MCP arthrodesis.
- Isolated injuries to the thumb MCP radial collateral ligament may occur after a forced flexion-ulnar deviation mechanism; most treated nonoperatively, although high-grade or complete tears may be associated with volar MCP subluxation and best suited for operative intervention.
- MCP joint dislocation
  - Classified as simple (reducible) or complex (irreducible)
  - Dorsal dislocations are most common.
    - Skin dimpling in distal palm is pathognomonic
  - Index, small fingers most frequently involved
  - In simple dislocation, P1 is perched on metacarpal and closed reduction usually possible
    - Longitudinal traction and MCP hyperextension avoided
    - Apply direct pressure over P1 with wrist in flexion to relax extrinsic flexors.
  - In complex dislocation, P1 and metacarpal are in bayonet position and interposition of volar plate and/or sesamoids likely
    - Usually irreducible by closed means
    - Open reduction through dorsal or volar approach
    - **Volar approach risks iatrogenic neurovascular injury.**
      - A1 pulley divided to loosen noose around metacarpal head, and volar plate extracted
- Boxer's knuckle
  - Most common hand injury in both amateur and professional fighters
  - The extensor hood of the MCP joint is ruptured, leading to increased risk of chondral injury and osteoarthrosis of the joint.
  - Presents with swelling, reduced ROM, and occasional extensor lag
  - Treatment is via direct repair of the extensor hood.
- P1 and P2 phalanges
  - Fractures of P1 deform with apex volar angulation.
    - Proximal fragment flexion (interossei)
    - Distal fragment extension (central slip)
  - Fractures of P2 deform with apex dorsal or volar angulation.
    - Apex dorsal if fracture proximal to FDS insertion
    - Apex volar if fracture distal to FDS insertion
  - Majority treated nonoperatively if less than 10 degrees of angulation and no rotational deformity
  - Three weeks of immobilization followed by aggressive motion recovery
  - Radiographic union lags behind clinical union by several weeks.
  - Irreducible or unstable fracture patterns may require surgery.

- Operative techniques:
  - Crossed Kirschner wires
  - Eaton-Belsky pinning through metacarpal head
  - Minifragment fixation:
    - Lag screws
    - Plate and screw construct
  - External fixation reserved for highly comminuted intraarticular fractures or those associated with gross contamination and segmental bone loss
- PIP joint dislocation
  - Dorsal dislocation most common
    - Injury to volar plate and at least one collateral ligament
    - "Simple" dislocation—middle phalanx in contact with condyles of proximal phalanx
      - Easily reduced with longitudinal traction
    - "Complex" dislocation—base of middle phalanx no longer in contact with condyle of proximal phalanx, giving a bayonet appearance
      - Volar plate acts as block to reduction if longitudinal traction applied
      - Reduction via hyperextension of middle phalanx followed by a volar-directed force
    - Short-term buddy taping is sufficient aftercare.
    - Persistent instability is rare but may be treated by dorsal block splinting.
    - Persistent swelling and soreness for months is common.
    - Irreducible complex dislocations require open reduction via a dorsal approach and incision between the central slip and lateral band.
  - Volar dislocation
    - Rare closed injury to central slip and at least one collateral ligament
    - Closed reduction with flexion followed by assessment of active extension
    - Stable injuries without excessive extensor lag are splinted temporarily.
    - **Significant extensor lag following reduction may necessitate central slip repair followed by 6 weeks of immobilization in full extension.**
    - **Inadequate treatment will lead to boutonnière deformity.**
  - Rotatory dislocation
    - One of the phalangeal condyles is buttonholed between central slip and lateral band
    - Unlike other PIP dislocations, this often requires open reduction.
- PIP joint fracture-dislocation
  - Dorsal dislocation accompanied by fracture at P2 base (Figures 7-27 and 7-28)
  - **Hastings classification based on amount of P2 articular surface involvement** (Table 7-3)
  - Treatment options include dorsal block splinting, dorsal block pinning, ORIF, and hemihamate reconstruction.
    - Regardless of treatment, maintenance of adequate joint reduction is the most important factor for favorable long-term outcome.
  - **Chronic PIP fracture-dislocations without severe posttraumatic osteoarthrosis are best treated with hemihamate reconstruction or volar plate arthroplasty, depending on demands of the patient.**

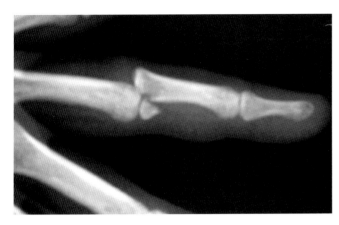

FIGURE 7-27 Dorsal subluxation of the proximal interphalangeal joint, with an impacted fracture at the base of the middle phalanx. (From Miller MD, Thompson SR, editors: *DeLee & Drez's orthopaedic sports medicine: principles and practice,* ed 4, Philadelphia, 2015, Elsevier Saunders, p 887.)

Table 7-3	**Classification of PIP Joint Fracture-Dislocations (Hastings)**	
TYPE	**AMOUNT OF P2 ARTICULAR SURFACE INVOLVED**	**TREATMENT**
I—Stable	<30%	Dorsally based extension block splint
II—Tenuous	30%-50%	If reducible in flexion, dorsally based extension block splint or dorsal blocking K-wire
III—Unstable	>50%	ORIF, hemihamate autograft, or volar plate arthroplasty

ORIF, Open reduction with internal fixation; *PIP,* proximal interphalangeal; *P2,* middle phalanx.

- Irreducible DIP dislocations are typically due to interposition of the volar plate; treatment is via open reduction and extraction of the volar plate.
- May accompany extensive soft tissue and/or nail bed disruption in severe fingertip injuries
- Open injuries initially treated with irrigation and débridement, reduction, nail bed repair (if necessary), antibiotics, tetanus prophylaxis, and splinting
- Unstable displaced fractures of the distal phalanx may require percutaneous pinning to support the nail bed repair.
- A stable tuft fracture is more common with these injuries and requires no specific treatment apart from temporary splinting.
- Soft tissue loss treated accordingly
- Highly comminuted injuries with significant soft tissue loss may be more amenable to revision amputation (shortening and closure).
- **Seymour fracture—a transverse physeal injury that may displace and require extraction of interposed nail matrix to prevent malunion**
- For further details see the section "Nail and Fingertip Injuries."

TENDON INJURIES AND OVERUSE SYNDROMES

■ Extensor tendon injury

- Description and treatment are based on zones of injury (see Figure 7-28).
- Most commonly injured digit is long finger
- **Partial lacerations less than 50% of tendon width do not require direct repair if patient can extend finger against resistance; treat with early protected motion to prevent tendon adhesions**
- After direct suture repair of complete lacerations or those constituting more than 50% of tendon width, rehabilitation is based on zone of injury.
- Specific injuries
  - Zone I injury (mallet finger)
    - Disruption of terminal extensor tendon at or distal to DIP joint
    - Sudden forced flexion of the extended fingertip
    - Patient cannot actively extend at DIP joint, and finger remains in flexed posture.
    - May be accompanied by bony avulsion injury from dorsal base of P3 (bony mallet)

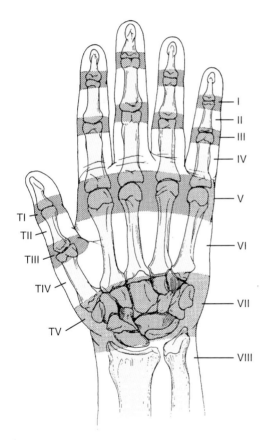

FIGURE 7-28 Zones of the extensor tendon system. (From Trumble TE et al, editors: *Core knowledge in orthopaedics: hand, elbow, and shoulder,* Philadelphia, 2006, Mosby, p 203.)

- Silicone arthroplasty or arthrodesis are salvage procedures for an arthritic PIP joint.
- **Highly comminuted "pilon" fractures are best handled with dynamic distraction external fixation for simple ligamentotaxis and early ROM.**
- DIP dislocation and distal phalanx fractures
  - DIP dislocation is treated with closed reduction followed by immobilization in slight flexion with a dorsal splint for 2 weeks.

- If detected within 12 weeks of injury, closed management with full-time DIP joint extension splinting for at least 6 weeks, followed by part-time splinting for an additional 4 to 6 weeks
- No consensus on best type of splint to use
- Hyperextension should be avoided because skin necrosis can occur.
- Noncompliance is common.
- Maintenance of PIP joint motion often overlooked
- A nondisplaced bony mallet finger may also be treated with extension splinting until fracture union.
- A relative surgical indication is a displaced bony mallet injury with significant volar subluxation of P3.
  - CRPP through DIP joint
  - Extension block pinning
  - ORIF if large fragment (>50% articular surface)
- Chronic mallet finger detected more than 12 weeks after injury
  - Closed treatment only if joint supple, congruent, and without arthritic changes
  - Dynamic splinting, serial casting for contracted joint
  - Operative—tenodermodesis
- Prolonged DIP flexion may lead to swan neck deformity caused by dorsal subluxation of lateral bands and corresponding PIP joint hyperextension.
  - Supple swan neck deformities may be treated with:
    - Fowler central slip tenotomy (maximum deformity 35 degrees)
    - Spiral oblique retinacular ligament (SORL) reconstruction
- A painful, stiff, arthritic DIP joint is treated with arthrodesis.
- Zone II injury
  - Occurs over middle phalanx of digit or over proximal phalanx of thumb
  - Mechanism of injury usually involves a dorsal laceration or crush component.
  - Partial disruptions (<50%) are treated nonoperatively with local wound care and early mobilization.
  - Direct repair may be attempted for greater than 50% lacerations.
  - Some surgeons will temporarily pin across terminal joint after direct repair.
- Zone III injury (boutonnière)
  - Occurs over PIP joint of digit (central slip) or MCP joint of thumb
  - Open injuries are directly repaired if possible.
    - Loss of tendon substance may require a free-tendon graft or extensor mechanism turndown flap.
  - For closed injuries, the **Elson test** is performed by flexing the patient's PIP joint 90 degrees over the edge of a table and asking patient to extend the PIP joint against resistance.
    - If the central slip is intact, the DIP joint will remain supple.
    - If the central slip is ruptured, the DIP joint will be rigid.
- An acute boutonnière deformity results from central slip disruption and volar subluxation of the lateral

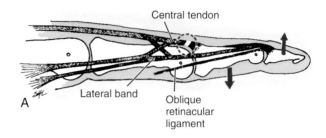

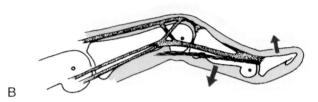

FIGURE 7-29 Pathomechanics of the boutonnière deformity. **A,** Attenuation of the central slip results in unopposed flexion at the proximal interphalangeal (PIP) joint. **B,** With PIP joint flexion, the lateral bands drift volar to the axis of rotation at the PIP joint. The lateral bands stay in the volar position owing to loss of dorsal support from the attenuated triangular ligament and contracture of the transverse retinacular ligament. (From Green DP et al, editors: *Green's operative hand surgery,* ed 6, Philadelphia, 2011, Churchill Livingstone, p 175.)

bands, resulting in DIP hyperextension (Figure 7-29).
- **Closed injuries are treated with full-time PIP extension splinting for at least 6 weeks, followed by part-time splinting for an additional 4 to 6 weeks.**
  - DIP flexion maintained to balance extensor mechanism
- Chronic (untreated) boutonnière deformity
  - May require dynamic splinting or serial casting to achieve maximal passive motion first
  - Terminal extensor tenotomy, PIP volar plate release
  - Central slip reconstruction techniques:
    - Tendon graft
    - Extensor turndown
    - Lateral band mobilization
    - Transverse retinacular ligament
    - FDS slip
- A painful, stiff, arthritic PIP joint is treated with arthrodesis.
- Zone IV injury
  - Occurs over proximal phalanx of digit or over the metacarpal of thumb
  - Treatment is similar to that for injuries in zone II.
  - A common complication in this zone is adhesion formation, with resulting loss of digital flexion.
    - Adhesion formation may be reduced with early protected ROM and dynamic splinting.
    - Failure of nonoperative management may require extensor tenolysis.
- Zone V injury
  - Occurs over MCP joint of digit or over CMC joint of thumb
  - Early mobilization and dynamic splinting is advocated

- A fight bite requires surgical débridement of the MCP joint with loose or delayed wound closure.
  - *Eikenella corrodens* is a commonly offending mouth organism.
  - Extensor lag and loss of flexion are common.
- **A sagittal band rupture ("flea-flicker" injury) may result from forced extension of flexed digit.**
  - Long finger most common
  - Rupture of the stronger radial fibers may lead to extensor tendon subluxation/dislocation.
  - Finger will be held in flexed position at MCP joint with no active extension
  - Passive extension of the MCP joint is possible, and the patient can then usually maintain the finger in an extended position.
  - Acute injuries may be treated with 4 to 6 weeks of extension splinting of the MCP joint (one of the only exceptions to splinting the MCP joints in flexion).
  - Failure of nonoperative management or missed injuries with delayed diagnosis may require repair or reconstruction of the sagittal band.
- Zone VI injury
  - Occurs over metacarpal and represents most frequently injured zone
  - Associated lacerations of superficial veins and nerves are likely.
  - Direct repair is indicated when the disruption constitutes more than 50% of the tendon substance.
  - Early protected motion advocated postoperatively
    - Dynamic splinting may offer better short-term ROM and strength, without increased complications, over static splinting.
  - The prognosis is good in the absence of concurrent skeletal injury.
- Zone VII and VIII injuries
  - Zone VII injury occurs at the level of the wrist joint, and zone VIII injury occurs in the distal forearm at the musculotendinous junction.
  - Lacerations at wrist level are usually associated with extensor retinaculum disruption, and postoperative adhesions are common.
  - The retinaculum should be repaired to prevent tendon bowstringing.
  - Static immobilization with the wrist held in extension and the MCP joints partially flexed is advised for the first 3 weeks, followed by protected motion.
  - The results of surgical repair in these zones are not as good as those in zones IV, V, and VI.

■ **Flexor tendon injury**
▨ Overview
- This injury usually results from volar lacerations, and concomitant neurovascular injury is common.
- Rather than attempting to probe wounds acutely, note the resting posture of the hand and check the tenodesis effect with passive wrist flexion and extension.
- Each digit is then tested in isolation for active DIP and PIP flexion, especially in setting of multiple digit trauma.
- Partial lacerations may be associated with gap formation or triggering with nonoperative treatment.

- Triggering may be alleviated by trimming tendon ends under flexor tendon sheath.
- Standard of care for lacerations greater than 60% of tendon width is simultaneous core and epitendinous repair within 3 weeks, but preferably within 7 to 10 days of injury.
- Basic surgical techniques of flexor tendon repair
  - Strength of repair proportional to number of suture strands that cross repair site
    - Six to eight strands have superior strength and stiffness.
  - High-caliber (e.g., 5-0 instead of 6-0) suture material decreases gap formation and increases strength and stiffness.
  - A locking-loop configuration decreases gap formation.
  - Epitendinous repair decreases gap size and increases overall strength by 10% to 50%.
  - *Purchase,* defined as the longitudinal distance from cut tendon end to transverse component of the core suture, should be 0.7 to 1.2 cm.
  - Dorsally placed core sutures are stronger.
  - Repair of the flexor tendon sheath has no effect on flexor tendon repair
- An atraumatic minimal-touch technique minimizes adhesions.
- **To prevent tendon bowstringing, A2 and A4 pulleys should be preserved in digits and oblique pulley preserved in thumb.**
- Risk of tendon rupture greatest 3 weeks after repair; failure typically occurs at suture knots
- **In general, early protected ROM is advocated to increase tendon excursion, decrease adhesion formation, and increase repair strength.**
  - Use of an active flexion protocol postoperatively requires a minimum four-strand repair with epitendinous suture.
  - **Young children cannot comply with protected motion protocols and require cast immobilization for 4 weeks.**
- Tendon healing factors
  - No repair tissue matches the strength and stiffness of a normal uninjured tendon.
  - Intrinsic healing is directed by tendon fibroblasts (tenocytes).
  - Extrinsic healing potential is limited
    - Only small contribution from repair cells within tendon sheath or from vascular invasion
  - Tendon healing is strongly influenced by biomechanical stimuli, and early mobilization has been shown to decrease adhesion formation and increase the strength of repair tissue.
  - Many recent studies have investigated the use of growth factor augmentation of flexor tendon repair, although no definitive conclusions can be made at this point.
- Treatment according to Verdan zones (Figure 7-30)
  - Zone I injury ("rugger jersey" finger)
    - Closed FDP avulsion occurring distal to the FDS insertion
    - Mechanism of injury is forced extension of the DIP joint during grasping.
    - The ring finger is involved in 75% of cases.
    - Leddy and Packer classification (Figure 7-31):

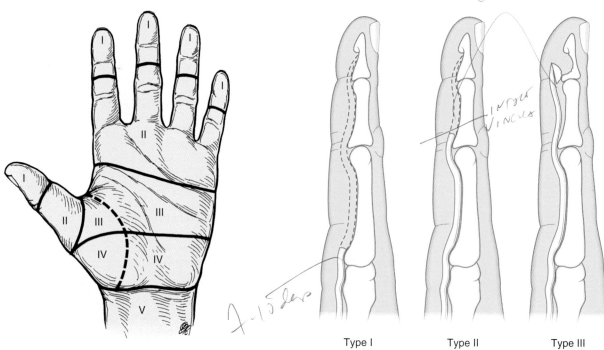

6 wurks

Type I   Type II   Type III

FIGURE 7-30 Zones of the flexor tendon system. (Copyright Elizabeth Martin.)

FIGURE 7-31 Classification of profundus tendon avulsions. (From Tang JB, editor: *Tendon surgery of the hand*, Philadelphia, 2012, Elsevier Saunders, p 220.)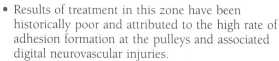

- Type I injuries, in which the FDP is retracted to the palm, require direct repair within 7 to 10 days.
- Type II injuries may be directly repaired up to 6 weeks later because the intact vincula prevent FDP retraction proximal to the PIP joint.
- Type III injuries are associated with small bony avulsion fragments with little retraction and may be successfully repaired up to 6 weeks after injury.
- Profundus advancement of 1 cm or more carries a risk of DIP joint flexion contracture or quadrigia.
  - The latter phenomenon occurs because the FDP tendons (middle, ring, small) share a common muscle belly, and distal advancement of one tendon will compromise flexion of the adjacent digits, resulting in forearm pain.
- If full PIP flexion is present, chronic injuries may be treated with observation or DIP arthrodesis in a functional position.
  - Two-stage flexor tendon reconstruction may be considered in young motivated patients.
- Zone II injury ("no man's land")
  - Occurs within the flexor tendon sheath between the FDS insertion and the distal palmar crease
  - Both the FDS and FDP may be injured in this zone.
  - Tendon lacerations may be at a different level than the skin laceration, depending on the position of the finger when the laceration occurred.
  - Direct repair of both tendons with a core and epitendinous suture technique followed by an early mobilization protocol is typically advocated.

- Results of treatment in this zone have been historically poor and attributed to the high rate of adhesion formation at the pulleys and associated digital neurovascular injuries.
- **Advances in postoperative rehabilitation have improved the clinical outcomes, although up to 50% of patients require subsequent tenolysis to enhance active motion at least 3 months after repair.**
- Zone III injury
  - Occurs between the distal palmar crease and the distal end of the carpal tunnel
  - Compared with zone II injuries, the results of direct repair are much better.
  - Lumbrical muscles originate from the radial aspect of FDP tendons in zone III.
- Zone IV injury
  - Occurs within the carpal tunnel
  - Transverse carpal ligament should be repaired in a lengthened fashion to prevent bowstringing and allow for immobilization of wrist in flexion.
- Zone V injury
  - Occurs between proximal end of carpal tunnel and musculotendinous junction
  - Direct repair in this zone has a favorable prognosis.
  - Results may be compromised by coexisting nerve injury.
- FPL injury
  - Zone I injuries—occur distal to interphalangeal joint
  - Zone II injuries—occur between interphalangeal and MCP joints
  - Zone III injuries—occur deep to thenar muscles
- Postoperative rehabilitation
  - Two most common postoperative rehabilitation protocols are those of Kleinert and Duran.

- Kleinert protocol employs dynamic splinting, which allows for active digit extension and passive digit flexion.
- Duran protocol requires strict patient compliance because other hand is used to perform passive digital flexion exercises.
- Both programs restrict active flexion for approximately 6 weeks.
  - Newer protocols add components of early active digital flexion with the hope of further reducing adhesion formation and increasing tendon excursion.
    - These protocols require stronger repair methods, such as the use of more than four core strands.
- Flexor tendon reconstruction
  - Indicated for failed primary repair or chronic, untreated injuries
  - Requirements include supple skin, a sensate digit, adequate vascularity, and full passive ROM of adjacent joints
  - The majority of cases require two-stage reconstruction.
    - In stage I, a temporary silicone (Hunter) rod is implanted, secured distally, and allowed to glide proximally.
      - A2 and A4 pulleys are either preserved or reconstructed.
    - Stage II is performed at least 3 months later, after full passive ROM has been attained and a sheath has formed around the silicone rod.
      - The rod is removed and a tendon autograft is passed through the sheath.
      - Extrasynovial graft choices such as palmaris longus or plantaris act as scaffolding and heal by tenocyte repopulation.
      - Intrasynovial grafts such as FDS retain their gliding surface and heal intrinsically.
  - Postoperative rehabilitation is intensive, and subsequent tenolysis is needed more than 50% of the time.

■ Stenosing tenosynovitis (trigger finger)

- Most common in women older than age 50
- Commonly associated with diabetes and inflammatory arthropathy
- May otherwise result from repetitive grasping activities (idiopathic form)
- Histologic finding: fibrocartilaginous metaplasia (pulley and/or FDS tendon)
- Initially characterized by pain/tenderness in the distal palm, progresses to mechanical catching/locking, and may become "fixed" (Green classification [Table 7-4])
- Patients often complain of referred pain at the dorsal MCP/PIP area.
- Middle and ring finger involvement most common in adults
- Concomitant trigger finger/carpal tunnel syndrome in 40% to 60% of patients at initial presentation
- Recent evidence shows the pulley system of the thumb to be composed of four components rather than the traditional view of three. Variable annular pulley (Av) found in approximately 75%; four types of arrangements possible; may contribute to stenosis.
- Many respond to corticosteroid injection into flexor tendon sheath.

Table 7-4	Classification of Trigger Digit (Green)
GRADE	**DESCRIPTION**
I	Pain and tenderness at the A1 pulley
II	Catching of digit
III	Locking of digit; passively correctable
IV	Fixed, locked digit

- Review of best evidence indicates that injection "curative" in about 60%
- Diabetic patients generally less responsive to injection
- No difference between soluble and insoluble preparations
- Failure of nonoperative management treated by surgical release of A1 pulley (open or percutaneous) with resection of ulnar FDS slip when necessary
  - Relatively high minor complication rate includes wound dehiscence, scar tenderness, decreased ROM
- Pediatric trigger digits
  - Trigger thumb
    - In contrast to adults, pathologic nodular tendon thickening (Notta node)
    - Presents with mechanical catching or fixed flexion deformity of interphalangeal joint in early childhood
    - More accurately deemed "developmental" rather than "congenital"
    - May initially be observed, but annular pulley release may be required between ages of 2 and 4 to prevent IP joint contracture
  - Trigger finger
    - In contrast to adults, usually caused by anatomic anomaly
    - Treatment on case-by-case basis, guided by intraoperative findings
    - A1 pulley release may not resolve triggering; additional A3 release or resection of ulnar FDS slip may be required

■ de Quervain tenosynovitis

- Attritional and degenerative condition affecting the first extensor compartment (APL/EPB)
- Commonly affects middle-aged women
- Other high-risk groups: new mothers, golfers, and racquet-sport athletes
- Dorsoradial wrist tenderness, swelling, crepitus
- Finkelstein test and/or Eichoff maneuver places first extensor compartment tendons under maximum tension and exacerbates symptoms.
- Nonoperative management includes rest, activity modification, thumb spica splinting/bracing, nonsteroidal antiinflammatory drugs (NSAIDs), and corticosteroid injections into the first dorsal extensor compartment.
  - Corticosteroid injections successful in more than 80% of patients
- When these measures fail, surgical release of the first extensor compartment may be performed.
  - Dorsal retinaculum is released to prevent volar tendon subluxation
  - Anatomic variation within the first extensor compartment is frequently encountered in recalcitrant cases.
    - **APL may have multiple slips (two to four), and EPB may have its own separate compartment.**
  - Outcomes generally excellent

- Complications of operative treatment include **iatrogenic injury to the superficial sensory radial nerve,** tendon subluxation, complex regional pain syndrome, and recurrence from incomplete release.

■ **Intersection syndrome**

▦ Tenosynovitis and/or bursitis occurring at the junction between the first and second extensor compartments where APL and EPB tendons cross ECRL and ECRB

▦ Affects rowers, weight lifters, football lineman, martial artists, and golfers

▦ Tenderness, swelling, and crepitus are localized to an area approximately 4 to 5 cm proximal to the radiocarpal joint.

▦ Initially treated with ice, splinting, NSAIDs, corticosteroid injection into the second extensor compartment

▦ When nonoperative measures fail, surgical release of the second extensor compartment and débridement of inflamed bursae may be effective.

■ **Acute calcific tendonitis**

▦ Overuse syndrome from repetitive resisted wrist flexion

▦ Most frequently described for FCU but may also involve FCR

▦ Acute onset of wrist pain, swelling, and discoloration that mimics infection or crystalline arthropathy in severity

▦ **Fluffy calcium deposits may be detected on plain radiographs.**

▦ Usually responds to short course of oral steroids or high-dose NSAIDs, ice, and immobilization

■ **ECU tendonitis and subluxation**

▦ ECU tendon held tightly within a groove in the distal ulna, tethered by a fibroosseous sheath

▦ Overuse tendinopathy often affects racquet-sport athletes.

▦ MRI may reveal thickening (hypertrophy), partial longitudinal tears, or generalized increased signal intensity within tendon and/or sheath.

▦ Nonoperative management with rest, activity modification, splinting, NSAIDs, and corticosteroid injections recommended first

▦ Traumatic subluxation of ECU tendon may result from forceful hypersupination and ulnar deviation of wrist.

- A painful audible snap or visible dislocation may be induced with reproduction of this mechanism on physical examination.
- If diagnosed early, long-arm cast immobilization (or Muenster splint) with the wrist held in pronation and slight radial deviation can be attempted.
- Chronic cases require either direct repair or reconstruction of the overlying extensor retinaculum, often accompanied by deepening of the ulnar groove.
- Wrist arthroscopy reveals concurrent triangular fibrocartilage complex (TFCC) tears in about 50% of cases.

DISTAL RADIOULNAR JOINT, TRIANGULAR FIBROCARTILAGE COMPLEX, AND WRIST ARTHROSCOPY

■ **Anatomy**

▦ Radius rotates around a fixed ulna at the DRUJ.

▦ *Ulnar variance* measures the distance in millimeters between the distal aspect of the ulnar head and the articular surface of the distal radius (Figure 7-32).

- Determined on posteroanterior radiograph of wrist with forearm in neutral

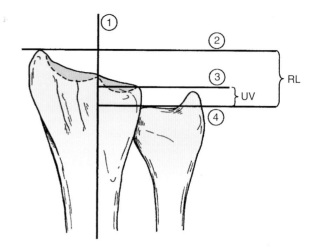

FIGURE 7-32 The relative length (RL) of the radius and ulna can be determined by measuring the distance from the tip of the radial styloid *(line 2)* drawn perpendicular to the long axis of the radius *(line 1)* and the distal end of the ulnar articular surface *(line 4)*. The ulnar variance (UV) is the distance between line 4 and *line 3*, the dense cortical line along the ulnar border of the distal radius articular surface. (From Trumble TE: Distal radioulnar joint and triangular fibrocartilage complex. In Trumble TE, editor: *Principles of hand surgery and therapy,* Philadelphia, 2000, WB Saunders.)

- There is relative positive ulnar variance with forearm in pronation and relative negative ulnar variance with forearm in supination.

▦ **The TFCC stabilizes the DRUJ and transmits 20% of axial load at the wrist (neutral ulnar variance).**

▦ **Components of the TFCC include the dorsal and volar radioulnar ligaments, the articular disc, a meniscus homologue, the ECU subsheath, and the origins of the ulnolunate and ulnotriquetral ligaments.**

▦ **Periphery is well vascularized, whereas the radial central portion is relatively avascular** (Figure 7-33).

▦ TFCC is composed of superficial and deep limbs.

- Ligamentum subcruentum—deep fibers inserting into the distal ulna fovea

■ **TFCC tears**

▦ Classified as traumatic (class I) or degenerative (class II)

▦ Further divided by Palmer into subtypes based on the specific location within the complex (Tables 7-5 and 7-6)

▦ Class and location of the tear have important implications for treatment.

▦ Value of MRI is increasing with regard to overall detection and localization of TFCC pathology.

▦ All acute traumatic TFCC injuries are initially managed with immobilization and NSAIDs.

▦ When nonoperative management fails to relieve persistent symptoms, wrist arthroscopy and/or open repair is indicated.

▦ Arthroscopic trampoline test performed to assess TFCC resiliency by balloting central portion with small probe

- Class I
  - Central class IA tears are inherently stable and may simply be débrided when persistently symptomatic.
    - A 2-mm peripheral rim must be maintained.
  - Peripheral class IB tears are amenable to arthroscopic or open repair.
    - Concurrent fractures of ulnar styloid with persistent instability are either excised or internally fixed

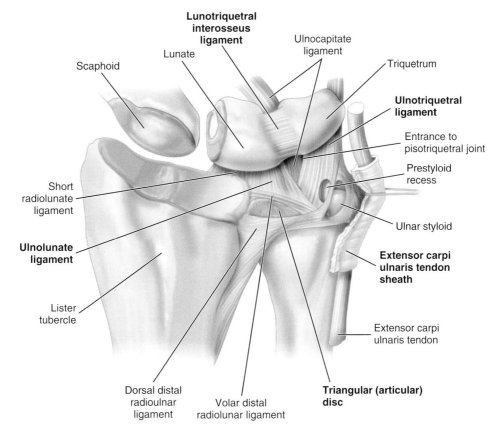

FIGURE 7-33 Anatomy of the triangular fibrocartilage complex. (From Cooney WP et al: *The wrist: diagnosis and operative treatment,* St Louis, 1998, Mosby.)

Table 7-5	**Class I (Traumatic) TFCC Injuries**	
CLASS	**CHARACTERISTICS**	**TREATMENT**
IA	Central perforation or tear	Resection of an unstable flap back to a stable rim
IB	Ulnar avulsion with or without ulnar styloid fracture	Repair of the rim to its origin at the ulnar styloid
IC	Distal avulsion (origins of UL and UT ligaments)	Advancement of the distal volar rim to the triquetrum (bone anchor)
ID	Radial avulsion (involving the dorsal and/or volar radioulnar ligaments)	Direct repair to the radius to preserve the TFCC contribution to DRUJ stability

DRUJ, Distal radioulnar joint; *TFCC,* triangular fibrocartilage complex; *UL,* ulnolunate; *UT,* ulnotriquetral.

Table 7-6	**Class II (Degenerative) TFCC Tears (Ulnocarpal Impaction Syndrome)**
CLASS	**CHARACTERISTICS**
IIA	TFCC wear (thinning)
IIB	IIA + lunate and/or ulnar chondromalacia
IIC	TFCC perforation + lunate and/or ulnar chondromalacia
IID	IIC + LT ligament disruption
IIE	IID + ulnocarpal and DRUJ arthritis

DRUJ, Distal radioulnar joint; *LT,* lunotriquetral; *TFCC,* triangular fibrocartilage complex.

- Rare class IC tears are managed by either arthroscopic or open repair.
- Class ID tears are frequently associated with distal radius fractures and often respond to reduction of radius.
- Patients who undergo repair of a traumatic TFCC tear within 3 months of injury should expect to regain 80% of wrist ROM and grip strength.
- Class II
  - Degenerative class II tears are associated with positive ulnar variance, increased ulnocarpal loading, and ulnocarpal impaction syndrome from abutment of the ulnar head into the proximal carpal row.
- Patients present with chronic ulnar-sided wrist pain, increased with forearm rotation and grip.
- Pain with loading wrist in extension and ulnar deviation
- In addition to detectable TFCC pathology, MRI may demonstrate focal increased T2-weighted signal in proximal ulnar corner of lunate and/or ulnar head at point of chronic impaction
- When conservative management fails, the goal of surgery is reduction of ulnocarpal loading.
  - In the absence of DRUJ osteoarthrosis, the most commonly performed procedure is an ulnar-shortening osteotomy.
  - Alternatively, a simple wafer resection of the ulnar head dome has been described.
  - Coexisting TFCC pathology is addressed by arthroscopic or open débridement.

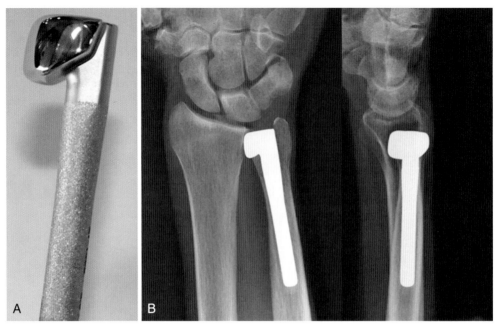

FIGURE 7-34 **A,** Partial ulnar head replacement. **B,** Posteroanterior and lateral radiographs of a partial ulnar head replacement. (From Green DP et al, editors: *Green's operative hand surgery,* ed 6, Philadelphia, 2011, Churchill Livingstone, p 556.)

■ **DRUJ instability and posttraumatic osteoarthritis**
▓ Instability
- Acute dislocation of DRUJ can occur alone or in combination with ulnar styloid (base), radial shaft (Galeazzi), or Essex-Lopresti injuries.
- Isolated dislocations may be treated by closed reduction and immobilization.
- Closed reduction may be impeded by interposition of the ECU tendon.
- Concurrent distal ulna fractures and TFCC tears may require open or arthroscopic treatment.
- **In a Galeazzi injury, ORIF of the radial shaft is followed by assessment of DRUJ stability.**
  - An unstable DRUJ may require TFCC repair and/or temporary radioulnar pinning proximal to the joint, with the forearm immobilized in relative supination.
- Chronic DRUJ instability may result from distal radius malunion, ulnar styloid nonunion, or large TFCC/ligamentous disruptions.
  - Subtle chronic instability of the DRUJ may be evaluated on sequential CT scans, with the forearm held in a neutral position, full supination, and full pronation and compared with the contralateral side (>50% translation is abnormal).
  - When chronic instability results from soft tissue incompetence, TFCC repair or ligament reconstruction (Adams) with a palmaris tendon autograft may be indicated.
  - A severely angulated distal radius malunion necessitates corrective osteotomy and appropriate treatment of resulting positive ulnar variance.
▓ Posttraumatic DRUJ osteoarthritis (Figure 7-34)
- Maximize nonoperative management
- Surgical options
  - Distal ulna resection (Darrach procedure) is typically reserved for low-demand elderly patients and may lead to painful proximal ulna stump instability.

- Hemiresection or interposition arthroplasty maintains the ulnar insertion of the TFCC and prevents radioulnar impingement by soft tissue (ECU tendon or capsular flap) interposition.
- Fusion of the DRUJ with creation of a proximal pseudarthrosis at the ulnar neck is termed the *Sauve-Kapandji procedure.*
- Early results of metallic ulnar head prosthetic replacement are promising, but no long-term studies have been performed to date.
- Creation of a one-bone forearm eliminates forearm rotation altogether and remains the ultimate salvage operation for persistent pain or other complications.

■ **Wrist arthroscopy**
▓ Indicated for the diagnosis of unexplained wrist pain
▓ Indications
- TFCC tears
- Osteochondral injuries
- Loose bodies
- Partial intracarpal ligament injuries
- Ganglions
▓ May assist in the treatment of distal radius and scaphoid fractures
▓ Traction tower, 2.7-mm 30-degree arthroscope
▓ Arthroscopic portals (Figure 7-35)
▓ Radiocarpal, ulnocarpal, and midcarpal joints inspected systematically
▓ **Injury to superficial sensory nerves (branches of superficial sensory radial, dorsal sensory ulnar, lateral antebrachial cutaneous) is most common complication.**

NAIL AND FINGERTIP INJURIES

■ **Introduction**
▓ Fingertip injuries are the most common hand injuries seen in emergency departments.
▓ Long finger is most commonly involved digit

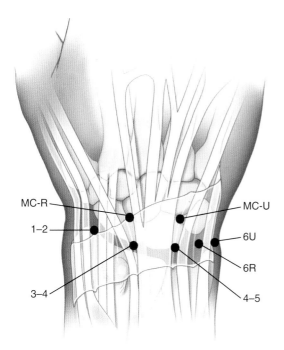

FIGURE 7-35 Arthroscopic wrist portals. Numbers indicate wrist extensor compartments and associated portals. *MC-R,* Midcarpal radial; *MC-U,* midcarpal ulnar; *R,* radial; *U,* ulnar. (From Miller MD et al, editors: *Orthopaedic surgical approaches,* Philadelphia, 2008, Elsevier.)

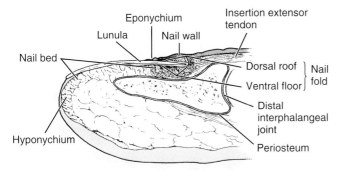

FIGURE 7-36 Sagittal depiction of nail bed anatomy. (From Green DP et al, editors: *Green's operative hand surgery,* ed 6, Philadelphia, 2011, Churchill Livingstone, p 333.)

▦ These injuries may be broadly classified as those with and those without soft tissue loss.
▦ Crush injuries without extensive soft tissue loss may result in nail plate avulsions, nail matrix lacerations, and distal phalanx (tuft) fractures.
▦ Distal phalanx fractures are typically reduced when the nail bed is repaired, but large displaced fragments may require percutaneous pinning.

■ Nail structure
▦ Nail plate composed of keratin and originates from germinal matrix proximal to nail fold
▦ Sterile matrix lies directly beneath nail plate and contributes keratin to increase plate thickness.
▦ Crescent-shaped white lunula is seen through proximal nail plate at junction of sterile and germinal matrices
▦ Hyponychium lies between distal nail bed and skin of fingertip, serving as a barrier to microorganisms
▦ Eponychium, also called the cuticle, is at distal margin of proximal nail fold
▦ Paronychium forms lateral margins (Figure 7-36)

■ Nail bed injury
▦ A small subungual hematoma constituting less than 50% of nail area may be treated without nail plate removal.
  • Nail plate should be perforated with a sterile needle.
▦ **Subungual hematomas greater than 50% of nail area require nail plate removal for repair of underlying nail matrix lacerations.**
  • Acute repair offers best results.
  • Remember tetanus prophylaxis and antibiotic coverage.
  • A digital block should be administered, and a clamped Penrose drain may be used as a temporary finger tourniquet.
  • If it is still available, the nail plate is removed and soaked in Betadine.
  • The wound is débrided and thoroughly irrigated.
  • Sterile and/or germinal matrix lacerations are repaired with 6-0 or smaller absorbable suture under loupe magnification.
  • The eponychial fold is then splinted open with the Betadine-soaked nail plate, piece of aluminum foil, or nonadherent gauze to allow new nail plate to grow distally from germinal matrix.
  • A single-institution randomized controlled trial demonstrated faster healing using 2-octylcyanoacrylate (Dermabond) compared to suture repair.
▦ If significant nail matrix has been lost, options include a split-thickness matrix graft from an adjacent injured finger or transfer of the nail matrix from second toe.
▦ Nail plate deformities, especially nail ridging, are very common after crush injuries but may be minimized by a flat nail bed repair.
▦ **A hook nail may result from a tight nail bed repair, distal advancement of the matrix, or loss of underlying bony support.**
▦ Patients should be counseled about high incidence of fingertip hypersensitivity and/or cold intolerance for up to 1 year.
▦ Nail growth occurs at about 0.1 mm/day, and complete growth of a new nail plate takes 3 to 6 months, depending on patient's age.

■ Fingertip injuries with tissue loss
▦ Treatment of these injuries may be time intensive and challenging.
▦ The general principles of treatment include preservation of digit length, maintenance of sensate fingertip pulp, prevention of joint contracture, and eventual pain-free use of digit.
▦ The correct characterization of the injury is critical and guides treatment.
  • Fingertip injuries without exposed bone
    • These may be allowed to heal by secondary intention if less than 1 cm² of the tip or pulp is involved.
    • Otherwise, skin or composite grafts may be required.
    • Full-thickness skin grafts are best for the fingertip because they provide better durability, minimal contraction, and superior sensibility compared with the split-thickness variety.
  • Fingertip injuries with exposed bone
    • Characterized by the orientation of tissue loss (Figure 7-37)
      • Volar oblique injury
        • Cross-finger flap

- Dorsal skin and subcutaneous tissue elevated superficial to the paratenon from adjacent digit to create a bed for the injured fingertip
- Donor site is covered with a split-thickness skin graft.

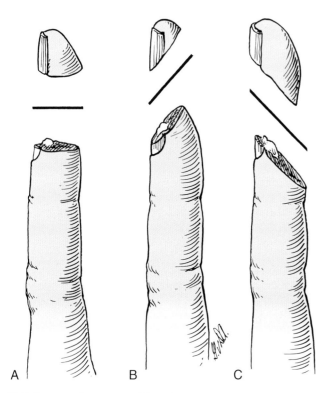

FIGURE 7-37 Orientation of fingertip amputations. **A,** Transverse. **B,** Dorsal oblique. **C,** Volar oblique. (Modified from Lister GD: The theory of the transposition flap and its practical application in the hand, *Clin Plast Surg* 8:115-128, 1981.)

- The flap is split during a separate procedure 2 to 3 weeks later (Figure 7-38).
- Thenar flap
  - Best reserved for volar oblique injuries to the index or long digits
  - Flap is lifted parallel to the proximal thumb crease and split after 2 to 3 weeks.
  - Potential complications include donor site tenderness and PIP contracture (especially in older patients).
- Homodigital island flap
  - Raised on digital artery of involved finger and may maintain sensory innervation to the fingertip
- Heterodigital island flap
  - Raised on ulnar aspect of the long or ring finger and typically tunneled in the palm to provide coverage to the thumb
- Other possible donor sites
  - Include distant flaps in the chest, abdomen, and groin, although they may be cumbersome and too bulky for the fingertip
- Transverse or dorsal oblique digit injury
  - V-Y advancement
    - May be performed to preserve length and cover transverse or dorsal oblique fingertip injuries
    - A wide volar flap is lifted off the distal phalanx, with a tapered base created at the level of the DIP flexion crease.
    - Flap is advanced over the fingertip toward the dorsal side, and a tension-free closure is made.
  - Kutler popularized two separate smaller V-Y advancements from the lateral aspects of the digit to cover transverse fingertip injuries.

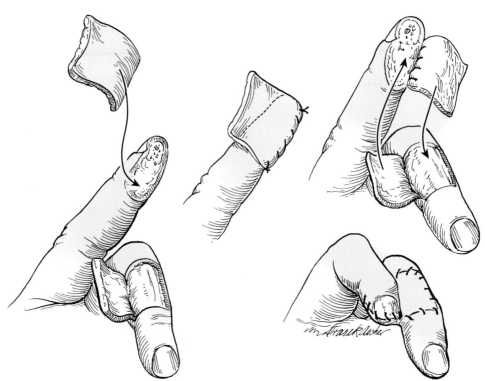

FIGURE 7-38 Cross-finger flap. (From the Christine Kleinert Institute for Hand and Microsurgery, Inc., with permission.)

- Alternatively, these injuries are treated by bone shortening and conversion to a volar coverage option.
- Shortening and closing an injury that acutely violates the FDP insertion may result in a lumbrical-plus finger.
  - FDP tendon retracts and creates tension on the extensor mechanism through its lumbrical, causing paradoxical interphalangeal joint extension with active digit flexion.
    - Treated with release of the radial lateral band
- Transverse or volar oblique thumb injury
  - Moberg advancement flap
    - Entire volar surface of thumb is advanced with its neurovascular bundles (Figure 7-39)
    - Potential complications include flap necrosis and thumb interphalangeal joint flexion contracture.
- Dorsal thumb injury
  - This injury may be covered with a first dorsal metacarpal artery "kite" flap or heterodigital island flap.
- Pediatric distal fingertip amputation
  - **Composite flaps** (reattachment of amputated tissue without vascular repair) for distal fingertip amputations may be attempted in patients younger than age 6, but parents must be willing to see it fail.

SOFT TISSUE COVERAGE AND MICROSURGERY

■ Upper extremity wounds
▦ Introduction

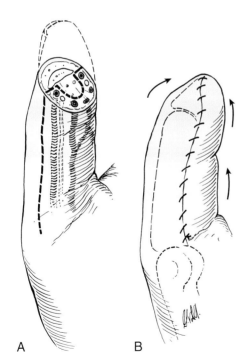

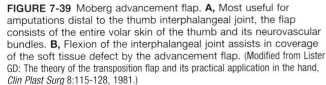

FIGURE 7-39 Moberg advancement flap. **A,** Most useful for amputations distal to the thumb interphalangeal joint, the flap consists of the entire volar skin of the thumb and its neurovascular bundles. **B,** Flexion of the interphalangeal joint assists in coverage of the soft tissue defect by the advancement flap. (Modified from Lister GD: The theory of the transposition flap and its practical application in the hand, *Clin Plast Surg* 8:115-128, 1981.)

- Management begins with thorough assessment of wound, including size, location, involvement of deep structures, and presence of contamination.
- Standard of care involves early débridement and administration of antibiotics guided by the degree of contamination, extent of involvement, and associated injuries.
- Complex wounds may require serial surgical débridements to remove nonviable tissue.
- A clean wound bed is essential before any definitive coverage procedure.
- Infection rates increase dramatically if coverage is delayed longer than 1 week after injury.
▦ Reconstructive ladder
- Goals of soft tissue reconstruction
  - Provide coverage of deep structures (e.g., bone, cartilage, tendons, nerves, blood vessels)
  - Create a barrier to microorganisms, restore dynamic function of the limb, and prevent joint contracture
  - Cosmetic appearance is a secondary priority.
- Options for soft tissue closure/reconstruction:
  - Primary closure
  - Secondary intention
  - Skin grafting
  - Flaps
- Choice of definitive procedure is guided by wound characteristics and patient factors.
- Primary closure of a traumatic wound is generally not advised unless the wound is minimally contaminated and is closed within about 6 hours of injury.
- Wounds may be allowed to heal by secondary intention, a process involving wound granulation, epithelialization, and contraction.
  - Deep neurovascular, tendinous or bony structures cannot be exposed.
  - Regular dressing changes or vacuum-assisted closure (VAC) devices are necessary to promote this type of healing.
  - Positive effects of VAC devices include dissipation of interstitial edema, reduction of bacterial counts, and stimulation of cell division by mechanical stretching of cells.
▦ Specific methods of soft tissue coverage
- Skin grafts
  - Autografts may be either split-thickness skin grafts or full-thickness skin grafts.
  - Both types require a clean wound bed without exposed bone or tendon.
  - **Skin grafts are prone to early failure from shear stress and hematoma formation.**
  - Split-thickness skin grafts
    - Preferred for dorsal hand wounds
    - Meshed grafts provide greater surface area and typically have a better "take" because of a lower incidence of hematoma formation and infection.
    - Anterolateral thigh is a common donor site, reepithelialization occurs in 2 to 3 weeks.
  - Full-thickness skin grafts
    - Preferred for volar hand and fingertip wounds
    - **Go through sequential process of plasma imbibition, inosculation and revascularization**
    - More durable, contract less, and provide better sensibility

- Less contraction with higher total percentage of dermis grafted, early grafting, and pressure application during remodeling phase
- Proximal forearm, medial arm, and hypothenar aspect of the hand are common donor sites.
- Allografts may be used as temporary measures to prepare a wound bed for later autografting.
- Xenografts are occasionally used as biologic dressings.
- Flaps
  - A flap is a unit of tissue supported by blood vessels and moved from a donor site to a recipient site to cover a defect.
  - This unit may be composed of one tissue type or a composite of several tissue types that may include skin, fascia, muscle, tendon, nerve, or bone.
  - Transfer of vascularized tissue promotes healing and lowers the secondary infection rate.
  - Flap reconstruction indicated when wound has exposed bone (stripped of periosteum), tendon (stripped of paratenon), cartilage, or an orthopaedic implant
  - Flaps may be classified by their vascular supply, tissue type, donor site, and method of transfer.
    - Flap classification by blood supply
      - Axial-pattern flaps
        - Single named arteriovenous pedicle
        - More predictable blood supply
        - Greater resistance to infection
        - Raised on their pedicle and transferred locally or pedicle can be divided and transferred to a distant site as a free flap
      - Random-pattern flaps
        - No single named arteriovenous pedicle
        - Depend on microcirculation
        - Examples are cross-finger and thenar flaps
    - Flap classification by tissue type
      - Single
        - Fascia
          - Lateral arm
        - Muscle
          - Latissimus, gastrocnemius
        - Bone
          - Medial femoral condyle
      - Composite
        - Cutaneous flaps include skin and subcutaneous tissue.
          - Thenar flap
        - Fasciocutaneous flaps include fascia with overlying skin and subcutaneous tissue.
          - Radial forearm flap (Figure 7-40)
        - Musculocutaneous flaps include muscle with the overlying skin, subcutaneous tissue, and fascia.
          - Gracilis
        - Osteocutaneous flap composed of a portion of bone with overlying soft tissue
          - Fibular, iliac crest
      - Innervated flaps preserve the nerve supply with the tissue unit.
        - Either motor or sensory nerves may be preserved, depending on their anatomic location and the choice of flap to be transferred.

- Flap classification by donor site
  - Local flap—provided by tissue adjacent to or near the defect
    - Transposition flaps are geometric in design and may be either axial or random pattern with regard to blood supply.
      - One example is **Z-plasty.**
      - Limbs should always be equal, but the flap cut angles may vary to change the amount of desired lengthening.
      - Theoretically 30 degrees, 45 degrees, 60 degrees yields 25%, 50%, 75% lengthening, respectively, along the line of the central limb (Figure 7-41).
    - Rotation flaps are not geometric and are universally random pattern with regard to blood supply.
      - Length of rotated flap should not exceed width of its base; doing so will exceed capacity of the microcirculation to maintain tissue viability

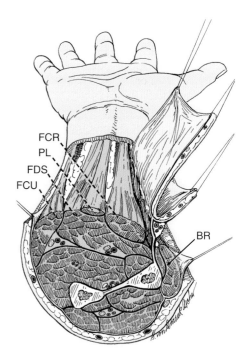

FIGURE 7-40 Radial forearm flap. Incision of fascia lifts the entire flap off the underlying forearm muscles. *BR,* Brachioradialis; *FCR,* flexor carpi radialis; *FCU,* flexor carpi ulnaris; *FDS,* flexor digitorum superficialis; *PL,* palmaris longus. (From the Christine Kleinert Institute for Hand and Microsurgery, Inc., with permission.)

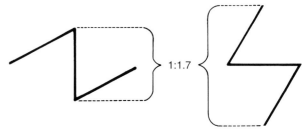

FIGURE 7-41 Standard 60-degree Z-plasty. (From Green DP et al, editors: *Green's operative hand surgery,* ed 6, Philadelphia, 2011, Churchill Livingstone, p 1668.)

- Advancement flaps such as V-Y and Moberg types proceed in straight line to fill defect
- Axial flag flaps are based on a digital artery.
  - Homodigital
  - Heterodigital
- Fillet flap, taken from an amputated digit, occasionally salvaged for initial coverage of a mangled hand
- Distant flap
  - Used when local flaps are either inadequate or unavailable for soft tissue coverage
  - For example, a degloved or burned hand may be placed in a raised pocket of tissue in the abdomen or groin.
    - Several weeks later, the flap is divided and the donor site either skin grafted or allowed to heal by secondary intention.
    - Alternatively, the defect site may be dissected away from the distant pocket of skin. In this case the donor site is primarily closed, and the defect may require a split-thickness skin graft over the vascularized granulation tissue.
- Flap classification by method of transfer
  - Flap reconstruction may be performed in a single stage or in two stages, like the previously mentioned abdominal or groin pocket flap.
  - In most instances, the donor tissue remains attached to the native vasculature.
  - Alternatively, free flaps (free tissue transfer) are distant axial-pattern flaps raised on a named arteriovenous pedicle.
  - Free flaps are then divided and reanastomosed to donor vessels near the defect but away from the zone of injury.
  - Most frequently used donors for use in the upper extremity include:
    - **Gracilis (medial femoral circumflex artery)**
    - **Latissimus dorsi (thoracodorsal artery)**
    - **Serratus anterior (serratus branch of subscapular artery)**
    - **Anterolateral thigh (descending branch of lateral femoral circumflex artery)**
    - **Lateral arm (posterior branch of radial collateral artery)**
  - Patients typically monitored postoperatively in intensive care unit
  - Room kept warm for vasodilation
  - Main cause of free-flap failure: inadequate arterial blood flow
  - Persistent vasospasm may lead to thrombosis at the anastomosis.
  - Hypotension must be avoided and the patient kept well hydrated.
  - Vasoconstrictive agents (e.g., nicotine, caffeine) restricted
  - Seroma or hematoma formation can also lead to flap demise.

Traumatic upper extremity amputation
- Indications and contraindications
  - **Primary indications to attempt replantation**
    - Thumb
    - Multiple digits
    - Wrist level or proximal
    - Any amputation in child
  - Relative indication is a level distal to the FDS insertion (zone I)
  - Primary contraindications to replantation
    - Single digit amputation, especially index
    - Crushed or mangled amputated parts
    - Prolonged ischemia
    - Segmental amputations
    - Level of amputation within zone II flexor tendon sheath
  - Patients with multisystem traumatic injuries and those with multiple medical comorbidities or disabling psychiatric conditions may be poor candidates for attempted replantation.
- Care of the amputated part
  - Part should be wrapped in moist gauze (normal saline or lactated Ringer solution) and placed within a sealed plastic bag, which is then placed in an ice-water bath.
  - **Although controversial, replantation is not recommended if warm ischemia time is more than 6 hours for an amputation level proximal to the carpus or more than 12 hours for an amputated digit.**
  - **Cold ischemia times of less than 12 hours for an amputation level proximal to the carpus or less than 24 hours for an amputated digit may still permit successful replantation, highlighting the importance of appropriate cooling of the amputated part.**
- **Operative sequence of replantation**
  - Bone stabilization, usually with shortening
  - Extensor tendon repair
  - Flexor tendon(s) repair
  - Arterial reanastomosis
  - Venous reanastomosis
  - Nerve repair
  - Skin approximation (loose)
    - If multiple digits, priority sequence is thumb, long, ring, small, and index
    - Surgeon preference and level of amputation may lead to variation in overall operative sequence.
    - Structure-by-structure technique faster and yields higher viability rate
    - Use of venous couplers may result in quicker operative times and less vasospastic collapse of the anastomosis.
- Postoperative care
  - Warm environment (≈80°F)
  - Adequate hydration
  - Aspirin
  - Dextran/heparin controversial
  - Thorazine acts as both vasodilator and anxiolytic (especially good for children)
  - Prohibit nicotine, caffeine, other vasoconstricting agents
- Replantation monitoring
  - Most reliable methods are close observation of color, capillary refill, and tissue turgor
  - Measuring oxygen saturation by pulse oximetry and measuring skin surface temperature are safe, noninvasive, reproducible monitoring methods.

- Either a drop in temperature of more than 2°C in 1 hour or a temperature of less than 30°C indicates decreased digital perfusion.
- Others advocate placement of implantable venous Doppler probe
- Flap monitoring may be discontinued after day 4 to 5.
- Complications
  - **Most frequent cause of early (within 12 hours) replantation failure is arterial thrombosis from persistent vasospasm**
    - Arterial insufficiency suggested by pale skin color, decreased or absent capillary refill, loss of Doppler-measurable signal
    - Consider releasing constricting bandages, place extremity in dependent position, administer heparin, perform stellate ganglion block.
    - If these measures fail, exploration and attempt at reanastomosis warranted
  - **Failure after 12 hours is typically secondary to venous congestion or thrombosis.**
    - Venous insufficiency suggested by ruborous skin color, increased capillary refill, tissue engorgement
    - May subsequently diminish arterial inflow
    - Remove dressings and elevate extremity.
    - Heparin-soaked pledgets
    - **Medicinal leeches (*Hirudo medicinalis*)**
      - Produce the anticoagulant hirudin, yield 8 to 12 hours of sustained bleeding (Figure 7-42)
      - May be required for up to 5 to 7 days
      - ***Aeromonas hydrophila* infection is risk; prophylactic antibiotics such as ceftriaxone or ciprofloxacin warranted during leech therapy**
    - Revision of venous anastomosis is last resort
  - Late complications include tendon adhesions, bone nonunion, and neuroma formation.
    - Tenolysis is the most commonly performed secondary procedure following successful replantation.
- Results
  - Factor most predictive of digit survival after replantation is mechanism of injury
  - Next most important factor is probably ischemia time.
  - Clean transverse amputations with cold ischemia time less than 8 hours survive replantation in more than 90% of cases.

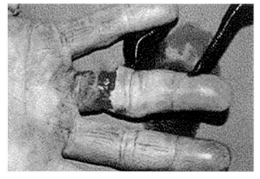

FIGURE 7-42 Class IIC ring avulsion injury of the ring finger, with venous insufficiency treated by leech therapy. (From Tuncali D et al: The value of medical leeches in the treatment of class IIC ring avulsion injuries: report of two cases, *J Hand Surg Am* 29:943–946, 2004.)

- After 8 hours, the success rate drops to approximately 75%.
- Replanted digits typically regain 50% total active motion and static two-point discrimination of approximately 10 mm.
- Long-term cold intolerance almost universal, regardless of whether amputated digit is replanted or revised
- Forearm and arm replantation
  - Arterial inflow established before skeletal stabilization (with use of shunts if necessary) to minimize ischemia time
  - Post-replantation fasciotomies performed to prevent reperfusion-induced compartment syndrome
  - Muscle necrosis may lead to myoglobinuria and life-threatening renal failure.
  - Elevated postoperative serum potassium level may be prognostic of replantation failure.
  - Late complications: infection, Volkmann ischemic contracture, insignificant functional recovery
- Hand allotransplantation
  - Controversial procedure that introduces potentially life-threatening complications from postoperative immunosuppression for a condition that is not itself life threatening
  - Occurring around the world with more frequency, including in United States, at specialized centers with abundant resources
  - Bilateral transplants have been performed with good survivorship, including several above the elbow.
  - Newer immunosuppressive protocols are less toxic and may lead to less long-term recipient morbidity.
  - Still debatable whether this tremendously expensive endeavor is superior to an upper limb prosthetic

- **Ring avulsion injuries**
- Forceful avulsion of overlying soft tissues from skeletal structures
- **Classified by Urbaniak:**
  - Class I—adequate circulation, digit salvage with standard soft tissue treatment
  - Class II—circulation compromised and inadequate, revascularization recommended if no accompanying severe bone or tendon injury
  - Class III—complete degloving treated with completion amputation
- **Thumb reconstruction**
- Traumatic thumb loss devastating to overall hand function
- Amputation through middle to proximal third of proximal phalanx
  - First web space deepening
  - Metacarpal lengthening with distraction external fixator
    - Average 3-cm gain
- More proximal amputation level
  - Index pollicization
  - Great or second toe transfer by microvascular reconstruction

VASCULAR DISORDERS

- **Anatomy**
- The hand is supplied by the radial and ulnar arteries.
- The ulnar artery is the main contributor to the superficial palmar arch.

- The radial artery is the main contributor to the deep palmar arch and the thumb via the princeps pollicis artery.
- **A complete arch, present in more than 80% of hands, provides arterial branches to all five digits, and if either the radial or ulnar artery is injured proximally, sufficient digital perfusion remains through the uninjured artery and the complete arch.**
- Individuals with an incomplete arch (≈20%) may have significant compromise of perfusion if the dominant artery is injured.
- Presence of an incomplete arch can be detected by an Allen test.
- In some studies up to 15% have a persistent median artery.
  - Associated with high median nerve division or bifid nerve

Evaluation of vascular dysfunction

- Allen test
  - Compress both radial and ulnar arteries at distal forearm, and ask patient to squeeze and release hand several times.
  - In sequential tests, one artery is released while the other remains compressed.
  - A positive test denotes absent arterial filling of the digits when either the compressed radial or ulnar artery is released at the wrist.
  - May also be performed with aid of Doppler probe
- Cold-stimulation testing
  - May demonstrate autonomic vascular dysfunction
  - Patients with arterial disease require more than 20 minutes to return to preexposure temperatures when submersed in ice water for 20 seconds, compared with normal subjects, who require approximately 10 minutes.
- Digital brachial index
  - Comparison of blood pressure between arm and digit
  - Less than 0.7 is abnormal for a digit.
- Color duplex ultrasonography
  - Excellent noninvasive study to help detect many forms of vessel pathology, with rates of sensitivity and specificity similar to those in arteriography (with experienced operators)
- Photoplethysmography (pulse volume recordings)
  - Demonstrates arterial insufficiency when there is loss of the dicrotic notch or a decreased rate of rise in the systolic peak
- Three-phase bone scan
  - May be useful adjunctive test in certain clinical scenarios
    - Phase 1 images taken 2 minutes after radiotracer injection provide information similar to arteriography.
    - Arterial occlusion, arteriovenous malformations, and vascular tumors can be detected during this phase.
    - After 5 to 10 minutes, phase II (soft tissue) images may show decreased perfusion when vasospastic disorders are present.
    - Delayed phase III (skeletal) images are obtained 2 to 3 hours after injection but are not particularly helpful in vascular disorders.
- Arteriography
  - Gold standard for elucidating the nature and extent of thrombotic and embolic disease of the hand vasculature
  - Provides a road map for surgical intervention

Occlusive vascular disease

- Etiologies include blunt or penetrating arterial trauma, atherosclerosis, aneurysm formation, emboli, and a variety of systemic diseases.
- Often presents with unilateral claudication (ischemic pain), paresthesias, and/or cold intolerance
- Ulcerations and gangrene are late findings of unrecognized vascular compromise.
  - **Hypothenar hammer syndrome**
    - Most common posttraumatic vascular occlusive condition of the upper extremity
    - Thrombosis or aneurysm formation of the distal ulnar artery occurs from blunt trauma to the hypothenar eminence (roofers, carpenters, etc.).
    - Clinical findings may include localized tenderness, cold intolerance, ischemic pain, and accompanying compression neuropathy of the ulnar nerve in the Guyon canal.
    - Noninvasive vascular studies or arteriography may help confirm the diagnosis.
    - Treatment may involve resection and ligation of the thrombosed ulnar artery or reconstruction with a reversed interposition vein graft or arterial conduit for better patency rate (Figure 7-43).
  - Small-vessel occlusive disease
    - May be seen in connective tissue diseases such as scleroderma, systemic lupus erythematosus (SLE), rheumatoid arthritis (RA), Sjögren syndrome, and dermatomyositis
    - Buerger disease is small-vessel arteritis, which affects predominantly male heavy smokers.
    - These conditions are often progressive despite treatments such as calcium channel blockers and periarterial sympathectomy.
  - Embolic disease
    - Majority of upper extremity emboli are of cardiac origin, with a smaller subset from the subclavian system in cases of vascular thoracic outlet syndrome
    - Emergency embolectomy is performed when feasible and followed by anticoagulation.
    - Smaller vessels are treated with thrombolytic agents such as tissue plasminogen activator (TPA), streptokinase, or urokinase if the diagnosis is made within 36 hours of occlusion.
    - Warfarin is given for 3 to 6 months.

Vasospastic disease

- Periodic digital ischemia may be induced by cold temperature or other sympathetic stimuli (e.g., pain, emotional stress)
- Digits initially turn white from vasospasm and cessation of flow, then blue from cyanosis and venous stasis, and finally red from rebound hyperemia.
- Last stage often accompanied by dysesthesia
- **Vasospastic disease with a known underlying cause (Box 7-1) is termed the Raynaud phenomenon (Table 7-7).**
  - Some degree of vascular occlusive disease is always present, giving a combined clinical picture.
  - Symptoms are usually asymmetric, and peripheral pulses are often absent.
  - Trophic changes may occur.
  - Treatment is focused on the underlying disease.

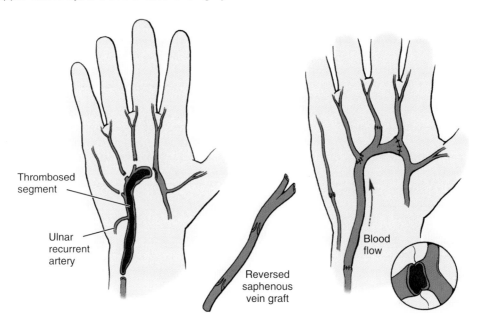

FIGURE 7-43 Complex reversed interposition vein grafts may be necessary to reconstruct extensive occlusive disease in the hand. (From Green DP et al, editors: *Green's operative hand surgery,* ed 6, Philadelphia, 2011, Churchill Livingstone, p 2224.)

Box 7-1	Causes of Secondary Vasospastic Disorder

- Connective tissue disease: scleroderma (incidence of Raynaud disease, 80%-90%), SLE (incidence, 18%-26%), dermatomyositis (incidence, 30%), RA (incidence, 11%)
- Occlusive arterial disease
- Neurovascular compression: thoracic outlet syndrome
- Hematologic abnormalities: cryoproteinemia, polycythemia, paraproteinemia
- Occupational trauma: percussion and vibratory tool workers
- Drugs and toxins: sympathomimetics, ergot compounds, β-adrenergic blockers
- CNS disease: syringomyelia, poliomyelitis, tumors/infarcts
- Miscellaneous: RSD, malignant disease

CNS, Central nervous system; *RA,* rheumatoid arthritis; *RSD,* reflex sympathetic dystrophy; *SLE,* systemic lupus erythematosus.

Table 7-7	Raynaud Disease versus Raynaud Phenomenon	
CHARACTERISTIC	DISEASE	PHENOMENON
HISTORY		
Triphasic color change	Yes	Yes
Age > 40 years	No	Yes
Progression rapid	No	Yes
Underlying disease	No	Yes
Female predominance	Frequent	Occasional
PHYSICAL EXAMINATION		
Trophic findings (ulcer, gangrene)	Infrequent	Frequent
Abnormal Allen test	No	Common
Asymmetric findings	Infrequent	Frequent
LABORATORY TESTING		
Blood chemistry	Normal	Frequently abnormal
Microangiology	Normal	Frequently abnormal
Angiography	Normal	Frequently abnormal

From Green DP et al, editors: *Green's operative hand surgery,* ed 5, Philadelphia, 2005, Churchill Livingstone, p 2304.

- When no underlying cause is present, the clinical condition is known as Raynaud disease (see Table 7-7).
  - Most commonly affected group: premenopausal women
  - Symptoms usually bilateral, peripheral pulses often present
  - Calcium channel blockers may provide transient relief of symptoms.
  - Biofeedback techniques may also be beneficial.
  - Digital sympathectomy is considered in severe cases.
- Smoking cessation and avoidance of cold exposure are imperative in both the Raynaud phenomenon and Raynaud disease.
- Recent interest in use of botulinum toxin type A for treatment of vasospastic digital ischemia

- **Acute compartment syndrome**
- Surgical emergency resulting from increased pressure within a closed anatomic space, leading to reduced capillary blood flow below the threshold for local tissue perfusion and oxygen delivery

- Prolonged ischemia secondary to a missed or delayed diagnosis may result in irreversible muscle or nerve damage within a compartment.
- **Three forearm compartments:**
  - Mobile wad of three (brachioradialis, ECRL, and ECRB)
  - Dorsal
  - Volar (deep muscles incur highest pressure)
- **Ten hand compartments:**
  - Thenar
  - Hypothenar
  - Adductor pollicis
  - Four dorsal interosseous
  - Three volar interosseous
- Compartment syndrome is a clinical diagnosis, and a high index of suspicion is critical after crush injuries and limb reperfusion.

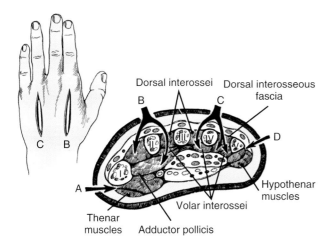

FIGURE 7-44 Both dorsal and volar interosseous compartments and the adductor compartment to the thumb can be released through two longitudinal incisions over the second and third metacarpals (B and C). The thenar and hypothenar compartments are opened through separate incisions (A and D). (From Green DP et al, editors: *Green's operative hand surgery,* ed 5, Philadelphia, 2005, Churchill Livingstone, p 1993.)

▦ **The most common cause in children is a supracondylar humerus fracture.**

▦ **Compartment pressures should be measured in equivocal cases or in unresponsive patients.**

▦ Compartment monitoring is also imperative after animal bites, high-energy trauma, and burn injuries.

▦ **Increased pain with passive stretch of the affected compartment is most sensitive finding on physical examination**

▦ **Paresthesias, pallor, pulselessness, and paralysis are late findings.**

▦ **Treatment is emergency fasciotomy of affected compartments.**
  • Forearm fasciotomies require three skin incisions over the three compartments.
  • Hand fasciotomies may be accomplished through five skin incisions.
    • Two dorsal incisions to release five interossei and the adductor pollicis.
    • Separate incisions over thenar and hypothenar musculature (Figure 7-44)
    • Transverse carpal ligament release often done in same setting, although the carpal tunnel is not a true compartment
  • Delayed wound closure and/or skin grafting recommended

▦ Most important prognostic factor is time between tissue compromise and surgical intervention

▦ Long-term sequelae of unrecognized and untreated acute compartment syndrome include muscle fibrosis and Volkmann ischemic contracture.

▦ **Volkmann ischemic contracture**

▦ Classical sequela of untreated acute compartment syndrome developing from advanced myonecrosis and muscle fibrosis in the forearm

▦ **FDP and FPL muscles most vulnerable**

▦ Mild, moderate, and severe forms have been described.

▦ Mild form is manifested as mild DIP flexion contractures, but patients often have normal strength and sensibility.

▦ Progressively worsening contractures and sensorimotor deficits are seen in the moderate and severe forms.

▦ Chronic pain and significant hand dysfunction are common.

▦ Patients with the severe form often have an insensate hand with an intrinsic-minus ("claw hand") deformity.

▦ Muscle slides, contracture releases, and tendon transfers are performed to help improve function, although the success of these procedures may be limited in severe cases.

▦ Nerve decompression may be necessary in patients with chronic neuropathic pain, especially when muscle fibrosis causes extrinsic compression on intrinsically compromised peripheral nerves.

▦ Free innervated gracilis muscle transfer used in selected severe cases

▦ **Frostbite**

▦ Damage to tissue from prolonged exposure to subfreezing temperatures

▦ Ice crystals form within extracellular fluid, causing subsequent intracellular dehydration and cell death.

▦ Increased wind chill, skin contact with metal or ice, and alcohol intoxication exacerbate cases of frostbite.

▦ **After initial resuscitative management, rapid rewarming of the affected body part is performed in a water bath kept at 40° to 42°C.**

▦ Intravenous (IV) analgesics or conscious sedation is usually necessary during this exquisitely painful process.

▦ Repeated freeze/thaw cycles are avoided.

▦ Local wound management with topical aloe vera, limb elevation, splinting, and early therapy are routine aspects of care.

▦ Surgical débridement and amputation should be delayed until unequivocal tissue demarcation occurs (1-3 months), although urgent escharotomy is required for constrictive circumferential digital involvement.

▦ **Bone scan or angiography used to evaluate severity of injury**
  • **IV TPA recommended if no digital blood flow exists**

▦ Chronic cold intolerance, neuropathy, and articular cartilage degradation are common.

▦ Calcium channel blockers or surgical sympathectomy may be required for late, persistent vasospastic disease.

▦ Children may have premature growth plate closure.

COMPRESSION NEUROPATHY

▦ **Introduction**

▦ Chronic condition that may involve any peripheral upper extremity nerve with sensory, motor, or mixed manifestations (Figure 7-45)

▦ First sensory perceptions to be lost are those of light touch, pressure, and vibration; last to be impaired are pain and temperature.

▦ Paresthesias result from early microvascular compression and neural ischemia.
  • Intraneural edema increases over time and exacerbates microvascular compression.
  • Pressure and vibratory thresholds are increased.

- Continued compression may lead to structural changes such as demyelination, fibrosis, and axonal loss.
  - These changes may cause weakness or paralysis of the motor nerve.
  - Abnormal two-point discrimination may also be evident after prolonged compression.
- Patient history may reveal night symptoms, dropping of objects, clumsiness, or weakness.
- If onset of symptoms was preceded by viral illness and shoulder pain, consider Parsonage-Turner syndrome, a self-limiting inflammatory brachial neuritis or plexopathy.
- Changes in skin color, temperature, texture, and moisture may result from sympathetic nervous system dysfunction.

- Other clues may indicate an associated systemic disease, such as diabetes, thyroid disease, inflammatory arthropathy, and vitamin deficiency (Box 7-2).
- Examine individual muscle strength (grades 0-5), pinch strength, and grip strength in cases of long-standing compression with complaints of weakness.
- Neurosensory testing performed in context of both dermatomal and peripheral nerve distributions
  - **Semmes-Weinstein monofilaments measure the cutaneous pressure threshold, a function of large nerve fibers (first to be affected in compression neuropathy).**
    - Sensing 2.83 monofilament is normal.

Peripheral Compression Neuropathies of the Upper Extremity

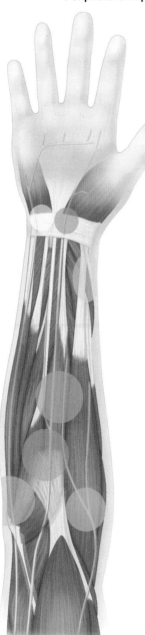

Carpal Tunnel Syndrome
Median nerve
Transverse carpal ligament

Ulnar Tunnel Syndrome
Ulnar nerve
Mass effects from ganglion, lipoma, hook of hamate nonunion, ulnar artery aneurysm, for example

Wartenberg Syndrome
Superficial sensory branch of the radial nerve
Between brachioradialis and ECRL, external compression from tight cast, wristwatch, bracelet, etc.

AIN Syndrome
Anterior interosseous branch of the median nerve
Same as pronator syndrome, also enlarged bicipital bursa, Gantzer muscle (accessory FPL head), association with Parsonage-Turner syndrome

Pronator Syndrome
Median nerve
Two heads of pronator teres, lacertus fibrosus, FDS aponeurotic arch, possible supracondylar process with ligament of Struthers

Radial Tunnel/PIN Syndromes
Posterior interosseous branch of the radial nerve
Recurrent leash of Henry, ECRB edge, Arcade of Frohse (proximal edge of supinator), distal edge of supinator

Cubital Tunnel Syndrome
Ulnar nerve
Arcade of Struthers, medial intermuscular septum, medial triceps, Osborne ligament, aponeurosis of FCU and proximal FDS, possible anconeus epitrochlearis

FIGURE 7-45 Composite image displaying common upper extremity peripheral compression neuropathies.

- Two-point discrimination should be performed with patient's eyes closed.
  - Inability to perceive a difference between points greater than 6 mm apart is considered abnormal and constitutes a late finding in compression neuropathy.
  - Pertinent provocative maneuvers are described for each nerve compression syndrome below.
- Electrodiagnostic testing
  - **Sensory and motor nerve function tested by electromyography (EMG) and nerve conduction study (NCS)**
    - Operator dependent but may provide only objective evidence of neuropathic condition
    - Most helpful in localizing point of compromise and distinguishing between several differential diagnoses in equivocal cases
    - High false-negative rate, especially in early disease
    - NCS measures nerve conduction velocity, distal latency, and amplitude
      - **Demyelination decreases conduction velocity (sensory fibers before motor fibers) and increases distal latency.**
      - **Decreased sensory and/or motor potential amplitude with axonal loss**
    - EMG measures electrical activity of muscle during voluntary contraction.
      - **With muscle denervation, EMG abnormalities include fibrillations, positive sharp waves, and fasciculations.**

Box 7-2 | Nerve Compression Associations

SYSTEMIC
Diabetes
Alcoholism
Renal failure
Raynaud
INFLAMMATORY
Rheumatoid arthritis
Infection
Gout
Tenosynovitis
FLUID IMBALANCE
Pregnancy
Obesity
ANATOMIC
Synovial fibrosis
Lumbrical encroachment
Anomalous tendon
Persistent median artery
MASS
Ganglion
Lipoma
Hematoma

- Compression neuropathy is characterized by phases of disease (Table 7-8).
  - Treatment decisions guided by history, physical examination, sensory threshold testing, and electrodiagnostic testing
- Double-crush phenomenon
  - Normal axonal function is dependent on factors synthesized in the nerve cell body.
  - Blockage of axonal transport at one point makes the entire axon more susceptible to compression elsewhere.
  - Cervical radiculopathy or proximal nerve entrapment may coexist with distal nerve compression in double-crush syndrome.
  - Outcome of surgical decompression may be disappointing unless all points of compression are addressed.
  - Logical to start with less complex distal releases first
- **Median nerve**
- Carpal tunnel syndrome (CTS)
  - Most common compressive neuropathy in the upper extremity
    - Approximately 500,000 cases per year in United States
  - Anatomy of the carpal tunnel
    - Volar boundary is TCL
      - Attaches to scaphoid tubercle/trapezium radially and to pisiform/hook of hamate ulnarly
    - Dorsal boundary (floor) formed by proximal carpal row and deep extrinsic volar carpal ligaments
    - Carpal tunnel contains the median nerve, flexor pollicis longus tendon, four FDS tendons, and four FDP tendons
    - Normal pressure approximately 2.5 mm Hg
    - When pressure exceeds 20 mm Hg, epineural blood flow decreases and nerve becomes edematous.
    - When pressure exceeds 30 mm Hg, nerve conduction decreases.
  - Forms of CTS
    - Idiopathic form most common in adults
      - Mucopolysaccharidosis is the most common cause in children.
    - May also be anatomic variation
      - Persistent median artery, small carpal canal, anomalous muscles, extrinsic mass effect
    - Common systemic risk factors include obesity, pregnancy, diabetes, thyroid disease, chronic renal failure, inflammatory arthropathy, storage diseases, vitamin deficiency, alcoholism, advanced age, and vibratory exposure during occupational activity.
    - Direct relationship between repetitive work activities (e.g., keyboarding) and CTS has never been established.

Table 7-8 | Compression Neuropathy

PHASE	SYMPTOMS	NCV	EMG	PATHOLOGY	TREATMENT
Early	Intermittent	Normal or ↑ sensory latency	Normal	Edema	Nonoperative
Intermediate	Constant	+	±	Edema	Surgery
Late	Sensory and motor deficit	+	+	Fibrosis and axonal loss	Surgery—less predictable outcome

↑, Increased; *EMG*, electromyography; *NCV*, nerve conduction velocity.

- Acute CTS occurs in the setting of high-energy trauma, hemorrhage, or infection.
  - Evolving paresthesias become severely intense.
  - Requires emergency decompression
- Diagnosis
  - Paresthesias and pain (often at night) in volar aspect of radial 3½ digits (thumb, index, long, and radial half of ring)
  - Most sensitive provocative test: carpal tunnel compression test (Durkan test)
    - Other provocative tests: Tinel and Phalen
  - Large sensory fibers (light touch, vibration) are affected before small fibers (pain and temperature).
  - **Semmes-Weinstein monofilament testing is sensitive for diagnosing early CTS.**
  - Weakness, loss of fine motor control, and abnormal two-point discrimination are later findings.
  - Thenar atrophy may be present in severe denervation.
  - Electrodiagnostic tests are not necessary for the diagnosis of CTS but may help confirm diagnosis in equivocal cases.
    - Distal sensory latencies of more than 3.5 milliseconds or motor latencies of more than 4.5 milliseconds are abnormal.
    - Decreased conduction velocity and decreased peak amplitude are less specific.
    - EMG may show increased insertional activity, positive sharp waves, fibrillation, and/or abductor pollicis brevis fasciculation.
  - Differential diagnoses include cervical radiculopathy, brachial plexopathy, thoracic outlet syndrome, pronator syndrome, ulnar neuropathy with Martin-Gruber anastomoses, and peripheral neuropathy of multiple etiologies.
- Treatment
  - Nonoperative treatment includes activity modification, night splints, and NSAIDs.
  - Single corticosteroid injection yields transient relief in approximately 80% after 6 weeks, but only 20% are symptom free by 1 year
    - Failure to improve after corticosteroid injection is poor prognostic sign; surgery less successful in these cases
  - Operative treatment options include open, mini-open, or endoscopic release of the TCL.
    - No additional benefit gained from internal median neurolysis or flexor tenosynovectomy
    - Ulnar neurovascular structures within Guyon canal can be injured if incision and approach are too ulnar.
    - Risk to recurrent motor branch of the median nerve increased if incision and approach is too radial (Figure 7-46)
      - Three main variations of the recurrent motor branch:
        - Extraligamentous—approximately 50%
        - Subligamentous—approximately 30%
        - Transligamentous—approximately 20%
    - Endoscopic carpal tunnel release associated with less early scar tenderness, improved short-term grip/pinch strength, shorter return to work and better patient satisfaction scores in some studies

- Long-term results compared to open release are largely equivalent.
- May have slightly higher complication rate, with most devastating being direct nerve injury and most common being incomplete TCL division
  - After standard open release, pinch strength returns to the preoperative level in 6 weeks and grip strength in 3 months.
  - Pillar pain adjacent to incision common for 3 to 4 months after open carpal tunnel release
  - Persistent symptoms after carpal tunnel release may be secondary to incomplete release of the TCL, iatrogenic median nerve injury, a missed double-crush phenomenon, concomitant peripheral neuropathy, or a space-occupying lesion.
- Preoperative symptom severity negatively impacts the degree of symptom relief after carpal tunnel release.
  - Depression and poor coping mechanisms shown to predict patient dissatisfaction
  - Pain catastrophizing also prolongs return to work.
- In elderly patients with chronic compression
  - Full sensory and motor function rarely recovered
  - Relief of painful nocturnal paresthesias more consistent
  - Improved activities of daily living, work performance, and overall hand function
    - Over 90% satisfied with outcome
- The success of revision carpal tunnel release relies on identifying the underlying cause of the failure.
  - Hypothenar or inguinal fat pad graft

- Pronator syndrome
  - Compression of the median nerve in the arm/forearm
  - Potential offending structures include (Figure 7-47):
    - Supracondylar process (anterior distal humerus seen on lateral radiograph), occurs in approximately 1% of the population
    - Ligament of Struthers (courses between the supracondylar process and medial epicondyle)
    - Bicipital aponeurosis (lacertus fibrosis)
    - Between the two heads of pronator teres muscle
    - FDS aponeurotic arch
  - Pronator syndrome differentiated from CTS by proximal volar forearm pain and sensory disturbances in distribution of palmar cutaneous branch of the median nerve
  - Test resisted elbow flexion with forearm supinated (bicipital aponeurosis), resisted forearm pronation with elbow extended (pronator teres), and resisted long finger PIP-joint flexion (FDS)
  - Electrodiagnostic tests may be inconclusive.
  - Nonoperative treatment consists of activity modification, splints, and NSAIDs.
  - When nonoperative management fails, surgery must address all potential sites of compression.
  - Success rate approximately 80% in most series
  - Pronator syndrome is associated with medial epicondylitis and tends to improve with its treatment.

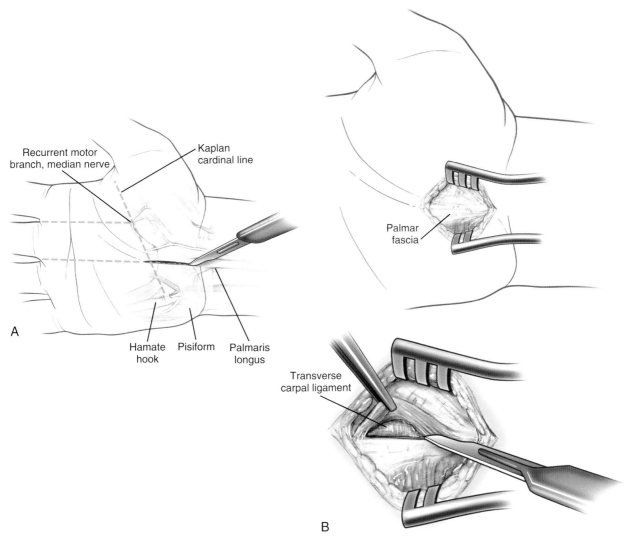

FIGURE 7-46 A, Landmarks for carpal tunnel release surgical approach. **B,** Exposure of the palmar fascia and transverse carpal ligament. (From Miller MD et al: *Orthopaedic surgical approaches,* Philadelphia, 2008, Saunders.)

▧ **Anterior interosseous nerve syndrome**
- Involves motor loss of FPL, index +/− long FDP, and pronator quadratus
- No sensory disturbance
- Index FDP and thumb FPL tested by asking patient to make an "OK" sign (precision pinch)
- Pronator quadratus involvement tested by resisted pronation with elbow maximally flexed
- Transient anterior interosseous nerve palsy is associated with **Parsonage-Turner syndrome (viral brachial neuritis),** especially if motor loss was preceded by intense shoulder pain.
- Electromyography may be helpful.
- Important to rule out isolated tendon disruption, such as FPL rupture in patients with RA (Mannerfelt syndrome)
- Apart from aforementioned sites in pronator syndrome, additional sites of compression include:
  - Enlarged bicipital bursa
  - **Gantzer muscle (accessory head of the FPL)**
- **Vast majority of patients recover with observation**
- Nonoperative treatment involves activity modification and elbow splinting in 90 degrees of flexion.

- Results of surgical decompression generally satisfactory if done within 3 to 6 months after onset of symptoms

▧ **Ulnar nerve**

▧ Cubital tunnel syndrome
- Second most common compression neuropathy of upper extremity
- Definition of the cubital tunnel
  - Deep (floor)—medial collateral ligament (MCL) and elbow joint capsule
  - Walls of the tunnel—medial epicondyle and olecranon
  - Roof—FCU fascia and arcuate ligament of Osborne (fibrous band that traverses cubital tunnel from medial epicondyle to olecranon)
- **Sites of compression include** (Figure 7-48):
  - Arcade of Struthers (fascial thickening at hiatus of medial intermuscular septum as the ulnar nerve passes from anterior to posterior compartment 8 cm proximal to the medial epicondyle)
  - Medial head of triceps
  - Medial intermuscular septum
  - Osborne ligament

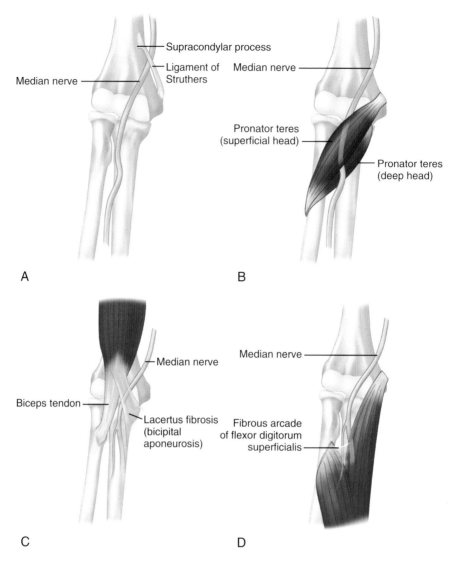

FIGURE 7-47 A, The ligament of Struthers bridges the supracondylar process of the humerus to the medial epicondyle or the origin of the humeral head of the pronator teres. **B,** The median nerve may be compressed between the two heads of the pronator teres. **C,** The lacertus fibrosis is an aponeurosis layer of the distal biceps, coursing obliquely in a distal and medial orientation. **D,** The most distal site of proximal median nerve compression occurs at the fibrous arcade of the flexor digitorum superficialis. (From Trumble TE et al, editors: *Core knowledge in orthopaedics: hand, elbow, and shoulder,* Philadelphia, 2006, Mosby, p 243.)

- Anconeus epitrochlearis (anomalous muscle originating from medial olecranon and inserting on medial epicondyle)
- Between two heads of FCU muscle/aponeurosis
- Aponeurosis of proximal edge of FDS
- Other potential external sources of compression: tumors, ganglions, osteophytes, heterotopic ossification, medial epicondyle nonunion
- Burns, cubitus varus or valgus deformities, medial epicondylitis, and repetitive elbow flexion/valgus stress during occupational or athletic activities are other associations.
- Symptoms include paresthesias of the ulnar 1½ digits (ulnar half of ring finger and small finger) and dorsal ulnar hand.
- Provocative tests include direct cubital tunnel compression, Tinel sign, and prolonged elbow hyperflexion, all of which may reproduce or intensify paresthesias.

- Check for subluxation of ulnar nerve over medial epicondyle during elbow flexion-extension arc
- Classical examination findings secondary to motor weakness
  - **Froment sign**
    - Compensatory thumb interphalangeal joint flexion (FPL) during key pinch due to weak adductor pollicis
  - Jeanne sign
    - Hyperextension of thumb MCP with key pinch due to weak adductor pollicis
  - **Wartenberg sign**
    - Persistent abduction and extension of small digit during attempted adduction due to weak third volar interosseous and small finger lumbrical
  - Masse sign
    - Flattening of palmar arch and loss of ulnar hand elevation due to weak opponens digiti quinti and decreased small digit MCP flexion

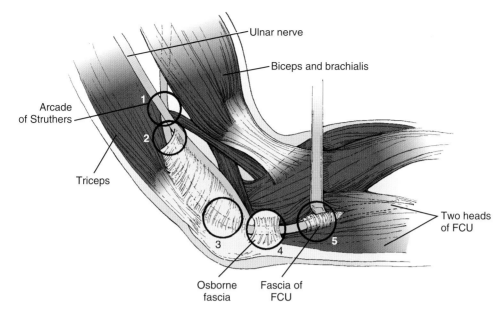

FIGURE 7-48 Sites of ulnar entrapment. The nerve may be entrapped by (1) the arcade of Struthers, (2) the medial intermuscular septum, (3) the distal transverse fibers of the arcade of Struthers, (4) the Osborne ligament, and/or (5) the fascia (aponeurosis) of the flexor carpi ulnaris (FCU) and fascial bands within the FCU. (From Miller MD et al: *Surgical atlas of sports medicine*, Philadelphia, 2003, Saunders, p 402.)

- Interosseous and/or first web space atrophy
- Ring and small digit clawing
- Electrodiagnostic tests are helpful for diagnosis and prognosis.
- Conduction velocity of less than 50 m/sec across elbow typical threshold for diagnosis; larger decreases in conduction velocity signal worse disease
- Nonoperative treatment includes activity modification, night splints (elbow held in relative extension), and NSAIDs.
- Numerous surgical techniques described
  - In situ decompression
  - Anterior transposition
    - Subcutaneous
    - Submuscular
    - Intramuscular
  - Medial epicondylectomy
- **Recent meta-analyses of techniques fail to show statistically significant difference in outcome between simple decompression and transposition.**
- Higher rate of recurrence as compared to carpal tunnel release
- Surgery should be performed before motor denervation.
- No long-term clinical data for endoscopic techniques
- Persistent postoperative medial/posterior elbow pain may be secondary to neuroma formation from iatrogenic injury to branches of the medial antebrachial cutaneous nerve.
- Ulnar tunnel syndrome
  - Compression neuropathy of ulnar nerve in the Guyon canal
  - **Most common cause of ulnar tunnel syndrome is ganglion cyst (80% of nontraumatic cases)**
    - Other causative factors may include hook-of-hamate nonunion, ulnar artery thrombosis, lipoma, palmaris brevis hypertrophy, or other anomalous muscle.
  - Borders of the Guyon canal are the volar carpal ligament (roof), the transverse carpal ligament (floor),

the hook of hamate (radial), and the pisiform and abductor digiti minimi muscle belly (ulnar).
- Ulnar tunnel divided into three zones
  - Zone I is proximal to bifurcation of ulnar nerve and associated with mixed motor/sensory symptoms.
  - Zone II includes the deep motor branch and is associated with pure motor symptoms.
  - Zone III includes the distal sensory branches and is associated with pure sensory symptoms.
- Useful adjunctive tests include CT for hamate hook fracture, MRI for ganglion cyst or other space-occupying lesion, and Doppler ultrasonography for ulnar artery thrombosis.
- Success of treatment depends on identifying the cause.
- Nonoperative treatment includes activity modification, splints, and NSAIDs.
- Operative treatment involves decompressing ulnar nerve by addressing underlying cause
- Guyon canal is adequately decompressed by release of the transverse carpal ligament when concurrent CTS exists.

- **Radial nerve**
- Proper radial nerve
  - Rarely compressed by lateral head of triceps, typically compromised in setting of humerus trauma or related surgical approaches
  - "Saturday night palsy"—intoxicated patient passes out with arm hanging over chair, wakes up with wrist drop
  - Clinical findings include weakness of proper radial nerve–innervated muscles such as triceps, brachioradialis, and ECRL, plus all muscles innervated by the PIN.
  - Sensory deficits may be present in the distribution of the superficial sensory branch.
  - EMG may be helpful to determine severity and prognosis.
  - May be initially observed but may be explored if no significant recovery evident at 3 months

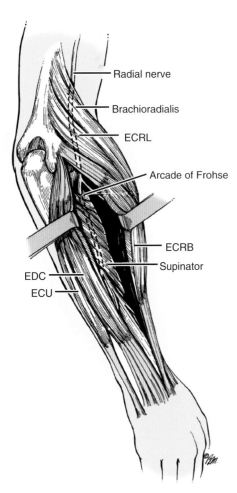

FIGURE 7-49 Extension of the dorsal Thompson approach to the radial tunnel. *ECRB*, Extensor carpi radialis brevis; *ECRL*, extensor carpi radialis longus; *ECU*, extensor carpi ulnaris; *EDC*, extensor digitorum communis. (From Green DP et al, editors: *Green's operative hand surgery,* ed 5, Philadelphia, 2005, Churchill Livingstone, p 1039.)

▓ **Posterior interosseous nerve compression syndrome**
- Symptoms include lateral elbow pain and distal muscle weakness.
- Radial deviation with active wrist extension, because ECRL innervated by proper radial nerve more proximally
- PIN innervates the ECRB, supinator, EIP, ECU, extensor digitorum communis (EDC), extensor digiti minimi, APL, EPB, and EPL.
- Patients may also have dorsal wrist pain where the terminal nerve fibers provide sensory innervation to the dorsal wrist capsule.
  - Terminal branch is located on the floor of the fourth extensor compartment.
- EMG may be helpful.
- **Anatomic sites of compression include** (Figure 7-49):
  - Fascial band at the radial head
  - Recurrent leash of Henry
  - Edge of the ECRB
  - Arcade of Frohse (most common site, at proximal edge of supinator)
  - Distal edge of the supinator
- Unusual causes include chronic radial head dislocation, Monteggia fracture-dislocation,

radiocapitellar rheumatoid synovitis, and space-occupying elbow mass (e.g., lipoma).
- PIN palsy is differentiated from extensor tendon rupture by a normal wrist tenodesis test.
- Nonoperative treatment includes activity modification, splinting, and NSAIDs.
- Operative intervention warranted if no recovery by 3 months
- Surgical decompression of anatomic sites of compression provides good to excellent results for 85% of patients.

▓ Radial tunnel syndrome
- Characterized by lateral elbow and radial forearm pain without motor or sensory dysfunction
- Provocative tests include resisted long-finger extension (positive if resistance reproduces pain at the radial tunnel) and resisted supination.
- **Lateral epicondylitis coexists in a small percentage of patients.**
- The point of maximum tenderness is several centimeters distal to the lateral epicondyle.
- Despite affecting the same nerve (PIN) and sites of compression, electrodiagnostic tests are typically inconclusive.
- Prolonged nonoperative treatment for up to 1 year with activity modification, splints, NSAIDs, and local modalities
- Success of surgical decompression less predictable than for PIN syndrome, with good to excellent results in only 50% to 80% after prolonged postoperative recovery.

▓ **Cheiralgia paresthetica (Wartenberg syndrome)**
- Compressive neuropathy of superficial sensory branch of the radial nerve
- Compressed between brachioradialis and ECRL with forearm pronation (by a scissor-like action between the tendons)
- Symptoms include pain, numbness, and paresthesias over the dorsoradial hand.
- Provocative tests include forceful forearm pronation for 60 seconds and a Tinel sign over the nerve.
- Initially treated by activity modification, splinting, and NSAIDs
- Surgical decompression warranted if 6-month trial of nonoperative treatment fails

▓ **Thoracic outlet syndrome**
▓ Vascular
- Subclavian vessel compression or aneurysm diagnosed by physical examination and angiography
- Adson test
  - Patient keeps arm at the side, hyperextends neck, and rotates head to the affected side, producing a diminished radial artery pulse with inhalation.
- Duplex ultrasonography has better than 90% sensitivity and specificity in the diagnosis of vascular thoracic outlet syndrome.
▓ Neurogenic
- Entrapment neuropathy of the lower trunk of the brachial plexus
- Often overlooked or undetected on history and physical examination
  - Fatigue is common, particularly when arm is used in a provocative position.

Table 7-9	Classification of Nerve Injury		
CLASSIFICATION			
SEDDON	**SUNDERLAND**	**INJURY**	**PROGNOSIS**
Neurapraxia	First degree	Demyelination injury	Temporary conduction block; resolves in 1-2 days
Axonotmesis	Second degree	Axonal injury	Regeneration is usually complete but may take several weeks or months.
	Third degree	Endoneurium injured	Regeneration occurs but is not satisfactory.
	Fourth degree	Perineurium injured	Spontaneous regeneration is unsatisfactory, resulting in neuroma in continuity.
Neurotmesis	Fifth degree	Severed nerve trunk	Spontaneous regeneration is not possible without surgery.

From Trumble TE et al, editors: *Core knowledge in orthopaedics: hand, elbow, and shoulder,* Philadelphia, 2006, Mosby, p 227.

- Nonspecific paresthesias are most common initial complaint; present in about 95% of patients
- Electrodiagnostic studies are rarely helpful.
- Sensory disturbance of medial brachial and antebrachial cutaneous nerves may differentiate the condition from cubital tunnel syndrome.
- Roos sign
  - Indicates heaviness or paresthesias in the hands after holding them above the head for at least 1 minute
- Cervical and chest radiographs obtained to rule out cervical rib or Pancoast tumor
- Physical therapy focuses on shoulder girdle strengthening and proper posture and relaxation techniques.
- Transaxillary first rib resection by thoracic surgeon yields good to excellent results when cervical rib is cause
  - Combined approach with anterior and middle scalenectomy also described

NERVE INJURIES AND TENDON TRANSFERS

- **Peripheral nerve injuries**
- Introduction
  - Peripheral nerve function may be compromised by compression, stretch, blast, crush, avulsion, transection, and tumor invasion.
  - Evaluation and treatment of traumatic peripheral nerve dysfunction are guided by mechanism of injury and presence of other injuries.
  - Most important prognostic factor for nerve recovery is age.
  - Prognosis also better in stretch injuries, clean wounds, and after direct surgical repair
  - Conversely, poor outcome expected in crush or blast injuries, infected or scarred wounds, and delayed surgical repair
- Classification
  - Seddon and Sunderland (Table 7-9)
    - **Neurapraxia**
      - Mild nerve stretch or contusion
      - Focal conduction block
      - No wallerian degeneration
      - Disruption of myelin sheath
      - Epineurium, perineurium, endoneurium intact
      - Prognosis excellent, recovery expected
    - **Axonotmesis**
      - Incomplete nerve injury
      - Focal conduction block

- Wallerian degeneration distal to injury
- Disruption of axons
- Sequential loss of axon, endoneurium, perineurium (Sunderland class 2, 3, and 4)
- May develop neuroma-in-continuity
- Recovery unpredictable
  - **Neurotmesis**
    - Complete nerve injury
    - Focal conduction block
    - Wallerian degeneration distal to injury
    - Disruption of all layers, including epineurium
    - Proximal nerve end forms neuroma
    - Distal end forms glioma
    - Worst prognosis
- **In axonotmesis and neurotmesis, the distal nerve segment undergoes wallerian degeneration.**
  - The degradation products are removed by phagocytosis.
    - Myelin-producing Schwann cells proliferate and align themselves along the basement membrane, forming a tube that will receive regenerating axons.
    - Nerve cell body enlarges as rate of structural protein production increases
    - Each proximal axon forms multiple sprouts that connect to the distal stump and migrate at a rate of 1 mm/day.
- Surgical repair
  - Best results achieved when performed within 10 to 14 days of injury
  - Repair must be free of tension.
  - Repair must be within clean, well-vascularized wound bed.
  - Nerve length may be gained by neurolysis or transposition.
  - Repair techniques:
    - Epineurial
    - Individual fascicular
    - Group fascicular
  - No technique deemed superior
  - **Use of nerve conduits** (Figure 7-50) **has gained popularity for digital nerve gaps greater than 8 mm (polyglycolic acid and collagen based).**
  - Larger gaps, especially of mixed nerves, require grafting.
    - Autogenous (e.g., sural, medial/lateral antebrachial cutaneous, terminal/PIN)
    - Vascularized
  - Limited data available on decellularized nerve allografts

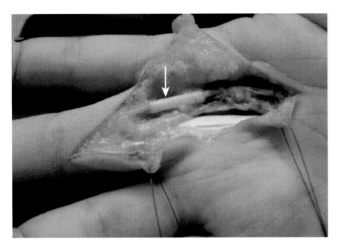

FIGURE 7-50 View of a collagen nerve guide *(arrow)* used to span a gap in the radial digital nerve of the right middle finger. (From Haug A et al: Sensory recovery 1 year after bridging digital nerve defects with collagen tubes, *J Hand Surg Am* 38:90–97, 2013.)

- Growth factor augmentation (e.g., insulinlike, fibroblast) studied in animal models and shown to promote nerve regeneration
- Chronic peripheral nerve injuries may be treated with nerve transfers and/or tendon transfers.
  - Use of nerve transfers for high radial and ulnar nerve injuries gaining popularity (Figure 7-51)

Traumatic brachial plexus injury

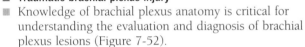

- Knowledge of brachial plexus anatomy is critical for understanding the evaluation and diagnosis of brachial plexus lesions (Figure 7-52).
- High-energy mechanisms are associated with more severe lesions such as nerve root avulsions and rupture of entire segments of the plexus.
  - Diagnosis
    - Location and severity of injury
    - Comprehensive motor and sensory evaluation
    - Supraclavicular versus infraclavicular
    - **Preganglionic (nerve root avulsions) have worst prognosis**
  - Signs of severe injury
    - Complete sensory loss
    - Global motor dysfunction
    - Neuropathic pain
    - **Horner sign—ptosis, miosis, anhidrosis**
  - Complete radiographic series should include cervical spine, chest, and shoulder girdle.
    - Inspiratory and expiratory chest radiographs may demonstrate a paralyzed hemidiaphragm, indicating a severe upper root injury.
    - Root avulsions may be indicated by the presence of corresponding fractures of transverse spinal processes.
    - Scapulothoracic dissociation is often linked to multiple root avulsions and major vascular injury.
  - MRI and CT myelography
  - EMG and NCS to monitor recovery
  - Somatosensory evoked potentials
- Timing of surgical treatment
  - Modern series reveal reverse relationship between time from injury to operative intervention and clinical outcome.

- Immediate surgical exploration may be indicated in certain cases of penetrating trauma or iatrogenic injury.
- On the other hand, one study showed that many patients with gunshot wounds to the plexus improved over time without surgical exploration.
- Reasonable to observe these patients for 3 months in the absence of major vascular injury
- **Early surgical intervention (3 weeks to 3 months after injury) is indicated in patients with complete or near-complete injuries resulting from a high-energy mechanism.**
- Patients with brachial plexus palsy resulting from low-energy mechanisms, especially in those with an incomplete upper plexus lesion, are best observed for at least 3 to 6 months for spontaneous recovery.
- Surgery may be warranted if recovery plateaus early.
- Nerve repair or reconstruction beyond 6 months from the time of injury has a less predictable clinical outcome.
- Most reliable clinical sign of nerve regeneration and recovery is an advancing Tinel sign.
- Muscle fibrosis occurs after 18 to 24 months.
- Tendon/nerve transfers
  - Isolated C8-T1 injury best treated with early tendon transfers
    - Full recovery unlikely because of distance between lesion and intrinsic muscles of hand
  - For other lesions, nerve repair or reconstruction prioritized
    - Elbow flexion
    - Shoulder stabilization
    - Hand function
  - Direct repair often compromised by excessive tension
    - Neuroma excision and nerve cable grafting favored methods
    - Donor sites: sural, medial brachial cutaneous, and medial antebrachial cutaneous nerves
    - Best outcomes obtained in young patients treated within 3 months of injury
  - Nerve transfers indicated when insufficient number of proximal axons available, such as occurs in multiple root avulsions
    - **Oberlin transfer—ulnar nerve motor branch (fascicle) to the FCU transferred to musculocutaneous nerve to help restore elbow flexion**
    - Descending branch of spinal accessory nerve (cranial nerve [CN] XI) transferred to suprascapular nerve to help restore shoulder abduction
    - Radial nerve motor branch to the triceps transferred to the axillary nerve to help restore shoulder abduction/forward elevation
  - Patients without meaningful recovery of shoulder and elbow function after 6 to 12 months may be good candidates for shoulder arthrodesis and tendon transfers.

Obstetric brachial plexopathy

- Associated with high birth weight, cephalopelvic disproportion, shoulder dystocia, and forceps delivery
- Muscle grading system
  - M0—no contraction
  - M1—contraction without movement
  - M2—contraction with slight movement
  - M3—complete movement

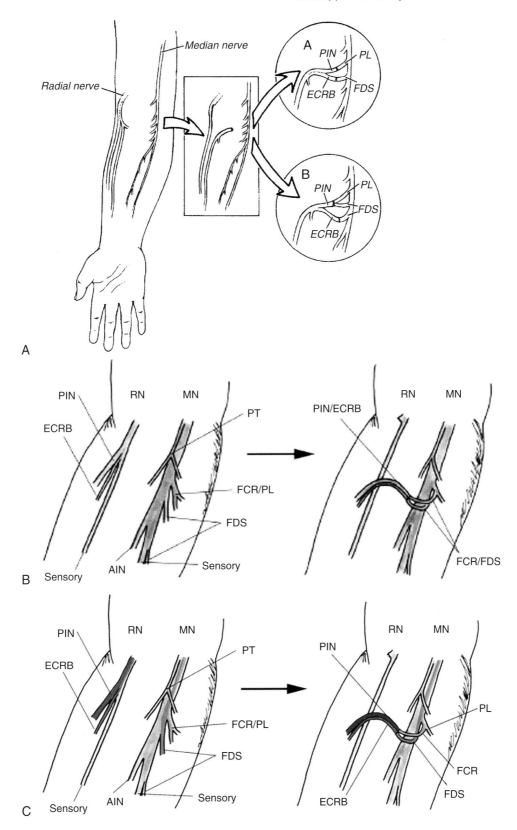

FIGURE 7-51 Median nerve–to–radial nerve transfers in the forearm for high radial nerve palsy. Branch of the median nerve (MN) to the flexor digitorum superficialis (FDS) transferred to extensor carpi radialis brevis (ECRB) branch of the radial nerve (RN), and branch of the median nerve to the flexor carpi radialis (FCR) transferred to the posterior interosseous nerve (PIN). *AIN,* Anterior interosseous nerve; *PL,* palmaris longus; *PT,* pronator teres. (From Ray WZ, Mackinnon SE: Clinical outcomes following median to radial nerve transfers, *J Hand Surg Am* 36:201–208, 2011.)

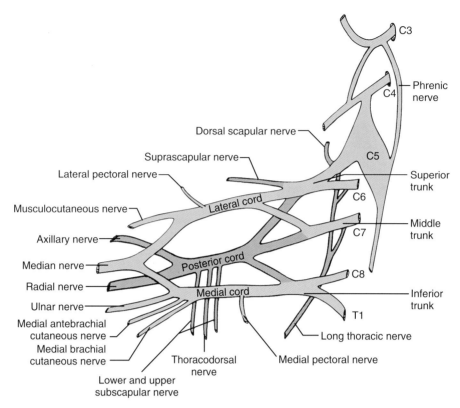

FIGURE 7-52 Brachial plexus anatomy. (From Brushart TM, Wilgus EF: Brachial plexus and shoulder girdle injuries. In Browner BD, Jupiter JB, editors: *Skeletal trauma*, ed 2, Philadelphia, 1998, WB Saunders, p 1696.)

▓ **Complete recovery possible if biceps and deltoid are M1 by 2 months**

▓ Incomplete recovery expected if biceps and deltoid do not contract within 3 to 6 months

▓ Surgery usually not recommended if biceps contraction evident by 6 months (some advocate sooner)

▓ Results of nerve grafting better in infants than adults, and reinnervation of the hand intrinsic muscles is possible

■ **Cerebral palsy**

▓ Introduction
  • Nonprogressive central nervous system insult
  • Typical upper extremity deformities
    • **Thumb-in-palm**
    • Clenched fist
    • Wrist flexion
    • Forearm pronation
    • Elbow flexion
    • Shoulder internal rotation

▓ Nonoperative treatment
  • Initially involves physical therapy and nighttime static splinting
  • Antispasticity medications such as diazepam, baclofen, tizanidine, and dantrolene
  • Intrathecal baclofen infusion pump
  • **Botulinum toxin A is transiently effective (3-6 months) and may be used periodically for severe spasticity.**

▓ Operative treatment
  • **Best performed on children with higher IQs (over 50-70), voluntary muscle control, and good sensibility**
    • Voluntary muscle control is the most important predictor of success.

• A thumb-in-palm deformity is corrected by release or lengthening of the adductor pollicis, first dorsal interosseous, flexor pollicis brevis, and FPL muscles, combined with first web space Z-plasty and tendon transfers to augment thumb extension and abduction.

• Fractional or Z-lengthening of tendon with or without ulnar motor neurectomy may improve digital flexor tightness and intrinsic spasticity in patients with a clenched fist.

• **Wrist flexion deformity may be treated early by FCU to ECRB/ECRL tendon transfer or wrist arthrodesis for fixed contractures in late stages.**
  • Concomitant proximal row carpectomy at the time of fusion may improve wrist positioning and help rebalance severe digital flexor tightness.

• Mild elbow flexion contractures may be improved by musculocutaneous neurectomy; severe contractures addressed by biceps/brachialis lengthening combined with anterior joint capsulotomy.

• Shoulder contractures may be addressed with derotational humeral osteotomy, lengthening of the subscapularis and pectoralis major muscles, or shoulder arthrodesis.

■ **Stroke**

▓ Cerebral vascular accident (CVA) may lead to significant upper extremity disability

▓ Spontaneous neurologic recovery 6 to 12 months after CVA

▓ Uncontrolled muscle spasticity may lead to typical joint contractures.
  • Shoulder adduction
  • Elbow flexion
  • Forearm pronation

- Wrist and digit flexion
- Thumb-in-palm
- Clenched fist
- Contracture releases and/or tendon transfers done for functional positioning
- Clenched fist deformity in patient without volitional control treated with superficialis-to-profundus (STP) tendon transfer to decrease pain and improve hygiene

 ■ **Tendon transfers**

- Indications
  - Replace irreparably injured tendons/muscles
  - Substitute for function of a paralyzed muscle
  - Restore balance to a deformed hand
- Timing of tendon transfers is controversial and depends on age, indication, and prognosis
- Tendon transfers are generally deferred until tissue equilibrium is achieved and passive joint mobility is restored.
  - Sometimes over 12 months after brachial plexus injury or until spasticity resolves in a tetraplegic hand
- Key concepts
  - **Force is proportional to the cross-sectional area of the muscle.**
    - The greatest force of contraction is exerted when the muscle is at its resting length.
  - **Amplitude or excursion is proportional to the length of the muscle.**
    - Smith 3-5-7 rule estimates excursion of wrist flexors/extensors (3 cm), MCP extensors (5 cm), and the FDP (7 cm)
  - Work capacity is force times length (F × L).
  - Power is the amount of work performed in a unit of time.
  - **Selection of a transfer**
    - What function is missing?
    - What muscle-tendon units are available?
    - What are the options for transfer?
  - **Basic tenets**
    - Donor must be expendable.
    - Donor must be of similar excursion and power.
    - One transfer should perform one function.
    - Synergistic transfers are easier to rehabilitate.
    - A straight line of pull is optimal.
    - One grade of motor strength will be lost after transfer.
- Classic transfers outlined in Table 7-10
- Most common complication of tendon transfer is development of motion-limiting adhesions, requiring aggressive hand therapy or secondary tenolysis if minimal improvement

ARTHRITIS

■ Osteoarthritis

- Primary idiopathic degenerative joint disease
- Commonly affects DIP joints and trapeziometacarpal joint of thumb
- Erosive form more commonly affects PIP joints.
- MCP joints not typically involved
- Osteoarthritis of wrist is usually posttraumatic
- Hallmark symptoms of osteoarthritis are pain, swelling, and decreased motion.
- **Classical radiographic findings are joint space narrowing, osteophytes, subchondral sclerosis, and subchondral cyst formation.**

- Nonoperative management includes activity modification, NSAIDs, and intraarticular corticosteroid injections.
- Specific joint findings and treatment
  - DIP joint
    - Often asymptomatic despite radiographic changes
    - Heberden nodes from marginal osteophytes
    - May be associated with symptomatic mucous cyst
      - The cyst may be excised, along with any accompanying osteophytes, for symptomatic relief.
      - Occasionally, skin coverage with a local rotational flap is necessary after cyst excision.
    - Definitive surgery may be warranted for unremitting pain, instability, or deformity.
      - Arthrodesis with Kirschner wires or headless cannulated screw with joint in 5 to 10 degrees of flexion
  - PIP joint
    - Bouchard nodes from marginal osteophytes
    - Surgical options include arthrodesis and arthroplasty.
    - Arthrodesis provides more predictable outcome for the index PIP joint, where lateral stresses associated with pinch may compromise the durability of arthroplasty.
    - **If arthrodesis is chosen, the joint should be fused in increasing degrees of flexion from radial to ulnar.**
      - Index—40 degrees
      - Long—45 degrees
      - Ring—50 degrees
      - Small—55 degrees
    - PIP arthroplasty is better reserved for the long, ring, and small digits, which are involved in power grasp.
      - Dorsal and volar approaches described
      - Silicone and pyrocarbon implants available
        - Use of pyrocarbon requires competent collateral ligaments to prevent instability.
      - Postoperative motion is most dependent on preoperative motion.
  - MCP joint
    - Primary cases rare
    - May be involved in patients with hemochromatosis
    - Silicone or pyrocarbon implants are preferred treatment
    - Arthrodesis severely limits hand function but may be necessary in setting of failed arthroplasty or septic arthritis
      - Index—25 degrees
      - Long—30 degrees
      - Ring—35 degrees
      - Small—40 degrees
  - Thumb MCP joint
    - Wide variability in ROM depending on metacarpal head morphology
    - Rarely involved in primary osteoarthritis
    - Pain is reliably relieved by arthrodesis, with the joint placed in 10 to 20 degrees of flexion.
  - **Thumb trapeziometacarpal joint**
    - Also termed *basal joint* or *CMC joint*
    - Theorized by Pellegrini to result from anterior oblique ligament ("beak" ligament) attenuation
      - Leads to instability, dorsoradial subluxation, and abnormal articular cartilage degeneration
    - Pain and/or crepitus may be elicited with the axial grind test, using combined axial compression and circumduction.

Table 7-10 | Classic Tendon Transfers

PALSY	LOSS	TRANSFER
Radial	Wrist extension	Pronator teres to ECRB
	Finger extension	FCU to EDC II-V, FCR to EDC II-V
		FDS III to EPL and EIP, FDS IV to EDC III-V
	Thumb extension	Palmaris longus to EPL
		FDS to radial lateral band
Low ulnar	Hand intrinsics	ECRL to lateral band
	(interosseous and	EDQ EIP to lateral band FCR + graft to lateral band
	ulnar lumbricals)	Metacarpal phalangeal capsulodesis
	Thumb adduction	ECRL + graft to adductor pollicis
		Brachioradialis + graft to adductor pollicis
	Index abduction	EIP to first dorsal interosseous
		Abductor pollicis longus to first dorsal interosseous
		ECRL to first dorsal interosseous
High ulnar	Low problems + FDP Ring and small fingers	Suture to functioning FDP index and long index and long finger
Low median	Opposition	FDS ring to abductor pollicis brevis (FCU pulley)
		EIP to thumb proximal phalanx (routed around the ulna for line of pull)
		Abductor digiti quinti to abductor pollicis brevis
		Palmaris longus to abductor pollicis brevis
High median	Thumb IP flexion	Brachioradialis to flexor pollicis longus
	Index- and long-finger flexion	Suture to functioning FDP ring and small finger or ECRL to FDP index and long finger if additional power is needed
Low median and ulnar	Thumb adduction	ECRB + graft to adductor tubercle of thumb
	Index abduction	Abductor pollicis longus to first dorsal interosseous
	Opposition	EIP to abductor pollicis brevis
	Clawed fingers	Brachioradialis + four-tailed free graft to the A2 pulley
	Volar sensibility	Neurovascular island flap from back of hand
High median and ulnar	Thumb adduction	ECRB + graft to adductor tubercle of thumb
	Thumb IP flexion	Brachioradialis to FPL
	Thumb abduction	EIP to abductor pollicis brevis
	Index abduction	Abductor pollicis longus to first dorsal interosseous
	Finger flexion	ECRL to FDP
	Clawed fingers	Tenodesis of all metaphalangeal joints, with free-tendon graft from dorsal carpal ligament routed deep to transverse metacarpal ligament to extensor apparatus
	Wrist flexion	ECU to FCU
	Volar sensibility	Neurovascular island flap from back of hand

ECRB, Extensor carpi radialis brevis; *ECRL,* extensor carpi radialis longus; *ECU,* extensor carpi ulnaris; *EDC,* extensor digitorum communis; *EDQ,* extensor digiti quinti; *EIP,* extensor indicis proprius; *EPL,* extensor pollicis longus; *FCR,* flexor carpi radialis; *FCU,* flexor carpi ulnaris; *FDP,* flexor digitorum profundus; *FDS,* flexor digitorum superficialis; *FPL,* flexor pollicis longus; *IP,* interphalangeal.

- Metacarpal adduction, first web space contracture, and compensatory MCP hyperextension are late findings.
- **Up to 50% of patients with thumb CMC osteoarthritis also have carpal tunnel syndrome.**
- Eaton and Littler staging (Figure 7-53 and Table 7-11)
- Many treatment alternatives exist, but all share at least partial excision of trapezium.
- Young laborers treated with arthrodesis may be antiquated concept
  - 20 degrees of radial abduction and 40 degrees of palmar abduction
- Arthroscopic hemitrapeziectomy recently described for early-stage disease
- Most commonly performed procedure for advanced thumb CMC osteoarthritis is trapezium excision with ligament reconstruction and tendon interposition
  - FCR and APL common choices for tendon graft
  - Status of scaphotrapezoidal joint assessed intraoperatively and treated accordingly
  - **Thumb MCP hyperextension is addressed with either volar capsulodesis or arthrodesis.**
  - **Proximal migration ("settling") of first metacarpal during pinch does not seem to correlate with clinical outcome in most series.**

- **There is evidence to support simple trapeziectomy alone for lowest complication rate and similar clinical outcome to more complex procedures.**
- Interposition of synthetic or allograft materials, as well as prosthetic arthroplasty, have been described but to date do not offer superior outcome to traditional procedures.
- Past use of silicone arthroplasty resulted in unacceptably high failure rate from silicone synovitis or instability.
- Use of off-label hyaluronic acid injection has not demonstrated a difference between placebo or corticosteroid injection.

■ **Rheumatoid arthritis**

▦ Overview
- Systemic autoimmune inflammatory disease that primarily affects the hand and wrist (Figure 7-54)
- Arthritis of hand joints lasting longer than 6 weeks is one of seven diagnostic criteria used by American College of Rheumatology.
- In contrast to osteoarthritis, the DIP joints are usually spared in RA.
- Emergence of more effective disease-modifying antirheumatic drugs (DMARDs) has dramatically

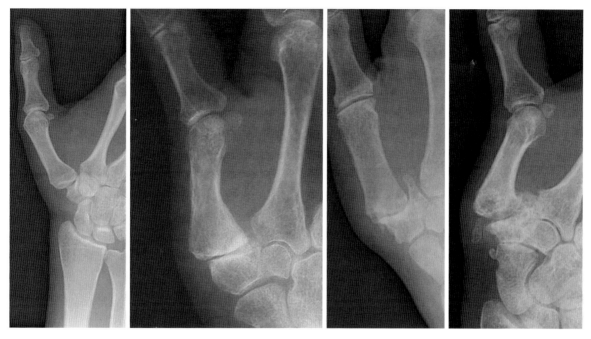

FIGURE 7-53 Eaton radiographic stages of trapeziometacarpal osteoarthritis. *Left to right,* Stages I through IV. (From Green DP et al, editors: *Green's operative hand surgery,* ed 6, Philadelphia, 2011, Churchill Livingstone, p 409.)

Table 7-11	Eaton Radiographic Stages of Trapeziometacarpal Osteoarthritis
STAGE	**DESCRIPTION**
I	Normal-appearing joint with the exception of possible widening from synovitis
II	Joint space narrowing, with debris and osteophytes < 2 mm
III	Joint space narrowing, with debris and osteophytes > 2 mm
IV	Joint space narrowing of scaphotrapezial and trapeziometacarpal articulations

From Trumble TE et al, editors: *Core knowledge in orthopaedics: hand, elbow, and shoulder,* Philadelphia, 2006, Mosby, p 330.

reduced the frequency of surgical intervention for these patients.

- Diagnosis
  - Symmetric complaints of pain, morning stiffness, hand swelling
  - **Tenosynovitis and tendon rupture are common.**
    - Digit triggering treated by tenosynovectomy in addition to A1 pulley release
    - May require ulnar FDS slip excision or debulking of flexor tendon to relieve triggering
  - **Tendon ruptures often require tendon transfer.**
  - Serologic studies may be positive (rheumatoid factor in 70%-90% of patients) within several months of disease onset.
  - Classic radiographic features, including diffuse osteopenia, periarticular erosion, and joint subluxation, may not appear for several years.
  - MRI with IV contrast more sensitive for detecting early disease, with findings of enhanced synovial proliferation, bone marrow edema, and periarticular erosion.

- Disability may be diminished by early diagnosis, referral to rheumatologist, and aggressive medical management with DMARDs and/or oral corticosteroids.
- Treatment
  - Rheumatoid nodules
    - Subcutaneous masses consisting of chronic inflammatory cells surrounded by collagenous capsule
    - Most common extraarticular manifestation of the disease
    - Occur over bony prominences on extensor surfaces
    - May erode through skin and cause chronic draining sinus
    - Excision may be indicated for diagnostic biopsy, pain relief, or improved cosmesis
  - Tenosynovitis
    - Hyperplasia and inflammatory cell infiltration of synovium-lined tendon sheaths that may precede joint manifestations
    - May involve flexor and/or extensor tendons of hand/wrist
    - Nonoperative management with rest, activity modification, splinting, and antiinflammatory medication is attempted for 4 to 6 months.
    - Tenosynovectomy reserved for cases that fail conservative treatment or when impending tendon rupture evident
  - Tendon rupture
    - May occur secondary to chronic tenosynovitis or mechanical abrasion over bony prominences
    - **Vaughan-Jackson syndrome** describes progressive rupture of extensor tendons, starting with extensor digiti minimi and continuing radially, from attrition over a prominent distal ulnar head (caput ulnae syndrome).
    - **EPL may rupture from same process at the Lister tubercle.**

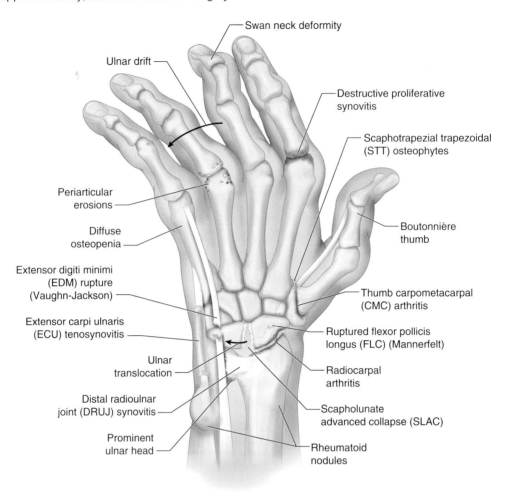

Swan neck deformity

Ulnar drift

Destructive proliferative synovitis

Scaphotrapezial trapezoidal (STT) osteophytes

Periarticular erosions

Diffuse osteopenia

Extensor digiti minimi (EDM) rupture (Vaughn-Jackson)

Extensor carpi ulnaris (ECU) tenosynovitis

Ulnar translocation

Distal radioulnar joint (DRUJ) synovitis

Prominent ulnar head

Boutonnière thumb

Thumb carpometacarpal (CMC) arthritis

Ruptured flexor pollicis longus (FLC) (Mannerfelt)

Radiocarpal arthritis

Scapholunate advanced collapse (SLAC)

Rheumatoid nodules

FIGURE 7-54 Composite image showing pathologic manifestations of rheumatoid disease in the hand and wrist.

- **Mannerfelt syndrome** results in FPL and/or index FDP rupture secondary to attrition over a volar STT joint osteophyte.
  - Direct repair prone to failure, so tendon transfer is preferred method of treatment (Figure 7-55)
- Caput ulnae syndrome
  - End-stage finding of DRUJ instability from chronic synovitis and surrounding capsular and ligamentous laxity
  - As the ECU subsheath stretches, the ECU tendon subluxes in ulnar and volar direction.
  - Subsequently, the carpus supinates on radius and further stretches the dorsal restraints.
  - Ulnar head subluxes dorsally ("piano-key sign").
  - Attritional rupture of extensor tendons (see earlier discussion of Vaughn-Jackson syndrome)
  - Treatment options include Darrach distal ulna resection, Sauve-Kapandji procedure, resection hemiarthroplasty, and ulnar head prosthetic replacement.
- Rheumatoid wrist
  - Extensive synovitis and pannus formation weakens the capsular and ligamentous structures that stabilize the radiocarpal joint and DRUJ.
  - Carpus subluxes in volar and ulnar direction.

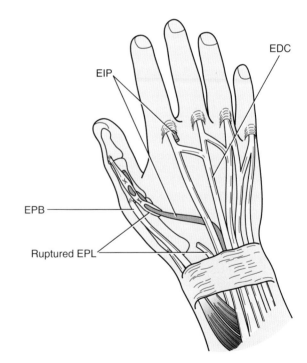

EDC

EIP

EPB

Ruptured EPL

FIGURE 7-55 Transfer of the extensor indicis proprius (EIP) for an extensor pollicis longus (EPL) rupture. *EDC,* Extensor digitorum communis; *EPB,* extensor pollicis brevis. (From Trumble TE et al, editors: *Core knowledge in orthopaedics: hand, elbow, and shoulder,* Philadelphia, 2006, Mosby, p 365.)

- Chronic scapholunate ligament disruption can lead to rotatory subluxation of the scaphoid and progressive carpal collapse (SLAC pattern).
- Early synovectomy may delay severe joint destruction and deformity in some cases.
- Intermediate-stage disease may benefit from radiolunate arthrodesis (Chamay), which centralizes the lunate and diminishes further carpal subluxation and ulnar translocation (preserves midcarpal motion).
- **Total wrist arthrodesis remains gold standard for advanced radiocarpal destruction** (Figure 7-56)
  - For bilateral procedures, fuse one wrist in slight extension and the other in slight flexion.
- **Total wrist arthroplasty is an option in low-demand patients with adequate bone stock, minimal deformity, and intact extensor tendon function** (Figure 7-57).
  - Newer-generation metal/polyethylene combination implants are helping decrease the historically high rate of complications associated with total wrist arthroplasty.
- Both total wrist arthrodesis and total wrist arthroplasty have been deemed cost-effective procedures for the treatment of rheumatoid wrist.
- It may be reasonable to consider an arthroplasty of the dominant wrist and a fusion of the nondominant wrist in selected patients.
- MCP joint involvement
  - Characteristic deformity pattern of ulnar deviation and volar subluxation
    - Initial presentation may be an extension lag.

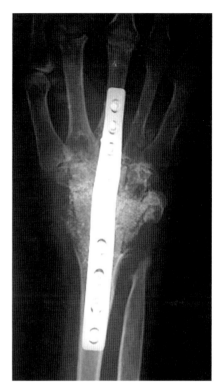

FIGURE 7-56 Posteroanterior wrist radiograph following total wrist arthrodesis with a dorsal plate. (From Wehbe MA, editor: Arthroplasty around the wrist: CMC, radiocarpal, DRUJ, *Hand clinics*, Philadelphia, 2013, Elsevier, p 88.)

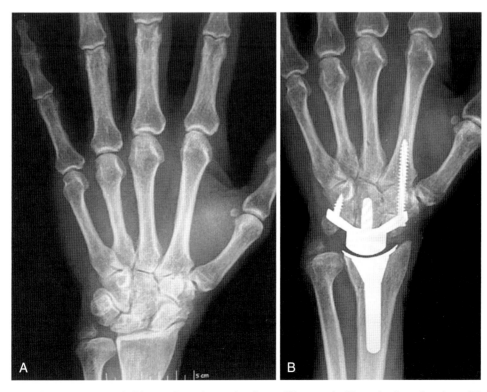

FIGURE 7-57 A 57-year-old man with scaphoid nonunion advanced collapse **(A)**, treated with total wrist arthroplasty **(B)**. (From Nydick JA et al: Clinical outcomes of total wrist arthroplasty, *J Hand Surg Am* 37:1580–1584, 2012.)

- Synovitis and pannus formation stretch the weaker radial sagittal bands, and extensor tendons subluxate ulnarly.
- Concurrent loss of volar plate and collateral ligament integrity
- Contracture of the intrinsic muscle tendons leads to ulnar deviation of fingers.
- Simultaneous wrist involvement leads to Z-deformity.
  - Ulnar translocation and supination of carpus
  - Radial deviation of metacarpals
  - Ulnar deviation of digits
- Early treatment with synovectomy and recentralization of the extensor tendons provides temporary solution.
- **Silicone MCP arthroplasty most common definitive treatment to relieve pain and improve cosmesis**
  - Ultimate function less predictable
  - **Complications may include infection, implant failure, and recurrent deformity.**
  - Concomitant correction of wrist deformity is paramount to the success of MCP arthroplasty.
- PIP joint involvement
  - Synovitis leads to attenuation of stabilizing structures and characteristic deformities.
    - **Boutonnière**—attenuation of central slip/triangular ligament leads to volar subluxation of lateral bands and consequent PIP hyperflexion and DIP hyperextension.
    - **Swan neck**—attenuation of volar plate leads to dorsal subluxation of lateral bands and consequent PIP hyperextension and DIP hyperflexion.
  - Rheumatoid thumb
    - Classified into six types by Nalebuff
    - Most common deformity is type I boutonnière thumb
    - Treatment dictated by deformity with options including synovectomy, soft tissue reconstruction, arthrodesis, and arthroplasty

■ **Juvenile rheumatoid arthritis**
▦ Age of onset before 16 years
▦ Other rheumatic diseases must be excluded.
▦ **A classic difference between juvenile rheumatoid arthritis (JRA) and adult form is radial deviation of the MCP joints and ulnar deviation of the wrist.**
▦ Nonoperative treatment favored to avoid damage to growing physes
▦ Three disease types—systemic (20%), polyarticular (40%), and pauciarticular (40%)
- **Systemic form (Still disease)**
  - May be associated with transient arthritis in the setting of fever, anemia, hepatosplenomegaly, uveitis, and lymphadenitis
  - **Rheumatoid factor is negative.**
  - Only one fourth of patients develop chronic disabling arthritis.
- Polyarticular form
  - Symmetric form affecting at least five joints
  - Small percentage have positive rheumatoid factor
  - More closely resembles adult form
  - Chronic progression likely

- **Pauciarticular form**
  - Asymmetric form affecting less than five joints
  - Produces more large-joint and lower extremity involvement
  - Female patients typically have earlier disease onset and may have positive antinuclear antibody.
  - An association with human leukocyte antigen (HLA)-B27 and sacroiliitis is more common in male patients.

■ **Psoriatic arthritis**
▦ Seronegative spondyloarthropathy affects approximately 20% of patients with psoriasis.
▦ Skin involvement precedes joint manifestations by several years.
▦ Classical clinical findings include nail pitting and sausage digits.
▦ PIP flexion and MCP extension contractures
▦ Radiographs may show DIP joint "pencil-in-cup" deformity.
▦ Operative treatment with DIP arthrodesis

■ **Systemic lupus erythematosus**
▦ Most often affects young women (age 15-25 years)
▦ Majority have rheumatoid-like presentation of inflammatory small joint hand and wrist arthritis
▦ Swan neck more common than boutonnière deformity in SLE
▦ MCP joints have characteristic ulnar deviation and volar subluxation.
▦ Other potential findings in SLE include marked joint laxity, Raynaud phenomenon, facial butterfly rash, positive antinuclear antibody, and anti-DNA antibodies.
▦ Radiographs largely normal
▦ DMARDs are mainstay of treatment
▦ When medical management is maximized, arthrodesis of affected joints is more reliable than arthroplasty.

■ **Scleroderma (systemic sclerosis)**
▦ Hand manifestations include Raynaud phenomenon, PIP flexion contractures, skin ulceration, fingertip pulp atrophy, and calcific deposits within digits (calcinosis cutis)
▦ Absorption of distal phalangeal tufts may be seen radiographically.
▦ Periadventitial digital sympathectomy may be necessary for refractory cases of Raynaud phenomenon with unremitting ischemic pain or signs of distal tissue ulceration or necrosis.
- Results of sympathectomy better for scleroderma than for atherosclerotic disease
▦ Arthrodesis is used for fixed PIP flexion contractures.
▦ Symptomatic calcific deposits may be excised.
▦ Fingertip ulcerations/necrosis are best treated with débridement and possible amputation.

■ **Gout**
▦ Caused by precipitation of **monosodium urate crystals,** which deposit in joints and/or tendon sheaths or may even coalesce as tophi in the soft tissues (Figure 7-58)
▦ Most cases (90%) occur in men.
▦ Elevated uric acid levels do not necessarily correlate with the prevalence of gout attacks.
▦ Gout may be associated with any state of high metabolic turnover (e.g., tumor lysis syndrome).
▦ **Radiographs may show periarticular erosions and soft tissue tophi in chronic cases.**

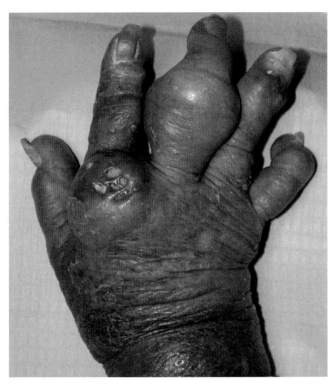

FIGURE 7-58 Tophaceous gout. (From Green DP et al, editors: *Green's operative hand surgery*, ed 6, Philadelphia, 2011, Churchill Livingstone, p 81.)

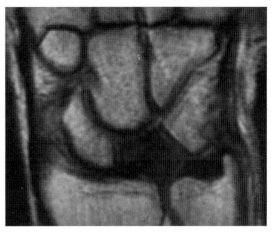

FIGURE 7-59 T1-weighted magnetic resonance image of the carpus, revealing decreased signal within the lunate. (From Trumble TE et al, editors: *Core knowledge in orthopaedics: hand, elbow, and shoulder,* Philadelphia, 2006, Mosby, p 179.)

▦ Aspiration yields negatively birefringent monosodium urate crystals.

▦ Acute attacks treated with high dose NSAIDs, oral steroids, or colchicine

▦ Allopurinol used for chronic prophylaxis against further attacks

◼ **Calcium pyrophosphate deposition disease (pseudogout)**

▦ Causes an acute monoarticular arthritis that mimics septic arthritis

▦ Wrist is second most commonly affected joint (knee)

▦ Aspiration yields positively **birefringent calcium pyrophosphate dihydrate crystals.**

▦ Radiographs may show chondrocalcinosis of the TFCC and/or other carpal ligaments.

▦ Treat acute attacks with high-dose NSAIDs.

▦ Chronic arthritis (scaphotrapeziotrapezoid, SLAC patterns) treated according to stage of disease

IDIOPATHIC OSTEONECROSIS OF THE CARPUS

 ◼ **Kienböck disease (idiopathic osteonecrosis of the lunate)**

▦ Overview

• Progressive, often debilitating disease

• Characterized by fragmentation and collapse of lunate

• Most common in men aged 20 to 40

• Rare in children but better prognosis

• Rarely bilateral

• Multifactorial etiology postulated

• Lunate geometry

• Anatomic variability of lunate blood supply

• Single arterial supply, limited intraosseous branching most susceptible

• Increased intraosseous pressure from venous stasis

• Negative ulnar variance

• Increased shear stress on marginally perfused lunate

• Decreased radial inclination

▦ Diagnosis

• Dorsal wrist pain, mild swelling, limited motion, weakness

• Ulnar variance determined with wrist posteroanterior in neutral rotation

• Radiographs may be initially normal or show a linear fracture.

• Subsequent involvement demonstrates lunate sclerosis followed by lunate collapse.

• Unexplained persistent, non–activity-related dorsal wrist pain in young adult with negative ulnar variance should prompt MRI evaluation.

• MRI findings in early Kienböck disease include diffuse low-signal intensity throughout lunate on T1- and T2-weighted images (Figure 7-59); increased signal intensity on T2-weighted images may indicate revascularization.

• **Lichtman classification** (Table 7-12)

• Modification using radioscaphoid angle greater than 60 degrees to distinguish between stage IIIA and B increases interobserver reliability.

▦ Treatment

• Based on Lichtman stage and ulnar variance

• A 3-month trial of cast immobilization is appropriate for stage I disease, but long-term success of nonoperative treatment is limited.

• Operative treatment is indicated for patients who present with radiographic abnormalities (stage II or higher) or those who fail a trial of immobilization.

• First-line surgical treatment is a joint-leveling procedure.

• In patients with ulnar-negative variance, radial-shortening osteotomy is preferred over ulnar lengthening with bone grafting (goal is neutral or 1-mm positive).

• Capitate shortening with capitohamate fusion is used for patients with ulnar-positive variance.

Table 7-12	Stages of Kienböck Disease
STAGE	**DESCRIPTION**
I	Normal radiographs or linear fracture
	Increased uptake on bone scan
	MRI shows low signal intensity in lunate on T1-weighted images
II	Lunate sclerosis
	One or more obvious fracture lines
	Possible early lunate collapse at radial border
IIIA	Lunate collapse with normal carpal alignment
IIIB	Lunate collapse with fixed scaphoid rotation (ring sign)
	Proximal capitate migration
IV	Severe lunate collapse
	Degenerative changes at midcarpal ± radiocarpal joints

Adapted from Allan CH et al: Kienböck's disease: diagnosis and treatment, *J Am Acad Orthop Surg* 9:128–136, 2001.

- **Core decompression of the radius and ulna has been described.**
  - Thought to incite local vascular healing response
- Vascularized bone grafting has been used for stages I to IIIA.
  - Preferred pedicle is from the fourth plus fifth extracompartmental artery (4+5 ECA)
  - May be combined with scaphocapitate pinning and/or external fixation to "unload" the lunate temporarily
  - Pedicled vascularized transfers from pisiform and index metacarpal have also been described, as well as free transfers from remote sites.
- There is little evidence to support one procedure over another for the treatment of stage I to IIIA disease.
- Treatment of stage IIIB Kienböck disease must address the associated carpal instability.
  - Options include scaphoid-trapezium-trapezoid fusion, scaphocapitate fusion, and proximal row carpectomy.
  - Stage IV disease with radiocarpal and/or midcarpal osteoarthrosis typically requires either proximal row carpectomy or wrist fusion.

■ **Preiser disease (idiopathic osteonecrosis of the scaphoid)**
▥ Rare diagnosis based on radiographic evidence of sclerosis and fragmentation of the scaphoid without evidence of prior fracture
▥ Predisposing vascular patterns have not been determined.
▥ Average age at onset is 45 years.
▥ Patients present with insidious dorsoradial wrist pain.
▥ Four-stage radiographic classification similar to Kienböck disease
▥ Preiser disease may also be simply classified into complete and partial involvement by MRI.
▥ Initially treated with cast immobilization
▥ Operative treatment may include core decompression, curettage, allograft replacement, vascularized bone grafting, proximal row carpectomy, scaphoid excision and four-corner fusion, or total wrist fusion.

DUPUYTREN DISEASE

■ **Introduction**
▥ Dupuytren disease is a benign fibroproliferative disorder of unclear etiology.

▥ Typically begins as a nodule in the palmar fascia and progresses insidiously to form diseased cords and finally digital flexion contractures involving the MCP and/or PIP joints
▥ Predominantly seen in white men of northern European descent
▥ Although an autosomal dominant inheritance pattern with variable penetrance is suspected, the offending gene has not been isolated, and sporadic cases are still more common.
▥ Dupuytren disease has been associated with tobacco and alcohol use, diabetes, epilepsy, chronic pulmonary disease, tuberculosis, and human immunodeficiency virus/acquired immunodeficiency syndrome (HIV/AIDS).
▥ No association with occupation has been determined.
■ **Pathophysiology**
▥ Cytokine-mediated (transforming growth factor [TGF]-β) transformation of normal fibroblasts into myofibroblasts has been implicated.
▥ Myofibroblast contractile properties are abnormal and exaggerated.
■ **Increase in ratio of type III to type I collagen**
■ Increase in free radical formation
■ Three stages of disease are recognized:
  - Proliferative, involutional, and residual
■ **Structural anomalies**
■ **Normal fascial structures that become involved** (Figure 7-60):
  - Pretendinous band
  - Natatory band
  - Spiral band
  - Retrovascular band
  - Grayson ligament
  - Lateral digital sheet
■ **Cleland ligaments are not involved.**
■ Normal bands become diseased cords (see Figure 7-60).
  - **Spiral cord**
    - Contributions from the pretendinous band, spiral band, lateral digital sheet, and Grayson ligament
    - **Leads to PIP contracture**
    - Put neurovascular bundle at risk during surgery by displacing it more centrally and superficially
  - Central cord
  - Lateral cord
  - Natatory cord
  - Retrovascular cord
  - Abductor digiti minimi cord
  - Intercommissural cord of first web space
■ **Diagnosis**
▥ May present early with tender palmar nodule or later with flexion contractures that impair simple activities (shaking hands, placing hand in a pocket, etc.)
▥ Distribution of digit involvement, in decreasing order of frequency, are the ring, small, long, thumb, and index digits.
▥ **"Dupuytren diathesis"** describes patients with early disease onset and rapid progression of joint contractures, often bilateral and including more radial digits.
▥ Additional extrapalmar locations may be involved, such as the dorsum of the PIP joint (Garrod knuckle pads), penis (Peyronie disease), and plantar surface of the foot (Ledderhose disease).

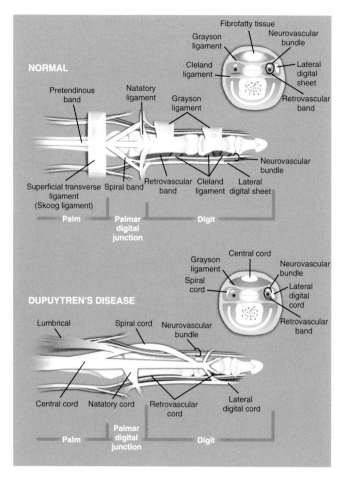

FIGURE 7-60 Normal fascial anatomy and pathoanatomy of fascial cords in Dupuytren disease. (*Courtesy of School of Medicine, SUNY Stony Brook, NY.*)

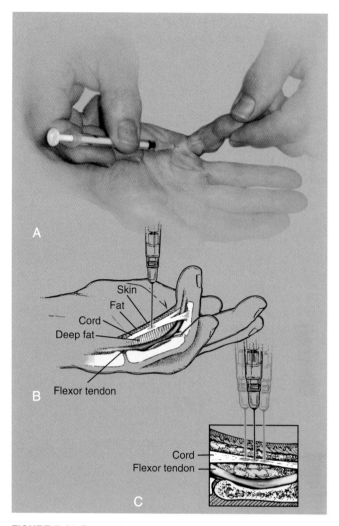

FIGURE 7-61 Enzymatic fasciectomy for Dupuytren disease. **A,** Collagenase injected into a central cord. **B,** Enzyme diffuses in cord. **C,** One third of collagenase dose disseminated in each of three different locations within a cord. (*Courtesy of School of Medicine, SUNY Stony Brook, NY.*)

▦ Patients with Dupuytren diathesis should be counseled about flare reactions and higher recurrence rates after surgical intervention.

▪ **Treatment**
▦ Nonoperative
  • Acceptance of office-based collagenase injection (derived from *Clostridium histolyticum*) as an alternative to surgery has become more widespread in the hand surgery community (Figure 7-61).
    • Cord is injected directly with enzyme, and patient returns the following day for manipulation of the contracture under digital block anesthesia.
    • Pooled results of open-label studies demonstrate average MCP correction of up to 85% and PIP correction of up to 60%.
    • Common adverse effects include temporary pain, swelling and bruising; other complications include skin tears (up to 12%) and flexor tendon rupture (rare).
▦ Operative
  • Indications include inability to place hand flat on tabletop (Hueston test), MCP flexion contracture greater than 30 degrees, or any PIP flexion contracture.
  • **Procedure of choice is typically open limited fasciectomy.**
    • Iatrogenic digital nerve injury in up to 7% of cases in some series

  • Tourniquet should be deflated prior to closure to assess digital perfusion after large contracture releases.
  • Total palmar fasciectomy no longer favored because of high complication rate
  • Percutaneous cord release under local anesthetic with a large-gauge needle is an alternative to formal open surgery and may be most favorable in an elderly patient with low demands and multiple comorbidities.
  • Open-palm McCash technique with skin healing by secondary intention may still be used to reduce hematoma formation, decrease edema, and allow early motion.
  • Skin deficits after contracture release may be addressed with Z-plasty, V-Y advancement, full-thickness skin grafting, or healing by secondary intention.
▦ Complications and postoperative care
  • **Most common complication after operative treatment is recurrence, with long-term rates as high as 50% (higher in Dupuytren diathesis).**
  • Judicious postoperative therapy with active ROM and static nighttime splinting to maintain extension

correction is critical for improved outcomes and the prevention or delay of recurrence.
- Early postoperative "flare reactions" are more common in women and may be treated with short courses of oral steroids or NSAIDs.
- Other potential complications include hematoma, infection, digital neurovascular injury, complex regional pain syndrome, and amputation.

HAND TUMORS

■ Benign soft tissue tumors
▨ Ganglion
- Most common soft tissue mass of the hand and wrist (Box 7-3)
- Contains either joint or tendon sheath fluid
- Encapsulating tissue does not have true epithelial lining.
- These masses often fluctuate in size over time.
- A traumatic etiology is suspected in many cases.
- Ganglions are often firm and well-circumscribed and may transilluminate on physical examination.
- **Site of 70% of cases is the dorsal wrist, usually originating from scapholunate articulation** (Figure 7-62).
  - Small (occult) dorsal ganglions may be more symptomatic than larger ones.

| **Box 7-3** | **Tumors of the Hand and Upper Extremity** |

Most common benign soft tissue tumor—GANGLION
Most common malignant soft tissue tumor—EPITHELIOID or SYNOVIAL SARCOMA
Most common skin malignancy—SQUAMOUS CELL CARCINOMA
Most common benign bone tumor—ENCHONDROMA
Most common malignant bone tumor—CHONDROSARCOMA
Most common primary site for acral metastases—LUNG

- **Majority of volar wrist ganglions originate from radioscaphoid or scaphotrapezial joints** (Figure 7-63)
  - These emerge in close proximity to radial artery and its branches.
  - Higher recurrence rate compared to dorsal ganglions
- Mucous cysts occur at dorsum of DIP joint in patients with osteoarthritis (Figure 7-64).
  - Surgery must address underlying osteophytes.
- Retinacular cysts form from herniated tendon sheath fluid.
- Overall recurrence rate after aspiration of ganglions is approximately 50%.

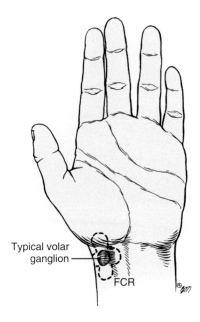

FIGURE 7-63 Typical location of a volar wrist ganglion. Possible subcutaneous extensions *(dashed lines)* are often palpable. (Copyright Elizabeth Martin.)

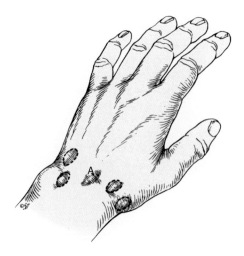

FIGURE 7-62 A few of the many locations of dorsal wrist ganglions. The most common site (A) is directly over the scapholunate ligament. (Copyright Elizabeth Martin.)

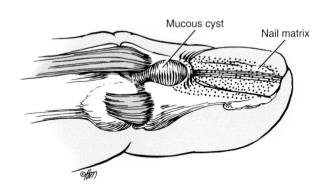

FIGURE 7-64 A mucous cyst originating from the distal interphalangeal joint may put pressure on the nail matrix and result in longitudinal grooving in the nail plate. (Copyright Elizabeth Martin.)

- Open excision is the surgical procedure of choice, although many dorsal ganglions can be effectively removed arthroscopically.
  - The cyst stalk and portion of capsule should be removed.
- A brief period of immobilization is recommended postoperatively.
- Giant cell tumor of tendon sheath
  - Second most common soft tissue mass of the hand
  - Other names include *xanthoma* and *localized nodular synovitis*.
  - Presents as slow-growing, nontender, nodular or multilobulated mass
  - Contains multinucleated giant cells, round stromal cells, and lipid-laden foam cells with hemosiderin deposits (histologic findings similar to pigmented villonodular synovitis)
  - Treatment is marginal excision.
  - Multilobulated lesions with extension into tendon or joint capsule associated with higher recurrence rate (≈45% in some series), but no cases of malignant transformation have been reported.
- Lipoma
  - Extremely common tumor of adipose cell origin
  - Though usually painless, they may reach substantial size over time.
  - Lipomas in the palm may compress the carpal tunnel or the Guyon canal, leading to neurologic deficits.
  - MRI may be helpful for preoperative planning in these cases.
  - Lesions have same bright signal characteristics as subcutaneous fat on T1-weighted images.
  - Treatment is either observation or marginal excision.
  - Low recurrence rate
- Epidermal inclusion cyst
  - Common painless, slow-growing mass arising after penetrating injury that drives keratinizing epithelium into subcutaneous tissue
  - Curative treatment is marginal excision.
- **Neurilemoma (schwannoma)**
  - Most common peripheral nerve tumor of the upper extremity
  - Typically painless mass that may have positive Tinel sign
  - Cell of origin is the myelin-forming Schwann cell.
    - The tumor is composed of Antoni A (cellular) and Antoni B (matrix) regions.
  - Treatment is marginal excision.
  - Because these tumors are eccentric and encapsulated, they can be shelled out of nerve without disrupting axons.
  - Neurologic injury in less than 5% of cases
  - Low recurrence rate
- Neurofibroma
  - Slow-growing, painless mass arising from nerve fascicle
  - May be solitary in hand and wrist (no history of neurofibromatosis)
  - Portion of nerve usually sacrificed during excision, and grafting may be necessary
- **Glomus tumor**
  - Smooth muscle tumor of perivascular temperature-regulating bodies
  - Usually occurs in subungual region and may cause nail ridging and erosions of the distal phalanx

- Also reported in palm
- Characterized by exquisite pain and cold intolerance
- MRI with gadolinium is a potentially helpful adjunctive diagnostic study.
- Treatment is marginal excision.
- Low recurrence rate
- Hemangioma
  - Vascular proliferations divided into capillary (superficial) and cavernous (deep) lesions
  - Many infantile hemangiomas become involuted by age 7, and those that arise during childhood are observed.
  - Kasabach-Merritt syndrome is a rare complication resulting from entrapped platelets and a potentially fatal coagulopathy.
  - In adults, MRI with gadolinium may help distinguish these benign vascular tumors from arteriovenous malformations and angiosarcomas.
  - Small and accessible lesions treated with marginal excision
  - Embolization may be more feasible alternative for larger lesions.
- Pyogenic granuloma (lobular capillary hemangioma)
  - Rapidly growing, pedunculated cutaneous lesion with friable tissue that bleeds easily (Figure 7-65)
  - Vascular tumor with lobules of endothelial cells and luminal structures in edematous stroma histologically
  - Many methods of treatment described, all with high recurrence rates.
  - Some evidence to support simple silver nitrate cauterization

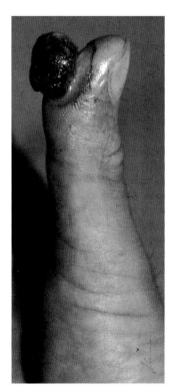

FIGURE 7-65 Pyogenic granuloma. (From Green DP et al, editors: *Green's operative hand surgery,* ed 6, Philadelphia, 2011, Churchill Livingstone, p 81.)

■ **Malignant soft tissue tumors**

▓ **Squamous cell carcinoma**

- Most common malignancy of the hand
- Usually seen in elderly men with premalignant conditions such as actinokeratosis or chronic osteomyelitis
  - Dorsum of hand is high-risk lesion
- Primary risk factor: excessive exposure to ultraviolet radiation
- Also most common subungual malignancy
- Higher metastatic potential than basal cell carcinoma
- Consultation with dermatologist recommended
- Mohs micrographic surgery has highest cure rate (highest for all nonmelanotic skin cancers)
- Excision of aggressive lesions that are poorly differentiated or greater than 2.5 cm requires at least 6-mm margin.
- Lymph node biopsy may be necessary.
- Adjuvant radiation for tumor recurrence, lesions over 2 cm wide and/or 4 mm deep, perineural invasion, lymph node metastases

▓ Sarcoma

- **Most common sarcomas are epithelioid and synovial.**
- Other common sarcomas of the upper extremity include liposarcoma and malignant fibrous histiocytoma.
- Evaluated by MRI
- Most soft tissue sarcomas metastasize to the lungs.
- Lymph nodes are the second most common area.
  - Epithelioid sarcoma
    - Firm, slow-growing mass presenting in young to middle-aged adults
    - Locations include digits, palm, or forearm.
    - May eventually ulcerate and drain
    - Commonly spreads to regional lymph nodes
    - Composed of malignant epithelial cells and central areas of necrosis
    - Treatment is wide or radical excision accompanied by sentinel lymph node biopsy.
    - Adjuvant chemotherapy or radiation therapy may be considered but is controversial for this tumor.
  - Synovial sarcoma
    - Firm, slow-growing mass presenting in young to middle-aged adults
    - Usually forms adjacent to the carpus
    - Composed of epithelial and spindle cells with multiple histologic patterns
    - Treatment is wide or radical excision, with 5-year survival rates of approximately 80%.
    - More recently, adjuvant chemotherapy and external beam radiation have proven successful in reducing local recurrence rates.

■ **Benign bone tumors**

▓ **Enchondroma**

- Most common benign bone tumor of the upper extremity
- Typically occurs in second to fourth decades
- Most cases asymptomatic and discovered incidentally
- Arises from metaphyseal medullary canal and spreads to diaphysis (Figure 7-66)
- Usually involves proximal phalanx or metacarpal (Figure 7-67)

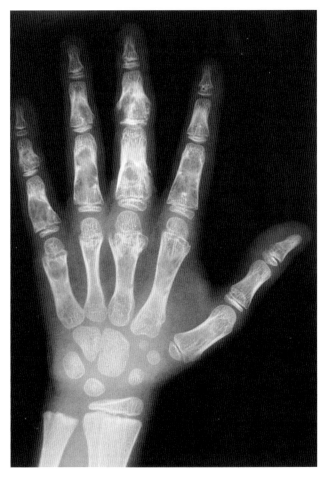

FIGURE 7-66 Multiple enchondromatosis (Ollier disease). (From Green DP et al, editors: *Green's operative hand surgery,* ed 6, Philadelphia, 2005, Churchill Livingstone, p 2179.)

- Symmetric fusiform expansion of bone with endosteal scalloping and intramedullary calcifications
- May present as pathologic fracture
- Hand enchondromas are distinguished histologically by their high cellularity.
  - Presence of mitotic figures may signal low-grade chondrosarcoma.
- Treatment is curettage.
  - Benefit of void augmentation with autograft, allograft, cement, and so forth not clearly shown in the literature

▓ Osteochondroma

- Benign tumor characterized by a bony surface outgrowth capped by cartilage
- Rarely seen in the hand except in multiple hereditary exostosis
- Distal aspect of P1 is most common location in hand
- May be seen near DRUJ or arising from shafts of radius/ulna
- Low chance of malignant transformation
- Asymptomatic lesions observed
- Symptomatic lesions may have associated bursitis/periostitis and are excised with low recurrence rate.

▓ **Osteoid osteoma**

- May present with swelling without pain in the hand
- Usually found in carpus (scaphoid) or proximal phalanx
- Radiolucent nidus within sclerotic lesion

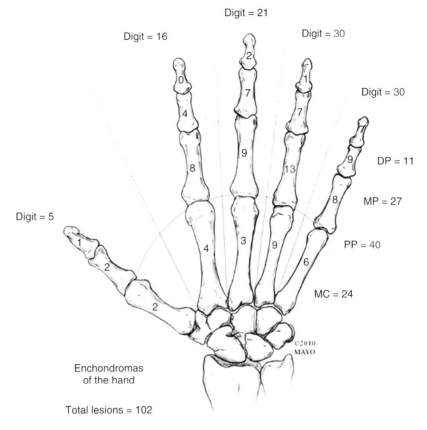

FIGURE 7-67 Location of enchondromas. (From Sassoon AA et al: Enchondromas of the hand: factors affecting recurrence, healing, motion and malignant transformation, *J Hand Surg Am* 37:1229–1234, 2012, Figure 1.)

- Nonoperative management with immobilization/NSAIDs
- Excision of nidus is curative.
- Radiofrequency ablation also effective
- Unicameral bone cyst
  - Common tumor in children
  - Occasionally seen in metacarpals, phalanges, or metaphyseal portion of distal radius
  - Most resolve spontaneously
  - Treatment with aspiration and injection of methylprednisolone acetate
- **Giant cell tumor**
  - Characterized as benign but may be locally aggressive
  - More common in young to middle-aged women
  - Presents with pain, swelling, and/or pathologic fracture
  - Distal radius is most common location (Figure 7-68)
  - An eccentric, lytic lesion is seen in metaphysis and epiphysis.
  - May cause cortical destruction and associated soft tissue mass
  - Osteoclast-like multinucleated giant cells and stromal cells with matching nuclei histologically
  - Treatment is wide excision (curettage alone yields high local recurrence rate).
  - Packing the lesion with polymethylmethacrylate (PMMA) has been successful.
  - Occasionally requires reconstruction with allograft or vascularized free fibula

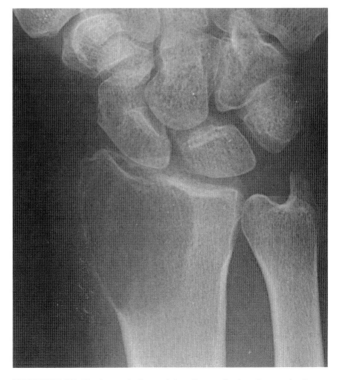

FIGURE 7-68 Posteroanterior wrist radiograph showing a giant cell tumor of the distal radius, characterized by an expansile, lytic epiphyseal lesion without a sclerotic rim. (From Green DP et al, editors: *Green's operative hand surgery*, ed 6, Philadelphia, 2011, Churchill Livingstone, p 2184.)

- Malignant bone tumors
- **Most common hand malignancy is metastatic lung carcinoma, usually involving distal phalanx**
- Breast and kidney metastases also reported
- Acral metastasis is poor prognostic sign, with less than 6-month survival expected at time of discovery
- **The three most common primary malignant bone tumors of the hand:**
  - Chondrosarcoma
  - Osteosarcoma
  - Ewing sarcoma
- Location usually metacarpal or phalanx
- Treatment for each tumor is the same as elsewhere in the body.

HAND INFECTIONS

- **Introduction**
- Hand infections can involve any tissue type and a variety of pathogens (Table 7-13)
- *Staphylococcus aureus*—**overall most common pathogen**
- *Streptococcus*—second most common
- Gram-negative and anaerobic bacteria are seen in intravenous drug abusers (IVDA), diabetic patients, and after farmyard injuries or bite wounds.
- **Community-acquired methicillin-resistant *S. aureus* (MRSA) is becoming more prevalent, especially in urban communities.**
  - Risk factors: antibiotic use in previous year, close and crowded living conditions, compromised skin integrity, shared items (towels, whirlpools, fitness equipment)
  - Risk groups: IVDA, homeless, children in daycare, prison inmates, military recruits, athletes in contact sports
  - High complication rate in diabetic patients
  - IV treatment with vancomycin or clindamycin, outpatient treatment with oral trimethoprim-sulfamethoxazole or clindamycin
- **Paronychia/eponychia**
- Infections involving the nail fold are most common in hand

- Typically *S. aureus*
- Treated by incision and drainage, partial or total nail plate removal, oral antibiotics, soaks, and dressing changes
- Important to preserve eponychial fold (cuticle) if possible
- **Chronic paronychia unresponsive to oral antibiotic therapy often secondary to fungal infection (*Candida albicans*)**
- In rare cases, marsupialization (excision of the dorsal eponychium) may be required to eradicate the infection.
- **Felon**
- Infection of the septated fingertip pulp
- *S. aureus* is most common pathogen
- Treated by incision and drainage through a central or midlateral incision
  - Important to break up the septae to adequately decompress the fingertip
  - Midlateral digital incisions are usually placed ulnarly, except for the thumb and small digit, where they are placed radially (Figure 7-69).
  - Incision should be left open to heal by secondary intention.
  - Delayed treatment may lead to concurrent flexor tenosynovitis, osteomyelitis, or digital tip necrosis.
- **Human bite**
- Potentially serious infection treated promptly with incision and drainage, especially if joint or tendon sheath is violated

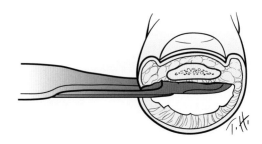

FIGURE 7-69 Decompression of an acute felon. (From Green DP et al, editors: *Green's operative hand surgery,* ed 6, New York, 2011, Churchill Livingstone, p 49.)

Table 7-13	Hand Infections			
TYPE	**LOCATION**	**PATHOGEN**	**ANTIBIOTIC**	**COMMENT**
Paronychia	Nail complex	*Staphylococcus aureus*	Dicloxacillin or clindamycin PO *or* Nafcillin IV	Partial or complete nail removal, release eponychial fold
Felon	Pulp space	*S. aureus*	Dicloxacillin or clindamycin PO *or* Nafcillin IV	Release all septae
Human bite	MCP and PIP	*Streptococcus* spp. *S. aureus* *Eikenella corrodens*	Ampicillin/sulbactam IV Penicillin for *E. corrodens*	Treatment failure with cephalosporins usually due to *E. corrodens*
Dog and cat bites	Varied	α-Hemolytic streptococci *Pasteurella multocida* *S. aureus* Anaerobes	Ampicillin/sulbactam IV followed by amoxicillin/clavulanate PO	Failure of oral treatment common; cat bites have higher rate of operative débridement
Necrotizing fasciitis	Varied	Clostridia Group A β-hemolytic streptococci	Broad-spectrum triple antibiotic—penicillin, clindamycin, gentamicin	High mortality, amputations frequent
Fungal	Cutaneous	*Candida albicans*	Topical antifungal	Common in diabetic patients with chronic paronychia
	Nail Subcutaneous	*Trichophyton rubrum* *Sporothrix schenckii* *Mycoplasma* spp.	Ketoconazole or itraconazole PO Based on culture	Pulse dosing 1 week per month

IV, Intravenous; *MCP,* metacarpophalangeal; *PIP,* proximal interphalangeal; *PO,* orally

- Most commonly involves the third or fourth MCP joint (fight bite)
- **Most frequently isolated organisms: group A streptococci, *S. aureus*, *Eikenella corrodens*, and *Bacteroides* spp.**
- Empirical antibiotics of choice are IV ampicillin/sulbactam and oral amoxicillin/clavulanate
- **Dog and cat bites**
- More than two million cases per year in the United States
- Vast majority are dog bites, with lower rate of serious infection
  - More likely to avulse or crush soft tissue but often amenable to local wound care
- Minority are cat bites, but with higher rate of serious infection
  - Deeper penetrance and longer time to initiation of treatment
- If patient presents immediately after bite, nonoperative treatment
  - Splinting, elevation, soaks, and antibiotics, followed by aggressive therapy once infection controlled
- Delayed treatment may lead to abscess formation and need for operative incision and drainage.
  - Further delay could lead to septic tenosynovitis, septic arthritis, and/or osteomyelitis.
- Ampicillin/sulbactam and amoxicillin/clavulanate are empirical antibiotics of choice (ciprofloxacin, doxycycline, or tetracycline if penicillin allergic).
  - **Covers *Pasteurella multocida* (part of animal oral flora), *S. aureus*, and *Streptococcus* spp.**
- **Pyogenic flexor tenosynovitis (FTS)**
- Infection of flexor tendon sheath
- May occur in delayed fashion after penetrating trauma

- *S. aureus* is most common pathogen
- Kanavel signs (four):
  - Flexed resting posture of digit
  - Fusiform swelling of digit
  - Tenderness of flexor tendon sheath
  - Pain with passive digit extension
- If infection recognized early, patient should be admitted and treated with splinting, IV antibiotics, and close observation
  - If signs improve within first 24 hours, surgery may be avoided.
- **Otherwise, the treatment of choice is incision and drainage of flexor tendon sheath.**
  - May be accomplished either by full open exposure using long midaxial or Bruner incision or with two small incisions placed distally (open A5 pulley) and proximally (open A1 pulley) using an angiocatheter (Figure 7-70)
  - Continuous-drip irrigation with an indwelling catheter carries a risk for extreme digit swelling.
- **Index and thumb FTS can spread to deep thenar space.**
- **Long, ring, and small finger FTS can spread to the midpalmar space.**
  - **Small finger FTS can also spread to the ulnar bursa.**
  - **Classical "horseshoe abscess" is based on proximal communication between the thumb and small finger flexor tendon sheaths in the Parona space, a potential space between the pronator quadratus and FDP tendons.**
  - Aggressive postoperative hand therapy is paramount because tendon adhesions and digital stiffness are likely.

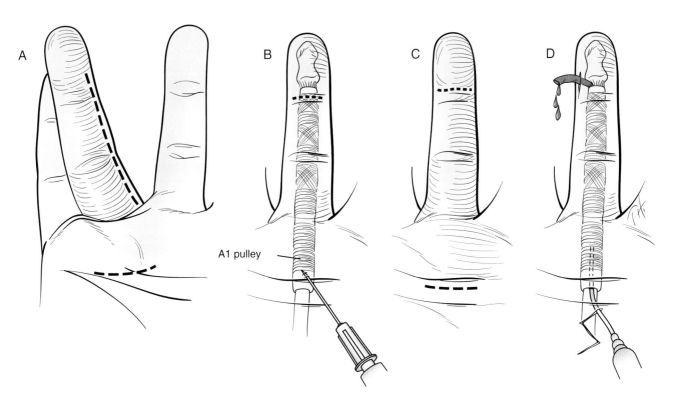

FIGURE 7-70 Incisions for drainage of septic digital flexor tenosynovitis. (From Neviaser R: Closed tendon sheath irrigation for pyogenic flexor tenosynovitis, *J Hand Surg* 3:462-466, 1978.)

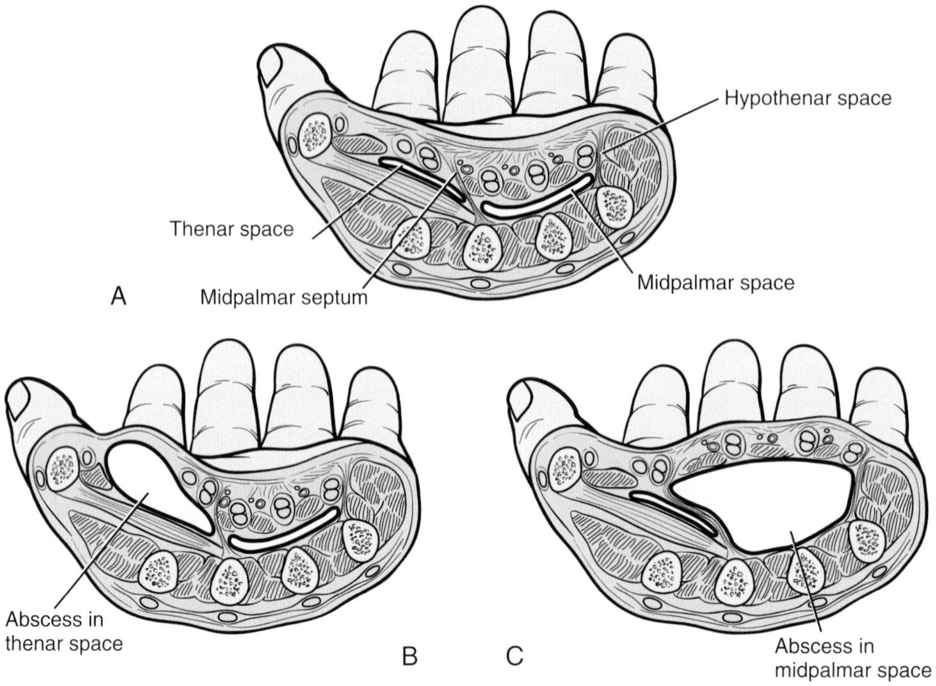

A diagram with labels:
- Hypothenar space
- Thenar space
- Midpalmar septum
- Midpalmar space
- **A**
- Abscess in thenar space
- **B**
- **C**
- Abscess in midpalmar space

FIGURE 7-71 A, Potential spaces of the deep palm. **B,** Thenar space abscess. **C,** Midpalmar space abscess. (From Green DP et al, editors: *Green's operative hand surgery,* ed 6, New York, 2011, Churchill Livingstone, p 58.)

▦ Herpetic whitlow
  • Caused by herpes simplex virus (HSV) type 1
  • Dental hygienists, healthcare workers, and toddlers at risk
  • Presents with digit pain and erythema, followed by formation of small vesicles that may coalesce into bullae
  • May be accompanied by fever, malaise, and lymphadenitis
  • Diagnosis confirmed by Tzanck smear and antibody titers
  • **Self-limiting, usually resolves within 7 to 10 days**
  • Incision and drainage are not recommended, because the rates of secondary bacterial infection are high.
  • Treatment with acyclovir may shorten the duration of symptoms.
  • Recurrence may be stimulated by fever, stress, and/or sun exposure.
▦ Deep potential-space infections
  • A *collar button abscess* occurs in the web space between digits.
    • Treated by incision and drainage with volar and dorsal incisions (avoiding the skin in the web itself) and IV antibiotics
  • Midpalmar space infections are rare.
    • Clinically, there is loss of midline contour of the hand.
    • Palmar pain elicited with flexion of the long, ring, and small fingers
  • Thenar and hypothenar space infections are also rare.
    • Present with pain and swelling over respective areas, exacerbated by flexion of the thumb or small finger
  • Incision and drainage and IV antibiotics are required for all of these deep potential-space infections (Figure 7-71).

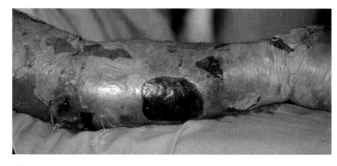

FIGURE 7-72 Characteristic appearance of necrotizing fasciitis. (From Green DP et al, editors: *Green's operative hand surgery,* ed 6, New York, 2011, Churchill Livingstone, p 78.)

■ **Necrotizing fasciitis**
▦ Severe infection with devastating outcomes and potential death when treatment delayed (Figure 7-72)
▦ **Group A β-hemolytic *Streptococcus* is the most common organism.**
▦ Groups at risk include immunocompromised patients (those with diabetes, cancer, or AIDS) as well as alcoholics and IVDA.
▦ Requires emergency radical débridement and broad-spectrum IV antibiotic coverage
▦ Intraoperative findings may include liquefied subcutaneous fat, dishwater pus, muscle necrosis, and venous thrombosis.
▦ Hemodynamic monitoring is critical.
▦ Amputation may be necessary when life threatening
▦ **Mortality rate is high and correlates with time to initiation of treatment.**
■ **Gas gangrene**
▦ Caused by ***Clostridium perfringens*** and other *Clostridium* spp. (gram-positive rods)

■ Condition occurs in devitalized contaminated wounds and leads to myonecrosis.

■ Extensive surgical débridement is necessary to prevent systemic infection.

■ **Fungal infection**

■ Serious infection usually seen in immunocompromised patients

■ Divided into cutaneous, subcutaneous, and deep locations

- Cutaneous infection
  - Chronic paronychia usually caused by *C. albicans* and treated with topical or oral antifungal agents and nail marsupialization
  - Onychomycosis is a destructive, deforming infection of the nail plate that is usually caused by *Trichophyton rubrum* and treated with topical or oral antifungal agents.
- Subcutaneous infection
  - Usually caused by **Sporothrix schenckii,** following penetrating injury while handling plants or soil (the rose thorn is the classical vehicle of transmission)
  - Starts with papule at site of inoculation, with subsequent lesions developing along the lymphatic vessels
  - Treatment is with potassium iodine solution.
- Deep infection
  - Several forms of deep infection exist, including tenosynovitis, septic arthritis, and osteomyelitis.
  - Treatment involves surgical débridement and culture-specific antifungal agents.
  - Endemic infections include histoplasmosis, blastomycosis, and coccidioidomycosis.
  - Opportunistic infections include aspergillosis, candidiasis, mucormycosis, and cryptococcosis.

■ **Atypical nontuberculous mycobacterial infections**

■ These organisms are widely distributed in the environment but are infrequent human pathogens.

■ Often indolent and fail to respond to usual treatments

■ Musculoskeletal manifestations (papules, ulcers, nodules) involve hand in majority of cases

■ May progress to tenosynovitis, septic arthritis, or osteomyelitis

■ Average incubation period 2 weeks; can be more than 6 months

■ Average time to diagnosis and appropriate treatment often more than 1 year

■ **Most common organism: *Mycobacterium marinum***

- Proliferates in freshwater and saltwater enclosures, especially in stagnant environment (e.g., aquarium)
- Patients come into contact with infected water, fish hooks, spiny sea creatures, and the like.

■ Granulomas are common on histopathologic studies; they may or may not show acid-fast bacilli.

■ **Cultures and sensitivities are critical and require a special medium (Lowenstein-Jensen) at exact temperatures (32°C).**

■ Treatment generally requires surgical débridement and oral antibiotics such as ethambutol, trimethoprim-sulfamethoxazole, clarithromycin, azithromycin, or tetracycline.

- Combination of agents often used
- Rifampin added for bone involvement
- Oral therapy continued 3 to 6 months

■ **Injection injury**

■ High-pressure injection injuries can be devastating.

■ High rate of digital amputation

- Organic solvents more toxic to tissue
- Oil-based paint worse than latex, water-based

■ Emergency wide surgical débridement recommended

CONGENITAL HAND DIFFERENCES

■ **Introduction**

■ Limb bud appears during fourth week of gestation

■ Hand begins as paddle, with digital separation occurring between 47 and 54 days

■ Development of lower limb lags behind by 48 hours.

■ All limb structures are present by end of embryogenesis at 8 weeks.

■ Most congenital anomalies occur by this time.

■ **Signaling centers that control limb development**

- Apical ectodermal ridge
  - Mediates proximal-to-distal growth
  - Fibroblast growth factor
- Zone of polarizing activity
  - Mediates radial-to-ulnar growth
  - **Sonic hedgehog protein**
- Wingless-type pathway
  - Mediates dorsal-to-volar growth
  - LMX-1 protein

■ Congenital hand anomalies occur at a rate of 1 in 600 live births.

- Three most common types:
  - Polydactyly (1 in 600)
  - Syndactyly (1 in 2000)
  - Bifid thumb (radial polydactyly) (1 in 3000)

■ Classification

- Failure of formation
- Failure of differentiation
- Duplication
- Overgrowth
- Undergrowth
- Amnion disruption sequence
- Generalized skeletal abnormalities

■ In general, surgical intervention to address congenital hand differences should be performed before the child establishes compensatory mechanisms and before starting school.

■ Cosmetic appearance should not be improved at the cost of further functional impairment.

■ Early genetic counseling is a critical part of the care of a child with congenital hand differences in the setting of other extraskeletal anomalies.

■ **Failure of formation**

■ Transverse absence

- Also termed *congenital amputation*
- Usually occur at proximal forearm level
- Majority are unilateral and thought to be result of vascular insult to apical ectodermal ridge rather than part of a syndrome
- Amputation through proximal third of forearm most common
- End of limb may have nubbins or dimpling
- Early prosthetic fitting before age 2 years is treatment of choice

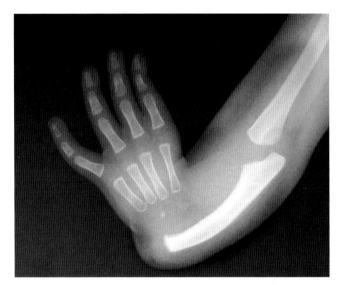

FIGURE 7-73 Type IV radial deficiency and absent thumb in an 18-month-old. (Courtesy of Shriners Hospitals for Children, Philadelphia.)

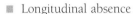

▦ Longitudinal absence
- Radial dysplasia (radial clubhand)
  - Characterized by deficiency of the radius and radial carpal structures (Figure 7-73)
  - Thumb dysplasia is included in the spectrum of presentation (see the section "Undergrowth").
  - Both extremities are affected in over 50% of cases.
  - Associated systemic syndromes
    - Thrombocytopenia with absent radius (TAR)
    - **VACTERL syndrome** (vertebral, anal, cardiac, tracheal, esophageal, renal, and limb anomalies)
    - Holt-Oram syndrome
    - Fanconi anemia
      - Life threatening, treated with bone marrow transplant
  - Four types recognized:
    - Type I—short radius
    - Type II—hypoplastic radius
    - Type III—partially absent radius
    - Type IV—completely absent radius
  - Early therapy to preserve passive ROM is critical.
  - A centralization procedure to realign the carpus on the distal ulna may be attempted when the child is between 6 and 12 months of age.
    - Inadequate elbow ROM is a contraindication to a centralization procedure.
- Ulnar dysplasia (ulnar clubhand)
  - Characterized by deficiency of the ulna or ulnar carpal structures
  - This type of dysplasia is 10-fold less common than its radial counterpart and is not associated with systemic syndromes.
  - Additional hand anomalies, however, such as a digit absence and syndactyly, are prevalent.
  - Elbow abnormalities are frequently evident.
  - Other musculoskeletal anomalies, including proximal femoral focal deficiency, fibula deficiency, phocomelia, and scoliosis, are also common.
  - Five types recognized:
    - Type 0—deficiencies of hand/carpus only
    - Type I—small ulna with both physes present

- Type II—partially absent ulna
- Type III—completely absent ulna
- Type IV—radiohumeral synostosis
  - General clinical considerations include the position of the hand, function of the thumb, stability of the elbow, and presence of syndactyly.
  - The condition of the thumb is the most important determinant of surgical intervention in ulnar dysplasia.
- Cleft hand
  - Also known as split hand-foot malformation
  - Often bilateral and familial, involves the feet, and has associated absent metacarpals, differentiating it from symbrachydactyly
  - Severity of this anomaly varies widely from a cleft between the middle and ring fingers to absent radial digits and syndactyly of the ulnar digits.
  - Cleft closure and thumb web construction are the top priorities.
  - Syndactyly should be released early.
  - Thumb reconstruction may require web space deepening, tendon transfer, rotational osteotomy, and/or toe-to-hand transfer.
    - Web deepening should not precede cleft closure; it may compromise the flaps for cleft closure.
  - Transverse bones should be removed because they widen the cleft as the child grows.

■ **Failure of differentiation**
▦ Radioulnar synostosis
- Bony bridge between proximal radius and ulna
- Bilateral in over 60%
- Associated with chromosomal abnormalities, particularly duplication of sex chromosomes
- Examination reveals a fixed pronation deformity.
- Radius is wide and bowed, whereas ulna is narrow and straight
- If significant pronation deformity exists, a rotational osteotomy may be done at approximately age 5 for better hand positioning.
▦ Symphalangism (congenital digital stiffness)
- Hereditary symphalangism is autosomal dominant and associated with correctable hearing loss.
  - More common in ulnar digits
- Nonhereditary symphalangism is seen in conjunction with syndactyly, Apert syndrome, and Poland syndrome.
- Appearance and function of the digits may be improved by angular osteotomies toward the end of adolescent growth.
▦ Camptodactyly (congenital digital flexion deformity)
- Classically occurs at small-finger PIP joint
  - Type I seen in infancy and affects the sexes equally
    - Responds to splinting and stretching
  - Type II seen in adolescent girls
    - Deformity results from either abnormal lumbrical insertion or an abnormal FDS origin and/or insertion.
    - If full PIP extension can be achieved actively with the MCP held in flexion, the digit can be explored and the abnormal tendon transferred to the radial lateral band.
  - Type III involves multiple digits with more severe flexion contractures and is usually associated with a syndrome.

- In general, nonoperative treatment is favored for all three types.
- If functional deficit exists after skeletal maturity, corrective osteotomy may improve alignment and function.
- Clinodactyly (congenital curvature of the digit in the radioulnar plane)
  - Small finger most common
  - Type I—most common, minor angulation, normal digit length
  - Type II—present in 25% of children with Down syndrome, minor angulation, short middle phalanx
  - Type III—marked angulation and a delta phalanx
    - C-shaped epiphysis and longitudinally bracketed diaphysis
    - Early excision is performed when the delta phalanx is a separate bone and involved digit is excessively long.
    - Otherwise, opening wedge osteotomy to correct angulation
- Flexed thumb
  - Two main causes: pediatric trigger thumb and congenital clasped thumb
    - Pediatric trigger thumb
      - Common developmental condition
      - Mechanical catching/locking of thumb, may progress to fixed flexion deformity at interphalangeal joint
      - Postural hyperextension of MCP joint
      - Some cases respond to early splinting or may resolve spontaneously.
      - May be surgically treated with A1 pulley release (similar to adult) with low recurrence rate
        - Thumb radial digital nerve in jeopardy as it crosses more centrally near MCP joint flexion crease
    - Congenital clasped thumb
      - Flexion-adduction thumb deformity at MCP joint
      - Typically caused by absent or hypoplastic EPB
      - Supple deformities may be treated by splinting or long/ring FDS tendon transfer to EPB.
      - Rigid variety associated with hypoplastic extensors, MCP joint contractures, UCL deficiency, thenar muscle hypoplasia, and first web space skin deficiency
      - Complex cases may require release of MCP capsule; release of adductor pollicis, flexor pollicis brevis, or first dorsal interosseous; Z-lengthening of the FPL; extensor or opposition tendon transfer; and/or deepening of the first web space.
- Arthrogryposis (congenital curved joints)
  - Results from defect in the motor unit and may be either neurogenic (90%) or myopathic (10%)
  - Immobility in the womb results in symmetric joint contractures.
  - Three types:
    - Type I—single localized deformity such as fixed forearm pronation or complex clasped thumb, which may be surgically corrected in usual fashion
    - Type II—full expression with absence of shoulder musculature, tubular limbs, elbow extension contractures, wrist flexion and ulnar deviation contractures, finger flexion contractures, and thumb adduction contractures
    - Type III—type II contractures plus polydactyly and other organ system involvement
  - Types II and III are treated with a combination of splinting, serial casts, and therapy to decrease the severity of joint contractures.
  - Once passive joint mobility is restored, tendon transfers may be performed.
  - An attempt is made to provide child with functional elbows and wrists; however, arthrodesis may provide improved ability to perform activities of daily living in certain cases.
- Syndactyly
  - Common congenital hand anomaly (1 in 2500 live births) that results from failure of apoptosis to separate digits
  - Classified based on absence (simple) or presence (complex) of bony connections between the involved digits and whether the bony connections are complete or incomplete (Figure 7-74)
  - *Acrosyndactyly* refers to fusion between more distal portions of the digit, often seen in constriction ring syndrome.
  - Pure syndactyly is autosomal dominant, with reduced penetrance and variable expression that yield a positive family history in 10% to 40% of cases.
  - Distribution of digit involvement:
    - Long-ring—50%
    - Ring-small—30%
    - Index-long—15%
    - Thumb-index—5%
  - Release performed at approximately 1 year of age.
  - Rays of unequal length should be released before 6 months.
  - Acrosyndactyly requires distal release in neonatal period.
  - Multiple-digit syndactyly releases are performed in two stages, with only one side of the digit released during one operation to reliably preserve circulation of digit.
  - Full-thickness skin grafting invariably required
  - Possible complications include web creep and nail deformities.
  - Poland and Apert syndromes are commonly tested conditions with associated syndactyly.
- **Duplication**
- **Preaxial polydactyly (thumb duplication)**
  - **Classified by Wassel** (Table 7-14)
    - Type IV is the most common (43%), characterized by duplicated proximal phalanx (Figure 7-75).
  - Thumb duplication usually unilateral, sporadic, and not associated with a syndrome except in type VII
    - Type VII associations include Holt-Oram syndrome, Fanconi anemia, Blackfan-Diamond anemia, hypoplastic anemia, imperforate anus, cleft palate, and tibial defects.
  - Best possible thumb is reconstructed from the available anatomic structures.
  - If duplicate thumbs are of equal size, preserve ulnar thumb to retain ulnar collateral ligament for pinch.
    - Soft tissue from ablated thumb should be preserved and used to augment retained thumb.
  - Most reconstructed thumbs have satisfactory length and girth, but nail deformity and interphalangeal joint angulation are reported problems.

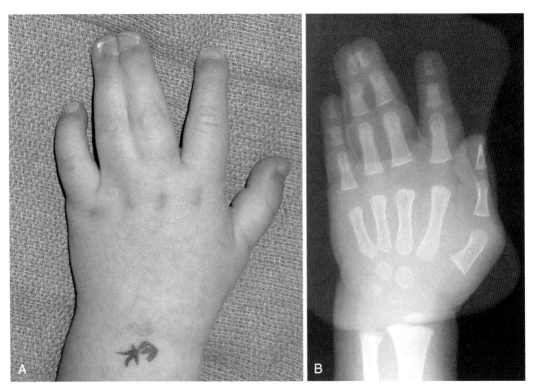

FIGURE 7-74 Clinical **(A)** and radiographic **(B)** images of complex syndactyly. (From Goldfarb CA: Congenital hand anomalies: a review of the literature, 2009-2012, *J Hand Surg Am* 38:1854–1859, 2013.)

Table 7-14	Preaxial Polydactyly Thumb Classification	
TYPE	**DESCRIPTION**	**FREQUENCY**
I	Bifid distal phalanx	2%
II	Duplicated distal phalanx	15%
III	Bifid proximal phalanx	6%
IV	Duplicated proximal phalanx	43% (most common)
V	Bifid metacarpal	10%
VI	Duplicated metacarpal	4%
VII	Triphalangia	20%

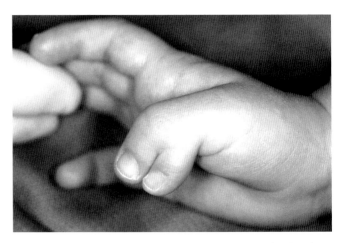

FIGURE 7-75 Type IV duplication with duplicated proximal and distal phalanges that articulate with a bifid metacarpal head. (Courtesy Shriners Hospitals for Children, Philadelphia.)

■ **Postaxial polydactyly (small-finger duplication)**
- Ten times more common in African Americans (1 in 143 live births) than whites (1 in 1339 live births)
  - Autosomal dominant inheritance
  - More extensive genetic workup mandatory in whites because of multiple known chromosomal abnormalities
- Type A is a well-formed duplicated digit.
  - Ulnar digit removed
- Type B is a rudimentary skin tag.
  - May be tied off shortly after birth

■ **Central polydactyly**
- Usually associated with syndactyly
- Early surgery indicated to prevent angular deformity with growth
- Impaired motion may result from interposed digits or symphalangism of adjacent digits.
- Tendons, nerves, and vessels may be shared to the point that only one finger from three skeletons may be obtainable.
- Angular deviation may require ligament reconstruction and/or osteotomy.

■ **Overgrowth**
▓ Macrodactyly
- Characterized by nonhereditary congenital digital enlargement
- Unilateral in 90% of cases; 70% of cases involve multiple digits
- Adult analogue is lipofibromatous hamartoma of the median or other peripheral nerves.
- Angular deviation, joint stiffness, and nerve compression syndromes also occur.
- Static macrodactyly is present at birth, and growth is linear with the adjacent digits.
- Progressive macrodactyly is not always evident at birth, but exponential growth occurs thereafter.

Table 7-15	Blauth Classification of Thumb Hypoplasia
TYPE	**CHARACTERISTICS**
I	Minor hypoplasia with all structures present
II	Normal articulations
	MCP ulnar collateral ligament instability
	Thenar hypoplasia
	Adduction contracture
IIIA	Extensive intrinsic and extrinsic musculotendinous deficiencies
	Normal CMC joint
IIIB	Extensive intrinsic and extrinsic musculotendinous deficiencies
	Abnormal or absent CMC joint
IV	Total or subtotal metacarpal aplasia
	Rudimentary phalanges
	Thumb attached to hand by a skin bridge (pouce flottant)
V	Complete absence of thumb

CMC, Carpometacarpal; *MCP,* metacarpophalangeal.

- Most favorable outcome for severely affected single digit is amputation
- When the thumb or multiple digits are involved, the following procedures may offer improvement:
  - Epiphyseal ablation, angular and/or shortening osteotomies, longitudinal narrowing osteotomies, nerve stripping, and debulking
- Stiffness and neurovascular compromise are common.

■ **Undergrowth**
▨ Thumb hypoplasia
- Classified by Blauth (Table 7-15)
- **Critical structure is CMC joint**
  - Separates type IIIA from type IIIB
  - Determines whether the thumb is reconstructable (II, IIIA) or whether it requires pollicization (IIIB, IV, V)
- Type I is a small thumb with slender bones and normal thenar musculature, which typically requires no treatment.
- Types II and IIIA are treated with stabilization of the MCP joint UCL, web deepening, and extrinsic extensor tendon reconstruction.
- **Types IIIB to V are best treated with index pollicization.**

■ **Amnion disruption sequence (constriction ring syndrome)**
▨ Sporadic occurrence with no evidence of hereditary predisposition
▨ Manifested in four ways:
- Simple constriction rings
- Rings with distal deformity, with or without lymphedema
- Acrosyndactyly
- Amputation
▨ Neonatal surgery is indicated when edema jeopardizes digital circulation.
▨ Release accomplished by multiple circumferential Z-plasties

■ **Generalized skeletal abnormalities**
▨ Congenital dislocation of the radial head
- May be distinguished from traumatic origin by bilateral involvement, other congenital anomalies (60%), and familial occurrence
- Typically irreducible by closed means

- Some helpful radiographic clues include:
  - Hypoplastic capitellum
  - Short ulna with long radius
  - Convex radial head
- Surgical indications include pain, limited motion, and cosmetic dissatisfaction.
  - Radial head excision performed at skeletal maturity
▨ Madelung deformity
- Disruption of volar ulnar physis of distal radius
  - Implicated tethering structure is the Vickers ligament
- As child grows, the distal radius exhibits excessive radial inclination and volar tilt (spectrum of abnormality seen).
- Hypothesized to be due to an X-linked dominant disorder, Léri-Weill dyschondrosteosis, which is a mutation in the short-stature homeobox-containing (*SHOX*) gene
- Early release of Vickers ligament advocated by some
- Often asymptomatic and found incidentally in adulthood after minor wrist injury prompts radiographic examination
- Symptoms arise from ulnocarpal impaction, restricted forearm rotation, and median nerve compression.
  - Corrective osteotomy of the radius with or without distal ulna resection

ELBOW

■ **Articular anatomy**
▨ Ulnohumeral, radiocapitellar, and proximal radioulnar joints
▨ Articular surface of distal humerus angled 30 degrees anterior to humeral shaft axis
▨ Distal humerus consists of medial and lateral columns.
▨ Normal range of elbow flexion/extension: 0 to 150 degrees
▨ Normal forearm pronosupination (rotation): 80 to 85 degrees each direction
▨ **Functional ROM—30 to 130 degrees flexion/ extension and 50 degrees pronosupination**
▨ Normal valgus carrying angle of the elbow is 5 to 10 degrees for men and 10 to 15 degrees for women.
▨ In full extension, 60% of axial load is transmitted through the radiocapitellar joint.

■ **Ligamentous anatomy**
▨ Medial (ulnar) collateral ligament (MCL)
- Anterior, posterior, and transverse bundles (Figure 7-76)
- **Anterior bundle is primary restraint to valgus stress within functional elbow ROM (secondary restraint is radial head)**
- Originates on posterior medial epicondyle, inserts on sublime tubercle of medial coronoid process
- **Posterior bundle is primary restraint to valgus stress with elbow in maximal flexion**
- Stability in full extension is provided by MCL, joint capsule, and ulnohumeral articulation
▨ Lateral collateral ligament (LCL) complex
- Composed of radial collateral ligament (RCL), lateral ulnar collateral ligament (LUCL), accessory collateral ligament, and annular ligament (Figure 7-77)
- LUCL originates on posterior lateral epicondyle and inserts on crista supinatoris of proximal ulna

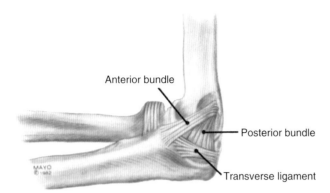

FIGURE 7-76 Anatomic distribution of the medial collateral ligament complex. (Courtesy the Mayo Foundation.)

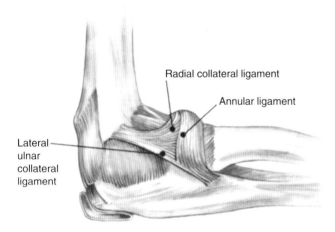

FIGURE 7-77 The lateral collateral ligament complex consists not only of the radial collateral ligament but also a lateral ulnar collateral ligament. (Courtesy the Mayo Foundation.)

- **LUCL is primary restraint to varus and external rotational stress throughout elbow motion**
- **Joint aspiration or injection**
- Best performed through anconeal soft spot laterally
- Between triangle of bony landmarks (Figure 7-78)
  - Radial head
  - Lateral epicondyle
  - Tip of olecranon
- Therapeutic aspiration of hemarthrosis after trauma
- Corticosteroid injection for diagnostic differentiation between intra- and extraarticular pain generators in some cases
- **Elbow imaging**
- Plain radiographs—anteroposterior, lateral, and oblique views
- CT—provides superior bony detail
  - Complex fractures of the distal humerus, radial head and coronoid process; ossified loose bodies, heterotopic ossification
- MRI—provides superior soft tissue detail
  - Ligamentous injuries, occult fractures, osteochondritis dissecans, nonossified loose bodies, tendinous injury, and soft tissue masses

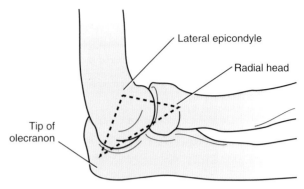

FIGURE 7-78 The anconeal soft spot (lateral infracondylar recess) is the most sensitive area in which to detect a joint effusion, aspirate a hemarthrosis, and/or inject corticosteroid. This triangular area located on the lateral aspect of the elbow is outlined by the radial head, tip of the olecranon, and lateral epicondyle. (From Trumble TE et al, editors: *Core knowledge in orthopaedics: hand, elbow, and shoulder,* Philadelphia, 2006, Mosby, p 489.)

- **Tendon disorders**
- Lateral epicondylitis (tennis elbow)
  - Common tendinopathy of ECRB origin
  - Degenerative rather than inflammatory process
    - Histologic finding: angiofibroblastic hyperplasia
  - Precipitated by repetitive wrist extension and forearm rotation
  - Related to vocation more often than racquet-sport play
  - Lateral elbow pain exacerbated by resisted wrist extension with the elbow extended and the forearm pronated
  - Grip strength diminished with elbow extended as compared to elbow flexed at 90 degrees
  - Treatment
    - Largely nonoperative: avoidance of aggravating activities, antiinflammatories, counterforce bracing, occupational therapy for local modalities (ice, heat, ultrasonography, iontophoresis)
    - Efficacy of corticosteroid injection recently debated
      - Prospective double-blind randomized clinical trial showed no more efficacy than placebo (pain, grip strength, Disabilities of the Arm, Shoulder, and Hand [DASH] score).
      - May actually have long-term detrimental effects
      - Depression and ineffective coping skills strongest predictors of perceived arm-specific disability
    - Extracorporeal shock wave therapy trials show no difference at 6 months compared to placebo.
    - Platelet-rich plasma (PRP) injection of recent interest
    - Operative treatment considered for recalcitrant cases with symptoms lasting longer than 1 year
    - Surgical intervention may be open or arthroscopic.
    - ECRB tendon débridement with or without lateral epicondylectomy
    - Nirschl scratch test—degenerative friable tendon
    - Avoid iatrogenic injury to LUCL.
    - Watertight deep closure to avoid synovial fistula
    - Other causes of lateral elbow pain if surgery fails: LUCL injury, osteochondritis dissecans, radiocapitellar osteoarthrosis, synovial plicae, radial tunnel syndrome

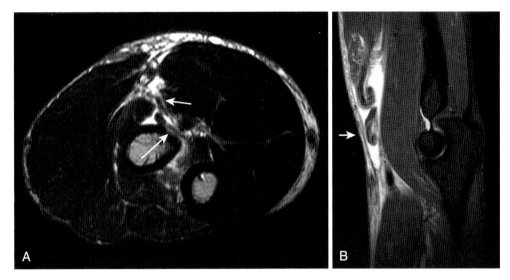

FIGURE 7-79 Distal biceps tendon rupture. **A,** Axial T2-weighted image shows disruption of the distal biceps tendon from its insertion at the radial tuberosity *(long arrow)*, accompanied by surrounding edema and increased fluid within the bicipitoradial bursa *(short arrow)*. **B,** Sagittal T2-weighted image shows a completely torn and retracted distal biceps tendon with surrounding high-intensity fluid and soft tissue edema *(arrow)*. (**A,** Modified from Brunton LM, et al: The elbow. In Khanna AJ, editor: *MRI for orthopaedic surgeons,* New York, 2010, Thieme. **B,** Modified from Brunton LM, et al: Magnetic resonance imaging of the elbow: update on current techniques and indications, *J Hand Surg Am* 31[6]:1001–1011, 2006.)

▦ Medial epicondylitis (golfer's elbow)
- Common tendinopathy of flexor-pronator mass origin
- Pain elicited with resisted forearm pronation and wrist flexion
- Prolonged conservative management recommended because success of surgical débridement is less predictable than it is in lateral epicondylitis
- Always evaluate for associated cubital tunnel syndrome.

▦ Distal biceps tendon injury
- Mechanism—eccentric loading of the flexed elbow during manual labor, weight lifting, or other poorly executed lifting activity
- Almost exclusively in middle-aged males
- Steroid and tobacco use are risk factors.
- Patients may experience a painful "pop" deep in proximal forearm.
- Supination strength is diminished more than flexion strength (biceps is main forearm supinator, brachialis is main elbow flexor).
  - If left untreated, only about 50% supination and 70% flexion strength regained by 1 year
- Biceps muscle belly unlikely to be proximally retracted if lacertus fibrosis (bicipital aponeurosis) remains intact
- Abnormal "hook test"
- MRI may help distinguish partial from complete injuries in equivocal cases (Figure 7-79).
  - May see associated bicipitoradial bursitis with chronic tendinopathy
  - Partial ruptures primarily occur on the radial side of the tuberosity footprint, owing to its function as a supinator.
- Partial injuries initially treated nonoperatively with rest, NSAIDs and therapy but may eventually require detachment, débridement, and reattachment.
- Surgical reattachment to radial tuberosity recommended in active individuals with complete rupture to regain strength

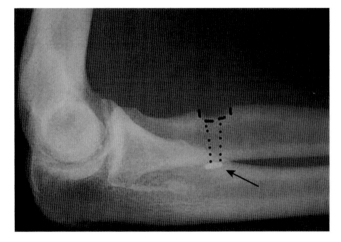

FIGURE 7-80 Lateral x-ray shows Endobutton *(arrow)* in the desired position and orientation on the posterior aspect of the proximal radius. Also visible on the x-ray is the trough *(dashed lines)* and the 4-mm-wide channel *(dotted lines)*. (From Greenberg JA: Endobutton repair of distal biceps tendon ruptures, *J Hand Surg Am* 34:1541–1548, 2009.)

- Single-incision and two-incision techniques described.
  - Classic single-incision risk is neurologic injury (lateral antebrachial cutaneous nerve in up to ≈ 25% of cases).
  - Classic two-incision risk is radioulnar synostosis.
- Bone trough/drill holes, suture anchors, interference screw, Endobutton are all described fixation methods (Figure 7-80).
  - Biomechanical studies have shown Endobutton to have superior strength.
- Chronic injuries (>6 weeks) may require tendon autograft or allograft augmentation; strength recovery diminished as compared to acute reattachment with native tendon.
- Avoid strengthening for approximately 8 to 10 weeks postoperatively.

- Distal triceps tendon injury
  - Less common injury caused by direct blow to posterior elbow or sudden forceful flexion of extended elbow
  - Patients describe posterior elbow pain and swelling and may have a palpable defect proximal to the olecranon tip.
  - Diminished elbow extension strength, although active extension still possible through intact anconeus
    - As many as 50% of these injuries are initially missed.
  - Rupture may occur at musculotendinous junction or olecranon insertion.
  - May be associated with anabolic steroid use, multiple local corticosteroid injections or chronic olecranon bursitis
  - Surgical repair/reattachment for high-grade partial (>50% of tendon width) and complete tears, typically through transosseous tunnels
  - Slow rehabilitation with progressive elbow flexion recovery
- **Elbow trauma**
- Distal humerus fractures
  - Anatomic morphology is two columns with a spool.
  - Most adult fractures involve both columns and articular surface.
  - High-energy trauma in younger patients, low-energy trauma in elderly patients with poor bone quality
  - CT scan helpful to better characterize fracture pattern
  - Nonoperative treatment only recommended for elderly patients with multiple comorbidities and low functional demands; goal is a stiff, painless elbow
  - Vast majority treated by ORIF
  - Approaches include triceps-splitting, triceps-sparing, and olecranon osteotomy.
  - Articular surface reconstructed with headless compression screws and/or lag screws across spool
  - Anatomically precontoured column locking plates available
  - Plates may be applied orthogonally (90-90—direct medial and posterolateral) or parallel with interdigitation of screw threads.
  - **Healthy, active elderly patients with severe articular comminution may be better served by semiconstrained total elbow arthroplasty (TEA) to allow early rehabilitation but are restricted to 10-pound weight-lifting limit for life.**
    - In patients older than age 65, higher Mayo Elbow Performance Score (MEPS) at 2-year follow-up for those randomized to TEA compared to ORIF
- Radial head fracture
  - Lateral elbow pain and swelling after trauma; may be occult on initial plain radiographs (check for fat pad sign)
  - May require aspiration of hemarthrosis and injection of local anesthetic to assess for mechanical block to forearm rotation
  - Classified by Mason, modified by Hotchkiss:
    - Type I—nondisplaced or minimally displaced, no mechanical block
    - Type II—less than 2 mm of articular displacement, with or without mechanical block
    - Type III—comminuted
    - Type IV—associated with elbow dislocation
  - Often difficult to characterize by plain radiographs alone
    - CT may be helpful in borderline cases.

- Associated injuries—MCL, other periarticular fractures
- Always assess forearm and wrist for Essex-Lopresti injury.
- Type I—managed nonoperatively with early motion
- Type II with mechanical block—may require ORIF
- Type III—either ORIF or metallic replacement
- Overstuffing leads to early capitellar wear/late instability.
- Excision contraindicated with incompetent MCL/interosseous membrane
- Essex-Lopresti injury
  - **Longitudinal radioulnar instability caused by sequential injury to the DRUJ, interosseous ligament, and radial head**
  - Radial head injury must either be internally fixed or replaced to prevent proximal migration of radius and resulting ulnocarpal impaction.
  - Treat TFCC pathology concurrently.
  - Notoriously difficult injury to treat
  - Multiple reconstructions of interosseous ligament described, but long-term results unavailable
- Coronoid fractures
  - Occur most often in setting of elbow dislocation
  - Regan and Morrey classification based on size of process fracture
  - O'Driscoll classification more comprehensive; recognizes fractures of the anteromedial facet that may lead to varus posteromedial rotatory instability if left untreated
  - Treat unstable fractures with ORIF.
    - Suture, screw, and miniplate fixation all described
- Olecranon fractures
  - Typically result from direct blow to proximal forearm
  - Proximal fragment displaced by triceps pull
  - Treatment depends on displacement and articular congruity.
  - **Tension band constructs work well for simple transverse fracture patterns but are associated with high rate of symptomatic hardware (>50%).**
  - **Comminuted fractures with articular displacement best treated with ORIF using plate-and-screw construct**
  - **Elderly patients with severely comminuted fractures may benefit from excision of the proximal fragment and reattachment of triceps tendon adjacent to the joint line.**
- Elbow dislocation
  - Most commonly posterolateral
  - Simple or complex (with associated fractures)
  - Closed reduction performed promptly after assessment of neurovascular status
  - Test elbow stability through flexion-extension arc after reduction and immobilize initially at 90 degrees with forearm in pronation.
  - Simple dislocations treated with early ROM within 3 weeks of injury
  - **Persistent instability within 30 degrees of full extension may be indication for acute ligamentous repair**
    - Lateral ligamentous complex always repaired, followed rarely by MCL if instability persists
  - Loss of terminal extension is the most common complication after closed treatment of a simple elbow dislocation.

- "Terrible triad" injury consists of:
  - Elbow dislocation
  - Radial head fracture
  - Coronoid process fracture
  - **Almost always treated with ORIF of coronoid process, ORIF or prosthetic radial head replacement, and lateral and/or medial ligamentous repair**
  - Persistent instability may require hinged external fixator or transarticular ulnohumeral pinning.
  - Early ROM starting with intraoperative arc of stability
    - LCL-repaired and MCL-intact elbow kept in forearm pronation to increase stability
    - LCL-repaired but MCL-deficient elbow kept in forearm supination to increase stability
    - LCL- and MCL-repaired elbow kept in neutral
- Monteggia fracture-dislocations
  - Proximal-third ulnar fracture accompanied by radial head subluxation/dislocation
  - Bado classification types I to IV
  - Anatomic reduction of the proximal ulna usually reduces the radial head.
  - Persistent proximal radioulnar instability may require annular ligament reconstruction.
- Elbow instability
- Posterolateral rotatory instability
  - Caused by incompetence of the LUCL
  - Patients relate history of previous elbow dislocation treated nonoperatively.
  - Pain and subjective instability
  - LCL-deficient elbow more stable in forearm pronation
  - Lateral pivot shift test
    - Reproduces instability with combination of supination, axial compression, and valgus loading as elbow is brought from full extension to 40 degrees of flexion
    - Ulna rotates externally on trochlea and produces posterior radial head subluxation.
    - With increasing flexion, the triceps becomes taut and the radial head reduces with palpable clunk.
    - Patient apprehension is common, and either intraarticular local anesthetic or examination under general anesthesia may be necessary to confirm diagnosis.
  - MRI shows LUCL pathology in approximately 50% of cases.
  - Chronic instability may require reconstruction of the LUCL with tendon autograft.
- Varus posteromedial rotatory instability
  - Increasingly recognized but poorly understood entity
  - Results from fracture of anteromedial coronoid process
  - Treatment requires ORIF of coronoid with buttress plate, assessment of MCL insertion
- Valgus instability
  - May be acute after elbow trauma or chronic from repetitive loading and attenuation of the MCL
    - In baseball, the late cocking and acceleration phases of throwing places the highest stress on the MCL.
  - Primary ligamentous repair or reattachment with suture anchors only possible in acute setting
  - Chronic instability and dysfunction common in overhead-throwing athletes such as baseball pitchers or javelin throwers

- Valgus extension overload
  - Pain during deceleration phase as elbow reaches terminal extension
  - Osteophytes of the posteromedial olecranon process block full extension.
- Surrounding muscle stabilizers may mask clinical valgus instability in 50% of cases; FCU is the primary dynamic stabilizer, and FDS is a secondary stabilizer.
- MRI to evaluate MCL, flexor-pronator mass, adjacent bone (especially in pediatric population) (Figure 7-81)
- Ulnar neuritis/cubital tunnel syndrome may also be present.
- May attempt gradual rehabilitation with symptomatic treatment, maintenance of elbow motion, local modalities, and gradual return to throwing protocol
- MCL reconstruction with tendon autograft may be indicated in competitive athletes (Tommy John surgery) who fail a trial of nonoperative treatment (Figure 7-82).
- Nearly 75% to 80% of patients return to sports at the same level or better 1 year after reconstruction
- Unrecognized or untreated MCL insufficiency may lead to capitellar wear, posteromedial impingement, olecranon osteophyte formation, and loose-body formation (valgus overload syndrome).
- Arthroscopic débridement of osteophytes and loose body removal may be effective.
- Elbow contracture
- Stiffness and loss of motion frequent complications after elbow injury
- Aggressive motion recovery started as soon as possible
- Loss of 30 degrees terminal extension well tolerated in general population
- Loss of flexion interferes with activities of daily living (<130 degrees)
- Intrinsic factors
  - Articular incongruity (malunion, OA, OCD), loose bodies, synovitis
- Extrinsic factors
  - Heterotopic ossification, muscle fibrosis, hardware impingement, ligamentous/capsular contracture
- Aggressive therapy
- Dynamic/static progressive splinting
- Arthroscopic versus open treatment depending on primary pathology
- Elbow arthritis
- Rheumatoid arthritis
  - Most prevalent type of elbow arthritis
  - Elbow affected in up to 50% of patients with RA
  - Chronic inflammation and synovitis lead to ligament attenuation, periarticular osteopenia, and joint contracture.
  - Medical management is mainstay
  - Synovectomy and radial head resection is historically good short term.
  - Semiconstrained total elbow arthroplasty for more permanent pain relief and preserved function
    - Complication rate must be considered.
    - Infection rate
    - Implant failure requiring revision
    - Periprosthetic fracture

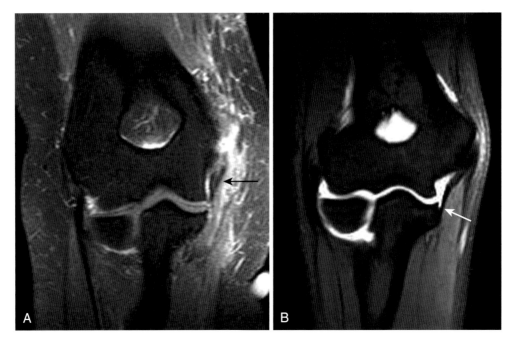

FIGURE 7-81 Tears of the medial collateral ligament. **A,** Complete tear of the medial collateral ligament. Coronal fat-suppressed T2-weighted image shows discontinuity of the ligament with surrounding edema and hemorrhage *(arrow)*. **B,** Partial tear of the medial collateral ligament. Coronal fat-suppressed T1-weighted arthrogram shows a "T sign," with leakage of intraarticular contrast material at the undersurface of the ligament at its distal insertion on the sublime tubercle *(arrow)*. (**A,** Modified from Brunton LM, et al: Magnetic resonance imaging of the elbow: update on current techniques and indications, *J Hand Surg Am* 31[6]:1001–1011, 2006. **B,** Modified from Brunton LM, et al: The elbow. In Khanna AJ, editor: *MRI for orthopaedic surgeons*, New York, 2010, Thieme.)

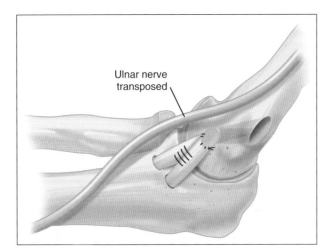

Ulnar nerve transposed

FIGURE 7-82 Medial collateral ligament reconstruction. A tendon graft is passed through tunnels and sutured in place. (From Miller MD, Thompson SR, editors: *Delee & Drez's orthopaedic sports medicine: principles and practice*, ed 4, Philadelphia, 2015, Elsevier Saunders, p 791.)

▓ Posttraumatic ulnotrochlear/radiocapitellar arthritis
  • Second most common type of elbow arthritis
  • Typically young patients who fail conservative management treated by:
    • Arthroscopic or open débridement of osteophytes, abrasion chondroplasty, and removal of loose bodies
    • Ulnohumeral arthroplasty, also known as Outerbridge-Kashiwagi (O-K) procedure, describes removal of anterior elbow osteophytes by trephination of the distal humerus from a posterior approach through the olecranon fossa (Figure 7-83).
    • Interposition arthroplasty with autograft (tensor fascia latae) or allograft (Achilles)

▓ Primary osteoarthritis
  • Least common form of elbow arthritis
  • Typically affects middle-aged male laborers
  • Pain at extremes of motion
  • Osteophyte formation may lead to mechanical block of motion.
  • Open or arthroscopic débridement to delay arthroplasty
  • Postoperative continuous passive motion not shown to add benefit postoperatively
▓ **Charcot elbow (neuroarthropathy)**
  • Associated with syringomyelia
  • MRI of the cervical spine and electrodiagnostic evaluation are paramount.
▓ Total elbow arthroplasty
  • Indications
    • Refractory RA
    • Advanced osteoarthritis (primary and posttraumatic)
    • Chronic instability
    • Complex distal humerus fractures in elderly patients
  • TEA is contraindicated in the setting of prior or chronic infection, in which primary arthrodesis is favored.
  • Patients have lifelong weight-lifting restriction of 10 pounds.
  • Two primary types:
    • Unconstrained (unlinked) and semiconstrained (linked)
      • Unconstrained TEA theoretically better for osteoarthritis with competent collateral ligaments and good bone quality
    • Semiconstrained TEA acts as "sloppy hinge" with limited rotational and coronal plane motion.
      • Best for RA, chronic instability, and distal humerus fractures in elderly patients

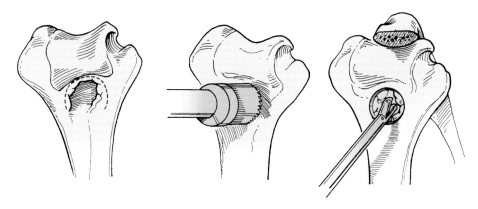

FIGURE 7-83 Outerbridge-Kashiwagi procedure (ulnohumeral arthroplasty) performed through a triceps-splitting approach. The coronoid is approached through a Cloward drill hole in the olecranon fossa. The olecranon can also be débrided with this approach. (From Miller MD et al: *Review of sports medicine and arthroscopy,* Philadelphia, 1995, WB Saunders, p 180.)

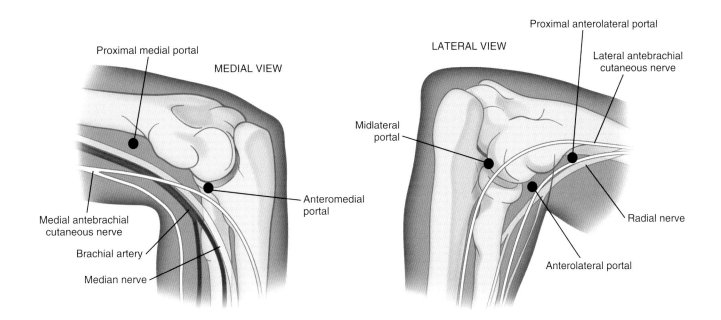

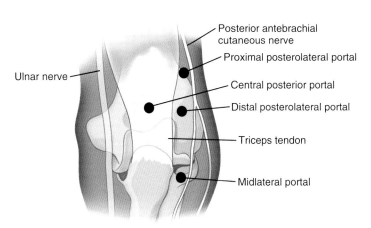

FIGURE 7-84 Arthroscopic portals for elbow arthroscopy. (From Miller MD et al: *Orthopaedic surgical approaches,* Philadelphia, 2008, Elsevier.)

- Pain relief is reliable.
- Surgical approaches may split or spare triceps; ulnar nerve transposed anteriorly and radial head often resected
- A competent extensor mechanism is critical for good functional outcome.
- Complications of TEA include infection, nerve injury, instability, periprosthetic fracture, and implant loosening from polyethylene wear.
- **Staged reimplantation after infection has a poor salvage rate.**

ELBOW ARTHROSCOPY

- Current indications include diagnosis of suspected pathology, removal of loose bodies, treatment of osteochondritis dissecans, osteophyte débridement, capsular release, synovectomy, assistance for intraarticular fracture fixation, and lateral epicondylitis.
- **Requires extreme caution because the potential for neurovascular injury is far higher at the elbow as compared to other joints treated arthroscopically**
- The most common transient nerve palsy after elbow arthroscopy is an ulnar nerve palsy. Meticulous care is taken in patients who have undergone prior ulnar nerve surgery and in patients with chronic elbow contractures.
- Superficial radial nerve, posterior interosseous nerve, medial antebrachial cutaneous nerve, and anterior interosseous nerve palsies have also been reported.
- The brachial artery and median nerve are also at risk during aggressive anterior capsular releases.
- The overall rate of neurologic injury is cited as 0% to 14%. Risk is minimized by keeping the elbow at 90 degrees of flexion, joint insufflation, using far proximal portals, avoiding posteromedial portals, using a nick-and-spread technique, and appreciating scenarios that are particularly dangerous, such as patients with distorted anatomy, inflammatory arthritis, or heterotopic ossification.
- **Commonly used portals** (Figure 7-84)
  - Anteromedial portal: placed under direct visualization 2 cm distal and 2 cm anterior to the medial epicondyle. The medial antebrachial cutaneous and median nerves are at risk.
  - Proximal anteromedial portal: placed 2 cm proximal to the medial epicondyle and 1 cm anterior to the medial intermuscular septum. The medial antebrachial cutaneous nerve is the most at risk.
  - Proximal anterolateral portal: placed 2 cm proximal and 1 to 2 cm anterior to the lateral epicondyle. The lateral antebrachial cutaneous and radial nerves are less at risk than a standard anterolateral portal, which is described as 3 cm distal and 1 cm anterior to the lateral epicondyle.
  - Straight posterior (transtriceps) portal: placed 3 cm proximal to the olecranon tip and centered to pass through the olecranon fossa
  - Posterolateral portals: variably placed just lateral to the triceps tendon and anywhere from 1 to 4 cm proximal to the olecranon tip. The closest nerve is the posterior antebrachial cutaneous.

SELECTED BIBLIOGRAPHY

The selected bibliography for this chapter can be found on https://expertconsult.inkling.com.

TESTABLE CONCEPTS

I. Anatomy

- Flexor tendon nutrition is via direct vascular supply (vincula) and synovial diffusion.
- The carpal tunnel contains the median nerve and nine flexor tendons (one FPL, four FDS and four FDP).
  - FPL is most radial, whereas the long and ring FDS tendons are volar to index and small FDS.
- Lumbrical muscles originate on the radial aspect of FDP tendons and pass volar to transverse metacarpal ligaments to insert on the radial aspect of the extensor hood lateral bands.
- Intrinsic tightness commonly occurs in cerebral palsy, rheumatoid arthritis (RA), and following trauma.
  - The intrinsic tightness test demonstrates decreased proximal interphalangeal (PIP) flexion with the metacarpophalangeal (MCP) held in extension.

II. Distal Radius Fractures

- Examination of a patient with a distal radius fracture should include evaluation for concurrent ulnar-sided and anatomic snuffbox tenderness, as well as assessment of median and ulnar nerve function.
  - Acute carpal tunnel syndrome (evolving paresthesias and disproportionate pain) requires emergency release.
- Radiographic evaluation follows the 11-22-11 guide:
  - Radial height-11 mm; radial inclination-22 degrees; volar tilt-11 degrees
  - Assess ulnar variance; load sharing across the radius and ulna is significantly altered in an ulnar-positive wrist (more force across ulna).
- Acceptable reduction parameters:
  - Radial shortening less than 3 mm
  - Dorsal articular tilt less than 10 degrees
  - Intraarticular step-off less than 2 mm
- Closed treatment is indicated for minimally displaced injuries, but joint stiffness, muscle atrophy, and disuse osteopenia may result from prolonged immobilization.
- Open reduction with internal fixation (ORIF) through a volar approach is best for volarly displaced fractures (Smith and volar Barton) but has also become standard for dorsally displaced fractures (Colles) and some intraarticular fracture patterns.
- Direct visualization of the articular surface is best from a dorsal exposure.
- The most common complication after distal radius fracture is median nerve dysfunction.
- EPL tendon rupture most commonly occurs as a late complication following closed treatment due to attritional wear and/or vascular insufficiency near the Lister tubercle.
  - Treat with EIP-to-EPL tendon transfer, because primary repair is not possible.
- FPL rupture is the most common flexor injury after volar plating, typically due to poor plate position (too distal and volar).
- EPL may also be injured by dorsally prominent screws.

III. Carpal Fractures and Instability

- Scaphoid fractures are the most commonly injured carpal bone and are at risk for nonunion, osteonecrosis, and posttraumatic osteoarthrosis if neglected or poorly treated.
  - Acute operative indications include more than 1 mm displacement, intrascaphoid angle greater than 35 degrees (humpback deformity), and trans-scaphoid perilunate dislocation.
  - Proximal pole fracture is a relative operative indication.

- Minimally displaced fractures may be treated with headless compression screw fixation, commonly performed by percutaneous or limited open incision methods.
- Formal ORIF is recommended for displaced injuries or those treated in a delayed fashion.
- Guide pin placement should be along the central axis of both the proximal and distal fragments.
- Volar approach potentially avoids disruption of the primary dorsal blood supply of the scaphoid.
- Scaphoid nonunion may be treated with ORIF and bone grafting (multiple techniques, vascularized vs. non-vascularized).
  - Untreated, chronic scaphoid nonunion may lead to posttraumatic osteoarthrosis (SNAC wrist).
  - The radioscaphoid joint is affected first, followed by the scaphocapitate and lunocapitate; the radiolunate joint is spared the longest.
- Hook-of-hamate fractures are due to blunt trauma to the palm, often associated with stick or racquet sports.
  - A carpal tunnel view or computed tomographic (CT) scan is diagnostic.
  - Failure of cast immobilization can be salvaged with fragment excision.
- Carpal instability can be broadly classified into four types:
  - Carpal instability dissociative
  - Dorsal intercalated segmental instability (DISI)
  - Volar intercalated segmental instability (VISI)
  - Carpal instability nondissociative
  - Carpal instability adaptive
  - Carpal instability complex
- DISI is the most common form of carpal instability (increased SL angle).
  - Scapholunate ligament disruption
  - Dorsal portion strongest
  - Untreated chronic instability may result in scapholunate advanced collapse (SLAC) wrist with stages of involvement similar to SNAC wrist.
- VISI is the second most common (decreased SL angle)
  - Lunotriquetral ligament disruption
  - Volar portion strongest
  - Natural history less clear
- Perilunate dislocations are an example of carpal instability complex.
  - Mayfield described four stages of progressive disruption:
  - I—scapholunate
  - II—midcarpal
  - III—lunotriquetral
  - IV—circumferential
- Prompt treatment with closed reduction (especially if acute carpal tunnel syndrome)
- Definitive treatment with ORIF using dorsal ± volar approach

IV. Metacarpal and Phalangeal Injuries

- The majority of metacarpal and phalangeal injuries can be treated nonoperatively.
- General indications for operative intervention include displaced fractures, intraarticular fractures, digit malrotation, open injuries and multiple fractures.
- Bennett fracture is an intraarticular fracture-dislocation of the thumb metacarpal base.
  - APL and thumb extensors cause proximal, dorsal and radial displacement of the metacarpal shaft.
  - The "beak" ligament keeps the volar-ulnar base fragment *reduced* to the trapezium.

TESTABLE CONCEPTS

- Skier's or gamekeeper's thumb describe acute and chronic injuries, respectively, to the thumb MCP joint ulnar collateral ligament (UCL).
  - Following radiograph, stress joint with radial deviation both at neutral and 30 degrees of flexion.
  - Instability in 30 degrees of flexion indicates injury to proper UCL.
  - In over 85% of cases, a complete injury is accompanied by a Stener lesion, in which the adductor pollicis aponeurosis is interposed between the avulsed UCL and its insertion site on the base of the proximal phalanx.
- PIP dislocations most commonly occur dorsally and result from volar plate and collateral ligament injury.
  - Volar PIP dislocation requires disruption of the central slip and must be splinted in full extension following reduction to prevent a boutonnière deformity.
  - Rotatory PIP dislocation occurs when one of the phalangeal condyles is buttonholed between the central slip and a lateral band.
- PIP fracture-dislocations are classified based on the amount of middle phalanx (P2) articular surface involvement.
  - A volar P2 base fragment with less than 30% involvement is usually stable enough for nonoperative management, initially in a dorsal block splint.
  - Unstable injuries with larger P2 base fragments often require operative intervention, such as dorsal block pinning, ORIF, hemihamate reconstruction, or volar plate arthroplasty.
- Irreducible MCP and DIP dislocations are typically due to interposition of the volar plate; treatment is via open reduction and extraction of the volar plate.

V. Tendon Injuries and Overuse Syndromes

- Mallet finger is treated with DIP extension splinting if detected within approximately 12 weeks of injury.
  - A relative surgical indication is a displaced bony mallet injury with significant volar subluxation of P3.
- Dorsal injury over the PIP may disrupt the central slip insertion.
  - Lateral bands subluxate volarly.
  - Acute boutonnière deformity results in a posture of PIP flexion and DIP hyperextension.
  - Chronic boutonnière deformity may be addressed by central slip reconstruction if the deformity is flexible.
- Open "fight bites" over the MCP extensor hood are best treated with surgical débridement and IV antibiotics, owing to concern for infection by oral flora.
- Partial flexor tendon lacerations should be trimmed if painful triggering occurs within the tendon sheath.
- Lacerations with over 60% involvement necessitate primary repair.
- Fundamental principles of flexor tendon repair:
  - Strength of repair proportional to number of core suture strands that cross repair site
  - A locking-loop configuration decreases gap formation.
  - Dorsally placed core sutures are stronger.
  - Epitendinous repair increases overall repair strength by up to 50%.
- Early protected ROM is advocated to increase tendon excursion, decrease adhesion formation, and increase repair strength.
  - Active flexion protocols require a minimum four-strand core repair.
  - Young children cannot comply with therapy and require cast immobilization for 4 weeks.

- Closed flexor tendon injury from forced DIP extension during grasping is termed a "jersey" finger (closed FDP avulsion in zone 1 distal to the FDS insertion).
  - Profundus advancement of 1 cm or more carries a risk of DIP joint flexion contracture or quadrigia.
  - Quadrigia occurs because the middle-ring-small FDP tendons share a common muscle belly, and distal advancement of one tendon will compromise flexion of the adjacent digits, resulting in forearm pain.
- Adult trigger finger (stenosing flexor tenosynovitis) should be treated surgically with release of A1 pulley when conservative management fails.
  - Preserve A2 pulley in digits and oblique pulley in thumb.
  - High association with diabetes and rheumatologic disease
  - Diabetics respond less favorably to corticosteroid injection management.
- Pediatric trigger thumb is more common than pediatric trigger finger.
  - May present with fixed flexion deformity of the thumb interphalangeal joint and generally requires release of the A1 pulley
  - Pediatric trigger finger may stem from aberrant anatomy, and A1 pulley release alone may not sufficiently resolve triggering (add FDS ulnar slip excision).
- de Quervain tenosynovitis of the first extensor compartment often affects middle-aged women, new mothers, and golfers.
  - Corticosteroid injection is successful in more than 80% of patients.
  - Intraoperative findings at the time of compartment release often reveal multiple slips of the APL tendon and a separate dorsal compartment for the EPB tendon.
- Intersection syndrome is a tendinopathy occurring at the junction between the first and second extensor compartments.
  - Commonly affects rowers and generally treated nonoperatively

VI. Distal Radioulnar Joint, Triangular Fibrocartilage Complex, and Wrist Arthroscopy

- Components of the triangular fibrocartilage complex (TFCC) include the dorsal and volar radioulnar ligaments, the articular disc, a meniscus homologue, the extensor carpi ulnaris (ECU) subsheath, and the origins of the ulnolunate and ulnotriquetral ligaments.
- Acute (class I) tears are most commonly avulsions at the ulnar periphery (type IB).
  - No clear clinical outcome differences between open and arthroscopic repair techniques
- Degenerative (class II) tears are associated with positive ulnar variance and ulnocarpal impaction syndrome.
  - In the absence of DRUJ osteoarthrosis, the most commonly performed procedure is arthroscopic débridement and ulnar shortening osteotomy.
- Posttraumatic DRUJ osteoarthritis may be treated with hemiresection interposition arthroplasty, Darrach resection, Sauve-Kapandji arthrodesis or prosthetic arthroplasty.

VII. Nail and Fingertip Injuries

- Nail bed injuries with less than 50% subungual hematoma may be treated without nail plate removal (nail trephination for pain relief).
- Nail bed injuries with greater than 50% subungual hematoma may be treated with nail plate removal and repair of underlying nail matrix lacerations.

TESTABLE CONCEPTS

- Fingertip injury treatment guided by orientation of amputation, degree of soft tissue loss and presence or absence of exposed bone
  - Secondary intention if wound less than 1 cm^2 without exposed bone
  - Larger wounds without exposed bone may require skin graft.
  - Exposed bone
  - Volar oblique injury treated by cross-finger or thenar flap
  - Transverse or dorsal oblique injury treated by V-Y advancement (digit) or Moberg advancement flap (thumb) to preserve skeletal length; alternative treatment is skeletal shortening and closure at level with available skin
  - Dorsal thumb injury may require kite flap from the index (based on first dorsal metacarpal artery).
- Shortening and closing an injury that acutely violates the FDP insertion may result in a lumbrical-plus finger.
  - FDP tendon retracts and creates tension on the extensor mechanism through its intact lumbrical origin, causing paradoxical PIP joint extension with active finger flexion.
  - Treat with release of the radial lateral band.

VIII. Soft Tissue Coverage and Microsurgery

- Full-thickness skin grafts are preferred for volar hand and fingertip wounds, because they are more durable, contract less, and provide better sensibility.
- Primary indications for replantation:
  - Level of amputation outside of zone II flexor tendon sheath, multiple digits, thumb, proximal amputations and any injury in a child
- Primary contraindications to replantation:
  - Level of amputation within zone II flexor tendon sheath, single digit amputation (except thumb), segmental, crush, prolonged ischemia, multisystem injuries
- Factor most predictive of digit survival after replantation is mechanism of injury
- Most frequent cause of early (within 12 hours) replantation failure is arterial thrombosis
  - Consider releasing constricting bandages, place extremity in dependent position, administer heparin, and perform stellate ganglion block.
- Failure after 12 hours is typically due to venous congestion or thrombosis.
  - Consider leech therapy and provide antibiotic prophylaxis against *Aeromonas hydrophila.*
- Tenolysis is the most commonly performed secondary procedure following successful replantation.

IX. Vascular Disorders

- Allen test is used to determine the presence or absence of a complete arch in the palm; approximately 20% of people have an incomplete arch.
- Hypothenar hammer syndrome is the most common posttraumatic vascular occlusive condition of the upper extremity, involving the ulnar artery in the proximal palm.
  - Treatment may include resection of the thrombosed segment and interposition vein graft or arterial conduit (better patency rate).
- Vasospastic disease with a known underlying cause is termed *Raynaud phenomenon.*
- Vasospastic disease *without* a known underlying cause is termed *Raynaud disease.*

- There are 10 hand compartments: thenar, hypothenar, adductor pollicis, four dorsal interosseous, and three volar interosseous (carpal tunnel is not a compartment).
- The FDP and FPL muscles are most vulnerable in Volkmann ischemic contracture.

X. Compression Neuropathy

Median Nerve

- Carpal tunnel syndrome is typically idiopathic in adults, but mucopolysaccharidosis is the most common association in children.
  - Single corticosteroid injection yields transient relief in approximately 80% after 6 weeks, but only 20% are symptom free by 1 year.
  - Operative techniques vary but common theme is division of transverse carpal ligament; neurolysis and flexor tenosynovectomy confer no additional benefit
  - Endoscopic carpal tunnel release may be associated with less early scar tenderness, improved short-term function, and better patient satisfaction scores in some studies; long-term results are largely equivalent to traditional open release.
  - Chronic severe cases in older adults may have incomplete neurologic recovery after surgery.
- *Pronator syndrome* is a compression of the median nerve in the arm/forearm.
  - Potential sites of compression: supracondylar process, ligament of Struthers (courses between the supracondylar process and medial epicondyle), lacertus fibrosis, between the two heads of pronator teres muscle, FDS aponeurotic arch
  - May be differentiated from carpal tunnel syndrome by presence of more proximal forearm pain and paresthesias that include the distribution of the palmar cutaneous branch of the median nerve
- Anterior interosseous nerve syndrome
  - Involves motor loss of FPL, index ± long FDP, and pronator quadratus

Ulnar Nerve

- Cubital tunnel syndrome may manifest as pain, numbness, weakness.
  - Potential sites of compression: arcade of Struthers, medial head of triceps, medial intermuscular septum, Osborne ligament, anconeus epitrochlearis, between two heads of FCU, aponeurosis of FDS proximal edge
  - Recent meta-analyses of techniques fail to show statistically significant difference in outcome between simple in situ decompression and transposition.
- Ulnar tunnel syndrome (compression in Guyon canal) is usually secondary to an extrinsic mass (e.g., ganglion, lipoma, aneurysm, etc.).

Radial Nerve

- Proper radial nerve palsy ("Saturday night palsy") is differentiated from PIN compression by additional weakness of proper radial nerve–innervated muscles, such as triceps, brachioradialis, and ECRL.
- PIN compression syndrome symptoms include distal muscle weakness
  - Potential sites of compression: fascial band at the radial head, recurrent leash of Henry, proximal edge of the ECRB tendon, arcade of Frohse (proximal edge of supinator), distal edge of supinator

TESTABLE CONCEPTS

- Radial tunnel syndrome is marked by lateral proximal forearm pain rather than distal motor weakness of the hand and wrist.
  - Sites of compression same as PIN syndrome
  - Outcome of surgical decompression less predictable than for PIN syndrome
- *Cheiralgia paresthetica* describes compressive neuropathy of the superficial sensory branch of the radial nerve.

Thoracic Outlet

- Vascular—subclavian vein compression
- Neurogenic—entrapment of the lower brachial plexus
  - Nonspecific paresthesias, fatigue
  - Rule out Pancoast tumor with chest radiograph.
  - Maximize nonoperative management.
  - Resection of cervical rib if present

XI. Nerve Injuries and Tendon Transfers

- Seddon classification divides nerve injury into neurapraxia, axonotmesis, and neurotmesis (increasing severity).
- Peripheral nerve repairs are best when performed early, free of tension, clean wound bed
  - No technique deemed superior
  - Gaps may be addressed with nerve conduit, decellularized nerve allograft, or autograft
- Nerve transfers considered for irreparable nerve injuries
  - Advantage is providing shorter innervation distance to end-target muscle
  - Classic nerve transfers for upper brachial plexus injury
- Ulnar motor branch to FCU coapted to musculocutaneous nerve (elbow flexion)
- Descending branch of spinal accessory nerve coapted to suprascapular nerve (shoulder abduction)
- Radial nerve motor branch to triceps coapted to axillary nerve (shoulder abduction)
- Volitional control most important predictor of success in cerebral palsy patients undergoing surgery to augment upper extremity function
- Basic tenets of tendon transfers:
  - Donor must be expendable.
  - Donor must be of similar excursion and power.
  - One transfer should perform one function.
  - Synergistic transfers are easier to rehabilitate.
  - A straight line of pull is optimal.
  - One grade of motor strength will be lost after transfer.
- Tendon transfers for high radial nerve palsy
  - Wrist extension—PT to ECRB
  - Finger extension—FCU or FCR to EDC
  - Thumb extension—PL to EPL
- Tendon transfer (opponensplasty) options for low median nerve palsy
  - FDS of ring, EIP, abductor digiti minimi, PL—all transferred to APB

XII. Arthritis

- Osteoarthritis of the hand commonly affects the DIP, PIP, and thumb CMC.
- Thumb CMC joint (basal joint or trapeziometacarpal) is theorized to result from anterior oblique ligament attenuation.
  - Trapeziectomy with ligament reconstruction and tendon interposition most common reconstructive surgery for late-stage disease

- Rheumatoid arthritis is a systemic autoimmune disease that often affects the synovium surrounding small joints of the hand and wrist.
  - Manifestations include rheumatoid nodules, tenosynovitis, tendon rupture, ulnar MCP drift, swan neck/ boutonnière deformities, caput ulnae, carpal subluxation, and SLAC wrist.
  - *Vaughan-Jackson syndrome* describes progressive rupture of extensor tendons, starting with EDM and continuing radially, from attrition over a prominent distal ulnar head.
  - *Mannerfelt syndrome* describes rupture of FPL and/or index FDP secondary to attrition over a volar STT osteophyte.
  - Common procedures include synovectomy/tenosynovectomy, tendon transfers, extensor centralization at MCP joints, silicone arthroplasty, and wrist arthrodesis versus wrist arthroplasty.

XIII. Idiopathic Osteonecrosis of the Carpus

- Kienböck disease (idiopathic osteonecrosis of the lunate) is most common in young men and presents with nontraumatic dorsal wrist pain and decreased grip strength.
- Unexplained dorsal wrist pain in a young adult with negative ulnar variance should prompt MRI evaluation.
  - Lichtman classification directs treatment, particularly between stage IIIA (lunate collapse with normal carpal alignment and height) and stage IIIB (fixed scaphoid rotation with decreased carpal height and proximal migration of capitate).
- First-line surgical treatment is a joint-leveling procedure.
  - In patients with ulnar-negative variance, radial-shortening osteotomy is preferred.
  - Supplemental vascularized bone grafting has been described.
- Treatment of symptomatic stage IIIB is a salvage procedure for associated carpal instability and/or degenerative osteoarthrosis (partial wrist fusion or proximal row carpectomy)

XIV. Dupuytren Disease

- Benign fibroproliferative disorder that is sometimes inherited and sometimes sporadic
- Myofibroblasts are the predominant cell type found histologically in Dupuytren fascia, and their contractile properties are abnormal and exaggerated.
- Cleland ligaments are not involved.
- Spiral cord is clinically most important leading to PIP contracture
  - Neurovascular bundle at risk during surgery from central and superficial displacement
- Surgical indications include inability to place hand flat on tabletop (Hueston test), MCP flexion contracture greater than 30 degrees, or any PIP flexion contracture.
- Open limited fasciectomy is generally the preferred technique.
- Emerging nonoperative treatment: collagenase injection and cord manipulation
  - Pooled studies show average MCP correction up to 85% and PIP correction up to 60%.
  - Pain, swelling, and bruising are likely temporary adverse effects of injection.
  - Skin tears are more common complications than flexor tendon rupture.

XV. Hand Tumors

- Ganglions are the most common soft tissue mass of the hand and wrist.
  - Dorsal wrist—scapholunate articulation
  - Volar wrist—radioscaphoid or STT joint

- IP joint—osteophyte
- Distal palm–flexor tendon sheath
- Giant cell tumor of tendon sheath is the second most common soft tissue tumor and presents as a slow-growing firm mass often on the volar aspect of a digit.
  - Treatment is marginal excision, but recurrence rate is relatively high.
- Other soft tissue tumors for differential diagnosis include epidermal inclusion cyst, lipoma, schwannoma, glomus, hemangioma, pyogenic granuloma.
- Must-know hand tumors:
  - Most common malignancy—squamous cell carcinoma
  - Most common sarcomas—epithelioid and synovial
  - Most common benign bone tumor—enchondroma
  - Most common malignant bone tumor—metastatic lung carcinoma
  - Most common malignant primary bone tumor—chondrosarcoma

XVI. Hand Infections

- *Staphylococcus aureus* is the most common pathogen.
- Gram-negative and anaerobic bacteria are seen in intravenous drug abusers (IVDAs), diabetic patients, and after farmyard injuries or bite wounds.
- Human bites are a potentially serious infection treated promptly with incision and drainage, especially if joint or tendon sheath is violated.
  - Most frequently isolated organisms are group A streptococci, *S. aureus, Eikenella corrodens,* and *Bacteroides* spp.
- Dog bites occur more frequently than cat bites, but cat bites more commonly result in serious infections that require surgical intervention.
  - Cover *Pasteurella multocida, Staphylococcus,* and *Streptococcus* with ampicillin/sulbactam and amoxicillin/clavulanate.
- Pyogenic flexor tenosynovitis is a suppurative infection of the flexor tendon sheath.
  - Kanavel signs: flexed resting posture of digit, fusiform swelling of the digit, tenderness of flexor tendon sheath, pain with passive digit extension
  - If recognized early, patient should be admitted and treated with splinting, IV antibiotics, and close observation
  - If signs improve within first 24 hours, surgery may be avoided.
  - Otherwise proceed with incision and drainage of flexor tendon sheath.
- Mortality rate of necrotizing fasciitis correlates with time to initiation of treatment.
- A herpetic whitlow is commonly seen in toddlers, dental hygienists, and healthcare workers and treated nonoperatively.
- Atypical mycobacterial infections such as *Mycobacterium marinum* commonly involve the hand.
  - Treatment generally requires surgical débridement and oral antibiotics such as ethambutol, trimethoprim-sulfamethoxazole, clarithromycin, azithromycin, or tetracycline.
- High-pressure injection injuries can be devastating, with a high rate of digital amputation when the solvent is organic or paint is oil-based.

XVII. Congenital Hand Differences

- The three signaling centers that control limb development are the apical ectodermal ridge, zone of polarizing activity formation, and wingless-type pathway.
  - The apical ectodermal ridge controls proximal-to-distal growth.

- The zone of polarizing activity formation controls radial-to-ulnar growth.
- Wingless-type controls dorsal-to-volar growth.
- Radial clubhand is associated with a variety of systemic problems, including TAR syndrome, Holt-Oram syndrome, VACTERL syndrome, and life-threatening Fanconi anemia.
  - Wrist centralization if elbow ROM adequate
- Radioulnar synostosis is associated with duplication of sex chromosomes.
- Duplication can be preaxial (radial) or postaxial (ulnar).
  - Preaxial polydactyly (thumb duplication) is most commonly Wassel type IV with duplicate proximal phalanx.
  - Postaxial polydactyly (small finger duplication) is 10 times more common in African Americans than whites.
- Syndactyly results from failure of apoptosis to separate digits.
  - Characterized as simple (soft tissue) or complex (bony), complete, or incomplete
  - Long-ring most common
  - Border digit syndactyly released earlier
  - Web creep is a frequent delayed complication following surgical separation.
  - Poland syndrome (absent pectoralis major and chest wall abnormalities) and Apert syndrome (acrosyndactyly and mental retardation) are commonly associated with syndactyly.
- Thumb hypoplasia treatment is based on the carpometacarpal (CMC) joint (separates Blauth type IIIA from IIIB).
- Absence of thumb CMC necessitates index pollicization.

XVIII. Elbow

- Anterior bundle of the medial (ulnar) collateral ligament is the primary restraint to valgus stress.
- Lateral ulnar collateral ligament (LUCL) is the primary restraint to varus and external rotational stress.
- Lateral epicondylitis is a degenerative tendinopathy of the ECRB origin.
  - Histologic examination demonstrates angiofibroblastic hyperplasia.
  - No clear benefit from corticosteroid injection in prospective randomized studies
  - Operative treatment for select recalcitrant cases that fail prolonged conservative management
- Distal biceps tendon rupture results in diminished supination strength more than flexion strength.
  - Partial ruptures primarily occur on the radial side of the tuberosity footprint, owing to its function as a supinator.
  - Treat complete tears with retraction expediently.
  - Single-incision technique risks the lateral antebrachial cutaneous nerve and PIN.
  - Two-incision technique risks radioulnar synostosis.
  - Endobutton has been shown to have superior fixation strength.
  - Chronic untreated tears may require autograft or allograft reconstruction; less predictable outcome.
- Terrible triad" injury consists of radial head fracture, coronoid fracture, and elbow dislocation.
- Posterolateral rotatory instability results from incompetence of the LUCL, a potentially delayed presentation following a previous dislocation episode.
- Varus posteromedial rotatory instability typically results from complex fracture of the anteromedial coronoid process.
- Valgus instability usually affects overhead throwers and is due to incompetence of the MCL.

TESTABLE CONCEPTS

- May require MCL reconstruction in elite athletes, with about 80% returning to sport at same level after at least 1 year of rehabilitation
- Valgus overload syndrome follows untreated chronic MCL incompetence, leading to posteromedial impinging osteophytes, capitellar wear, loose body formation, and other complications.
- Elbow contracture may be due to intrinsic or extrinsic factors.
- Elbow osteoarthritis usually affects middle-aged manual laborers.

- Operative management of elbow arthritis—arthroscopic versus open osteophyte débridement, loose body removal, interposition arthroplasty, total elbow arthroplasty
- Indications for total elbow arthroplasty:
  - Refractory RA
  - Advanced osteoarthritis (primary and posttraumatic)
  - Chronic instability
  - Complex distal humerus fractures in elderly patients

SPINE

Francis H. Shen

CONTENTS

INTRODUCTION*

■ **History (Table 8-1)**
▦ Localized pain (tumor, infection), especially pain radiating to the extremity (radicular symptoms)
▦ Mechanical pain (instability, discogenic disease)
▦ Radicular pain (herniated nucleus pulposus [HNP], stenosis), night pain (tumor)
▦ Systemic symptoms such as fever or unexplained weight loss (infection, tumor)
▦ History of an acute injury or precipitating event should be investigated (trauma).
▦ Complete review of symptoms (including psychiatric history)
 • The finding of an "inverted-V" triad of hysteria, hypochondriasis, and depression on the Minnesota Multiphasic Personality Inventory has been identified as a significant adverse risk factor for lumbar disc surgery.
 • Psychosocial evaluation, pain drawings, and psychological testing are helpful in some cases.
▦ Social history
 • Occupational risks: jobs requiring prolonged sitting and repetitive lifting
 • Smoking may increase disc degeneration.

---

*The practice of medicine continues to evolve and advance, and our knowledge and treatment of the spine are no different. Perhaps two of the greatest rewards in my field are understanding and caring for patients with disorders of the spine and also having the opportunity to teach this practice to others. I remember Dr. Lauerman, who came to the University of Virginia as a visiting professor to prepare me and my fellow residents for the boards and the in-training examination several years ago. His breath of knowledge and enthusiasm for the topic made understanding the complexities of the spine much easier. Since that time, I have become a spine surgeon myself at the University of Virginia. The Spine chapter would not have been possible without Dr. Lauerman, who wrote this chapter for the first six editions. I have tried to follow his work as closely as possible, while updating and expanding the text with some of the newer techniques. Dr. Lauerman is greatly missed, but his legacy continues to live on, not just through his work on this textbook but also through all of the medical students, residents, and fellows that he helped train, teach, and mentor.

Table 8-1	Examination of Patients with Disorders of the Spine	
COMPONENT	**FEATURES**	
Inspection	Overall alignment in sagittal and coronal planes (sciatic scoliosis)	
Gait	Wide-based (myelopathy), forward-leaning (stenosis), antalgic	
Palpation	Localized posterior swelling (trauma), acute gibbus deformity, tenderness	
Range of motion	Flexion/extension, lateral bend, full versus limited	
Neurologic function	Motor, sensory, reflexes, assessment of long-tract signs (see also Table 8-3)	
Special tests	Straight-leg raise, Spurling test, Waddell signs of inorganic pathology	

■ **Physical examination (Figure 8-1; Tables 8-2 and 8-3)**
▦ Observe for muscle atrophy (rare), postural changes, gait, hair distribution, and so forth.
▦ Palpation of posterior spine (spasm, localized tenderness)
▦ Motor examination, motor grading (Table 8-4)
▦ Sensory examination
▦ Reflexes
▦ Rectal examination
 • Should evaluate for perianal sensation, rectal tone, and presence or absence of bulbocavernosus reflex
 • **Bulbocavernosus reflex (BCR)**
 • **Tests for presence of spinal shock** and is performed by monitoring for anal sphincter contraction in response to squeezing the glans penis or clitoris or tugging on an indwelling Foley catheter.
 • Presence of anal sphincter contraction is a normal or present BCR, whereas absence of anal sphincter contraction in the 24- to 48-hour period after a spinal cord injury is abnormal and implies the presence of spinal shock.
▦ Assess surrounding joints and associated neurovascular structures.
 • Localized hip and shoulder pathology may simulate spine disease and must also be evaluated.
 • Vascular evaluation (distal pulses)

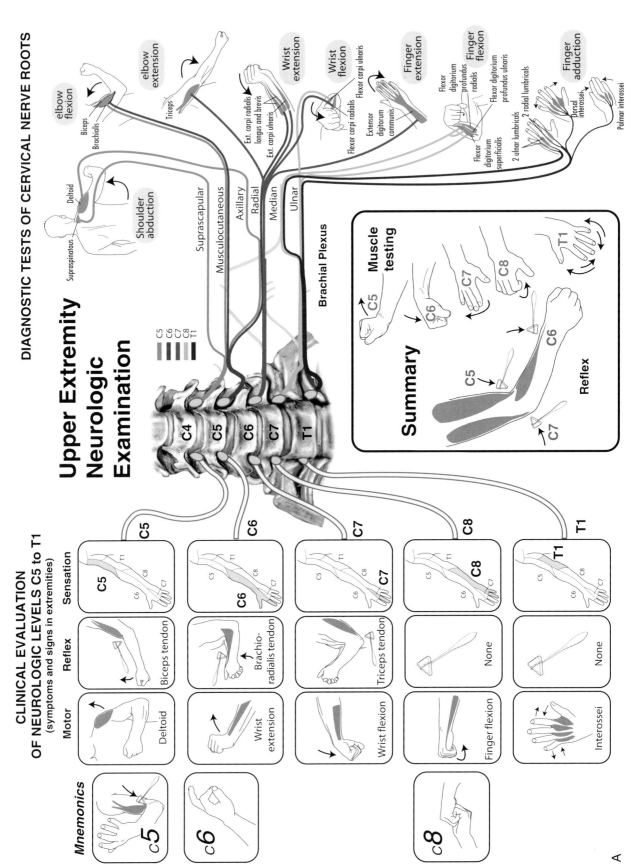

FIGURE 8-1 Upper and lower extremity neurologic examination.

Lower Extremity Neurologic Examination

DIAGNOSTIC TESTS OF LUMBOSACRAL NERVE ROOTS

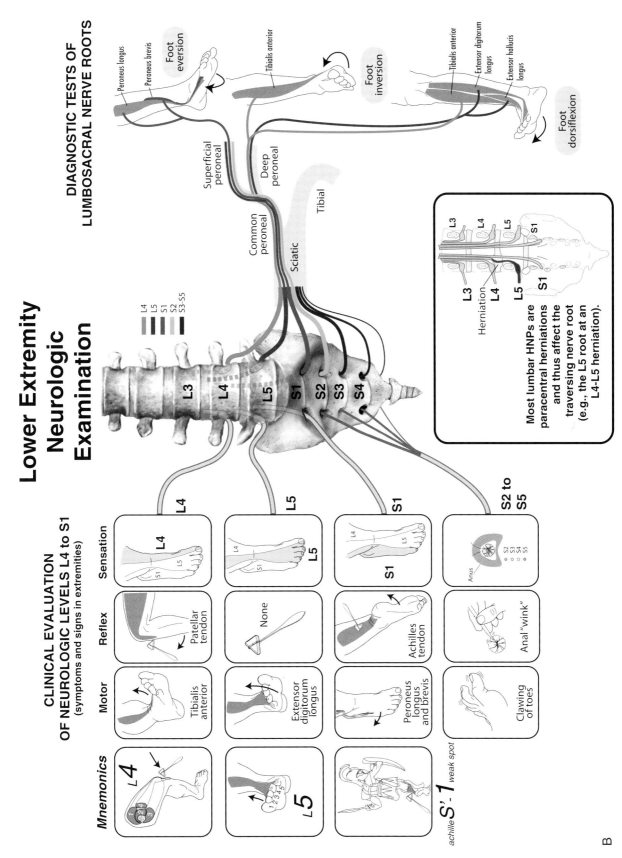

Peroneus longus
Peroneus brevis
Foot eversion

Tibialis anterior
Foot inversion

Tibialis anterior
Extensor digitorum longus
Extensor hallucis longus
Foot dorsiflexion

Superficial peroneal
Deep peroneal
Common peroneal
Tibial
Sciatic

L4
L5
S1
S2
S3-S5

L3
L4
L5
S1
S2
S3
S4

L3
L4
L5
S1

L3
Herniation
L4
L5
S1

Most lumbar HNPs are paracentral herniations and thus affect the traversing nerve root (e.g., the L5 root at an L4-L5 herniation).

CLINICAL EVALUATION OF NEUROLOGIC LEVELS L4 to S1
(symptoms and signs in extremities)

Mnemonics	Motor	Reflex	Sensation	
L4	Tibialis anterior	Patellar tendon	L4 / L5 / S1	**L4**
L5	Extensor digitorum longus	None	L4 / L5	**L5**
achille *S'1* *weak spot*	Peroneus longus and brevis	Achilles tendon	L4 / L5	**S1**
	Clawing of toes	Anal "wink"	Anus — S2 S3 S4 S5	**S2 to S5**

FIGURE 8-1, cont'd

B

Table 8-2	Findings in Cervical Nerve Root Compression			
LEVEL	**ROOT**	**MUSCLES AFFECTED**	**SENSORY LOSS**	**REFLEX**
C3-C4	C4	Scapular	Lateral neck, shoulder	None
C4-C5	C5	Deltoid, biceps	Lateral arm	Biceps
C5-C6*	C6	Wrist extensors, biceps, triceps (supination)	Radial forearm, thumb, index finger	Brachioradialis
C6-C7	C7	Triceps, wrist flexors (pronation)	Middle finger	Triceps
C7-T1	C8	Finger flexors, interossei	Ulnar hand, ring, and small finger	None
T1-T2	T1	Interossei	Ulnar forearm	None

*Most common level.

Table 8-3	Findings in Lumbar Nerve Root Compression			
LEVEL	**NERVE ROOT**	**SENSORY LOSS**	**MOTOR LOSS**	**REFLEX LOSS**
L1-L3	L2, L3	Anterior thigh	Hip flexors	None
L3-L4	L4	Medial calf	Quadriceps, tibialis anterior	Knee jerk
L4-L5	L5	Lateral calf, dorsal foot	EDL, EHL	None
L5-S1	S1	Posterior calf, plantar foot	Gastrocnemius/soleus	Ankle jerk
S2-S4	S2, S3, S4	Perianal	Bowel/bladder	Cremasteric

EDL, Extensor digitorum longus; *EHL,* extensor hallucis longus.

- Abdominal (bruits and pulsatile masses) and rectal examination
- ◼ Imaging
- ◼ Plain radiographs
  - Should be obtained 4 to 6 weeks after onset of symptoms
  - "Red flag" symptoms warrant immediate radiographs.
  - **Upright x-rays may simulate spinal alignment and identify subtle instability better than supine films and should be obtained whenever possible.**
  - **Flexion-extension radiographs for suspected instability**
  - Low specificity of plain radiographs. By age 65, 95% of men and 70% of women have degenerative changes.
- ◼ Magnetic resonance imaging (MRI)
  - Excellent for further imaging of HNP, stenosis, soft tissue, tumor, and infection (Figure 8-2)
  - MRI with gadolinium is the best study for a recurrent HNP
  - False-positive MRIs are common:
    - On cervical MRI, 25% of asymptomatic patients older than age 40 will have findings of either HNP or foraminal stenosis.
    - Correlation with history and physical examination is critical.
  - MRI is also useful for detecting intrinsic changes in the spinal cord and disc degeneration.
  - **Myelomalacia**—area of bright signal in the cord on T2-weighted imaging (Figure 8-3)
- ◼ Computed tomography (CT) with fine cuts with or without myelographic dye is used to examine bony anatomy after previous surgery and the quality of fusion. Because CT myelograms can be reformatted in multiple planes they can also be helpful in patients with sagittal or coronal plane deformity to better define the areas of stenosis.
- ◼ Bone scan is helpful in evaluating metastatic disease and may be negative with multiple myeloma.

Table 8-4	Motor Grading
GRADE	**DESCRIPTION**
0	No movement, no contractions
1	Flicker; contraction without movement
2	Movement with gravity removed
3	Movement against gravity
4	Movement against gravity and against some resistance
5	Full motor strength against resistance

- ◼ Laboratory evaluation
- ◼ C-reactive protein (CRP) and erythrocyte sedimentation rate (ESR) for infection
- ◼ Metabolic screening, serum/urine protein electrophoresis for myeloma
- ◼ Complete blood cell count (often a high-normal white blood cell [WBC] count with infection or anemia with myeloma).
- ◼ Electromyogram (EMG) and nerve conduction studies (NCS)
- ◼ Frequently performed together as EMG/NCS
  - EMG can help assess for diseases that damage muscle tissue, nerves, or the junction between the two; measures electrical activity of muscles at rest and during contraction
  - NCS help identify injury to peripheral nervous system; measure how well and how fast nerves can send electrical signals
- ◼ Can be useful for differentiating peripheral nerve compression from radiculopathy and for detecting systemic neurologic disorders such as amyotrophic lateral sclerosis (ALS).
- ◼ Evaluation of spine for presence of nerve root pathology should include evaluation of paraspinous muscles.
- ◼ Have a high false-negative rate, therefore correlation with history, clinical examination, and imaging important
- ◼ **Differential diagnosis—physical examination, imaging studies, and laboratory tests assist with differential diagnosis (Table 8-5).**

CERVICAL SPINE

■ **Cervical degenerative disc disease (also known as cervical spondylosis)**—chronic disc degeneration and associated facet arthropathy that can result in four clinical entities:
- Discogenic neck pain (axial pain)
- Radiculopathy (root compromise)
- Myelopathy (cord compression)
- Myeoloradiculopathy (combinations of spinal cord and root compromise)

▥ Epidemiology
- Peaks between age 40 and 50 years
- Men affected more than women
- C5-C6 level most frequently involved, followed by C6-C7
- Risk factors
  - Frequent lifting
  - Cigarette smoking
  - History of excessive driving

▥ Pathoanatomy
- Degenerative spinal cascade
  - First described in 1970s by Kirkaldy-Willis; emphasis on interdependence of intervertebral disc and two facet joints in the thoracolumbar spine
  - In cervical spine, is the result of interplay of intervertebral disc and four other articulations (Figure 8-4)
    - Two uncovertebral joints (of Luschka)
    - Two facet joints—facet joint capsules known to have sensory receptors that may play a role in pain and proprioceptive sensation in cervical spine
  - Progressive collapse of cervical discs, resulting in loss of normal lordosis of cervical spine and chronic anterior cord compression across the kyphotic spine/anterior chondroosseous/discoosteophytic spurs
  - Subsequent loading of facet and uncovertebral joint, resulting in spondylotic changes in foramina that may restrict motion and lead to spinal cord and/or nerve root compression

- Clinical relevance
  - "Soft" disc herniation
    - Nonspecific terminology often used to describe herniation of nucleus pulposus of intervertebral disc without bony osteophytes
    - Usually posterolateral, between the posterior edge of the uncinate process and the lateral edge of the posterior longitudinal ligament, it may result in acute radiculopathy.

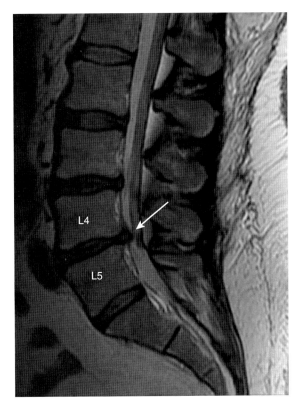

FIGURE 8-2 Sagittal T2-weighted lumbar MRI demonstrating herniated disc *(arrow)* at L4-L5.

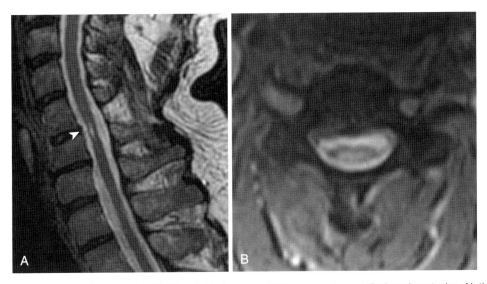

FIGURE 8-3 Myelomalacia. Sagittal **(A)** and axial **(B)** T2-weighted cervical MRI months after a spinal cord contusion. Notice there is focal thinning and volume loss of the spinal cord and a central small myelomalacic area in the spinal cord, displaying well-defined high T2 cerebrospinal fluid–like signal *(arrowhead)*. (From Cianfoni A, Colosimo C: Imaging of spine trauma. In Law M et al, editors: *Problem solving in neuroradiology*, Philadelphia, 2011, Elsevier, p 494.)

Table 8-5	Differential Diagnosis in Disorders of the Spine						
	DISORDER						
PARAMETER	**HNP**	**SPINAL STENOSIS**	**SPONDYLOLISTHESIS/ INSTABILITY**	**TUMOR**	**SPONDYLOARTHROPATHY**	**METABOLIC ABNORMALITY**	**INFECTION**
Predominant pain (leg vs. back)	Leg	Leg	Back	Back	Back	Back	Back
Constitutional symptoms				+	+		+
Tension sign	+						
Neurologic examination		+	+ After stress				
Plain radiographic studies		+	+	±	+	+	±
Lateral motion radiographic studies				+			
CT	+	+		+			+
Myelogram	+	+					
Bone scan				+	+	+	+
ESR				+	+		+
Ca/P/alk phos				+			

Modified from Weinstein JN, Wiesel SW: *The lumbar spine,* Philadelphia, 1990, WB Saunders, 1990, p 360.
+, Present; ±, present or absent; *Ca/P/alk phos,* calcium, phosphorus, alkaline phosphatase; *CT,* computed tomography; *ESR,* erythrocyte sedimentation rate; *HNP,* herniated nucleus pulposus.

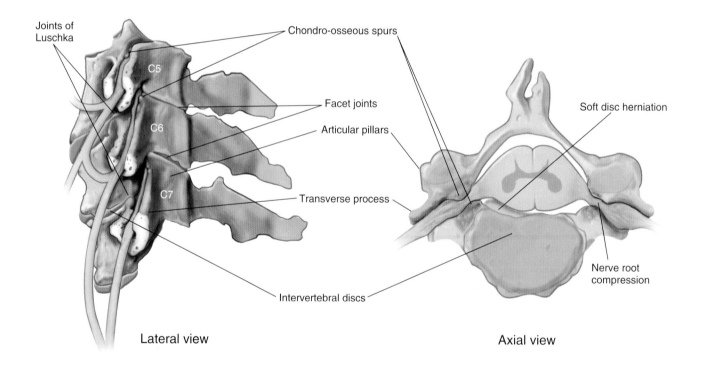

FIGURE 8-4 Cervical root impingement due to cervical spondylosis.

- Anterior herniation may cause dysphagia (rare).
- Myelopathy may be seen with large central herniation or spondylotic bars with a congenitally narrow canal.
- "Hard" disc herniation
  - Nonspecific terminology often used to describe HNP with associated discoosteophytic spur
  - Can result in similar symptomatology as soft disc herniations, including spinal cord and/or nerve root compression; rarely dysphagia with anterior osteophytes

- Cord compromise as canal diameter decreases
  - Congenital versus acquired (traumatic, degenerative)
  - **Measured on plain lateral radiograph from posterior aspect of vertebral body to spinolaminar line** (Figure 8-5); **concern when diameter is less than 14 mm**
    - Normal 14 mm or greater
    - Relative stenosis: less than 14 mm (10-13 mm)
    - Absolute stenosis: less than 10 mm

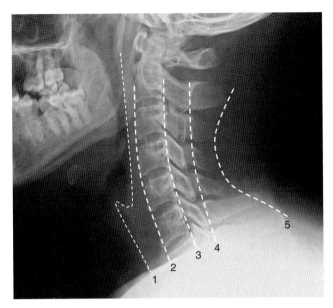

FIGURE 8-5 Five vertebral lines of the lateral cervical radiograph. *1,* Prevertebral soft tissue line. *2,* Anterior vertebral line. *3,* Posterior vertebral line. *4,* Spinolaminar line. *5,* Spinous process line. (Adapted from Shen FH: Spine. In Miller MD et al, editors: *Orthopaedic surgical approaches,* ed 2, Philadelphia, 2015, Elsevier, p 166.)

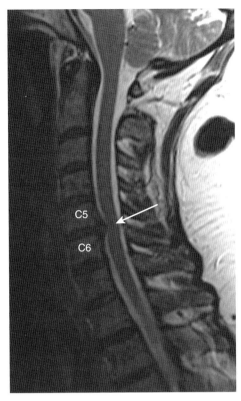

FIGURE 8-6 Sagittal T2-weighted cervical MRI demonstrating a C5-C6 herniated disc *(arrow)* resulting in C6 nerve root compression.

- Pavlov (Torg) ratio (canal/vertebral body width)
  - Clinical significance debated
  - Normal ratio should be 1.0.
  - Ratio of less than 0.8 considered abnormal and may be a risk factor for later neurologic involvement (debated)
- Dynamic compression
  - Neck extension—cord is compressed between degenerative disc and spondylotic bar anteriorly and the hypertrophic facets and infolded ligamentum flavum posteriorly
  - Neck flexion results in slight increase in canal diameter and relief of cord compression.

▥ Discogenic neck pain

▦ Secondary to intervertebral disc degeneration without other pathologic entities, such as spinal instability, fractures, dislocations, or neural compression

▦ Symptoms
- May present as insidious onset of neck pain without neurologic signs or symptoms, exacerbated by excess vertebral motion
- Occipital headache common but not necessary as part of diagnosis

▦ Examination
- Typically benign; normal motor and sensory examination, normal reflexes
- May have decreased cervical range of motion secondary to pain but no pathologic evidence of mechanical instability

▦ Imaging
- Radiographs—typically normal without evidence of instability; may demonstrate disc space narrowing
- MRI typically demonstrates intervertebral disc degeneration; decreased signal in the disc on T2-weighted imaging (dark disc), with or without annular tear or high-intensity zone (HIZ).

▦ Treatment
- **Nonoperative therapy: antiinflammatories, symptomatic care**
- **Patient education emphasizing the self-limiting nature of symptoms is important.**

▥ Cervical radiculopathy

▦ Nerve root compromise without reference to specific pathologic entity
- Can be due to herniated disc, discoosteophytic complex, facet arthropathy, thickened ligamentum flavum, uncovertebral osteophyte, and others
- Can involve one or multiple roots (polyradiculopathy)
- Commonly shoulder and arm pain, paresthesias, and numbness
- Overlapping findings because of intraneural intersegmental connections of sensory nerve roots

▦ **Caudal nerve root at a given level is usually affected (see Table 8-2)**
- **Cervical nerve roots exit above their corresponding vertebrae (e.g., C5 exits at C4-C5 neural foramen).**
- **Consequently, disc herniation at C5-C6 involves the C6 nerve root** (Figure 8-6).
- **Recognize that disc herniation at C7-T1 involves the C8 root.**

▦ Symptoms
- May initially present as neck pain then develop radicular symptoms
- Pain, numbness, paresthesia in a dermatomal distribution to upper extremity

▦ Physical examination
- Motor—weakness uncommon but when present is associated with the myotome

- Sensory—pain, numbness, or dysesthesias along dermatomal distribution is common.
- Reflexes—typically normal or hyporeflexic
- **Spurling test**—suggestive for nerve root pain when radicular symptoms occur with rotation and lateral bend of the neck, with vertical compression on the head
- **Shoulder abduction sign**—relief of radicular pain with shoulder abduction (placing hand on top of patient's head) is suggestive of a cervical etiology.
- Treatment
  - Nonsurgical treatment—nonsteroidal antiinflammatory drugs (NSAIDs), cervical epidural injections, isometric exercises, traction, and occasionally temporary collar immobilization
  - Surgical indications—progressive motor weakness, persistent disabling pain despite conservative measures
  - Procedures
    - Anterior cervical discectomy and fusion (ACDF)—removal of herniated disc with excision of associated osteophytes followed by strut graft fusion with or without instrumentation; can be single level or multilevel ACDF
    - Anterior cervical corpectomy and fusion (ACCF)—if neural compression is due to pathology behind the vertebral body, then removal of vertebral body (corpectomy) may be necessary, with subsequent bony fusion with or without instrumentation.
    - Application of anterior plating may increase the fusion rate in multilevel discectomies with fusion and will protect a strut graft in multilevel corpectomies.
    - Posterior keyhole laminoforaminotomy—less commonly performed but option for radiculopathy secondary to posterior compression (facet hypertrophy) or for lateral soft disc herniations.

 ■ **Cervical myelopathy** (Figure 8-7)
- Spinal cord compromise without reference to specific pathologic entity
- Presenting symptoms can be subtle:
  - Finger clumsiness, deterioration of handwriting, difficulty in fine motor control of hands
  - Ataxia with wide-based gait, leg heaviness, and inability to perform tandem walk
  - Urinary retention, urgency, or frequency
  - Lower extremity weakness (corticospinal tracts) can be associated with worse prognosis.
 ■ Natural history of cervical spondylotic myelopathy is characterized by one of three presentations:
  - **Stepwise deterioration in symptomatology followed by a period of stability** (most common, 65%-80%)
  - **Slowly progressive decline** (over months to years, 20%-25%)
  - **Rapidly progressive decline** (over days to weeks, 3%-5%)
- Physical examination
  - Upper motor neuron findings in myelopathy
  - "Myelopathy hand" and the "finger escape sign" (small finger spontaneously abducts because of weak intrinsic muscles)
  - **Hyperreflexia, Hoffmann sign, clonus, or Babinski sign**

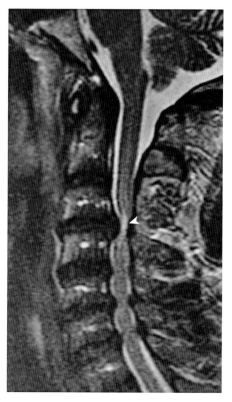

FIGURE 8-7 Disc-related myelopathy. Fast T2-weighted sagittal image of the cervical spine. The C3-C4 disc is protruding into the spinal canal, and there is compression of the cord with high signal within it *(arrowhead)*. The cord abnormality is the result of cord ischemia with myelomalacia. The discs are protruding to a lesser extent at lower levels, causing multilevel canal stenosis.

- Inverted radial reflex (ipsilateral finger flexion when eliciting brachioradialis reflex)
- Funicular pain—central burning and stinging with or without the Lhermitte sign (radiating lightning-like sensations down the back with neck flexion)
- Upper motor neuron findings not always present in all patients
- Upper extremities may have radicular (lower motor neuron) signs along with evidence of distal myelopathy.
- Treatment
  - Nonsurgical treatment—NSAIDs, cervical epidural injections, isometric exercises, traction, and occasionally temporary collar immobilization
  - **Surgical indications—natural history of myelopathy is typically progressive, therefore surgical decompression is frequently indicated.**
  - Procedures
    - Anterior procedures include ACDF versus ACCF or combination (hybrid). Anterior-based procedures are options for patients with either kyphotic or lordotic cervical sagittal alignment.
    - Posterior options include laminectomy and fusion versus laminoplasty. Posterior-based options are contraindicated in patients with fixed cervical kyphosis owing to the inability to indirectly decompress the spinal cord.
    - Combined anterior and posterior procedures (circumferential surgery). Consider for patients requiring multilevel corpectomy resection with strut reconstructions (highly unstable spine).

Table 8-6	Ranawat Classification of Neurologic Impairment in Rheumatoid Arthritis
GRADE	**CHARACTERISTICS**
I	Subjective paresthesias, pain
II	Subjective weakness; upper motor neuron findings
III	Objective weakness; upper motor neuron findings
IIIA	Ambulatory
IIIB	Nonambulatory

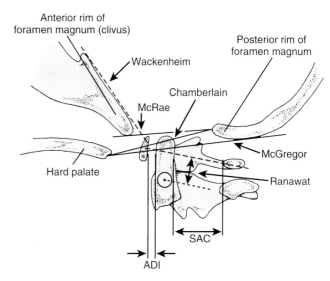

FIGURE 8-8 Common measurements in C1-C2 disorders. *ADI,* Atlantodens interval; *SAC,* space available for the cord.

■ Rheumatoid spondylitis

▦ Overview
- Less common owing to improvement and increased use of disease-modifying antirheumatic drugs (DMARDs)
- Patients with rheumatoid arthritis (RA) should have flexion/extension films before elective surgery.
- When spine is involved, the cervical spine, more specifically occipitoatlantoaxial joint (O-C2), is site most commonly involved
  - Atlantoaxial subluxation (AAS)—typically the first manifestation of cervical instability in rheumatoid patient
  - Atlantoaxial invagination (AAI)—typically follows next after AAS
  - Subaxial subluxation (SAS)—usually occurs after AAS and AAI
- Occurring in up to 90% of patients and is more common with long-standing disease and multiple joint involvement

▦ Presenting complaints
- Axial neck pain
- Stiffness
- Occipital headaches
  - Due to erosion of the C1-C2 joint, with subsequent compression of greater occipital branch of C2 nerve
  - Results more specifically in pain in posterior aspect of base of skull that is typically relieved with manual traction
- Myelopathy, radiculopathy, or myeloradiculopathy depending on neurologic structures at risk

▦ Physical examination
- Look for subtle signs of neurologic involvement.
- Neurologic impairment (weakness, decreased sensation, hyperreflexia) in patients with RA usually occurs gradually and is often overlooked or attributed to other joint disease.
- Neurologic impairment with RA has been classified by Ranawat (Table 8-6).

▦ Imaging
- Assess radiographic markers for impending neural compression (Figure 8-8).
  - Anterior atlantodens interval (AADI) or frequently referred to as simply atlantodens interval (ADI)
  - Posterior ADI (PADI) sometimes also referred to as space available for the cord (SAC)
- MRI
  - Cervicomedullary angle (CMA) (Figure 8-9) measured by drawing a line along anterior aspect of cervical spinal cord and the medulla
  - Normal: 135 to 175 degrees. In patients with progressive superior migration of the odontoid, the

CMA decreases owing to draping of the brainstem over the odontoid.

▦ Atlantoaxial subluxation (AAS)
- Typically first stage of cervical spine involvement in the rheumatoid patient
  - Occurs in 50% to 80% of patients with RA
  - Often the result of pannus formation at synovial joints between the dens and ring of C1, resulting in destruction of transverse ligament, dens, or both
  - Results in instability between C1 and C2, with subsequent subluxation
- Diagnosis
  - Anterior subluxation of C1 on C2 is the most common finding, but posterior and lateral subluxation can also occur.
  - Findings on examination may include limitation of motion, upper motor neuron signs, and weakness.
  - Plain radiographs that include patient-controlled flexion and extension views are evaluated to determine AADI as well as PADI.
  - Instability is suggestive with AADI motion of more than 3.5 mm on flexion and extension views, although radiographic instability in RA is common and not necessarily an indication for surgery.
- Surgical indications
  - Intractable pain
  - Progressive neurologic instability, cervical myelopathy
    - Can be due to mechanical instability
    - Direct compression for pannus of C2
  - Mechanical instability; evaluate C1-C2 motion/relationship
    - AADI of more than 9 to 10 mm
    - PADI of less than 14 mm
      - PADI may be more sensitive for identifying patients at increased risk of neurologic injury
      - PADI of less than 14 mm usually requires surgical treatment.
  - Surgery is less successful in Ranawat grade IIIB patients but should still be considered.

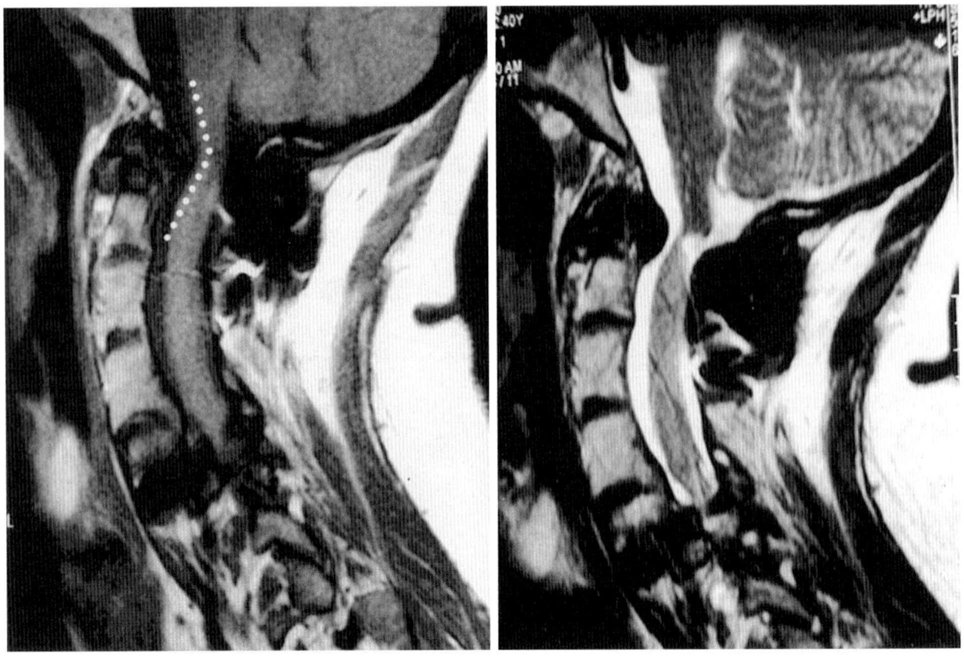

FIGURE 8-9 Cervicomedullary angle (CMA). Magnetic resonance images of a myelopathic rheumatoid patient with a CMA measuring 130 degrees *(dotted white line)*. Notice the effect of progressive cranial settling combined with an increasing retrodental pannus on the craniocervical junction. (From Shen FH et al: Rheumatoid arthritis: evaluation and surgical management of the cervical spine, *Spine J* 4:689–700, 2004.)

- Treatment
  - Surgical fixation
    - Gallie fusion—mostly of historical significance
    - Brooks fusion—mostly of historical significance and rarely used alone
    - C1-C2 transarticular screw fixation (Magerl)
      - Still used but less commonly since advent of C1-C2 Harms construct (see below)
      - Requires preoperative CT to evaluate position of vertebral arteries
      - Requires reduction of C1-C2 joint
      - Increased risk for vertebral artery and C2 nerve injury
    - C1 lateral mass—C2 pedicle/pars fixation (Harms construct)
      - Lower rate of vertebral artery and C2 nerve injury
      - **Biomechanically strongest construct of C1-C2 fixation techniques**
      - Does not require C1-C2 joint to be reduced
    - Odontoidectomy
      - Should be reserved as a secondary procedure
      - Anterior cord compression because of pannus often resolves after posterior spinal fusion.
- **Atlantoaxial invagination (AAI)**
  - Also known as *cranial settling, basilar invagination, cranial invagination,* and other names.
  - Second most common manifestation of RA in cervical spine
  - Occurs in 40% of patients with RA
  - **Results in cranial migration of the dens from erosion and bone loss between the occiput and C1-C2**
    - Often seen in combination with fixed atlantoaxial subluxation
    - Measurements are shown in Figure 8-8.
      - Landmarks may be difficult to identify.
      - Ranawat line is most reproducible.

- Diagnosis
  - Progressive cranial migration of dens
  - Findings on examination may include limitation of motion, upper motor neuron signs, weakness, and in severe cases bulbar symptoms.
- Surgical indications
  - Intractable pain
  - Progressive cranial migration or neurologic compromise may require operative intervention (occiput to C2 fusion).
  - **Cervicomedullary angle less than 135 degrees (on MRI) suggests impending neurologic impairment.**
- Treatment
  - Occipitocervical fusion
    - Typically from occiput to C2
    - Gentle traction to help bring odontoid process out of foramen magnum
  - Transoral or retropharyngeal odontoid resection for brainstem compression
- **Subaxial subluxation (SAS)**
  - Occurs in 20% of cases of RA
  - Seen in combination with upper cervical spine instability
  - Pathoanatomy
    - Pannus formation in uncovertebral joints (joints of Luschka) and facet joints. Subluxation may occur at multiple levels.
    - Radiographic markers of instability
      - Subaxial subluxation of greater than 4 mm or more than 20% of the body is indicative of cord compression.
      - A cervical height index (cervical body height/width) of less than 2.00 approaches 100% sensitivity and specificity in predicting neurologic compromise.

- Surgical indications
  - Intractable pain
  - Progressive neurologic compromise, cervical myelopathy
  - Mechanical instability—subluxation greater than 4 mm
- Procedure
  - Posterior spinal fusion with or without decompression
    - Fuse to the most distal unstable level.
    - Include occiput and/or C1-C2 joint if AAI or AAS exists.
  - Anterior spinal fusion
    - May be required to restore sagittal alignment
    - May be necessary to increase fusion rate on multilevel PSF
  - Surgery may not reverse significant neurologic deterioration, especially if a tight spinal canal is present, but it can stabilize it.

■ Ankylosing spondylitis (AS)

- Introduction
  - Chronic inflammation as part of group of conditions known as *spondyloarthropathies.*
  - Etiology unknown; association with HLA-B27. However, not all patients with HLA-B27 develop AS.
- Presentation and assessment
  - Symptoms most frequently start in sacroiliac joint (sacroiliitis) or lumbar spine
  - Patients with AS who present with complaint of spine pain, with or without a history of trauma, must be carefully evaluated for occult fracture.
    - In particular, AS patients with neck pain have a presumed fracture unless proven otherwise.
    - Concerns with pseudarthrosis and progressive kyphotic deformity
    - Undiagnosed cervical fractures in AS patients are at high risk for neurologic compromise.
  - Plain x-rays
    - Ossification of intervertebral disc
      - Marginal syndesmophytes
      - "Bamboo spine"
    - Plain radiographs frequently negative or can miss occult fractures. Results can be devastating if fractures missed in AS patients (Figure 8-10).
  - Advanced imaging should be strongly considered.
    - CT scan
    - MRI
  - In addition to occult fractures, AS patients are at risk for developing epidural hematomas.
  - Frequently AS patients can present with loss of horizontal gaze, inability to look straight ahead. (See Adult Deformity, Kyphotic deformity in ankylosing spondylitis.)
    - Chin-on-chest deformity
    - Associated with severe hip flexion contracture
    - Flexion deformity of the lumbar spine
    - Increased cervical, thoracic, and lumbar kyphosis common
- Treatment
  - Nonoperative: reduce pain, stiffness, and inflammation
  - Surgical (See Adult Deformity, "Kyphotic deformity in ankylosing spondylitis.")
    - Careful intraoperative positioning

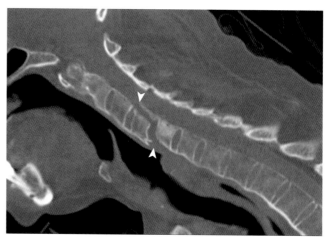

FIGURE 8-10 Parasagittal cervical CT reconstruction demonstrating classic changes consistent with ankylosing spondylitis with loss of cervical lordosis and marginal syndesmophytes. An oblique fracture entering through the ossified C4-C5 disc and then extending vertically through the vertebral body of C4 is identified *(arrowheads).*

- Ankylosed cervical spine can make intubation and airway management challenging
- Correction of hip and lumbar disorder first
- May require cervicothoracic laminectomy, osteotomy, and fusion for correction of the neck deformity
  - Typically performed at a C7-T1 pedicle subtraction osteotomy
  - C8 nerve root frequently at risk during this procedure
  - May require a staged anterior approach to obtain anterior column support at C7-T1 in patients that sustain substantial distraction and opening of the anterior column during completion of the osteotomy (osteoclasis)
- Postoperative immobilization may require addition of halo cast/vest.
  - Internal fixation should be as secure as possible in the attempt to avoid halo immobilization if possible.
  - Role of traction and halo immobilization as the primary treatment of cervical spine fractures in AS is controversial and being used less and less.
  - Traction and halo immobilization as the primary treatment is not well tolerated in AS.

■ Ossification of the posterior longitudinal ligament (OPLL)

- Introduction
  - Ectopic endochondral ossification of posterior longitudinal ligament
  - Typically cervical spine followed by thoracic spine and least frequently lumbar spine
  - Common in Asians, particularly Japanese population, but also seen in non-Asians
  - Men-to-women ratio, 2 : 1
  - Associated with other spondyloarthropathies, such as AS and diffuse idiopathic skeletal hyperostosis (DISH)
- Presentation and assessment
  - Majority can be asymptomatic
  - If symptomatic can present with symptoms of cervical stenosis with myelopathy and/or radiculopathy.

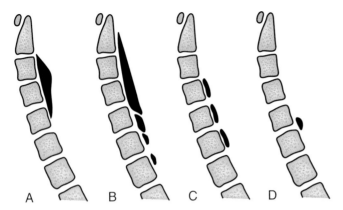

FIGURE 8-11 Classification of ossification of posterior longitudinal ligament. **A,** Continuous type. **B,** Mixed type. **C,** Segmental type. **D,** Localized type. (From Takeshita K: Ossification of the posterior longitudinal ligament. In Shen FH et al, editors: *Textbook of the cervical spine,* Maryland Heights, Mo., 2015, Elsevier, p 157.)

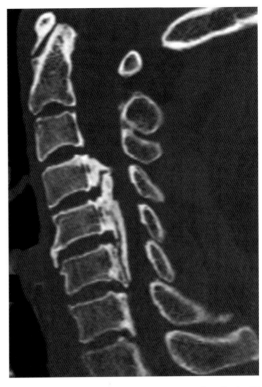

FIGURE 8-12 Sagittal reconstruction CT scan of patient with mixed-type ossification of the posterior longitudinal ligament. (From Takeshita K: Ossification of the posterior longitudinal ligament. In Shen FH et al, editors: *Textbook of the cervical spine,* Maryland Heights, Mo., 2015, Elsevier, p 160.)

- Imaging
  - Linear ossification immediately posterior to vertebral body in spinal canal (Figure 8-11). Classification:
    - Continuous—long lesions extending over several vertebrae
    - Mixed—combination of continuous and segmental
    - Segmental—one or several separate lesions
    - Localized (also known as *circumscribed*)—lesions mainly located at the level of the intervertebral disc space
  - OPLL can be hard to identify on MRI; can be misidentified as multilevel herniated disc
  - **Ossification is better defined on CT scan** (Figure 8-12).
- Treatment
  - Nonoperative
    - Important to recognize that majority of patients with OPLL are asymptomatic.
    - Prophylactic surgery in the asymptomatic patient is not necessary.
  - Operative
    - **Posterior approach**
      - **Relies on indirect decompression of spinal canal**
      - **Requires lordotic or neutral sagittal alignment**
      - **Laminectomy alone not performed as frequently; higher associated rate of post-laminectomy kyphosis**
      - **Laminectomy and fusion, typically with instrumentation**
      - **Laminoplasty**
        - **Requires neutral to lordotic sagittal alignment**
        - **Contraindicated in kyphotic spine**
    - Anterior approach
      - More directly addresses the pathology
        - Anterior cervical discectomy and fusion (ACDF)
        - Anterior cervical corpectomy and fusion (ACCF)
        - Hybrid of ACDF and ACCF combination
      - **However, OPLL is frequently associated with dural ossification.**
        - **Therefore anterior-based approaches may be associated with higher incidence of dural leaks.**

- Anterior floating technique has been described. OPLL is thinned down but not removed. Stenosis is decompressed laterally around the OPLL, allowing it to become "free-floating."
- **Sports-related cervical spine injuries**
- **Neurapraxia ("burners" and "stingers")**
  - Commonly associated with stretching of the upper brachial plexus
    - Bending the neck away from the depressed shoulder
    - Neck extension toward the painful shoulder in the setting of foraminal stenosis
  - Symptoms include burning dysesthesia and weakness in the involved extremity.
    - Typically unilateral
    - Bilateral symptoms or lower extremity symptoms suggestive of spinal cord injury
  - Fracture or acute HNP should be ruled out.
  - The athlete with a neck injury should be further evaluated for cervical pain, tenderness, or persisting neurologic symptoms.
  - **Use of steroids not indicated; neurapraxia due to peripheral nerve lesions**
- **Transient quadriplegia**
  - Usually seen after axial load injury (spearing) but may also be seen after forced hyperextension or hyperflexion
  - Presents as bilateral burning paresthesia and weakness or paralysis
  - Risk factors
    - Cervical stenosis
    - Torg ratio
      - Ratio width of sagittal canal diameter divided by with of vertebral body

- Normal 1.0
- Less than 0.8 indicates stenosis
- Poor positive predictive value; should not be used as screening tool
- Preexisting instability
- HNP
- Congenital fusions (Klippel-Feil syndrome)
- Third and fourth cervical levels are the most commonly affected.
- No definitive association with future permanent neurologic injury
- Patients with concurrent pathologic conditions, including instability, HNP, degenerative changes, and symptoms that last more than 36 hours, should be prohibited from participating in contact sports.

THORACIC SPINE

- ◼ **Thoracic disc disease**
- ▦ Epidemiology
  - **Radiographic evidence of disc degeneration is relatively common; however, symptomatic disc herniation is very uncommon (1% of all surgical HNPs).**
  - Typically involves the middle to lower thoracic levels
    - Most herniations occur at T11-T12.
    - 75% occur at T8-T12.
- ▦ Diagnosis
  - Presents as the onset of back or chest pain
  - May include radicular symptoms
    - Band-like chest or abdominal discomfort, numbness, paresthesias, leg pain
    - Myelopathy may be present.
    - Sensory changes, paraparesis, bowel/bladder/sexual dysfunction
  - Physical examination may be subtle and difficult to elicit
    - Localized tenderness
    - Thoracic radiculopathy—dermatomal sensory changes
    - **Thoracic myelopathy—patient will present with upper motor neuron signs of the lower extremity, with leg hyperreflexia, weakness, and normal upper extremity findings**
    - Abnormal rectal examination (rarely present)
  - Imaging
    - Radiographs may show disc narrowing and calcification or osteophytic lipping.
    - CT myelography or MRI should demonstrate thoracic HNP.
    - MRI is useful for ruling out cord disorder, but there is a high false-positive rate, requiring close clinical correlation.
- ◼ **Thoracic HNP**
- ▦ Pathophysiology
  - Disc degeneration
    - Aging results in loss of water content.
    - Tearing of the anulus
    - Myxomatous changes, resulting in herniation of nuclear material
  - Thoracic HNP can be divided into central, posterolateral, and lateral herniations.
  - Underlying Scheuermann disease may predispose patients to develop HNP.

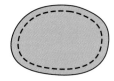

A Diffuse Disc Bulge

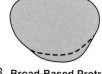

B Broad-Based Protrusion
(or focal disc bulge)

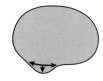

C Focal Disc Protrusion
AP < Mediolateral dimension

D Disc Extrusion
AP ≥ Mediolateral dimension

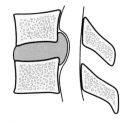

E Disc Extrusion
Disc migrates above and/or
below parent disc,
maintaining continuity with it

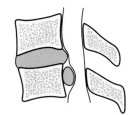

F Sequestered Disc
Separate from parent disc

FIGURE 8-13 Types of disc herniation.

- ▦ Disc herniation (Figure 8-13)
  - Discs can protrude (bulging nucleus, intact anulus).
  - Disc extrusion (through anulus but confined by posterior longitudinal ligament)
  - Disc sequestration (disc material free in canal)
  - HNP usually a disease of young and middle-aged adults; in older patients the nucleus desiccates and is less likely to herniate.
- ▦ Treatment
  - **Nonsurgical**
    - **Most thoracic disc herniations resulting in radiculopathy are managed symptomatically and nonoperatively.**
    - Immobilization, analgesics, and nerve blocks are sometimes helpful for radiculopathy.
  - **Surgical indications**
    - **Progressive thoracic myelopathy (worsening gait instability, ataxia, bowel or bladder dysfunction, etc.)**
    - Persistent unremitting radicular pain (uncommon)
  - Procedures
    - Anterior transthoracic approach—typically for midline or central HNP. Anterior discectomy (hemicorpectomy as needed) and fusion with or without instrumentation.
    - Posterior transpedicular/lateral extracavitary approach—for lateral HNP
      - Can be used for central disc herniations as well but can be more technically challenging
      - Depending on the degree of bony facet resection, typically requires fusion with or without instrumentation

- Thoracoscopic discectomy can also be employed; can be technically challenging.
- **Laminectomy—contraindicated**
  - **Listed mostly for historical interest**
  - **Associated with high rate of neurologic injury**
  - **Laminectomy does not allow safe access to the HNP without spinal cord retraction and manipulation.**

LUMBAR SPINE

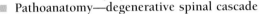

■ Lumbar disc disease (also known as *lumbar spondylosis*)

- Major cause of morbidity, with a major financial impact in the United States
  - Spectrum of symptoms that can result in several clinical entities, including discogenic back pain, lumbar disc herniations, spondylolisthesis, and lumbar spinal stenosis
  - Usually involves the L4-L5 disc (the "backache disc"), followed closely by L5-S1
- ■ **Pathoanatomy—degenerative spinal cascade**
  - **First described in 1970s by Kirkaldy-Willis.** Emphasis on interdependence of intervertebral disc and two facet joints in the thoracolumbar spine.
  - Progressive collapse of the lumbar intervertebral disc, resulting in loss of normal lordosis of the lumbar spine and chronic anterior cord compression, resulting in anterior chondroosseous/discoosteophytic spurs
  - Subsequent loading of facet joint resulting in spondylotic changes in the foramina
  - Can result in segmental instability (spondylolisthesis) due to collapse of the disc and incompetence of the facet joint

■ Discogenic back pain

- Secondary to intervertebral disc degeneration without other pathologic entities, such as spinal instability, fractures, dislocations, or neural compression
- Diagnosis
  - Examination
    - Paucity of physical findings
    - Back pain greater than leg pain
    - No radiculopathy—negative tension signs
  - Imaging
    - Radiographs are negative for instability but may show disc space narrowing or other stigmata of spondylosis.
    - MRI typically reveals decreased signal intensity in the disc space on T2-weighted imaging (dark disc), with or without annular tear or high intensity zone (HIZ) (Figure 8-14).
  - Discography
    - Controversial study
    - Designed as a preoperative study to correlate MRI findings with a clinically significant pain generator
      - Needle placed into intervertebral disc space and contrast dye injected
      - Extra fluid in disc increases pressure in the disc. To be considered reliably positive, the procedure should elicit pain after injection similar to that usually described by the patient (concordant pain).

- The study should involve at least one minimally painful, nonconcordant level.
- Study should be performed at multiple levels to include all abnormal levels and one or more normal levels on MRI.
- Evidence suggests that annular tears created by the needle during discography may accelerate the rate of symptomatic disc degeneration.

■ Treatment

- **Almost always conservative treatment**
  - More than half of patients who seek treatment for low back pain recover in 1 week, and 90% recover within 1 to 3 months.
  - NSAIDs, physical therapy, and conditioning
  - Patient education about the self-limiting nature of discogenic back pain is important.
- Surgical interventions
  - Controversial; surgery should be avoided whenever possible for discogenic back pain.
    - Conservative measures should be exhausted before any consideration of surgical intervention.
    - Currently no good surgical option available that reliably reduces symptoms of discogenic back pain
  - Options available include:
    - Interbody fusion
      - Anterior retroperitoneal approach, or direct lateral, or through a posterior midline lumbar, or posterior transforaminal lumbar interbody fusion approach
      - Fusion is performed with structural constructs (femoral ring allografts or interbody fusion cages) in the disc space.

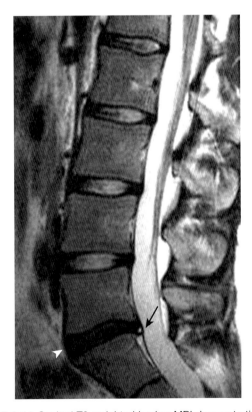

FIGURE 8-14 Sagittal T2-weighted lumbar MRI demonstrating a degenerative dark disc *(white arrowhead)* with associated annular tear *(black arrow),* also known as a *high-intensity zone* (HIZ).

- Intradiscal electrothermy—involves percutaneously heating the fibers of the anulus fibrosus to reconfigure the collagen fibers, thus restoring the mechanical integrity of the disc.
  - This may be effective in early conditions (<50% loss of disc height) but not in more advanced disease.
  - Long-term follow-up suggests that symptomatic improvement often lasts less than 1 year, and this procedure has been largely abandoned.
- Total disc arthroplasty
  - Another surgical option for patients with degenerative disc disease at a single level (L4-L5 or L5-S1) in the lumbar spine with the absence of spondylolisthesis and no relief from 6 months of nonoperative therapy
  - In direct comparison with anterior interbody fusion, total disc arthroplasty showed equivalent clinical results and no catastrophic failures at 2-year follow-up.
  - Significant concerns include long-term results, design issues, cost, and the safety of revision procedures.

■ **Lumbar herniated disc**
▨ Pathophysiology
  - **Most herniations are posterolateral (where the posterior longitudinal ligament is the weakest) and may present as back pain and nerve root pain/ sciatica involving the lower nerve root at that level (L5 nerve at the L4-L5 level).**
  - **Herniations lateral to the neural foramen (also called "far lateral" disc herniations) involve the upper nerve root (L4 nerve at the L4-L5 level).**
  - **Central herniations are often associated with back pain only; however, acute insults may precipitate a cauda equina compression syndrome** (Figure 8-15).
▨ Diagnosis (See I. Introduction.)
  - History
    - Typically presents initially as back pain with or without history of trauma
    - Subsequent development of leg pain that is worse with sitting and better with standing and lying

Pain:
Backs of thighs and legs

Numbness:
Buttocks, backs of legs, soles of feet

Weakness:
Paralysis of legs and feet

Atrophy:
Calves

Paralysis:
Bladder and bowel

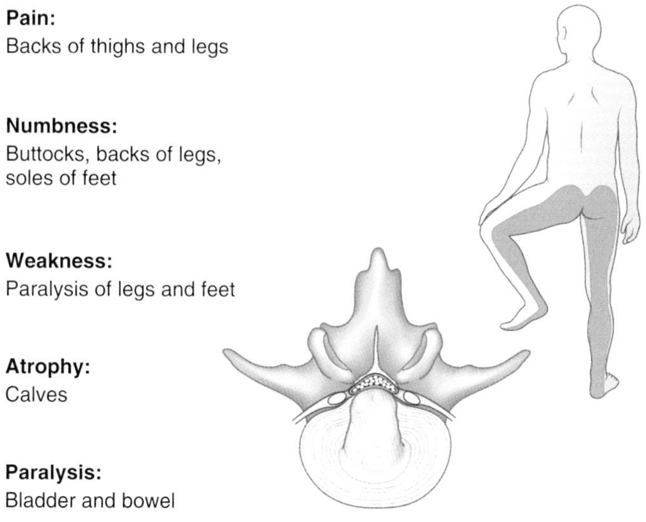

FIGURE 8-15 Cauda equina syndrome.

- Pain or numbness radiating beyond the knee, typically in a dermatomal distribution
- Weakness and bowel and bladder dysfunction less common, but should be elicited during history.
- Red flag signs (fever, chills, nausea, vomiting, weight loss, night sweats, etc.) typically negative
- **Examination** (see Table 8-3)
  - Motor—typically normal but weakness may be present depending on nerve root involved.
  - Sensory examination—typically presents with pain, numbness, and/or dysesthesia radiating down leg in a dermatomal pattern
  - Reflexes—typically normal but may be hyporeflexic at level of involved nerve root
  - **Provocative maneuvers:**
    - **Supine straight leg test**—patient supine and raising leg with knee straight between 30 and 70 degrees reproduces and/or exaggerates symptoms radiating down leg. Sensitive for L4, L5, and S1 nerve root irritation but not very specific.
    - **Seated straight leg test**—variation of straight leg raise; performed while patient in seated position. Hip flexion with knee extension reproduces and/or exaggerates symptoms radiating down leg. Less sensitive than supine straight leg raise.
    - **Contralateral straight leg test**—raising contralateral asymptomatic leg with knee straight results in pain radiating down the symptomatic leg. More specific for an axillary disc herniation.
    - **Lasegue sign**—relief of radiating leg symptoms with knee flexion while hip is flexed
    - **Femoral tension sign**—patient prone and knee is passively flexed with the hip extended; reproduces and/or exaggerates symptoms radiating down anterior thigh. Sensitive for L2, L3, and L4 nerve root irritation but not very specific.
- Imaging
  - Plain radiographs
    - Upright x-rays may simulate spinal alignment and identify subtle instability better than supine films and should be obtained whenever possible.
    - **Flexion-extension radiographs should be obtained, assessing for instability, particularly if surgical intervention is considered.**
  - MRI
    - **False-positive MRIs are very common; clinical correlation between history, examination, and imaging is vital to achieve a successful surgical outcome.**
    - **MRI with gadolinium is the best study for recurrent disc herniations.**
  - CT myelogram can be obtained if MRI contraindicated; useful in patients with previous surgery to better define bony anatomy.
▨ Treatment
  - Nonsurgical treatment—physical therapy, NSAIDs, activity modification, and spinal steroid injections
  - Surgical indications—progressive motor weakness, persistent disabling pain despite conservative measures
  - Procedures
    - Surgical discectomy
      - Patients with positive study results, neurologic findings, tension signs, and predominantly sciatic

symptoms without mitigating psychosocial factors are the best candidates for surgical discectomy.
- Open, limited open, microscope-assisted, or endoscopic approaches are all equally effective. Visualization and localization of herniated disc and neural structures remains most important aspect of the surgical approach.
  - Hemilaminotomy and discectomy are the most commonly performed surgical procedures.
  - Total laminectomy may be necessary to access large central herniations and allow for adequate safe retraction of the common dural sac.
  - Paramedian/muscle splitting (Wiltse) approach may be necessary for far-lateral disc herniations.
- **Operative positioning requires the abdomen to be free to decrease pressure on the inferior vena cava and consequently on the epidural veins.**
- Fusion with or without instrumentation
  - Typically NOT required for surgical decompression of a herniated disc
  - Performed in presence of instability in conjunction with surgical decompression, not instead of it
  - **Indications of fusion**
    - **Preoperative evidence of segmental spinal instability at level of disc herniation, such as spondylolisthesis and/or increased translational or angular mobility on flexion/ extension films.**
    - **Intraoperative iatrogenic instability secondary to resection of over 50% of bilateral facet, 100% of unilateral facet joint, or excessive resection of pars intraarticularis**
- ■ **Spinal stenosis (Figure 8-16)**
- ▦ Introduction
  - *Spinal stenosis* is narrowing of the spinal canal or neural foramina, producing nerve root compression, root ischemia, and a variable syndrome of back and leg pain.
  - Classification:
    - Central stenosis
    - Lateral recess stenosis/subarticular stenosis/entry zone stenosis
    - Foraminal stenosis
  - Stenosis is not usually symptomatic until patients reach late middle age; men are affected somewhat more often than women.
  - **"Tandem stenosis"** is the occurrence of both cervical and lumbar stenosis and can present as neurogenic claudication, radiculopathy, and myelopathy.
- ■ **Central stenosis—thecal sac compression**
  - Introduction
    - The *central canal* is defined as the space posterior to the posterior longitudinal ligament, anterior to the ligamentum flavum and laminae, and bordered laterally by the medial border of the superior articular process.
    - Soft tissue structures, including the hypertrophied ligamentum flavum, facet capsule, and bulging disc, may contribute as much as 40% to thecal sac compression.
    - *Absolute stenosis* is defined as a cross-sectional area of less than 100 mm^2 or less than 10 mm of anteroposterior diameter as seen on CT cross section.

- Central stenosis is more common in men because their spinal canal is smaller at the L3-L5 level than in women.
- It affects an older population more than lateral recess stenosis does.
- Etiology—congenital versus acquired
  - Congenital (idiopathic or developmental in achondroplastic dwarfism)
  - Acquired stenosis (most common) is usually:
    - Degenerative secondary to enlargement of osteoarthritic facets with medial encroachment
    - Degenerative secondary to spondylolisthesis
    - Posttraumatic
    - Iatrogenic (postsurgical)
    - Secondary to systemic disease processes such as Paget disease, AS, acromegaly, fluorosis, and others
- History
  - Symptoms include insidious pain and paresthesias with ambulation and are relieved by sitting or flexion of the spine.
  - Patients commonly complain of lower extremity pain, usually in the buttock and thigh, with numbness or "giving way."
  - History of radiating leg pain in a true dermatomal distribution is relatively uncommon in those with spinal stenosis.
  - **Neurogenic claudication**
    - **Differentiate from vascular claudication**
    - **Pain starts proximal (buttock) and extends distal.**
    - **Pain relieved only when sitting, not with standing**
    - **Normal vascular examination**

- Physical examination
  - Few neurologic findings; abnormal neurologic examination found in fewer than 50%. Tension signs are rarely positive.
  - Primary finding is typically limited extension, which may exacerbate pain
  - Normal extremity perfusion and pulses
  - Standing treadmill tests can be a sensitive (>90%) provocative evaluation of neurogenic claudication (Table 8-7).
- Diagnostic studies—further workup may include:
  - Plain radiographs
    - Interspace narrowing due to disc degeneration
    - Medially placed facets
    - Flattening of the lordotic curve
    - Subluxation and degenerative changes of the facet joints may also be seen.
  - CT myelogram
    - Osteophyte formation
    - Axial CT of axial canal morphology may demonstrate Trefoil canal.
  - **MRI—test of choice** (Figure 8-17)
    - Hypertrophy of ligamentum flavum
    - Foraminal stenosis and nerve root entrapment
    - Evaluation for malignancy
  - EMG/nerve conduction velocity testing may be used.
    - Sensitivity is variable and depends on the examiner.

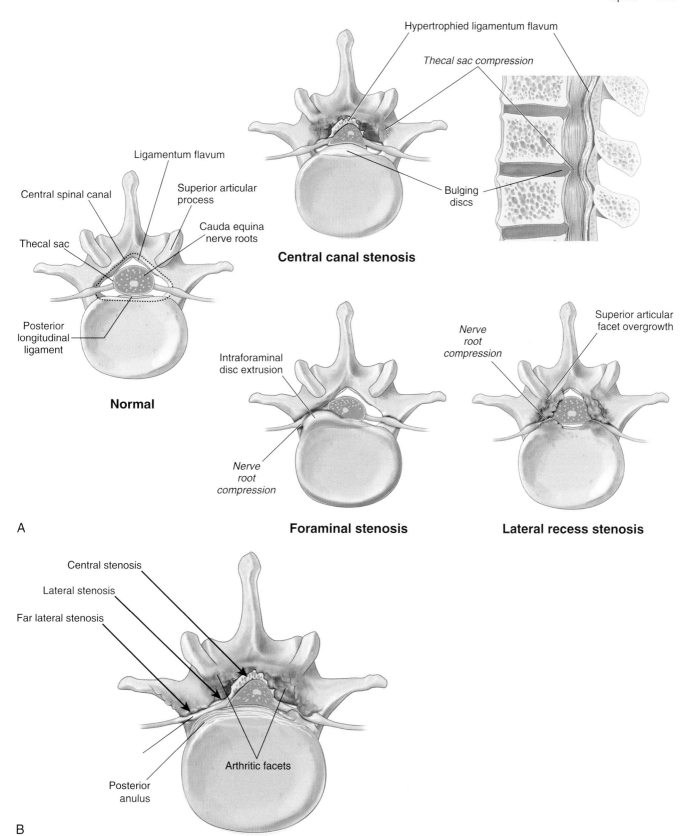

Hypertrophied ligamentum flavum

Thecal sac compression

Bulging discs

Central canal stenosis

Ligamentum flavum

Central spinal canal

Superior articular process

Cauda equina nerve roots

Thecal sac

Posterior longitudinal ligament

Normal

Intraforaminal disc extrusion

Nerve root compression

Foraminal stenosis

Nerve root compression

Superior articular facet overgrowth

Lateral recess stenosis

A

Central stenosis

Lateral stenosis

Far lateral stenosis

Arthritic facets

Posterior anulus

B

FIGURE 8-16 Pathoanatomy of spinal stenosis. Comparison of central, lateral/foraminal, and far lateral/lateral recess stenosis.

- Nerve conduction velocity testing is sometimes helpful in differentiating radiculopathy from peripheral neuropathy.
- Treatment
  - Nonoperative:
    - Rest, Williams flexion exercises, NSAIDs, weight reduction
    - Lumbar epidural steroids may be helpful for short-term relief but have shown variable results in controlled studies.
    - Transforaminal nerve block can be effective when the involved roots can be identified.
  - Surgery indications:
    - Positive study results and a persistent unacceptably impaired quality of life

Table 8-7	Findings on Treadmill Tests in Neurogenic Claudication	
	FINDING	
ACTIVITY	**VASCULAR CLAUDICATION**	**NEUROGENIC CLAUDICATION**
Walking	Distal-proximal pain, calf pain	Proximal-distal thigh pain
Uphill walking	Symptoms develop sooner	Symptoms develop later
Rest	Relief with sitting or bending	
Bicycling	Symptoms develop	Symptoms do not develop
Lying flat	Relief	May exacerbate symptoms

- Progressive motor weakness and/or bowel and bladder dysfunction (uncommon)
- Techniques:
  - **Adequate decompression of the identified disorder typically includes laminectomy and partial medial facetectomy, which can usually be done without destabilizing the spine, thus avoiding fusion.**
  - Residual foraminal stenosis is a common reason for persistent radicular pain after laminectomy.
  - Indications for fusion:
    - Surgical instability (removal of one facet or more)
    - Pars defects (including those that are postsurgical) with disc disease
    - Symptomatic radiographic instability
    - Degenerative or isthmic spondylolisthesis
    - Degenerative scoliosis
- **Outcomes—Spine Patient Outcomes Research Trial (SPORT)**
  - At 4-year follow-up, significant improvement in primary outcome measures for operative compared with nonoperative groups (SF-36 Bodily Pain and Physical Function and Oswestry Disability Index)
  - Both operative and nonoperative groups had improvement from baseline.
- **Lateral recess stenosis—nerve root compression**
  - Introduction
    - Lateral recess stenosis is also known as *subarticular stenosis* or *entry zone stenosis*.
    - The lateral recess is defined by the superior articular facet posteriorly, the thecal sac medially, the pedicle

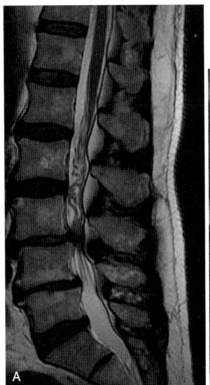
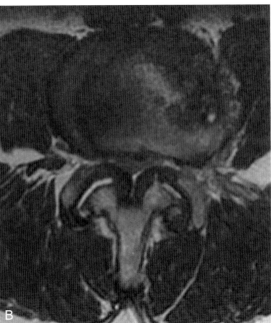

FIGURE 8-17 Spinal stenosis. Sagittal **(A)** and axial **(B)** T2-weighted MRI demonstrating central stenosis (particularly at L2-L3) due to a combination of anterolisthesis, disc herniation, thickened ligamentum flavum, and facet hypertrophy. Note the classic appearance of curly nerve roots above the stenosis known as *redundant nerve roots*. (From Van Goethem JWM et al: Spine and lower back pain. In Law M et al, editors: *Problem solving in neuroradiology,* Philadelphia, 2011, Elsevier, p 610.)

laterally, and the posterolateral vertebral body anteriorly.
- Compression of individual nerve roots by medial overgrowth of the superior articular facet at a given facet joint
- Etiology
  - Impingement of nerve roots lateral to thecal sac as they pass through the lateral recess and into the neural foramen
  - Associated with facet joint arthropathy (superior articular process enlargement) and disc disease (see Figure 8-16, *B*)
  - Subarticular compression—compression between medial aspect of a hypertrophic superior articular facet and posterior aspect of vertebral body and disc
  - Hypertrophy of the ligamentum flavum and/or ventral facet joint capsule and vertebral body osteophyte/disc exacerbates the stenosis.
  - **Affects the traversing (lower) nerve root (L5 root at L4-L5)**
- Treatment
  - After failure of nonoperative treatment, decompression of the hypertrophied lamina and ligamentum flavum and partial facetectomy are usually successful.
  - Nerve root compression can occur at more than one level and must be completely decompressed to relieve the symptoms.
  - Fusion may be necessary if instability is present or created.
- Foraminal stenosis—nerve root compression
  - Introduction
    - The intervertebral foramen is bordered superiorly and inferiorly by the adjacent level pedicles, posteriorly by the facet joint and lateral extensions of the ligamentum flavum, and anteriorly by the adjacent vertebral bodies and disc.
    - Normal foraminal height is 20 to 30 mm; superior width is 8 to 10 mm.
  - Etiology
    - Intraforaminal disc protrusion
    - Impingement of the tip of the superior facet
    - Lower lumbar areas (L4-L5 and L5-S1) are usually involved because the foramina decrease in size as the size of the nerve root increases.
    - Foraminal stenosis affects the exiting (upper) root (L4 at L4-L5) at a motion segment.
    - Pain may be the result of intraneural edema and demyelination.
  - History and physical examination
    - More consistent with nerve root compression, as with radiculopathy from herniated disc
    - Pain, numbness, and/or dysesthesia typically follow a dermatomal distribution.
    - Motor and reflex examination typically normal but in the presence of weakness will follow myotome; reflexes typically normal or hyporeflexic
    - Tension signs can be positive.
  - Imaging studies are analogous to those for other lumbar conditions.
  - Treatment
    - Nonoperative should remain the mainstay of management.
    - Surgical indications:

- Positive study results and a persistent unacceptably impaired quality of life
- Progressive motor weakness and/or bowel and bladder dysfunction (uncommon)
- Techniques:
  - Identify area of and source of stenosis.
  - **Typically partial medial facetectomy and resection of medial process of superior articular process**
  - **Care should be taken to preserve greater than 50% of facet joint and pars intraarticularis to preserve stability.**
  - **Fusion and stabilization should be considered if evidence of preoperative instability or iatrogenic intraoperative instability.**

- **Spondylolysis and spondylolisthesis**
- Spondylolysis—defect in the pars interarticularis
  - **One of the most common causes of low back pain in children and adolescents**
    - **Typically symptoms aggravated with extension**
    - **Improved with flexion**
    - May or may not be associated with radicular symptoms and nerve root irritation
  - Fatigue fracture from repetitive hyperextension stresses
    - Most common in gymnasts and football linemen
    - Probable hereditary predisposition
  - Imaging
    - Plain lateral radiographs demonstrate 80% of the lesions.
    - **Another 15% are visible on oblique radiographs, which show a defect in the neck of the "Scottie dog."**
    - **CT, bone scanning, and (more recently) single-photon emission computed tomography (SPECT) may be helpful in identifying subtle defects.**
    - **Increased uptake on SPECT is more compatible with acute lesions that have the potential to heal.**
  - Treatment
    - Usually aimed at symptomatic relief rather than fracture healing in spondylolysis without spondylolisthesis
      - Activity restriction
      - Flexion exercises
      - Bracing
    - Nonunion is common and may not show on scans.
  - Prognosis—unilateral defects rarely have progression of the slippage (-olisthesis).
- Spondylolisthesis—forward slippage of one vertebra on another ("-olisthesis")
  - **Classification—six types (Newman, Wiltse, McNab) (Figures 8-18 and 8-19; Table 8-8)**
  - **Grading—five grades according to severity (Meyerding); severity of the slip based on amount or degree (compared with S1 width) (Figure 8-20)**
    - Grade I: 0% to 25%
    - Grade II: 25% to 50%
    - Grade III: 50% to 75%
    - Grade IV: greater than 75%
    - Grade V: greater than 100% (spondyloptosis)
  - Other relevant measurements (see Figure 8-20)
    - Sacral inclination (normally > 30 degrees)
    - Slip angle (normally < 0 degrees, signifying lordosis at the L5-S1 disc)
      - Means for quantifying lumbopelvic deformity

"Scottie dog"

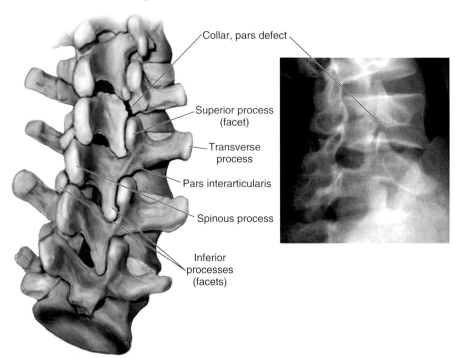

Collar, pars defect

Superior process
(facet)

Transverse
process

Pars interarticularis

Spinous process

Inferior
processes
(facets)

FIGURE 8-18 Spondylolysis. Note disruption of the neck of the "Scottie dog."

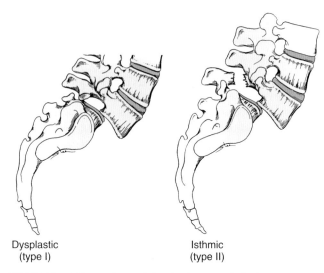

Dysplastic
(type I)

Isthmic
(type II)

FIGURE 8-19 Comparison of dysplastic versus isthmic spondylolisthesis. (Adapted from Rothman RH, Simeone FA: *The spine,* ed 2, Philadelphia, 1982, WB Saunders, p 264.)

Table 8-8	Types of Spondylolisthesis	
TYPE	**AGE**	**PATHOLOGY/OTHER**
I—Dysplastic	Child	Congenital dysplasia of S1 superior facet
II—Isthmic*	5-50 yr	Predisposition leading to elongation/fracture of pars (L5-S1)
III—Degenerative	>40 yr	Facet arthrosis leading to subluxation (L4-L5)
IV—Traumatic	Any age	Acute fracture other than pars
V—Pathologic	Any age	Incompetence of bony elements
VI—Postsurgical	Adult	Excessive resection of neural arches/facets

*Most common type.

- Predicts intervention and affects cosmesis as well as prognosis
- **Pelvic incidence (normally 50 degrees)**
- The natural history of the disorder is that unilateral pars defects almost never slip and that the progression of spondylolisthesis slows over time.
- **However, in adulthood, degeneration and narrowing of the disc (usually L5-S1) are common and lead to narrowing of the neural foramen and compression of the exiting (L5) root that causes the radicular symptoms.**
- ▪ Pediatric/adolescent considerations
  - Presentation

- Typically back pain (instability), hamstring tightness, palpable step-off, **alteration in gait ("pelvic waddle")**
- Although symptoms may begin at any time in life, screening studies identify the slippage as occurring most commonly at age 4 to 6 years.
- Severe slips are rare and may be associated with radicular findings (L5), cauda equina dysfunction, kyphosis of the lumbosacral junction, and "heart-shaped" buttocks.
- Epidemiology
  - Usually at L5-S1 and typically grade II
  - Occurs most often in whites, boys, and children who participate in hyperextension activities
  - Remarkably frequent in some Eskimo tribes (>50%)
- Etiology
  - **Thought to result from shear stress at the pars interarticularis and to be associated with repetitive hyperextension**

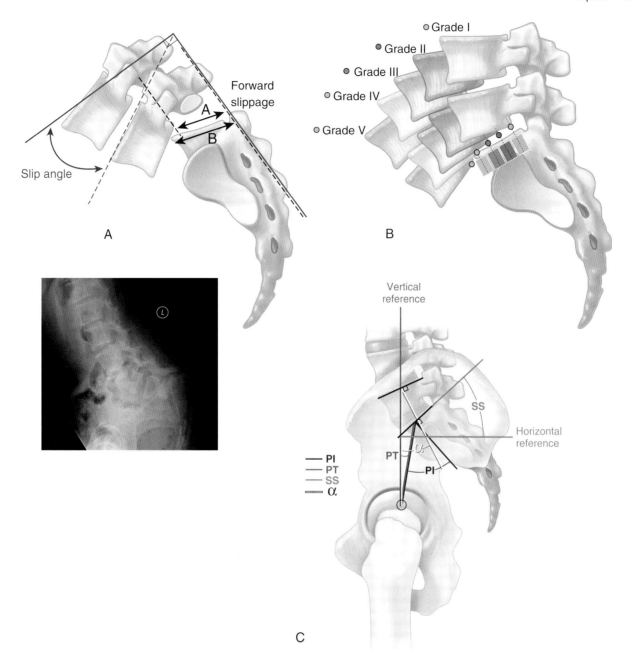

FIGURE 8-20 Spondylolisthesis. **A, Slip angle** and percentage of forward slippage. The slip angle is measured from the superior border of L5 and a perpendicular line from the posterior edge of the sacrum. **B, Meyerding grades I to V.** The grade of spondylolisthesis is determined by dividing the sacral body into four segments, with grade V as spondyloptosis. **C, Pelvic incidence (PI).** A line perpendicular to the midpoint of the sacral end plate is drawn. A second line connecting the same sacral midpoint and the center of the femoral heads is drawn. The angle subtended by these lines is the pelvic incidence. Should the femoral heads not be superimposed, the center of each femoral head is marked and the point halfway between the two centers serves as the femoral head center. **Pelvic tilt (PT).** A line from the midpoint of the sacral end plate is drawn to the center of the femoral heads. The angle subtended between this line and the vertical reference line is the pelvic tilt. **Sacral slope (SS).** A line parallel to the sacral end plate is drawn. The angle subtended between this line and the horizontal reference line is the sacral slope. α **Angle–L5 incidence.** A line from the midpoint of the upper end plate of L5 is connected to the center of the femoral heads. A second line perpendicular to the upper L5 end plate is drawn from the midpoint of the end plate. The angle subtended by these two lines (α) is the L5 incidence. (Modified from Herring J: *Tachdjian's pediatric orthopaedics,* ed 4, Philadelphia, 2007, Elsevier.)

- **Patients with type I or dysplastic spondylolisthesis are at a higher risk for slip progression and the development of cauda equina dysfunction because the neural arch is intact.**
- Spina bifida occulta, thoracic hyperkyphosis, and Scheuermann disease have been associated with spondylolisthesis.

- Treatment
  - Nonoperative
    - Most treated conservatively with symptomatic care
      - Usually responds to nonoperative treatment consisting of activity modification and exercise
      - Adolescents with a grade I slip may return to normal activities, including contact sports, once asymptomatic.

- Those with asymptomatic grade II spondylolisthesis are restricted from activities such as gymnastics or football.
- Careful observation must be maintained to assess for progression of slip in the pediatric and adolescent patient.
- Risk factors for progression: young age at presentation, female sex, slip angle of greater than 10 degrees, high-grade slip
- Dysplastic types include dome-shaped or significantly inclined sacrum (>30 degrees beyond vertical position), trapezoid-shaped L5, sagittally shaped or dysplastic facets of S1.
- **Surgical indications**
  - Progression of slip
  - Weakness (uncommon), persistent severe back or leg pain despite conservative measures
- Operative
  - **Low-grade spondylolisthesis (grades I and II)**
    - **Surgery for patients with a low-grade slip generally consists of L5-S1 posterolateral fusion in situ and is usually reserved for those with intractable pain in whom nonoperative treatment has failed or those demonstrating progressive slippage.**
    - Wiltse has popularized a paraspinal muscle–splitting approach to the lumbar transverse process and sacral alae that is frequently used in this setting.
    - L5 radiculopathy is uncommon in children with low-grade slips and rarely if ever requires decompression.
    - Repair of the pars defect with the use of a lag screw (Buck) or tension band wiring (Bradford) with bone grafting has been reported. Indicated in young patients with slippage less than 10% and a pars defect at L4 or above
  - **High-grade disease (grades III through V)**
    - Commonly cause neurologic abnormalities
    - L5-S1 isthmic spondylolisthesis causes an L5 radiculopathy (contrast to S1 radiculopathy in L5-S1 HNP).
    - Prophylactic fusion is recommended in growing children with slippage of more than 50% (grade III, IV, V).
    - **Often requires in situ bilateral posterolateral fusion, usually at L4-S1 (L5 is too far anterior to effect L5-S1 fusion), with or without instrumentation**
    - Nerve root exploration is controversial but usually limited to children with clear-cut radicular pain or significant weakness.
    - Other surgical procedures described include posterior decompression, fibular interbody fusion, and posterolateral fusion without reduction, with excellent long-term results (Bohlman), as well as L5 vertebrectomy and fusion for spondyloptosis (Gaines resection).
  - Considerations for reduction of spondylolisthesis:
    - Reduction of spondylolisthesis has been associated with a 20% to 30% incidence of L5 root injuries (most are transient) and should be used cautiously.
    - A cosmetically unacceptable deformity and L5-S1 kyphosis so severe that the posterior fusion mass from L4 to the sacrum would be under tension without reversal of the kyphosis are the most commonly cited indications.
    - **In situ fusion leaves a patient with a high-grade slip and lumbosacral kyphosis with such severe compensatory hyperlordosis above the fusion that long-term problems frequently ensue.**
    - **Reduction in this setting is gaining widespread acceptance.**
    - Close neurologic monitoring is needed during the procedure and for several days afterward to identify postoperative neuropathy.

- **Degenerative spondylolisthesis considerations**
  - Epidemiology
    - More common in African Americans, persons with diabetes, and women older than age 40
    - Most frequent at the L4-L5 level
    - Reported to be more common in patients with transitional (sacralized) L5 vertebrae and sagittally oriented facet joints
  - **Presentation**
    - **Central stenosis results in neurogenic claudication.**
      - Decreased ambulatory status
      - Leg heaviness and cramping
      - Improved with flexion, exacerbated with extension (positive "shopping cart" sign)
      - Bowel and bladder dysfunction (uncommon)
    - **Lateral recess stenosis results in nerve root compression.**
      - Typically traversing nerve root compression
      - Due to compression between the hypertrophic and subluxated inferior facet of superior vertebra and the posterosuperior body of inferior vertebra
      - L4-L5 degenerative spondylolisthesis typically compresses on the L5 nerve root.
  - Treatment
    - Nonoperative—same as for stenosis
    - Operative—decompression of the nerve roots and stabilization by fusion (traditionally posterolateral), with or without instrumentation
      - Outcomes (SPORT trial)
      - At 4-year follow-up there is significant improvement in primary outcome measures (SF-36 Bodily Pain and Physical Function, Oswestry Disability Index) for operative compared with nonoperative groups.
      - Both operative and nonoperative groups had improvement from baseline.
- **Adult isthmic spondylolisthesis considerations**
  - Introduction
    - Familial association
    - **Associated increased pelvic incidence**
      - As pelvic incidence increases, sacral slope increases, necessitating an increasing in lumbar lordosis to maintain sagittal balance.
      - Normal individuals have a pelvic incidence of 50 to 55 degrees, whereas patients with spondylolisthesis have 70 to 80 degrees.

- However, pelvic incidence does not predict progression of listhesis.
- L5-S1 most common level for isthmic spondylolisthesis
- **Presentation**
  - **Low back pain—typically aggravated with extension and due to posterior element compression**
  - **Radiculopathy—typically exiting nerve root and due to compression from the fibrocartilaginous reparative pars (Gill nodule).**
    - **L5-S1 isthmic spondylolisthesis results in L5 (exiting nerve root) radicular pain.**
- Treatment
  - Nonoperative—hamstring stretching, core strengthening, lumbar flexion-based exercises, NSAIDs (etc.)
  - Operative options
    - Foraminal decompression
    - **In situ posterolateral L5-S1 fusion for grade I/II slips versus posterolateral L4-S1 fusion for grade III/IV/V slips**
    - **Reduction controversial—may result in L5 nerve root palsy**
    - **Interbody fusion controversial—may increase fusion rates, improve neuroforaminal height, help restore lumbar lordosis, and avoid fusion to L4 in high grade slips**

■ **Cauda equina syndrome**
- Secondary to large extruded disc, surgical trauma, and/or hematoma
- Suspected in patients with postoperative urinary retention
- **Presents as bilateral buttock and lower extremity pain as well as bowel or bladder dysfunction (usually urinary retention), saddle anesthesia, and varying degrees of loss of lower extremity motor or sensory dysfunction**
- **Digital rectal examination is used for the initial diagnosis.**
  - **Should check for presence of rectal tone, perianal sensation, and volitional control/contraction. In particular, evaluation of perianal sensation is important for immediate diagnosis.**
- **Urgent/emergent MRI can help assess for compression of the cauda equina.**
- Timing of surgical decompression remains controversial, but in general earliest possible decompression is indicated to arrest progression of neurologic loss.
- Although the prognosis for recovery is guarded in most cases, surgical decompression within the first 48 hours was reported to lead to best outcomes.

■ **Surgical complications**
- **Recurrent herniation** (usually acute recurrence of signs/symptoms after a 6- to 12-month pain-free interval)
  - Herniation at another level
  - Unrecognized lateral stenosis (may be the most common)
- Vascular injury—may occur during attempts at disc removal if curettes or pituitary rongeurs are allowed to penetrate the anterior longitudinal ligament
  - Intraoperative pulsatile bleeding due to deep penetration is treated with rapid wound closure, intravenous (IV) administration of fluids and blood, repositioning the patient, and a transabdominal approach to find and stop the source of bleeding.

- Mortality may exceed 50%.
- Late sequelae of vascular injuries may include delayed hemorrhage, pseudoaneurysm, and arteriovenous fistula formation.
- Nerve root injury—more common with anomalous nerve roots
- Iatrogenic vertebral instability
- Pseudarthrosis—may be reduced with use of instrumentation
- Epidural fibrosis occurs at about 3 months postoperatively and may be associated with back or leg pain.
  - Responds poorly to reexploration
  - Scarring can be differentiated from recurrent HNP with a gadolinium-enhanced MRI.
- **Dural tear—1% to 4% incidence**
  - Primary repair necessary to avoid the development of a pseudomeningocele or spinal fluid fistula (Figure 8-21)
  - **More common during revision surgery (up to 47%)**
  - Fibrin adhesive sealant may be a useful adjunct for effecting dural closure.
  - Bed rest and subarachnoid drain placement are advocated if cerebrospinal fluid (CSF) leak is suspected postoperatively.
  - If tear is adequately repaired, clinical outcomes are generally unaffected.
- Wound infection (≈1% in open discectomy)—increased risk in diabetics
- **Discitis (3-6 weeks postoperatively, with rapid onset of severe back pain). (Also see Spinal Infections.)**
  - **MRI with gadolinium is the best diagnostic modality.**
  - Needle biopsy followed by empirical use of antibiotics
  - Surgery usually not needed

ADULT DEFORMITY

■ **Adult scoliosis—coronal plane deformity**
- Usually defined as scoliosis in patients older than age 20; more symptomatic than its childhood counterpart (see Chapter 3, Pediatric Orthopaedics).
- Classification
  - Idiopathic—progression of untreated adolescent scoliosis
  - De novo
    - Neuromuscular
    - Degenerative (secondary to degenerative disc disease or osteoporosis)
    - Posttraumatic
    - Iatrogenic
- Diagnosis
  - Association between pain and scoliosis in the adult is controversial.
  - Progression of symptoms to side of curve convexity indicates poor prognosis.
  - Lumbar stenosis, in particular in the concavity of the curve
  - Cosmetic deformity may be present.
  - Cardiopulmonary problems (thoracic curves > 60 to 65 degrees may alter pulmonary function tests; curves > 90 degrees may affect mortality)
  - Myelography with CT or MRI is useful for evaluation of nerve root compression in stenosis.

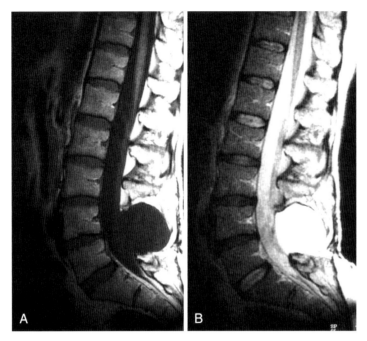

FIGURE 8-21 Postoperative pseudomeningocele. Sagittal T1-weighted **(A)** and T2-weighted **(B)** MRI and axial T1-weighted MRI demonstrating a large cystic mass that is visible in the laminectomy defect. It has signal intensities identical to cerebrospinal fluid and shows no enhancement. (From Van Goethem JWM et al: Spine and lower back pain. In Law M et al, editors: *Problem solving in neuroradiology,* Philadelphia, 2011, Elsevier, p 610.)

- MRI, facet injections, and/or discography may be used to evaluate symptoms in the lumbar spine.
- **Curve progression**
  - There is no demonstrated association between curve progression and pregnancy.
  - **Progression is unlikely in curves of less than 30 degrees.**
  - **Right thoracic curves of greater than 50 degrees are at the highest risk for progression (usually 1 degree/yr), followed by right lumbar curves.**
- Treatment
  - Nonoperative treatment:
    - Uncertain correlation between adult scoliosis and back pain makes conservative management essential.
    - Nonoperative treatment includes NSAIDs, weight reduction, therapy, muscle strengthening, facet joint injections, and orthoses (used with activity).
  - Operative indications:
    - Young adults (<30 years) with curves of greater than 50 to 60 degrees
    - Older patients with refractory pain
    - Sagittal plane imbalance is a strong predictor of disability.
    - Progressive curves
    - Cardiopulmonary compromise (worsening pulmonary function tests in severe curves)
    - Refractory spinal stenosis
  - Operative techniques:
    - Selective posterior fusions for flexible thoracic curves
    - Combined anterior release and fusion and posterior fusion and instrumentation may be beneficial for large (>70 degree), more rigid curves (as determined on side-bending films) or curves in the lumbar spine.

- Fusion to L5
  - Associated with development of L5-S1 degenerative disc disease
  - Associated with progressive sagittal imbalance
- Fusion to sacrum
  - Increases stability of long lumbar fusion
  - Increased incidence of pseudarthrosis and potential for postoperative gait disturbances
- Fixation to ilium
  - Indicated in lumbosacral fusions involving more than three levels
  - Potential for prominent implants
- Anterior interbody fusion
  - Achieve anterior column support
  - Increases stability of long fusions including L5-S1
  - Helps maintain corrections of sagittal and coronal deformities
  - Increased fusion rates
- Outcomes
  - Nonsurgically treated adults with late-onset idiopathic scoliosis are highly productive at 50-year follow-up, with a slightly increased risk of shortness of breath with activity and chief complaints of back pain and poor cosmesis.
  - Operative risk for these patients is high (up to a 25% complication rate in older patients).
- Complications
  - Pseudarthrosis (15% with posterior fusion only; the highest risk at the thoracolumbar junction and at L5-S1)
  - Urinary tract infection, instrumentation problems, infection (up to 5%), and neurologic deficits
  - Preservation of normal sagittal alignment with fusion is critical to outcomes
- **Kyphosis—sagittal plane deformity**
- Etiology

- Idiopathic (old Scheuermann disease [since adolescence])
- Posttraumatic (missed posterior ligamentous complex injury)
- AS
- Metabolic bone disease
  - Progressive kyphosis secondary to multiple osteoporotic compression fractures
  - Treated with exercise, bracing, and medical management of the underlying bone disease
- Nontraumatic adult kyphosis
  - Severe idiopathic or congenital kyphosis may be a source of back pain in the adult, particularly when it is present in the thoracolumbar or lumbar spine.
  - When the symptoms fail to respond to nonoperative management (see preceding discussion on adult scoliosis), posterior instrumentation and fusion of the entire kyphotic segment with a compression implant may be indicated.
  - Anterior fusion is considered for curves not correcting to 55 degrees or less on hyperextension lateral radiographs.
- **Kyphotic deformity in ankylosing spondylitis (AS)**
  - Introduction
    - Frequently seen in patients with AS
    - Progressive inflammation and ossification of the spine results in kyphotic deformity of the spine.
    - Results in loss of horizontal gaze
    - Can also be associated with hip flexion contractures
  - Spinal involvement can involve any level of the spine.
    - Frequently direct cervical and cervicothoracic involvement
      - Chin-on-chest deformity
      - Measurements include chin-brow angle.
    - Progressive deformity of the thoracolumbar spine can result in loss of horizontal gaze as well.
  - Nonsurgical management should include prevention with careful exercise and use of medications.
  - Surgical management
    - Should be undertaken only if deformity is debilitating—surgical correction of kyphotic deformity in AS patients associated with high risk of complications
    - **Careful assessment of location of deformity, including hip and knees**
      - If present these should corrected first.
      - May eliminate the need for surgical management of the spine
    - **Spinal osteotomies**
      - Typically performed at level of greatest deformity
      - Lumbar osteotomies are below the level of the spinal cord and may be safer to perform—traditionally performed at L3.
      - **Cervicothoracic pedicle subtraction osteotomy (PSO) typically performed at C7-T1**
        - Typically vertebral artery has not entered cervical spine at C7
        - Perform PSO (described later)
        - Careful examination of C8 root postoperatively
        - Staged anterior procedure may be necessary to achieve anterior column support at C7-T1 if there is a large anterior defect after osteoclasis.

- Posttraumatic kyphosis
  - Present after fractures of the thoracolumbar spine treated without surgery, particularly in setting of posterior ligamentous complex injury
  - Fractures treated by laminectomy without fusion and also fractures for which fusion has been performed unsuccessfully
  - Progressive kyphosis may produce pain at the fracture site, with radiating leg pain and/or neurologic dysfunction if there is associated neural compression.
- **Postlaminectomy deformity**
  - Progressive deformity (usually kyphosis) resulting from a prior wide laminectomy
  - In children this procedure is followed by a high risk (90%) of deformity.
  - Fusion plus internal fixation may be considered prophylactic for young patients who require extensive decompression.
  - Fusion using pedicle screw fixation is best for reconstruction in the adult lumbar spine.
- Operative options:
  - Posterior fusion with compression instrumentation for milder deformities
  - Combined anterior and posterior osteotomies, instrumentation, and fusion for more severe deformities
  - Anterior spinal cord or cauda equina decompression combined with posterior instrumentation and fusion for cases involving neurologic dysfunction
  - **Osteotomies**
    - **Smith-Petersen osteotomy (SPO)—5 to 10 degrees of sagittal plane correction**
      - Excision of superior and inferior articular facet at level of osteotomy
      - Removal of inferior lamina, spinous process, and ligamentum flavum at level of osteotomy (typically chevron-shaped osteotomy)
      - Osteotomy is typically closed through intact flexible disc space.
      - In AS, DISH, and ankylosed patients, osteotomy closure may require aggressive opening of the intervertebral disc anteriorly (known as *osteoclasis*).
        - Osteoclasis is becoming less commonly used, because it is a spinal column–lengthening procedure that can result in traumatic vascular injury of the great vessels and create a void anteriorly, with loss of anterior column support.
    - **Pedicle subtraction osteotomy (PSO)—30 degrees of sagittal plane correction**
      - Wide extensive laminectomy required
      - Pedicles isolated at the level of the osteotomy by resecting superior and inferior articular facets bilaterally
      - Transverse process disarticulated from pedicle
      - Pedicles resected back to the level of the posterior vertebral body
      - Vertebral body decancellated through pedicles with curettes
      - Lateral walls of vertebral body carefully isolated with vertebral body retractors
      - Osteotomy completed by removing wedge-shaped cortical bone of lateral wall

- Care is taken not to complete the osteotomy through anterior vertebral body, which can result in extremely unstable spine and parallel collapse of the vertebral body with undercorrection.
- Temporary rods are frequently placed during osteotomy to reduce risk of vertebral body translation.
- Once osteotomy is closed, the dural sac and exiting and traversing nerve roots are checked to ensure excessive compression or dural buckling are not present.
- **Vertebral body resection (VBR)—30 to 40 degrees of sagittal plane correction**
  - Posterior elements removed as during PSO (see first four steps)
  - Vertebral body can be removed piecemeal or en bloc
    - En bloc—vertebral retractors are carefully inserted around vertebral body; intervertebral disc is removed above and below vertebral body; vertebral body is carefully rotated around the common dural sac.
    - Piecemeal—vertebral body retractors are carefully inserted around vertebral body; decancellation of vertebral body with curettes through pedicles; vertebral body removed with curettes, pituitary, and rongeurs.

■ **Metabolic bone disease**
▥ Introduction
- Osteopenia and osteoporosis remain common causes for vertebral body compression fractures, with subsequent kyphosis and positive sagittal balance.
- Prevention of compression fractures has been successful with bisphosphonate treatment, with a decreased incidence of vertebral fractures of 65% at 1 year and 40% at 3 years.
- An underlying malignancy as a cause of the osteopenia should be considered; evaluation with MRI is sensitive for determining the presence of tumor.
- Surgical attempts at correction and stabilization are marked by a high complication rate.
▥ Cement augmentation—vertebroplasty and kyphoplasty
- Percutaneous techniques designed to relieve pain typically use polymethylmethacrylate (PMMA).
  - Vertebroplasty uses low-volume, high-pressure, low-viscosity cement.
  - Kyphoplasty has also been proposed to correct deformity (controversial); uses high-volume, low-pressure, higher-viscosity cement.
- Indications:
  - Subacute injuries, although precise indications are poorly defined
  - To respond to either technique, a fracture must still be in the active healing phase, which is best demonstrated on MRI (spin tau inversion recovery [STIR] sequences).
  - A patient with a painful but healed fracture is unlikely to improve.
  - Improvement in pain and quality of life has been questioned in recent studies.
- Complications:
  - Hypotensive reaction to cement

- Extravasation of cement into canal, resulting in compression of neural elements
- Pulmonary embolization of cement (debated)

SACROPELVIS

■ **Sacroiliac joint dysfunction**
▥ Diagnosis
- Gaenslen test—elicited with patient lying on affected side without support
- FABER test—*f*lexion, *ab*duction, and *e*xternal *r*otation of involved extremity
- Direct compression with reproduction of symptoms or with flexion, abduction, and external rotation (FABER) test of involved extremity
▥ Treatment
- Local injections may have diagnostic and therapeutic roles.
- Orthotic management (trochanteric cinch) can be helpful.
- Fusion is not indicated unless an infection is present.

■ **Coccygodynia**
▥ Diagnosis
- Pain and point tenderness over coccyx
- More common in women and may occur after pregnancy or minor trauma or idiopathically
- Occasionally associated with a fracture
- Plain radiographs may demonstrate fracture or an increased angular deformity to coccyx but can frequently be normal.
▥ Treatment
- Symptoms may last 1 to 2 years but are almost always self-limiting.
- Treatment should be conservative and may include a sitting donut, NSAIDs, stretching exercises, and local injection.
- Surgery is associated with a high failure rate and significant risk of complications.
- Consider MRI or CT scan of pelvis and/or spine if symptoms persist despite conservative measures.

■ **Sacral insufficiency fracture**
▥ Diagnosis
- Occurs in older patients with osteopenia
- Often without a history of trauma
- Complaints include low back and groin pain.
- This fracture is diagnosed with a technetium bone scan (H-shaped uptake pattern is diagnostic) or with CT.
▥ Treatment
- Nonoperative: rest, analgesic medication, and ambulatory aids until symptoms resolve
- Evaluation and management should include an evaluation and workup for osteopenia and osteoporosis.

SPINAL TUMORS

■ **Introduction—spine is a frequent site of metastasis; certain tumors with a predilection for the spine have unique manifestations in vertebrae.**
▥ **Tumors of the vertebral body**
- Histiocytosis X
- Giant cell tumor
- Chordoma
- Osteosarcoma
- Hemangioma

- Metastatic disease
- Marrow cell tumors
- **Tumors of the posterior elements**
  - Aneurysmal bone cysts
  - Osteoblastoma
  - Osteoid osteoma
- Imaging studies
  - Radiographic changes:
    - Most tumors are osteolytic and not demonstrated on plain films until over 30% destruction of the vertebral body has occurred.
    - **Absent pedicle (winking owl sign on anteroposterior radiograph)**
    - Cortical erosion or expansion
    - Vertebral collapse
  - Bone scans can be helpful in cases of protracted back pain or night pain.
  - MRI is the diagnostic test of choice.
    - Malignant tumors have decreased T1 and increased T2 signal intensity.
    - **Sensitivity of MRI is increased with use of gadolinium.**
    - Malignant tumors occur more frequently in the lower spinal levels (lumbar > thoracic > cervical) and in the vertebral body.
  - CT scan can provide information on bony involvement and mechanical stability.
  - In cases where primary tumor is unknown, CT-guided needle biopsy is often possible and may avoid need of surgical open biopsy.
- General treatment considerations
  - **Multispecialty involvement important**
  - Prognosis dependent on several factors; considerations should include:
    - Primary versus metastatic lesion
    - Tumor pathology
    - Location in cephalad-caudal direction (cervical vs. thoracic vs. lumbar vs. sacrum vs. pelvis)
    - Location within vertebral body (vertebral body vs. posterior element)
    - Presence of neurologic involvement and length time of deficit
    - Mechanical stability
  - Complete surgical excision (en bloc) can be difficult but may be an option in selected cases; however, surgical excision frequently consists of tumor debulking and stabilization.
  - Consideration for preoperative embolization should be considered, in particular for renal cell and thyroid carcinomas.
  - Adjuvant therapy (chemotherapy, external beam radiation therapy) should be considered and can be an important part of therapy for many spinal primary and metastatic tumors.
  - For more details on these tumors, refer to Chapter 9, Orthopaedic Pathology.
- **Metastasis—the most common tumors of the spine, spreading to the vertebral body first and later to the pedicles**
- Diagnosis
  - History of cancer
    - Breast, lung, thyroid, renal, gastrointestinal, and prostate metastases are the most common tumors to metastasize to bone.
    - Lymphoma, myeloma

- Recent unexplained weight loss
- Night pain
- Age older than 50 years
- Examination—careful physical and neurologic examination vital
- Imaging
  - Should include plain radiographs of entire spine
  - **MRI with gadolinium of suspected levels; may require imaging entire neuraxis**
  - **CT scan of chest, abdomen, and pelvis can help identify possible primary lesion.**
  - Bone scan can assist in assessing for primary lesion and remote sites of involvement (but can be negative in up to 25% of cases).
  - Percutaneous biopsy of spinal lesion may avoid need for surgical open biopsy and can confirm diagnosis.
- Treatment
  - **Regardless of surgical or nonsurgical intervention, treatment should include multispecialty involvement.**
  - Nonsurgical treatment
    - Tumors that are radiosensitive, chemosensitive, or hormonal responsive should be considered for nonoperative treatment.
    - Radiosensitivity varies among primary tumor types, but newer techniques have made traditionally radioresistant tumors radioresponsive.
    - Patients with mechanical instability or evolving/progressive neurologic deficit should be considered for surgical intervention along with adjuvant radiation and/or chemotherapy.
    - In the case of epidural spinal cord compression, radiation therapy should be combined with direct surgical decompression for the best clinical outcomes.
  - Surgical treatment
    - Indications:
      - Progressive neurologic dysfunction that is unresponsive to radiation therapy
      - Persistent pain despite radiation therapy
      - Need for an open diagnostic biopsy
      - Pathologic mechanical instability
      - Radioresistant tumor
      - Life expectancy should play an important role with regard to whether surgical treatment is performed.
    - Techniques:
      - Vertebroplasty is gaining favor in cases of metastatic disease of the spine (myeloma, breast) without instability or neurologic compromise and represents a minimally invasive alternative to open surgery.
      - In cases of neurologic deficit and/or spinal instability, anterior decompression and stabilization (preserving intact posterior structures) may result in recovery of neurologic function.
      - Posterior stabilization or a circumferential approach is indicated in cases of multiple levels of destruction, involvement of both the anterior and posterior columns, or translational instability.
- **Primary tumors**
- **Osteoid osteoma (<2 cm in size) and osteoblastoma (≥2 cm in size)**
  - Diagnosis

- Common in the spine
- May present with painful scoliosis in a child
- Pain typically relieved by aspirin and/or NSAIDs
- Osteoblastomas typically occur in the posterior elements in older patients, with neurologic involvement in more than half.
- Imaging
  - Bone scan can help localize the level.
  - Thin-cut CT can direct surgical excision.
  - MRI is sensitive but not specific; surrounding hyperemic soft tissue may be misidentified as an aggressive lesion.
- Treatment
  - Scoliosis (lesion is typically at apex of convexity) resolves with early resection (within 18 months) in a child younger than age 11.
  - **If there is no scoliosis, aspirin and/or NSAIDs are the mainstay of treatment.**
  - Surgery is done if nonoperative treatment fails.
  - En bloc resection versus marginal or intralesional excision
  - CT-guided radiofrequency ablation (controversial)
  - May require posterior spinal fusion depending on degree of resection
- Aneurysmal bone cyst
  - Diagnosis
    - May represent degeneration of more aggressive tumor
    - Presents during second decade of life
    - Arises in the posterior elements, but possibly also involves the anterior elements
  - Treatment
    - Marginal or wide excision if possible
    - Alternatively, curettage and bone grafting
    - Radiation therapy if lesion inaccessible
- Hemangioma
  - Diagnosis
    - Common; typically seen in asymptomatic patients
    - Symptomatic patients older than 40 years may seek treatment after small spinal fractures.
    - The classic patient with hemangioma has "jailhouse striations" on plain films and "spikes of bone" demonstrated on CT.
    - Vertebrae are typically of normal size and not expanded (as in Paget disease).
  - Treatment
    - Observation or radiation therapy in cases of persistent pain after pathologic fracture
    - Anterior resection and fusion are reserved for refractory cases or pathologic collapse and neural compression, but massive bleeding may be encountered.
- Eosinophilic granuloma
  - Diagnosis
    - Usually seen in children younger than age 10
    - More common in thoracic spine
    - May present with progressive back pain
    - **Classically results in vertebral flattening (vertebra plana** [Calvé disease]**) seen on lateral radiographs**
    - Biopsy may be required for diagnosis unless the radiographic picture is classic.
  - Treatment
    - Symptoms are usually self-limiting.

- Chemotherapy is useful for the systemic form.
- Bracing may be indicated in children to prevent progressive kyphosis.
- Low-dose radiation therapy may be indicated in the presence of neurologic deficits.
- At least 50% reconstitution of vertebral height may be expected.
- Giant cell tumor
  - Diagnosis
    - Usually seen in the fourth and fifth decades of life
    - Destruction of the vertebral body in an expansile fashion
  - Treatment
    - Surgical excision and bone grafting
    - High recurrence rate is reported.
    - Radiation therapy should be avoided because of the possibility of malignant degeneration of the tumor.
- Plasmacytoma/multiple myeloma
  - Diagnosis
    - Shown as osteopenic lytic lesions on radiographs
    - Workup includes skeletal survey.
    - **Lesions are cold on bone scans.**
    - Pain secondary to pathologic fractures
    - Increased calcium level and decreased hematocrit levels as well as abnormal protein studies are common.
  - Treatment
    - Radiation therapy (3000-4000 cGy) with or without chemotherapy
    - Surgery is reserved for patients with spinal instability and those with refractory neurologic symptoms.
- **Chordoma**
  - Diagnosis
    - **Slow-growing lytic lesion in the midline of the anterior sacrum or the base of the skull**
    - May occur in other vertebrae (cervical spine next most common)
    - Patients with these tumors may present with intraabdominal complaints and a presacral mass.
    - **Physaliferous cells on biopsy specimens**
  - Treatment
    - **Surgical excision—treatment of choice (radioresistant tumor)**
    - **Typically requires resection of sacral nerve roots to achieve margin**
    - **If half of the sacral roots (i.e., all roots on one side) are preserved, patient may still maintain bowel and bladder function.**
    - **High recurrence rate**
    - Although a complete cure is rare, patients typically survive 10 to 15 years after diagnosis.
    - Lumbopelvic reconstruction is required after surgical resection.
- **Osteochondroma**
  - Arises in the posterior elements and is frequently seen in the cervical spine
  - Treatment is by excision, which may be necessary to rule out sarcomatous changes.
- Neurofibroma
  - Benign tumor of neural origin
  - Can present with enlarged intervertebral foramina seen on oblique radiographs
  - Malignant degeneration to fibrosarcoma can occur, which may present as new-onset neurologic deficit.

- Malignant primary skeletal lesions
  - Diagnosis
    - Osteosarcoma, Ewing sarcoma, and chondrosarcoma are uncommon in the spine.
      - When they occur they are associated with a poor prognosis.
  - Treatment
    - Chemotherapy and irradiation are the mainstays of treatment, but aggressive surgical excision may have a role.
    - The lesions may actually be metastases, which are treated palliatively.
- Lymphoma
  - **Can present as "ivory" vertebrae**
  - Usually associated with a systemic disease
  - Lymphoma typically treated with radiation and/or chemotherapy
  - Surgery typically only necessary if pathologic fracture is present
- Fibrous dysplasia
  - At least 60% of patients with polyostotic fibrous dysplasia will have spinal involvement, mostly in the posterior elements.
  - There is a strong correlation between the presence of a lesion and scoliosis, making scoliosis screening very important in the population with polyostotic disease.

SPINAL INFECTIONS AND INFLAMMATORY ARTHRITIDES

- **Osteodiscitis—disc space infection**
- Introduction
  - Bloodborne infection can primarily invade the disc space in children.
  - *Staphylococcus aureus* is the most common offender, but gram-negative organisms are common in older patients.
- Diagnosis
  - Although all age groups are affected, children (mean age, 7 years) are affected more often.
  - Presentation
    - History—may or may not have history of recent spinal procedure such as spinal injection
    - Inability to walk, stand, or sit
    - Back pain/tenderness
    - Restricted range of motion
  - Laboratory studies—elevated ESR, CRP, and WBC count (often high normal or mildly elevated)
  - **Imaging**
    - Radiographic findings
      - Loss of normal lumbar lordosis—earliest finding
      - Disc space narrowing
      - End plate erosion
      - Findings do not occur until 10 days to 3 weeks after onset, and their absence is unreliable.
    - **MRI with gadolinium is the diagnostic test of choice.**
    - Bone scan may be useful in the diagnosis as well.
  - **Treatment**
    - **Typically medical**

      - Obtain percutaneous biopsy if possible.
      - Hold IV antibiotics prior to biopsy (if possible) to reduce incidence of negative biopsy/culture.
      - Targeted antibiotic therapy once culture and sensitivity completed

- **Surgical indications:**
  - Patient medically systemically ill (uncommon for osteomyelitis)
  - Evidence of epidural abscess
  - Failed medical treatment
  - Unable to obtain percutaneous biopsy
  - No known diagnosis
- **Pyogenic vertebral osteomyelitis**
- Introduction
  - Seen with increasing frequency
  - Frequently still associated with a significant (6- to 12-week) delay in diagnosis
  - Organism usually hematogenous (*S. aureus* in 50%-75% of cases)
- Diagnosis
  - History and physical examination
    - Older, debilitated patients
    - IV drug users are at increased risk.
    - History of unremitting spinal pain at any level is characteristic, and tenderness, spasm, and loss of motion are seen.
    - More common in patients with a history of pneumonia, urinary tract infection, skin infection, or immunologic compromise (transplant, RA, diabetes mellitus, human immunodeficiency virus [HIV with CD4$^+$ counts < 200])
    - Fungal spondylitis can be seen in patients with immunologic compromise.
    - Neurologic deficits—40% seen in older patients, patients with infections at more cephalic levels of the spine, patients with debilitating systemic illnesses such as diabetes or RA, and those with delayed diagnoses
  - Laboratory studies—elevated ESR, CRP, and WBC count (often high normal or mildly elevated)
  - Imaging
    - Plain radiographic findings
      - Osteopenia
      - Paraspinous soft tissue swelling (loss of a psoas shadow)
      - Erosion of the vertebral end plates
      - Disc destruction (disc space preserved in metastatic disease)
    - Bone scanning is sensitive for a destructive process.
    - **MRI**
      - Sensitive for detecting infection and specific in differentiating infection from tumor
      - **Gadolinium enhances MRI sensitivity** (Figure 8-22).
    - Tissue diagnosis via blood cultures or aspirate of the infection is mandatory.
- Treatment
  - **Nonoperative**
    - **After tissue diagnosis, 6 to 12 weeks of IV antibiotics is the treatment of choice.**
    - Bracing may be used adjunctively.
  - Operative
    - Open biopsy is indicated when a tissue diagnosis has not been made.
    - Anterior débridement and strut grafting are reserved for refractory cases that are associated with abscess formation or cases involving neurologic

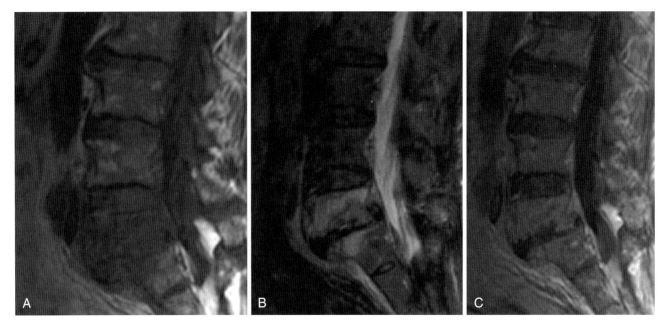

FIGURE 8-22 Pyogenic spondylodiscitis at L5-S1 in an intravenous drug abuser. Sagittal T1-weighted MRI **(A),** T2-weighted spin tau inversion recovery **(B),** and gadolinium-enhanced T1-weighted MRI **(C)** showing characteristic appearance of pyogenic osteodiscitis with end plate and disc space involvement. (From Kim PE et al: Spine: tumors and infections. In Law M et al, editors: *Problem solving in neuroradiology,* Philadelphia, 2011, Elsevier, p 589.)

deterioration, extensive bony destruction, or marked deformity.
- Posterior surgery is usually ineffective for débridement; posterior stabilization may occasionally be required after anterior débridement and strut grafting.

 ■ **Epidural abscess**
▦ Introduction
- Bacterial infection that results in accumulation of purulent material within the epidural space
- Most located posteriorly in the thoracic and lumbar spine
▦ Diagnosis
- History
  - Back pain is the most common presenting symptom, followed by neurologic deficit and fever.
  - Diagnosis is delayed in half of patients.
  - Patients are frequently more systemically ill than patients with osteodiscitis and osteomyelitis.
  - Risk factors include IV drug abuse, diabetes, and multiple medical problems.
- Laboratory studies—elevated ESR and CRP values (often more elevated than in osteodiscitis)
- Imaging
  - **MRI—modality of choice; supplementation with gadolinium allows differentiation between epidural abscess and CSF.**
  - Abscess and CSF have high signal intensity on T2-weighted images.
  - **Gadolinium enhances the pus on T1-weighted images, whereas CSF remains low signal.**
▦ Management
 - **Typically surgical—urgent evaluation and treatment**
- Laminectomy is performed if the epidural abscess is predominately posterior.

- If there is concomitant vertebral osteomyelitis, anterior and posterior decompression is performed.

■ **Spinal tuberculosis**
▦ Introduction
- **Most common extrapulmonary location of tuberculosis**
- May be seen in HIV-positive population with a CD4⁺ counts of 50 to 200
- Originates in the metaphysis of the vertebral body and spreads under the anterior longitudinal ligament (Figures 8-23 and 8-24)
- This leads to destruction of several contiguous levels or results in skip lesions (15%) or abscess formation (50%).
▦ Diagnosis
- On early plain radiographs, anterior vertebral body destruction with preservation of the disc distinguishes tuberculosis from pyogenic infection.
- About two thirds of patients have abnormal chest radiographs, and 20% have a negative test for purified protein derivative of tuberculin or are anergic.
- Severe kyphosis, sinus formation, and (Pott) paraplegia are late sequelae.
- Spinal cord injury may occur secondary to direct pressure from the abscess, bony sequestra, or (rarely) meningomyelitis (poor prognosis).
▦ Treatment
- **Nonoperative—chemotherapy is the mainstay of treatment.**
- **Surgical indications:**
  - Neurologic deficit
  - Spinal instability
  - Progressive kyphosis
  - Failed medical management
  - Advanced disease with caseation, fibrosis, and avascularity that limits antibiotic penetration

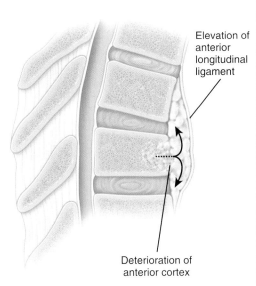
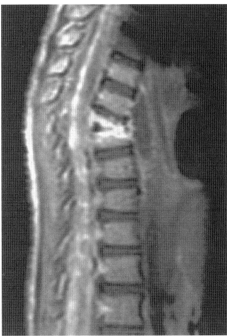

Elevation of
anterior
longitudinal
ligament

Deterioration of
anterior cortex

FIGURE 8-23 Pathogenesis of spinal tuberculosis. (From Herring JA: *Tachdjian's pediatric orthopaedics,* ed 3, Philadelphia, 2002, WB Saunders, p 1832.)

- Surgical
  - Radical anterior débridement of the infection followed by uninstrumented autogenous strut grafting (Hong Kong procedure) is the accepted surgical treatment.
  - Advantages include less progressive kyphosis, earlier healing, and a decrease in sinus formation.
  - Adjuvant chemotherapy beginning 10 days before surgery has been recommended (controversial) but is not always possible.
  - Use of antitubercular medications after surgery is mandatory.
- ▰ **Destructive spondyloarthropathy**
- ▰ Seen in hemodialysis patients with chronic renal failure
- ▰ Typically involves three adjacent vertebrae and two intervening discs
- ▰ Changes include subluxation, degeneration, and narrowing of the disc height.
- ▰ Although the process may resemble infection, it probably represents crystal or amyloid deposition.
- ▰ **Diffuse idiopathic skeletal hyperostosis (DISH)—also known as *Forestier disease* (Figure 8-25)**
- ▰ **DISH is defined by the presence of nonmarginal syndesmophytes (differentiated from AS, which has marginal syndesmophytes) at three successive levels.**
- ▰ Syndesmophytes are vertical outgrowths that extend across the disc space and represent calcification of the anulus fibrosus and anterior and posterior longitudinal ligaments.
- ▰ DISH can occur anywhere in the spine but usually in the thoracic region and is more often seen on the right side.
- ▰ DISH is associated with chronic low back pain and is more common in patients with diabetes and gout.
- ▰ The prevalence of DISH has been found to be as high as 28% in autopsy specimens.
- ▰ DISH is associated with extraspinal ossification at several joints, including an increased risk of heterotopic ossification after total hip surgery.

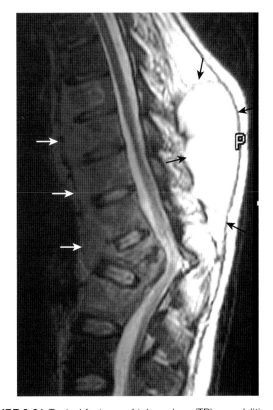

FIGURE 8-24 Typical features of tuberculous (TB) spondylitis. Sagittal T1-weighted MRI demonstrating many hallmarks of TB spondylitis: relative sparing of discs, subligamentous spread to multiple contiguous levels *(white arrows),* extensive vertebral body destruction and deformity, including gibbus deformity, and large paraspinous "cold abscesses" *(black arrows).* (From Kim PE et al: Spine: tumors and infections. In Law M et al, editors: *Problem solving in neuroradiology,* Philadelphia, 2011, Elsevier, p 589.)

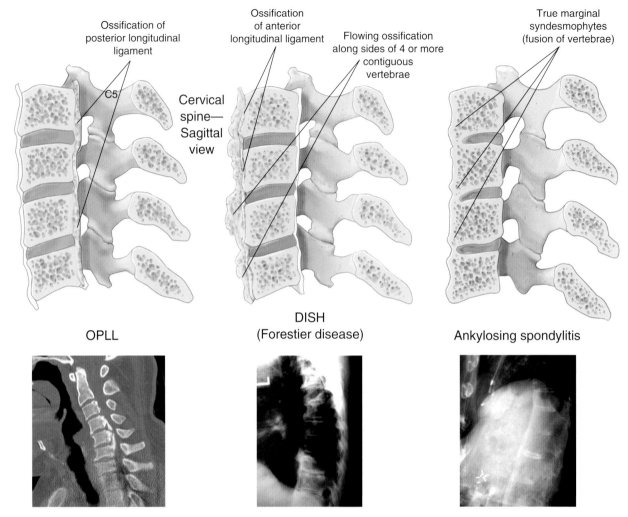

Ossification of
posterior longitudinal
ligament

Ossification
of anterior
longitudinal ligament

Flowing ossification
along sides of 4 or more
contiguous
vertebrae

True marginal
syndesmophytes
(fusion of vertebrae)

C5

Cervical
spine—
Sagittal
view

OPLL

DISH
(Forestier disease)

Ankylosing spondylitis

FIGURE 8-25 Schematic drawings and corresponding radiographic appearance of ossification of the posterior longitudinal ligament (OPLL), diffuse idiopathic skeletal hyperostosis (DISH), and ankylosing spondylitis.

■ **Ankylosing spondylitis** (see Figure 8-25)
▦ Introduction
- 95% of patients with AS are positive for human leukocyte antigen (HLA)–B27
- Usually young men present with insidious onset of back and hip pain during the third or fourth decade of life.
▦ Imaging
- Sacroiliac joint obliteration (iliac side affected first) and marginal syndesmophytes allow radiographic differentiation from DISH.
- *Bamboo spine* is the descriptive term applied to multiple vertebral levels ankylosed by marginal syndesmophytes.
- May result in fixed kyphotic deformities, leading to sagittal imbalance
▦ Assessment
- Assessment of the patient for hip flexion contractures or cervicothoracic kyphosis is mandatory.
- Assessment of global and focal alignment, including chin-brow angle
▦ Management
- Extension osteotomy and fusion of the lumbar spine with compression instrumentation can successfully balance the head over the sacrum.

- The cervical spine may be corrected by a C7-T1 osteotomy and fusion under local anesthesia.
▦ Complications
- Nonunion
- Loss of correction
- Neurologic injury, especially C8 nerve root
- Aortic injury
▦ Associated medical conditions
- Anterior uveitis
- Restrictive lung disease and pulmonary fibrosis
- Aortic regurgitation and stenosis
- Ileitis or colitis

SPINAL TRAUMA

■ **General considerations**
▦ Spinal trauma can be the result of high-energy trauma with associated injuries.
▦ **Adherence to Advanced Trauma Life Support (ATLS) protocols remains imperative.**
- **Primary survey (ABCs, with D and E)**
  - **A—Airway maintenance with cervical spine protection**
  - **B—Breathing and ventilation**
  - **C—Circulation with hemorrhage control**

- D—Disability and neurologic assessment
- E—Exposure of patient
- Initial radiologic workup performed during primary survey or shortly after
  - A rapid radiologic workup that includes at a minimum anteroposterior (AP) chest, AP pelvis, and lateral cervical spine views is standard.
  - **Lateral cervical radiograph must include C7-T1 junction or is considered an inadequate imaging exam. Assess radiographic lines for continuity.**
    - **Anterior soft tissue shadows**
      - **At C2: 6 mm**
      - **At C6: 20 mm**
    - **Anterior spinal line**
    - **Posterior spinal line**
    - **Spinolaminar line**
    - **Spinous process line**
  - CT scan
    - Availability and increased processing speed is leading to CT of cervical spine replacing lateral cervical spine radiography for trauma evaluation.
    - Sagittal views detect 85% of cervical spine fractures.
    - CT is useful for evaluating C1 fractures and assessing bone in the canal but may miss an axial plane fracture (type II odontoid).
  - MRI
    - Has advantages for demonstrating soft tissue abnormalities:
      - Integrity of posterior ligamentous complex (PLC)
      - Disc herniation
      - Canal compromise
      - Spinal cord injury and edema
    - Increasingly used in cervical spine "clearance" (controversial)
- Secondary survey performed once primary survey and initial imaging complete.
  - Head-to-toe evaluation—each region fully examined
    - Facial injuries, hypotension, and localized tenderness or spasm should be investigated.
    - Careful neurologic examination to document the lowest remaining functional level and to assess patient for the possibility of sacral sparing (sparing of posterior column function, indicating an incomplete spinal cord injury) is essential (see Figure 8-1).
    - The neurologic level, as defined by the standards of the **American Spine Injury Association (ASIA)**, is the most cephalad level with normal bilateral motor and sensory function (Figure 8-26).
  - Additional x-rays as indicated from secondary survey
    - Complete cervical spine series (C1-T1)
    - Multiple-level injuries occur in 10% to 20% of cases.
  - If patient status deteriorates at any point during secondary survey, primary survey is reinitiated.
- **Shock and resuscitation**
  - **Hemorrhagic or hypovolemic shock**
    - The physiologic state of loss of intravascular volume leading to hypotension and tachycardia
    - Most common cause of hypotension of the trauma patient (even in those with spinal fracture)

- Treatment—aggressive fluid resuscitation and management/control of the source of hemorrhage
- Swan-Ganz monitoring is helpful in the setting of spine trauma because neurogenic and hypovolemic shock often occur concurrently.
- Neurogenic shock
  - **Hypotension with bradycardia**
    - **Due to disruption of the sympathetic pathway within the spinal cord**
    - **Most common in patients who sustain a cervical or upper thoracic spinal cord injury**
    - **Hypotension due to decreased systemic vascular resistance**
    - **Bradycardia due to unopposed vagal activity**
    - **Can be differentiated from hypovolemic shock based on presence of relative bradycardia in neurogenic shock**
  - Treatment
    - Initial management remains volume, particularly if there is concomitant hemorrhagic shock.
    - However, once initial resuscitation is complete, vasopressors are frequently required (fairly quickly) to help restore systemic vascular resistance.

■ Spinal cord injury (SCI) (Figure 8-27)

- General concepts
  - **The first goal of treatment is stabilization.**
    - Cervical in-line traction and cervical collar
    - Logroll patients for examination and transport.
    - Backboard
      - Used for transportation only
      - Remove patients from backboards as soon as clinically safe.
        - Decubitus ulcers can occur after only 30 to 60 minutes on backboard.
  - Skeletal traction
    - Halo vest immobilization
      - Indications
        - May be effective in controlling spinal motion in the upper cervical spine (O-C2); control of subaxial spine may be less effective.
        - Does not control axial distraction well
      - Not well tolerated, particularly by elderly patients, so use is declining.
      - **Safe zone for anterior pin placement: above the eyebrow in the middle to lateral third to avoid the supraorbital nerve** (Figure 8-28)
      - Adults: 4 pins (6 to 8 inch-lb pressure pins), children: 8 to 10 pins (2 inch-lb pressure pins)
      - Complications—pin loosening, pin infection, pressure sores, nerve injury, dural penetration
    - Gardner-Wells (GW) tongs
      - Can be used more acutely to realign the spine in the presence of a displaced fracture with or without neurologic injury
      - Pins parallel to the external auditory meatus approximately 1-cm above pinna
  - High-dose methylprednisolone
    - Role of steroids is unclear and controversial.
      - Efficacy has been questioned, and many centers have discontinued its use.
      - Currently considered a treatment option at best and certainly not "standard of care"

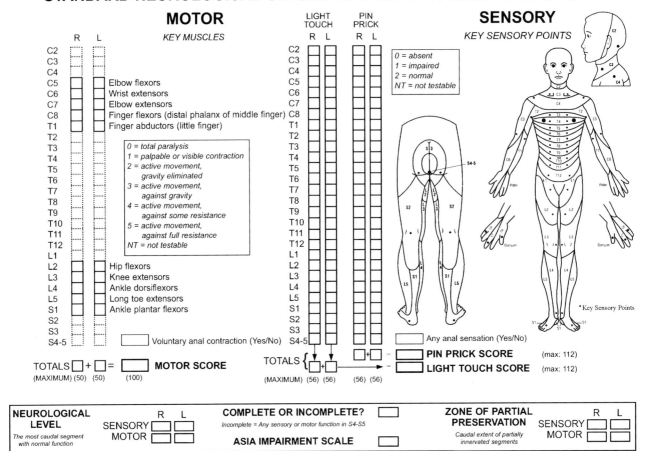

STANDARD NEUROLOGICAL CLASSIFICATION OF SPINAL CORD INJURY

FIGURE 8-26 American Spinal Injury Association neurologic classification of spinal cord injury. (From Kim DH et al: *Atlas of spine trauma: adult and pediatric,* Philadelphia, 2008, Elsevier, p 24.)

- Consider for cord injuries (not root injuries) with accompanying neurologic deficit (National Acute Spinal Cord Injury Studies [NASCIS] II and III)
  - A bolus of 30 mg/kg methylprednisolone over 15 minutes, with a maintenance infusion of 5.4 mg/kg/h
  - If given within 3 hours, administer for 24 hours.
  - If given within 3 to 8 hours, administer for 48 hours.
  - Consideration for administration of gastrointestinal prophylaxis to reduce risk of ulcer bleeds
- **Contraindications to use of high-dose steroids:**
  - Penetrating spinal wounds, particularly gunshot wounds
  - Injury more than 48 hours before
  - Peripheral nerve injuries such as brachoplexopathy, stingers, root level injuries, cauda equina (etc.)
  - Pregnancy
  - Age younger than 13 years
  - Concomitant infection
  - Uncontrolled diabetes
- **American Spinal Injury Association (ASIA) classification**

- A—0/5 motor score, complete sensory deficit
- B—0/5 motor score, incomplete sensory deficit
- C—less than 3/5 motor score, incomplete sensory deficit
- D—greater than 3/5 motor score, incomplete sensory deficit
- E—5/5 motor score, no sensory deficit
- **Complete spinal cord injuries**
  - No function below a given level
  - With complete injuries, an improvement of one nerve root level can be expected in 80% of the patients, and approximately 20% recover two functioning root levels.
  - Can not be determined until the end of spinal shock, which is signified by return of the bulbocavernosus reflex, or 48 hours after the time of injury
- **Incomplete spinal cord injuries**
  - **Defined as some sparing of distal motor or sensory function**
  - Three important generalizations regarding prognosis:
    - The greater the sparing, the greater recovery.
    - The more rapid the recovery, the greater recovery.
    - When recovery plateaus, no further recovery will happen.

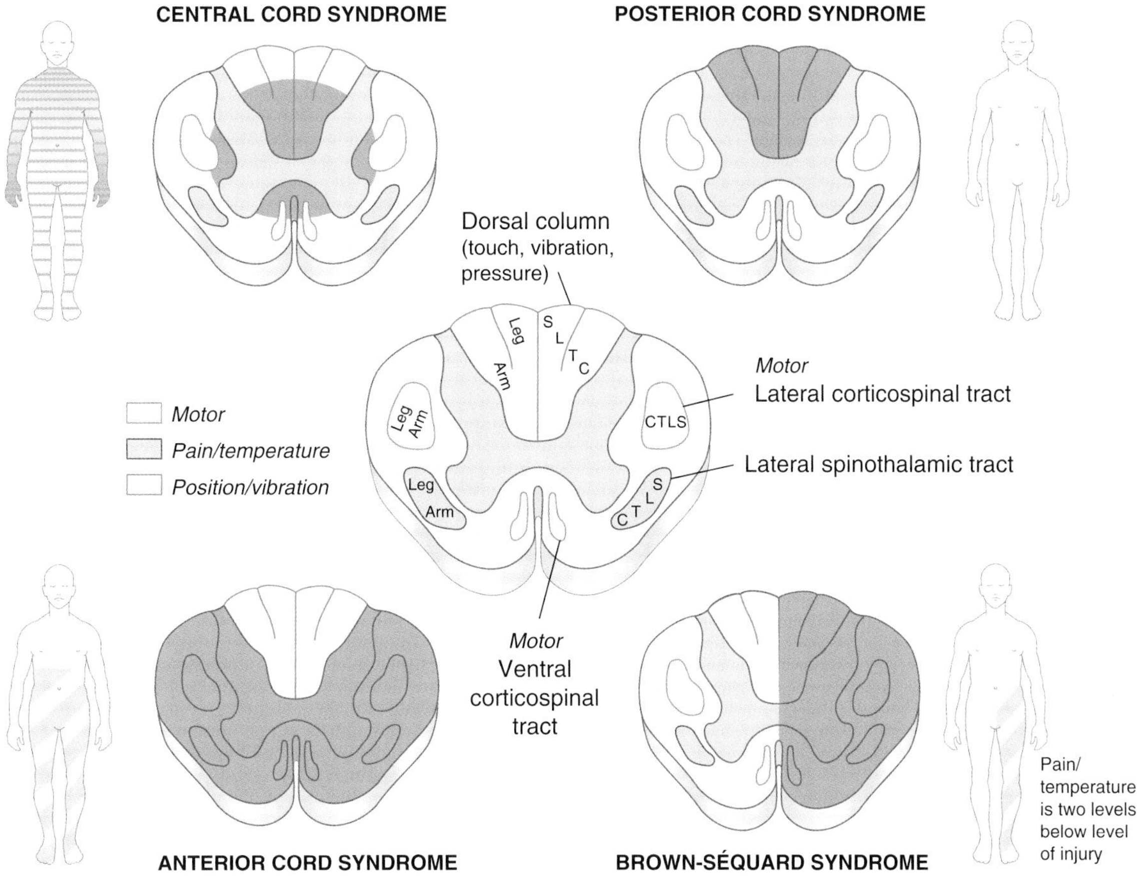

CENTRAL CORD SYNDROME

POSTERIOR CORD SYNDROME

Dorsal column
(touch, vibration,
pressure)

□ *Motor*
□ *Pain/temperature*
□ *Position/vibration*

Leg
Arm
Leg
Arm
S
L
T
C

Motor
Lateral corticospinal tract

CTLS

Motor
Ventral
corticospinal
tract

Leg
Arm

C
T
L
S

Lateral spinothalamic tract

ANTERIOR CORD SYNDROME

BROWN-SÉQUARD SYNDROME

Pain/
temperature
is two levels
below level
of injury

FIGURE 8-27 Incomplete spinal cord injury syndromes.

- **Spinal shock**
  - **Spinal shock usually involves a 24- to 72-hour period of paralysis, hypotonia, and areflexia.**
  - **Return of the bulbocavernosus reflex (anal sphincter contraction in response to squeezing the glans penis or tugging on the Foley catheter) signifies the end of spinal shock.**
  - Injuries at or below the thoracolumbar level (conus or cauda equina) may permanently interrupt the bulbocavernosus reflex.
  - **In complete injuries, further neurologic improvement is minimal.**
  - Phases of spinal shock (variable)
    - Phase 1—areflexic/hyporeflexic phase
      - Typically first 24 to 48 hours
      - Loss of reflexes below level of SCI
      - Due to loss of basal level of excitatory stimulation from brain to neurons involved in the reflex arc
      - As a result, there is less responsiveness to stimuli and therefore hyporeflexia or areflexia.
    - Phase 2—initial reflex return
      - Next 1 or 2 days
      - Return of some but not all reflexes below level of SCI
      - First reflexes to return are polysynaptic; bulbocavernosus is polysynaptic and typically the first reflex to return.
      - Monosynaptic reflexes such as deep tendon reflexes (DTRs) typically do not return until phase 3.

- Phase 3—initial hyperreflexia
  - Next 1 to 4 weeks
  - Abnormal strong reflexes
  - Increased expression of neurotransmitter receptors results in increased reflex response with minimal stimulation.
- Phase 4—final hyperreflexia/spasticity
  - Next 1 to 12 months
  - In addition to hyperreflexia, this phase results in altered skeletal muscle performance and hypertonia.
  - Loss of inhibitory input to motor neuron below level of SCI
- **Clinical syndromes** (Table 8-9)
  - **Central cord syndrome**
    - **Most common incomplete spinal cord syndrome**
    - Typical mechanism is hyperextension with preexisting canal stenosis.
    - Cord is compressed anteriorly by osteophytes and posteriorly by the infolded ligamentum flavum.
    - **Cord is injured in the central gray matter, resulting in proportionately greater loss of motor function to upper extremities than to lower extremities.**
    - **The upper extremity is affected more than the lower extremity.**
    - **Variable sensory sparing**
    - **The prognosis is good for the recovery of ambulation, but the patient is less likely to recover upper extremity function.**
  - **Anterior cord syndrome (spinothalamic tract injury)**

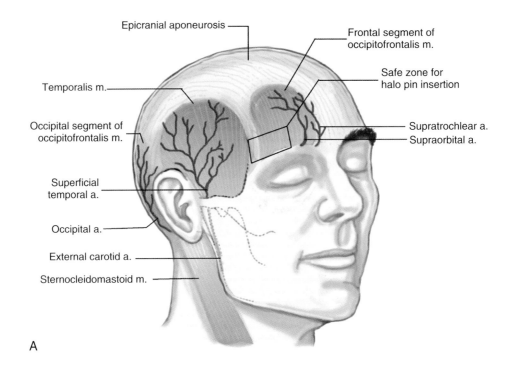

A

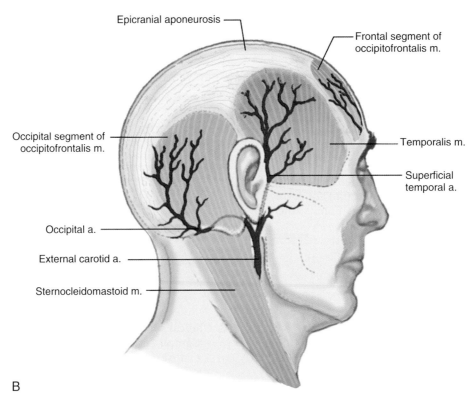

B

FIGURE 8-28 "Safe zones" for placement of skull pins. **A,** Anterior view. **B,** Posterolateral view with relevant anatomy. (From Kim DH et al: *Atlas of spine trauma: adult and pediatric,* Philadelphia, 2008, Elsevier, p 99.)

- The second most common incomplete cord injury
- No typical mechanism for injury
  - Direct compression to anterior spinal cord
  - Less commonly vascular injury to anterior spinal artery, or spinal cord ischemia (e.g. anterior spinal artery, artery of Adamkiewicz)
- **Damage is primarily in the anterior two thirds of the cord.**

- Loss of motor response, pain reception, and temperature reception below the level of injury
- Patients demonstrate greater motor loss in the legs than the arms.
- Preservation of posterior/dorsal column; vibration sensation, proprioception, and deep pressure sensation intact
- The prognosis for motor recovery is poor.
- **Brown-Séquard syndrome (spinal cord hemisection)**

Table 8-9	Spinal Cord Injury Syndromes		
SYNDROME	**PATHOLOGY**	**CHARACTERISTICS**	**PROGNOSIS**
Central	Age > 50, extension injuries	Affects upper > lower extremities; motor and sensory loss	Fair
Anterior	Various mechanisms; may include flexion-compression injury, possible vascular insult	Incomplete motor and some sensory loss	Poor
Brown-Séquard	Penetrating trauma	Loss of ipsilateral motor function, contralateral pain, and temperature sensation	Best
Root	Foramina compression/herniated nucleus pulposus	Based on level (weakness)	Good
Complete	Burst/canal compression	No function below injury level	Poor

- Typical cause is penetrating trauma.
  - Ipsilateral loss of motor and loss of position/proprioception function on the side of injury
  - Contralateral loss of pain and temperature to the side of injury (usually one to two levels below the insult)
  - Best prognosis for recovery of ability to walk (90%)
- Posterior cord syndrome
  - Very rare; least common incomplete spinal cord pattern
  - Injury to posterior/dorsal column—loss of proprioception, vibrator sensation, and deep pressure sensation
  - Preservation of anterior column; motor response, pain reception, and temperature reception intact
- **Autonomic dysreflexia**
  - **Most commonly follows spinal cord injuries above T6 and encompasses a constellation of symptoms**
    - Pounding headache (from severe hypertension)
    - Anxiety
    - Profuse head and neck sweating
    - Nasal obstruction
    - Blurred vision
  - **Due to sympathetic overdrive**
    - **Most commonly triggered by bladder distension or fecal impaction**
    - **Undiagnosed orthopaedic injuries such as femur or ankle fracture**
- Rehabilitation after spinal cord injury
  - Functional level determined by both sensory and motor level as determined by:
    - Most distal intact functional sensory level AND
    - Most distal motor level where motor grade is 4 or greater
  - Respiratory function by level of cord injury
    - C1-C2 injury
      - Vital capacity only 5% to 10% of normal
      - Ventilator dependent
      - Cough absent
    - C3-C5 injury
      - Vital capacity 20% of normal
      - Cough weak and ineffective
    - Lower cervical and upper thoracic
      - Vital capacity 30% to 50% of normal
      - Cough weak but may be effective
    - T11 and below
      - Respiratory dysfunction minimal
      - Vital capacity near normal
      - Cough strong
  - Mobility and function determined by highest motor level

- C3 or above—respiratory dependent
- C4—transfer dependent
- C5—transfer assist
- C6—independent transfers
- Activities of daily living
  - C6—independent grooming and dressing; can operate flexor hinge wrist-hand orthosis
  - C7—able to use knife to cut food

- **Syringomyelia (syrinx)**
- Introduction
  - Confluent collection of abnormal CSF within the spinal cord
    - In regards to orthopaedic spine, most common etiology is posttraumatic syrinx and secondary to herniated disc.
    - Other primary causes of spinal syringomyelia include postinflammatory, secondary to arachnoid abnormalities (arachnoid cyst), tumor, and idiopathic.
    - Syringomyelia can also be related to abnormalities of the foramen magnum: tonsilar descent (Chiari malformation), arachnoid veil with fourth ventricle outlet obstruction.
  - **Differentiate syringomyelia from hydromyelia**
    - Hydromyelia—confluent CSF cavity within spinal cord that is a remnant of central canal of spinal cord
      - Typically considered a normal variant
      - Spinal cord typically not expanded by hydromyelia and therefore not associated with symptoms and not considered a pathologic entity
  - **Differentiate syringomyelia from spinal cord edema**
    - Spinal cord edema is increased fluid that is interstitial, and not as a confluence of fluid.
    - This can be secondary to spinal cord contusion or tumor-associated cyst.
- Presentation
  - Variable but typically due to the etiology of the syrinx and its associated pathophysiology
  - Symptoms associated with partial CSF obstruction (e.g., tussive headaches, strain-related activities)
  - Symptoms related to brainstem compression (e.g., swallowing difficulty, voice changes, nystagmus, ataxia, sleep apnea)
  - Symptoms related to syringomyelia (e.g., sensory loss [upper greater than lower typically], upper extremity weakness, hand and upper extremity atrophy, gait impairment, lower extremity spasticity, bowel and bladder dysfunction, dysesthetic pain)
- Imaging
  - MRI is study of choice
    - Does not disrupt CSF dynamics

- T1-weighted image demonstrates intramedullary fluid-filled cavity.
- MRI with gadolinium necessary to rule out presence of associated spinal tumor.
- T2-weighted images may help identify anatomic detail such as septa in the subarachnoid space.
- CT myelogram
  - May have a role in determining obstructive arachnoid disease
    - In these cases, performing myelography puncture at C1-C2 rather than lumbar route may allow for pooling of the contrast at the level of the web.
    - This may not be seen if contrast is introduced from lumbar route, owing to obstructive subarachnoid web acting as a one-way valve.

■ **Upper cervical spine injuries**
■ Occipitocervical dissociation (OCD) (Figure 8-29)
  - Head is disconnected from C1.
  - Frequently fatal
  - Diagnosis challenging on plain films (CT/MRI ≈ 85% sensitive)
  - Radiologic measurements
    - **Powers ratio** (Figure 8-30)
      - **Measure distance from basion to posterior arch of atlas; divide by distance of anterior arch of atlas to opisthion.**
      - **Greater than 1.0 indicates instability of the atlantoaxial junction (from possible dislocation)**
      - **Only good for anterior occipitocervical dislocations. Can miss posterior OCD.**
    - Harris method
      - Basion-axial interval—distance from basion to line drawn tangential to posterior border of C2 (normal, 4-12 mm)

- Basion dental interval—distance from basion to odontoid
  - The distance between the odontoid and basion is 4 to 5 mm in adults and up to 10 mm in children.
  - More than 12 mm is abnormal.
- **Classification**—Harborview classification
  - Stage I—MRI evidence of injury to ligamentous stabilizers, alignment within 2 mm of normal, and distraction of 2 mm or less on manual traction radiograph
  - Stage II—same as stage I, except distraction of less than 2 mm on a manual-traction radiograph
  - Stage III—distraction of more than 2 mm on static radiographs
- Treatment
  - Nonoperative treatments typically not options
  - Operative treatment indications—stage II or III injuries or any injury with associated neurologic deficit
  - Operative procedure—posterior occipitocervical fusion (O-C2)

■ Occipital fracture
- Classification—Anderson-Montesano classification
  - Type I—comminuted impaction fracture of occiput; generally stable
  - Type II—shear or compression fracture extending into base of the skull; variably stable
  - Type III—avulsion injuries that have a transverse fracture component; generally unstable—may be associated with occipitocervical dissociation
- Treatment
  - Operative indication
    - Evidence of mechanical instability
    - Presence of neurologic deficit
  - Stable injuries—cervical collar
  - Posterior occipitocervical fusion stabilization for unstable injuries

■ C1 ring fractures
- Classification—Levine and Edwards
  - Posterior arch fractures—hyperextension
  - Lateral mass fractures—axial load with lateral bend
  - Isolated anterior arch fractures—hyperextension
  - **Burst fractures (Jefferson)—axial load**

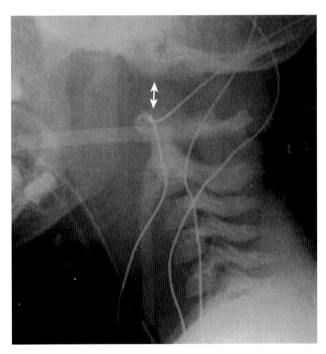

FIGURE 8-29 Lateral radiograph of a skeletally immature cervical spine demonstrating complete occipitocervical dissociation *(double-headed arrow)*. (From Cianfoni A, Colosimo C: Imaging of spine trauma. In Law M et al, editors: *Problem solving in neuroradiology*, Philadelphia, 2011, Elsevier, p 477.)

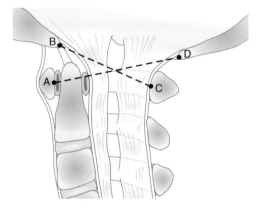

FIGURE 8-30 Powers ratio. The distance from the basion (B) to the posterior arch of the atlas (C) divided by the distance of the anterior arch of the atlas (A) to the opisthion (D) should equal 1 or less. If greater than 1, the patient may have an anterior occipitocervical subluxation or dislocation.

- Treatment—based predominantly on stability of transverse ligament
  - Indications
    - Combined lateral mass displacement of greater than 6.9 mm (8.1 mm with standard radiographic magnification) indicates transverse ligament rupture (Figure 8-31).
    - Atlantodens interval (ADI)
      - If greater than 3.5 mm, indicates transverse ligament is damaged
      - If greater than 5 mm, indicates both the transverse and alar ligaments are damaged
    - Residual combined lateral mass displacement of greater than 6.9 mm or ADI of more than 3.5 mm after halo stabilization
  - Operative procedures
    - Halo vest stabilization for 6 to 12 weeks for fractures with an intact transverse ligament
    - Posterior spinal fusion (C1-C2 or occiput-C2) if the transverse ligament is incompetent
- Atlantoaxial instability
  - Classification—Fielding and Hawkins
    - Type I—rotationally unstable but transverse alar ligament intact; odontoid is the pivot point.
    - Type II—rotationally unstable, with transverse alar ligament incompetence; one facet acts as the pivot.
    - Type III—both facets subluxed anteriorly, atlantodens interval greater than 5 mm
    - Type IV—both facets subluxed posteriorly
    - Type V—frank dislocation
  - Treatment
    - Nonoperative options:
      - Limited in true traumatic atlantoaxial instability versus patients with instability due to chronic conditions
      - Consider external immobilization if transverse ligament intact (type I) and possibly type II. Careful follow-up and conversion to surgical decompression if progression of deformity.
    - Operative indications:
      - Presence of neurologic deficits or failed closed treatment
    - Procedure:
      - Posterior C1-C2 posterior fusion; include the occiput if instability is associated with occipitocervical dislocation.

- Odontoid fracture
  - Classification—Anderson-D'Alonso (Figure 8-32)
    - Type I—avulsion of alar ligaments from the tip
    - Type II—fracture at the base of odontoid
    - Type IIA—comminuted fracture of the base of odontoid
    - Type III—fractures that extend into the body of C2
  - Treatment
    - Operative indications—based on risk of developing nonunion. Risk factors for nonunion in type II:
      - Displacement greater than 5 mm
      - Posterior displacement
      - Age older than 40 years
      - Delayed treatment
      - Angulation greater than 10 degrees
    - Type I—immobilization in rigid cervical orthosis
    - Type II and IIa
      - Nondisplaced—immobilization in rigid cervical orthosis (controversial)
      - Displaced types II and IIA fractures are generally considered operative because of the high rate of nonunion with nonoperative treatment.
    - Type III—typically high incidence of union; most will heal in rigid external cervical orthosis. Consider operative treatment if initial displacement is greater than 5 mm.

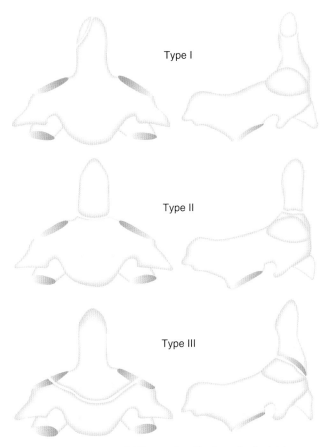

Type I

Type II

Type III

FIGURE 8-32 Anderson-D'Alonso classification of odontoid fractures. Type I is an oblique avulsion fracture from the upper portion of the dens. Type II is a fracture of the odontoid process at its base. Type III is an odontoid fracture through body of C2.

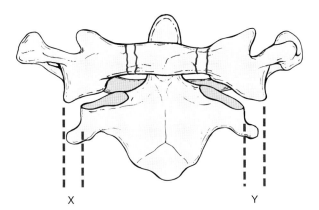

X   Y

FIGURE 8-31 Lateral mass overhang. If X + Y is greater than 6.9 mm, this is suggestive of rupture of the transverse ligament.

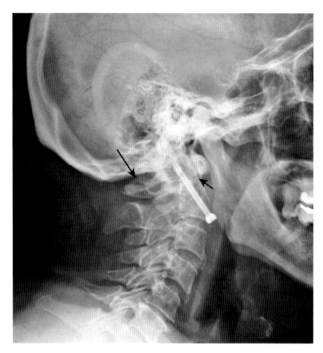

FIGURE 8-33 Direct osteosynthesis of type 2 dens fracture. Lateral cervical radiograph demonstrating a postoperative anterior odontoid screw for direct osteosynthesis of type 2 dens fracture. Arrows identify combined anterior and posterior C1 ring fractures. (From Kim DH et al: *Atlas of spine trauma: adult and pediatric*, Philadelphia, 2008, Elsevier, p 178.)

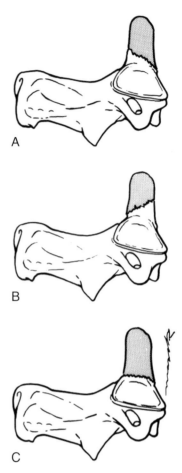

FIGURE 8-34 Subclassification of type II odontoid fractures based on fracture line orientation. **A,** Anterior oblique. **B,** Posterior oblique. **C,** Horizontal. Fracture lines that are anterior oblique **(A)** are the most difficult to treat with anterior odontoid screw and are most likely to result in screw cut out. Conversely, posterior oblique **(B)** is the fracture line more amenable to direct osteosynthesis, since the screw can be placed perpendicular to the fracture orientation. (From Kim DH et al: *Atlas of spine trauma: adult and pediatric*, Philadelphia, 2008, Elsevier, p 205.)

- Procedures:
  - Posterior C1-C2 fusion
  - Direct osteosynthesis—anterior odontoid screw (Figure 8-33)
    - Fracture must be reducible. **Nonreduced fracture is a contraindication to anterior odontoid screw.**
    - Fracture geometry must be favorable, which is anterior superior to posterior inferior ("anterior oblique pattern") (Figure 8-34)
    - This procedure is associated with a higher failure rate than posterior fusion but theoretically preserves atlantoaxial motion.
- Complications:
  - Overall nonunion rate for type II is approximately 32%.
  - Patients older than age 80 do poorly, regardless of operative or nonoperative management.
  - Airway problems postoperatively or with halo vest immobilization
- ■ C2 fracture (traumatic spondylolisthesis of the axis or hangman fracture)
  - Classification—Levine (Figure 8-35)
  - Type I—minimally displaced fracture of the pars secondary to hyperextension and axial loading (<3 mm displacement, no angulation)
  - Type IA—same as type I except fracture lines are asymmetric
  - Type II—displaced fractures (>3 mm) of the pars, with subsequent flexion after hyperextension and axial loading
  - Type IIa—flexion without displacement; *be careful* not to mistake this for a type I fracture,

which represents total disc avulsion, because traction may worsen fracture.
  - Type III—bilateral pars fracture with bilateral facet dislocations (rare)—has flexion-distraction then hyperextension mechanism
- Treatment
  - Type I—rigid cervical orthosis
  - Type II—operative; typically C1-C2 fixation, or direct osteosynthesis
  - Type IIA—halo vest or surgery (no traction!)
  - Type III—generally operative, usually C2-C3 fusion (may require C1-C3 fixation depending on comminution of pars and quality of fixation into C2)
- Complications—vascular injury; vertebral artery injury is rare but increasingly diagnosed by magnetic resonance angiogram (MRA).
- ■ **C1-C2 posterior cervical fixation techniques** (Table 8-10)
  - **C1-C2 Modified Gallie**
    - Autograft iliac crest placed over C2 spinous process and against posterior arch of C1

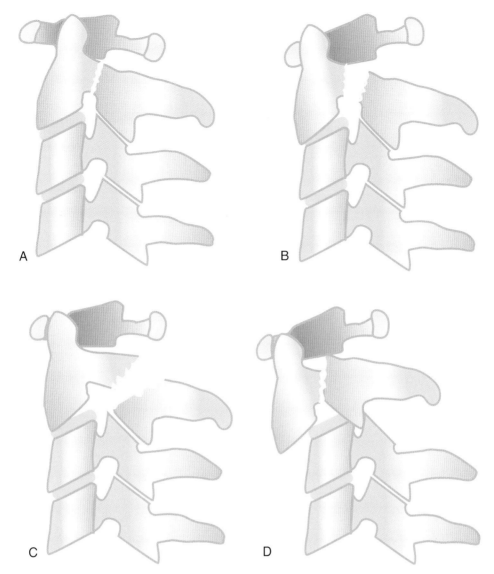

FIGURE 8-35 Levine-Edwards classification for C2 traumatic spondylolisthesis fractures. (From Kim DH et al: *Atlas of spine trauma: adult and pediatric,* Philadelphia, 2008, Elsevier, p 214.)

Table 8-10	Biomechanics of C1-C2 Posterior Cervical Fixation Techniques		
	FLEXION	**EXTENSION**	**ROTATION**
Modified Gallie	Good	Poor	Poor
Brooks fusion	Good	Good	Poor
C1-C2 transarticular screws	Better	Better	Better
C1–lateral mass/ C2–pedicle screw	Best	Best	Best

- Held in place by sublaminar wire under arch of C1 and under spinous process of C2 (total of one sublaminar wire)
- **C1-C2 Brooks fusion**
  - Two separate iliac crest autografts placed between C1 and C2
  - One sublaminar wire is placed on either side (total of two sublaminar wires).
- **C1-C2 transarticular (Magerl) screws**

- Preoperative CT scan to assess for location of vertebral artery at C1-C2 junction is imperative.
- Adequate intraoperative radiographs are required, or the technique should not be used.
- Cannulated screw is placed under fluoroscopy-assisted guidance over a guidewire.
- Screw is placed through the C1-C2 facet joint (transarticular), thereby coupling C1-C2.
- **C1 lateral mass–C2 pedicle (Harms) screws**
  - C1 screws are placed through the lateral masses. Starting point of the screw is the center of the lateral mass.
  - C2 screws are placed traditionally as pedicle screw. In the case of aberrant vertebral artery a shorter, more straight-ahead pars screw can be used in C2 instead.
- **Complications**
  - **Vertebral artery runs in transverse foramen of C2 then onto superior aspect of C1 in the groove/ sulcus of the vertebral artery.**

- C2 (greater occipital) nerve lies just dorsal to the C1-C2 joint. Injury can result in numbness in the posterior aspect of the skull.
  - Neurologic injury
  - Dural leaks
  - Nonunion/malunion
- **Subaxial cervical spine (C3-C7)**
  - Classification
    - **Allen-Ferguson** (based on mechanism)—descriptive classification
      - Based on position of the head and neck at the time of injury (flexion/extension) and the mode of failure (distraction/compression) (Table 8-11)
        - Compressive flexion
        - Distractive flexion
        - Compressive extension
        - Vertical compression
        - Distractive extension
        - Lateral flexion
      - Decision for surgery can be difficult using mechanistic classification; however, general considerations include:
        - Patient with associated neurologic instability
        - Disruption of posterior ligamentous complex
        - Fracture dislocations and distractive flexion injuries (jumped facets)
        - Burst fracture without neurologic injury and intact posterior ligamentous complex and acceptable alignment can be considered to be treated with external immobilization (controversial).
    - **Subaxial Cervical Spine Injury Classification System (SLIC)** (Table 8-12)
      - Based on three separate injury axes:
        - Fracture morphology
        - Discoligamentous complex (DLC) integrity
        - Neurologic status
      - Scoring
        - Each axis considered an independent determinant to prognosis and management
        - Each axis receives numerical score, with increasing severity receiving a high numerical value
        - No set value defined as surgical; however, higher numerical values suggestive of increased need for operative intervention
  - Treatment goals
    - Address neurologic deficits.
      - Typically, approach is selected based on location of compression.
      - Anterior cervical discectomy and/or corpectomy for anterior compression
      - Posterior laminectomy for posterior compression
      - Restoring spinal alignment can help through indirect decompression.
    - Achieve immediate stability and long-term fusion. Approach varies depending on injury pattern and presence of associated neurologic instability.
    - Restore spinal alignment.
  - Special considerations: MRI in facet fracture-dislocations (jumped facets) remains controversial.
    - The role of MRI to evaluate the disc before or after closed reduction is controversial, particularly as it relates to neurologic status.

- The purpose is to identify potential anterior causes of impingement to the spinal cord during the reduction maneuver.
  - **Closed reduction before MRI**
    - Patient must be awake, alert, and cooperative.
    - Patient must be able to comply with a thorough neurologic exam during reduction.
  - **MRI before closed reduction**
    - Patient unable to cooperative with a thorough neurologic examination during reduction
    - Presence of alcohol or drugs in system, obtunded patient (etc.)
    - Neurologically intact
- Closed reduction is with Gardner-Wells tongs or halo and slow progressive application of traction.
  - Neurologic exam performed after each successive addition of weight.
  - Lateral cervical radiographs obtained after each successive addition of weight
- **MRI is generally required before open reduction.**
- **If patient is obtunded, develops neurologic symptoms, or fails closed reduction, obtain MRI to evaluate disc.**
- **Thoracic and lumbar spine injuries** (see Table 8-11)
  - General considerations
    - **Anatomic considerations**
      - Upper thoracic spine (T1-T10) is stabilized by ribs, facet joint orientation, and sternum and may provide additional stability and is less susceptible to trauma.
      - Thoracolumbar junction is a transition zone from relatively rigid thoracic spine to relatively mobile lumbar spine.
      - Middle thoracic spine is a vascular "watershed" area, and vascular insult can lead to cord ischemia.
      - Spinal cord ends and the cauda equina begins at level of L1-L2, so lesions below L1 (in general) have a better prognosis because the nerve roots (not the cord) are affected.
    - **Column theory**
      - Originally described by Denis as three columns
        - **Anterior column—equivalent to the anterior longitudinal ligament, anterior one third of the vertebral body with corresponding portion of the intervertebral disc and anulus**
        - **Middle column—equivalent to the posterior longitudinal ligament, posterior two thirds of the body with corresponding portion of the intervertebral disc and anulus**
        - **Posterior column—equivalent to the spinous process, lamina, pedicles, transverse process, and ligamentum flavum; interspinous ligament; supraspinous ligament; and facets**
      - More recently, the "fourth column" has been described in the thoracic spine.
        - Intact sternum and rib complex may impart additional stability to the thoracic spine.
        - Clinical significance still not completely known in trauma
    - Associated injuries
      - Adynamic ileus is common.
      - Calcaneus fractures are associated in approximately 10% of cases.

Table 8-11   Subaxial Cervical Spine Injury Classification (Allen-Ferguson)

LEVEL	INJURY TYPE	CLASSIFICATION	COMMON NAME	MECHANISM OF INJURY	RISK OF NEUROLOGIC INJURY	TREATMENT	INDICATION FOR SURGERY	IMPORTANT POINTS
Occipitocervical dislocation	I	Traynelis et al.	Anterior	Anterior translation	Very high	Occipitocervical fusion	Surgery indicated	Very unstable; rarely survive injury
	II		Distraction	Pure distraction	Very high	Occipitocervical fusion	Surgery indicated	Very unstable; rarely survive injury
	III		Posterior	Posterior translation	Very high	Occipitocervical fusion	Surgery indicated	Very unstable; rarely survive injury
Occipital condyle fracture	I	Anderson-Montesano	Impacted condyle fracture	Compression of skull	Low	Collar	Usually not required	Alar ligament and tectorial membrane usually intact
	II		Occipital condyle and basilar skull fracture	Compression of skull	Low	Collar	Usually not required	Alar ligament and tectorial membrane usually intact
	III		Avulsion fracture of alar ligament	Distraction of skull	Moderate to high	Collar, halo, or surgery, depending on stability	More than 1 mm of displacement	Potential for ligament disruption
C1 ring fracture	Posterior arch fracture		Lamina fracture	Hyperextension	Low	Immobilization	Not indicated	Hyperextension
	Two- and three-part fractures		Lateral mass fracture	Lateral compression	Low	Immobilization	Not indicated	
	Four-part fracture		Jefferson fracture	Axial compression	Low	Immobilization, sometimes traction	Optional for widely displaced lateral masses	>7-mm offset of lateral mass indicates transverse ligament rupture
C2 fracture	Traumatic spondylolisthesis	Levine	Hangman fracture	Hyperextension	Low	Collar		Prove stable with supervised flexion-extension radiographs
	I or IA		IA called atypical hangman					
	II or IIA			Hyperextension with secondary flexion	Low to moderate	Immobilization; avoid traction with IIA	Osteosynthesis optional	Type II, use traction; type IIA, avoid traction
	III		Bilateral facet dislocation	Hyperextension with secondary flexion/distraction	High	Surgical reduction of facet dislocation and C2-C3 fusion	Surgery required to reduce facets	Open reduction of facets required
	Odontoid fracture	Anderson-D'Alonso	Avulsion fracture	Hyperextension of distraction	Low	Collar	None	Watch for associated occipitocervical instability
	II		Fracture at junction of odontoid and body	Multiple mechanisms	Moderate	Halo vs. internal fixation	Unstable fracture or nonunion	Most common; high rate of nonunion
	III		Fracture into C2 body	Multiple mechanisms	Moderate	Halo vest immobilization	Displacement, instability	Usually stable

Continued

Table 8-11 Subaxial Cervical Spine Injury Classification (Allen-Ferguson)—cont'd

LEVEL	INJURY TYPE	CLASSIFICATION	COMMON NAME	MECHANISM OF INJURY	RISK OF NEUROLOGIC INJURY	TREATMENT	INDICATION FOR SURGERY	IMPORTANT POINTS
C2 body fracture				Similar to subaxial cervical spine	Low			
Transverse ligament disruption			C1-C2 instability	Severe flexion	Moderate to high	C1-C2 fusion	ADI > 3-5 mm	Often associated with dizziness, syncope, respiratory problems, and blurred vision Many causes; infection and trauma most common
C1-C2 rotatory subluxation	I	Fielding-Hawkins	Rotatory fixation	Rotational trauma	Low	Immobilization/traction/surgery	Indicated for chronic cases with fixed deformity and spasm or instability	
	II		Rotatory fixation with 3-5 mm of anterior displacement	Rotational trauma	Moderate	Immobilization/traction/surgery	Indicated for chronic cases with fixed deformity and spasm or instability	
	III		Rotatory fixation with >5 mm anterior displacement	Rotational trauma	Moderate	Immobilization/traction/surgery	Indicated for chronic cases with fixed deformity and spasm or instability	
	IV		Rotatory fixation with posterior displacement	Rotational trauma	Moderate to high	Immobilization/traction/surgery	Indicated for chronic cases with fixed deformity and spasm or instability	
Subaxial cervical spine		Allen-Ferguson		Mechanisms implied by name	Depends on stage of injury	Depends on stage of injury		
	Compressive flexion			Compression and flexion	Low to high		Instability or neurologic deficit with cord compression	
	Distractive flexion			Distraction and flexion	Low to high		Instability or neurologic deficit with cord compression	
	Axial compression			Axial compression	Low to high		Instability or neurologic deficit with cord compression	
	Compressive extension			Compression and extension	Low to high		Instability or neurologic deficit with cord compression	
	Distractive extension			Distraction and extension	Low to high		Instability or neurologic deficit with cord compression	
	Lateral flexion			Lateral bending	Low to moderate		Instability or neurologic deficit with cord compression	
	Compression		Compression	Flexion	Low	Collar		Watch for signs of posterior ligament

		Injury	Mechanism	Stability	Treatment	Indication	Comments
cervical spine (cont'd)		Flexion teardrop	Compression and flexion	High	Halo vs. anterior decompression/fusion	Cord compression	Very unstable
		Facet dislocation	Flexion and distraction	High	Reduction of facet, fusion	Bilateral facet dislocation	Possible disc herniation; consider MRI before reduction
	Posterior element fracture	Spinous process	Extension (sometimes flexion or rotation)	Low	Collar	Floating lateral mass	Most are stable
Thoracolumbar spine	Denis	Compression	Flexion and axial loading		Bracing	>50% anterior collapse or widening of spinous process	Osteoporotic compression fracture requires workup and treatment of underlying condition; watch for ileus
		Burst Stable	Axial loading		Bracing	Progressive deformity or neurologic compromise	Watch for any signs of posterior ligament rupture vs. MRI; watch for ileus
		Unstable			Surgery	>30 degrees kyphosis; incomplete cord injury with cord compromise	Cord decompression required if neurologic deficit present
		Seatbelt injury	Chance fracture (bony injury) — Distraction and flexion		Surgery for posterior ligament ruptures, bracing for postoperative treatment	>17% kyphosis with bony injury, posterior ligament injury	High rate of associated intraabdominal injury
		Fracture-dislocation	Rotation and shear		Surgical alignment, fusion, instrumentation	All require surgery	Long segmental posterior construct

decompression specifically indicated in cases of incomplete cord injury

ADI, Atlantodens interval; *MRI,* magnetic resonance imaging.

Table 8-12	Subaxial Cervical Spine Injury Classification System (SLIC)
CATEGORY	**POINTS**
MORPHOLOGY	
No abnormality	0
Compression	1
Burst	+1 = 2
Distraction (e.g., facet perch, hyperextension)	3
Rotation/translation (e.g., facet dislocation, unstable teardrop or advanced-stage flexion compression injury	4
DISCOLIGAMENTOUS COMPLEX (DLC)	
Intact	0
Indeterminate (e.g., isolated interspinous widening, MRI signal change only)	1
Disrupted (e.g., widening of disc space, facet perch, or dislocation)	2
NEUROLOGIC STATUS	
Intact	0
Root injury	1
Complete cord injury	2
Incomplete cord injury	3
Continuous cord compression in setting of neurologic deficit (neurologic modifier)	+1

From Vaccaro AR et al: The subaxial cervical spine injury classification system: a novel approach to recognize the importance of morphology, neurology, and integrity of the disco-ligamentous complex, *Spine (Phila Pa 1976)* 32:2365–2374, 2007.

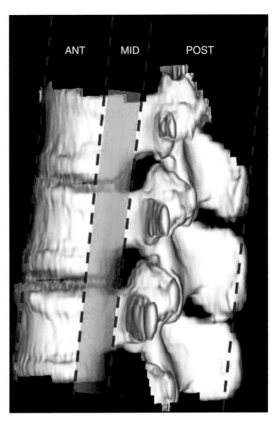

FIGURE 8-36 Three-column theory for spinal trauma as demonstrated on lateral 3D CT reconstruction. The original classification highlighted the significance of the middle column *(red shading)* in regard to neurologic involvement and potential mechanical instability. Newer classifications focus on the involvement of the posterior ligamentous complex as well. (From Cianfoni A, Colosimo C: Imaging of spine trauma. In Law M et al, editors: *Problem solving in neuroradiology,* Philadelphia, 2011, Elsevier, p 476.)

 ■ **Classifications**
- **Denis**—based on three-column theory described earlier (Figure 8-36). Four main types of spinal injuries described:
  - Compression fractures involve only the anterior column; by definition, middle column not involved.
  - Burst fractures involve the middle and anterior column; posterior column may or may not be involved.
  - Flexion-distraction (Chance) injuries involve failure of the posterior and middle columns in tension. Axis of rotation is at anterior longitudinal ligament.
  - Fracture-dislocations involve failure of all three columns; high rate of associated neurologic injuries.
- **AO Classification** (Figure 8-37)
  - Type A—compression fractures caused by axial loading
  - Type B—distraction injuries with ligamentous (B1) or osseoligamentous (B2) injury posteriorly
  - Type C—multidirectional injuries, often fracture-dislocations; very unstable with very high likelihood of neurologic injury
- **Thoracolumbar Injury Severity Score (TLISS)** (Table 8-13)
  - Based on three separate injury axes:
    - Injury mechanism
    - Integrity of posterior ligamentous complex (PLC)
    - Neurologic status
  - Scoring:
    - Score is total of three components
    - Score of 3 or less suggests nonoperative treatment.
    - Score of 4, operative or nonoperative
    - Score of 5 or greater suggests operative treatment.
■ **Treatment**
- General
  - No clear agreement on indications for surgery
  - Typically, presence of neurologic deficits and disruption of PLC increase likelihood for surgery
- Compression fracture
- Stable fracture
- Most compression managed in an orthosis or symptomatically
- **Burst fractures**
  - **May be treated in a hyperextension orthosis if there is no neurologic deficit and PLC remains intact**
  - **Disruption of PLC**
    - **Typically posterior approach and posterior spinal fusion with instrumentation to reconstruct PLC**
    - **Traditionally three levels above and two levels below injury; however, newer instrumentation may allow for short segment fixation.**
  - **Presence of neurologic deficit**
    - **Consider anterior approach for decompression of retropulsed middle column.**
    - **Consider posterior approach if presence of lamina fracture.**
      - Lamina fractures with neurologic deficits associated with possible nerve root entrapment with corresponding dural tear. Typically requires stabilization.
    - **Laminectomy alone typically contraindicated owing to the high risk of progressive kyphosis.**

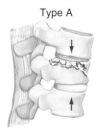

Type A

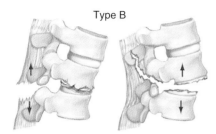

Type B

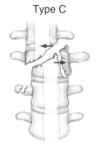

Type C

FIGURE 8-37 Thoracolumbar spine injuries based on AO classification. (From Kim DH et al: *Atlas of spine trauma: adult and pediatric,* Philadelphia, 2008, Elsevier, p 271.)

Table 8-13	Thoracolumbar Injury Severity Score (TLISS)
MECHANISM	**POINTS**
Compression	1
Lateral angulation > 15 degrees	+1
Burst	+1
Translational/rotational	3
Distraction	4
Neurologic injury	
Nerve root	2
Spinal cord or conus injury	
Complete	2
Incomplete	3
Cauda equina	3
Posterior ligamentous complex	
Intact	0
Indeterminate	2
Injured	3

Adapted from Vaccaro AR et al: The thoracolumbar injury severity score: a proposed treatment algorithm, *J Spinal Disord Tech* 18:209-215, 2005.

- Flexion-distraction (Chance)
  - Bony flexion-distraction injury—hyperextension external orthosis
  - Ligamentous flexion-distraction injury
    - High rate of posttraumatic kyphosis due to incompetent PLC
    - Posterior spinal fusion
- Fracture-dislocations
  - Frequently associated with neurologic injury

Table 8-14	Frankel Classification for Grading of Functional Motor Recovery After Spinal Cord Injury
FRANKEL GRADE	**FUNCTION**
A	Complete paralysis
B	Sensory function only below injury level
C	Incomplete motor function (grades 1-2 of 5) below injury level
D	Fair to good (useful) motor function (grades 3-4 of 5) below injury level
E	Normal function (grade 5 of 5)

- Most are highly unstable and require operative stabilization with multiple points of fixation above and below the injury level.
  - May require anterior approach for decompression and/or achieve anterior column support for additional stability.
- Complications
  - Potentially negative outcomes are numerous and include neurologic injury, nonunion, and malunion.
  - Delayed instability
    - Associated with greater than 3.5 mm of subluxation
    - Greater than 11 degrees of difference in angulation between adjacent motion segments
- Prognosis—Frankel classification useful when assessing functional recovery from spinal cord injury (Table 8-14)

■ **Gunshot wounds to the spine**

■ Typically mechanically stable injures that do not require surgery for mechanical instability

■ Progressive neurologic decline and retained projectile in canal—consider surgical removal.

■ Neurologically intact or stable and projectile retained in spinal canal
- L1 and below—consider removal of projectile.
- T12 and above—removal of projectile controversial; may result in worsening neurologic deficit

■ Penetrating spine injuries accompanied by injury to abdominal content
- Associated hollow viscera injury (gastrointestinal perforation)—tetanus prophylaxis and IV antibiotics for 7 to 14 days
- Associated solid viscera injury (kidney, liver, etc.)—treat with oral antibiotics

■ **Considerations in pediatric spine trauma**

■ Many pediatric spinal injuries are analogous those occurring in the adult population.

■ Notable differences include:
- Bony skeleton more ductile in pediatric population than in adults
- Head is relatively larger than body.
  - Therefore pediatric torso must be elevated 2 to 3 cm to maintain inline cervical alignment.
  - Special pediatric spine board can be used, or if not available, blankets or towels can be placed under torso to create necessary elevation.
- Thickness of skull is thinner in pediatric patient population.
  - Pediatric skull tongs and halo require more pins at lower torque.
  - Total 6 to 8 pins at 2 to 4 inch-lb
- Spinal cord and vertebral body relationship varies with increasing age.

- Spinal cord begins at approximate level of L3 at birth.
- Spinal cord stops growing around infancy.
- Final spinal cord length ends with conus medullaris, typically ending around T12-L1/L1-L2.
- Therefore in adult, lumbar spine houses cauda equina, spinal nerve roots.

▪ **Spinal cord injury without radiographic abnormality (SCIWORA)**
- Clinical entity primarily occurring in children
- Thought to be secondary to tenuous spinal cord blood supply and greater elasticity in vertebral column than in spinal cord
- Original description by Pang and Wilberger in 1982 defined SCIWORA as objective findings of spinal cord injury/myelopathy without evidence of ligamentous injury or fractures on plain x-rays or tomographic studies.
  - Original description did not include MRI as a diagnostic modality.
  - Original description excluded penetrating trauma, electric shock, obstetric complications, and congenital spinal spine abnormalities.
  - More recent imaging studies including MRI have identified ligamentous and disc injury, complete spinal cord transections, and spinal core hemorrhage; however, normal MRI findings have also been described.

▪ **C2 pediatric dens fracture**
- **Most common pediatric cervical spine fracture**
- **Typically occurs in patients younger than age 6**
- **Frequently fractures through basilar synchondrosis (residual disc) of dens**
- **Treatment**
  - Avoid traction; can result in distraction of dens.
  - Reduction in hyperextension followed by Minerva or compression halo vest.

▪ Pediatric atlantoaxial (C1-C2) rotatory subluxation
- Similar to adults, except in pediatric population typically due to loss of ligamentous stability between C1 and C2. Results in rotation with lateral tilt.
  - Can occur spontaneously
  - Secondary to trauma
- Etiology in pediatric population includes:
  - Atlantoaxial instability secondary to pharyngeal infections (Grisel syndrome)
  - Down syndrome
  - Morquio syndrome
  - Achondroplasia
  - Klippel-Feil syndrome
  - Spondyloepiphyseal dysplasia
  - Larsen syndrome
- Differentiate from torticollis
  - Torticollis is secondary to fibrosis of sternal head of sternocleidomastoid (SCM).
  - Typically palpable mass within SCM for congenital torticollis

▪ **Pseudosubluxation of cervical spine in the pediatric population**
- Cervical spine mobility, particularly in flexion and extension, is physiologically increased in pediatric population.

- Most commonly occurs at C2-C3 followed by C3-C4 in pediatric population
- Excess motion in children younger than 8 years is considered normal.
- Radiographic evaluation
  - **Anterior ADI can be up to 5 mm in pediatric patients.**
  - Up to 4 mm or 40% anterior displacement of C2 on C3 can be seen.
  - Subluxation can be accentuated if child's head in slight flexion.
  - Normal prevertebral soft tissue shadow on lateral radiograph
  - Absence of anterior soft tissue swelling
  - **Swischuk line—line drawn through posterior arch of C2 should be within 2 mm of the spinolaminar line drawn at C1-C3.**

▪ Pediatric flexion-distraction injuries (Chance fracture)
- Mechanism analogous to adult flexion-distraction injuries
  - Axis of rotation is anterior to vertebral body at anterior longitudinal ligament.
  - **High association with intraabdominal injuries**
- Adult flexion-distraction injuries typically occur between T11-L1, but pediatric flexion distraction injuries can occur lower at L1-L2 and L2-L3, owing to different center of gravity.
- **Treatment**
  - **Bony flexion-distraction injuries and neurologically intact can be treated closed with extension bracing.**
  - **Purely ligamentous flexion-distraction injuries frequently require surgery, owing to late ligamentous instability.**

▪ Apophyseal ring spine avulsion fractures
- Introduction
  - Avulsion of apophyseal ring in association with disc herniation
  - Pathophysiology unclear; associated with relative weakness of apophyseal ring during childhood
  - May have association with Scheuermann disease (debated)
  - Typically adolescent and young-adult age group
  - Acute spinal trauma is not always identified.
  - Must be differentiated from posterior longitudinal ligament, anulus, or calcified herniated disc, and posterior discoosteophytic ridge.
- Imaging
  - Although in some reports can be identified on plain radiographs in up to 70%, can still be missed in up to one third of cases or greater
  - CT scan able to identify injury in nearly all cases.
  - MRI does not identify bone as well as CT, and apophyseal avulsion can be missed on MRI.

SELECTED BIBLIOGRAPHY

The selected bibliography for this chapter can be found on www.expertconsult.com.

TESTABLE CONCEPTS

I. Introduction

- Careful history is vital to accurate diagnosis and management of spinal pathology.
- Physical examination should include motor, sensory, reflexes, and when appropriate rectal examination.
- In the absence of trauma and "red-flag" signs, plain radiographs are not required unless symptoms have persisted longer than 4 to 6 weeks.
- False-positive MRIs are common, and imaging should be correlated carefully with the history and physical examination.

II. Cervical Spine

- Cervical spondylosis most commonly occurs at C5-C6.
  - Cervical nerve roots exit above their corresponding vertebrae (e.g., C5 exits at the C4-C5 neural foramen). Consequently, disc herniation at C5-C6 involves the C6 nerve root.
  - The natural history of cervical spondylotic myelopathy is characterized by stepwise deterioration in symptomatology followed by a period of stability.
  - False-positive MRIs are common, with 25% of asymptomatic patients older than 40 years demonstrating a herniated nucleus pulposus or foraminal stenosis.
  - Operative indications include myelopathy with motor/gait impairment and radiculopathy with persistent disabling pain that has failed nonoperative measures.
  - Anterior cervical discectomy and fusion complications include recurrent laryngeal nerve injury, dysphagia, airway obstruction, nonunion, and adjacent segment disease. Nonunion should be treated with posterior fusion.
  - Canal-expansive laminoplasty is used for multilevel spondylosis, congenital cervical stenosis, and ossification of the posterior longitudinal ligament. It is contraindicated in the setting of fixed kyphosis.
- In cervical stenosis, a Pavlov (Torg) ratio of less than 0.80 or a sagittal diameter of less than 13 mm are considered significant risk factors for later neurologic involvement. *Absolute stenosis* is defined as an anteroposterior canal diameter less than 10 mm.
- Rheumatoid spondylitis most commonly presents as an occipital headache due to compression of the greater occipital branch of C2.
  - Progressive cervical instability secondary to pannus formation and erosion of the joints and capsular structures occurs in up to 90% of patients. This can manifest as (1) atlantoaxial instability, (2) cranial settling (basilar invagination), and (3) subaxial subluxation.
  - Atlantoaxial subluxation is most common. A posterior atlantodens interval (ADI) less than 14 mm is associated with an increased risk of neurologic injury and usually requires surgical treatment. Transarticular screw fixation (Magerl) across C1-C2 eliminates the need for halo immobilization associated with wiring alone. Surgery is less successful in Ranawat grade IIIB patients but should be considered.
  - Always obtain flexion/extension films before elective surgery in patients with rheumatoid arthritis.
- Patients with ankylosing spondylitis (AS) with neck pain should be carefully evaluated for an occult cervical spine fracture.
- Cervical spine injury can be associated with spinal shock and/or neurogenic shock.
  - Spinal shock is over when the bulbocavernosus reflex returns.
  - Neurogenic shock is secondary to loss of sympathetic tone and can be recognized by relative bradycardia.

- Incomplete spinal cord syndromes are anatomically classified, and all involve some sparing of distal function.
  - Central cord syndrome is most common, affecting elderly patients with a spondylotic cervical spine. It presents as motor and sensory loss greater in the upper than the lower extremity. Independent ambulation is regained in approximately half of elderly patients and almost always in young patients.
  - Anterior cord syndrome is the second most common and has the worst prognosis. It presents as greater motor loss in the legs than in the arms.
  - Brown-Séquard syndrome presents as motor weakness on the side of injury and contralateral loss of pain and temperature. It has the best prognosis.
- Autonomic dysreflexia is a syndrome of uncontrolled sympathetic nervous output occurring in patients with a spinal cord injury above T6. It presents as hypertension, pupillary dilation, headache, pallor, and reflex bradycardia. Treat with urinary catheterization, fecal disimpaction, antihypertensives, and atropine in severe cases.

III. Thoracic Spine

- Most thoracic herniated discs are treated nonsurgically.
  - Indications for surgery include progressive thoracic myelopathy and persistent unremitting radicular pain.
- Thoracic HNP is typically treated via an anterior transthoracic approach for midline or central herniations. Anterior discectomy and hemicorpectomy are performed as needed. A transpedicular approach is used for a lateral herniation.
  - Posterior approach and laminectomy are contraindicated because of an inability to retract the spinal cord and high rate of neurologic injury.

IV. Lumbar Spine

- The differential diagnosis of thoracolumbar disease can be (over) simplified based on whether leg pain or back pain are predominant and whether the pain is worse with flexion or extension:
  - Back pain predominant
    - Worse with flexion → discogenic back pain
    - Worse with extension → spondylolisthesis or facet arthropathy
  - Leg pain predominant
    - Worse with flexion → lumbar disc disease
    - Worse with extension → spinal stenosis

Lumbar Disc Disease

- Most herniations are posterolateral (where the posterior longitudinal ligament is the weakest) and may present as back pain and nerve root pain/sciatica involving the lower nerve root at that level (L5 at the L4-L5 level).
- Far lateral herniation or foraminal stenosis involves the exiting nerve root (L4 at the L4-5 level).
- A positive contralateral straight-leg raising test (pain in the affected buttock/leg when the opposite leg is raised) is the most specific test for HNP.
- More than half of patients who seek treatment for low back pain recover in 1 week, and 90% recover within 1 to 3 months. Half of patients with sciatica recover in 1 month. Conservative treatment is with NSAIDs and physical therapy.
- Failure to improve within 6 weeks warrants further investigation. Radiographs are generally performed at this point.
- Standard partial laminotomy and discectomy are the most commonly performed surgical procedures.
- Outcomes from the SPORT trial (2-year follow-up):

- No significant differences in primary outcome measures for operative compared with nonoperative groups
- However, trends favoring surgical intervention in primary outcome measures
- Statistically significant improvement in secondary outcome measures for surgical intervention: sciatica bothersomeness, self-rated improvement
- Workers' compensation patients are more likely to continue to receive disability compensation and have worse symptoms, functional status, and satisfaction outcomes.
- Complications include vascular injury, nerve root injury, infection (1% but increased in diabetics), discitis, cauda equina syndrome, and dural tear.
  - Treatment of a dural tear includes bed rest and subarachnoid drain placement. If adequately repaired, clinical outcomes are generally unaffected.

Spinal Stenosis
- Spinal stenosis can be classified anatomically into central, lateral recess, and foraminal stenosis. Tandem stenosis is said to occur when there is both cervical and lumbar stenosis.
  - Central → narrowing of central spinal canal from one edge of dural tube to the other
  - Lateral → narrowing of subarticular recess, bounded by takeoff of nerve root from dural tube to the medial border of the pedicle
  - Foraminal → narrowing of neural foramen, bounded by disc anteriorly, pars articularis posteriorly, and pedicles superiorly and inferiorly
- Central stenosis that fails nonoperative management should be treated with laminectomy and partial medial facetectomy. Surgical instability (via removal of a facet), a pars defect, spondylolisthesis (degenerative or isthmic), degenerative scoliosis and radiographic instability are indications for fusion.
  - Residual foraminal stenosis is a common reason for persistent radicular pain after laminectomy
  - Outcomes from the SPORT trial (4-year follow-up):
    - Significant improvement in pain and function for operative compared with nonoperative groups
- Lateral recess stenosis that fails nonoperative management should be treated with decompression of the hypertrophied lamina and ligamentum flavum and partial facetectomy.
- The use of alendronate has been shown to decrease spinal fusion rates in animal models. Administration should be held in the postoperative period.

Spondylosis and Spondylolisthesis
- Spondylosis is a defect in the pars interarticularis. Unilateral defects almost never progress to "-olisthesis."
- Spondylolisthesis is divided into six types. The most common is isthmic (L5-S1 level), followed by degenerative (L4-L5 level).
- Isthmic spondylolisthesis can present in childhood or in adults.
  - Pediatric
    - Low-grade disease (<50% slip) typically responds to nonoperative treatment.
    - High-grade disease should be treated with prophylactic fusion. This often requires in situ bilateral posterolateral fusion from L4-S1.
  - Adult
    - Associated with an increased pelvic incidence
    - Operative treatment includes in situ L4 or L5-S1 posterolateral fusion.
- Degenerative spondylolisthesis is four to five times more common in women and more common in African Americans and diabetics.

- It presents as symptoms of central and lateral recess spinal stenosis.
- Operative treatment for degenerative spondylolisthesis involves decompression of the nerve roots and stabilization by posterolateral fusion.
  - Outcomes from the SPORT trial (4-year follow-up):
    - Significant improvement in pain and function for operative compared with nonoperative groups

Cauda Equina
- Typically secondary to large extruded disc, surgical trauma, and/or hematoma.
- Presents with bowel and bladder dysfunction, saddle anesthesia, and varying degrees of lower extremity weakness
- Urgent/emergent MRI can help assess for compression of the cauda equina, with surgical decompression as soon as possible.

V. Adult Deformity

Scoliosis—Coronal Plane Deformity
- Adult scoliosis is typically lumbar/thoracolumbar and more symptomatic than its childhood counterpart.
- Right thoracic curves of greater than 50 degrees are at the highest risk for progression (usually 1 degree/yr), followed by right lumbar curves.
- Sagittal plane imbalance is a strong predictor of disability, and preservation of normal sagittal alignment with fusion is critical.
- Whether to end a fusion at L5 or S1 is controversial. Fusion to L5 is associated with development of L5-S1 degenerative disc disease and progressive sagittal imbalance. Fusion to the sacrum is associated with increased incidence of pseudarthrosis and gait disturbance.

Kyphosis—Sagittal Plane Deformity
- Kyphosis is a sagittal plane deformity and can occur with or without an associated coronal plane deformity (scoliosis).
- Can occur secondary to variety of sources; however, common causes include osteoporotic compression fractures, postlaminectomy kyphosis, and junctional kyphosis above or below a previous surgical site.

VI. Sacropelvis
- Sacroiliac joint dysfunction and coccygodynia are typically self-limiting and therefore managed nonoperatively.
- Sacral insufficiency fractures can occur in patients with osteopenia/osteoporosis and should therefore be part of the evaluation and management.

VII. Spinal Tumors
- Metastatic disease is the most common malignancy of the spine and most commonly involves the vertebral body.
- "Red flags" for metastatic disease include a history of cancer, unexplained weight loss, night pain, and age older than 50.
- Wide excision is typically performed for primary bone tumors without known metastases and solitary metastases with likelihood of prolonged survival.
- Decompressive surgery techniques:
  - Upper cervical spine → posterior approach
  - Posterior element tumor of lower cervical, thoracic, or lumbar spine → posterior approach
  - Majority of lower cervical, thoracic or lumbar spine → anterior approach because most tumors are located in the body
  - Multilevel involvement or en bloc spondylectomy → combined anterior/posterior approach

VIII. Spinal infections and Inflammatory Arthritides

- Osteodiscitis most commonly presents as pain and elevated erythrocyte sedimentation rate and C-reactive protein level.
  - Radiographs are often negative, with loss of lumbar lordosis and disc space narrowing the earliest findings.
  - Treatment is with IV antibiotics, and C-reactive protein should be used to monitor response.
  - Anterior débridement and strut grafting are reserved for refractory cases. Isolated laminectomy is generally avoided.
- Pyogenic vertebral osteomyelitis is usually from hematogenous spread and involves *Staphylococcus aureus* in 50% to 75% of cases.
- Epidural abscess typically presents with patients being more systemically ill than osteodiscitis and osteomyelitis patients.
- Management is typically surgical, with irrigation and débridement of infected tissue.
- Tuberculosis spondylitis differs from pyogenic infections in four ways:
  - Originates in metaphysis of vertebral body and spreads under the anterior longitudinal ligament
  - Large anterior abscesses
  - Discs are preserved.
  - Severe kyphosis more common
  - AS is associated with HLA-B27, but only 2% of patients with HLA-B27 have AS; therefore it is not used in the diagnosis.
  - Sacroiliac joint obliteration (iliac side affected first) and marginal syndesmophytes allow radiographic differentiation from diffuse idiopathic skeletal hyperostosis.
  - The spine often becomes fused in kyphosis. Posterior extension osteotomies are performed, followed by posterior fusion.
- Diffuse idiopathic skeletal hyperostosis is typically seen in older patients and more common in the thoracic spine. It is differentiated on radiographs by undulating "nonmarginal syndesmophytes."

IX. Spinal Trauma

Upper Cervical Spine Injuries

- ASIA classification of spinal cord injury is based on motor strength and complete versus incomplete sensory deficit. An ASIA C grade represents less than 3/5 motor score and incomplete sensory deficit.
- C1 burst fractures (Jefferson) may be stable or unstable, depending on the integrity of the transverse ligament. Combined lateral mass displacement greater than 7 mm indicates transverse ligament disruption. Posterior spinal fusion is recommended.
- Odontoid fracture treatment is based on the risk of developing nonunion.
  - Type I—rigid cervical orthosis
  - Generally, type II fractures are considered operative, particularly in those older than 50. For a posterior C1-C2 fusion, an anterior screw may be used unless body habitus or anterior oblique fracture orientation prevents it.
  - Risk factors for type II nonunion: displacement greater than 5 mm, angulation greater than 10 degrees, posterior displacement, age older than 40 years, delayed treatment
  - Nondisplaced type II—rigid cervical orthosis versus halo
  - Type III—halo vest
- Hangman fracture acceptable reduction: less than 4 mm translation and less than 10 degrees angulation
- Halo vest orthosis is effective in controlling most spinal motions except axial distraction.
  - The safe zone for anterior pins is the middle to lateral third above the eyebrow to avoid the supraorbital nerve.
  - Adults require 4 pins at 6 to 8 inch-lb pressure. Children need 8 to 10 pins with 2 inch-lb pressure.

Lower Cervical Spine Injuries

- Bilateral facet joint dislocations demonstrate greater than 50% translation and are often associated with spinal cord injury.
- The role of MRI in reducing facet dislocations is controversial.
- Most authors recommend obtaining an MRI before closed reduction in an obtunded patient.
- Closed reduction before MRI can be considered in an awake, alert, and cooperative patient who can participate in a full neurologic examination.

Thoracolumbar and Lumbar Spine Injuries

- Flexion-distraction injuries involve failure of the posterior and middle columns in tension.
  - These injuries are routinely treated with surgical stabilization via posterior approach. Occasionally they require additional anterior decompression and stabilization.
- Burst fractures may be treated in an orthosis if kyphosis if patient is neurologically intact and the posterior ligamentous complex remains intact.

CHAPTER **9**

ORTHOPAEDIC PATHOLOGY

Ginger E. Holt

CONTENTS

SECTION 1 INTRODUCTION

CLINICAL EVALUATION

- **History: patient age. Certain diseases are common in particular age groups (Table 9-1).**
- **Physical examination: patients with suspected bone tumors should be examined carefully.**
- Site is inspected for soft tissue masses, overlying skin changes, adenopathy, and general musculoskeletal condition.
- When metastatic disease is suspected, the thyroid gland, abdomen, prostate, and breasts should be assessed.
- **Laboratory studies: results of blood tests are often nonspecific. For musculoskeletal neoplasms, studies that may be diagnostic include:**
- Prostate-specific antigen (PSA) for prostate cancer
- **Serum or urine electrophoresis (SPEP or UPEP) for myeloma**
- Erythrocyte sedimentation rate (ESR) or C-reactive protein (CRP) for infection

IMAGING

- **Radiographs in two planes are the first imaging studies to be performed. Enneking's 4 questions: (1) Location (epiphyseal, metaphyseal, diaphyseal, etc.), (2) tumor-bone interaction, (3) bone-tumor interaction (refers to the interplay between host bone and tumor described by Lodwick [Table 9-2]), and (4) matrix (i.e., what are the tumor cells producing?—bone, cartilage, etc. [Figures 9-1 through 9-3; Table 9-3]).**

- Technetium-labeled bone scan is an excellent modality to search for occult bone involvement. In patients with myeloma for whom scan results may be negative, a skeletal survey is more sensitive.
- Magnetic resonance imaging (MRI) is excellent for assessing the primary tumor site and for screening the spine for occult metastases, myeloma, or lymphoma.
- A chest radiograph should be obtained to assess for primary lung disease or metastases in patients of any age when the clinician suspects a malignant lesion.
- Radiographs must be carefully inspected to formulate a working diagnosis, which then guides the clinician during further evaluation and treatment. Formulation of the differential diagnosis is based on several clinical and radiographic parameters:
  - Number of bone lesions: is the process monostotic or polyostotic? **If there are multiple destructive lesions in middle-aged and older patients (age >40), the most likely diagnosis is metastatic bone disease, multiple myeloma, or lymphoma.** In young patients (<age 30), multiple lytic and oval lesions in the same extremity are probably vascular tumors (hemangioendothelioma). In children younger than 5 years, multiple destructive lesions may represent metastatic disease such as neuroblastoma or Wilms tumor or Langerhans cell histiocytosis (LCH). Fibrous dysplasia and Paget disease may manifest with multiple lesions in all age groups.

Table 9-1	Bone Lesion by Age		
	AGE		
	<5	**<30**	**>30**
Malignant	LCH (Letter-Siwe) LCH (Hand-Schüller-Christian) Metastatic rhabdomyosarcoma Metastatic neuroblastoma	Ewing sarcoma Osteosarcoma	Chondrosarcoma Metastases Lymphoma Myeloma Chordoma Adamantinoma
Benign	Osteomyelitis Osteofibrous dysplasia	Osteoid osteoma Osteoblastoma Chondroblastoma Aneurysmal bone cyst LCH Osteofibrous dysplasia Nonossifying fibroma	Giant cell tumor Paget disease

LCH, Langerhans cell histiocytosis.

Table 9-2	Tumor-Bone Interaction (From Lodwick)		
LESION	**TYPE I**	**TYPE II**	**TYPE III**
Radiographic appearance	Geographic A: sclerotic B: distinct C: indistinct	Moth eaten	Destructive
Examples	A: nonossifying fibroma B: unicameral bone cyst C: giant cell tumor	Osteomyelitis Metastases	Ewing sarcoma
Image			

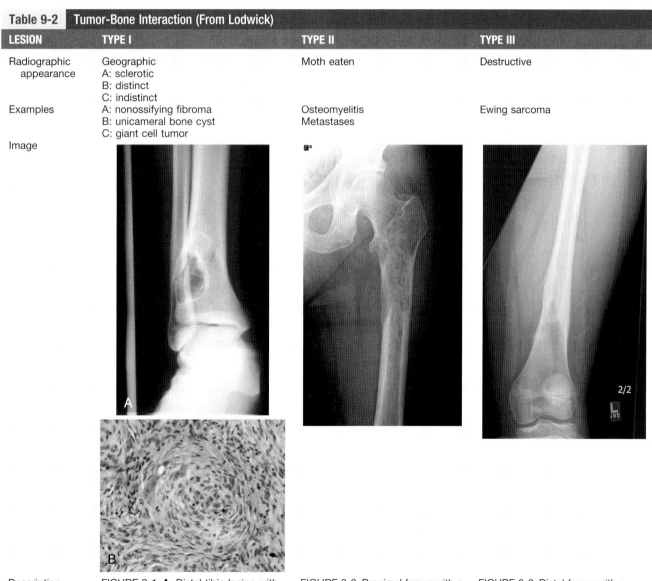

| Description | FIGURE 9-1 **A,** Distal tibia lesion with a geographic border and a sclerotic rim. **B,** Nonossifying fibroma. | FIGURE 9-2 Proximal femur with a "moth-eaten" appearance; metastatic carcinoma. | FIGURE 9-3 Distal femur with a destructive lesion. There is an aggressive lesion creating a large soft tissue mass and minimal cortical response; Ewing sarcoma. |

Table 9-3	Classification of Primary Tumors of Bone and Bone Matrix*	
HISTOLOGIC TYPE	**BENIGN**	**MALIGNANT**
Hematopoietic		Myeloma
		Lymphoma
Chondrogenic	Osteochondroma	Primary chondrosarcoma
	Chondroma	Secondary chondrosarcoma
	Chondroblastoma	Dedifferentiated chondrosarcoma
	Chondromyxoid fibroma	Mesenchymal chondrosarcoma
		Clear cell chondrosarcoma
Osteogenic	Osteoid osteoma	Osteosarcoma
	Osteoblastoma	Parosteal osteosarcoma
		Periosteal osteosarcoma
Unknown origin	Giant cell tumor (fibrous) histiocytoma	Ewing tumor
		Malignant giant cell tumor
		Adamantinoma
Fibrogenic	Fibroma	Fibrosarcoma
	Desmoplastic fibroma	Malignant fibrous histiocytoma
Notochordal		Chordoma
Vascular	Hemangioma	Hemangioendothelioma
		Hemangiopericytoma
Lipogenic	Lipoma	Liposarcoma
Neurogenic	Neurilemoma	Malignant peripheral nerve sheath tumor (MPNST)

*Classification is based on that advocated by Lichtenstein L: Classification of primary tumors of bone, *Cancer* 4:335–341, 1951.

Table 9-4	Tumors by Location

EPIPHYSEAL
Chondroblastoma
Giant cell tumor
Clear cell chondrosarcoma (femoral head)
METAPHYSEAL
Osteosarcoma
Chondrosarcoma
Metastatic disease
DIAPHYSEAL
A = adamantinoma
E = eosinophilic granuloma
I = infection
O = osteoid osteoma/osteoblastoma
U = Ewing sarcoma
Y = myeloma, lymphoma, fibrous dysplasia
Metastatic disease
FLAT BONES
Chondrosarcoma
Fibrous dysplasia
Hemangioma
Paget disease
Ewing sarcoma
SPINE
Anterior column
　Giant cell tumor
　Metastatic disease
Posterior column
　Osteoid osteoma/osteoblastoma
　Aneurysmal bone cyst
SACRUM
Midline
　Chordoma
Eccentric
　Aneurysmal bone cyst/giant cell tumor/metastatic disease

- Anatomic location within bone: Certain lesions have a predilection for occurring within a certain bone or a particular part of the bone (Table 9-4).

BIOPSY (BONE AND SOFT TISSUE)

- Determines tumor type and grade. Biopsy is generally performed after complete evaluation of the patient. A narrow working diagnosis is of great benefit to both the

Table 9-5	Principles of Musculoskeletal Biopsy	
PRINCIPLE	**RATIONALE**	
Make longitudinal incision in line with future resection.	Longitudinal incision is extensile.	
Biopsy through a single compartment.	Biopsy tract can be excised with final resection remaining extensile.	
Avoid critical structures (i.e., neurovascular bundles).	Contamination of critical structures precludes limb salvage.	
Biopsy the soft tissue component when present.	Bone is weakened when its cortex is disrupted. Bone requires decalcification for evaluation, and this process may affect pathology.	
Maintain strict hemostasis. Use a drain in line with the incision when needed.	Avoid increased contamination outside of the biopsy tract by iatrogenic tumor spread.	

pathologist and the surgeon because it allows accurate interpretation of the frozen-section analysis, and definitive treatment of some lesions can be based on the frozen section. Clinicians must follow several surgical principles (Table 9-5):

- **Orientation and location of the biopsy tract are critical.** If the lesion proves to be malignant, the entire biopsy tract must be removed with the underlying lesion. Transverse incisions should be avoided.
- The surgeon must maintain meticulous hemostasis to prevent hematoma formation and subcutaneous hemorrhage. When possible, biopsy incisions are made through muscles so the muscle layer can be closed tightly. Neurovascular structures should be avoided. Tourniquets are used to obtain tissue in a bloodless field and then are released so bleeding points can be controlled. Hemostatic agents are used as necessary. If hemostasis cannot be achieved, a small drain should be placed at the corner of the wound to prevent hematoma formation. A compression dressing is routinely used on the extremities.

Table 9-6 Immunohistochemistry

MARKER	PATHOLOGY	TUMOR
SMA (smooth muscle actin)	Smooth muscle	Leiomyosarcoma
Desmin	Skeletal muscle	Rhabdomyosarcoma
MyoD1/myogenin (myf-4)	Skeletal muscle	Rhabdomyosarcoma
S-100	Neural	Schwannoma, MPNST
CD34/CD31	Endothelial cells/vascularity	Hemangioma, hemangioendothelioma, angiosarcoma
β-Catenin	Membrane marker Wnt signaling pathway	Fibromatosis
CD99		Ewing sarcoma, PNET
Keratin		Epithelioid sarcomas, synovial sarcoma, carcinoma, adamantinoma
EMA (epithelial membrane antigen)		Epithelioid sarcomas, synovial sarcoma
Vimentin		Soft tissue sarcoma
CD20, CD45		Lymphoma
CD138		Myeloma

MPNST, Malignant peripheral nerve sheath tumor; *PNET,* peripheral neuroectodermal tumor.

Table 9-7 Common Chromosomal Translocations

DIAGNOSIS	CHROMOSOMAL ABNORMALITY	GENES
Ewing sarcoma/PNET	t(11;22)	*EWS-FLI1*
Myxoid liposarcoma	t(12;16)	*TLS-CHOP*
Alveolar rhabdomyosarcoma	t(2;13)	*PAX3-FKHR*
Clear cell sarcoma	t(12;22)	*EWS-ATF1*
Synovial sarcoma	t(x;18)	*SSX1-SYT*
Myxoid chondrosarcoma (extraskeletal)	T(9;22)	*EWS-CHN*
Osteosarcoma	None	None

PNET, peripheral neuroectodermal tumor.

■ A frozen-section analysis is performed on all biopsy samples to ensure adequate diagnostic tissue is obtained. When possible, the soft tissue component rather than the bony component should be sampled.

■ All biopsy samples should be submitted for bacteriologic analysis if the frozen section does not reveal a neoplasm. Antibiotics should not be delivered until cultures are obtained.

■ Needle biopsy is an excellent method for achieving a tissue diagnosis and providing minimum tissue disruption. Careful correlation of the small tissue sample with the radiographs often yields the correct diagnosis. When the nature of the lesion is obvious on the basis of the radiographic features and when adequate tissue can be obtained with a needle, the needle biopsy technique is safe to use. The pathologist must be experienced and comfortable with the small sample of tissue. When the diagnoses of needle biopsy and imaging studies are not concordant, an open biopsy should be performed to establish the diagnosis. Open biopsy is often necessary with low-grade tumors and when the needle biopsy does not provide a definitive diagnosis. Immunostains are helpful in diagnosis (Table 9-6).

MOLECULAR BIOLOGY (BONE AND SOFT TISSUE)

■ **Chromosomes—sarcoma-associated translocations. The most well-known is Ewing sarcoma, balanced translocation of chromosomes 11 and 22. The gene fusion product from this balanced translocation is the *EWS-FLI1* gene. A gene with a sequence that causes cancer is an oncogene. *EWS-FLI1* and *SSX1-SYT* genes are oncogenes.**

■ Tumor suppressor genes: genes that inhibit cell proliferation. Mutations allow for unregulated tumor growth. **Examples are *Rb* (retinoblastoma), mutated in 35% of osteosarcomas, and *p53,* mutated in 50% of all tumors and 20% to 65% of osteosarcomas** (Table 9-7).

■ Hereditary cancer syndromes—associated with tumor-suppressor genes or specific genetic defects. **Most common associated with osteosarcoma are Li-Fraumeni (*p53* gene) and congenital bilateral retinoblastoma (*Rb* gene); with chondrosarcoma, multiple hereditary exostoses (*EXT 1, EXT 2, EXT 3)*; and with malignant peripheral nerve sheath tumor, *NF1*** (Table 9-8).

GRADING (BONE AND SOFT TISSUE)

Grading is based on nuclear atypia (degree of loss of structural differentiation), pleomorphism (variations in size and shape), and nuclear hyperchromasia (increased nuclear staining). Grading of tumors covers a morphologic range.

■ Most grading systems are based on three grades.
■ The grade of the tumor is most strongly correlated with the potential for metastasis.
■ Most malignant bone lesions are high grade (grade G_2); low-grade malignant (grade G_1) lesions are less common.
■ Soft tissue tumors have a greater range of grade (Table 9-9).

STAGING (BONE AND SOFT TISSUE)

Staging systems are used for communicating, planning treatment, and predicting prognosis. The staging systems of the Musculoskeletal Tumor Society (MSTS), also called the *Enneking system,* and the American Joint Commission on Cancer (AJCC) are the most common for musculoskeletal diseases. Staging systems exist for both bone and soft tissue sarcomas.

■ Enneking system: benign and malignant bone and soft tissue tumors (Table 9-10)
■ Benign—stages 1, 2, 3
■ Malignant—stages I, II, III
■ AJCC system for bone: listed in order of importance (Table 9-11)
■ Stage (presence of metastases = stage IV)
■ Discontinuous tumor (stage III)
■ Grade (I = low, II = high)
■ Size (> or < 8 cm)

Table 9-8	Musculoskeletal Syndromes, Genes, and Neoplasms		
SYNDROME	**DISEASE**	**MUSCULOSKELETAL NEOPLASM**	**GENETIC ASSOCIATION**
Li-Fraumeni	SBLA syndrome	Osteosarcoma	P53
Retinoblastoma	Bilateral malignant tumor of the eye in children	Osteosarcoma	RB1
Rothmund-Thomson	Sun-sensitive rash with prominent poikiloderma and telangiectasias	Osteosarcoma	RECQL4
Multiple hereditary exostoses	Multiple osteochondromas	Chondrosarcoma	EXT1, EXT2
Ollier disease	Enchondromas	Chondrosarcoma	PTHR1
Maffucci syndrome	Enchondromas + angiomas and CNS, pancreatic, and ovarian malignancies	Chondrosarcoma and/ or angiosarcomas	PTHR1
McCune-Albright	Polyostotic fibrous dysplasia, precocious puberty, and café au lait spots		GNAS1
Mazabraud	Fibrous dysplasia + soft tissue myxomas		GNAS1
Jaffe-Campanacci	Multiple nonossifying fibromas with café au lait skin patches		
POEMS	**P**olyneuropathy (peripheral nerve damage) **O**rganomegaly (abnormal enlargement of organs) **E**ndocrinopathy (damage to hormone-producing glands) **M** protein (an abnormal immunoglobulin) **S**kin abnormalities (hyperpigmentation)	Myeloma	
Hand-Schüller-Christian disease (<5 years old)	Multifocal LCH and exophthalmos, diabetes insipidus, and lytic skull lesions	LCH	
Letterer-Siwe disease (infants)	Multifocal LCH, visceral and bone disease, and is fatal	LCH	
Stuart-Treves	Chronic lymphedema	Angiosarcoma	
Neurofibromatosis type 1	Multiple neurofibromas	MPNST	NF1
Familial adenomatous polyposis	Multiple intestinal polyps, colon cancer, hepatoblastomas	Desmoid tumors	APC

CNS, Central nervous system; *LCH*, Langerhans cell histiocytosis; *MPNST*, malignant peripheral nerve sheath tumor; *SBLA*, sarcoma, breast, leukemia, and adrenal gland.

Table 9-9	Histologic Grading of Soft Tissue Tumors*	
GRADE	**DIFFERENTIATION**	**METASTATIC POTENTIAL**
I	Well	<10%
II	Moderately	10-30%
III	Poorly	>50%

*Based on FNCLCC grading system.

- **AJCC system for soft tissue sarcoma: listed in order of importance (Table 9-12)**
  - Stage (presence of metastases = stage IV)
  - Grade
  - Size (>5 cm)
  - Depth (deep to fascia)

TREATMENT (BONE AND SOFT TISSUE)

- **Surgical procedures: treatment goal for malignant bone tumors is to remove the lesion, with minimal risk of local recurrence Table 9-13).**
  - Limb salvage is performed when two essential criteria are met:
    - Local control of the lesion must be at least equal to that of amputation surgery.
    - The limb that has been saved must be functional. A wide-margin surgical resection (excising a cuff of normal tissue around the tumor) is the operative goal.
  - Surgical margins are graded according to MSTS system (Figure 9-4).
    - **Intralesional margin:** plane of dissection goes directly through the tumor. When the surgery involves malignant mesenchymal tumors, an intralesional margin results in 100% local recurrence.
    - **Marginal margin:** a marginal line of resection goes through the reactive zone of the tumor; the reactive zone contains inflammatory cells, edema, fibrous tissue, and satellites of tumor cells. When malignant mesenchymal tumors are resected, a plane of dissection through the reactive zone probably results in a local recurrence rate of 25% to 50%. A marginal margin may be safe and effective if the response to preoperative chemotherapy has been excellent (95%-100% tumor necrosis).
    - **Wide margin:** a wide line of surgical resection is accomplished when entire tumor is removed with a cuff of normal tissue. Local recurrence rate drops below 10% when such a surgical margin is achieved.
    - **Radical margin:** achieved when the entire tumor and its compartment (all surrounding muscles, ligaments, and connective tissues) are removed
- **Adjuvant therapy**
  - Chemotherapy (Table 9-14)
    - **Multiagent chemotherapy has a significant effect on both the efficacy of limb salvage and disease-free survival for bone sarcomas and is used in the following scenarios: osteosarcoma, nonosteogenic osteosarcoma (malignant fibrous histiocytoma [MFH] of bone, fibrosarcoma, etc.), periosteal osteosarcoma, Ewing sarcoma, dedifferentiated chondrosarcoma, mesenchymal chondrosarcoma.**
    - The common mechanism of action of drugs is the induction of programmed cell death (apoptosis).
    - Most protocols entail preoperative regimens (neoadjuvant chemotherapy) for 8 to 24 weeks. The tumor is then restaged and, if appropriate, limb salvage is performed.

Table 9-10 Staging System of the Musculoskeletal Tumor Society (Enneking System)

STAGE	GRADE, TUMOR SIZE, AND METASTASIS STATUS	DESCRIPTION	NOTE ABOUT ENNEKING SYSTEM
IA	$G_1T_1M_0$	Low grade Intracompartmental No metastases	High-grade (G_2) lesions are intermediate between low-grade (G_1), well-differentiated tumors and high-grade, undifferentiated tumors. The size of the tumor is determined through specialized imaging, including radiography, tomography, nuclear studies, CT, and MRI. Compartments are specified to describe the tumor site. These compartments are usually defined on the basis of fascial borders in the extremities. Of note, the skin and subcutaneous tissues are classified as a compartment, and the potential periosseous space between cortical bone and muscle is often considered a compartment as well. T_0 lesions are confined within the capsule and within its compartment of origin. T_1 tumors have extracapsular extension into the reactive zone around it, but both the tumor and the reactive zone are confined within the compartment of origin. T_2 lesions extend beyond the anatomic compartment of origin by direct extension or some other means (e.g., trauma, surgical seeding). Tumors that involve major neurovascular bundles are almost always classified as T_2 lesions. Both regional and distal metastases have ominous prognoses; therefore, the distinction is simply between the absence of metastases (M_0) and the presence of metastases (M_1).
IB	$G_1T_2M_0$	Low grade Extracompartmental No metastases	
IIA	$G_2T_1M_0$	High grade Intracompartmental No metastases	
IIB	$G_2T_2M_0$	High grade Extracompartmental No metastases	
IIIA	$G_{1/2}T_1M_1$	Any grade Intracompartmental With metastases	
IIIB	$G_{1/2}T_2M_1$	Any grade Extracompartmental With metastases	

Table 9-11 American Joint Committee on Cancer Staging System for Primary Malignant Tumors of Bone for Those Tumors Diagnosed on or after January 1, 2010

Stage IA	T1	N0	M0	G1,2 low grade, GX
Stage IB	T2	N0	M0	G1,2 low grade, GX
	T3	N0	M0	G1,2 low grade, GX
Stage IIA	T1	N0	M0	G3,4 high grade
Stage IIB	T2	N0	M0	G3,4 high grade
Stage III	T3	N0	M0	G3,4
Stage IVA	Any T	N0	M1a	Any G
Stage IVB	Any T	Any N1	Any M	Any G
	Any T	Any N	M1b	Any G

From AJCC: Soft tissue sarcoma. In: Edge SB, et al, eds: *AJCC Cancer Staging Manual,* 7th ed. New York: Springer, 2010, pp 281-287.

TX	Primary tumor cannot be assessed
T0	No evidence of primary tumor
T1	Tumor 8 cm in greatest dimension
T2	Tumor more than 8 cm in greatest dimension
T3	Discontinuous tumors in the primary bone site
NX	Regional lymph nodes cannot be assessed
N0	No regional lymph node metastasis
N1	Regional Lymph node metastasis
N0	No regional lymph node metastasis
M0	No distant metastasis
M1	Distant metastasis
M1a	Lung
M1b	Other distant sites
GX	Grade cannot be assessed
G1	Well-differentiated–low-grade
G2	Moderately differentiated–low-grade
G3	Poorly differentiated
G4	Undifferentiated

Table 9-12 American Joint Committee on Cancer Staging System for Primary Malignant Tumors of Soft Tissue for Those Tumors Diagnosed on or after January 1, 2010

Stage IA	T1a	N0	M0	G1, GX
	T1b	N0	M0	G1, GX
Stage IB	T2a	N0	M0	G1, GX
	T2b	N0	M0	G1, GX
Stage IIA	T1a	N0	M0	G2, G3
	T1b	N0	M0	G2, G3
Stage IIB	T2a	N0	M0	G2
	T2b	N0	M0	G2
Stage III	T2a, T2b	N0	M0	G3
	Any T	N1	M0	Any G
Stage IV	Any T	Any N	M1	Any G

Adapted from AJCC: Soft tissue sarcoma. In: Edge SB, et al, eds: *AJCC Cancer Staging Manual,* 7th ed. New York, NY: Springer, 2010, pp 291-298.

TX	Primary tumor cannot be assessed.
T0	No evidence of primary tumor.
T1	Tumor ≤5 cm in greatest dimension. (Size should be regarded as a continuous variable, and the measurement should be provided.)
T1a	Superficial tumor.
T1b	Deep tumor.
T2	Tumor >5 cm in greatest dimension.
T2a	Superficial tumor.
T2b	Deep tumor.
NX	Regional lymph nodes cannot be assessed.
G1	Low grade
G2	Intermediate grade
G3	High grade
GX	Any grade
N0	No regional lymph node metastasis.
N1[b]	Regional lymph node metastasis.
M0	No distant metastasis.
M1	Distant metastasis.

- Patients undergo maintenance chemotherapy for 6 to 12 months.
- Patients with localized osteosarcoma or Ewing tumor have up to a 60% to 70% chance for long-term disease-free survival with the combination of multiagent chemotherapy and surgery.

- **The role of chemotherapy for soft tissue sarcoma remains more controversial. Chemotherapy is used for rhabdomyosarcoma.**
- Radiation therapy (Table 9-15)
  - External beam irradiation produces free radicals and direct genetic damage and is used for the following:

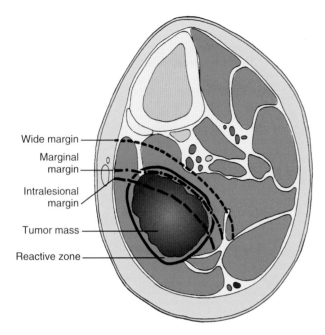

FIGURE 9-4 Types of surgical margins. An intralesional line of resection enters the substance of the tumor. A marginal line of resection travels through the reactive zone of the tumor. Wide-margin surgical resection removes the tumor, along with a cuff of normal tissue. (From Sim FH et al: Soft tissue tumors: diagnosis, evaluation and management, *Am Acad Orthop Surg* 2:209, 1994. ©1994 American Academy of Orthopaedic Surgeons. Reprinted with permission.)

Table 9-13	Treatment Regimens
TREATMENT	**DISEASE**
Chemotherapy + surgery	Ewing sarcoma, osteosarcoma
Radiation + surgery	Soft tissue sarcoma
Limb salvage surgery/wide excision	Chondrosarcoma, adamantinoma, chordoma, parosteal osteosarcoma
ORIF (+ radiation/ chemotherapy)	Metastases, lymphoma, myeloma
Intralesional resection	GCT, ABC, NOF, LCH, osteoblastoma, chondroblastoma
Radiofrequency ablation	Osteoid osteoma

ABC, Aneurysmal bone cyst; *GCT*, giant cell tumor; *LCH*, Langerhans cell histiocytosis; *NOF*, nonossifying fibroma; *ORIF*, open reduction and internal fixation.

- Local control of Ewing tumor, lymphoma, myeloma, and metastatic bone disease
- As an adjunct in the treatment of soft tissue sarcomas, in which it is used in combination with surgery
- Radiation may be delivered preoperatively (5000 cGy), followed by resection of the lesion with increased risk of wound healing.
- Postoperative external beam radiation (6600 cGy) yields equal local control rates, with a lower postoperative wound complication rate but a higher incidence of postoperative fibrosis.
- There are several complications of radiation therapy:
  - Postirradiation sarcoma: a devastating complication in which a spindle sarcoma occurs within the field of irradiation for a previous malignancy (e.g., Ewing tumor, breast cancer, Hodgkin disease). Histologic

Table 9-14	Chemotherapy Treatment for Bone Sarcomas	
CHEMOTHERAPY AGENT	**TOXICITY**	**DISEASE**
Doxorubicin (Adriamycin)	Cardiotoxic	OGS EWS
Cisplatin	Audiotoxic Nephrotoxic Neurotoxic (peripheral)	OGS
Methotrexate	Oral cavity toxicity	OGS
Ifosfamide	Nephrotoxic Neurotoxic (central encephalopathy)	EWS
Vincristine	Neurotoxic (peripheral)	EWS
Cyclophosphamide (Cytoxan)	Secondary leukemia/ lymphoma Cystitis Bladder cancer	EWS
Etoposide	Secondary leukemia	EWS

EWS, Ewing sarcoma; *OGS*, osteogenic sarcoma.

Table 9-15	Radiation Therapy for Soft Tissue Sarcomas	
RADIOTHERAPY	**PREOPERATIVE**	**POSTOPERATIVE**
Dose	50 Gy	66 Gy
Field Size	Smaller field (only includes tumor volume)	Larger field (includes tumor volume and entire post op surgical field)
Complications	Short term— wound healing	Long term—soft tissue fibrosis Bone necrosis and fracture

Table 9-16	Most Common Musculoskeletal Tumors
TUMOR TYPE	**TUMOR NAME**
Soft tissue tumor (children)	Hemangioma
Soft tissue tumor (adults)	Lipoma
Malignant soft tissue tumor (children)	Rhabdomyosarcoma
Malignant soft tissue tumor (adults)	Undifferentiated pleomorphic sarcoma (UPS)
Primary benign bone tumor	Osteochondroma
Primary malignant bone tumor	Osteosarcoma
Secondary benign lesion	Aneurysmal bone cyst
Secondary malignancies	Malignant fibrous histiocytoma Osteosarcoma Fibrosarcoma
Phalangeal tumor	Enchondroma
Soft tissue sarcoma of the hand and wrist	Epithelioid sarcoma
Soft tissue sarcoma of the foot and ankle	Synovial sarcoma

Courtesy Luke S. Choi, MD, Resident, Department of Orthopaedic Surgery, University of Virginia.

features are usually those of an osteosarcoma, a fibrosarcoma, or MFH. Postirradiation sarcomas are probably more frequent in patients who undergo intensive chemotherapy (especially with alkylating agents) and irradiation.
- Late stress fractures: also may occur in weight-bearing bones to which high-dose irradiation has been applied. The subtrochanteric region and the diaphysis of the femur are common sites.
- It can be beneficial to recognize tumors that are more common (Table 9-16).

SECTION 2 SOFT TISSUE TUMORS

INTRODUCTION

Soft tissue tumors are common. They may appear as small lumps or large masses.

■ **Clinical presentation: presents with an enlarging painless or painful mass.**

■ Masses are deceptively painless and commonly inappropriately assumed to be lipomas.

■ **A mass greater than 5 cm, growing, deep to the superficial fascia should be presumed to be a soft tissue sarcoma until proven otherwise, and assessed with three-dimensional imaging first.**

■ **Classification: soft tissue tumors can be broadly classified as benign or malignant (sarcoma) or characterized by reactive tumorlike conditions. Lesions are classified according to the direction of differentiation of the lesion: the tumor tends to produce collagen (fibrous lesion), fat, or cartilage.**

■ Benign soft tissue tumors: may occur in all age groups. The biologic behavior of these lesions varies from asymptomatic and self-limiting to growing and symptomatic. On occasion, benign lesions grow rapidly and invade adjacent tissues.

■ Malignant soft tissue tumors (sarcomas): rare tumors of mesenchymal origin. In the United States, there are approximately 12,000 new cases of soft tissue sarcoma each year.

  • Diagnosis: often an enlarging painless or painful soft tissue mass, which is the most common reason for seeking medical attention.
    • **Most sarcomas are large (>5 cm), deep, and firm.**
    • In some instances, they are small and may be present for a long time before they are recognized as tumors (synovial sarcoma, rhabdomyosarcoma, epithelioid sarcoma, and clear cell sarcoma).
    • Poor prognostic factors include the presence of metastases, high grade, size greater than 5 cm, and location below the deep fascia.
    • **MRI is the best imaging modality for defining the anatomy and helping characterize the lesion.**
    • **Computed tomography (CT) scan of the chest is required to evaluate for metastasis.** CT scan of the abdomen and pelvis is obtained for liposarcoma because of synchronous retroperitoneal liposarcoma.
  • Treatment: radiation therapy is an important adjunct to surgery in the treatment of soft tissue sarcomas.
    • Ionizing radiation can be delivered preoperatively, perioperatively with brachytherapy after loading tubes, or postoperatively.
    • Treatment regimens most commonly use external beam irradiation.

■ **Diagnosis: evaluation of patients with soft tissue tumors must be systematic to avoid errors.**

■ **Unplanned removal of a soft tissue sarcoma is the most common error.**
  • **Residual tumor may exist at the site of the operative wound, and repeat excision for all patients with an unplanned removal should be performed.**

■ Delay in diagnosis may also occur if the clinician does not recognize that the lesion is malignant.

■ **Patients who have a new soft tissue mass or one that is growing or causing pain should undergo MRI.**

■ The MRI scan should be carefully reviewed to characterize the nature of the mass. If it can be determined that the lesion is a benign process such as a lipoma, ganglionic cyst, or muscle tear, then it is classified as a *determinate lesion,* and treatment can be planned without a biopsy. In contrast, if the exact nature of a lesion cannot be determined, the lesion is classified as *indeterminate,* and a biopsy is necessary to determine the exact diagnosis. Then treatment can be planned.

■ **Excisional biopsy should not be performed when the clinician does not know the origin of a soft tissue tumor.**

■ **Metastasis: most soft tissue sarcomas metastasize to the lung.**

■ **Lymph node metastasis occurs with 5% of soft tissue sarcomas. ESARC tumors (epithelioid sarcoma, synovial sarcoma, angiosarcoma, rhabdomyosarcoma, and clear cell sarcoma) most commonly metastasize via lymphatic vessels** (Table 9-17).

TUMORS OF FIBROUS TISSUE

Fibrous tumors are common, and their characteristics range widely, from small, self-limiting, benign conditions to aggressive, invasive, benign tumors. The malignant fibrous tumors are fibrosarcoma and MFH.

■ **Calcifying aponeurotic fibroma**

■ Manifests as a slow-growing, painless mass in the hands and feet in children and young adults 3 to 30 years of age

■ Radiographs may reveal a faint mass with stippling.

■ Histologic examination reveals a fibrous tumor with centrally located areas of calcification and cartilage formation.

■ After local excision, the tumor often recurs (in up to 50% of cases); however, the condition appears to resolve with maturity.

■ **Fibromatosis**

■ Palmar (Dupuytren) and plantar (Ledderhose) fibromatosis: disorders consisting of firm nodules of fibroblasts and collagen that develop in the palmar and

Table 9-17	Soft Tissue Sarcomas with Lymph Node Metastases—ESARC	
TUMOR	**CHARACTERISTIC**
Epithelioid sarcoma	Occurs in young adults
	Most common: hand STS
Synovial sarcoma	Translocation t(x;18) and SYT-SSX fusion product
Angiosarcoma	Associated with Stewart-Treves syndrome
	Cutaneous spread
Rhabdomyosarcoma	Most common: pediatric STS
Clear cell sarcoma	Occurs in young adults
	Common lower extremity/foot tumor

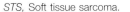

STS, Soft tissue sarcoma.

plantar fascia. Nodules and fascia become hypertrophic, producing contractures.

- ▥ Extraabdominal desmoid tumor
  - Most locally invasive of all benign soft tissue tumors
  - Commonly occurs in adolescents and young adults
    - **Patients with Gardner syndrome (familial adenomatous polyposis) have colonic polyps and a 10,000-fold increased risk of developing desmoid tumors.**
  - On palpation, the tumor has a distinctive "rock-hard" character.
  - Multiple lesions may be present in the same extremity (10%-25%).
  - Histologically, the tumor consists of well-differentiated fibroblasts and abundant collagen. The lesion infiltrates adjacent tissues. Immunohistochemistry study reveals positivity for estrogen receptor β, and inhibitors have been used for treatment.
  - Surgical treatment is aimed at resecting the tumor with a wide margin.
  - Local recurrence is common.
  - Radiotherapy has been used as an adjunctive treatment to prevent recurrence and progression.
  - Behavior of the tumor is capricious; recurrent nodules may remain dormant for years or grow rapidly for some time and then stop growing.
- ◼ Nodular fasciitis
- ▥ A common reactive lesion that manifests as a painful, *rapidly enlarging* mass in a young person (15-35 years of age)
- ▥ Half of these lesions occur in the upper extremity.
- ▥ Short, irregular bundles and fascicles; a dense reticulum network; and only small amounts of mature collagen characterize the lesion histologically. Mitotic figures are common, but atypical mitoses are not a feature.
- ▥ Treatment consists of excision with a marginal line of resection.
- ◼ Malignant fibrous soft tissue tumors: undifferentiated pleomorphic sarcoma (previously MFH) and fibrosarcoma are the two malignant fibrous lesions.
- ▥ Diagnosis
  - Similar clinical and radiographic manifestations; similar treatment methods
  - Patients are generally between age 30 and 80 years.
  - Most common manifestation is an enlarging, generally painless mass.
  - **MRI often shows a deep-seated inhomogeneous mass with low signal on T1-weighted images and high signal on T2-weighted images.** The two lesions may be similar histologically, but there are distinctive features:
    - *Undifferentiated pleomorphic sarcoma:* spindle and histiocytic cells are arranged in a storiform (cartwheel) pattern. Short fascicles of cells and fibrous tissue appear to radiate about a common center around slitlike vessels. Chronic inflammatory cells may also be present.
    - *Fibrosarcoma:* fasciculated growth pattern with fusiform or spindle-shaped cells, scanty cytoplasm, and indistinct borders; cells are separated by interwoven collagen fibers. In some cases, the tissue is organized into a herringbone pattern that consists of intersecting fascicles in which the nuclei in one

fascicle are viewed transversely but in an adjacent fascicle are viewed longitudinally.
- Treatment is by wide-margin local excision. Radiation therapy is employed in many cases when the size of the tumor exceeds 5 cm.

- ◼ Dermatofibrosarcoma protuberans
- ▥ Rare nodular cutaneous tumor that occurs in early to middle adulthood
- ▥ Low grade, with a tendency to recur locally; only rarely metastasizes (often after repeated local recurrence)
- ▥ In 40% of the cases, it occurs on the upper or lower extremities. The tumor grows slowly but progressively.
- ▥ The central portion of the nodules shows uniform fibroblasts arranged in a storiform pattern around an inconspicuous vasculature.
- ▥ Wide-margin surgical resection is the best form of treatment.

TUMORS OF FATTY TISSUE

There is a wide spectrum of benign and malignant tumors of fat origin. Each has a particular biologic behavior that guides evaluation and treatment.

- ◼ Lipomas: common benign tumors of mature fat
- ▥ Occur in a subcutaneous, intramuscular, or intermuscular location
- ▥ History of a mass is long, but sometimes the mass was only recently discovered.
- ▥ Not painful
- ▥ Radiographs may show a radiolucent lesion in the soft tissues if the lipoma is deep within the muscle or between muscle and bone.
- ▥ **CT scan or MRI shows a well-demarcated lesion with the same signal characteristics as those of mature fat on all sequences. On fat suppression sequences, the lipoma has a uniformly low signal. If the patient experiences no symptoms and the radiographic features are diagnostic of lipoma, no treatment is necessary** (Figure 9-5).
- ▥ If the mass is growing or causing symptoms, excision with a marginal line of resection or an intralesional margin is all that is necessary.
- ▥ Local recurrence is uncommon.
- ▥ Differential is liposarcoma (Table 9-18)
- ▥ Several variants:
  - Spindle cell lipoma
    - Commonly occurs in men (45-65 years of age)
    - Manifests as a solitary, painless, growing, firm nodule
    - Histologically characterized by a mixture of mature fat cells and spindle cells. There is a mucoid matrix with a varying number of birefringent collagen fibers.
    - Treatment is excision with a marginal margin.
  - Pleomorphic lipoma
    - Occurs in middle-aged patients
    - Manifests as a slow-growing mass
    - Histologically characterized by lipocytes, spindle cells, and scattered bizarre giant cells
    - May be confused with different types of liposarcoma
    - Treatment is by excision with a marginal margin.
  - Angiolipoma
    - The only lipoma that is very painful when palpated
    - Manifests with small nodules in the upper extremity that are intensely painful

Table 9-18	Fat Tumors		
	LIPOMA	**LIPOSARCOMA**	**DEDIFFERENTIATED LIPOSARCOMA**
History	Slowly enlarging mass May be incidentally found	Slowly enlarging mass May be incidentally found	Mass that has been present begins to grow Enlarging mass Pain
Imaging	Consistent with fat on all imaging	Consistent with fat on all imaging May have areas of heterogeneity	Areas consistent with fat and other areas appear similar to soft tissue sarcoma
Pathology	Fat	Fat Immature lipoblasts MDM2 (+)	Fat juxtaposed to high grade elements
Treatment	Marginal excision	Marginal excision +/– radiation	Wide excision and radiation
Image	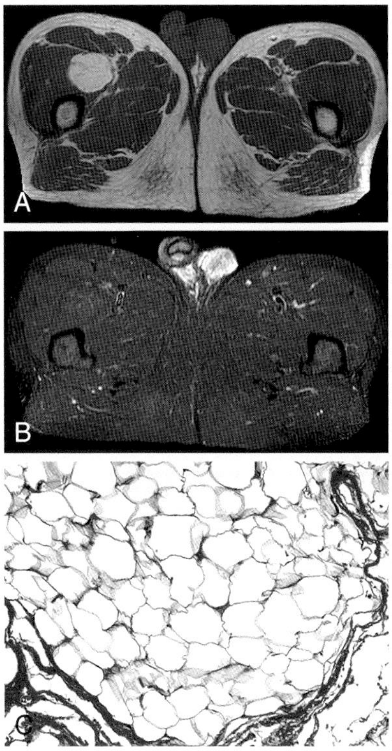	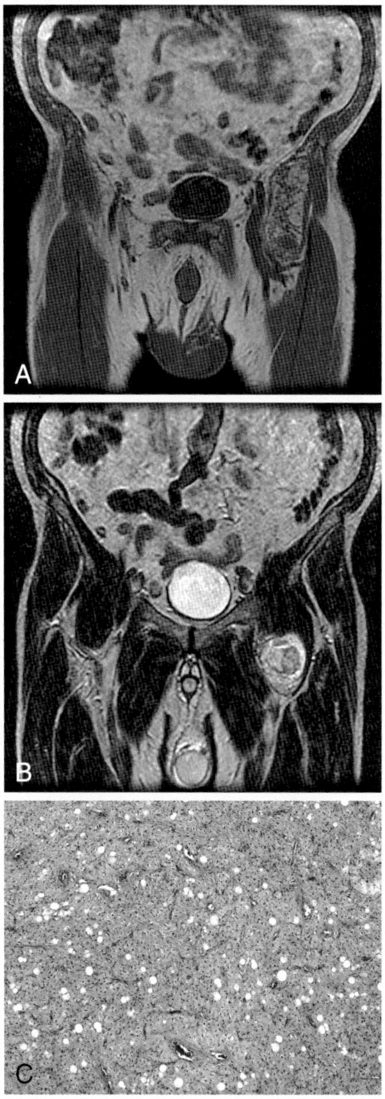	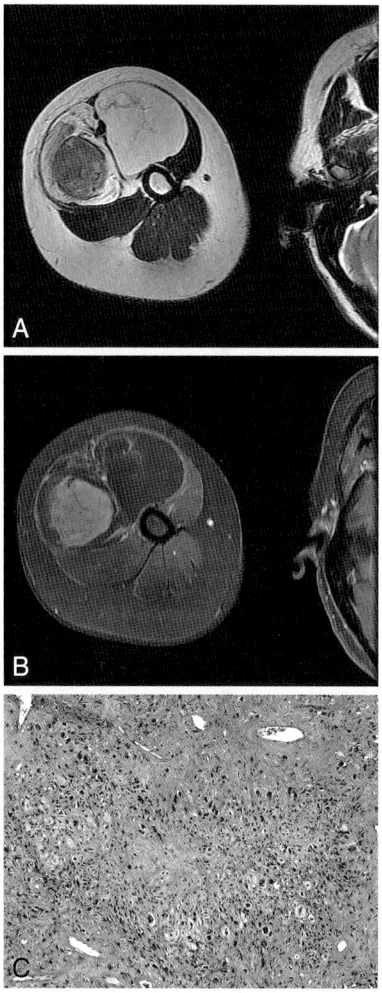
Description	FIGURE 9-5 **A,** T1-weighted image shows a lipoma in the vastus intermedius. **B,** On T2 suppression the lesion completely suppresses and appears identical to fat on both images. **C,** Histology shows acellular, mature fat consistent with a benign lipoma.	FIGURE 9-6 **A,** T1 weighted image shows a left rectus lesion that is consistent with fat in some areas. **B,** With signal suppression the low-grade fat areas suppress but the liposarcoma regions do not. **C,** Histology shows immature lipoblasts intermixed with spindle cells.	FIGURE 9-7 **A,** T1-weighted image and a lesion that is mostly fat, but the lobule on the left has a clearly demarcated area that does not suppress on fat images **(B).** **C,** Histology confirms a highly malignant lesion with highly cellular elements with high mitotic rate and large, bizarre cells characteristic of a dedifferentiated liposarcoma.

- MRI may show a small fatty nodule or completely normal appearance.
- Consists of mature fat cells (as in a typical lipoma) and nests of small arborizing vessels

■ **Liposarcomas**

■ Type of sarcoma; direction of differentiation is toward fatty tissue

■ Heterogeneous group of tumors, having in common the presence of lipoblasts (signet ring–shaped cells) in the tissue

■ **Liposarcomas virtually never occur in the subcutaneous tissues.**

■ They are classified into the following types:
  - Well-differentiated liposarcoma (low grade) (Figure 9-6)
    - Lipoma-like
    - Sclerosing
    - Inflammatory
  - Myxoid liposarcoma (intermediate grade)
  - Dedifferentiated (high grade) (Figure 9-7)
  - Round-cell liposarcoma (high grade)
  - Pleomorphic liposarcoma (high grade)

■ **Liposarcomas metastasize according to the grade of the lesion:**
  - **Well-differentiated liposarcomas have a very low rate of metastasis (<10%).**
  - **The metastasis rate of intermediate-grade liposarcomas is 10% to 30%.**
  - **The metastasis rate of high-grade liposarcomas is more than 50%.**

TUMORS OF NEURAL TISSUE

The two benign neural tumors are neurilemoma and neurofibroma. Their malignant counterpart is neurofibrosarcoma.

■ **Neurilemoma (benign schwannoma)**

■ Benign nerve sheath tumor

■ Occurs in young to middle-aged adults (20-50 years of age)

■ Patients have no symptoms except for the presence of the mass.

■ Tumor grows slowly and may wax and wane in size (cystic changes).

■ **MRI studies may demonstrate an eccentric mass arising from a peripheral nerve, or they may show only an indeterminate soft tissue mass (low signal on T1-weighted images and high signal on T2-weighted images).**

■ Histologically, the lesion is composed of Antoni A and B areas.
  - Antoni A area:
    - Compact spindle cells usually having twisted nuclei, indistinct cytoplasm, and occasionally clear intranuclear vacuoles
    - There may be nuclear palisading, whorling of cells, and Verocay bodies.
    - When the lesion is predominantly cellular (Antoni A), the tumor may be confused with a sarcoma.
    - Treatment: removing the eccentric mass while leaving the nerve intact
  - Antoni B area:
    - Less orderly and cellular

- Arranged haphazardly in the loosely textured matrix (with microcystic changes, inflammatory cells, and delicate collagen fibers)
- Vessels are large and irregularly spaced.

■ **Neurofibroma**

■ Solitary or multiple (neurofibromatosis)

■ Superficial, slow-growing, and painless

■ When they involve a major nerve, they may expand it in a fusiform manner.

■ Histologic study shows interlacing bundles of elongated cells with wavy dark-staining nuclei.

■ Cells are associated with wirelike strands of collagen.

■ Small to moderate amounts of mucoid material separate the cells and collagen.

■ Treatment: excision with a marginal margin

■ **Neurofibromatosis (von Recklinghausen disease)**

■ Autosomal dominant trait (both peripheral and central forms)

■ Café au lait spots (smooth) and Lisch nodules (melanocytic hamartomas in the iris)

■ Variable skeletal abnormalities (metaphyseal fibrous defect [nonossifying fibroma], scoliosis, and long-bone bowing)

■ Malignant changes occur in 5% to 30% of affected patients.

■ Pain and an enlarging soft tissue mass may herald conversion to a sarcoma.

■ **Neurofibrosarcoma/malignant peripheral nerve sheath tumor (MPNST)**

■ Tumor that may arise in a de novo manner or in the setting of neurofibromatosis

■ High-grade sarcoma; treated in a manner similar to that for other high-grade sarcomas

TUMORS OF MUSCLE TISSUE

■ **Leiomyosarcoma**

■ Manifests as a small nodule or a large extremity mass

■ May or may not be associated with blood vessels

■ Low or high grade

■ **Rhabdomyosarcoma**

■ **The most common sarcoma in young patients; may grow rapidly**

■ Composed of spindle cells in parallel bundles, multinucleated giant cells, and racquet-shaped cells

■ Cross-striations within the tumor cells (rhabdomyoblasts)

■ **Rhabdomyosarcomas are sensitive to multiagent chemotherapy and wide-margin surgical resection after induction of chemotherapy. External beam irradiation plays a prominent role in treatment.**

VASCULAR TUMORS

■ **Hemangioma**

■ Commonly seen in children and adults

■ Cutaneous, subcutaneous, or intramuscular location

■ Large tumors have signs of vascular engorgement (aching, heaviness, swelling).

■ MRI scans demonstrate a heterogeneous lesion with numerous small blood vessels and fatty infiltration.

■ It is important to examine the patient in both the supine and standing positions (lower extremity often fills with blood after several minutes).

■ Radiographs may reveal small phleboliths.

- Nonoperative treatment: nonsteroidal antiinflammatory drugs (NSAIDs), vascular stockings, and activity modification if local measures adequately control discomfort
- Can be treated with an intralesional sclerosing agent (e.g., alcohol)
- **Angiosarcoma**
- Cells resemble the endothelium of blood vessels.
- Highly malignant
- Lymph node and cutaneous metastases are common.
- Infiltrative; with local excision, the rate of failure is high.
- Amputation may be necessary to achieve local control.
- Pulmonary metastases are common.

SYNOVIAL DISORDERS

- **Ganglia**
- Outpouching of the synovial lining of an adjacent joint
- Common locations: wrist, foot, and knee
- Filled with gelatinous mucoid material
- Paucicellular connective tissue without a true epithelial lining
- MRI: homogeneously low signal on T1-weighted images and a very bright signal on T2-weighted images. Contrast agent such as gadolinium is useful in differentiating a cyst from a solid neoplasm because cysts do not enhance (except for a small rim at the periphery) but active neoplasms usually do.
- **Pigmented villonodular synovitis (PVNS)**
- Reactive condition (not a true neoplasm) characterized by an exuberant proliferation of synovial villi and nodules
- May occur locally (within a joint) or diffusely
- Knee affected most often, followed in frequency by hip and shoulder
- Manifests with pain and swelling in affected joint
- Recurrent atraumatic hemarthrosis is the hallmark (arthrocentesis demonstrates a bloody effusion).
- Cystic erosions may occur on both sides of the joint.
- Highly vascular villi are lined with plump hyperplastic synovial cells, hemosiderin-stained multinucleated giant cells, and chronic inflammatory cells.
- **Treatment is aimed at complete synovectomy by arthroscopy for resection of all the intraarticular disease, followed by open posterior synovectomy to remove the posterior extraarticular extension.**
- **The local form of PVNS may be treated with partial synovectomy.**
- Local recurrence is common (30%-50% of cases) despite complete synovectomy.
- External beam irradiation (3500-4000 cGy) can reduce the rate of local recurrence to 10% to 20%.
- **Giant cell tumor of tendon sheath**
- Benign nodular tumor occurs along the tendon sheaths (hands/feet).
- Moderately cellular (sheets of rounded or polygonal cells) zones, hypocellular collagenized zones; multinucleated giant cells are common, as are xanthoma cells.
- Treatment: resection with a marginal margin
- Local recurrence is common (usually treated with repeat excision).
- **Synovial chondromatosis**

- Synovial proliferative disorder that occurs within joints or bursae, ranging in appearance from metaplasia of the synovial tissue to firm nodules of cartilage
- Typically affects young adults, who present with pain, stiffness, and swelling
- The knee is the most common location.
- Radiographs may demonstrate fine, stippled calcification.
- Treatment: removal of loose bodies and synovectomy

OTHER RARE SARCOMAS

- **Synovial sarcoma**
- Highly malignant high-grade tumor
- **Although the name implies that it arises from synovial cells, it rarely arises from an intraarticular location.**
- Typically manifests between the ages of 15 and 40 years
- May be present for years or may manifest as a rapidly enlarging mass
- Lymph nodes may be involved.
- **Synovial sarcoma is the most common sarcoma in the foot.**
- **Radiographs or CT scans may show mineralization within the lesion in up to 25% of cases (spotty mineralization may even resemble the peripheral mineralization seen in heterotopic ossification).**
  - Irregular contour differentiates these lesions from hemangioma.
- Tumor is often biphasic, with both epithelial and spindle cell components.
  - Epithelial component may show epithelial cells that form glands or nests, or they may line cystlike spaces.
- Tumor may also be composed of a single type of cell (monophasic); the monophasic fibrous type is much more common than the monophasic epithelial type.
- **Translocation between chromosome 18 and the X chromosome—t(X;18)—is always present in tumor cells; staining of tumor cells yields positive results for keratin and epithelial membrane antigen.**
- **Balanced translocation results in gene fusion products. The two most common are SYT-SSX1 and SYT-SSX2.**
- Wide-margin surgical resection with adjuvant radiotherapy is the most common method of treatment.
- Metastases develop in 30% to 60% of cases.
- Larger tumors (>5 to 10 cm) are more prone to distant spread.
- **Epithelioid sarcoma**
- Rare nodular tumor that commonly occurs in the upper extremities of young adults
- May also occur about the buttock/thigh, knee, and foot
- **Most common sarcoma of the hand**
- May ulcerate and mimic a granuloma or rheumatoid nodule
- Lymph node metastases are common.
- Cells range in shape from ovoid to polygonal, with deeply eosinophilic cytoplasm (cellular pleomorphism is minimal).
- Often misdiagnosed as benign processes
- Wide-margin surgical resection is necessary to prevent local recurrence.
- **Clear cell sarcoma**
- Manifests as a slow-growing mass in association with tendons or aponeuroses

- Usually occurs about the foot and ankle but may also involve the knee, thigh, and hand
- Lymph nodes may be involved.
- Characterized by compact nests or fascicles of rounded or fusiform cells with clear cytoplasm; multinucleated giant cells are common.
- Wide-margin surgical resection with adjuvant irradiation is the treatment of choice.

■ **Alveolar cell sarcoma**
- Manifests as a slow-growing painless mass in young adults (15-35 years of age)
- Occurs in the anterior thigh
- Dense fibrous trabeculae dividing the tumor into an organoid or nestlike arrangement; cells are large and rounded and contain one or more vesicular nuclei with small nucleoli.
- Treatment: wide-margin surgical resection with adjuvant irradiation in selected cases

POSTTRAUMATIC CONDITIONS

■ **Hematoma**
- Hematoma may occur after trauma to the extremity.
- Organizes and resolves with time
- Sarcomas may spontaneously hemorrhage into the body of the tumor or after minor trauma and masquerade as a benign process. A lack of fascial plane tracking and subcutaneous ecchymosis suggests bleeding is contained by a pseudocapsule; this is an important physical examination finding.
- Clinicians should monitor patients with hematomas at 6-week intervals until the mass resolves.
- MRI scanning is often not able to distinguish a simple hematoma from a sarcoma with spontaneous hemorrhage.

■ **Myositis ossificans (heterotopic ossification)**
- Develops after single or repetitive episodes of trauma; occasionally patients cannot recall the traumatic episode.

Table 9-19	Soft Tissue Sarcoma Pearls
Prognostic factors	Size (≥5 cm)
	Grade (high)
	Depth (deep to superficial fascia)
Imaging (MRI)	Decreased signal on T1 weight
	Increased signal on T2 weight
Genetics	Synovial sarcoma—t(x;18) SYT-SSX
	Myxoid liposarcoma—t(12:16) (q13:p11)
	Rhabdomyosarcoma (Alv)—t(2:13)
Unique metastatic patterns—to lymph nodes + lungs (ESARC)	Epithelioid
	Synovial sarcoma
	Angiosarcoma
	Rhabdomyosarcoma
	Clear cell sarcoma
Treatment	LSS (+) XRT > 5 cm
	LSS (−) XRT < 5 cm and subcutaneous location
	Chemo +/− LSS = rhabdomyosarcoma
Syndromes	NF1—MPNST
	Stuart Treves—angiosarcoma
Characteristic locations	Hand—epithelioid sarcoma
	Foot—clear cell sarcoma; synovial sarcoma

- Most common locations are over the diaphyseal segment of long bones (in the middle aspect of the muscle bellies).
- As maturation progresses, radiographs show peripheral mineralization with a central lucent area.
- Lesion is not attached to the underlying bone, but in some cases, it may become fixed to the periosteal surface.
- Histology shows a zonal pattern with mature trabecular bone at the periphery and immature tissue in the center.
- Treatment is nonoperative.

SOFT TISSUE TUMOR PEARLS

■ (See Table 9-19).

SECTION 3 BONE TUMORS

PRESENTATION

■ Clinical presentation: pain, mass, fracture, or incidentally found. Most patients with bone tumors present with musculoskeletal pain. However, the most common presentation of a benign bone tumor in childhood is as an incidental finding.
- Pain is typically deep-seated and persistent.
  - Pain may be from mechanical disruption of the bone
    - Stress fracture
    - Impending displacement of a pathologic fracture
  - Pain may be from compression due to expanding tumor volume.
- Pain usually progresses in intensity and becomes constant and eventually is not relieved by NSAIDs or narcotics.
- Patients with a high-grade sarcoma present with a 1- to 3-month history of pain.

- With low-grade tumors (e.g., chondrosarcoma, adamantinoma, chordoma) there may be a long history of mild to moderate pain (6-24 months).
- **Osteoid osteoma has a characteristic night pain or diurnal pain pattern relieved with aspirin or NSAIDS.**

NOMENCLATURE

A common classification system for bone tumors is shown in Table 9-18.

■ **Sarcomas**
- Malignant neoplasms of connective tissue (mesenchymal) origin
- Exhibit rapid growth in a centripetal manner and invade adjacent normal tissues
- Each year in the United States, about 2800 new bone sarcomas are diagnosed.

- Malignant bone tumors manifest most commonly with pain. This is in contrast to soft tissue tumors, which most commonly manifest as a painless mass.
- High-grade malignant bone tumors tend to destroy the overlying cortex and spread into soft tissues.
- Low-grade tumors are generally contained within the cortex or surrounding periosteal rim.
- **Bone sarcomas metastasize primarily via the hematogenous route; lungs are the most common site.**
- **Osteosarcoma and Ewing sarcoma may also metastasize to other bone sites either at initial manifestation or later in the disease.**
- **Benign bone tumors**
- May be small and have limited growth potential or be large and destructive
- **Tumor simulators and reactive conditions**
- These processes occur in bone but are not true neoplasms (e.g., osteomyelitis, aneurysmal bone cyst, bone island).

BONE-PRODUCING LESIONS

There are three lesions in which tumor cells produce osteoid: osteoid osteoma, osteoblastoma, and osteosarcoma.

- **Osteoid osteoma**
     Self-limiting benign bone lesion that produces pain in young patients (<30 years of age)
- Diagnosis
- **Pain at night, or diurnal that increases with time**
  - Classically relieved by salicylates and other NSAIDs
  - Pain may be referred to an adjacent joint, and when the lesion is intracapsular, it may simulate arthritis.
  - May produce painful nonstructural scoliosis, growth disturbances, and flexion contractures
    - Scoliosis caused by an osteoid osteoma results in a curve with the lesion on the concave side. This is thought to result from marked paravertebral muscle spasm.
  - Common locations include diaphyseal bone, proximal femur, tibia, and spine.
  - Radiographs usually show intensely reactive bone and a radiolucent nidus (Figure 9-8). Because of the intense reactive sclerosis, it may only be possible to detect the nidus with CT or MRI.
  - **The nidus is by definition always less than 1 cm in diameter, although the area of reactive bone sclerosis may be greater.**
  - Technetium-labeled bone scans always yield positive findings and show intense focal uptake.
  - **CT is superior to MRI in detecting and characterizing osteoid osteomas; CT demonstrates better contrast between the lucent nidus and reactive bone.**
  - There is a distinct demarcation between the nidus and the reactive bone (nidus consists of an interlacing network of osteoid trabeculae with variable mineralization), trabecular organization is haphazard, and the greatest degree of mineralization is in the center of the lesion.
  - **Histology shows mineralized woven bone with regularly shaped nuclei containing little chromatin but abundant cytoplasm and appears similar to osteoblastoma.**

- Patients can be treated with three different methods: NSAIDs, CT scan–guided radiofrequency ablation (RFA), and open surgical removal.
  - In about 50% of patients treated with NSAIDs, the lesions burn out over time (several years), with no further medical or surgical treatment necessary.
  - **CT scan–guided RFA is the dominant method of treatment.**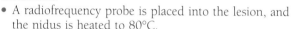
    - A radiofrequency probe is placed into the lesion, and the nidus is heated to 80°C.
    - A lesion close to a critical structure (i.e., neurovascular bundle or spinal cord) is a contraindication to RFA. Surgery is preferred.
- **Osteoblastoma**
- Rare bone-producing tumor that can attain a large size and is not self-limiting (Figure 9-9)
- Manifests with pain; when lesion involves spine, neurologic symptoms may be present.
- Common locations include spine, proximal humerus, and hip.
- Causes bone destruction, with or without the characteristic reactive bone formation in osteoid osteoma
- Area of bone destruction occasionally has a moth-eaten or permeative appearance simulating a malignancy; is greater than 2 cm.
- Histology shows mineralized woven bone with regularly shaped nuclei containing little chromatin but abundant cytoplasm and appears similar to osteoid osteoma.
- Tumor does not permeate the normal trabecular bone but instead merges with it.
- Treatment: curettage or excision with a marginal line of resection

Osteoid osteoma and osteoblastoma are easily confused; a comparison is provided in Table 9-20.

- **Osteosarcoma**
- Spindle cell neoplasms that produce osteoid are arbitrarily classified as osteosarcoma.
- There are many types of osteosarcoma (Box 9-1).
- **Lesions that must be recognized include high-grade intramedullary osteosarcoma (ordinary or classic osteosarcoma), parosteal osteosarcoma, periosteal osteosarcoma, telangiectatic osteosarcoma, osteosarcoma occurring with Paget disease, and osteosarcoma after irradiation.**
- Historically, osteosarcoma was treated by amputation; long-term studies demonstrated a survival rate of only 10% to 20%, the pulmonary system being the most common site of failure.

Table 9-20	Osteoid Osteoma versus Osteoblastoma	
	OSTEOID OSTEOMA	**OSTEOBLASTOMA**
Presentation	Diurnal pain pattern/night pain Pain relieved by aspirin/NSAIDs	Random pain pattern Pain not relieved by aspirin/NSAIDs
Imaging	Central radiolucent nidus < 1 cm Large secondary bone reaction Characteristic "target" appearance	Central radiolucent nidus > 2 cm Minimal secondary bone reaction gives lesion a more aggressive appearance
Location	Diaphyseal (typical)	Diaphyseal or metaphyseal Posterior spine elements
Growth pattern	Self-limited growth pattern	Unlimited growth pattern
Pathology	Same as osteoblastoma NO associated aneurysmal bone cyst	Same as osteoid osteoma 40% can have associated aneurysmal bone cyst
Treatment	Radiofrequency ablation (RFA) Surgery if tumor is close to nerve or vessels (e.g., spine)	Intralesional excision
Image	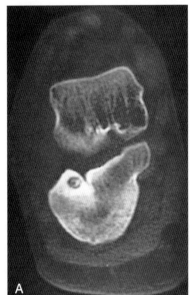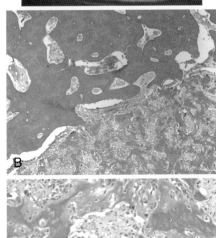	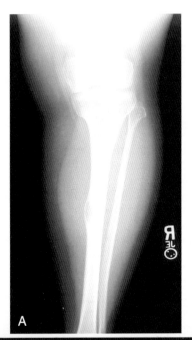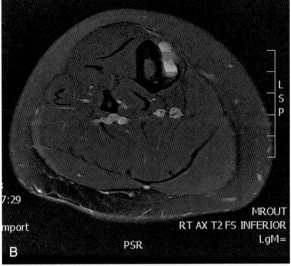
Description	FIGURE 9-8 Osteoid osteoma of the calcaneus. **A,** Radiograph shows a well-circumscribed lytic lesion with dense surrounding bone and a central nidus. **B,** Low-power photomicrograph (×25) shows the nidus. **C,** Higher-power photomicrograph (×160) shows mineralizing new bone with a loose fibrovascular stroma.	FIGURE 9-9 **A,** Plain radiograph with a diaphyseal, cortically based lesion with a nidus larger than 2 cm, confirmed on **(B)** T2-weighted MRI scan, where lesion is greater than 2 cm. Histology is the same as osteoid osteoma (see Figure 9-8).

▦ Multiagent chemotherapy has dramatically improved long-term survival and the potential for limb salvage.
  • Doxorubicin (cardiac toxicity)
  • Cisplatin (neurotoxicity)
  • Methotrexate (for cases of myelosuppression, also administer leucovorin)
▦ Chemotherapy both kills the micrometastases that are present in 80% to 90% of patients at presentation and sterilizes the reactive zone around the tumor.
▦ Preoperative chemotherapy is delivered for 8 to 12 weeks, followed by resection of the tumor.
  • Osteosarcoma metastasizes most commonly to the lung and next most commonly to bone.
▦ Rate of long-term survival is approximately 60% to 70%.
▦ Prognostic factors that adversely affect survival include (1) expression of P-glycoprotein, high serum level of alkaline phosphatase, high lactic dehydrogenase level, vascular invasion, and no alteration of DNA ploidy after chemotherapy, (2) the absence of anti–shock protein-90 antibodies after chemotherapy, and (3) a poor response to chemotherapy as seen on histologic tumor necrosis (<90%).
▦ **Osteosarcoma is associated with an abnormality in the tumor suppressor genes *Rb* (retinoblastoma) and *p53* (Li-Fraumeni syndrome).**
  • **High-grade intramedullary osteosarcoma**
    • **Also called "classic" osteosarcoma, this neoplasm is the most common type of osteosarcoma and usually occurs about the knee in children and young adults, but its incidence has a second peak in late adulthood.**
    • Other common sites include the proximal humerus, proximal femur, and pelvis.
    • Patients present primarily with pain.
    • **More than 90% of intramedullary osteosarcomas are high grade and penetrate the cortex early to form a soft tissue mass (stage IIB lesion).**
    • About 10% to 20% of affected patients have pulmonary metastases at presentation.
    • Radiographs demonstrate a lesion in which there is bone destruction and bone formation (Figure 9-10). On occasion, the lesion is purely sclerotic or lytic. MRI and CT are useful for defining the anatomy of the lesion with regard to intramedullary extension, involvement of neurovascular structures, and muscle invasion.
    • **Diagnosis depends on two histologic criteria: (1) tumor cells produce osteoid and (2) stromal cells are frankly malignant.**
    • **Treatment: neoadjuvant chemotherapy (i.e., before surgery), followed by wide-margin surgical resection and adjuvant chemotherapy (i.e., after surgery)**
  • Parosteal osteosarcoma (low-grade surface)
    • Low-grade osteosarcoma that occurs on the surface of the metaphysis of long bones
    • Affected patients often present with a painless mass.
    • Most common sites are the posterior aspect of the distal femur, proximal tibia, and proximal humerus.
    • Characteristic radiographic appearance: a heavily ossified, often lobulated mass arising from the cortex (Figure 9-11)

• Most prominent feature is regularly arranged osseous trabeculae; between the nearly normal trabeculae are slightly atypical spindle cells, which typically invade skeletal muscle found at the periphery of the tumor.
  • **Treatment: resection with a wide margin, which is usually curative**
    • **Low-grade lesion: chemotherapy *not* required**
  • Of the lesions that appear radiographically to be parosteal osteosarcoma, approximately 17% are high-grade malignancies (dedifferentiated parosteal osteosarcoma).
• Periosteal osteosarcoma (intermediate grade surface)
  • Rare surface form of osteosarcoma occurs most often in the diaphysis of long bones (typically femur or tibia).
  • Radiographic appearance is fairly constant: a sunburst-type lesion rests on a saucerized cortical depression (Figure 9-12).
  • Histologic characteristics: lesion is predominantly chondroblastic; grade of lesion is intermediate (grade II). Highly anaplastic regions are not found.
  • **Prognosis for periosteal osteosarcoma is intermediate between those of very low-grade parosteal osteosarcoma and high-grade intramedullary osteosarcoma. Preoperative chemotherapy, resection, and maintenance chemotherapy constitute the preferred treatment. The risk of pulmonary metastasis is 10% to 15%.**
• High-grade surface osteosarcoma
  • Extremely rare form of surface osteosarcoma
  • Imaging is a mixed lytic sclerotic aggressive surface lesion in the metaphysis or diaphysis.
  • Treatment is the same as conventional osteosarcoma.
  • Prognosis is the same as conventional osteosarcoma.
• Telangiectatic osteosarcoma
  • Tissue of the lesion can be described as a bag of blood with few cellular elements.
  • Radiographic features of telangiectatic osteosarcoma are those of a destructive, lytic, expansile lesion. Telangiectatic osteosarcomas occur in the same locations as aneurysmal bone cysts; radiographic appearances of both can be confused.

Comparison of common osteosarcoma varieties is presented in Table 9-21.

CHONDROGENIC LESIONS

Comparison of these lesions is shown in Table 9-22.

▦ Chondroma
▦ Histologic and radiographic features
  • When benign cartilage tumors occur on the surface of the bone, they are called *periosteal chondroma*.
  • Occur on surfaces of distal femur, proximal humerus, and proximal femur (Figure 9-16)
  • Appearance: usually a well-demarcated shallow cortical defect and a slight periosteal reaction
    • Buttress of cortical bone at the edges of the lesion
    • One third of the periosteal chondromas exhibit a mineralized cartilaginous matrix on the radiograph, whereas two thirds have no apparent radiographic mineralization.

Table 9-21	Comparison of Osteosarcomas		
	CONVENTIONAL (INTRAMEDULLARY)	**PAROSTEAL**	**PERIOSTEAL**
Age	<30 and > 60	<45	<30
Presentation	Pain	Painless mass	Pain
Imaging	Mixed lytic/destructive aggressive intramedullary bone producing lesion	Ossified lobulated surface lesion	Sunburst saucerized surface lesion
		Metaphyseal	Diaphyseal
	Common location metaphyseal	Characteristic location posterior distal femur	Characteristic location femur or tibia
Histology	Poorly arranged osseous trabeculae with malignant rimming osteoblasts	Regularly arranged osseous trabeculae	Osseous trabeculae
	Atypical spindle cells	Minimally atypical spindle cells	Chondroblastic elements
Biology	65% 5-year survival	95% 5-year survival	80% 5-year survival
Treatment	Chemotherapy	Limb salvage surgery	Chemotherapy
	Limb salvage surgery		Limb salvage surgery
Image	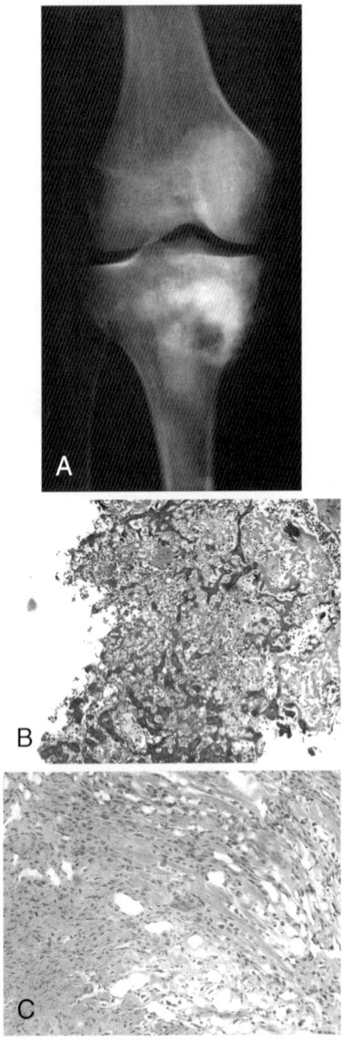	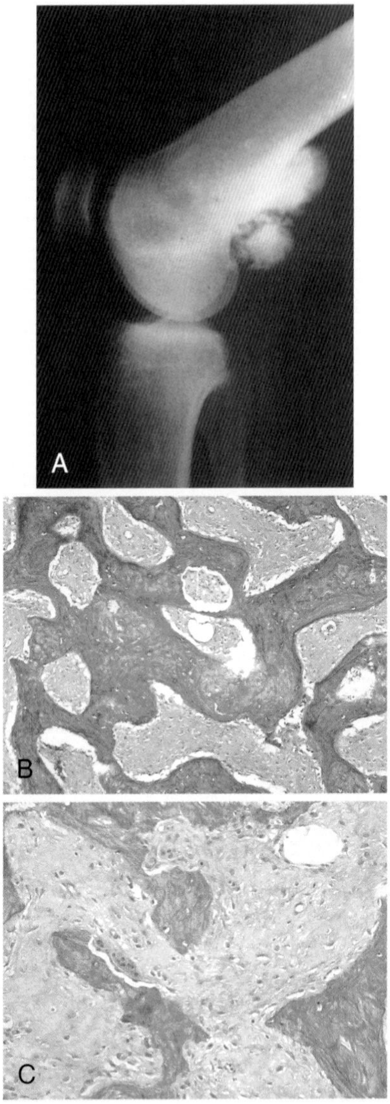	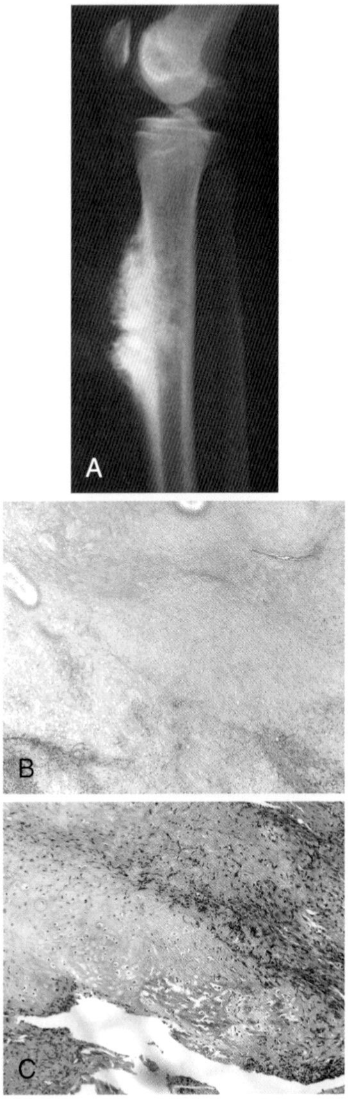
Description	FIGURE 9-10 Conventional osteoblastic osteosarcoma of the proximal tibia. **A,** Radiograph shows a poorly defined osteoblastic lesion in the proximal tibial metaphysis. **B,** Low-power photomicrograph (×160) shows lacelike mineralizing osteoid surrounding atypical osteoblasts. **C,** Higher-power photomicrograph (×400) shows pleomorphism and bone formation.	FIGURE 9-11 Parosteal osteosarcoma of the distal femur. **A,** Radiograph shows an exophytic bony mass in the posterior distal femur. **B,** Low-power photomicrograph (×160) shows plates of new bone in a fibrous matrix. **C,** Higher-power photomicrograph (×400) shows a fibrous stroma with atypical cells.	Figure 9-12 Periosteal osteosarcoma of the diaphysis of the tibia. **A,** Lateral radiograph showing a surface lesion with bone formation. **B,** Low-power photomicrograph (×160) showing cartilage and bone formation. **C,** Higher-power photomicrograph showing pleomorphism and direct production of osteoid by the tumor cells.

Table 9-22	Cartilage Tumors		
	ENCHONDROMA	OSTEOCHONDROMA	CHONDROSARCOMA
Age	Any	Any	>50
Symptoms	Incidental	Mechanical	Pain
Imaging	No change in bone architecture No endosteal scalloping or erosion	Sessile or pedunculated lesion is confluent with the intramedullary canal.	Bone architecture is altered. Endosteal scalloping and erosion Bone destruction Soft tissue mass
Pathology	Bland cartilage with minimal cellular elements	Mature bone stalk with a benign, mature cartilage cap	Differing degrees of cellular atypia and a high rate of mitotic figures
Treatment	Observation	Observation unless mechanical pain is significant	Wide surgical resection
Caveats	Pathology may have high degree of cellularity in the hands and feet and can be confused with chondrosarcoma.	Lesions should mature with the patient; a cartilage cap >2 cm requires observation.	Chemotherapy is added with dedifferentiated and mesenchymal chondrosarcoma.
Syndrome association	Ollier disease Maffucci syndrome	Multiple hereditary exostoses (MHE)	Ollier disease Maffucci syndrome MHE
Image	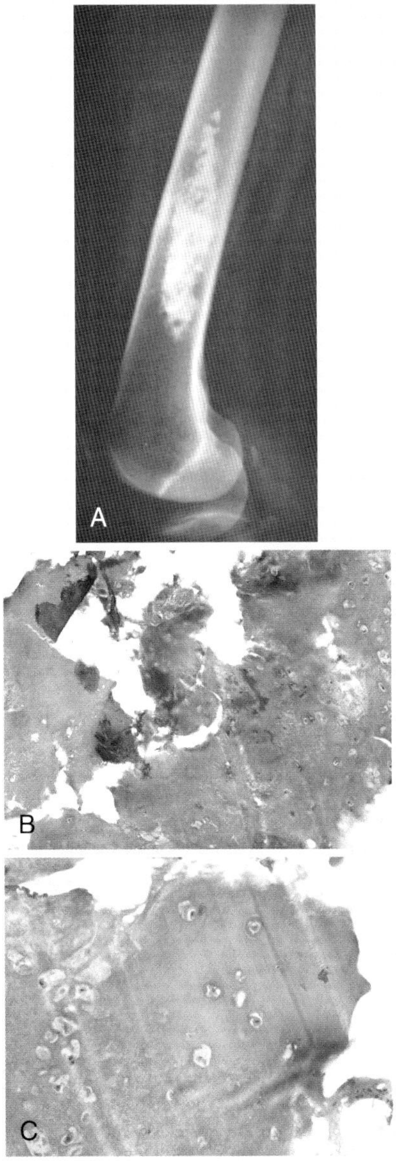	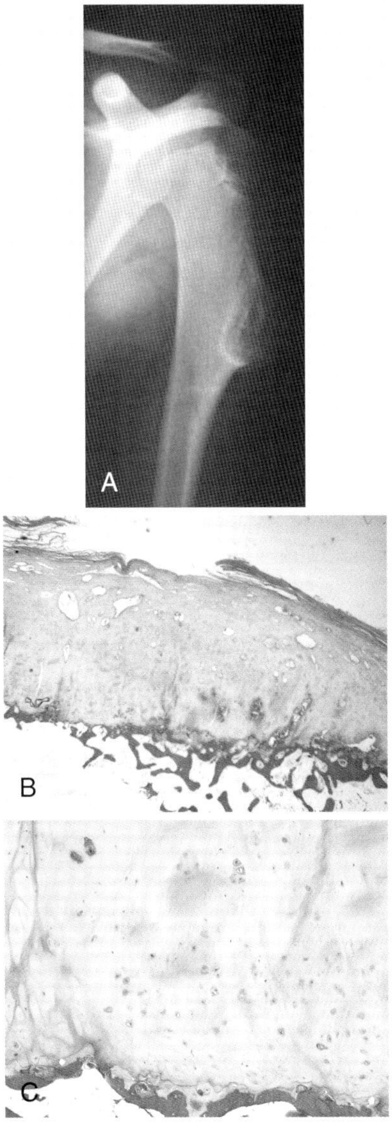	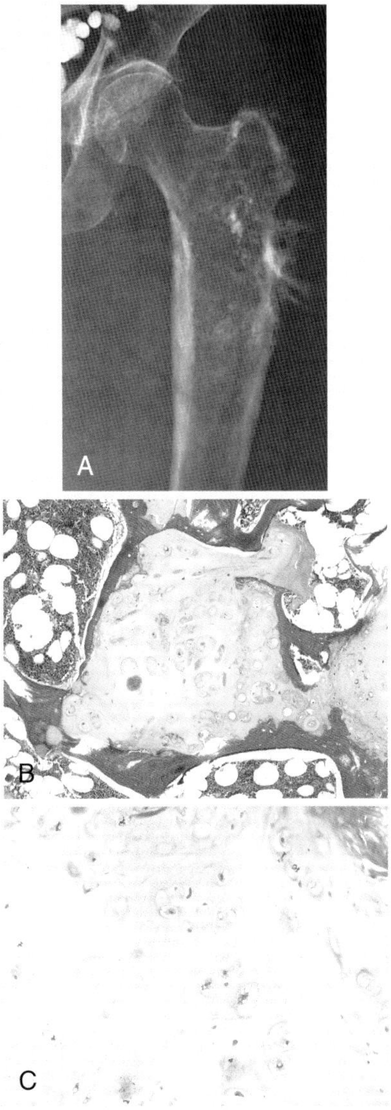
Description	FIGURE 9-13 Enchondroma of the distal femur. **A,** Radiograph shows densely mineralized medullary lesion. **B,** Low-power (×160) photomicrograph shows mineralized hyaline cartilage. **C,** Higher-power (×250) photomicrograph shows bland chondrocytes in lacunae.	FIGURE 9-14 Osteochondroma of the proximal humerus. **A,** Radiograph shows sessile osteochondroma of the proximal humerus. **B,** Photomicrograph (×6) shows the osteochondroma with a cartilaginous cap. **C,** Higher-power photomicrograph (×25) is a close-up view of the cartilage cap, which is undergoing endochondral ossification.	FIGURE 9-15 Central (intramedullary) chondrosarcoma of the proximal femur. **A,** Radiograph shows an expansile lytic lesion in the proximal femur with stippled calcifications. **B,** Low-power photomicrograph (×40) shows cartilage with a permeative growth pattern. **C,** Higher-power photomicrograph (×250) shows cellular cartilage.

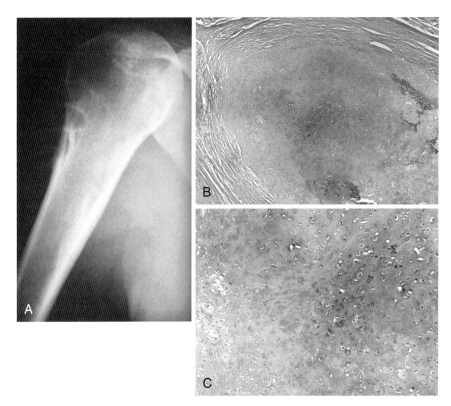

FIGURE 9-16 Periosteal chondroma of the proximal humerus. **A,** Radiograph shows surface lesion with stippled calcifications scalloping the cortex. **B,** Low-power photomicrograph (×100) shows bland hyaline cartilage. **C,** Higher-power photomicrograph (×250) shows cartilage cells and matrix.

- In the medullary cavity in the metaphysis of long bones, especially the proximal femur and humerus and the distal femur, they are called *enchondromas*.
- **Enchondromas are also common in the hand, where they usually occur in the diaphysis and metaphysis. Lesions in the hand may be hypercellular and display worrisome histologic features, and pathologic fractures in the hand are common.**
- Most enchondromas in long bones are asymptomatic.
- Radiographically there may be a prominent stippled or mottled calcified appearance (Figure 9-13).
- Tumor is composed of small cells that lie in lacunar spaces; it is hypocellular, and the cells have a bland appearance (no pleomorphism, anaplasia, or hyperchromasia).
- When lesions are not causing pain, serial radiographs are obtained to ensure that the lesions are inactive (not growing). Radiographs are obtained every 3 to 6 months for 1 to 2 years and then annually as necessary.
- **Enchondroma can be distinguished from low-grade chondrosarcoma on serial plain radiographs. In low-grade chondrosarcomas, cortical bone changes (large erosions [>50%] of the cortex, cortical thickening, and destruction) or lysis of the previously mineralized cartilage is visible.**
- Ollier disease/Maffucci syndrome
  - When there are many lesions, the involved bones are dysplastic, and the lesions tend toward unilaterality, the diagnosis is multiple enchondromatosis, or Ollier disease.

- Inheritance pattern is sporadic.
- If soft tissue angiomas are also present, the diagnosis is Maffucci syndrome.
- **Patients with multiple enchondromatosis are at increased risk of malignancy (in Ollier disease, 30%; in Maffucci syndrome, 100%).**
- **Patients with Maffucci syndrome also have a markedly increased risk of visceral malignancies, such as astrocytomas and gastrointestinal malignancies.**
- **For most enchondromas, no treatment other than observation is required. When surgical treatment is necessary, enchondromas are treated by curettage and bone grafting. Periosteal chondromas are usually excised with a marginal margin.**

■ **Osteochondroma**
▨ Features
- Benign surface lesions probably arise secondary to aberrant cartilage (from the perichondrial ring) on the surface of bone.
- They manifest with a painless mass after trauma, or the mass is discovered incidentally.
- Osteochondromas usually occur about the knee, proximal femur, and proximal humerus.
- Characteristic appearance: a surface lesion in which the cortex of the lesion and the underlying cortex are continuous and the medullary cavity of the host bone also flows into (is continuous with) the osteochondroma (Figure 9-14).
- Osteochondromas may have a narrow stalk (pedunculated) or a broad base (sessile).

- Typically occur at the site of tendon insertions; affected bone is abnormally wide.
- **Underlying cortex is covered by a thin cap of cartilage (usually only 2-3 mm thick; in a growing child, the cap thickness may exceed 1-2 cm).**
- Chondrocytes are arranged in linear clusters, with an appearance resembling that of the normal physis.
- When asymptomatic, these lesions are treated with observation only.
- Surgery is considered when patients experience pain secondary to muscle irritation, mechanical trauma (contusions), or an inflamed bursa over the lesion.
- Malignant transformation
  - Pain in the absence of mechanical factors is a warning sign of malignant change.
  - Development of a sarcoma in an osteochondroma is rare, occurring in far fewer than 1% of cases.
  - Destruction of the subchondral bone, mineralization of a soft tissue mass, and an inhomogeneous appearance are radiographic changes of malignant transformation.
  - A low-grade chondrosarcoma is usually present, although a dedifferentiated chondrosarcoma may occur in rare cases.
  - The lesion is termed a "secondary chondrosarcoma."
  - The prognosis is usually excellent; these low-grade tumors seldom metastasize.

- **Multiple hereditary exostoses**
  - **The osteochondromas are often sessile and large. This is an autosomal dominant condition with mutations in the *EXT1* and *EXT2* gene loci. Approximately 10% of patients with multiple exostoses develop a secondary chondrosarcoma. The *EXT1* mutation is associated with a greater burden of disease and higher risk of malignancy.**
- ■ **Chondroblastoma**
- **Centered in the epiphysis in young patients, usually with open physes; may also occur in an apophysis (vs. GCT [Table 9-23])**
- Most common locations: distal femur, proximal tibia, and proximal humerus
- Manifests with pain referable to the involved joint
- Causes a central region of bone destruction that is usually sharply demarcated from the normal medullary cavity by a thin rim of sclerotic bone (Figure 9-17)
- Mineralization may or may not occur within the lesion.
- The basic proliferating cells are thought to be chondroblasts.
  - Scattered multinucleated giant cells are found throughout the lesion.
  - Zones of chondroid substance are present.
  - Mitotic figures may be found.
- **Treatment: curettage (intralesional margin) and bone grafting**
- Lung metastasis occurs in 2% of benign chondroblastomas.
- ■ **Chondromyxoid fibroma**
- Rare benign cartilage tumors that contain variable amounts of chondroid, fibromatoid, and myxoid elements
- More common in boys and men
- Tend to involve long bones (especially tibia); pelvis and distal femur are other common locations.
- Manifest with pain of variable duration (months to years).

- There is a lytic destructive lesion that is eccentric and sharply demarcated from adjacent normal bone (Figure 9-19).
- Grows in lobules; often a condensation of cells at the periphery of the lobules (concentration of chondroid element may vary from light to heavy).
- Treatment: intralesional curettage
- ■ **Chondrosarcoma**
- Intramedullary chondrosarcoma
  - **This malignant neoplasm of cartilage occurs in older adults.**
  - Most common locations include the shoulder and pelvic girdles, knee, and spine.
  - Patients may have pain or a mass.
  - **Radiographs usually show diagnostic findings, with bone destruction, thickening of the cortex, and mineralization consistent with cartilage within the lesion (Figure 9-15; see Table 9-22).**
  - Prominent cortical changes are present in 85% of affected patients.
  - Differentiating malignant cartilage may be extremely difficult on the basis of histologic features alone.
  - Clinical, radiographic, and histologic features of a particular lesion must be considered in combination to avoid incorrect diagnosis. Criteria for the diagnosis of malignancy include:
    - Many cells with plump nuclei
    - More than an occasional cell with two such nuclei
    - Especially large cartilage cells with large single or multiple nuclei containing clumps of chromatin
    - Infiltration of the bone trabeculae
  - **Chondromas of the hand (enchondromas)—the lesions in patients with Ollier disease and Maffucci syndrome—and periosteal chondromas may have atypical histopathologic features.**
  - **Treatment: wide-margin surgical resection**
  - **Chemotherapy has *not* been shown to improve survival.**

- Dedifferentiated chondrosarcoma
  - Most malignant cartilage tumor
  - Most common locations include the distal and proximal femur and the proximal humerus.
  - Bimorphic histologic and radiographic appearances
  - Low-grade cartilage component that is intimately associated with a high-grade spindle cell sarcoma (osteosarcoma, fibrosarcoma, MFH)
  - More than 80% of the lesions are typical chondrosarcomas with a superimposed highly destructive area (Figure 9-20).
  - Manifestations are similar to those of low-grade chondrosarcoma, including pain and decreased function.
  - **Prognosis is poor; rate of long-term survival is less than 10%.**
  - **Treatment: wide-margin surgical resection and multiagent chemotherapy**

FIBROUS LESIONS

- ■ **Metaphyseal fibrous defect (also known as *nonossifying fibroma, nonosteogenic fibroma,* and *xanthoma*)**
- Occurs in young patients
- Most such lesions resolve spontaneously and are probably not true neoplasms.

Table 9-23	Epiphyseal Lesions—Chondroblastoma versus Giant Cell Tumor	
	CHONDROBLASTOMA	**GIANT CELL TUMOR**
Patient age	<30	>30
Imaging	Plain x-ray—skeletally immature	Plain x-ray—skeletally mature
	Well-circumscribed lytic lesion	Poorly circumscribed eccentric, lytic lesion
	Stippled calcifications	MRI—lesion may contain fluid-fluid levels (ABC collision)
	MRI—edema surrounding lesion greatly out of proportion to the lesion	
Histology	Chondroblasts	Multinucleated giant cells within a background of mononuclear stromal cells
	"Chicken-wire" calcifications in a lacelike pattern	Frequent ABC component
Biology	Lung metastases in <1% of patients	Lung metastases in 5% of patients
Treatment	Intralesional curettage	Intralesional curettage
		For pathologic fracture, ORIF or resection and reconstruction
Image	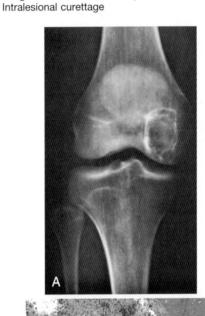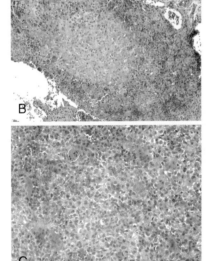	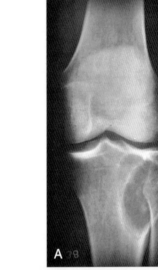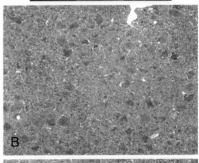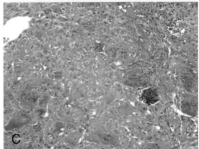
Description	FIGURE 9-17 Chondroblastoma of the distal femur. **A,** Radiograph shows a well-circumscribed lytic lesion with a sclerotic rim in the distal femoral epiphysis. **B,** Low-power photomicrograph (×160) shows cellular stroma in a chondroid matrix. **C,** Higher-power photomicrograph (×400) shows rounded stromal cells with multinucleated giant cells.	FIGURE 9-18 Giant cell tumor of the proximal tibia. **A,** Radiograph shows a well-circumscribed lytic lesion involving both the epiphysis and the metaphysis. **B,** Low-power photomicrograph (×160) shows sheets of multinucleated giant cells. **C,** Higher-power photomicrograph (×300) shows giant cells and mononucleic cells.

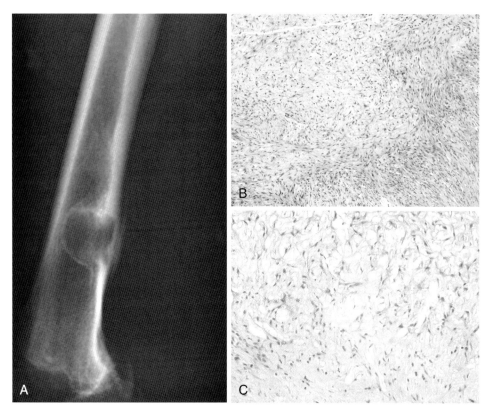

FIGURE 9-19 Chondromyxoid fibroma of the femur. **A,** Radiograph shows a well-circumscribed lytic lesion in the distal femur, with a rim of sclerotic bone. **B,** Low-power photomicrograph (×100) shows lobules of fibromyxoid tissue. **C,** Higher-power photomicrograph (×250) shows myxoid stroma with stellate cells.

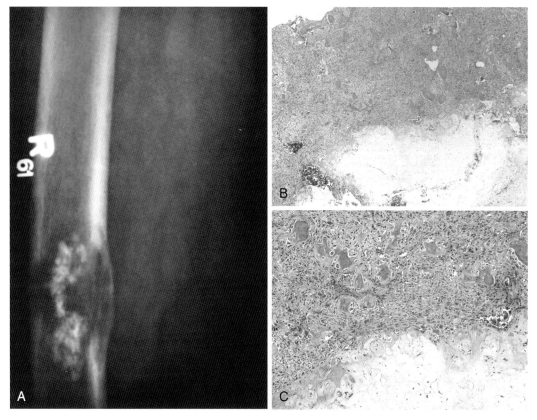

FIGURE 9-20 Dedifferentiated chondrosarcoma of the femur. **A,** Radiograph shows focal dense mineralization surrounded by a poorly defined lytic lesion. **B,** Low-power photomicrograph (×100) shows an island of hyaline cartilage surrounded by a cellular neoplasm. **C,** Higher-power photomicrograph (×250) shows hyaline cartilage adjacent to pleomorphic rounded cells.

- Most common locations are the distal femur, distal tibia, and proximal tibia.
- These lesions are usually asymptomatic and discovered incidentally.
- Characteristic radiographic appearance: a lucent lesion that is metaphyseal, eccentric, and surrounded by a sclerotic rim (Figure 9-21). The overlying cortex may be slightly expanded and thinned.
- Cellular fibroblastic connective tissue background, with cells arranged in whorled bundles (numerous giant cells, lipophages, and various amounts of hemosiderin pigmentation)
- Treatment: observation if the radiographic appearance is characteristic and the risk of pathologic fracture is not excessive
- If more than 50% to 75% of the cortex is involved and the patient has symptoms, curettage and fixation are performed.
- **Desmoplastic fibroma**
- Rare and low-grade but aggressive fibrous tumor of bone
- Lesion is purely lytic.
- When process is low grade, residual or reactive trabeculated (or corrugated) bone is often present.
- Lesion is composed of abundant collagen and mature fibroblasts with no cellular atypia.
- With wide-margin surgical resection, the risk of local recurrence is lowest.
- **Fibrosarcoma**

- Presentation and localization are similar to those of osteosarcoma.
- This tumor affects primarily older persons but does occur during all decades of life.
- Lytic bone destruction is often in permeative pattern (Figure 9-22).
- Spindle cells, variable collagen production, and a herringbone pattern
- Treatment: wide-margin surgical resection and chemotherapy

MALIGNANT FIBROUS HISTIOCYTOMA

- Most common locations include the distal femur, proximal tibia, proximal femur, ilium, and proximal humerus.
- Also known as *nonosteogenic osteosarcoma.* This is a primary bone osteosarcoma with a mesenchymal origin and cellular pattern, but no osteoid is produced or seen in histology.
- Malignant bone tumors that have proliferating cells with a histiocytic quality
- Nuclei are often indented, cytoplasm is usually abundant and may be slightly foamy, nucleoli are often large, and multinucleated giant cells are usually a prominent feature.
- Variable amounts of fibrous tissue found within the lesion, and fibrogenic areas have a storiform appearance.
- Patients present with pain and swelling.
- This lesion is destructive, with either purely lytic bone destruction or a mixed pattern of bone destruction and formation (Figure 9-23).

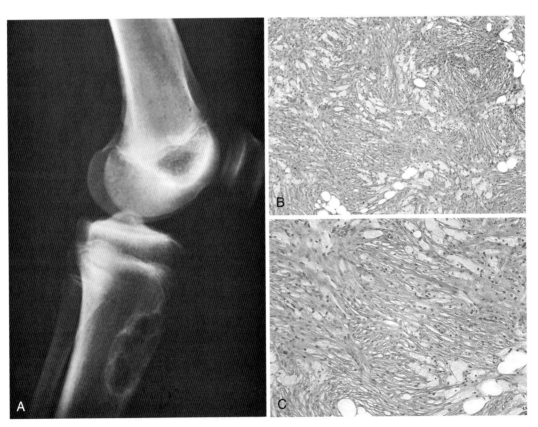

FIGURE 9-21 Metaphyseal fibrous defect (nonossifying fibroma) of the proximal tibia. **A,** Radiograph shows a scalloped, well-circumscribed lesion with a sclerotic rim in the proximal tibial metaphysis. **B,** Low-power photomicrograph (×160) shows spindle cells in a storiform pattern and occasional multinucleated giant cells. **C,** Higher-power photomicrograph (×250) of photomicrograph in **B.**

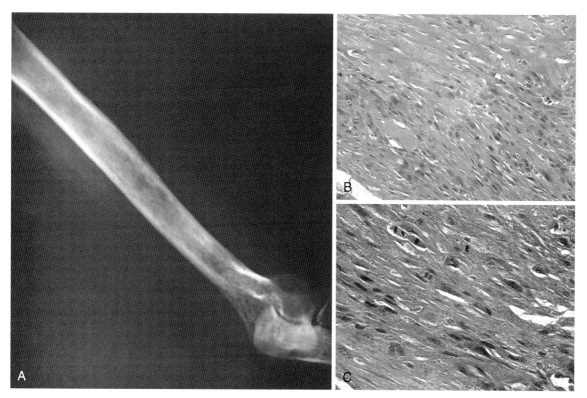

FIGURE 9-22 Fibrosarcoma of the humerus. **A,** Radiograph shows a permeative lesion in the midshaft of the humerus. **B,** Low-power photomicrograph (×250) shows atypical spindle cells. **C,** Higher-power photomicrograph (×400).

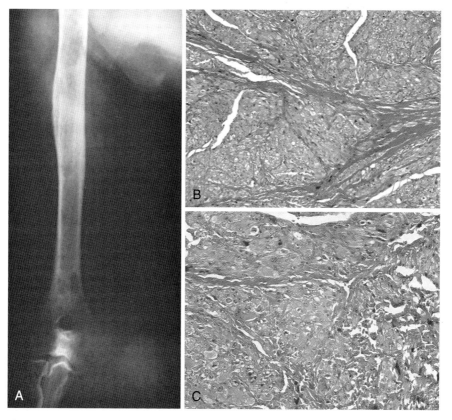

FIGURE 9-23 Malignant fibrous histiocytoma of the humerus. **A,** Radiograph shows poorly defined lytic lesions in the proximal and distal humerus. **B,** Low-power photomicrograph (×200) shows spindle cells arranged in a storiform pattern. **C,** Higher-power photomicrograph (×400) shows a uniform population of pleomorphic cells.

■ Treatment: same as osteogenic sarcoma—chemotherapy and surgery

NOTOCHORDAL TISSUE

■ *Chordoma* is a malignant neoplasm in which the cell of origin is derived from primitive notochordal tissue.
■ Occurs predominantly at the ends of the vertebral column clivus of the skull or sacrum (sacrococcygeal)
■ About 10% of chordomas occur in the vertebral bodies (cervical, thoracic, and lumbar regions).
■ Patients present with an insidious onset of pain. Lesions in the sacrum may manifest as pelvic pain, low-back pain, or hip pain or with primarily gastrointestinal symptoms (obstipation, constipation, loss of rectal tone). When vertebral bodies are involved, neurologic symptoms may vary widely because of nerve compression.
■ Radiographs often do not reveal the true extent of sacrococcygeal chordomas. The sacrum is difficult to evaluate on plain radiographs because of overlying bowel gas and fecal material and the angulation of the sacrum away from the x-ray beam on the anteroposterior view. In addition, the anteroposterior pelvic view reveals bone destruction only at the sacral cortical margins and neural foramina; these areas are not typically involved early.
■ CT scans show midline bone destruction and a soft tissue mass (Figure 9-24).
■ MRI is an excellent modality for both detecting a chordoma and defining the anatomic features of the tumor.
▦ Low signal on T1-weighted images
▦ Very bright signal on T2-weighted images
▦ Sacrum is often expanded, and the soft tissue mass may exhibit irregular mineralization.
▦ In the vertebral bodies, areas of lytic bone destruction or a mixed pattern of both bone formation and bone destruction are often observed.
■ The tumor grows in distinct lobules.
▦ Chordoma cells sometimes have a vacuolated appearance and are called *physaliferous* cells.
▦ Often arrayed in strands in a mass of mucus
▦ Treatment: wide-margin surgical resection
▦ Radiation therapy may be added if a wide margin is not achieved.
■ Chordomas metastasize late in the course of the disease, and local extension can be fatal.

VASCULAR TUMORS

■ Hemangioma (Figure 9-25)
▦ These tumors usually occur in vertebral bodies.
▦ Patients may present with pain or pathologic fracture (often asymptomatic).
▦ Vertebral hemangiomas have a characteristic appearance, with lytic destruction and vertical striations or a coarsened honeycomb appearance. On occasion, more than one bone is involved.
▦ There are numerous blood channels. Most lesions are cavernous, although some may be a mixture of capillary and cavernous blood spaces.
■ Hemangioendothelioma
▦ May occur in any age group, and affected patients present with pain

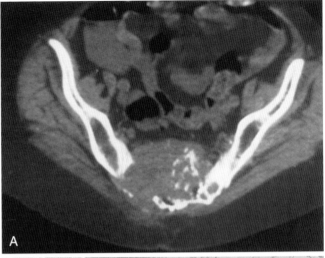
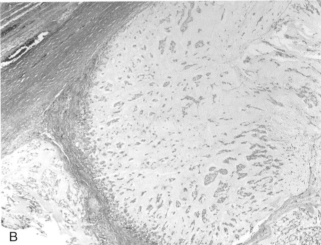
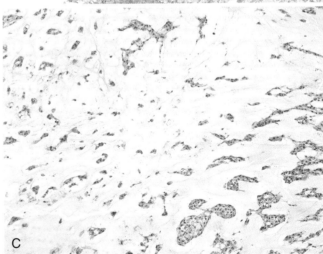

FIGURE 9-24 Chordoma of the sacrum. **A,** CT scan shows a destructive lesion in the sacrum. **B,** Low-power photomicrograph (×100) shows a lobular arrangement of tissue. **C,** Higher-power photomicrograph (×250) shows nests of physaliferous cells.

▦ Multifocal involvement of the bones of the same extremity is common
▦ Predominantly oval lytic lesion with no reactive bone formation
▦ Tumor cells form vascular spaces. Lesions range in structure from very well differentiated (easily

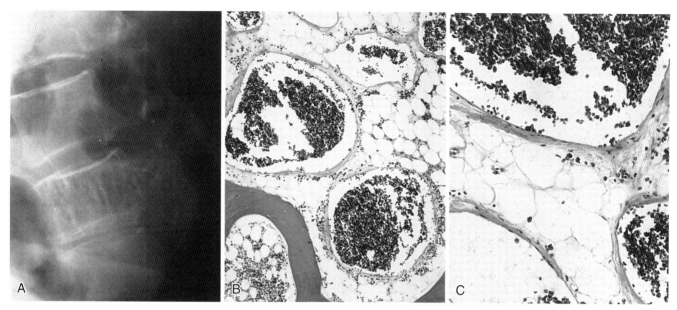

FIGURE 9-25 Hemangioma of the vertebra. **A,** Radiographic view shows vertical strictions. **B,** Low-power photomicrograph shows dilated vascular spaces in the marrow (×50). **C,** Higher-power photomicrograph (×100) shows endothelium-lined spaces.

Table 9-24	Blue Cell Tumors—Lernm (Learn 'EM)		
TUMOR	**MOLECULAR MARKER**	**AGE**	**IMAGING**
Lymphoma	CD45+ CD20+ LCA+ (leucocyte common antigen)	>30	*Plain x-ray*—minimal bone destruction *MRI*—large soft tissue mass out of proportion to bone destruction
Ewing sarcoma	CD99+ FLI-1+ t(11;22) translocation	<30	*Plain x-ray*—onion skinning and Codman triangle *MRI*—large soft tissue mass out of proportion to bone destruction
Rhabdomyosarcoma	Desmin+	<30	*Plain x-ray*—normal *MRI*—soft tissue mass
Neuroblastoma	NSE+ (neuron-specific enolase)	<30	*Plain x-ray*—normal *MRI*—soft tissue mass
Myeloma	Kappa/lambda light chain+ Monoclonal spike on SPEP/UPEP CD138+	>30	*Plain x-ray*—punched-out bone lesion with no host response *MRI*—visible lesion with small zone of surrounding edema

Histologically, these tumors appear as small blue cells on H&E staining due to a prominent nucleus and a small amount of surrounding cytoplasm. Molecular markers are utilized to distinguish tumor type.

recognizable vascular spaces) to very undifferentiated (difficult to recognize their vasoformative quality).
- Low-grade multifocal lesions may be treated with radiation alone.

HEMATOPOIETIC TUMORS

Hematopoietic tumors are small round blue cell tumors (SRBCTs) that are often difficult to distinguish from a number of SRBCTs (Table 9-24).
- **Lymphoma**
- **Lymphoma of bone is uncommon and occurs in three scenarios:**
  - **As a solitary focus (primary lymphoma of bone)**
  - **In association with other osseous sites and nonosseous sites (nodal disease and soft tissue masses)**
  - **As metastatic foci**
- Most common locations: distal femur, proximal tibia, pelvis, proximal femur, vertebra, and shoulder girdle

- Occurs at all ages
- Affected patients generally present with pain.
- Images often show a lesion that involves a large portion of the bone (long lesion; Figure 9-26).
  - Bone destruction is common and often has a mottled appearance.
  - Reactive bone formation admixed with bone destruction is often observed. The cortex may be thickened.
- A mixed cellular infiltrate is usually present. Most lymphomas of bone are diffuse, large B-cell lymphomas.
- **Treatment generally combines multiagent chemotherapy and consolidative irradiation.**
- **Surgery is generally used only to stabilize fractures.**
- **Myeloma**

Plasma cell dyscrasias represent a wide range of conditions from monoclonal gammopathy of undetermined significance (MGUS; Kyle disease) to multiple myeloma. There are three plasma cell dyscrasias with which orthopaedists must be familiar: multiple myeloma, solitary plasmacytoma of bone, and osteosclerotic myeloma.

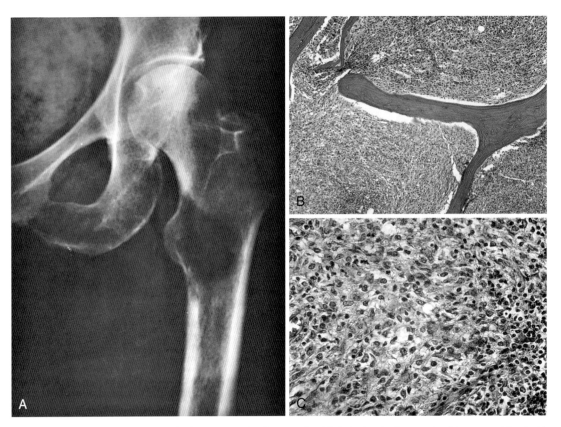

FIGURE 9-26 Lymphoma of bone. **A,** Radiograph shows a poorly circumscribed lytic lesion in the proximal femur and the ischium. **B,** Low-power photomicrograph (×200) shows marrow replacement by a uniform population of lymphoid cells. **C,** Higher-power photomicrograph (×400) shows uniform cell population.

▪ Multiple myeloma
- **Malignant plasma cell disorder that commonly occurs in patients between 50 and 80 years of age**
- Manifests with bone pain, usually in the spine and ribs, or a pathologic fracture
- Fatigue is a common complaint secondary to the associated anemia.
- Symptoms may be related to complications such as renal insufficiency, hypercalcemia, and the deposition of amyloid.
- Serum creatinine levels are elevated in about 50% of affected patients.
- Hypercalcemia is present in about 33% of affected patients.
- **Radiographic appearance is of punched-out lytic lesions (Figure 9-27), which may show expansion and a "ballooned" appearance.**
- **Classic histologic appearance: sheets of plasma cells that appear monoclonal with immunostaining.**
  - **Well-differentiated plasma cells have an eccentric nucleus and a peripherally clumped, chromatic "clock face."**
  - There is a perinuclear clear zone (halo) that represents the Golgi apparatus.
- Treatment:
  - **Systemic therapy and bisphosphonates**
  - **Surgical stabilization with irradiation is used for impending and complete fractures.**
  - Radiotherapy is also used for palliation of pain and treatment of neurologic symptoms.

- Prognosis is related to stage of disease; overall median survival time is 18 to 24 months.

▪ Solitary plasmacytoma of bone
It is important to differentiate solitary myeloma from multiple myeloma because of the more favorable prognosis in patients with the solitary form. Diagnostic criteria include:
- A solitary lesion on skeletal survey
- Histologic confirmation of plasmacytoma
- Bone marrow plasmacyte count of 10% or less
- Patients with serum protein abnormalities and Bence Jones proteinuria (protein levels < 1 g/24 h) at presentation are not excluded if they meet the aforementioned criteria.
- Treatment:
  - External beam irradiation of the lesion (4500-5000 cGy)
  - When necessary, prophylactic internal fixation
- In approximately 50% to 75% of affected patients, solitary myeloma progresses to multiple myeloma.

▪ Osteosclerotic myeloma
- Rare variant in which bone lesions are associated with a chronic inflammatory demyelinating polyneuropathy.
- Diagnosis of osteosclerotic myeloma is not generally made until the polyneuropathy is recognized and evaluated.
- Sensory symptoms (tingling, pins and needles, coldness) are noted first, followed by motor weakness.
  - Sensory and motor changes begin distally, are symmetric, and proceed proximally.
  - Severe weakness is common, but bone pain is not characteristic.

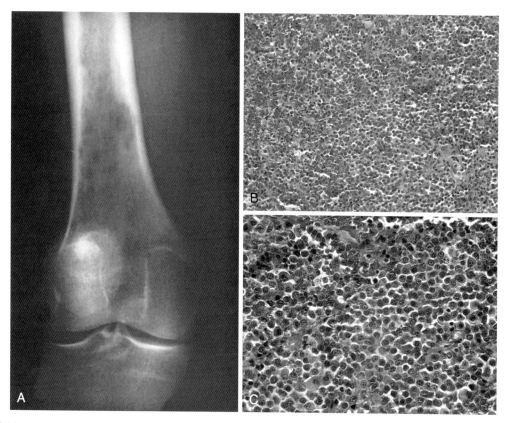

FIGURE 9-27 Multiple myeloma in the femur. **A,** Radiograph shows a poorly circumscribed lytic lesion in the distal femur. **B,** Low-power micrograph shows marrow replacement by a uniform population of cells. **C,** Higher-power photomicrograph (×400) shows sheets of atypical plasma cells.

- Radiographs may show a spectrum from pure sclerosis to a mixed pattern of lysis and sclerosis. Lesions usually involve the spine, pelvic bones, and ribs; extremities are generally spared.
- **Affected patients may have abnormalities outside the nervous system and have a constellation of findings termed *POEMS* syndrome (*p*olyneuropathy, *o*rganomegaly, *e*ndocrinopathy, M-protein, and skin changes). Treatment is with a combination of chemotherapy, radiotherapy, and plasmapheresis. Neurologic changes may not improve with treatment.**

TUMORS OF UNKNOWN ORIGIN

◼ Giant cell tumor
◻ Benign form
- Distinctive neoplasm that has poorly differentiated cells
- Benign but aggressive
- Confusion in diagnosis results from the fact that in rare cases (<5%), this benign tumor metastasizes to the lungs (benign metastasizing giant cell tumor).
- **Most common in the epiphysis and metaphysis of long bones; about 50% of lesions occur about the knee. Vertebra, sacrum, and distal radius are involved in about 10% of cases.**
- **The sacrum is the most common axial location of giant cell tumors of bone.**

- Unlike most bone tumors, which occur more often in boys and men, giant cell tumors are more common in girls and women.
- They are uncommon in children with open physes.
- Manifest with pain that is usually referable to the joint involved
- **A purely lytic destructive lesion in the metaphysis that extends into the epiphysis and often borders the subchondral bone** (see Figure 9-18)
- Early in the symptomatic phase, radiographs may appear normal; a small lytic focus is difficult to detect.
- **Basic proliferating cell has a round to oval or even spindle-shaped nucleus (giant cells appear to have the same nuclei as the proliferating mononuclear cells). Mitotic figures may be numerous.**
- **Giant cell tumors may undergo a number of secondary degenerative changes, such as aneurysmal bone cyst formation, necrosis, fibrous repair, foam cell formation, and reactive new bone.**
- **Treatment is aimed at removing the lesion, with preservation of the involved joint.**
  - Extensive exteriorization (removal of a large cortical window over the lesion)
  - Curettage with manual and power instruments
  - Chemical cauterization may be used (phenol, peroxide).
  - Area of defect is usually reconstructed with subchondral bone grafts, methylmethacrylate, or both.

- Local control with this treatment regimen has a success rate of 85% to 90%.
- Malignant forms: primary and secondary malignant giant cell tumors
  - With primary malignant giant cell tumor of bone, a benign giant cell tumor coexists with a high-grade sarcoma (occurs with ≈ 1% of giant cell tumors)—most commonly aneurysmal bone cysts.
  - Secondary malignant giant cell tumor occurs after irradiation to treat a giant cell tumor or after multiple local recurrences.

■ **Ewing tumor**
- Diagnosis
  - Distinctive small round cell sarcoma that occurs most often in children and young adults; most affected children are older than 5 years.
  - **When a small blue cell tumor is found in a child younger than 5 years, metastatic neuroblastoma and leukemia should be confirmed or ruled out. In patients older than 30 years, metastatic carcinoma must be confirmed or ruled out** (see Table 9-24).
  - Most common locations include the pelvis, distal femur, proximal tibia, femoral diaphysis, and proximal humerus.
  - Manifests with pain; fever may be present.
  - Affected patients may exhibit an elevated ESR, leukocytosis, anemia, and an elevated white blood cell count.
  - Radiographs often show a large destructive lesion that involves the metaphysis and diaphysis.
  - Lesion may be purely lytic or may have variable amounts of reactive new bone formation (Figure 9-28).
  - Periosteum may be lifted off in multiple layers, which produces a Codman triangle and an onionskin appearance.
  - Soft tissue component is often large.
  - Immunohistochemistry studies reveal CD99 positivity.
- **Classic 11:22 chromosomal translocation produces the *EWS/FLI1* fusion gene.**
- Bone marrow biopsy is performed for staging purposes.
- Treatment: a multimodality approach with multiagent chemotherapy, irradiation, and surgical resection
  - **Standard treatment includes chemotherapy.**
  - **Local tumor control may be irradiation or surgery.**
  - **Major benefits of wide-margin surgical resection are a decrease in the risk of local recurrence and avoidance of the potential for postirradiation sarcoma.**
  - **Radiation may be used primarily for pelvic and spine disease where resection is morbid, or as an adjunct to surgery to maintain function while sparing critical structures.**
- Survival
  - Rate of long-term survival with multimodality treatment may be as high as 60% to 70%.
    - There is a consistent chromosomal translocation (11;22) with the formation of a fusion protein (EWS-FLI 1).

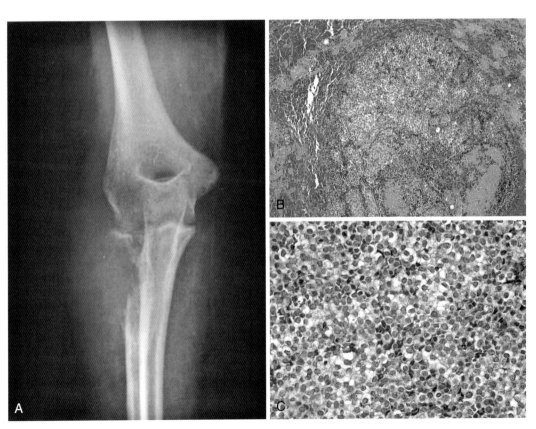

FIGURE 9-28 Ewing sarcoma of the proximal radius. **A,** Radiograph shows a destructive expansile lesion in the proximal radius. **B,** Low-power photomicrograph (×100) shows bone surrounded by a highly cellular neoplasm. **C,** Higher-power photomicrograph (×400) shows sheets of rounded cells.

- Metastatic disease involves the lungs (50%), bone (25%), and bone marrow (20%).
- Poor prognostic factors include:
  - Spine and pelvic tumors
  - Tumors larger than 100 cm^3 in diameter
  - A poor response to chemotherapy (<90% tumor cell necrosis)
  - Elevated lactic dehydrogenase levels (Temple)
  - The *P53* mutation and gene fusion products other than EWS-FLI 1

■ **Adamantinoma**
▨ **Rare low-grade malignant tumor of long bones that contains epithelium-like islands of cells**
▨ **Tibia is the most common site, although other long bones are infrequently involved (fibula, femur, ulna, radius).**
▨ **Affected patients are young adults and experience pain over months to years.**
▨ Radiographic appearance: multiple sharply circumscribed, lucent defects of different sizes, with sclerotic bone interspersed between the zones and extending above and below the lucent zones (Figure 9-29; see Table 9-26). One of the lesions in the midshaft is the largest and is associated with cortical bone destruction).
▨ Cells have an epithelial quality and are arranged in a palisading or glandular pattern; epithelial cells occur in a fibrous stroma.
▨ **Treatment: wide-margin surgical resection**
▨ Tumor may metastasize either early or after multiple failed attempts at local control.

TUMORLIKE CONDITIONS

There are many lesions that simulate primary bone tumors and must be considered in the differential diagnosis (Box 9-2). These lesions range from metastases to reactive conditions (Table 9-25).

■ **Aneurysmal bone cyst**
▨ Nonneoplastic reactive condition that may be aggressive in its ability to destroy normal bone and extend into the soft tissues
▨ **May arise primarily in bone or be found in association with other tumors (e.g., giant cell tumor, chondroblastoma, chondromyxoid fibroma, fibrous dysplasia)**

Box 9-2	**Tumorlike Conditions (Tumor Simulators)**

YOUNG PATIENT
Eosinophilic granuloma
Osteomyelitis
Avulsion fractures
Aneurysmal bone cyst
Fibrous dysplasia
Osteofibrous dysplasia
Heterotopic ossification
Unicameral bone cyst
Giant cell reparative
  granuloma
Exuberant callus
ADULT
Synovial chondromatosis
Pigmented villonodular
  synovitis
	Stress fracture
	Heterotopic ossification
	Ganglionic cyst
	OLDER ADULT
	Mastocytosis
	Hyperparathyroidism
	Paget disease
	Bone infarcts
	Bone islands
	Ganglionic cyst
	Cyst secondary to joint
	  disease
	Epidermoid cyst

▨ Some 75% of patients with an aneurysmal bone cyst are younger than 20 years.
▨ Affected patients experience pain and swelling.
▨ **Characteristic radiographic finding: an eccentric lytic, expansile area of bone destruction in the metaphysis**
▨ In classic cases, there is a thin rim of periosteal new bone surrounding the lesion (Figure 9-30).
▨ Radiograph may demonstrate the periosteal bone if it is mineralized.
▨ MRI usually shows the periosteal layer surrounding the lesion.
  - Fluid-fluid levels visible on T2-weighted MRI scans are characteristic of aneurysmal bone cysts.
▨ Essential histologic feature: cavernous blood-filled spaces without an endothelial lining
  - There are thin strands of bone present in the fibrous tissue of the septa.
  - Benign giant cells may be numerous.
▨ **Treatment: careful curettage and bone grafting**
▨ **Local recurrence is common in children with open physes.**

■ **Unicameral bone cyst (simple bone cyst)**
▨ Occurs most often in the proximal humerus; other sites are proximal femur and distal tibia
▨ Symmetric cystic expansion with thinning of the involved cortices
▨ Manifests with pain, usually after a fracture caused by minor trauma (e.g., sporting event, throwing a baseball, wrestling)
▨ Central lytic area and symmetric thinning of the cortices (Figure 9-31)
  - Affected bone is often expanded; however, the bone is generally no wider than the physis.
  - Often appears trabeculated
  - When the cyst abuts the physeal plate, the process is called *active;* when normal bone intervenes, the cyst is termed *latent.*
  - Thin fibrous lining contains fibrous tissue, giant cells, hemosiderin pigment, and a few chronic inflammatory cells.
  - Treatment: aspiration to confirm the diagnosis, followed by methylprednisolone acetate injection
  - Unicameral bone cysts of the proximal femur are often treated with curettage, grafting, and internal fixation to avoid fracture and osteonecrosis.

■ **Langerhans cell histiocytosis (LCH)**
▨ Lichtenstein originally divided this disorder into three entities: eosinophilic granuloma (monostotic bone disease), Hand-Schüller-Christian disease (multiple bone lesions and visceral disease), and Letterer-Siwe disease (a fulminating condition in young children).
  - This disorder is now usually referred to as *LCH.*
  - **The cellular abnormality is a proliferation of the Langerhans cells of the dendritic system.**
▨ Eosinophilic granuloma of bone is analogous to monostotic LCH, whereas Hand-Schüller-Christian disease could be called *polyostotic LCH with visceral involvement.*
  - LCH of bone is the most common manifestation; only a single bone (on occasion, multiple bones) involved.
  - Patients present with pain and swelling.

Table 9-25	Aneurysmal Bone Cyst versus Unicameral Bone Cyst
ANEURYSMAL BONE CYST	**UNICAMERAL BONE CYST**

ANEURYSMAL BONE CYST	UNICAMERAL BONE CYST

Occurs with other lesions, "collision lesion"
NO fallen leaf sign
X-ray—eccentric
Width of the tumor is greater than the width of the physis.
  Initial TREATMENT OPEN curettage.
	Does NOT occur with other lesions
	Fallen leaf sign
	X-ray—central
	Width of the tumor is NOT greater than the width of the physis.
	  Initial TREATMENT is aspiration/injection.

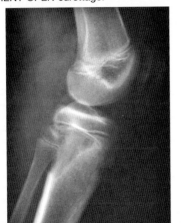

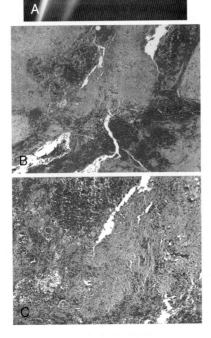

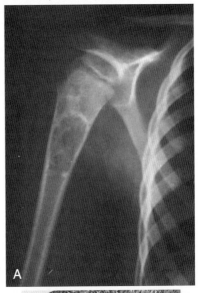

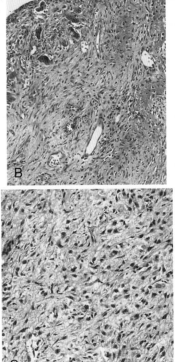

FIGURE 9-30 Aneurysmal bone cyst of the proximal tibia.
A, Radiograph shows a well-defined lytic lesion in the posterior tibial metaphysis. **B,** Low-power photomicrograph (×25) shows blood-filled lakes. **C,** Higher-power photomicrograph (×50) shows the wall of the cyst, with fibroblasts and occasional multinucleated giant cells.

FIGURE 9-31 Unicameral bone cyst of the humerus.
A, Radiograph shows a symmetric, midline, well-circumscribed, lytic lesion in the humeral metaphysis. **B,** Low-power photomicrograph (×160) shows the fibrous tissue membrane, with reactive bone and occasional multinucleated giant cells.
C, High-power photomicrograph shows a uniform population of spindle cells without nuclear atypia.

Table 9-26	Comparison of Osteofibrous Dysplasia, Fibrous Dysplasia, and Adamantinoma		
	ADAMANTINOMA	**FIBROUS DYSPLASIA**	**OSTEOFIBROUS DYSPLASIA**
Age	<30	Any	<30
Imaging	Lytic, mixed lytic/sclerotic, cortically based lesion	Ground-glass appearance Bone deformity/bowing	Multilocular, eccentric, lytic defects of cortex with a well-defined sclerotic border
Location	Tibia characteristic	Any bone	Tibia common
Histology	Nests of epithelioid cells in a background fibrous stroma	Fibroosseous lesion WITHOUT rimming osteoblasts	Fibroosseous lesion WITH rimming osteoblasts
Biology		Benign	Benign
Treatment	Wide excision with negative margins	Observe Treat pathologic fractures surgically.	Observe
Image	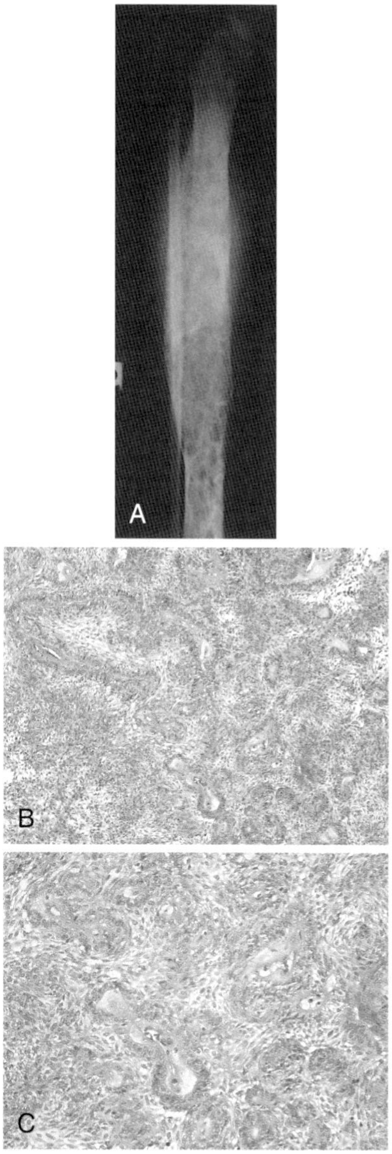	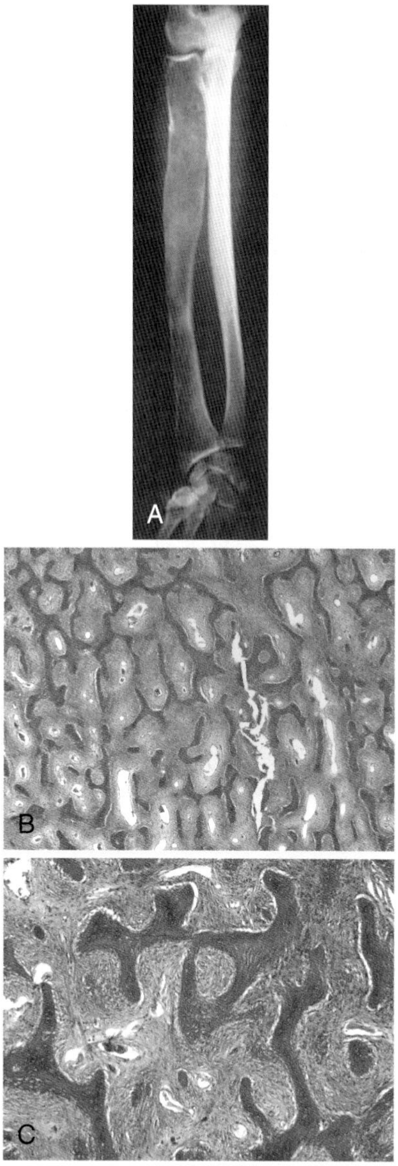	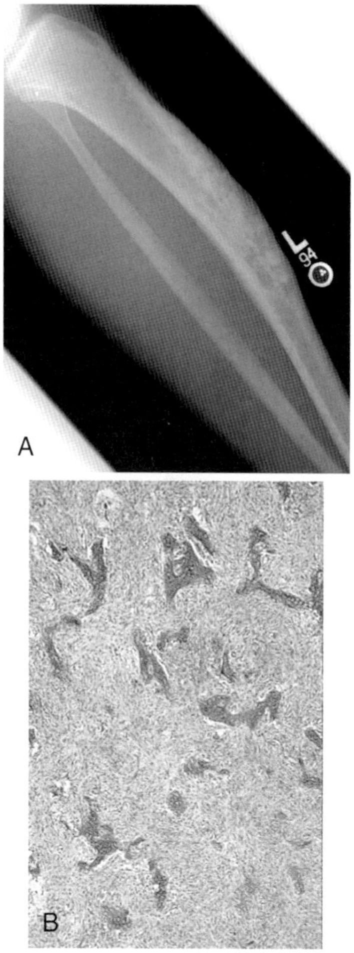
Description	FIGURE 9-29 Adamantinoma of the tibia. **A,** Radiograph shows a bubbly, symmetric, lytic lesion in the tibial diaphysis. **B,** Low-power photomicrograph (×250) shows biphasic differentiation, with spindle cells and epithelioid cells. **C,** Higher-power photomicrograph (×400) shows epithelial cells forming glands and spindle cells.	FIGURE 9-33 Fibrous dysplasia of the radius. **A,** Radiograph shows a long, symmetric lytic lesion of the radius with a ground-glass appearance. **B,** Low-power photomicrograph (×50) shows seams of osteoid in a fibrous background. **C,** Higher-power photomicrograph (×160) shows osteoid surrounded by bland fibrous tissue.	FIGURE 9-34 **A,** Plain x-ray shows a cortically based lesion with cortically based lytic areas with sclerotic rimming. **B,** Histology shows osteoid lakes in a fibrous stroma WITH rimming osteoblasts.

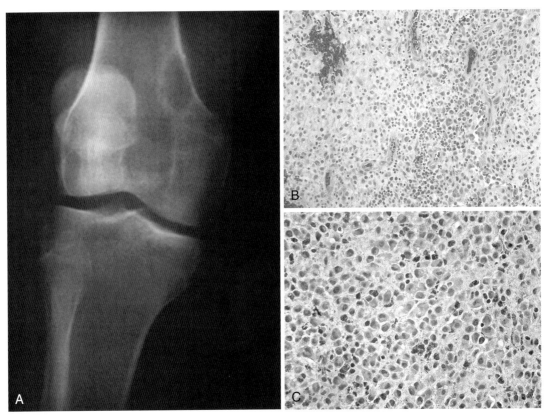

FIGURE 9-32 Eosinophilic granuloma of the distal femur. **A,** Radiograph shows a well-circumscribed lesion with a sclerotic rim in the femoral metaphysis. **B,** Low-power photomicrograph (×160) shows a heterogeneous population of inflammatory cells, with an aggregation of histiocytes. **C,** Higher-power photomicrograph (×400) shows nests of Langerhans histiocytes.

- The lesion is highly destructive and has well-defined margins (Figure 9-32).
- Cortex may be destroyed, and a periosteal reaction with a soft tissue mass simulating a malignant bone tumor may be present.
- Often different amounts of bone destruction of the involved cortices, resulting in the appearance of a bone within a bone
- There may be expansion of the involved bone.
- Any bone may be involved.
- Characteristic cell is a proliferating Langerhans cell with an indented or grooved nucleus.
  - Cytoplasm is eosinophilic.
  - Nuclear membrane has a crisp border.
  - Mitotic figures may be common.
  - Bilobed eosinophils with bright, granular, eosinophilic cytoplasm are present in large numbers.
  - Electron microscopy shows a tennis racquet–shaped Birbeck granule.
- Treatment:
  - **Eosinophilic granuloma is a self-limiting process.**
  - **Treatments such as corticosteroid injection, low-dose irradiation (600-800 cGy), curettage and bone grafting, and observation have been successful.**
  - **If the articular surface is in jeopardy or an impending fracture is a possibility, concomitant curettage and bone grafting is a logical treatment.**
  - **Low-dose irradiation is effective for most lesions that cannot be injected and is associated with low rates of morbidity.**

- Hand-Schüller-Christian disease:
  - Bone lesions and visceral involvement
  - Classic triad (occurs in fewer than one fourth of patients) includes exophthalmos, diabetes insipidus, and lytic skull lesions.
  - Multifocal disease is usually treated with chemotherapy.
- Letterer-Siwe disease occurs in young children and is usually fatal.

■ **Fibrous dysplasia**
■ Developmental abnormality of bone that is characterized by monostotic or polyostotic involvement
■ Yellow or brown patches of skin (café au lait spots with irregular borders) may accompany the bone lesions.
■ Failure of the production of normal lamellar bone
■ **Genetic mutation is an activating mutation of the GSα surface protein—*GNAS1***
  - **Increased production of cyclic adenosine monophosphate (cAMP)**
■ **When endocrine abnormalities (especially precocious puberty) accompany multiple bone lesions and skin abnormalities, the condition is called *McCune-Albright syndrome*.**
■ Any bone may be involved; proximal femur is most commonly affected.
■ Variable appearance (looks highly lytic or like ground glass [Figure 9-33])
  - Well-defined rim of sclerotic bone
  - Proliferation of fibroblasts (produces a dense collagenous matrix)
  - Trabeculae of osteoid and bone within the fibrous stroma

- Cartilage may be present in variable amounts.
- **Bone fragments are present in a disorganized manner, and their appearance has been likened to "alphabet soup" and "Chinese letters."**
  - Treatment: predicated on the presence of symptoms and the risk of fracture
    - Internal fixation and bone grafting are used in areas of high stress in which nonoperative treatment would not be effective.
    - Most affected patients do not need surgical treatment.
    - **Autogenous cancellous bone grafting is *never* used; transplanted bone is quickly transformed into the woven bone of fibrous dysplasia.**
    - Cortical or cancellous allografts are usually used.
    - Bisphosphonate therapy has been shown to be effective in decreasing pain and reducing bone turnover in patients with polyostotic fibrous dysplasia.
- **Osteofibrous dysplasia (also called *ossifying fibroma* or *Jaffe-Campanacci lesion*)**
- **Primarily involves the tibia and is usually confined to the anterior tibial cortex (Figure 9-34)**
- Bowing is very common, and affected children may develop pathologic fractures.
- Lesion typically manifests in children younger than 10 years.
- Biopsy is not necessary.
- **Biopsy, when performed, reveals fibrous tissue stroma and a background of bone trabeculae with osteoblastic rimming.**
- **Nonoperative treatment is preferred until the child reaches maturity.**
- **These lesions usually regress and do not cause problems in adults.**

Adamantinoma, osteofibrous dysplasia, and fibrous dysplasia are compared in Table 9-26.

- **Paget disease**
- Characterized by abnormal bone remodeling
- Usually diagnosed during the fifth decade of life
- Monostotic or polyostotic
- Radiographs demonstrate coarsened trabeculae and remodeled cortices.
- Coarsened trabeculae give the bone a blastic appearance.
- **Characteristic features: irregular broad trabeculae, reversal or cement lines, osteoclastic activity, and fibrous vascular tissue between the trabeculae**
- **Manifests with pain**
- Medical treatment: aimed at retarding activity of osteoclasts
- Agents used include diphosphonates and calcitonin (pamidronate and Zometa).
- Affected patients may present with degenerative joint disease, fracture, or neurologic encroachment; joint degeneration is common in the hip and knee.
- Patients undergoing arthroplasty should be treated with bisphosphonates to decrease bleeding at the time of surgery.
- Fewer than 1% of patients with Paget disease develop malignant degeneration with the formation of a sarcoma within a focus of a Paget lesion.
  - Symptoms of Paget sarcoma are abrupt onset of pain and swelling.
  - Radiographs usually demonstrate cortical bone destruction and the presence of a soft tissue mass.
  - Paget sarcoma is a deadly tumor with a poor prognosis (rate of long-term survival <20%).

- **Osteomyelitis**
- Bone infections that often simulate primary tumors
- Occult infections may occur in all age groups.
- Affected patients may present with fever, chills, bone pain, or a combination of these symptoms.
- Affected patients usually present with bone pain but without systemic symptoms.
- Radiograph findings may be nonspecific:
  - Bone destruction and formation are the characteristic findings of chronic infections.
  - Acute infections often produce cortical bone destruction and periosteal elevation.
  - **Serpiginous tracts and irregular areas of bone destruction are suggestive of infection rather than neoplasm.**
  - Lesion is usually apparent with the following:
    - Edema of granulation tissue
    - Numerous new blood vessels
    - **A mixed-cell population of inflammatory cells, plasma cells, polymorphonuclear leukocytes, eosinophils, lymphocytes, and histiocytes**
- A chronic infection with long-standing wound drainage is occasionally complicated by a squamous cell carcinoma.
- Material that has been sent for culture should be subjected to biopsy, and material that has been sent for biopsy should be subjected to culture.
- Treatment: removal of all dead tissue and appropriate antibiotic therapy

METASTATIC BONE DISEASE

- **Most common entity that destroys the skeleton in older patients**
- **When a destructive bone lesion is found in a patient older than 40 years, metastases must be considered first.**
- **Five carcinomas most likely to metastasize to bone: breast, lung, prostate, kidney, and thyroid. (Mnemonics: "BLT and a Kosher Pickle" or "PT Barnum Likes Kids")**
- **Most common locations of metastasis: pelvis, vertebral bodies, ribs, and proximal limb girdles**
- Pathologic fractures secondary to metastatic disease occur most commonly in the proximal femur.
- **Pathogenesis is probably related to Batson vertebral vein plexus.**
- Venous flow from the breast, lung, prostate, kidney, and thyroid drains into the vertebral vein plexus (Figure 9-35).
- The plexus has intimate connections to the vertebral bodies, pelvis, skull, and proximal limb girdles.
- **Radiographs demonstrate a destructive lesion that may be purely lytic, may have a mixed pattern of bone destruction and formation, or may be purely sclerotic (Figure 9-36).**
- **Histologic hallmark: appearance of epithelial cells in a fibrous stroma; epithelial cells are often arranged in a glandular pattern.**
- **Bone destruction is caused not by the tumor cells themselves but by activation of osteoclasts (Figure 9-37).**
- **Tumor cells secrete parathyroid hormone–related peptide (PTHrP), which stimulates release of the receptor activator for nuclear factor κB ligand (RANKL) from osteoblasts and marrow stromal cells.**
- **RANKL attaches to the receptor activator for nuclear factor κ (RANK) receptor on osteoclast precursor cells.**
- In the presence of granulocyte colony-stimulating factor (G-CSF), the osteoclast precursor cells differentiate into

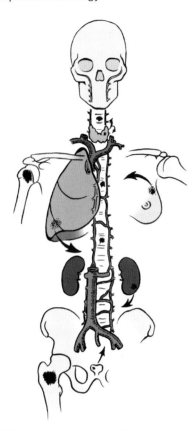

FIGURE 9-35 Batson venous plexus. This plexus is longitudinal and valveless and extends from the sacrum to the skull. The breast, lung, kidney, prostate, and thyroid glands connect to this system. Tumor cells can enter this system and spread to the vertebrae, ribs, pelvis, and proximal limb girdle. (From McCarthy EF, Frassica FJ: *Pathology of bone and joint disorders,* Philadelphia, 1998, WB Saunders.)

active osteoclasts that resorb the trabecular and cortical bone.

■ With bone resorption, transforming growth factor (TGF)-β, insulinlike growth factor (IGF)-1, and calcium are released, and these factors stimulate the tumor cells to multiply and release more PTHrP.

■ This process has been called the "vicious cycle" of metastatic bone disease.

■ **To combat osteoclastic bone destruction, many patients are now treated with antiresorptive agents (bisphosphonates) such as intravenous pamidronate and zoledronic acid.**

■ Treatment: aimed at controlling pain and maintaining patient's independence

■ Prophylactic internal fixation is performed when impending fracture is deemed likely.
  ● In comparison with treatment of completed pathologic fractures, prophylactic fixation results in less blood loss, shorter hospital stays, greater likelihood of discharge to home, and greater likelihood of independent ambulation.

■ **There are many suggested criteria for fixation. The following conditions put the patient most at risk for fracture:**
  ● **More than 50% destruction of diaphyseal cortices**
  ● **Permeative destruction of subtrochanteric femoral region**
  ● **More than 50% to 75% destruction of the metaphysis**
  ● **Persistent pain after irradiation**
  ● **Pain on weight bearing (especially in lower extremity with every footstep)**

■ **Treatment of pathologic fractures is almost always surgical, inasmuch as these fractures rarely have the potential to heal.**

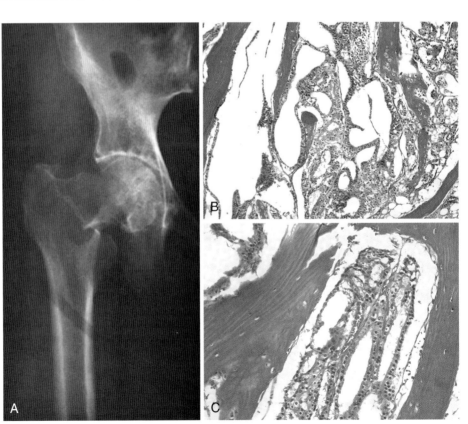

FIGURE 9-36 Metastatic carcinoma. **A,** Radiograph shows a lytic lesion in the femoral neck and the ilium. **B,** Low-power photomicrograph (×100) shows the glandular arrangement of cells in the marrow space. **C,** Higher-power photomicrograph (×400) shows epithelial cells in an organoid pattern.

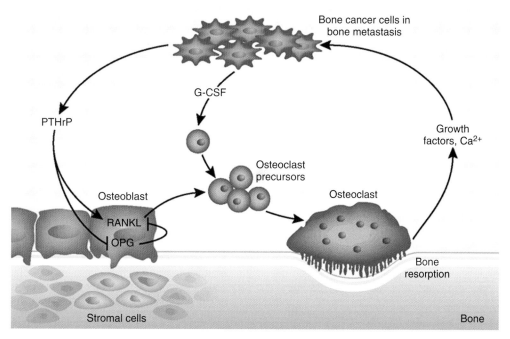

FIGURE 9-37 Breast cancer cells produce factors such as parathyroid hormone–related peptide (PTHrP) and granulocyte colony-stimulating factor (G-CSF), which enhance the formation of osteoclasts. *OPG,* Osteoprotegerin; *RANKL,* receptor activator for nuclear factor κB ligand. (From Roodman GD: Bone breaking cancer treatment, *Nat Med* 13:25–26, 2007, Figure 1.)

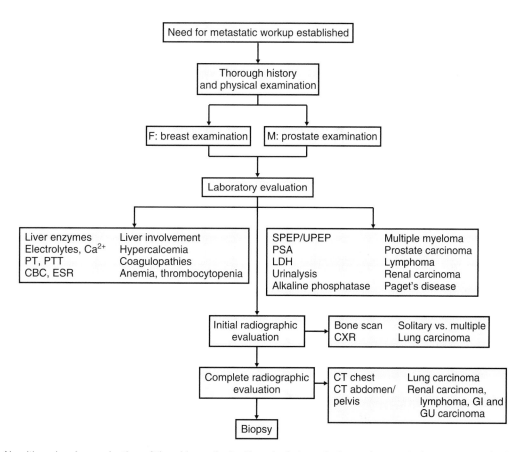

FIGURE 9-38 Algorithm showing evaluation of the older patient with a single bone lesion and suspected metastases of unknown origin. *CBC,* Complete blood cell count; *CT,* computed tomography; *CXR,* chest radiograph; *ESR,* erythrocyte sedimentation rate; *F,* female patient; *GI,* gastrointestinal; *GU,* genitourinary; *LDH,* lactate dehydrogenase; *M,* male patient; *PSA,* prostate-specific antigen; *PT,* prothrombin time; *PTT,* partial thromboplastin time; *SPEP,* serum protein electrophoresis; *UPEP,* urine protein electrophoresis. (From Damron TA: *Orthopaedic surgery essentials, oncology and basic science,* Philadelphia, 2008, Lippincott Williams & Wilkins, p 233.)

- **Surgical procedures should not rely on bony healing.**
- Most proximal femur fractures should be treated with cemented endoprostheses. To protect the femoral shaft in patients with relatively long life expectancy, consideration should be given to using a long stem.
- Risk factors for sudden death during insertion of a long-stem prosthesis: presence of breast cancer, hypovolemia, reduced pulmonary function
- **In patients older than 40 years with a single destructive bone lesion but without a known primary tumor, metastatic disease must be considered present. Simon outlined a** diagnostic strategy that identifies the primary lesion in up to 80% to 90% of patients (Figure 9-38).
- Histologically confirmed metastatic cancer for which a definitive primary site is not identified after a detailed medical examination is known as a *carcinoma, unknown primary* (CUP).

SELECTED BIBLIOGRAPHY

The selected bibliography for this chapter can be found on www.expertconsult.com.

TESTABLE CONCEPTS

SECTION 1 INTRODUCTION

- Prognostic factors in bone tumor staging, in order, are presence of metastases, discontinuous tumor, grade, and size.
- Prognostic factors in soft tissue tumor staging, in order, are presence of metastases, grade, size, and depth.
- The most common site of metastases from bone and soft tissue sarcomas is the lung.
- Chemotherapy is used to reduce or eliminate pulmonary metastases by inducing programmed cell death (apoptosis).
- Chemotherapy is commonly used with limb salvage surgery for osteosarcoma and Ewing sarcoma.
- Rhabdomyosarcoma and synovial sarcoma are two soft tissue tumors in which chemotherapy is used.
- Radiotherapy is used to reduce or eliminate local recurrence by inducing DNA damage.
- Radiation is used in combination with limb salvage surgery for soft tissue sarcomas and alone for metastatic bone disease, lymphoma, myeloma and in selected cases of Ewing sarcoma. Radiation therapy is associated with late stress fractures and postirradiation sarcoma.
- Radiation may be pre- or postoperative. Postoperative external beam irradiation yields equal local control rates, with a lower rate of postoperative wound complications but a higher incidence of postoperative fibrosis.
- Wide excision alone is used for chondrosarcoma, adamantinoma, parosteal osteosarcoma, and chordoma.
- Intralesional resection/curettage is used for GCT, ABC, NOF, LCH, osteoblastoma, and chondroblastoma.
- Benign bone tumors in children are most commonly an incidental finding.
- Different lesions occur in typical age ranges. Classic age associations are as follows:
  - Age <5 years: rhabdomyosarcoma, osteofibrous dysplasia, leukemia
  - Age <30 years: metaphyseal fibrous defect (nonossifying fibroma), enchondroma, unicameral bone cyst, osteosarcoma, Ewing sarcoma, osteoid osteoma, chondroblastoma, fibrous dysplasia, giant cell tumor
  - Older than 50 years: metastatic bone disease, fibrosarcoma, malignant fibrous histiocytoma, metastatic bone disease, myeloma, lymphoma, chondrosarcoma, Paget disease
- Some lesions have classic anatomic locations:
  - Anterior cortex of tibia: adamantinoma, osteofibrous dysplasia
  - Posterior cortex of distal femur: parosteal osteosarcoma, periosteal desmoid
  - Epiphysis: giant cell tumor, chondroblastoma, osteomyelitis (Brodie abscess), clear cell chondrosarcoma (femoral head)
  - Metaphysis: metaphyseal fibrous defect (nonossifying fibroma), aneurysmal bone cyst, giant cell tumor, osteosarcoma

- Diaphysis: Ewing sarcoma, fibrous dysplasia, eosinophilic granuloma (histiocytosis), multiple myeloma, osteoid osteoma/osteoblastoma, infection.
- Principles of biopsy:
  - Use longitudinal incisions and excise biopsy tracts if the lesion is malignant.
  - Approach lesions through muscles wherever possible. However, avoid functionally important structures and neurovascular structures.
  - Maintain meticulous hemostasis and—only in rare cases—use a small drain at the corner of the wound to prevent hematoma formation.
  - Frozen-section analysis should be performed intraoperatively to ensure that adequate diagnostic tissue is obtained.
  - Samples should be sent for bacteriologic analysis.
- There are four surgical margins of tumor excision: intralesional, marginal (through reactive zone), wide (including a cuff of normal tissue), and radical (entire tumor and its compartment, including surrounding muscles, ligaments, and connective tissues).
- Two essential criteria for limb salvage surgery: local control is at least equal to that of amputation; limb must be functional.
- Common tumor-associated genetic associations:
  - Osteosarcoma: tumor suppressor genes *Rb* (retinoblastoma) and *p53* (Li-Fraumeni syndrome)
  - Ewing sarcoma: t(11;22); gene product is EWS-FLI1
  - Synovial sarcoma: t(X;18); gene products are SYT-SSX1 and SYT-SSX2
  - Myxoid liposarcoma: t(12;16); gene product is FUS-CHOP
  - Alveolar rhabdomyosarcoma: t(2;13); gene product is PAX3-FKHR
  - Fibrous dysplasia: GNAS1-activating mutation of the GSα surface protein

SECTION 2 SOFT TISSUE TUMORS

I. Introduction

- The most common presentation of a soft tissue sarcoma is an enlarging painful or painless soft tissue mass.
- On MRI, most soft tissue malignancies are well defined (pseudocapsule) and heterogeneous. Any large (>5 cm) soft tissue mass deep to fascia should be considered a sarcoma.
- Soft tissue sarcomas are low intensity on T1-weighted sequences and high intensity on T2-weighted images.
- Metastatic workup includes CT scan of the chest. For liposarcoma, a CT scan of the abdomen and pelvis is required because of synchronous retroperitoneal liposarcoma.
- Unplanned removal of a soft tissue sarcoma is the most common error. Residual tumor may exist, and repeat excision should be performed.

TESTABLE CONCEPTS

- The most common soft tissue sarcoma of the hand is epithelioid sarcoma
- The most common soft tissue sarcoma of the foot is synovial sarcoma
- The primary site of metastases from soft tissue sarcomas is the lung. Lymphatic metastasis occurs in 5% of cases; tumors with a predilection for lymph node metastases are ESARC (epithelioid sarcoma, synovial sarcoma, angiosarcoma, rhabdomyosarcoma, clear cell sarcoma) and are the most common.

II. Tumors of Fibrous Tissue

- Extraabdominal desmoid tumors are "rock-hard." Patients with Gardner syndrome (familial adenomatous polyposis) have a 10,000-fold increased risk for such tumors. Estrogen receptor β inhibitors can be used for treatment. Wide-margin surgical resection is recommended, but local recurrence is common.
- Nodular fasciitis is a painful rapidly enlarging mass in a person 15 to 35 years of age. Perform a resection with a marginal margin.
- Undifferentiated pleomorphic sarcoma, previously known as *malignant fibrous histiocytoma,* is the most common malignant sarcoma of soft tissue in adults. It appears on MRI as a deep-seated inhomogeneous mass that has a low signal on T1-weighted images and a high signal on T2-weighted images. Treatment is with wide-margin local excision and adjuvant radiotherapy.
- Fibrosarcoma follows the same imaging patterns on MRI and has the same treatment as any high-grade soft tissue sarcoma, with limb salvage surgery, perioperative radiotherapy, and long-term surveillance.

III. Tumors of Fatty Tissue

- Lipomas appear on MRI as well-demarcated lesions with the same signal characteristics as those of mature fat on all sequences. On fat-suppression sequences, the lipoma has a uniformly low signal. Treatment of asymptomatic lesions is observation, whereas that for expanding or symptomatic lesions is marginal excision.
- Myxoid liposarcoma has a classic 12;16 chromosomal translocation.
- Liposarcoma is the second most common soft tissue sarcoma in adults. It virtually never occurs in the subcutaneous tissues. MRI demonstrates thicker and more irregular septa than for lipomas, which also appear bright on T2-weighted images.

IV. Tumors of Neural Tissue

- Neurofibromatosis can manifest with more than one neurofibroma or one plexiform neurofibroma, with café au lait spots, with Lisch nodules (melanocytic hamartomas in the iris), and with anterolateral tibial bowing.
- Patients with NF1 have a 5% chance of malignant degeneration of a neurofibroma to a malignant peripheral nerve sheath tumor (MPNST)
- MPNST follows the same imaging patterns on MRI and has the same treatment as any high-grade soft tissue sarcoma, with limb salvage surgery, perioperative radiotherapy, and long-term surveillance.

V. Tumors of Muscle Tissue

- Rhabdomyosarcoma is the most common soft tissue sarcoma in children. It most commonly manifests in the head and neck, genitourinary tract, and retroperitoneum. Extremity involvement is associated with the alveolar subtype; it involves a translocation of chromosomes 2 and 13, and the gene product is PAX3-FKHR.
- Rhabdomyosarcomas are sensitive to multi-agent chemotherapy. Wide-margin surgical resection and irradiation are used in treatment.
- Leiomyosarcoma follows the same imaging patterns on MRI and has the same treatment as any high-grade soft tissue sarcoma, with limb

salvage surgery, perioperative radiotherapy, and long-term surveillance.

VI. Vascular Tumors

- Hemangiomas are common in children and adults. Radiographs may reveal phleboliths. Multiple hemangiomas are associated with Maffucci syndrome.
- Angiosarcoma is associated with Stuart-Treves syndrome, cutaneous and lymph node metastases. It is treated with radiation and wide surgical excision.

VII. Synovial Disorders

- PVNS most commonly affects the knee, followed by the hip and shoulder. Recurrent atraumatic hemarthrosis with associated pain is the most common manifestation. Radiographs may show cystic erosions on both sides of the joint. Histologic study reveals highly vascular villi lined with plump hyperplastic synovial cells, hemosiderin-stained multinucleated giant cells, and chronic inflammatory cells.
- On both T1- and T2-weighted MRI sequences, PVNS appears as low-signal lesions.
- Treatment of PVNS is complete synovectomy except in highly localized forms of PVNS.

VIII. Other Rare Sarcomas

- Synovial sarcoma rarely arises from an intraarticular location. It most commonly occurs about the knee and is the most common sarcoma of the foot. Spotty mineralization on radiographs is highly characteristic.
- Histologic study of synovial sarcoma reveals a biphasic pattern: epithelial cells (resembling carcinoma) and spindle cells (resembling fibrosarcoma).
- All cells of synovial sarcomas have a translocation between chromosome 18 and the X chromosome that produces two gene fusion products (SYT-SSX1 and SYT-SSX2). Staining of tumor cells yield appearances positive for keratin and epithelial membrane antigen.
- Epithelioid sarcoma is the most common sarcoma of the hand. Lymph node metastases are common.
- Clear cell sarcoma is a melanin-producing lesion, but its cells have a t(12;22) translocation not present in melanoma cells. Lymph node metastases are common.

IX. Posttraumatic Conditions

- Sarcomas may spontaneously hemorrhage. On advanced imaging, the appearance of "hematomas" that do not have fascial plane tracking or subcutaneous ecchymosis suggests that the bleeding is contained by a pseudocapsule, and this finding is suspect for a sarcoma.
- For myositis ossificans, radiography reveals peripheral mineralization with a central lucent area.

SECTION 3 BONE TUMORS

II. Nomenclature

- Malignant bone tumors manifest most commonly with pain. This is in contrast to soft tissue tumors, which most commonly manifest as painless masses.
- Bone sarcomas metastasize primarily via the hematogenous route. The lung is the most common site of metastasis.
- Osteosarcoma and Ewing sarcoma commonly metastasize to other bone sites.

III. Bone-Producing Lesions

Osteoid Osteoma

- Classically manifests with increasing pain that is relieved by salicylates and other NSAIDs
- Radiographs show intensely reactive bone and a radiolucent nidus. CT scans provide better contrast between the lucent nidus and the reactive bone than does MRI.
- This lesion may produce a painful nonstructural scoliosis. This results in a curve with the osteoid osteoma on the concave side and is thought to result from marked paravertebral muscle spasm.
- CT scan–guided radiofrequency ablation is the dominant method of treatment; however, in 50% of patients treated with NSAIDs alone, the symptoms resolve.
- Osteoblastoma may be confused with osteoid osteoma. The self-limited nidus in osteoid osteoma is <1 cm and in osteoblastoma >2 cm, with unlimited growth and pain not relieved by salicylates/NSAIDS; both have the same histology.

Osteosarcoma

- Osteosarcoma is the most common malignant bone tumor in children.
- There are many types of osteosarcoma. The most commonly recognized are high-grade intramedullary osteosarcoma (ordinary or classic osteosarcoma), parosteal osteosarcoma, periosteal osteosarcoma, telangiectatic osteosarcoma, osteosarcoma occurring with Paget disease, and postradiation osteosarcoma.
- Classic high-grade intramedullary osteosarcoma is the most common type and usually occurs about the knee in children and young adults, but its incidence has a second peak in late adulthood.
  - Treated with neoadjuvant chemotherapy followed by resection of the tumor and adjuvant chemotherapy
  - Chemotherapy both kills the micrometastases that are present in 80% to 90% of affected patients at presentation and sterilizes the reactive zone around the tumor.
  - The rate of long-term survival is approximately 60% to 70%.
- Parosteal osteosarcoma is a low-grade osteosarcoma. It most commonly arises on the posterior aspect of the distal femur.
  - Histologic study reveals regularly arranged osseous trabeculae. Between the nearly normal trabeculae are slightly atypical spindle cells, which typically invade skeletal muscle found at the periphery of the tumor.
  - Treatment is by wide-margin surgical resection. Because this lesion is low grade, chemotherapy is not required.
  - Long-term survival is 95%.
- Periosteal osteosarcoma is a surface form that appears radiographically as a sunburst-type lesion resting on a saucerized cortical depression.
- Treatment is chemotherapy and wide surgical resection.
- Long-term survival is 85%.
- Telangiectatic osteosarcoma is described as a "bag of blood." Radiographic features are similar to those of aneurysmal bone cysts. Treatment is chemotherapy and wide surgical resection.

IV. Chondrogenic Lesions

Chondroma

- Benign cartilage tumors on the surface of bone are called *periosteal chondromas*. When they are in the medullary cavity, they are called *enchondromas*.
- Enchondromas appear radiographically as areas of stippled calcifications. Radiographic distinction between low-grade chondrosarcoma and enchondromas can be difficult. Serial plain radiographs show cortical bone changes or lysis of the previously mineralized cartilage in chondrosarcoma. Patients with chondrosarcoma have pain.
- Most enchondromas necessitate no treatment.
- Syndromes of multiple enchondromas include Ollier disease and Maffucci syndrome.
  - Ollier disease:
    - Multiple enchondromas
    - Dysplastic bones (particularly a shortened ulna)
    - 30% risk of transformation to chondrosarcoma
    - Random spontaneous mutation
  - Maffucci syndrome:
    - Multiple enchondromas and soft tissue hemangiomas (extremity and visceral)
    - 100% risk of malignancy

Osteochondroma

- Characteristic appearance is a surface lesion in which the cortex of the lesion and the underlying cortex are continuous and the medullary cavity of the host bone also flows into (is continuous with) the osteochondroma.
- When asymptomatic, these lesions are monitored with observation only.
- Malignant transformation into a secondary chondrosarcoma is rare, occurring in far fewer than 1% of cases. Thickness of the cartilage cap (>2 cm) may increase the risk of malignancy.
- Multiple hereditary exostosis is an autosomal disorder manifesting in childhood with multiple osteochondromas. Mutations are found in the *EXT1, EXT2,* and *EXT3* gene loci; the *EXT1* mutation is associated with a greater burden of disease and higher risk of malignancy. Approximately 5% to 10% of affected patients develop a secondary chondrosarcoma, which is low grade.

Chondroblastoma

- Centered in the epiphysis in young patients, usually with open physes
- Radiographs show a central region of bone destruction that is usually sharply demarcated from the normal medullary cavity by a thin rim of sclerotic bone. MRI shows edema far out of proportion to the lesion.
- Treatment is with curettage.

Chondrosarcoma

- Occurs in older persons; pelvis is the most common location.
- May be primary or arise secondarily in a previous lesion (enchondroma, osteochondroma)
- It may be extremely difficult to differentiate malignant cartilage on the basis of histologic features alone. The clinical, radiographic, and histologic features of a particular lesion must be considered in combination to avoid incorrect diagnosis.
- Treatment consists of wide-margin surgical resection.
- Chemotherapy is only used as an adjunct with dedifferentiated and mesenchymal types.
- Dedifferentiated chondrosarcoma is the most malignant cartilage tumor and has a bimorphic histologic and radiographic appearance. In typical cases, a high-grade spindle cell carcinoma is intimately associated with the low-grade cartilage component. Treatment is with wide-margin surgical resection and chemotherapy.

V. Fibrous Lesions

- Metaphyseal fibrous defect (nonossifying fibroma) is an extraordinarily common lesion, occurring in approximately 30% to 40% of children. The characteristic radiographic appearance is of a lucent lesion that is metaphyseal, eccentric, and surrounded by a sclerotic rim. The overlying cortex may be slightly expanded and thinned.

TESTABLE CONCEPTS

- Histologic study reveals a cellular fibroblastic connective tissue background, with the cells arranged in whorled bundles. Numerous giant cells and hemosiderin deposits are visible.
- Treatment is with observation. Curettage and bone grafting are indicated in symptomatic lesions with more than 50% of cortical involvement.

VII. Notochordal Tissue

- Chordoma is a malignant neoplasm that arises from primitive notochordal tissue.
- The most common location is the sacrococcygeal region, and second most common is the spheno-occipital region.
- CT scans show midline bone destruction.

IX. Hematopoietic Tumors

- Multiple myeloma is the most common primary tumor of bone.
- Light-chain subunits of immunoglobulins G and A are found in the urine.
- Radiographic appearance of multiple myeloma is punched-out lytic lesions.
- The classic histologic appearance is sheets of plasma cells that appear monoclonal with immunostaining. Well-differentiated plasma cells have an eccentric nucleus and a peripherally clumped, chromatic "clock face."
- Treatment is multimodal and includes chemotherapy, radiation therapy, and surgery.

X. Tumors of Unknown Origin

Giant Cell Tumor
- This is a benign but aggressive neoplasm that in rare cases metastasizes to the lung.
- It most commonly occurs about the knee and sacrum. Pain is referred to the involved joint.
- Radiographs demonstrate a purely lytic destructive lesion in the metaphysis that extends into the epiphysis and often borders the subchondral bone.
- Treatment is aimed at removal of the lesion with preservation of the involved joint. Curettage and subsequent reconstruction with subchondral bone grafts or methylmethacrylate is frequently performed.

Ewing Sarcoma
- This distinctive small round cell sarcoma occurs most often in children and young adults; most affected children are older than 5 years.
- Radiographs show a large destructive lesion that involves the metaphysis and diaphysis. Periosteum may be lifted off in multiple layers, which results in a characteristic but uncommon onionskin appearance.
- Immunohistochemistry studies reveal CD99 positivity. There is a consistent chromosomal translocation—t(11;22)—with the formation of a fusion protein (EWS-FLI1).
- Bone marrow biopsy is performed for staging purposes.
- Most lesions have traditionally been treated with chemotherapy and irradiation, but the role of surgery is evolving.
- Metastatic disease occurs in the lung (50%), bone (25%), and bone marrow (20%).

Adamantinoma
- Adamantinoma is rare tumor that classically manifests in the anterior cortex of the tibial diaphysis. Treatment is with wide-margin surgical resection.

XI. Tumorlike Conditions

Aneurysmal Bone Cyst
- This lesion is nonneoplastic but aggressive in its ability to destroy normal bone and extend into soft tissue.
- Characteristic radiographic finding is an eccentric, lytic, expansile area of bone destruction in the metaphysis. Fluid-fluid levels are characteristically visible on T2-weighted MRI.
- Treatment is with curettage and bone grafting. Local recurrence is common in children.

Unicameral Bone Cyst (Simple Bone Cyst)
- These most commonly involve the proximal humerus and manifest either with pain or with a pathologic fracture.
- Characteristic radiographic finding is symmetric cystic expansion with thinning of the involved cortices.
- Aneurysmal bone cyst in comparison with unicameral bone cyst (simplified):
  - Aneurysmal bone cyst manifests with pain and swelling. Unicameral bone cyst manifests with pathologic fracture and pain.
  - Aneurysmal bone cyst commonly occurs in the distal femur and proximal tibia. Unicameral bone cyst occurs in proximal humerus and proximal femur.
  - Aneurysmal bone cyst is eccentric and can expand wider than the growth plate. Unicameral bone cyst is central and does not expand wider than the growth plate.

Langerhans Cell Histiocytosis (Histiocytosis X)
- This lesion manifests as entities:
  - Eosinophilic granuloma
    - Monostotic
    - Highly destructive lesion with well defined margin
    - Self-limiting
  - Hand-Schüller-Christian disease
    - Multiple bone lesions and visceral disease (skull defects, exophthalmos, and diabetes insipidus)
  - Letterer-Siwe disease (a fulminating condition in young children)
    - Typically fatal

Fibrous Dysplasia
- This condition is caused by a genetic activating mutation of the GSα surface protein (GNAS1), which results in increased production of cAMP.
- Its radiographic appearance is variable but classically referred to as "ground glass."
- Its histologic appearance has been likened to "alphabet soup" and "Chinese letters."
- Autogenous cancellous bone grafting is never used for this disorder because the transplanted bone is quickly transformed into the woven bone of fibrous dysplasia.
- Polyostotic fibrous dysplasia is less common but more symptomatic and diagnosed earlier (before the age of 10 years) than monostotic fibrous dysplasia.
- Polyostotic fibrous dysplasia with endocrinopathy is termed *McCune-Albright syndrome* (café au lait spots, precocious puberty, and polyostotic fibrous dysplasia).

Osteofibrous Dysplasia
- This condition manifests in a similar manner but in children younger than 10 years.

Paget Disease
- This disorder is characterized by abnormal bone remodeling, which results in coarsened trabeculae and remodeled cortices.
- Medical treatment of Paget disease is aimed at retarding the activity of the osteoclasts. Agents used include diphosphonates and calcitonin.

- Fewer than 1% of patients with Paget disease develop malignant degeneration with the formation of a sarcoma within a focus of Paget disease.
- Paget sarcomas are deadly tumors with a poor prognosis (rate of long-term survival is < 20%).

XII. Metastatic Bone Disease

- Patients older than 40 with a destructive bone lesion should be presumed to have metastatic disease.
- History, physical, and radiographic staging (CT scan chest, abdomen, and pelvis) will identify the primary source of metastasis in 85% of cases; biopsy is necessary for definitive diagnosis.

- The five carcinomas most likely to metastasize to bone are those of the prostate, thyroid, breast, lung, and kidney.
- Pathologic fractures secondary to metastatic disease occur most commonly in the proximal femur.
- Histologic hallmark is the appearance of epithelial cells in a fibrous stroma; epithelial cells are often arranged in a glandular pattern.
- Bone destruction in metastatic disease results from activation of osteoclasts. Tumor cells secrete PTHrP, which stimulates RANKL release and results in activation of osteoclasts.

CHAPTER 10

REHABILITATION: GAIT, AMPUTATIONS, PROSTHESES, ORTHOSES, AND NEUROLOGIC INJURY

MaCalus Vinson Hogan and Ermias S. Abebe

CONTENTS

SECTION 1 GAIT

WALKING

■ **Definitions**
▥ **Walking** describes an energy-efficient process of synchronized repetitive lower limb motion used to move the body from one location to another while maintaining upright stability.
▥ During walking the motion of the two legs is coordinated so that one supporting foot is in contact with the ground at all times (single-limb support), with a period when both limbs are in contact with the ground (double-stance support) (Figure 10-1).

▥ A **step** is the distance between initial swing and initial contact of the same limb.
▥ **Stride** is the distance between initial contact and initial contact of the same limb (each stride compromises two steps) (Figure 10-2).
▥ **Velocity** defines steps per unit of time.
▥ **Running** differs from walking; involves a period when neither limb is in contact with the ground.
■ **Phases: normal gait cycle divided into stance and swing phases (See Figure 10-1).**
▥ Stance phase occupies **60%** of cycle
  • **Initial contact:** the instant reference foot contacts the ground

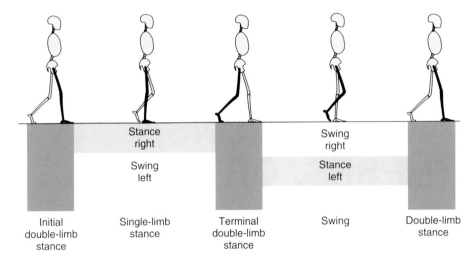

FIGURE 10-1 Subdivisions of gait and their relationships to the pattern of bilateral floor contact. (Adapted from Perry J: *Gait analysis: normal and pathological function,* New York, 1992, Slack Inc.)

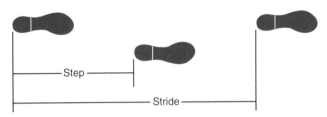

FIGURE 10-2 Step versus stride. (Adapted from Perry J: *Gait analysis: normal and pathological function,* New York, 1992, Slack Inc.)

- **Loading response** starts with initial contact of reference (swing) foot and ends with toe-off of contralateral foot.
- **Midstance** begins with toe-off of swing foot and ends when center of gravity is directly over body's center of gravity of the reference foot now in support phase.
- **Terminal stance** starts when center of gravity is directly over supporting (reference) foot and ends when this heel rises.
- **Preswing** begins with initial contact of contralateral limb and toe-off of reference foot.
- Swing phase is **40%** of the cycle.
  - **Initial swing** begins at toe-off, ending when knee is maximally flexed (60 degrees)
  - **Midswing** period from maximum knee flexion until tibia perpendicular/vertical to ground
  - **Terminal swing** begins from period when tibia is perpendicular/vertical to ground until initial contact of swing foot (Figure 10-3)
- Important characteristics of gait cycle
  - Normal gait cycle requires stance-phase stability, swing-phase ground clearance, correct position of the foot before initial contact, and energy-efficient step length and speed.
  - Throughout stance phase, **12% of time is spent in double-limb support.**
  - 38% of stance spent in single-limb support
  - During normal walking, the body's center of gravity is subject to both vertical and lateral displacement. Minimizing trunk displacement optimizes energy expenditure during bipedal gait.

- In the sagittal plane of the body, **vertical displacement follows a sinusoidal curve with amplitude of 5 cm.**
- Lateral displacement also follows a sinusoidal curve, with an amplitude of 6 cm.

GAIT DYNAMICS

- ■ The combined phases of gait contribute to an energy-efficient process by lessening excursion of the center of body mass.
- ■ Head, neck, trunk, and arms account for 70% of body weight.
- ■ The trunk center of gravity of body mass is located just anterior to t10, which is 33 cm above the hip joints in an individual of average height (184 cm).
- ■ The **body's line of gravity is anterior to s2** and provides a reference for the moment arm to the center of joint under consideration. the resulting gait pattern resembles a sinusoidal curve.

DETERMINANTS OF GAIT (MOTION PATTERNS)

- ■ In mechanical terms, there are six determinants of gaits that work in concert to minimize vertical and lateral displacement during normal walking. **these six determinants also represent the six degrees of freedom of gait and are defined by the flexion and extension of each of the three joints involved in gait (i.e., hip, knee, ankle [3 joints × 2 degrees of motion = 6]).**
- ■ Pelvic rotation: During forward motion, the pelvis externally rotates from initial contact to onset of preswing, and internally during preswing and swing. This symmetric net rotation minimizes the total vertical plane displacement needed for limb retraction and advancement in swing and stance.
- ■ **Pelvic list (tilt): non–weight-bearing contralateral side drops 5 degrees, reducing superior deviation.**
- ■ Knee flexion at loading: stance-phase limb is flexed 15 degrees to dampen the impact of initial loading.
- ■ Foot and ankle motion: through subtalar joint, damping of loading response occurs, leading to stability during midstance and efficiency of propulsion at push-off.
- ■ Knee motion: knee works together with foot and ankle to decrease necessary limb motion. The knee flexes at initial contact and extends at midstance.

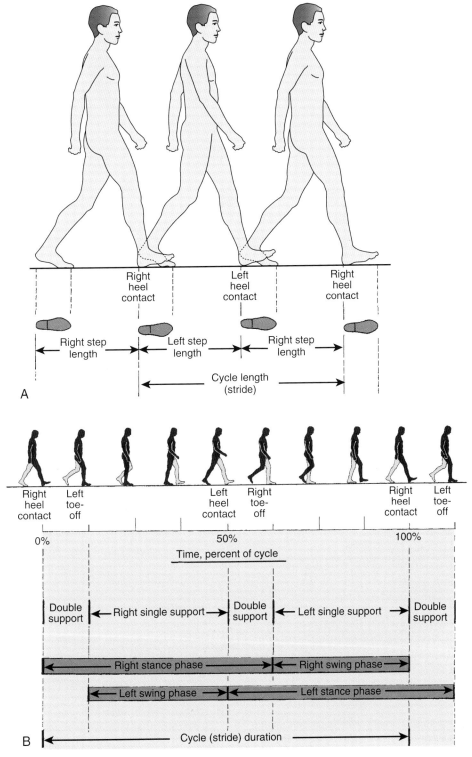

FIGURE 10-3 Dimensions of the walking cycle: distance **(A)** and time (duration) **(B).** (From Inman VT et al: *Human walking,* Baltimore, 1982, Williams & Wilkins, p 26.)

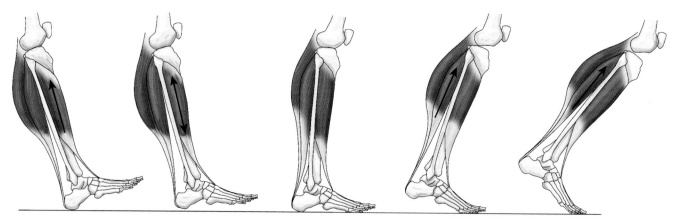

FIGURE 10-4 Effect of ankle motion, controlled by muscle action, on the pathway of the knee. The smooth and flattened pathway of the knee during the stance phase is achieved by forces acting from the leg on the foot. Foot slap is restrained during initial lowering of the foot; afterward, the plantar flexors raise the heel. (From Inman VT et al: *Human walking,* Baltimore, 1982, Williams & Wilkins, p 11.)

Table 10-1	Muscle Action and Function	
MUSCLE	**ACTION**	**FUNCTION**
Gluteus medius	Eccentric	Controls pelvic tilt (midstance)
Gluteus maximus	Concentric	Powers hip extension
Iliopsoas	Concentric	Powers hip flexion
Hip adductors	Eccentric	Control lateral sway (late stance)
Hip abductors	Eccentric	Control pelvic tilt (midstance)
Quadriceps	Eccentric	Stabilizes knee at heel strike
Hamstrings	Eccentric	Control rate of knee extension (stance)
Tibialis anterior	Concentric	Dorsiflexes ankle at swing
	Eccentric*	Slows plantar flexion rate during heel strike
Gastrocnemius-soleus	Eccentric	Slows dorsiflexion rate (stance)

*Predominant role.

Lateral pelvic displacement: relates to transfer of body weight onto limb. Length of motion is 5 cm over the weight-bearing limb, narrowing the base of support and increasing stance-phase stability.

MUSCLE ACTION

- Agonist and antagonist muscle groups work in concert during the gait cycle to effectively advance the limb through space.
- Hip flexors advance the limb forward during swing phase and are opposed during terminal swing, before initial contact by the decelerating action of the hip extensors.
- **Most muscle activity is *e*ccentric, which is muscle lengthening (aka *e*longation) while it contracts and allows an antagonist muscle to dampen the activity of an agonist and act as a "shock absorber" (Figure 10-4).**
- Isocentric contraction is muscle length's remaining constant during contraction (Table 10-1)
- Some muscle activity can be concentric, in which the muscle shortens to move a joint through space.

- Tibialis anterior has both eccentric (heel strike) and concentric (swing) muscle actions during normal gait

PATHOLOGIC GAIT

- Factors that lead to abnormal gait include muscle weakness, neurologic conditions, pain, limb deformity, and joint disease.
- Muscle weakness or paralysis: decreases ability to normally move a joint through space. Walking strategies develop on the basis of the specific muscle or muscle groups involved and the ability of the individual to acquire a substitution pattern to replace that muscle's action (Table 10-2).
- Neurologic conditions: may alter gait by producing muscle weakness, loss of balance, reduced coordination between agonist and antagonist muscle groups (i.e., spasticity), and joint contracture.
  - Hip scissoring is associated with overactive adductors, and knee flexion may be caused by hamstring spasticity.
  - Equinus deformity of the foot and ankle may result in steppage gait and backwards setting of the knee.
- **Pain in a limb: creates an antalgic gait pattern in which the individual shortens stance phase to lessen the time the painful limb is loaded.** The contralateral swing phase is more rapid.
- Joint abnormalities: alter gait by changing the range of motion of that joint or producing pain.
  - A hip and knee with arthritis may have joint contractures and reduced range of motion.
  - **An anterior cruciate–deficient knee has quadriceps-avoidance gait,** which represents a decreased quadriceps moment during **midstance.**
- Hemiplegia: characterized by prolongation of stance and double-limb support
  - Gait impairment may be excessive plantar flexion, weakness, and balance problems.
  - Associated problems are ankle equinus, limitation of knee flexion, and increased hip flexion.
  - Equinus deformity is surgically corrected 1 year after onset.

Table 10-2	Gait Abnormalities Caused by Muscle Weakness			
WEAK MUSCLE	**PHASE**	**DIRECTION**	**TYPE OF ABNORMAL GAIT**	**TREATMENT**
Gluteus medius	Stance	Lateral	Abductor lurch	Cane
Gluteus maximus	Stance	Backward	Lurch (hip hyperextension)	
Quadriceps	Stance	Forward	Lurch/back knee gait	AFO
Swing	Forward	Abnormal hip rotation		
Gastrocnemius/soleus	Stance	Forward	Flatfoot (calcaneal) gait	±AFO
Swing	Forward	Delayed heel rise		
Tibialis anterior	Stance	Forward	Foot drop/slap	AFO
Swing	Forward	Steppage gait		

±, With or without; *AFO,* ankle-foot orthosis.

- Crutches and canes: devices that ameliorate instability and pain, respectively
  - Crutches increase stability by providing two additional load points.
  - A cane helps shift the center of gravity to the affected side when the cane is used in the opposite hand. This decreases the joint reaction of the lower limb and reduces the pain. (**See Chapter 5, Adult Reconstruction.**)
- Arthritis: forces across knee may be four to seven times those of the body weight; 70% of load across knee occurs through medial compartment
- Water walking: significant decrease in joint moments and total joint contact forces as a result of buoyancy

SECTION 2 AMPUTATIONS

INTRODUCTION

- All or part of a limb may be amputated to treat peripheral vascular disease, trauma, tumor, infection, or a congenital anomaly.
- Should be considered a reconstructive procedure, often performed as an alternative to limb salvage
- A multidisciplinary team approach should be employed to help patient deal with psychologic implications and alteration of body self-image.

METABOLIC COST OF AMPUTEE GAIT

- Metabolic cost of walking is increased with proximal-level amputations and inversely proportional to length of residual limb and number of functional joints preserved.
- With a proximal amputation, patients have a decreased self-selected maximum walking speed.
- The higher the level of amputation (or the shorter the residual), the higher the oxygen consumption; thus the transfemoral amputee with peripheral vascular disease uses close to maximum energy expenditure during normal walking at self-selected velocity (Table 10-3). *(commonly tested exception to this rule: A Syme amputation is more energy efficient than the more distal midfoot [Chopart] amputation.)*
- Of note is that the required increase in energy expenditure for ambulation in bilateral transtibial amputation (41%) is less than that of unilateral transfemoral amputation (65%).

LOAD TRANSFER

- Soft tissue acts as an interface between the bone of the residual limb and prosthetic socket.
- The optimal soft tissue interface is composed of a well-attached mobile mass covering the bone end, and full-thickness skin that tolerates the direct pressures and "pistoning" (mobility) within the prosthetic socket.

- It is hard to achieve a perfect intimate fit. Some degree of mobility between the skin-and-muscle/prosthetic interface is desirable and eliminates the shear forces that produce tissue breakdown and ulceration.
- Load transfer (i.e., weight bearing) occurs either directly or indirectly.
- **Direct load transfer** (i.e., terminal weight bearing) occurs in knee (through-knee) or ankle disarticulation (Syme); intimacy of prosthetic socket is necessary only for suspension.
- **Indirect load transfer** occurs in transosseous amputation through a long bone (i.e., transfemoral or transtibial). The end of the stump does not take all the weight, and the load is transferred indirectly by the total contact method. The process requires an intimate fit of the prosthetic socket.

AMPUTATION WOUND HEALING

- Healing of amputation wounds depends on several factors, including nutrition, adequate immune status, and vascular supply. **transcutaneous partial pressure of oxygen [TcPO₂] is the factor most predictive of successful wound healing.**
- Nutrition and immune status:
  - Patients with malnutrition or immune deficiency have a high rate of wound failure or infection. A **serum albumin level of less than 3.5 g/dL** indicates that a patient is malnourished. An **absolute lymphocyte count of less than 1500/mm³** is a sign of immune deficiency.
  - If possible, amputation surgery should be delayed in patients with stable gangrene until these values can be improved by nutritional support, usually in the form of oral hyperalimentation.
  - In severely affected patients, nasogastric or percutaneous gastric feeding tubes are sometimes essential.

Table 10-3	Energy Expenditure for Ambulation		
AMPUTATION LEVEL	**ENERGY ABOVE BASELINE (%)**	**SPEED (m/min)**	**O₂ COST (mL/kg/m)**
Long transtibial	10	70	0.17
Average transtibial	25	60	0.20
Short transtibial	40	50	0.20
Bilateral transtibial	41	50	0.20
Transfemoral	65	40	0.28
Wheelchair	0-8	70	0.16

- When infection or severe ischemic pain necessitates urgent surgery, open amputation at the most distal viable level, followed by open-wound management, can be accomplished until wound healing can be optimized.

■ Vascular supply: oxygenated blood is a prerequisite for wound healing, and a hemoglobin concentration of **more than 10 g/dL** is necessary. Amputation wounds generally heal by collateral flow; thus, arteriography is rarely useful for predicting the success of wound healing.

- Standard Doppler ultrasonography helps measure arterial pressure and has been used as the measure of vascular inflow to predict the success of wound healing in the ischemic limb.
  - **An absolute Doppler pressure of 70 mm Hg was originally described as the minimum inflow pressure to support wound healing.**
  - The ischemic index is the ratio of the Doppler pressure at the level being tested to the brachial systolic pressure. It is generally accepted that patients require an **ischemic index of 0.5 or greater** at the surgical level to support wound healing. The ischemic index at the ankle (i.e., the ankle-brachial index) is the most accepted method for assessing adequate inflow to the ischemic limb.
  - In the normal limb, the area under the Doppler waveform tracing is a measure of flow. In at least 15% of patients with diabetes and peripheral vascular disease, those values are falsely elevated and not predictive because of the incompressibility and loss of compliance of calcified peripheral arteries. The ischemic index for toe pressure is more accurate in such patients and, if greater than 0.45, is usually predictive of adequate blood flow.
- Transcutaneous partial pressure of oxygen [TcPO₂] is the current gold standard for measurement of vascular inflow. It reflects the oxygen-delivering capacity of the vascular system to the level of contemplated surgery.
  - **Values higher than 40 mm Hg (ideally 45 mm Hg) are correlated with acceptable uneventful wound healing rates, without the false-positive values seen in noncompliant diseased peripheral vascular vessels.**
    - **Values higher than 30 mm Hg are also associated with healing.**
  - Pressures lower than 20 mm Hg are predictive of poor healing potential.

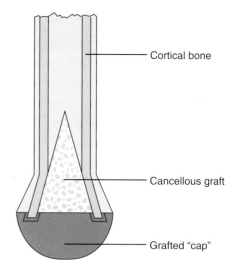

FIGURE 10-5 Diagram of the stump-capping procedure. The bone end has been split longitudinally. (Adapted from Bernd L et al: The autologous stump plasty: treatment for bony overgrowth in juvenile amputees, *J Bone Joint Surg Br* 73:203–206, 1991.)

PEDIATRIC AMPUTATION

■ Pediatric amputations are usually undertaken because of congenital limb deficiencies, trauma, or tumors.
■ Congenital amputations are the result of failure of formation.
■ Deficiencies are either longitudinal or transverse, with the potential for intercalary deficits.
■ Amputation is rarely indicated in congenital upper limb deficiency; even rudimentary appendages can be functionally useful. in the lower limb, amputation of an unstable segment may allow direct load transfer and enhanced walking (e.g., Syme amputation for fibular hemimelia).
■ In a growing child, disarticulations should be performed only when it is possible to maintain maximum residual limb length and prevent terminal bony overgrowth.
■ Such overgrowth usually occurs in the humerus, fibula, tibia, and femur, in that order; it is typical in diaphyseal amputations.
■ Numerous surgical procedures have been described to resolve this problem, but the best method is surgical revision of the residual limb with adequate resection of bone or autogenous osteochondral stump capping (Figure 10-5).

AMPUTATION AFTER TRAUMA

■ The grading scales for evaluating mangled extremities are not absolute predictors but provide reasonable guidelines for determining whether salvage is appropriate. **the extent of soft tissue injury has the greatest impact on the decision-making process.** outcomes following amputation are improved with psychological counseling and coping mechanisms.
■ Indications
  - The absolute indication for amputation after trauma is an ischemic limb with a vascular injury that cannot be repaired.
  - The guidelines for immediate or early amputation of mangled upper limbs differ from those for mangled lower limbs.
  - Early amputation in appropriate scenarios may prevent emotional, marital, financial, and addiction problems.

- Most grades IIIB and IIIC tibia fractures occur in young men who are laborers and may be more likely to return to gainful employment after amputation and prosthetic fitting.
- Sensation is not as crucial in the lower limb as in the upper limb, and current prostheses more closely approximate normal function.
- Disadvantages of limb salvage:
  - Severe open tibia fractures that are managed by limb salvage rather than amputation are often associated with high rates of mortality and morbidity as a result of infection, increased energy expenditure for ambulation, and decreased potential to return to work.
  - Limb salvage for Gustilo-Anderson grades IIIB and IIIC open fractures of the tibia and fibula generally has poor functional outcomes and multiple complications, and multiple surgical procedures may be needed.
  - The salvaged lower extremity with an insensate plantar weight-bearing surface (loss of posterior tibial nerve), with associated major functional muscle and bone loss, is unlikely to provide a durable limb for stable walking and is a potential source of early or late sepsis.
- Contraindications
  - Upper limb
    - When a salvaged upper limb remains sensate and has prehensile function, it will often function better than an amputated limb with prosthetic replacement.
    - Maintaining as much length as possible is the key to subsequent prosthetic use.
  - Lower limb
    - **Lack of plantar sensation is not an absolute indication to amputate, because it may result from neurapraxia, which has been shown to resolve over long-term follow-up.**
    - In the absence of other major factors, amputation should not be performed.

RISK FACTORS

- **Cognitive deficits**
- For patients to learn to walk with a prosthesis and care for their stumps and prostheses, they must possess certain cognitive capacities: memory, attention, concentration, and organization.
  - Patients with cognitive deficits or psychiatric disorders have a low likelihood of using prostheses successfully.
- **Diabetes**
- A majority of patients who undergo amputation are diabetic with inherent immune deficiency.
- The most important risk factors in amputation in diabetic patients are the presence of peripheral neuropathy and development of deformity and infection.
- **Peripheral vascular disease**
- Most of the other patients who undergo amputation are malnourished patients with peripheral vascular disease of sufficient magnitude to necessitate amputation, and their coronary and cerebral arteries are diseased.
- Appropriate consultation with physical therapy, social work, and psychology departments is important to determine rehabilitation potential.

- Medical consultation helps determine cardiopulmonary reserve. The vascular surgeon should determine whether vascular reconstruction is feasible or appropriate.
- The biologic amputation level is the most distal functional amputation level with a high probability of supporting wound healing.
  - This level is determined by the presence of adequate viable local tissue to construct a residual limb capable of supporting weight bearing, an adequate vascular inflow, and serum albumin level and a total lymphocyte count sufficient to aid surgical wound healing.
  - Selection of an appropriate amputation level is determined by combining the biologic amputation level with the rehabilitation potential in order to choose the level that maximizes ultimate functional independence.
- Morbidity and mortality rates have remained unchanged for several decades; 30% of patients with peripheral vascular disease die in the first 3 months after amputation, and nearly 50% die within the first year. The overall rate of prosthetic use is 43%.

MUSCULOSKELETAL TUMORS

- **Goal of surgery: to remove the tumor with adequate surgical margins**
- **Amputation versus limb salvage:**
- Advances in chemotherapy and allograft or prosthetic reconstruction have made limb salvage a viable option in extremity sarcomas.
- If adequate margins can be achieved with limb salvage, the decision can then be based on expected functional outcome.
- The advantage of limb salvage over amputation—with regard to energy expenditure to ambulate, quality-of-life measures, and function with activities of daily living—is controversial in the literature.
- Expected functional outcome should include the psychosocial and body image values associated with limb salvage.
  - These concerns should be balanced with improved task performance and lesser concern for late mechanical injury associated with amputation and fitting of prosthetic limbs.

TECHNICAL CONSIDERATIONS

- **Skin flaps should be of full thickness, and dissection between tissue planes should be avoided.**
- **Periosteal stripping should be sufficient to allow for bone transection; this minimizes regenerative bone overgrowth.**
- **Wounds should not be sutured under tension. muscles are best secured directly to bone at resting tension (myodesis) rather than to antagonist muscle (myoplasty).**
- **Stable residual limb muscle mass can improve function by reducing atrophy and providing a stable soft tissue envelope over the end of the bone.**
- **All transected nerves form neuromata. the nerve end should come to lie deep in a soft tissue envelope, away from potential pressure areas. Crushing the nerve may contribute to postoperative phantom or limb pain.**
- **Rigid dressings (postoperative) help reduce swelling, decrease pain, and protect the stump from trauma.**

- Early prosthetic fitting is done within 5 to 21 days after surgery in selected patients.

COMPLICATIONS

■ Pain
- Phantom limb sensation—the feeling that all or part of the amputated limb is present—occurs in almost all adults who have undergone amputation. It usually decreases with time.
- Phantom pain is a burning, painful sensation in the part having undergone amputation. It is diminished by prosthetic use, physical therapy, compression, and transcutaneous nerve stimulation.
- A common cause of residual pain is complex regional pain syndrome (reflex sympathetic dystrophy) or causalgia. Amputation should not be performed for this condition.
- Localized stump pain is often related to bony or soft tissue problems.
- Pain referred to the limb occurs in a frequent number of cases.

■ Edema
- Postoperative edema occurs after amputation. It may impede wound healing and place significant tension on the tissues.
- Rigid dressings and soft compression help reduce the problem.
- Swelling occurring after stump maturation is usually caused by poor socket fit, medical problems, or trauma.
- Persistence of chronic swelling may lead to verrucous hyperplasia, a wartlike overgrowth of skin with pigmentation and serous discharge.
  - It should be treated by a total-contact cast, which is changed regularly to accommodate the reduced edema.

■ Joint contractures
- These complications are usually noted as hip and knee flexion contractures, which can be produced at the time of surgery by anchoring of the respective muscles with the joints in a flexed position.
- They can be avoided by correct positioning of the amputated limb.

■ Wound failure to heal
- This outcome occurs most often in patients with diabetes and those with vascular disease.
- If the wound is not amenable to local care, wedge excision of soft tissue and bone, with closure and without tension, is the preferred treatment.

UPPER LIMB AMPUTATIONS (FIGURE 10-6)

■ Wrist disarticulation
- Advantages
  - Wrist disarticulation has two advantages over transradial amputation:
    - Preservation of more forearm rotation because of preservation of the distal radioulnar joint
    - Improved prosthetic suspension because of the flare of the distal radius
  - Effective function can be obtained at this level of amputation. Forearm rotation and strength are directly related to the length of the transradial (below-elbow) residual limb.

- Disadvantages
  - Wrist disarticulation provides challenges to the prosthetist that may outweigh its benefits.
  - Cosmetic disadvantage
    - The prosthetic limb is longer than the contralateral limb.
    - If myoelectric components are used, the motor and battery cannot be hidden within the prosthetic shank.

■ Transradial amputation or elbow disarticulation
- Complete brachial plexus injury and a nonfunctioning hand and forearm may be best treated by a transradial amputation or elbow disarticulation, which can be fitted with a prosthesis.
- The optimal length of the residual limb is at the junction of the middle and distal thirds of the forearm, where the soft tissue envelope can be repaired by myodesis and the components of a myoelectric prosthesis can be hidden within the prosthetic shank.
- Because the patient can maintain function at this level prosthetically only by being able to open and close the terminal device, retention of the elbow joint is essential.
- The length and shape of elbow disarticulation provides improved suspension and lever-arm capacity.
- To enhance suspension and reduce the need for shoulder harnessing, a 45- to 60-degree distal humeral osteotomy is performed.
- Gangrene of the upper limb, when it is not due to Raynaud or Buerger disease, represents end-stage disease, especially in diabetic patients. Such patients usually do not survive beyond 24 months.
  - Localized finger amputations are unlikely to heal. When surgery becomes necessary, amputation should be performed at the transradial level to achieve wound healing during the final months of the patient's life.

LOWER LIMB AMPUTATIONS (SEE FIGURE 10-6)

■ Toe and ray amputation
- Patients with ischemia generally ambulate with a propulsive gait pattern, so they suffer little disability from toe amputation.
- Patients with traumatic amputations lose some stability after toe amputation in the late-stance phase.
- The great toe should be amputated distal to the insertion of the flexor hallucis brevis.
- Isolated second-toe amputation should be performed just distal to the proximal phalanx metaphyseal flare, leaving the stump to act as a buttress and prevent late hallux valgus.
- Patients who undergo single outer (first or fifth) ray resections function well in standard shoes.
- Resection of more than one ray leaves the forefoot narrow, which is difficult to fit in shoes and often results in a late equinus deformity.
- Central ray resections are complicated by prolonged wound healing and rarely achieve better results than does midfoot amputation.

■ Transmetatarsal and Lisfranc tarsal-metatarsal amputation
- There is little functional difference in the outcomes of these two procedures. The long plantar flap acts as a myocutaneous flap and is preferred to fish-mouth dorsal-plantar flaps.

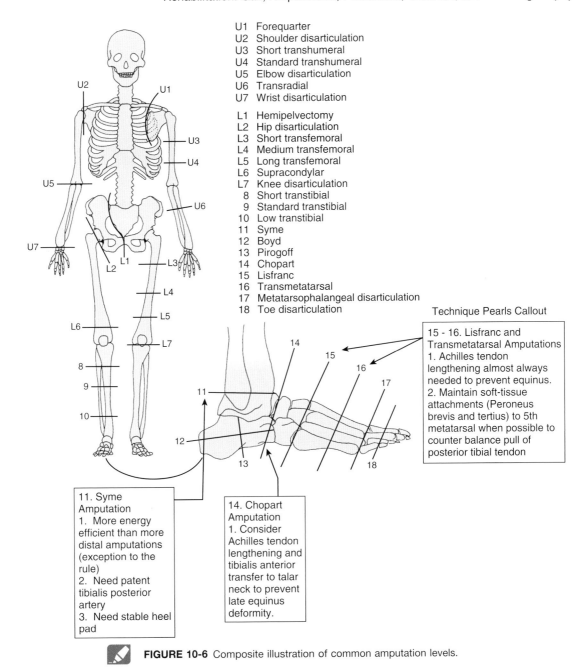

U1 Forequarter
U2 Shoulder disarticulation
U3 Short transhumeral
U4 Standard transhumeral
U5 Elbow disarticulation
U6 Transradial
U7 Wrist disarticulation

L1 Hemipelvectomy
L2 Hip disarticulation
L3 Short transfemoral
L4 Medium transfemoral
L5 Long transfemoral
L6 Supracondylar
L7 Knee disarticulation
8   Short transtibial
9   Standard transtibial
10 Low transtibial
11 Syme
12 Boyd
13 Pirogoff
14 Chopart
15 Lisfranc
16 Transmetatarsal
17 Metatarsophalangeal disarticulation
18 Toe disarticulation

Technique Pearls Callout

15 - 16. Lisfranc and Transmetatarsal Amputations
1. Achilles tendon lengthening almost always needed to prevent equinus.
2. Maintain soft-tissue attachments (Peroneus brevis and tertius) to 5th metatarsal when possible to counter balance pull of posterior tibial tendon

11. Syme Amputation
1. More energy efficient than more distal amputations (exception to the rule)
2. Need patent tibialis posterior artery
3. Need stable heel pad

14. Chopart Amputation
1. Consider Achilles tendon lengthening and tibialis anterior transfer to talar neck to prevent late equinus deformity.

FIGURE 10-6 Composite illustration of common amputation levels.

- Transmetatarsal amputation should be performed through the proximal metaphyses to prevent late plantar pressure ulcers under the residual bone ends.
- **Percutaneous Achilles tendon lengthening should be performed with transmetatarsal and Lisfranc amputations to prevent late development of equinus or equinovarus deformity.**
- Late varus deformity can be corrected with transfer of the tibialis anterior tendon to the neck of the talus.
  - The second tarsometatarsal joint should be osteotomized to preserve midfoot stability.
  - **The soft tissue at the fifth metatarsal base should be preserved because this represents the insertion site of peroneus brevis and tertius, which act as antagonists to the posterior tibial tendon.**

- Failure to preserve these tissues results in inversion during gait.
- Some authors have reported reasonable functional outcomes with hindfoot amputation (i.e., Chopart or Boyd amputations), but most experts recommend avoiding amputation at these levels if possible in patients with diabetes or vascular disease.
- Although children have been reported to function reasonably well, adults retain an inadequate lever arm and are prone to experience fixed equinus deformity of the heel if Achilles tendon lengthening and tibialis anterior tendon transfer are not performed.

■ **Ankle disarticulation (Syme amputation)**
- Often performed for forefoot trauma, this amputation allows direct load transfer and is rarely complicated by late residual limb ulcers or tissue breakdown.

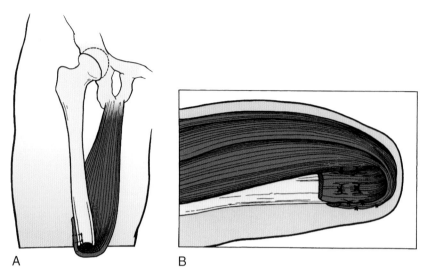

FIGURE 10-7 A, Diagram showing attachment of the adductor magnus to the lateral part of the femur. **B,** Diagram depicting attachment of the quadriceps over the adductor magnus. (From Gottschalk F: Transfemoral amputation. In Bowker J, Michael J, editors: *Atlas of limb prosthetics*, St Louis, 1992, Mosby–Year Book, pp 479–486.)

▓ It provides a stable gait pattern that rarely necessitates prosthetic gait training after surgery.

▓ **The outcome is more energy efficient than that of a midfoot amputation, despite the fact that it is a more proximal level** (*commonly tested exception to the rule of energy efficiency and amputations*).

▓ Surgery should be performed in one stage, even in ischemic limbs with insensate heel pads.

▓ **The posterior tibial artery must be patent to ensure healing.**

▓ The malleoli and metaphyseal flares should be removed from the tibia and fibula, but the remaining tibial articular surface should be retained to provide a resilient residual limb.

▓ The heel pad should be secured to the tibia either anteriorly through drill holes or posteriorly by securing the Achilles tendon.

■ Transtibial (below-knee) amputation

▓ **A long posterior myocutaneous flap is the preferred method of creating a soft tissue envelope, especially in patients with vascular disease, in as much as the direction of blood flow is from posterior to anterior.**

▓ The optimum bone length is at least 12 cm below the knee joint or longer if adequate amounts of the gastrocnemius or soleus muscle can be used to construct a durable soft tissue envelope.

▓ The posterior muscle should be secured to the beveled anterior tibia by myodesis.

▓ Rigid dressings are preferred during the early postoperative period, and early prosthetic fitting may be started 5 to 21 days after surgery if the residual limb is capable of transferring load and if the patient has a satisfactory physical reserve.

■ Knee disarticulation (through-knee amputation)

▓ The current technique involves the use of a long posterior flap, with the gastrocnemius muscle as end padding.
  • The alternative is to use sagittal skin flaps and cover the end of the femur with the gastrocnemius muscle to act as a soft tissue envelope end pad.

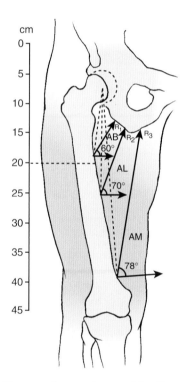

FIGURE 10-8 Diagram of moment arms of the three adductor muscles. Loss of the distal attachment of the adductor magnus (AM) will result in a loss of 70% of the adductor pull. *AB,* Adductor brevis; *AL,* adductor longus. (From Gottschalk FA et al: Does socket configuration influence the position of the femur in above-knee amputation? *J Prosthet Orthot* 2:94–102, 1989.)

▓ The patella tendon is sutured to the cruciate ligaments in the notch, leaving the patella on the anterior femur.
  • This level is generally used in nonambulatory patients who can support wound healing at the transtibial or distal level.
  • **Data from the Lower Extremity Assessment Project (LEAP) study have demonstrated that knee**

disarticulations resulted in the slowest walking speed and produced the least self-reported satisfaction.

▦ Knee disarticulation is muscle balanced and provides an excellent weight-bearing platform for sitting and a lever arm for bed-to-chair transfer. When this type of amputation is performed in a potential walker, it provides a residual limb for direct bed-to-chair transfer (end bearing).

■ **Transfemoral (above-knee) amputation**

▦ This form of amputation increases the energy cost for walking.

▦ Patients with transfemoral amputations who have peripheral vascular disease are unlikely to become efficient walkers; thus salvaging the limb at the knee disarticulation (transtibial level) is crucial for maintaining functional walking independence.

▦ With greater femoral length, the lever arm, suspension, and limb advancement are optimized. The optimum transfemoral bone length is 12 cm above the knee joint to accommodate the prosthetic knee.

▦ **Adductor myodesis** is important for maintaining femoral adduction during the stance phase to allow optimal prosthetic function (Figure 10-7).

▦ The major deforming force is toward abduction and flexion. Adductor myodesis at normal muscle tension eliminates the problem of adductor roll in the groin. Transecting the adductor magnus results in a loss of 70% of the adductor pull (Figure 10-8).

▦ Rigid dressings are difficult to apply and maintain at this level. Elastic compression dressings are used and may be suspended about the opposite iliac crest.

■ **Hip disarticulation**

▦ This procedure is infrequently performed, and of the patients who undergo this amputation, only a few make meaningful use of prostheses because of the high energy requirements for walking.

▦ Patients who have suffered trauma or who have tumors occasionally use the prosthesis for limited activity. These patients sit in their prostheses and must use the torso to achieve momentum for "throwing" the limb forward to advance it.

SECTION 3 PROSTHESES

UPPER LIMB

■ **Upper limb biomechanics**

▦ The shoulder provides the center of the radius of the functional sphere of the upper limb. The elbow acts as the caliper to position the hand at a workable distance from that center in order to perform its tasks.

▦ In a normal arm, tasks performed with the use of multiple joint segments usually occur simultaneously, whereas upper limb prostheses perform these same tasks sequentially; thus joint and residual-limb-length salvage is directly correlated with functional outcome.

▦ Motion at the retained joints is essential for maximizing that function.

▦ Residual limb length is important for suspending the prosthetic socket and providing the lever arm necessary to "drive" the prosthesis through space.

■ **Benefits of limb salvage**

▦ Limb salvage is more important for the upper limb, where sensation is crucial for function.
  • An insensate prosthesis provides less function than a partially sensate, partially functional salvaged limb.

■ **Timing of prosthetic fitting**

▦ Prosthetic fitting should be undertaken as soon as possible after amputation, even before complete wound healing has occurred.

▦ For transradial amputation, the outcomes for prosthetic limb use vary from 70% to 85% when prosthetic fitting occurs within 30 days of amputation, in contrast to less than 30% when the fitting starts later.

■ **Types of prostheses for different levels of amputation**

▦ Midlength transradial amputation:
  • Myoelectric prostheses provide good cosmesis and are used for sedentary work. They can be used in any position, including overhead activity, and are the most successful for patients with midlength transradial amputations, for whom only the terminal device needs to be activated.

  • Body-powered prostheses are used for heavy labor. The terminal device is activated by shoulder flexion and abduction. For optimal mechanical efficiency of figure-8 harnesses, the harness ring must be at the spinous process of C7 and slightly to the nonamputated side.

▦ Elbow disarticulation and transhumeral (above-elbow) amputations
  • When the residual forearm is so short that it precludes an adequate lever arm for driving the prosthesis through space, supracondylar suspension (Munster socket) and step-up hinges can be used to augment function.
  • In elbow disarticulation and transhumeral (above-elbow) amputations, two motions are needed to develop prehension; thus these levels of amputation have significantly less efficient outcomes, and the prostheses are heavier than they are for amputation at the transradial level.
  • Elbow flexion and extension are controlled by shoulder extension and depression. Amputations at these levels provide minimal function because the patient must sequentially control two joints and a terminal device.
  • The best function with the least weight at the lowest cost is provided by hybrid prosthetic systems in which myoelectric, traditional body-powered, and body-driven switch components are combined.

▦ Proximal transhumeral and shoulder disarticulation amputations
  • When the lever-arm capacity of the humerus is lost in proximal transhumeral or shoulder disarticulation amputations, limited function can be achieved with a manual universal shoulder joint positioned with the opposite hand and combined with lightweight hybrid prosthetic components.

LOWER LIMB

- ■ **Prosthetic feet: Several designs are available, divided into five classes:**
  - ▥ Single-axis foot
    - • Based on an ankle hinge that provides dorsiflexion and plantar flexion
    - • Disadvantages include poor durability and cosmesis.
  - ▥ Solid-ankle, cushioned-heel (SACH) foot
    - • This has been the standard for decades and was appropriate for general use in patients with low levels of activity.
    - • It may lead to overload problems on the nonamputated foot, and its use is being discontinued.
  - ▥ Dynamic-response foot
    - • Selection of the correct dynamic prosthetic foot depends on patient's height, weight, activity level, access for maintenance, cosmesis, and funding.
    - • The dynamic-response foot prostheses, including the Seattle foot, Carbon Copy II/III, and Flex Foot, allow amputees to undertake most normal activities (Figure 10-9).
    - • Dynamic-response foot prostheses may be grouped into articulated and nonarticulated.
      - • **Articulated dynamic-response foot**
        - • Allow inversion/eversion and rotation of the foot and are **useful for activities on uneven surfaces**
        - • May absorb loads and decrease shear forces to the residual limb
        - • Most dynamic-response feet have a flexible keel and are the standard for general use (Figure 10-10). The keel deforms under load, becoming a spring and allowing dorsiflexion, thereby decreasing loading on the normal side and providing a springlike response for push-off.
        - • Posterior projection of the keel provides a response at heel strike for smooth transition through the stance phase. A sagittal split allows for moderate inversion or eversion.

- • **Nonarticulated dynamic-response foot**
  - • These can have short or long keels. Shortened keels are not as responsive and are indicated for the moderate-activity ambulator, whereas long keels are for very high-demand activities.

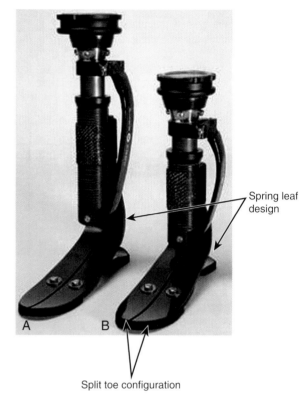

FIGURE 10-9 A, Flex Foot with carbon-fiber leaf and posterior projection of the keel for heel strike. **B,** Flex Foot with split-toe configuration and spring-leaf design. (Courtesy Flex Foot, Inc, Aliso Viejo, California.)

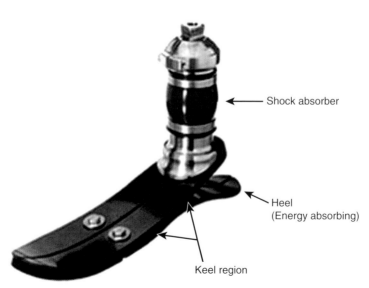

FIGURE 10-10 Ceterus prosthetic foot with leaf spring and shock absorber. (Courtesy Ossur Americas, Aliso Viejo, California.)

- Separate prosthetic feet for running and lower-demand activities may be indicated.

■ **Prosthetic shanks**

▥ These shanks provide the structural link between or among prosthetic components.

▥ Two varieties exist: endoskeletal, with a soft exterior and load-bearing tubing inside (the most common), and exoskeletal, with a hard load-bearing exterior shell.

▥ Rotator units are sometimes added for patients involved in twisting activities (e.g., golf) or for sitting.

■ **Prosthetic knees** (Table 10-4)

▥ Prosthetic knees provide controlled knee motion in the prosthesis.

▥ These components are used in transfemoral and knee disarticulation and are chosen on the basis of the patient's needs.

▥ Alignment stability (position of the prosthetic knee in relation to the patient's line of weight bearing) is important in the design and fitting of prosthetic knees. Placing the knee center of rotation posterior to the line of weight bearing allows control in the stance phase but makes flexion difficult. Alternatively, with the knee center of rotation anterior to the line of weight bearing, flexion is made easier but at the expense of control.

▥ Only the polycentric knee component offers the possibility of both options by having a variable center of rotation. Six basic types of knees are available:

- Polycentric (four-bar linkage) knee: has a moving instant center of rotation that provides for different stability characteristics during the gait cycle and may allow increased flexion for sitting. It is recommended for patients with transfemoral amputations, those with knee disarticulations, and those with bilateral amputations (Figure 10-11).

Table 10-4	Characteristics of Various Prosthetic Knees			
	CHARACTERISTICS			
KNEE TYPE	**ACTION**	**ADVANTAGES**	**DISADVANTAGES**	
Constant-friction	Limits flexion	Durable, long resistance	Decreased stability	
Variable- friction	Varies with flexion	Variable cadence	Poor durability	
Stance-control	Friction brake	Stability during stance	Poor durability, difficult to use on stairs	
Polycentric	Instant center moves	Stable, increased flexion	Poor durability, heavy	
Manual locking	Must unlock to sit	Maximum stability	Abnormal gait	
Fluid-control	Deceleration in swing	Variable cadence	Weight, cost	

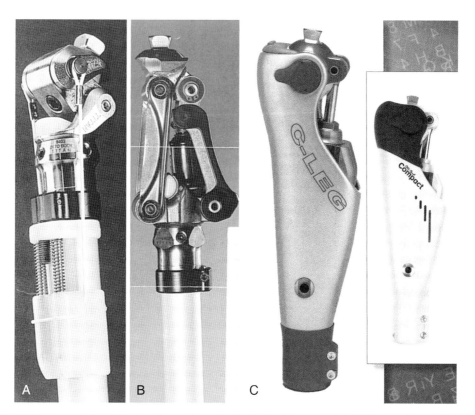

FIGURE 10-11 A, Stance-phase control unit for transfemoral prosthesis. **B,** Modular endoskeletal four-bar knee with hydraulic swing-phase control unit. **C,** Microprocessor knee unit. (Courtesy Otto Bock Orthopaedic Industries, Minneapolis.)

- Stance-phase control (weight-activated [safety]) knee: functions like a constant-friction knee during the swing phase but "freezes" by application of high-friction housing when weight is applied to the limb. Its use is reserved primarily for older patients, those with very proximal amputations, or those walking on uneven terrain.
- Fluid-control (hydraulic and pneumatic) knee: allows adjustment of cadence response by changing resistance to knee flexion by means of a piston mechanism. The design prevents excessive flexion and is extended earlier in the gait cycle, allowing a more fluid gait. The knee is best used in active patients who prefer greater utility and variability at the expense of more weight.
- Constant-friction knee: essentially a hinge designed to dampen knee swing by a screw or rubber pad that applies friction to the knee bolt. It is designed for general utility and may be used on uneven terrain. It is the most common knee prosthesis for children. Its major disadvantages are that it allows only single-speed walking and relies solely on alignment for stance-phase stability; therefore it is not recommended for older, weaker patients.
- Variable-friction (cadence control) knee: allows resistance to knee flexion to increase as the knee extends by employing a number of staggered friction pads. This knee allows walking at different speeds but is neither durable nor available in endoskeletal systems.
- Manual locking knee: consists of a constant-friction knee hinge with a positive lock in extension that can be unlocked to allow functioning similar to that of a constant-friction knee. The knee is often left locked in extension for more stability. It has limited indications and is used primarily in weak, unstable patients, those just learning to use prostheses, and blind amputees.

■ Suspension systems: Suspension is provided in modern lower extremity prostheses primarily through socket design and suspension sleeves. straps and belts are usually used for supplementation.

■ Sockets are prosthetic components designed to provide comfortable functional control and even pressure distribution on the amputated stump. Sockets can be hard (rigid or unlined) or soft (lined with a resilient material and/or flexible shell). In general, the suction-and-socket contour is the primary suspension modality used. The suction socket provides an airtight seal by means of a pressure differential between the socket and atmosphere. Total-contact support of the residual limb surface prevents edema formation. In total-contact support, different areas have different loads.

- Transfemoral or quadrilateral sockets in which the posterior brim provides a shelf for the ischial tuberosity have been the classic suspension system. **However, the design made it difficult to keep the femur in adduction.** Narrow mediolateral (ischial containment) transfemoral sockets distribute the proximal and medial concentrations of forces more evenly, as well as enhance rotational control of the socket. The ischium and ramus are contained within the socket of these more anatomic, comfortable, and functional designs. **Socket design for transfemoral prostheses allows for 10 degrees of adduction of the femur (to stretch the gluteus medius, allowing adequate strength for midstance stability) and 5 degrees of flexion (to stretch the gluteus maximus, allowing greater hip extension).**

- Transtibial sockets: weight bearing by the patella tendon loads all areas of the residual limb that tolerate weight (i.e., patella tendon, medial tibial flare, anterior compartment, gastrocnemius muscle, and fibular shaft). Weight-intolerant areas include the tibial crest and tubercle, distal fibula and fibular head, peroneal nerve, and hamstring tendons. The patella tendon–bearing supracondylar/suprapatellar socket has proximal extensions over the distal femoral condyles and patella. Total-surface weight bearing is different from total-contact weight bearing. With total-surface weight bearing, pressure is distributed more equally across the entire surface of the transtibial residual limb, and the interface liner material in the socket is important. Urethane liners cope with multidirectional forces by easy material distortion and recovery to the original shape. Another liner is made of mineral oil gel with reinforcing fabric. These liners provide good shock absorption and reduce skin problems. The anterior wedge shape of the socket helps control rotation of the socket on the limb.
- A supracondylar suspension system is recommended when the residual limb is less than 5 cm long. The socket is designed to increase the surface area for pressure distribution by raising the medial and lateral socket brim. A wedge may be used in the soft liner.
- A supracondylar-suprapatellar suspension system encloses the patella in the socket and has a bar proximal to the patella. This design also provides mediolateral stability, and no additional cuffs or straps are required. Corset-type prostheses can lead to verrucous hyperplasia and thigh atrophy, but they reduce socket loads, control the direction of swing, and provide some additional weight support.

■ **In prosthetic sleeves, friction and negative pressure are used for suspension.** The sleeves fit snugly to the upper third of the tibial prosthesis and are made from neoprene, latex, silicone, or thermoplastic elastomers.
- Transtibial suspension
  - Gel liner suspension systems with a locking pin constitute the preferred method of suspension.
  - Liners are made from silicone, urethane, or thermoplastic elastomer.
  - The sleeve rolls onto the stump, and the locking pin is then locked into the socket (Figure 10-12).
  - The liners provide suspension through suction and friction and act as the socket interface.
  - Prosthetic socks worn over the liner accommodate volume fluctuation.
  - This suspension allows unrestricted knee flexion and minimal piston action.
- Transfemoral suspension:
  - Vacuum (suction) suspension is frequently used.
  - It relies on surface tension, negative pressure, and muscle contraction.
  - A one-way expulsion valve helps maintain negative pressure, and no belts or straps are required. Stable body weight is required for this intimate fit.
  - Roll-on silicone or thermoplastic liners may be used with or without locking pins.

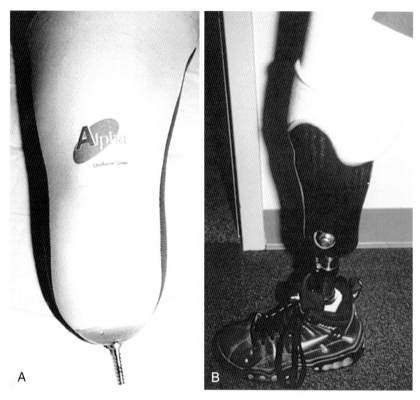

FIGURE 10-12 A, Gel liner suspension with locking pin. **B,** Transtibial prosthesis with liner locked in place.

- The total-elastic suspension belt, which is made of neoprene, fastens around the waist and spreads over a larger surface area (Figure 10-13). It is an excellent auxiliary suspension.

■ **Common prosthetic problems** (Table 10-5)

▨ Transtibial prostheses
- Pistoning during the swing phase of gait is usually caused by an ineffective suspension system.
- Pistoning in the stance phase results from a poor socket fit or volume changes in the stump (a change in thickness of the stump sock may be needed).
- Alignment problems are common (see Table 10-5).
- Pressure-related pain or redness should be corrected, with relief of the prosthesis in the affected area.
- Other problems may be related to the foot: too soft a heel results in excessive knee extension, whereas too hard a heel causes knee flexion and lateral rotation of the toes.

▨ Transfemoral prostheses
- Excessive prosthetic length and weak hip abductors or flexors can lead to circumduction, vaulting, and lateral trunk bending.
- Hip flexion contractures and insufficient anterior socket support can lead to excessive lumbar lordosis (compensatory).
- Inadequate prosthetic knee flexion can lead to a terminal knee snap.
- A medial whip (heel-in, heel-out) can be caused by a varus knee, excessive external rotation of the knee axis, or muscle weakness.
- A lateral whip (heel-out, heel-in) is caused by the opposite problem: valgus knee, internal rotation at knee, or muscle weakness. Table 10-6 summarizes common transfemoral prosthetic gait problems.

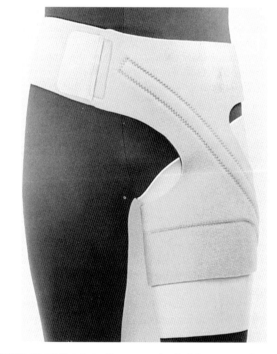

FIGURE 10-13 Total-elastic suspension belt for suspending a transfemoral socket. (Courtesy Syncor Manufacturers, Green Bay, Wisconsin.)

▨ Stair climbing
- In general, amputees ascend stairs by leading with the normal limb and descend by leading with the prosthetic limb ("the good goes up and the bad comes down").

✎ Table 10-5	Prosthetic Foot Gait Abnormalities
FOOT POSITION	**GAIT ABNORMALITY**
Inset	Varus strain, pain (proximomedial, distolateral), circumduction
Outset	Valgus strain, pain (proximolateral, distomedial), broad-based gait
Forward placement	Increased knee extension (patellar pain) but stable
Posterior placement	Increased knee flexion/instability
Dorsiflexed foot	Increased patellar pressure
Plantar-flexed foot	Drop-off, patellar pressure

Table 10-6	Transfemoral Prosthetic Gait Abnormalities
GAIT ABNORMALITY	**PROSTHETIC PROBLEM**
Lateral trunk bending	Short prosthesis, weak abductors, poor fit
Abducted gait	Poor socket fit medially
Circumducted gait	Prosthesis too long, excess knee friction
Vaulted gait	Prosthesis too long, poor suspension
Foot rotation at heel strike	Heel too stiff, loose socket
Short stance phase	Painful stump, knee too loose
Knee instability	Knee too anterior, foot too stiff
Mediolateral whip	Excessive knee rotation, tight socket
Terminal snap	Quadriceps weakness, unsure patient
Foot slap, knee hyperextension	Heel too soft
Knee flexion	Heel too hard
Excessive lordosis	Hip flexion contracture, socket problems

SECTION 4 ORTHOSES

INTRODUCTION

- The primary function of an orthosis is control of the motion of certain body segments.
- Orthoses are used to protect long bones or unstable joints, support flexible deformities, and occasionally substitute for a functional task. they may be static, dynamic, or a combination of these.
- With few exceptions, orthoses are not indicated for correction of fixed deformities or for spastic deformities that cannot be easily controlled manually.
- Orthoses are named according to the joints they control and the method used to obtain/maintain that control (E.G., a short-leg, below-the-knee brace is an ankle-foot orthosis [AFO]).

SHOES

- Specific shoes can be used by themselves or in conjunction with foot orthoses.
- Extra-depth shoes with a high toe box designed to dissipate local pressures over bony prominences are recommended for diabetic patients.
- The plantar surface of an insensate foot is protected by use of a pressure-dissipating material. a paralytic or flexible foot deformity can be controlled with more rigid orthoses.
- Sach heels absorb the shock of initial loading and lessen the transmission of force to the midfoot as the foot passes through the stance phase.
- **A rocker sole can lessen the bending forces on an arthritic or stiff midfoot during midstance as the foot changes from accepting the weight-bearing load to pushing off.** It is useful in treating metatarsalgia, hallux rigidus, and other forefoot problems. For the rocker sole to be effective, it must be rigid.
- Medial heel out-flaring is used to treat severe flatfoot of most causes. A foot orthosis is also necessary.

FOOT ORTHOSES

- Most foot orthoses are used to align and support the foot; prevent, correct, or accommodate foot deformities; and improve foot function.

- Three main types of foot orthosis are used: rigid, semirigid, and soft.
  - Rigid foot orthoses limit joint motion and stabilize flexible deformities.
  - Semirigid orthoses have hinges and allow dorsiflexion plantar flexion of the ankle, or both.
  - Soft orthoses have the best shock-absorbing ability and are used to accommodate fixed deformities of the feet, especially neuropathic, dysvascular, and ulcerative disorders.

ANKLE-FOOT ORTHOSES

- The most commonly prescribed lower limb orthosis (AFO) is used to control the ankle joint. It may be fabricated with metal bars attached to the shoe or thermoplastic elastomer. The orthosis may be rigid, preventing ankle motion, or it can allow free or spring-assisted motion in either plane.
- After hindfoot fusions, the primary orthotic goals are absorption of the ground reaction forces, protection of the fusion sites, and protection of the midfoot.
- The thermoplastic foot section achieves mediolateral control with high trimlines.
- When subtalar motion is present, an articulating AFO permits motion by a mechanical ankle joint design.
- Primary factors in selection of an orthotic joint include range of motion, durability, adjustability, and the biomechanical effect on the knee joint. A posterior leaf-spring AFO provides stability in stance phase.

KNEE-ANKLE-FOOT ORTHOSIS

- The knee-ankle-foot orthosis (KAFO) extends from the upper thigh to the foot. It is generally used to control an unstable or paralyzed knee joint. It provides mediolateral stability with the prescribed amounts of flexion or extension control.
- A subset of KAFOs are knee orthoses, which can be made of elastic for the treatment of patellar disease or made of metal and plastic for the treatment of an unstable anterior cruciate ligament.

HIP-KNEE-ANKLE-FOOT ORTHOSIS

- The hip-knee-ankle-foot orthosis (HKAFO) provides hip and pelvic stability but is rarely used by paraplegic adults because of the cumbersome nature of the orthosis and the magnitude of effort in achieving minimum gains.
- In experimental studies, it is being used in conjunction with implanted electrodes and the computerized functional stimulation of paraplegic patients.
- In children with upper-level lumbar myelomeningocele, the reciprocating gait orthoses are modified HKAFOs that can be used for standing and simulated walking.

ELBOW ORTHOSES

- Hinged-elbow orthoses provide minimum stability in the treatment of ligament instability.
- Dynamic spring-loaded orthoses have been successfully used in the treatment of flexion and extension contractures.

WRIST-HAND ORTHOSES (WHOs)

- The most common use of wrist and hand orthoses today is for postoperative care after injury or reconstructive surgery. these devices are static or dynamic.
- The opponens splint is successful in prepositioning the thumb but impairs tactile sensation.
- Wrist-driven hand orthoses are used in lower cervical quadriplegics. they may be body powered by tenodesis action or motor driven. Weight and cumbersomeness are the major limiting factors.

FRACTURE BRACES

- Fracture bracing remains a valuable treatment option for isolated fractures of the tibia and fibula.
- Prefabricated fracture orthoses can be used in simple foot and ankle fractures, ankle sprains, and simple hand injuries.

PEDIATRIC ORTHOSES

- Many dynamic orthoses are used by children to control motion without total immobilization.
- The Pavlik harness has become the mainstay for early treatment of developmental dislocation of the hip.
- Several dynamic orthoses have been used for containment in Perthes disease.

SPINE ORTHOSES

- Cervical spine:
- Numerous orthoses are used to immobilize the cervical spine.
- Effective immobilization ranges from the various types of collars, to posted orthoses that gain purchase about the shoulders and under the chin, to the halo vest, which achieves the most stability by the nature of its fixation into the skull.
- Thoracolumbar spine:
- Orthoses used to mechanically stabilize the back, thus reducing back pain, rely on increasing body cavity pressure.
- Three-point orthoses achieve their control by the length of their lever arm and the subsequent limitation of motion.

SECTION 5 SURGERY FOR STROKE AND CLOSED-HEAD INJURY

INTRODUCTION

- The orthopaedic surgeon can play a role in early management of adult-acquired spasticity secondary to stroke or closed-head brain injury when spasticity interferes with the rehabilitation program.
- Nonsurgical treatment:
  - Interventional modalities may include orthotic prescription, serial casting, and motor point nerve blocks with short-acting (bupivacaine HCl) or long-acting (phenol 6% in glycerol or botulinum toxin type A [Botox]) agents.
  - Splinting a joint (e.g., the ankle) in the neutral position is not sufficient to prevent development of a contracture (e.g., equinus contracture).
  - When functional joint ranging is insufficient to control the deformity, intervention is often indicated.
  - Local anesthetic injection to the posterior tibial nerve or sciatic nerve before casting relieves pain and allows for maximum correction of the deformity.
  - Open nerve blocks may be warranted to avoid injecting mixed nerves with large sensory contributions.
- Prerequisites for surgical treatment:
  - Surgical intervention in adult-acquired spasticity should be delayed until the patient achieves maximal spontaneous motor recovery (6 months for stroke and 12 to 18 months for traumatic brain injury).

- When patients reach a plateau in functional progress or the deformity impedes further progress, intervention may be considered.
- Invasive procedures in this population should be an adjunct to a standard functional rehabilitation program, not an alternative.
- When surgery is considered as a method of improving function, patients should be screened for cognitive deficits, motivation, and body image awareness.
  - Patients should not be confused and must have adequate short-term memory and the capacity for new learning.
  - In addition to specific cognitive strengths, motivation is necessary for patients to use functional gains and participate in their rehabilitation program.
  - Body image awareness is essential for surgical intervention to become meaningful and potentially beneficial. Patients who lack awareness of a limb or its position in space should undergo therapy directed toward ameliorating these deficits before undergoing surgical intervention.

LOWER LIMB

- **Balance is the best predictor of a patient's ability to ambulate after acquired brain injury.** the mainstay of treatment for the dynamic ankle equinus component of this gait deviation is to achieve ankle stability in the neutral position during initial floor contact (i.e., initial contact and stance) as well as floor clearance during the swing phase.

■ An adjustable AFO with ankle dorsiflexion and a plantar flexion stop at the neutral position is often used during the recovery period, followed by a rigid AFO once the patient has reached a plateau in recovery.

■ When the dynamic equinus overcomes the holding power of the orthosis and patients are unable to keep the brace in place, motor-balancing surgery is indicated.

■ **The equinus deformity is treated by percutaneous lengthening of the Achilles tendon.**

■ The dynamic varus-producing force in adults is the result of out-of-phase tibialis anterior muscle activity during the stance phase. This dynamic varus deformity is corrected by either split or complete lateral transfer of the tibialis anterior muscle.

UPPER LIMB

■ There is a paucity of literature dealing with acquired spasticity in the upper limb. invasive intervention can be considered for nonfunctional and functional goals.

▦ Nonfunctional goals: surgical release of static contracture; generally performed to complement nursing care or hygiene when the fixed contracture or spastic component results in skin maceration or breakdown.

▦ Functional goals: one functional use of static contracture release is to improve upper extremity "tracking" (i.e., arm swing) during walking. Most upper extremity surgery performed in this patient population has the goal of increasing prehensile hand function. The goal may be simply to improve placement, enabling use of the hand as a "paperweight," or to achieve improved fine motor control. In patients with prehensile potential, surgery may allow the "one-handed" patient to be "two-handed" by increasing involved hand function from no function to assistive or from assistive to independent.

- **Screening.** When the goal of surgery is to improve function, patients must first be screened for cognitive capacity, motivation, and body image awareness.
  - Patients must have the cognitive skills and learning capability to participate in their therapy after surgery and to functionally make use of their newly acquired skills at completion of their rehabilitation program.
  - If they are not motivated, they will not participate in the prolonged effort necessary to achieve meaningful functional improvement.
  - Patients with poor stereognosis or neglect (i.e., poor body image awareness) find that the involved hand "drifts" in space and is not "available" for use if they have not been carefully trained in visual compensation techniques.
- **Grading.** Once it has been determined that the patient has the potential to make functional upper extremity gains with surgery, he or she is graded on the basis of hand placement, proprioception and sensibility, and voluntary motor control. Dynamic electromyography is used when delineation of phasic motor activity is essential.
- **Methods.** By means of fractional musculotendinous or step-cut methods, muscle unit lengthening of the agonist-deforming muscle units is combined with motor-balancing tendon transfers of the antagonists to achieve muscle balance and improve prehensile hand function.

SECTION 6 POSTPOLIO SYNDROME

CAUSE

■ Polio is a viral disease affecting the anterior horn cells of the spinal cord. postpolio syndrome is *not* a reactivation of the poliovirus but rather an aging phenomenon by which more nerve cells become inactive.

■ The syndrome occurs after middle age, usually 30 to 40 years following the original polio illness.

■ Symptoms include progressive muscle and joint weakness and pain, general fatigue and exhaustion with minimal activity, muscle atrophy, breathing or swallowing problems, sleep-related breathing disorders (e.g., obstructive sleep apnea), and decreased tolerance of cold temperatures.

■ In most patients the syndrome progresses slowly, with symptomatic periods followed by periods of stability.

▦ Affected patients use a high proportion of their capacity for normal activities of daily living. With aging and the drop-off of muscle units, they no longer have the reserves to perform their daily activities.

▦ Risk factors for developing postpolio syndrome include severity of the initial polio illness, initial diagnosis as an adolescent or adult, greater recovery from initial illness, and physical activity to the point of exhaustion or fatigue.

TREATMENT

■ Treatment comprises prescribed limited exercise combined with periods of rest so that muscles are maintained but not overtaxed.

■ Standard polio surgeries, combining contracture release, arthrodesis, and tendon transfer, are indicated when the deformity overcomes functional capacity.

■ The use of lightweight orthoses is important in helping patients remain functionally independent.

SELECTED BIBLIOGRAPHY

The selected bibliography for this chapter can be found on www.expertconsult.com.

TESTABLE CONCEPTS

SECTION 1 GAIT

- Stance phase comprises 60% of the gait cycle; swing phase comprises 40% of the gait cycle.
- Double-limb support represents 12% of stance phase. The body's center of gravity (COG) while being propelled forward is also subject to 5 cm vertical and 6 cm lateral displacements. Most muscle activity is **e**ccentric; that is, muscle lengthens (**e**longates) while contracting. This allows an antagonist muscle to dampen the activity of an agonist and act as a "shock absorber." Eccentric muscle contraction is the main form of muscle activity for normal daily activities.
- Antalgic gait results in **decreased stance phase** to lessen the time the painful limb is loaded.
- Water walking results in a significant decrease in joint moments and total joint contact forces as a result of the effect of buoyancy.

SECTION 2 AMPUTATIONS

- The metabolic cost of walking is increased with proximal-level amputations and is inversely proportional to the length of the residual limb and the number of functional joints preserved.
- The required increase in energy expenditure for ambulation in bilateral transtibial amputation (41%) is less than that of unilateral transfemoral amputation (65%).
- Transcutaneous partial pressure of oxygen [TcPO$_2$] is the factor most predictive of successful wound healing after amputation. Albumin is the most important laboratory value.
- Bony overgrowth is common in children, particularly in the humerus, fibula, tibia, and femur. Autologous stump-capping can prevent this complication.
- Percutaneous Achilles tendon lengthening should be performed with transmetatarsal and Lisfranc amputations to prevent late development of equinus or equinovarus deformity.
- In Lisfranc amputations, the soft tissue at the fifth metatarsal base should be preserved because this represents the insertion site of peroneus brevis and tertius, which act as antagonists to the posterior tibial tendon. **Failure to preserve these tissues results in inversion during gait.**
- **Syme amputation is more energy efficient than a midfoot amputation, despite the fact that it is at a more proximal level. The posterior tibial artery must be patent to ensure healing. The heel pad must be secured.** *(Commonly tested exception to the energy efficiency of amputation rule)*
- Transtibial amputations should be closed with a long posterior myocutaneous flap. The optimal bone length is at least 12 cm below the knee joint.
- Knee disarticulation is generally used in nonambulatory patients, inasmuch as it is muscle balanced and provides an excellent weight-bearing platform for sitting and a lever arm for transfer from bed to chair. However, data from the LEAP trial have demonstrated this amputation to result in the slowest walking speed and produce the least self-reported satisfaction.
- Transfemoral amputation should be performed 12 cm above the knee joint to accommodate the prosthetic knee.
- In transfemoral amputation, adductor myodesis is crucial for maintaining femoral adduction during gait with a prosthesis. Transecting the adductor magnus results in a loss of 70% of the adductor pull.

SECTION 3 PROSTHESES

- Myoelectric prostheses are commonly used for midlength transradial amputation.

- Body-powered prostheses are used for heavy labor. The terminal device is activated by shoulder flexion and abduction.
- Short forearm amputations, elbow disarticulations, and above-elbow amputations necessitate supracondylar suspension (Munster socket) and step-up hinges to augment function.
- The SACH prosthetic foot is being discontinued because it results in overload problems in the nonamputated foot.
- A dynamic-response prosthetic foot can be either articulated or nonarticulated. **Articulated feet are useful for uneven terrain.** Nonarticulated long-keel feet are used for very high-demand activities.
- Prosthetic knees are used in transfemoral and knee disarticulations. Alignment stability is crucial.
- Knee center of rotation posterior to line of weight bearing promotes control in stance phase, but flexion is difficult.
- Knee center of rotation anterior to weight bearing makes flexion easier, but control is poor.
- Microprocessor knees with polycentric (four-bar linkage) configuration should be used for most ambulatory patients with transfemoral amputations.
- Stance-phase control (safety) knee prostheses are used for older patients.
- The constant-friction knee is the most common prosthetic knee in children. Its major disadvantages are that it allows only single-speed walking and relies solely on alignment for stance-phase stability; therefore it is not recommended for older, weaker patients.
- The preferred method of suspension for transtibial prosthetic sleeves is the gel liner with locking pin.
- Transfemoral suspension can be with or without belts and straps. Vacuum suspension requires stable body weight but avoids belts. Silesian belts prevent socket from slipping off when suction sockets are fitted to short transfemoral stumps.
- Problems are common in prosthetics. Foot placement too anterior results in increased knee extension and patellar pain. Too soft a heel results in excessive knee extension, whereas too hard a heel causes knee flexion and lateral rotation of the toes.

SECTION 4 ORTHOSES

- A rocker sole can lessen the bending forces on an arthritic or stiff midfoot during **midstance** as the foot changes from accepting the weight-bearing load to pushing off.
- After hindfoot fusions, the primary orthotic goals are absorption of the ground reaction forces, protection of the fusion sites, and protection of the midfoot.
- A posterior leaf-spring AFO provides ankle stability in stance phase.

SECTION 5 SURGERY FOR STROKE AND CLOSED-HEAD INJURY

- Surgical intervention in adult-acquired spasticity should be delayed until the patient achieves maximal spontaneous motor recovery (6 months for stroke and 12 to 18 months for traumatic brain injury).
- Equinus deformity is treated by percutaneous Achilles tendon lengthening.
- Weak peroneal tendons accentuate dynamic varus deformities.
- Dynamic varus-producing force in adults is the result of out-of-phase tibialis anterior muscle activity during the stance phase. This dynamic varus deformity is corrected by either split (SPATT) or complete lateral transfer of the tibialis anterior muscle.

SECTION 6 POSTPOLIO SYNDROME

- Postpolio syndrome is not a reactivation of the polio virus. It is an aging phenomenon by which more nerve cells become inactive.

TESTABLE CONCEPTS

- Symptoms include progressive muscle and joint weakness and pain, general fatigue and exhaustion with minimal activity, muscle atrophy, breathing or swallowing problems, sleep-related breathing disorders (e.g., obstructive sleep apnea), and decreased tolerance of cold temperatures
- Risk factors for developing postpolio syndrome include severity of initial polio illness, initial diagnosis as an adolescent or adult, greater recovery from initial illness, and physical activity to the point of exhaustion or fatigue.
- Treatment comprises prescribed limited exercise combined with periods of rest so that muscles are maintained but not overtaxed.

CHAPTER 11

TRAUMA

David J. Hak and Cyril Mauffrey

CONTENTS

SECTION 1 CARE OF THE MULTIPLY INJURED PATIENT

PRINCIPLES OF TRAUMA CARE

- Primary assessment—begins with the primary survey, which seeks to identify any life-threatening injuries. A rapid assessment of airway, breathing, and circulation (the ABCs) is performed.
  - The airway is often managed by intubation, especially in patients experiencing a great deal of pain or obtundation. The initial survey should include placement of intravenous lines and treatment of any life-threatening injuries that are encountered.
- Fluid resuscitation
  - Aggressive fluid resuscitation should begin immediately in most cases with the placement of two large-bore intravenous cannulas.
  - Two liters of lactated Ringer solution or normal saline should be administered.
  - If the patient remains hemodynamically unstable after initial crystalloid infusion, begin infusion of blood products.
    - Typically requires greater than 30% blood loss
  - Blood products
    - Universal donor
      - Group O negative
      - Used in severe shock when specific blood products are not yet available
    - Type-specific blood
      - Crossmatched for ABO and Rh type
      - Typically available within 10 minutes

- Fully typed and crossmatched
  - Minor antibodies are crossmatched.
  - Typically available within 60 minutes
- Fresh frozen plasma
  - Contains coagulation factor proteins, immunoglobulins, and complement
- Platelets
  - Typically prepared from whole blood and should be stored at 20° to 24°C with continuous gentle agitation
  - Platelets stored in the cold become activated and lose their normal discoid shape.
  - Transfusion
    - If a patient does not respond to 2 L of crystalloid, 2 units of packed red blood cells should be administered.
    - Patients become coagulopathic and thus require both fresh frozen plasma and platelets.
      - The amount administered is controversial.
      - **Recent literature supports administration of packed red blood cells, fresh frozen plasma, and platelets in a 1 : 1 : 1 ratio.**
        - May prevent early coagulopathy
    - The most common complication of massive transfusion is a dilutional thrombocytopenia, followed by hypothermia and metabolic alkalosis.
    - Increased citrate from packed red blood cells binds calcium directly and can cause hypocalcemia.

Table 11-1	Classification and Treatment of Hemorrhagic Shock				
	PARAMETERS				
CLASS	BLOOD VOLUME LOSS	HEART RATE (beats/min)	BLOOD PRESSURE	URINE OUTPUT (mL/hr)	TREATMENT
I	Up to 15%	<100	Normal	>30	Fluid replacement
II	15%-30%	>100	Decreased	20-30	Fluid replacement
III	30%-40%	>120	Decreased	5-15	Fluid and blood replacement
IV	>40% (emergently life threatening)	>140	Decreased	Negligible	Fluid and blood replacement

From Browner BD, on behalf of the American College of Surgeons Committee on Trauma: *Advanced trauma life support: skeletal trauma: basic science, management, and reconstruction,* ed 8, Chicago, 2008, American College of Surgeons.

▓ Hemodynamic instability may result from internal injury or fractures and is the most important consideration for the orthopaedic surgeon.
  • Once the airway and breathing are controlled, problems with circulation remain the biggest threat to life.
  • Rapid application of splints and reduction of fractures when possible can decrease bleeding and relieve pain.
▓ The end points of adequate resuscitation are not clear; use of hemodynamic parameters is inadequate.
  • **Base deficit**, as measured by **lactate level**, is a proxy for the amount of anaerobic metabolism by the body and is the **best measure of patient's resuscitation.**
  • Lactate levels and base deficit are frequently used in trauma to guide the adequacy of resuscitation.
    • In general, lactate levels less than 2.5 indicate adequate resuscitation.
▓ Shock
  • **Hemorrhagic** (Table 11-1)
    • Divided into four classes
    • Class III/IV requires administration of blood products.
    • Presents as:
      • Increased heart rate and increased systemic vascular resistance
      • Decreased cardiac output, decreased pulmonary capillary wedge pressure, decreased central venous pressure, and decreased mixed venous oxygen saturation
    • Treat with fluids and blood products.
  • Neurogenic
    • Due to a loss of sympathetic tone in setting of a spinal cord injury
    • Presents as low heart rate, low blood pressure, and warm skin
    • Treat with dobutamine and dopamine.
  • Septic
    • Typically a hyperdynamic state with a massive loss of systemic vascular resistance
    • Cardiac index is increased and central venous pressure is decreased.
    • Treat with antibiotics and norepinephrine (causes vasoconstriction without increasing cardiac output).
  • Hemodynamic
    • Tension pneumothorax; pericardial tamponade prevents diastolic filling.
      • Pulmonary embolism
    • Adrenal insufficiency
      • Cardiovascular collapse unresponsive to fluids or pressors

▓ The systemic inflammatory response syndrome (SIRS) is a generalized response to trauma characterized by an increase in cytokines, complement, and many hormones. These changes are seen in varying degrees after trauma, and there is probably a genetic predisposition to an intense form of these changes. Patients are considered to have SIRS if they have two or more of the following criteria:
  • Heart rate greater than 90 beats per minute
  • White blood cell count (WBC) less than $4/mm^3$ or greater than $10/mm^3$
  • Respiration greater than 20 breaths per minute, with $PaCO_2$ less than 32 mm
  • Temperature less than 36°C or greater than 38°C
▓ SIRS is associated with disseminated intravascular coagulopathy, acute respiratory distress syndrome (ARDS), renal failure, shock, and multisystem organ failure.
▓ **Tranexamic acid** is a synthetic analogue of lysine that can be used to prevent excessive bleeding. It's **mechanism of action is competitive inhibition of plasminogen activation.**
■ **Radiologic workup**
▓ A rapid radiologic workup that includes at a minimum anteroposterior (AP) chest, AP pelvis, and lateral cervical spine views is standard.
▓ Availability and increased processing speed of computed tomographic (CT) scanners is leading to CT of cervical spine replacing lateral cervical spine radiography for trauma evaluation.
▓ Care should be taken not to focus on obvious radiographic findings (e.g., open-book pelvic injury) and miss other important findings such as a widened mediastinum.
▓ Pelvic fractures can be life threatening. The orthopaedic surgeon may be called on to stabilize pelvic fractures in the emergency department and should be prepared to **immediately place a pelvic binder or sheet.**
▓ Pelvic bleeding that does not respond rapidly to pelvic compression with a sheet or binder should be evaluated by angiography and embolization, if indicated.
■ **Trauma scoring systems—numerous systems seek to quantify the injury a patient sustained (Tables 11-2 through 11-4). Although some may yield prognostic value, none is perfect; a thorough workup is needed to identify all injuries and prioritize their management. Although it may be desirable to repair all fractures on the day of admission, it may be inherently dangerous to do so because of hemodynamic instability and the added trauma surgery creates.**

Table 11-2	Glasgow Coma Scale
RESPONSE TO ASSESSMENT	**SCORE**
BEST MOTOR RESPONSE	
Obeys commands	6
Localizes pain	5
Normal withdrawal (flexion)	4
Abnormal withdrawal (flexion)—decorticate	3
Extension—decerebrate	2
None (flaccid)	1
VERBAL RESPONSE	
Oriented	5
Confused conversation	4
Inappropriate words	3
Incomprehensible sounds	2
None	1
EYE OPENING	
Spontaneous	4
To speech	3
To pain	2
None	1

To calculate a Glasgow Coma Scale score, add the score for Eye Opening with the scores for Best Motor Response and Verbal Response. The best possible score is 15, and the worst possible score is 3.

 ■ **Damage control orthopaedics.** Principles of damage control have been applied to orthopaedic surgery and are now widely accepted. Damage control orthopaedics involves staging the definitive care of the patient to avoid adding to the overall trauma the patient has undergone.

▦ Trauma is associated with a surge in inflammatory mediators, which peak 2 to 5 days after trauma.

▦ After the initial burst of cytokines and other mediators, leukocytes are "primed" and can be activated easily with further trauma such as surgery. This may lead to multisystem organ failure or ARDS.

▦ To minimize the additional trauma added with surgery, traumatologists will often treat only potentially life-threatening injuries during this acute inflammatory window.

  • In the *severely injured* polytrauma patient or one with significant chest trauma, only emergent and urgent conditions should be treated.

    • Compartment syndrome, fractures associated with vascular injury, unreduced dislocations, long bone fractures, open fractures, or unstable spine fractures should be stabilized acutely.

▦ Acute stabilization is achieved primarily via external fixation.

  • Femur fractures may be converted from an external fixator to an intramedullary (IM) nail within 3 weeks.

  • Tibia fractures should be converted within 7 to 10 days. If longer periods of time are necessary, a staged removal of the external fixator and subsequent nailing several days later is recommended.

▦ The definitive treatment of pelvic and acetabular fractures may be delayed for 7 to 10 days in polytrauma patients to allow consolidation of the pelvic hematoma and resolution of the acute inflammatory response.

■ **Care of the pregnant patient**

▦ Trauma is the most common cause of death in pregnancy.

▦ Place all pregnant patients at more than 20 weeks' gestation in the left lateral decubitus position.

  • The vena cava may be compressed by the uterus, reducing maternal cardiac output 30%.

Table 11-3	Abbreviated Injury Score
EXAMPLES OF ABBREVIATED INJURY SCORE	**SCORE**
HEAD	
Crush of head or brain	6
Brainstem contusion	5
Epidural hematoma (small)	4
FACE	
Optic nerve laceration	2
External carotid laceration (major)	3
Le Fort III fracture	3
NECK	
Crushed larynx	5
Pharynx hematoma	3
Thyroid gland contusion	1
THORAX	
Open chest wound	4
Aorta, intimal tear	4
Esophageal contusion	2
Myocardial contusion	3
Pulmonary contusion (bilateral)	4
Two or three rib fractures	2
ABDOMINAL AND PELVIC CONTENTS	
Bladder perforation	4
Colon transaction	4
Liver laceration with > 20% blood loss	3
Retroperitoneal hematoma	3
Splenic laceration—major	4
SPINE	
Incomplete brachial plexus	2
Complete spinal cord, C4 or below	5
Herniated disc with radiculopathy	3
Vertebral body compression > 20%	3
UPPER EXTREMITY	
Amputation	3
Elbow crush	3
Shoulder dislocation	2
Open forearm fracture	3
LOWER EXTREMITY	
Amputation	
Below knee	3
Above knee	4
Hip dislocation	2
Knee dislocation	2
Femoral shaft fracture	3
Open pelvic fracture	3
EXTERNAL	
Hypothermia 31° to 30°C	3
Electrical injury with myonecrosis	3
Second- to third-degree burns—20%-29% of body surface area	3

From Browner BD et al, editors: *Skeletal trauma,* ed 3, Philadelphia, 2003, Saunders, p 135.

▦ Most diagnostic radiographs are below the threshold of risk to the fetus.

  • The first-trimester fetus is most at risk.

■ **Psychologic sequelae**

▦ Polytrauma has a major impact on quality of life.

▦ Women are more affected than men, and at **10 or more years after severe polytrauma women show higher rates of posttraumatic stress disorder and take more sick leave time.**

CARE OF INJURIES TO SPECIFIC TISSUES

■ **Soft tissue injuries**

▦ Vascular injury—may be due to penetrating or blunt trauma

Table 11-4	Variables for the Mangled Extremity Severity Score	
COMPONENT		**POINTS**
SKELETAL AND SOFT TISSUE INJURY		
Low energy (stab, simple fracture, "civilian" gunshot wound)		1
Medium energy (open or multiplex fractures, dislocation)		2
High energy (close-range shotgun or "military" gunshot wound, crush injury)		3
Very high energy (same as above, plus gross contamination, soft tissue avulsion)		4
LIMB ISCHEMIA (score doubled for ischemia > 6 hr)		
Pulse reduced or absent but perfusion normal		1
Pulseless, paresthesias, diminished capillary refill		2
Cool, paralyzed, insensate (numb)		3
SHOCK		
Systolic blood pressure always > 90 mm Hg		0
Transient hypotension		1
Persistent hypotension		2
AGE (yr)		
<30		0
30-50		1
>50		2

From Johansen K et al: Objective criteria accurately predict amputation following lower extremity trauma, *J Trauma* 30:568, 1990.

- Diagnosis—orthopaedic surgeon should recognize the injury and refer the patient to a vascular surgery specialist or a microsurgeon as indicated.
  - Vascular injury can be present when pulses are palpable; a change in pulse or a difference from the contralateral side may be the only harbinger of a serious vascular injury.
  - If pulses are not equal to the uninjured side, a workup is indicated.
  - Vascular compromise may develop over the course of hours in the case of knee dislocations and must be recognized promptly.
  - Hard signs of arterial injury—mandate immediate operative treatment. Observed pulsatile bleeding, rapidly expanding hematoma, palpable thrill, audible bruit, obvious arterial occlusion after reduction/realignment of fracture (6 *P*'s: pulselessness, pallor, paresthesia, pain, paralysis, poikilothermia).
  - Soft signs of arterial injury—consider arteriogram, serial examination, duplex examination. History of arterial bleed at scene, penetrating wound or blunt trauma in proximity to major artery, diminished unilateral pulse, small nonpulsatile hematoma, evolving neurologic deficit, ankle-brachial index (ABI) less than 0.9, abnormal flow velocity waveform on Doppler ultrasound.
  - Treatment: reduction of fracture will often restore vascularity in the case of long bone fractures.
- Compartment syndrome
  - Diagnosis: intracompartmental pressure exceeds capillary pressure, thus preventing exchange of waste and nutrients across vessel walls. One of the most frequently missed complications of trauma.
    - Unless treated within 4 to 6 hours, permanent injury will ensue; diagnosis is clinical or made using a pressure monitor.

- Clinical hallmarks are pain out of proportion to the injury and pain with passive stretching of the muscle.
  - Paresthesias and motor weakness are late findings.
  - Pulselessness and pallor are not commonly seen in compartment syndrome and suggest arterial compromise.
- Intracompartmental pressure measurement is abnormal if pressure is within 30 mm of the diastolic pressure (ΔP) *or* greater than 30 mm of the absolute pressure (criteria are debated).
- Intraoperative diastolic blood pressure during anesthesia is approximately 18 mm Hg lower than "baseline," potentially giving spurious ΔP values.
- Treatment: emergent decompression via fasciotomy
  - In the medial approach of a two-incision fasciotomy, the soleus must be released to allow access to the deep posterior compartment.
- Sequelae of untreated compartment syndrome are common and include claw toes and contractures in the hand.
- Rhabdomyolysis
  - May occur from crush injury, untreated compartment syndrome, and even strenuous endurance exercise
  - Myoglobin released into the bloodstream from damaged muscle can lead to renal failure. Initially urine will be dark owing to presence of myoglobin.
  - Elevated serum creatine kinase—levels five times normal upper limit indicate rhabdomyolysis
  - Treatment includes supportive care; intravenous sodium bicarbonate, glucose, and insulin for treatment of hyperkalemia; sodium bicarbonate to alkalinize urine and reduce risk of acute tubular necrosis; diuretics (mannitol and furosemide) may be used to maintain urine output.
  - Complications include hyperkalemia with associated electrocardiograph abnormalities and disseminated intravascular coagulation (DIC)
- Nerve injury
  - Cause
    - Blunt trauma—direct impact, crush injury, or shock wave from missile injury
    - Laceration—sharp edge of bone or penetrating trauma
  - Most common form is nerve palsy (neurapraxia) caused by stretching of the nerve, which will recover over time (1 mm/day)
  - **Following gunshot wounds, ulnar nerve injuries exhibit the worst functional recovery.**
  - Treatment
    - Nerve laceration (neurotmesis)—may be treated by repair or grafting. Results vary according to the specific nerve injured and the degree of injury to the nerve.
    - **Radial nerve injuries in high-energy open humeral shaft fractures have been shown to be more frequently due to neurotmesis than neuropraxia in some studies.**
    - Disruption of the nerve axon with an intact epineurium (axonotmesis) may be treated initially by observation
  - Motor recovery potential after repair
    - Excellent
      - Radial, musculocutaneous, femoral

- Moderate
  - Median, ulnar, tibial
- Poor
  - Peroneal nerve
- Bites
  - Snake bites
    - Tend to occur in certain regions of the United States. Envenomation occurs in only 25% of cases. Venom may be neurotoxic (coral snakes) or hemotoxic (rattlesnake, cottonmouth).
    - Treatment and complications
      - Treatment is symptomatic and expectant: antivenin in a monitored setting, débridement of necrotic tissue, and fasciotomy. Antivenin is available for all endemic snakes, but there is a high incidence of anaphylaxis or serum sickness associated with its use.
      - Complications can include severe local tissue necrosis, compartment syndrome, coagulopathies, and arrhythmias.
  - Human and animal bites
    - Pathogens—despite association of certain bites with specific bacteria, *Staphylococcus* and *Streptococcus* remain most prevalent pathogens. Others include:
      - Cat bites—*Pasteurella*
      - Dog bites—*Eikenella*
      - Human bites—variable, including *Eikenella*
    - Treatment—broad-spectrum antibiotic is commonly given, although regional variations are also common.
- Thermal injury
  - Hypothermia
    - Cause: injury caused by ice crystals forming outside cell(s)
    - Treatment: rapid rewarming and attention to arrhythmias are the current treatments. Amputation may be necessary.
  - Burns—generally treated by burn surgeons, but extremity burns may be treated by orthopaedic surgeons. Débridement of deep dermal burns and skin grafting are hallmarks of treatment after early aggressive fluid resuscitation. Antibiotic prophylaxis and tetanus are routine.
- Electrical injury—may cause bone necrosis and massive soft tissue necrosis. Extent of tissue injury may not be apparent for days after injury because skin may not be broken despite significant injury underneath.
  - Treatment is similar to that of burns; débridement followed by reconstruction with amputation, a flap, or a skin graft is required.
- Chemical burns—first rule: avoid contamination from other people and further damage to the victim.
  - Initial treatment: dilution with copious irrigation. After initial irrigation, the degree of necrosis is assessed, with débridement of necrotic tissue. Hydrofluoric acid is extremely toxic, causing profound hypocalcemia and cardiac death with little exposure; calcium gluconate may be used to treat skin exposure.
- High-pressure injury (water, paint, grease)—hand injuries most common. There may be extensive damage to underlying soft tissues despite a small entrance wound. Wide débridement of necrotic tissue and foreign material is required.
- Hyperbaric oxygen—can be used to provide enhanced oxygen delivery to peripheral tissues damaged by trauma

Table 11-5	Gustilo Classification of Open Fractures
FRACTURE TYPE	**DESCRIPTION**
I	Skin opening of ≤ 1 cm, quite clean; most likely from inside to outside; minimum muscle contusion; simple transverse or short oblique fractures
II	Laceration > 1 cm long, with extensive soft tissue damage, flaps, or avulsion; minimum to moderate crushing component; simple transverse or short oblique fractures with minimum comminution
III	Extensive soft tissue damage, including muscles, skin, and neurovascular structures; often a high-velocity injury with severe crushing component
IIIA	Extensive soft tissue laceration, adequate bone coverage; segmental fractures, gunshot injuries
IIIB	Extensive soft tissue injury, with periosteal stripping and bone exposure; usually associated with massive contamination; requires soft tissue coverage
IIIC	Vascular injury requiring repair

From Gustilo et al: Problems in the management of type III (severe) open fractures: a new classification of type III open fractures, *J Trauma* 24:742, 1984.

- Pressure-sensitive implanted medical devices (e.g., insulin pump) are a contraindication to use of hyperbaric therapy.
- **Joint injuries—may be caused by penetrating or blunt trauma**
- Dislocations—orthopaedic emergencies that should be reduced as soon as possible to avoid injury to the nerve and vessels and the articular cartilage; general anesthesia may be needed. Neurovascular status should be assessed and documented both before and after reduction.
- Open joint injuries
  - Antibiotics—penetrating trauma such as gunshot wounds may be treated with oral antibiotics if there is no debris in the joint; however, foreign matter is often carried into the joint as it is penetrated, even in "clean" gunshot wounds.
  - Reverse arthrocentesis/saline load test
    - Performed by injecting saline into the joint and observing the injured area for signs of extravasation
    - **At least 155 mL must be injected into the knee**.
    - This may miss a small puncture wound.
- Fractures involving the joints—must be reduced as anatomically as possible to reduce unequal wear
- **Fractures**
- Open fractures
  - Classification—Gustilo and Anderson grading system is widely used (Table 11-5). There is considerable interobserver variability, and the type may change over time with further débridement. Absolute wound length is less important than energy of injury.
    - Type I—no periosteal stripping, minimum soft tissue damage, small skin wound (1 cm)
    - Type II—little periosteal stripping, moderate muscle damage, skin wound (1-10 cm)
    - Type IIIA—contaminated wound (high-energy gunshot wound, farm injury, shotgun) or extensive periosteal stripping with large skin wound (>10 cm)

Table 11-6	Orthopaedic Trauma Association Classification of Open Fractures
Skin	1. Can be approximated 2. Cannot be approximated 3. Extensive degloving
Muscle	1. No muscle in area, no appreciable muscle necrosis, some muscle injury with intact muscle function 2. Loss of muscle but the muscle remains functional, some localized necrosis in the zone of injury that requires excision, intact muscle-tendon unit 3. Dead muscle, loss of muscle function, partial or complete compartment excision, complete disruption of a muscle-tendon unit, muscle defect does not approximate
Arterial	1. No injury 2. Arterial injury without ischemia 3. Arterial injury with distal ischemia
Contamination	1. None to minimal contamination 2. Surface contamination (easily removed, not embedded in bone or deep soft tissues) 3. a. Imbedded in bone or deep soft tissues b. High-risk environmental conditions (barnyard, fecal, dirty water, etc.)
Bone loss	1. None 2. Bone missing or devascularized but still some contact between proximal and distal fragments 3. Segmental bone loss

From Orthopaedic Trauma Association, Open Fracture Study Group: A new classification scheme for open fractures, *J Orthop Trauma* 24:742, 2010.

- Type IIIB—same as IIIA but will **require flap coverage**
- Type IIIC—same as IIIA but with vascular injury that requires repair
- Classification—Orthopaedic Trauma Association (OTA) Open Fracture Classification (Table 11-6)
  - Developed to address shortcomings of Gustilo and Anderson classification, which was designed only for open tibia fractures and uses treatment (i.e. type of wound closure) to determine classification. Ideal classification should guide treatment rather than treatment guiding classification.
  - Assesses five factors associated with open fractures using specific identifiable subcategories:
    - Skin
    - Muscle
    - Arterial
    - Contamination
    - Bone loss
- Treatment
  - Antibiotics—usually started immediately. Antibiotic bead pouch with methylmethacrylate, tobramycin, and/or vancomycin may be used to initially manage highly contaminated wounds.
    - Types I and II—first-generation cephalosporin (cefazolin) for 24 hours
    - Type III—cephalosporin and aminoglycoside for 72 hours after last incision and drainage
    - Heavily contaminated wounds and farm wounds—cephalosporin, aminoglycosides, and high-dose penicillin

- Freshwater wounds—fluoroquinolones (ciprofloxacin, levofloxacin) or third- or fourth-generation cephalosporin (ceftazidime)
- Saltwater wounds—doxycycline and ceftazidime *or* a fluoroquinolone
- Tetanus prophylaxis
  - Tetanus is caused by the exotoxin of *Clostridium tetani*, which produces convulsion and severe muscle spasms with a 30% to 40% mortality rate.
  - Required tetanus prophylaxis treatment is based on the characteristics of the wound and the patient's immunization status.
  - Tetanus-prone wounds are more than 6 hours old, more than 1 cm deep, have devitalized tissue, and are grossly contaminated.
  - Patients with an unknown tetanus immunization status or who have received fewer than three tetanus immunizations and who have a tetanus-prone wound should receive tetanus and diphtheroid toxoid and human tetanus immunoglobulins (intramuscular injection of toxoid and immunoglobulin should occur at different sites).
  - Patients with unknown tetanus immunization states or who have received fewer than three tetanus immunizations and who have a non–tetanus-prone wound should receive only tetanus toxoid.
  - Fully immunized patients should receive tetanus toxoid if the wound is severe, more than 24 hours old, or if the patient has not had a booster in the past 5 years.
- Débridement—initial treatment should consist of local wound débridement that is adequate to clean the wound and débride all necrotic tissue.
- Stabilization of bony injuries—will decrease further damage to soft tissue
- Early coverage (goal: <5 days). However, zone of injury must be well defined before coverage (Figure 11-1).
  - Gastrocnemius flap—for proximal-third tibial fractures
  - Soleus flap—for middle-third tibial fractures
  - Fasciocutaneous flap or free-tissue transfer—for distal-third fractures
- Negative-pressure therapy is commonly used to treat wounds but is not a substitute for definitive coverage.
- Stabilization with external fixation
  - Immediate treatment: most fractures should be reduced and splinted promptly to avoid further soft tissue damage. External fixation may be used to treat grossly contaminated wounds and fractures that will require time for soft tissues to heal before definitive fixation.
  - Definitive treatment: external fixation may be used definitively for periarticular fractures, articular fractures that cannot be reconstructed, and segmental fractures, but internal fixation is far more common.
- Perioperative complications
  - Thromboembolic disease—incidence very high in pelvic, spine, hip, and lower extremity fractures. Pulmonary embolus develops in as many as 5% of those who have deep venous thrombosis (DVT).

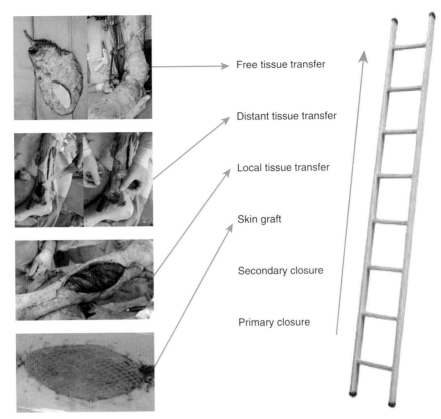

Free tissue transfer

Distant tissue transfer

Local tissue transfer

Skin graft

Secondary closure

Primary closure

FIGURE 11-1 Soft tissue defect ladder of reconstruction. Complexity of the treatment and expertise required increase throughout the ladder.

- Diagnosis of DVT is by Doppler ultrasound, magnetic resonance venography, or D-dimer titers.
- Treatment: all patients with these injuries should receive some form of thromboembolic disease prophylaxis (mechanical or pharmacologic). Risks of pharmacologic prophylaxis include prolonged bleeding from surgical or traumatic wounds or a cerebral bleed.
- Fat embolus syndrome—associated with reaming of long bones but can occur with any long bone fracture. Hypoxia, a petechial rash on the chest, and tachycardia are the hallmarks. Treatment is supportive.
- ARDS—patients with chest trauma and multiple fractures at high risk. It is unclear whether reamed nailing of long bone fractures causes it directly, but may be implicated in the "second hit" phenomenon. Treatment is supportive (O_2, ventilator).
- Fracture complications
  - Cast treatment complications
    - Pressure sore—care to pad bony prominences and perform more frequent skin inspections in patients with diminished sensory capacity
    - **Cast burn**; can be **minimized by not dipping plaster in hot water (use water temperature 20° to 24°C [68° to 75.2°F])**, not resting cast on a pillow while setting, not using excessive layers, and not overwrapping with fiberglass while plaster cast is curing
    - Delayed union—defined as no progression of healing over serial radiographs. Treatment may include bone grafting and external bone stimulation.

- Nonunion
  - Classification (Figure 11-2)
  - Biologic treatments—many new treatments, but scanty literature to support any one over the others
    - Bone morphogenetic protein—expensive, indicated in some acute tibia fractures, and possibly useful in nonunions
  - Traditional treatment
    - Identify infection and treat appropriately.
    - Address patient factors including vitamin D deficiency and nutrition.
    - Correct any deformity.
    - Provide stability for hypertrophic nonunions.
    - Provide improved biology (autogenous bone graft, muscle flap) for atrophic nonunions.
    - Preserve native biology.
  - Bone stimulator—no strong evidence for effectiveness of one method over another
    - Ultrasound—delivers small cumulative doses of ultrasound energy; thought to induce microfracture and healing response; **30 mW/cm² pulsed wave ultrasound has been shown effective for healing acute fractures**
    - Electromagnetic—attempts to promote healing by directing integral ion flow at cellular level of bone
  - Segmental bone loss—treatment includes bone graft, induced membrane technique followed by bone graft, interposition free tissue transfer (free-fibula transfer), bone transport (ring fixation), and amputation.
  - Heterotopic ossification

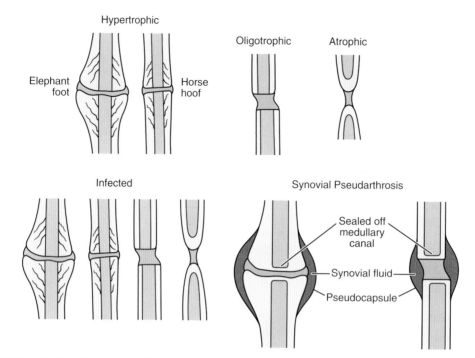

FIGURE 11-2 Classification of nonunions. (From Browner BD et al, editors. *Skeletal trauma,* ed 4, Philadelphia, 2008, Elsevier.)

- Diagnosis: common in head-injured patients and in hip, elbow, and shoulder fractures. Any fracture associated with extensive muscle damage is at risk.
- Prophylaxis: indomethacin 25 mg orally three times a day, or indomethacin sustained-release 75 mg orally daily for 6 weeks has been recommended. Efficacy of indomethacin is debatable and may increase nonunion rate.
- Radiation therapy (600-700 cGy) given 24 hours before or up to 72 hours after surgery; equal to indomethacin in effectiveness (but no issues with compliance with medication regimen)
- Treatment: early active range of motion (ROM) for elbow and shoulder. Excision of problematic heterotopic ossification can be considered when no further growth (controversial how to assess—"quiet" bone scan, stable disease shown on radiographs, time > 1 year).
- Osteomyelitis
  - Diagnosis
    - Definitive diagnosis—by bone biopsy. Bone culture and microscopic pathology. Bone culture may have high false-negative rate. Microscopic pathology to evaluate for inflammatory changes consistent with infection.
    - Other tests—may be used in combination with physical examination (draining wound, pain) to confirm diagnosis
    - Chronic draining wounds can differentiate into squamous cell carcinoma and should undergo histologic analysis when excised.
      - Magnetic resonance imaging (MRI)—95% sensitive and 90% specific
      - Technetium 99m (^{99m}Tc) study—85% sensitive and 80% specific
      - Indium study—95% sensitive and 85% to 90% specific
  - Treatment—based on grade and host type (Cierny/Mader)
    - Grade
      - Grade I—intramedullary; débridement by intramedullary reaming
      - Grade II—superficial, involves cortex, often seen in diabetic wounds; curettage
      - Grade III—localized, involves cortical lesion with extension into medullary canal; requires wide excision, bone grafting, and perhaps stabilization
      - Grade IV—diffuse, indicates spread through cortex and along medullary canal; wide sequestrectomy, muscle flap, bone graft, and stabilization
    - Host
      - A—normal healthy patient
      - B—locally compromised (vasculopathic)
      - C—not considered a medical candidate for surgery; may require suppressive antibiotics
- Fractures caused by gunshot wounds
  - Velocity is the most important determinant of the energy imparted to soft tissues.
  - High-energy gunshot and shotgun wounds—considered grade III open fractures because they are often associated with considerable soft tissue injury (Table 11-7). They require extensive surgical débridement of necrotic tissue and require surgical stabilization of the fracture.
  - Low-energy gunshot wounds—can be treated as a closed fracture but should get single-dose, first-generation cephalosporin and local wound care
  - Bullets that pass through colon—may contaminate any fracture caused by the bullet after perforation (pelvis, spine). Bony fractures may be managed with antibiotics alone if extraarticular and the fracture pattern is stable.

■ Principles of lower extremity amputation
  • Maintain knee joint and stump length when soft tissues permit, even if free flap is required for coverage
  • Lower Extremity Assessment Project (LEAP)
    • Multicenter prospective study of severe lower extremity trauma in the U.S. civilian population. Key findings and recommendations include:
    • Injury severity scoring systems do not provide valid predictive value to guide amputation decision.
    • Absence of plantar sensation on presentation is not predictive of extremity function or return of plantar sensation at 2-year follow-up.
    • At 2- and 7-year follow-up, no difference in functional outcome between patients who underwent either limb salvage surgery or amputation
    • Outcomes found to be more affected by patient's economic, social, and personal resources than by the injury treatment method
    • Patients with mangled extremity injuries have poor outcomes at 2 years. Outcomes continue to worsen between 2 and 7 years' follow-up. Factors associated with poor outcome include older age, females, nonwhite race, lower level of education, current or prior smoking history, poor economic status, low self-efficacy, poor health status prior to injury, and involvement in legal system to obtain disability.
    • Patients presenting with mangled lower extremity injuries are less agreeable, more likely to drink alcohol, smoke, be poor and uninsured, be neurotic and extroverted compared to population norms.
    • Patients who underwent below-knee amputation functioned better than those undergoing above-knee amputation. Patients undergoing through-knee amputation had the poorest function.

▓ Osteoporotic fractures
  • **World Health Organization Fracture Risk Assessment Tool (FRAX) calculates the 10-year risk of hip fracture**
  • **Low-energy stress fractures associated with bisphosphonate use in patients treated for osteoporosis; fracture characterized by cortical thickening, mostly transverse pattern, minimal comminution**
  • **Fracture of the proximal humerus consistently predicts patient's risk for a subsequent low-energy hip fracture.**

BIOMECHANICS OF FRACTURE HEALING (ALSO SEE CHAPTER 1, BIOMECHANICS.)

■ **Stability and fracture healing (Table 11-8)**
▓ Stability determines strain
  • Absolute stability
  • Relative stability
▓ Strain determines type of healing (Figure 11-3)
  • Strain less than 2% results in primary bone healing (endosteal healing).
  • Strain 2% to 10% results in secondary bone healing (enchondral ossification).
  • Strain greater than 10% does not permit bone formation.
    • *Strain* is defined as change in fracture gap divided by the fracture gap ($\Delta L/L$).
      • **Highest fracture site strain is seen in a simple fracture that is fixed with a gap (incompletely reduced).**

Table 11-7	Classification of Closed Fractures with Soft Tissue Damage
FRACTURE TYPE	**DESCRIPTION**
0	Minimum soft tissue damage; indirect violence; simple fracture patterns *Example:* torsion fracture of tibia in skiers
I	Superficial abrasion or contusion caused by pressure from within; mild to moderately severe fracture configuration *Example:* pronation fracture-dislocation of ankle joint, with soft tissue lesion over medial malleolus
II	Deep, contaminated abrasion associated with localized skin or muscle contusion; impending compartment syndrome; severe fracture configuration *Example:* segmental "bumper" fracture of tibia
III	Extensive skin contusion or crush injury; underlying muscle damage may be severe; subcutaneous avulsion; decompensated compartment syndrome; associated major vascular injury; severe or comminuted fracture configuration

From Tscherne H, Oestern HJ: Die Klassifizierung des Weichteilschadens bei offenen und geschlossenen Frakturen, *Unfallheilkunde* 85:111–115, 1982. ©Springer-Verlag.

Table 11-8	Type of Bone Healing with Different Stabilization Methods	
TYPE OF STABILIZATION	**PREDOMINANT TYPE OF HEALING**	**COMMENTS**
Cast	Secondary bone healing with periosteal callus	Exchondral ossification
Compression plate	Primary bone healing	Osteonal cutting cone with subsequent remodeling
Bridge plate	Secondary bone healing with periosteal bridging callus	
Intramedullary nail	Early periosteal bridging callus Late medullary callus	Bone healing through both intramembranous and enchondral ossification
External fixator	Secondary bone healing with periosteal bridging callus	
Inadequate fixation with adequate blood supply	Hypertrophic nonunion	Failed enchondral ossification with predominance of type II collagen
Inadequate fixation without adequate blood supply	Atrophic nonunion	

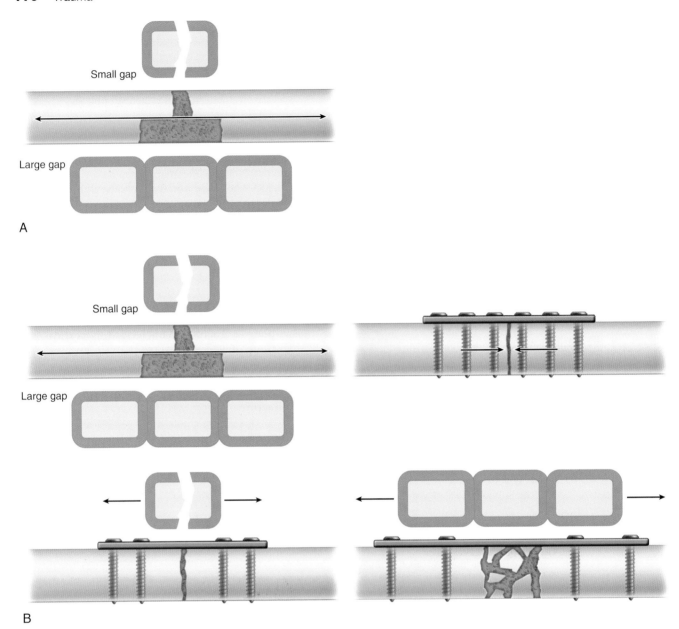

FIGURE 11-3 A, Simple fractures have limited ability to tolerate motion without disruption of healing and should generally be treated with compression. **B,** In contrast, multifragmentary fracture can tolerate more motion because it is shared along multiple sites. In this case, bridge plating, which will permit motion at the fracture site has been used.

- **Relative stability**
- Micromotion at fracture site under physiologic load leads to callus formation.
- Strain decreases as callus matures, leading to increased stability.
- If there is too much motion, callus becomes hypertrophic as it tries to spread out force, and hypertrophic nonunion can result.
- Examples: casts, external fixators, IM nails, bridge plates
- **Absolute stability**
- No motion at fracture site under physiologic load
- Bone heals through direct healing (no callus).
- Strain is low or zero.
- Healing times are longer and more difficult to confirm by radiography.
- Implants must have longer fatigue life.

- Examples: **single interfragmentary screw and neutralization plate** in oblique fracture pattern, compression plating in transverse fracture pattern
- **Healing in different bone types**
- Diaphyseal (cortical)
  - Decreased blood supply leads to longer healing times.
  - Bone is more amenable to compression techniques (in short oblique/transverse fractures).
  - Strain is concentrated over a smaller surface area.
- Cancellous (metaphyseal)
  - Larger surface area and better blood supply
  - Strain is lower as forces spread out over larger area.
  - Healing is more rapid.
  - However, joint surfaces tolerate very little malreduction (<2 mm), so there is often increased time to bear weight versus diaphyseal fractures.

BIOMECHANICS OF OPEN REDUCTION AND INTERNAL FIXATION (ORIF [ALSO SEE CHAPTER 1, BIOMECHANICS.])

- **Lag screws**
  - Provide rigid interfragmentary compression (absolute stability)
  - Force is concentrated over a small area (around screw), so typically a plate is needed to protect/neutralize the deforming forces.
- **Position screws**
  - Compress plate to bone but will not provide interfragmentary compression
  - Friction between screw, plate, and bone resists pullout or bending.
- **Plating (Figure 11-4)**
  - Plate length matters more for bending stability than number of screws in plate.
  - Torsional stability is more affected by position of screws (need end hole filled).
  - Longer plates spread the strain over more area (working length).
  - **To increase bending stiffness of a plate, decrease the working length** by placing screws closer to the fracture site (a 10-hole plate centered at a fracture with screws in holes 1, 5, 6, and 10 has a higher bending stiffness than one with screws in holes 1, 3, 8 and 10).
  - Plates are load bearing—will stress shield area covered by plate; important to protect area temporarily if plate removed after healing
- **Compression plate function**
  - Plate design (oval holes) or use of compression device allows plate to apply compressive forces across fracture.
  - Provides absolute stability when properly applied
  - Relies on friction between plate and bone (needs at least some nonlocking screws)
  - May need **pre-bend to achieve compression of both near and far cortex**
  - Insertion order is neutral position, then compression on opposite side of fracture, then lag screw (if placing through plate).
  - Tight contact of plate to bone when initially applied causes decreased periosteal blood flow and temporary osteopenia.
- **Bridge plate function**
  - Primarily for comminuted fracture patterns
  - Plate "bridges" area of comminution with fixation above and below fracture.
  - Allows some elastic deformation (relative stability)
  - Avoid use of screws too close to fracture.
  - Number and types of screws to insert are fracture dependent—no clear, widely accepted guidelines.
  - Nonlocking screws compress plate to bone and can be used to lag in fragments; locking screws provide angular stability in short metaphyseal segments or in osteoporotic bone.
- **Buttress plate function**
  - Plate provides support at 90-degree angle to fracture—typically in depressed metaphyseal/articular fractures that have been reduced
  - Can provide absolute stability to metaphyseal fragments
- **Submuscular/percutaneous plating**
  - To preserve biology at fracture site, plate may be placed in submuscular plane by sliding through small incisions

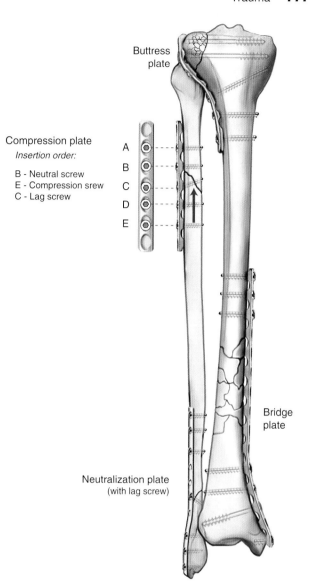

Compression plate
Insertion order:

B - Neutral screw
E - Compression srew
C - Lag screw

FIGURE 11-4 Plate function for various fracture patterns.

proximal or distal to fracture and avoiding exposure of fracture site.
  - Typically used in bridge mode, although not exclusive
  - Advantage: decreased soft tissue and biologic compromise
    - Medullary and periosteal perfusion are better retained.
  - Disadvantage: more prone to malreduction/malrotation
- **Locked plating**
  - Screws have threads in head that lock into corresponding holes in plate
    - Fail simultaneously rather than sequentially
  - Does not depend on friction between plate and bone for stability
  - Provides fixed-angle construct—similar to blade plate
  - Most useful in unstable short-segment metaphyseal fractures and osteoporotic bone
  - **Fractures in which locking plate use is supported by data include:**
    - Periprosthetic fractures
    - Proximal humerus fracture
    - Intraarticular distal femur and proximal tibia
    - Humeral shaft nonunion in the elderly

- **Unicortical locked screws**
  - Typically for metaphyseal bone
  - Similar pullout strength to bicortical locked screws in good-quality diaphyseal bone (but rare indications for use there)
  - **Weaker in torsion compared with bicortical screws**
- Bicortical locked screws: biggest advantage is in osteoporotic diaphyseal bone
- Multiaxial screws
  - May increase options for fixation in working around periprosthetic fractures
  - No advantage in strength or pullout
- "Hybridization" describes the use of both locking and nonlocking screws in combination. This allows for both compression and fixed-angle support.
- **IM nails**
- Load-sharing devices—relative stability
- Stiffness depends on:
  - Material
    - Stainless is greater than titanium.
  - Size

- Increased diameter leads to increased stiffness at a ratio of radius to the power of:
  - 3 in bending
  - 4 in torsion
- Wall thickness
  - Larger = stiffer nail
- Radius of curvature of femoral nails is typically less than anatomic, improving frictional fixation.
  - A large mismatch of curvature, however, results in difficult insertion, increased risk of intraoperative fracture, and malreduction in extension.
- Nails resist bending very well and require interlocks to resist torsion or compression loads.
- Working length is the portion of the nail that is unsupported by bone when loaded.
  - Increased working length produces increased interfragmentary motion and may delay union.
- Advantage of intramedullary position is decreased lever arm for bending forces (especially useful in peritrochanteric fractures versus plate-and-screw construct).

SECTION 2 UPPER EXTREMITY

SHOULDER INJURIES (TABLES 11-9 AND 11-10)

- **Sternoclavicular dislocation—"serendipity" view or CT scan reveals dislocation of sternoclavicular joint**
- Anterior dislocation—more common, treated by closed reduction. The majority will remain unstable regardless of initial treatment modality, but these are typically asymptomatic.

- Posterior dislocation—more serious—30% associated with significant compression of posterior structures. May cause dysphagia or difficulty breathing and sensation of fullness in the throat. Treated by closed reduction with a towel clip in the operating room. A thoracic surgeon should be on standby.

Table 11-9	Adult Shoulder Dislocations/Ligamentous Injuries			
INJURY	**EPONYM/OTHER NAME**	**CLASSIFICATION**	**TREATMENT**	**COMPLICATIONS**
Anterior (GH) dislocation (most common)		Subcoracoid > subglenoid (also subclavicular and intrathoracic)	Must get axillary view of GH joint; reduce, immobilize (young patient, 4 wk; old patient, 2 wk); passive > active (Rockwood 7)	Axillary nerve neurapraxia, axillary artery injury, cuff injury (>40 yr old), recurrence (85% in <20 yr old), bone injury (head [Hill-Sachs], greater tuberosity, glenoid)
Recurrent/ multidirectional		Anterior dislocation/ subluxation atraumatic	Prolonged rehabilitation (rotator cuff strengthening); if failure, consider surgery (inferior capsular shift)	Look for generalized laxity; AMBRI
	Bankart repair: anterior capsule → anterior rim	Late instability		
	Staple capsulorrhaphy: capsule → glenoid	Late DJD, migration		
	Putti-Platt repair: subscapularis imbrication	Late DJD, ↓ ER		
	Magnuson-Stack repair: subscapularis → lesser tuberosity	Late DJD, ↓ ER		
	Bone block: crest graft, anterior	↓ Range of motion, migration		
	Bristow repair: coracoid transfer	Nonunion, ↓ ER, migration		
	Capsular shift: redundant capsule, advanced	Minimum procedure of choice with multidirectional instability		

Table 11-9	Adult Shoulder Dislocations/Ligamentous Injuries—cont'd			
INJURY	**EPONYM/OTHER NAME**	**CLASSIFICATION**	**TREATMENT**	**COMPLICATIONS**
Posterior dislocation	Subacromial (seizures and shocks) (most common)	Reduce, immobilize for 3-6 wk; rotator cuff strengthening; operate if recurrent (glenoid osteotomy, bone block, posterior capsular shift)	Lesser tuberosity fracture, late recognition (may require advancement of lesser tuberosity into defect or total shoulder arthroplasty [place in less retroversion]); avoid by checking axial view	
Inferior GH	Luxatio erecta		Reduce and immobilize; rotator cuff strengthening, rehabilitation	Neurovascular injury can resolve after reduction; axillary artery thrombosis; watch for rotator cuff tear
AC injury		I—AC sprain	7-10 days rest/immobilization, sling	Joint stiffness, deformity, CC ligament and soft tissue calcification, AC DJD, associated fractures, distal clavicle osteolysis
		II—AC tear, CC sprain	Sling for 2 wk, rehabilitation, late-excision arthroplasty if required	
		III—AC tear, CC tear	Conservative vs. repair (athletes, laborers); Weaver-Dunn	
		IV—clavicle through trapezius posteriorly	Reduce and repair	
		V—clavicle 100%-300% elevated; trapezius, deltoid detached	Reduce and repair (Weaver-Dunn)	
		VI—clavicle inferior to coracoid	Reduce and repair	
Sternoclavicular injury		Anterior dislocation	Evaluate with "serendipity" view or computed tomography closed reduction with traction	Bump (cosmetic), DJD, mediastinal impingement (dysphagia, throat fullness), hardware migration (with operative treatment)
		Posterior dislocation	Closed reduction with towel clip or open; thoracic surgeon on standby	
		Chronic dislocation	Medial clavicle resection or ligament reconstruction (thoracic surgeon on standby)	
		Spontaneous atraumatic subluxation	Nonoperative	

AC, Acromioclavicular; *AMBRI,* atraumatic, multidirectional, bilateral, treated by rehabilitation instability; *CC,* coracoclavicular; *DJD,* degenerative joint disease; *ER,* external rotation; *GH,* glenohumeral.

Table 11-10	Adult Shoulder Fractures			
INJURY	**EPONYM**	**CLASSIFICATION**	**TREATMENT**	**COMPLICATIONS**
Proximal humerus fracture		Neer (parts > 1 cm or 45-degree displacement)		Missed dislocation, adhesive capsulitis (moist heat, gentle range of motion), malunion (reconstruction or TSA required), avascular necrosis (TSA required), nonunion (surgical neck, tuberosity fractures: ORIF), disrupted rotator cuff
		One-part (most common); impaction of the humeral neck	Sling for comfort, early motion; isometrics initially, advancing to progressive resistance	
		Two-part; displacement of the greater tuberosity > 1 cm	Closed reduction unless articular segment (ORIF), shaft (impacted and angulated: traction, Velpeau; unimpacted: closed reduction, CRPP or ORIF), greater tuberosity (repair cuff), tuberosity with block to internal rotation (ORIF)	

Continued

Table 11-10	Adult Shoulder Fractures—cont'd			
INJURY	**EPONYM**	**CLASSIFICATION**	**TREATMENT**	**COMPLICATIONS**
		Three-part; displacement of the greater or lesser tuberosities > 1 cm	ORIF in younger, ORIF/prosthesis in older; repair of rotator cuff	
		Four-part; displacement of lesser and greater tuberosities > 1 cm head splitting is variant	Same as three-part; nonoperative in elderly/diabetic/impacted four-part valgus pattern	
Proximal humerus		Anterior (greater tuberosity displacement)	Closed reduction; if > 1 cm after reduction, open repair	As above, with the addition of axillary nerve or plexus injury, myositis ossificans (wait > 1 yr to excise heterotopic bone)
Fracture-dislocation		Posterior (lesser tuberosity displacement)	Closed reduction, ORIF if three-part; treatment for fracture as above	
Impression/impaction of humeral head	Hill-Sachs	Stable (<20% articular surface)	Closed treatment	Avascular necrosis, DJD (TSA)
		Unstable (20%-50%)	Transfer of lesser tuberosity → defect (McLaughlin)	
Scapula fracture		Unstable (>45%) Zdravkovic and Damholt	Prosthesis vs. rotational osteotomy	Associated injuries (clavicle, rib, pulmonary contusion, pneumothorax), axillary artery injury, plexus palsy, pressure symptoms, vascular and plexus injuries
		I—body	Most treated nonoperatively	
		II—coracoid and acromion	Associated injury common; ORIF of large displaced fragments	
		III—neck and glenoid	ORIF of large unstable fractures (glenoid with displaced clavicle fracture)	
Clavicle fracture		Middle third (most common)	Nonoperative: sling, figure-eight brace ORIF: displacement, ipsilateral displaced glenoid neck fracture	Vascular injury/ pneumothorax, ligament injury (CC or AC), skin necrosis, malunion (osteotomy for young active patient); nonunion (ORIF and bone graft), nerve injury (rare); muscle fatigue/weakness, DJD (if articular)
		Distal third (Neer)	TSA if symptomatic	
		I—minimum interligamentous displacement (CC, AC)	Nonoperative; sling for comfort	
		II—fracture medial to CC ligaments	Nonoperative if nondisplaced; consider ORIF for displaced fracture	
		IIA—both ligaments attached to distal fragment	ORIF	
		IIB—conoid torn, trapezoid attached to distal fragment	ORIF	
		III—AC joint	Closed treatment; late-excision arthroplasty if required	
		Proximal third	Closed treatment	
Glenoid fracture		Ideberg	Nonoperative treatment if nondisplaced	
		I—anterior avulsion fracture	>25% of surface: ORIF if head is subluxated with major fragment; posterior approach	
		II—transverse/oblique fracture, inferior glenoid free		
		III—upper third of glenoid and coracoid		
		IV—horizontal glenoid through body		
		V—combination of II-IV		
Scapulothoracic dissociation (seen on scapular lateral or chest radiograph)			Closed reduction, sling immobilization	Vascular and brachial plexus injuries, associated clavicle fracture

AC, Acromioclavicular; *CC,* coracoclavicular; *CRPP,* closed reduction with percutaneous pinning; *DJD,* degenerative joint disease; *ORIF,* open reduction and internal fixation; *TSA,* total shoulder arthroplasty.

- Chronic dislocation—treated by resection of the medial clavicle, with preservation and reconstruction of costoclavicular ligaments
- Pseudodislocation—medial clavicular epiphysis is the last to close (mean age, 25 years). In patients younger than this, sternoclavicular dislocation is often a Salter-Harris type I or II fracture.

■ Clavicle fracture (Figure 11-5)

- Classification—classified by thirds
  - Middle—80%
  - Distal—15%
  - Medial—5%
- Diagnosis—AP and 15-degree cephalad-oblique radiographic views
- Associated injuries—open clavicle fractures associated with high rates of pulmonary and closed-head injuries
- Treatment
  - Nonoperative treatment: midthird fractures have traditionally been treated nonoperatively in a sling.
    - No difference in outcome between regular sling and figure-eight bandage
    - Risk of nonunion after midshaft fractures is higher in females and elderly and those fractures that are displaced, shortened more than 2 cm, or comminuted.
    - Lateral fractures have higher rates of nonunion compared with midshaft fractures.
  - Operative treatment
    - Middle third
      - Have higher rates of nonunion and decreased shoulder strength and endurance (≈15%)
      - Absolute surgical indications: open fracture, displaced fractures with skin compromise, associated neurovascular injury

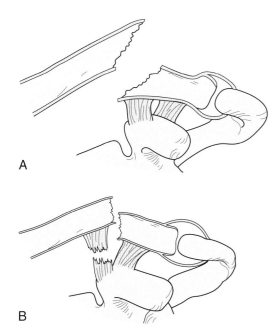

- Relative surgical indications: floating shoulder (associated scapular neck fracture), shortening greater than 15 to 20 mm, complete displacement, comminution
- Prospective randomized study comparing operative versus nonoperative treatment of displaced midthird clavicle fractures: operative treatment group had a 10-point improvement in Constant and DASH scores at all time points, earlier time to union, and statistically fewer nonunions, symptomatic malunions, and complications compared to the nonoperative treatment group.
  - Distal third
    - Some authors recommend operative treatment of distal fractures that extend into the acromioclavicular joint, whereas others recommend a late Mumford procedure.
    - Type II distal clavicle fractures, which involve displacement, have the highest nonunion incidence, but many nonunions are asymptomatic. Nonoperative and operative management provide similar results. Operative decision based on amount of displacement and individual patient demands. For example, **sling and early ROM is best treatment for middle-aged woman with 100% displacement of a distal clavicle fracture.**
  - Fixation options
    - Plate—typically dynamic compression plate; apply to superior aspect (better biomechanical strength but more prominent = hardware removal) or to anterior-inferior aspect (less hardware removal).
    - IM rod and screw—may be inserted percutaneously; higher rates of hardware irritation and complication
    - Avoid Steinmann pins, especially nonthreaded—can migrate.

■ Acromioclavicular dislocation

- Classification—classified by extent of involvement of the ligamentous support and direction and magnitude of displacement (Figure 11-6). Coracoclavicular (CC) and acromioclavicular (AC) ligaments may be ruptured.
  - Type I—sprain of AC joint
  - Type II—rupture of AC ligaments and sprain of CC ligaments
  - Type III—rupture of both AC and CC ligaments
  - Type IV—clavicle is buttonholed through trapezius posteriorly
  - Type V—trapezius and deltoid detached
  - Type VI—Clavicle is translocated beneath coracoid
- Treatment
  - Types I and II—always treated with brief immobilization in a sling
  - Type III—may be treated nonoperatively, but many would advocate early operative treatment in patients who are heavy laborers and throwers. Weaver-Dunn procedure is the treatment of choice.
  - Types IV to VI—usually treated operatively

■ Scapula fracture—associated with pulmonary contusion, pneumothorax, clavicle fracture (i.e., floating shoulder), rib fracture, head injury, brachial plexus injury, upper extremity vascular injury, pelvic or acetabular fracture and spine fracture. Scapula body fractures are generally treated in a sling for 7 to 10 days and then with early ROM.

■ Glenoid fracture

- Nonoperative treatment—used for nondisplaced fractures

FIGURE 11-5 When the distal end of the clavicle is fractured, the ligaments may either **(A)** remain intact and maintain apposition of the fracture fragments (type I) or **(B)** rupture, allowing wide displacement of the fragments (type II). (Redrawn from Rockwood CA, Green DP, editors: *Fractures,* ed 4, vol 1, Philadelphia, 1996, JB Lippincott.)

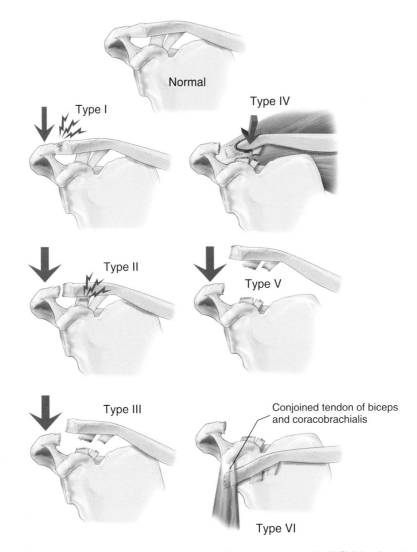

FIGURE 11-6 Classification of the ligamentous injuries that can occur to the acromioclavicular (AC) joint. In a type I injury, a mild force applied to the point of the shoulder does not disrupt either the AC or coracoclavicular (CC) ligament. In a type II injury, a moderate to heavy force applied to the point of the shoulder disrupts the AC ligaments but the CC ligaments remain intact. In a type III injury, when a severe force is applied to the point of the shoulder, both the AC and the CC ligaments are disrupted. In a type IV injury, not only are the ligaments disrupted but the distal end of the clavicle is also displaced posteriorly into or through the trapezius muscle. In a type V injury, a violent force applied to the point of the shoulder not only ruptures the AC and CC ligaments but also disrupts the muscle attachments and creates a major separation between the clavicle and acromion. A type VI injury is an inferior dislocation of the distal clavicle in which the clavicle is inferior to the coracoid process and posterior to the biceps and coracobrachialis tendons. The AC and CC ligaments have also been disrupted. (From Rockwood CA Jr et al: Disorders of the acromioclavicular joint. In Rockwood CA Jr et al, editors: *The shoulder,* ed 3, Philadelphia, 2004, Saunders.)

- Operative treatment—indicated for intraarticular fractures that are displaced more than 2 mm or widely displaced extraarticular fractures. Approach is usually through a posterior portal, although the Neviaser portal may be used to place a superoinferior screw in the glenoid.

■ **Glenoid neck fracture**

- Nonoperative treatment—advocated by many authors in almost all cases.
- Operative treatment—indicated when glenoid neck and humeral head are translocated anterior to the proximal fragment or are medially displaced. Reduction and plating is through a posterior approach between infraspinatus (suprascapular nerve) and teres minor (axillary nerve). The suprascapular nerve and artery are at risk from excessive superior retraction, whereas the circumflex scapular artery is at risk during the approach.

■ **Scapulothoracic dissociation—result of significant trauma to chest wall, lung, and heart. Severe cases are treated essentially with a closed forequarter amputation.**

- Associated with:
  - Brachial plexus avulsion
  - Subclavian or axillary artery injury
  - AC dislocation, clavicle fracture, and sternoclavicular dislocation
  - Mortality rate of 10%
- Diagnosis should be suspected when there is a neurologic and/or vascular deficit. Lateral displacement of the scapula more than 1 cm on a chest radiograph is also suggestive.
- Management
  - Hemodynamically stable: angiography before surgery. Vascular injury may potentially be treated nonoperatively owing to the extensive collateral network around the shoulder.

- Hemodynamically unstable: high lateral thoracotomy or median sternotomy to control bleeding
- Musculoskeletal injury treatment is controversial but is often nonoperative if vascular repair is not undertaken.
- Functional outcome is based on severity of associated neurologic injury.
- ■ **Floating shoulder—fracture of the glenoid neck and clavicle**
- Some authors recommend fixation when a clavicle fracture is associated with a displaced glenoid neck fracture, whereas others do not consider it necessary (depends on stability of superior shoulder suspensory complex [SSSC]).

- ■ **Proximal humerus fracture (Figure 11-7)**
- Neer classification (Neer define "part" as displacement of > 1 cm or angulation of > 45 degrees); parts are articular surface, greater tuberosity, lesser tuberosity, shaft
  - One-part—nondisplaced or minimally displaced fracture (often of the humeral neck)
  - Two-part—displacement of tuberosity of more than 1 cm; or surgical neck with head/shaft angled or displaced
  - Three-part—displacement of the greater or lesser tuberosities and articular surface
  - Four-part—displacement of shaft, articular surface, and both tuberosities. "Head splitting" is a variant, with split through the articular surface (usually requires replacement for treatment).
- Treatment
  - One-part—sling for comfort and early mobilization
  - Two-part—repair of the displaced tuberosity with sutures or tension band wiring; surgical neck fractures can normally be managed nonoperatively. Unstable, unimpacted fractures may be treated with closed reduction with percutaneous pinning (CRPP), ORIF with locking plate fixation, or IM nailing
    - Varying humeral nail designs. Straight nails are placed through a more central entry point (through superior articular cartilage) that can provide additional point of fixation. Nails with proximal bend are placed through an entry point just medial to the rotator cuff insertion.
    - Immediate physical therapy during nonoperative management results in faster recovery.
      - Greater tuberosity fractures are displaced superiorly and posteriorly owing to deforming pull of supraspinatus, infraspinatus, and teres minor. Healing in a displaced position will block abduction and external rotation. Surgery is indicated for displacement greater than 5 mm. In young patients with good bone can fix with screws alone, but nonabsorbable suture technique should be used in older patients.
  - Three-part
    - ORIF for young patients, with repair of the tuberosities or rotator cuff
      - Screw cutout is the most common complication following ORIF with a periarticular locking plate.
    - Hemiarthroplasty for older patients, with repair of the rotator cuff/tuberosities
  - Four-part—same as for three-part
    - Humeral height can be judged most reliably using the superior border of the pectoralis major insertion.
      - Nonanatomic placement of the tuberosities leads to significant impairment in external rotation

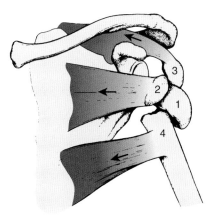

FIGURE 11-7 Proximal humeral fracture. There are four parts: *1*, head; *2*, lesser tuberosity; *3*, greater tuberosity; and *4*, humeral shaft. (From Neer CS, Rockwood CA: Fractures and dislocations of the shoulder. In Rockwood CA, Green DP, editors: *Fractures in adults*, ed 2, Philadelphia, 1984, JB Lippincott, p 696.)

kinematics and an eightfold increase in torque requirements.
- Complications
  - Avascular necrosis (AVN)
    - Factors associated with humeral head ischemia (Hertel criteria):
      - Disruption of the medial periosteal hinge
      - Medial metadiaphyseal extension less than 8 mm
      - Increasing fracture complexity
      - Displacement greater than 10 mm
      - Angulation greater than 45 degrees
  - Neurovascular injury
    - Axillary nerve injury
      - Lateral pins placed during CRPP place the nerve most at risk.
      - Anterior pins placed during CRPP risk the biceps tendon, cephalic vein, and musculocutaneous nerve.
  - Hardware failure
    - The most common complication after locking plate fixation is screw cutout.
  - Nonunion
    - Most common after two-part fracture of surgical neck
    - Nonunion of greater tuberosity following arthroplasty—loss of active shoulder elevation

- ■ **Shoulder dislocation**
- **TUBS**: *t*raumatic, *u*nidirectional, *B*ankart lesion, requires *s*urgical treatment. **AMBRI**: *a*traumatic, *m*ultidirectional, often *b*ilateral, *r*ehabilitation is primary initial treatment, *i*nferior capsular shift indicated for failed conservative therapy.
- Anterior (Figure 11-8)—*most common shoulder dislocation*
  - **Most commonly caused by fall on an abducted, externally rotated shoulder**
  - Diagnosis
    - Apprehension sign
    - Axillary view is diagnostic.
    - Usually traumatic and unilateral
    - Usually painful
  - Treatment: reduction (multiple maneuvers available)
    - Sling for 2 weeks in the elderly and 4 weeks in the young, followed by rotator cuff strengthening

AP in scapular plane.

Arm supported in sling.

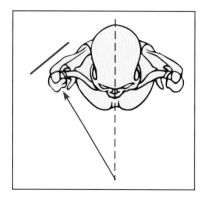

No overlap of head and glenoid.

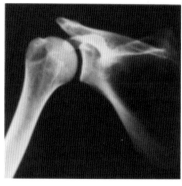

Lateral in scapular plane.

Arm supported in sling.

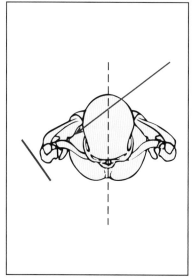

90 to AP.

Head in center of glenoid.

Identify anterior and posterior displacement.

Identify greater tuberosity displacement.

Evaluate shape of acromion for cause of impingement or cuff tears.

Emergency axillary.

Arm is gently abducted.

Tube at the hip.

Involved shoulder supported on pad.

Arm holds IV pole or is supported by assistant.

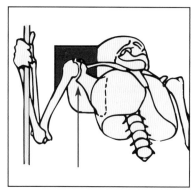

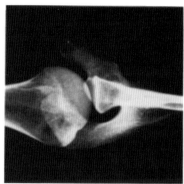

Evaluate glenoid for uneven wear or rim fractures.

Identify anterior and posterior dislocation.

Identify displaced tuberosities.

Identify unfused acromial epiphysis.

FIGURE 11-8 Trauma series views. (From Norris TR: In Chapman MW, Madison M, editors: *Operative orthopaedics,* Philadelphia, 1988, JB Lippincott, pp 203-220.)

- Consider operative treatment in cases of recurrence or rotator cuff tear.
  - The most common associated injury at arthroscopy after acute dislocation is anterior labral tear, followed by anterior capsular insufficiency and Hill-Sachs lesion.
  - High recurrence rate (≈50%) in young patients (owing to unstable labral tear)
  - High incidence of rotator cuff injury in older patients (>45 years)
- Multidirectional
  - Diagnosis
    - Often bilateral
    - Often atraumatic, not painful

- Examination of the shoulder reveals subluxation posteriorly as well as anteriorly and inferiorly.
  - Generalized ligamentous laxity
- Treatment
  - Rotator cuff strengthening
  - Inferior capsular shift is indicated if instability is refractory to nonoperative treatment.
- Posterior (Figure 11-9)
  - Diagnosis
    - Associated with seizures and electric shock
    - Often missed but easily seen on axillary view
    - **Lack of external rotation is key physical examination finding in fixed posterior dislocations**

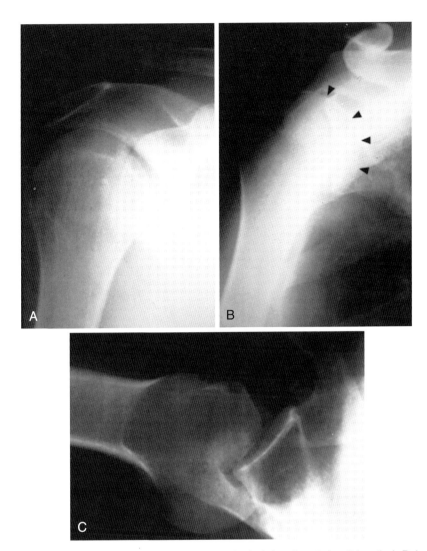

FIGURE 11-9 Anteroposterior radiographs. **A,** In the sagittal plane of the body (missed posterior dislocation). **B,** In the sagittal plane of the scapula, overlap of the head and glenoid *(arrowheads)* indicates a dislocation. **C,** Axillary or computed tomography scans are the best views for diagnosing posterior dislocation or fracture-dislocation. (From Browner BD et al, editors: *Skeletal trauma,* ed 4, Philadelphia, 2008, Elsevier.)

- May have fracture of lesser tuberosity or reverse Hill-Sachs lesion
- Treatment
  - Immobilization for 3 to 6 weeks
  - Rotator cuff strengthening
  - Possible open bone grafting of humeral head defect and repair of posterior labral tear
  - Allograft, coracoid transfer, or resurfacing for large defects
- Inferior (luxatio erecta)
  - Diagnosis
    - Associated with motor vehicle collision or sporting injury
    - **Arm is typically abducted between 100 and 160 degrees.**
    - Diminished or absent pulses
  - Treatment
    - Closed reduction successful in 50%
    - Capsular reconstruction if unstable

HUMERAL INJURIES

Shaft fracture (Table 11-11)
- Classification by location and fracture pattern
- Treatment
  - Nonoperative treatment: functional brace if there is less than 20 degrees of anterior angulation, less than 30 degrees of valgus/varus angulation, or less than 3 cm of shortening; **contraindicated in patients with associated brachial plexus palsy**
  - Operative treatment: open fracture, floating elbow, polytrauma, pathologic fracture, associated brachial plexus injury
    - ORIF
      - Probably the gold standard
        - Anterolateral approach—proximal two thirds
        - Distal half—posterior approach
        - Need for radial nerve exploration—lateral approach

Table 11-11	Adult Humeral Shaft Fractures			
INDICATIONS	**EPONYM**	**CLASSIFICATION**	**TREATMENT**	**COMPLICATIONS**
Pathologic fracture, open fracture, floating elbow *Relative indications:* segmental fracture, distal spiral with nerve injury (Holstein-Lewis), obesity, thoracic trauma, polytrauma	Holstein-Lewis (distal third)	Based on location/ fracture pattern	*Nonoperative:* coaptation splint or cast brace if < 20-degree anterior angulation, < 30-degree varus/valgus, < 3-cm shortening *Operative:* consider ORIF (compression plate) vs. IM nail	Nonunion (treat with compression plate and bone graft), malunion, radial nerve injury (5%-10% incidence; observe unless open fracture or persisting for 3-4 months), vascular injury; shoulder pain (IM nail)

IM, Intramedullary, *ORIF,* open reduction and internal fixation.

- Higher union rates and decreased secondary operations
- **Weight bearing to tolerance is safe after plate fixation.**
- IM nail
  - Possibly better for segmental or shaft/proximal humerus combination as well as pathologic fracture
  - Complication rate may be higher and associated with higher rates of reoperation compared with plate fixation.
  - Distal locking screw risks:
    - Radial nerve with lateral to medial screw
    - Musculocutaneous nerve with anteroposterior screw
- Complications
  - Radial nerve palsy (5%-10%)
    - When to observe:
      - The vast majority (up to 92%) resolve with observation for 3 to 4 months.
      - Brachioradialis followed by extensor carpi radialis longus **(wrist extension in radial deviation) are the first to return,** whereas extensor pollicis longus and extensor indicis proprius are last to return.
    - When to explore:
      - Open fracture
        - A higher likelihood of transection
        - Perform ORIF of fracture at time of exploration.
    - Controversial whether to observe or explore:
      - Secondary nerve palsy (i.e., after fracture manipulation)
      - Spiral or oblique fracture of distal third (Holstein-Lewis fracture)
    - Management of palsy that does not recover is also controversial as to timing of electromyography, nerve exploration, and tendon transfers.
  - Nonunion—treat with compression plate with bone graft if atrophic.
  - Shoulder pain; some papers report a high incidence of shoulder pain, whereas others do not. Overall incidence is higher with IM nails.
- **Supracondylar fracture—rare injury in adults**
- Classification
  - AO (Arbeitsgemeinschaft für Osteosynthesefragen)/ OTA distal humerus classification
    - Type A—extraarticular
    - Type B—intraarticular, single column
    - Type C—intraarticular, with both columns fractured and no portion of the joint contiguous with the shaft

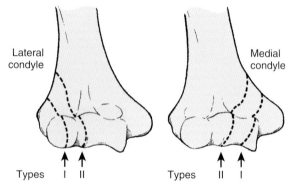

FIGURE 11-10 Humeral condyle fractures. (From Gelman MI: *Radiology of orthopedic procedures: problems and complications,* vol 24, Philadelphia, 1984, WB Saunders, p 56, reprinted by permission.)

- Treatment: ORIF
- Complications: neurovascular injury, nonunion, malunion, loss of motion (contracture, fibrosis, bony block)
- **Distal single-column (condyle) fracture**
- Classification
  - Classified as Milch types I and II lateral condyle fractures (more common) and types I and II medial condyle fractures. In type I lateral condyle fractures the lateral trochlear ridge is intact, and in type II lateral condyle fractures there is a fracture through lateral trochlear ridge (Figure 11-10).
  - AO/OTA distal humerus classification (see earlier)
- Treatment—type I nondisplaced: immobilize in supination (lateral condyle fracture) or pronation (medial condyle fracture); otherwise, CRPP or ORIF
- Complications: cubitus valgus (lateral) or cubitus varus (medial), ulnar nerve injury, and degenerative joint disease (DJD)
- **Distal two-column fracture**
- Presentation: five major articular fragments identified: capitellum/lateral trochlea, lateral epicondyle, posterolateral epicondyle, posterior trochlea, medial trochlea/epicondyle
- Classification
  - Jupiter classification
    - High T—proximal or at level of olecranon fossa
    - Low T (common)—transverse component just proximal to the trochlea
    - Y—oblique portion through both columns with distal vertical fracture
    - H—trochlea is free fragment (AVN)

- Medial lambda—proximal fracture exits medially
- Lateral lambda—proximal fracture exits laterally
- Multiplane—T type with additional fracture in coronal plane
- AO/OTA distal humerus classification (see earlier)
▪ Treatment (goal is early ROM with < 3 weeks of immobilization)
  - ORIF using a posterior approach with two plates applied to either column
    - Biomechanical studies support both parallel placement (one plate medial, one plate lateral) and perpendicular placement (one plate medial, one plate posterolateral) configurations
    - Used with olecranon osteotomy or triceps split/peel (final muscle strength similar with both)
    - In an open fracture, use ORIF by means of a triceps split through the defect, producing better results than osteotomy.
    - Low-T fractures are more difficult and frequently require reoperation (almost 50%) for stiffness, but they can have good results.
    - **No benefit from ulnar nerve transposition during ORIF**
  - "Bag-of-bones" technique—reasonable for demented patients and those who have severe medical comorbidities that prevent surgical treatment
  - **Total elbow arthroplasty—useful for comminuted fractures in low-demand patients older than 65 years, particularly with osteoporosis or rheumatoid arthritis**
▪ Complications
  - Stiffness
    - Most common complication
    - Initially treat with static-progressive splinting
  - Loss of elbow muscle strength of 25%
  - Ulnar nerve injury
    - Treat with anterior transposition
  - Heterotopic ossification (4%)
  - Infection
- ■ **Capitellum fracture**
▪ Classification
  - Bryan-Morrey (Figure 11-11)
    - Type I—Hahn-Steinthal; complete fracture of capitellum

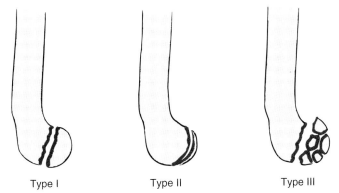

Type I   Type II   Type III

FIGURE 11-11 Fractures of the capitellum can be divided into type I, a complete capitellar fracture; type II, the more superficial lesion of Kocher-Lorenz; and type III, a comminuted capitellar fracture. (From Browner BD et al, editors: *Skeletal trauma,* ed 2, Philadelphia, 1998, WB Saunders, p 1511.)

- Type II—Kocher-Lorenz; shear fracture of articular cartilage
- Type III—comminuted
  - McKee modification
    - Type IV—coronal shear fracture including capitellum and trochlea
▪ Treatment
  - Type I—if nondisplaced, splint for 2 to 3 weeks and then allow motion; if displaced more than 2 mm, use ORIF.
  - Type II—if nondisplaced, splint for 2 to 3 weeks and then allow motion; if displaced, excise fragments.
  - Type III—if displaced, excise fragments.
  - Type IV—ORIF; lateral approach recommended
▪ Complications: nonunion (1%-11% with ORIF), olecranon osteotomy nonunion, ulnar nerve injury, heterotopic ossification (4% with ORIF), and AVN of capitellum

ELBOW INJURIES (TABLE 11-12)

- ■ **Olecranon fracture**
▪ Classification—Colton (Figure 11-12)
  - Type I—avulsion
  - Types IIA to IID—oblique fractures with increasing complexity
  - Type III—fracture-dislocation
  - Type IV—atypical, high-energy, comminuted fractures
▪ Treatment
  - Less than 1 to 2 mm displaced—splint at 60 to 90 degrees for 7 to 10 days, followed by gentle active ROM exercises.
  - Tension band—use stainless steel wire or braided cable, not braided suture material.
    - The wire loop should be dorsal to the midaxis of the ulna, thus transforming tensile forces at the fracture site into compressive forces at the articular surface.
    - Bury Kirschner wires in anterior cortex for increased stability. Protrusion through the anterior cortex, however, is associated with reduced forearm rotation.
    - Migration of Kirschner wires and prominent or painful hardware occurs in 71%.
    - **Compared to Kirschner wires that are positioned into the intramedullary canal, wires that penetrate the volar ulna cortex are associated with a higher potential risk of diminished forearm rotation.**
  - IM screw fixation—inadequate by itself, but a properly placed 7.3-mm partially threaded screw with tension band wiring works well.
  - Plate fixation (dorsal or tension side)—preferred technique for oblique fractures that extend distal to the coronoid process; more stable than tension band wiring
  - Excision with **triceps advancement**—used for **nonreconstructible proximal olecranon fractures in elderly low-demand patients.** Reattach close to the articular surface. Avoid resecting more than 50% of the olecranon.
▪ Complications: decreased ROM, DJD, nonunion, ulnar nerve neurapraxia, and instability

Table 11-12	Adult Elbow Fracture-Dislocations			
INJURY	**EPONYM**	**CLASSIFICATION**	**TREATMENT**	**COMPLICATIONS**
Supracondylar fracture		AO/OTA classification of distal humerus Type A—extraarticular Type B—intraarticular single column Type C—intraarticular with both columns fractured and no portion of the joint contiguous with the shaft	Displaced: ORIF (double plating)	Neurovascular injury, nonunion, malunion, contracture, pain, decreased ROM (fibrosis, bony block)
Bicolumn fracture		Jupiter I—high T pattern (at level of olecranon fossa) II—low T pattern (proximal to trochlea) III—Y pattern (through both columns, distal vertical fracture) IV—H pattern (trochlea is free fragment) V—medial lambda pattern (proximal fracture exits medially) VI—lateral lambda pattern (proximal fracture exits laterally) VII—multiplane: T type with additional fracture in coronal plane	Nondisplaced: immobilize for 2 wk, then gentle motion Displaced: ORIF (posterior approach, olecranon osteotomy or triceps split/peel): fix condyles first, then epitrochlear ridge to humeral metaphysis Arthroplasty (total elbow arthroplasty) in elderly (consider > 6 "bag-of-bones" technique for demented patients or those medically unfit for surgery)	Stiffness, heterotopic ossification, infection, ulnar neuropathy (treat with anterior transposition), AVN
Transcondylar fracture	Kocher	Intraarticular (fragment posterior to humerus)	ORIF	↓ROM
	Posadas	Intraarticular (fragment anterior to humerus)	ORIF	
Capitellar fracture	Bryan-Morrey			Nonunion (1%-11% with ORIF), olecranon osteotomy nonunion, ulnar nerve injury, heterotopic ossification (4% with ORIF), AVN of capitellum
	Hahn-Steinthal Kocher-Lorenz	I—complete fracture of capitellum, large trochlear piece II—minimum subchondral bone (shear fracture of articular cartilage) III—comminuted fracture IV (McKee modification)—coronal shear fracture, including capitellum and trochlea	Nondisplaced: splint for 2-3 wk, then motion; displaced > 2 mm: ORIF Nondisplaced: splint for 2-3 wk, then motion; displaced: excise displaced fragment Excise if displaced and unsalvageable ORIF	
Condylar fracture		Milch (lateral ≫ medial) I—lateral trochlear ridge intact II—fracture through lateral trochlear ridge	Nondisplaced: immobilize in supination (lateral condyle), pronation (medial condyle) Displaced: CRPP vs. ORIF	Cubitus valgus (lateral), cubitus varus (medial), ulnar nerve neurapraxia, DJD
Trochlear fracture	Laugier	Rare	Nondisplaced: splint for 3 wk Displaced: ORIF	
Epicondylar fracture	Granger	Medial ≫ lateral	Manipulation, immobilization for 10-14 days	Painful, unsightly fragment or ulnar nerve symptoms—late excision
Coronoid fracture	Regan and Morrey	Type I—fracture of the tip Type II—fracture of <50% of coronoid Type III—fracture of >50% of coronoid	Early motion if stable; ORIF with cerclage wire or suture if unstable ORIF ORIF	Instability (medial) and DJD
Olecranon fracture	Colton (modified)	Type I—avulsion Type II (A-D)—oblique fractures with increasing complexity Type III—fracture-dislocations Type IV—atypical high-energy, multifragmented fractures	Minimally displaced (<1-2 mm): splint at 60-90 degrees for 7-10 days, then motion Displaced: ORIF Tension band: use stainless steel wire or braided cable; migration of wire/prominent hardware in 71% Intramedullary 7.3-mm screw and tension band Plate fixation for oblique and comminuted fractures Excision for unreconstructible proximal olecranon fractures; reattach close to articular surface; avoid > 50% resection	↓ROM, DJD, nonunion, ulnar nerve neurapraxia, instability (with removal of > 80% of olecranon), symptomatic hardware/need for hardware removal

Table 11-12	Adult Elbow Fracture-Dislocations—cont'd			
INJURY	**EPONYM**	**CLASSIFICATION**	**TREATMENT**	**COMPLICATIONS**
Radial head fracture	Mason (and Johnston)	I—nondisplaced	Nonoperative; splint for 7 days, then early motion with or without aspiration	Loss of motion, posterior interosseous nerve injury; intraosseous membrane rupture; distal radioulnar joint disruption; Essex-Lopresti (distal radioulnar joint disruption); synovitis if Silastic radial head implant
		II—partially articular with displacement	If elbow stable and no block to motion: splint and early motion; otherwise, ORIF vs. arthroplasty	
		III—comminuted fractures involving the entire head of the radius	Arthroplasty; ORIF if < three pieces, good bone quality; excise in elderly, low functional demands	
		IV—fractures associated with ligamentous injury (elbow dislocation) or other associated fractures	Reduce dislocation and then address fracture surgically (arthroplasty for stability)	
Dislocation (pure ligamentous)		Posterolateral (most common), posterior, anterior, medial, lateral, divergent; simple (no fracture) or complex (fracture)	Closed reduction; check ROM/ stability; splint for 2-7 days and then gentle active ROM; open reduction unstable/interposed soft tissue ORIF complex (fracture) dislocations	Irreducibility, median and ulnar nerve injury, brachial artery injury, flexion contracture, heterotopic ossification, fractures (medial epicondyle, radial head, coronoid)

AVN, Avascular necrosis; *CRPP,* closed reduction with percutaneous pinning; *DJD,* degenerative joint disease; *ORIF,* open reduction and internal fixation; *ROM,* range of motion.

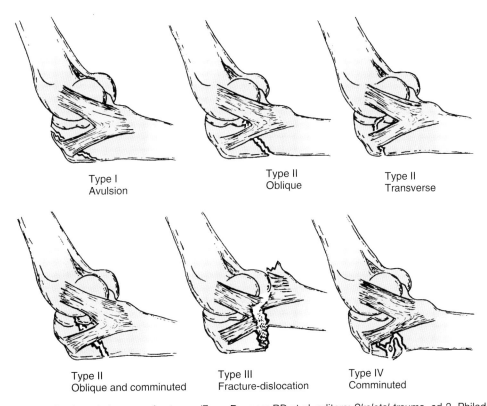

Type I
Avulsion

Type II
Oblique

Type II
Transverse

Type II
Oblique and comminuted

Type III
Fracture-dislocation

Type IV
Comminuted

FIGURE 11-12 Colton classification of olecranon fractures. (From Browner BD et al, editors: *Skeletal trauma,* ed 2, Philadelphia, 1998, WB Saunders, p 1469.)

■ **Coronoid fracture**
▦ Classification
  • Regan and Morrey classification
    • Type I—fracture of the tip of the coronoid process
    • Type II—fracture of 50% or less of coronoid

  • Type III—fracture of > 50% of coronoid
• O'Driscoll classification
  • Tip
  • **Anteromedial process**—caused by a varus posteromedial rotatory force and may be associated

with posteromedial instability. **Injury is at the attachment site of the anterior bundle of the medial collateral ligament.**
  • Basal
▥ Treatment
  • Type I—associated with episodes of elbow instability. If instability persists, apply cerclage wire or No. 5 suture through drill holes; if instability does not persist, no operation.
  • Types II and III—ORIF helps restore elbow stability; must confirm stability before nonoperative treatment begins
▥ Complications: instability (particularly medial) and DJD
■ **Radial head fracture**
▥ Classification (Figure 11-13)
  • Type I—nondisplaced
  • Type II—partial articulation with displacement
  • Type III—comminuted fractures involving the entire head of the radius
  • Type IV—fractures associated with ligamentous injury or other associated fractures
▥ Treatment
  • Type I—Splint for no more than 7 days, and then allow motion.

Type I

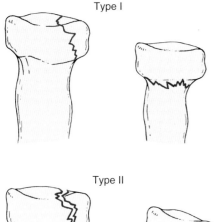

Type II

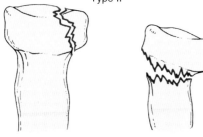

Type III

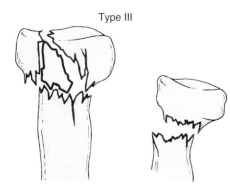

FIGURE 11-13 Modified Mason classification system for radial head fractures. (From Browner BD et al, editors: *Skeletal trauma*, ed 4, Philadelphia, 2008, Elsevier.)

  • Type II—nonsurgical treatment with analgesics and active ROM as symptoms resolve if elbow is stable and there is no block to motion with good reduction. Otherwise, use ORIF. Surgery provides better results (90%-100% good or excellent).
  • Type III—replace the radial head, usually with a metal implant. Use ORIF if fewer than three pieces. Excise only in elderly patients with low functional demands.
  • Type IV—requires surgical repair: must use either ORIF or metallic radial head replacement. Do not excise without adding radial head implant.
    • Safe zone for ORIF of radial head/neck is 110-degree arc (i.e., 25%) along lateral side, defined by radial styloid and Lister tubercle.
▥ Complications
  • Loss of motion
  • Posterior interosseous nerve injury
    • Pronate arm to avoid injury.
  • Radial shortening if Essex-Lopresti injury
  • Synovitis if a Silastic radial head implant is used
■ **Dislocation**
▥ Classification
  • 80% are posterolateral; rest are posterior, anterior, medial, lateral, or divergent
  • Simple (no associated fracture) or complex (fracture)
    • Associated injuries
      • Avulsion fracture of medial or lateral epicondyle
      • Radial head and neck fractures
      • Coronoid fractures
      • Osteochondral injury
▥ Mechanism of injury in elbow dislocation: disruption of circle of Horii; begins laterally and progresses medially in three stages
  • Stage 1 (posterolateral rotational instability)—lateral collateral ligament partially or completely disrupted
  • Stage 2 (perched ulna)—additional anterior and posterior disruption. Incomplete posterolateral dislocation with subluxation/dislocation of radial head, medial edge of ulna resting on the trochlear, and coronoid perched on the trochlear.
  • Stage 3 (complete dislocation)—elbow dislocates and coronoid lies posterior to trochlear.
  • Stage 3A—all soft tissue sleeve including posterior part of medial collateral ligament disrupted (anterior medial collateral ligament intact)
  • Stage 3B—entire MCL (including anterior bundle) disrupted. Varus, valgus, and rotatory instability all present following reduction. Immobilize in cast in 90-degree flexion.
  • Stage 3C:—soft tissues stripped off entire distal humerus (including flexor-pronator and common extensor origins). Grossly unstable even in flexion.
▥ Treatment
  • Simple—brief immobilization (1 week) for most and then allow motion. Long-term results are good.
  • Complex—surgical treatment is indicated. Anterior or divergent dislocations are usually high-energy injuries with a much higher incidence of open wounds, neurovascular injury, fracture, and recurrent instability.
▥ Complications
  • Stiffness and flexion contracture
    • Directly correlated with period of immobilization greater than 3 weeks

- Heterotopic ossification (collateral ligaments)
- Ulnar or median nerve injury
- Brachial artery injury

■ "Terrible triad" of the elbow
▓ Elbow dislocation with lateral collateral ligament injury, radial head fracture, and coronoid fracture
- The lateral collateral ligament injury is typically a ligamentous avulsion from the origin on the distal humerus.
▓ Always unstable and requires treatment
▓ Treatment
- Coronoid ORIF
- Radial head ORIF or replacement
- Lateral collateral ligament repair (typically to distal humerus)
- Possible medial collateral ligament repair depending on stability

FOREARM FRACTURES (TABLE 11-13)

■ Monteggia fractures
▓ Diagnosis/classification
- Bado classification (Figure 11-14)
  - Type 1 (60%)—anterior radial head dislocation and apex anterior proximal-third ulna fracture
  - Type 2 (15%)—posterior radial head dislocation and apex posterior proximal-third ulna fracture. Annular ligament is disrupted in posterior Monteggia fracture dislocations.
  - Type 3—lateral radial head dislocation and proximal ulnar metaphyseal fracture
  - Type 4—anterior radial head dislocation and proximal-third radius and ulna fractures
  - "Monteggia-equivalent or variant"—radial head fracture instead of dislocation

Table 11-13	Adult Radial and Ulnar Shaft Fractures and Dislocations			
INJURY	**EPONYM/ OTHER NAME**	**CLASSIFICATION**	**TREATMENT**	**COMPLICATIONS**
Radius and ulna fractures	"Both-bone"	Degree of displacement	ORIF with six-hole DCP; external fixation for type III open fracture, bone graft if > one-third (shaft) comminution	Malunion/nonunion, vascular injury, posterior interosseous nerve (PIN) injury, compartment syndrome, synostosis, infection, refracture (after plate removal)
Ulna fracture	Nightstick	Nondisplaced	Distal two thirds, <50% displaced, <10-degree angulation: long-arm cast to functional brace with good interosseous mold	Malunion, nonunion
		Displaced	Proximal third, >50% displaced, >10-degree angulation: ORIF; look for wrist/elbow injury	
Proximal ulna and radial head fracture	Monteggia	Bado		Posterior intraosseous nerve injury (usually spontaneously resolves), redislocation/ subluxation (inadequate reduction), synostosis, loss of motion
		Type I (60%)—radial head dislocation, anterior and apex anterior proximal-third ulna fracture	ORIF of ulna (DCP), closed-reduction head, immobilize; if radial head irreducible, ulna fracture reduction may be nonanatomic	
		Type II (15%)—radial head dislocation, posterior and apex posterior proximal-third ulna shaft fracture	ORIF of ulna (DCP), closed reduction head, immobilize at 70 degrees	
		Type III—radial head dislocation, lateral and proximal ulnar metaphyseal fracture	ORIF of ulna (DCP), closed reduction head, immobilize	
		Type IV—radial head dislocation, anterior fracture and forearm fracture of both bones	ORIF of radius and ulna, closed reduction head, immobilize	
Proximal radius fracture		Nondisplaced	Long-arm cast in supination, close follow-up	
		Displaced	Proximal one fifth: closed; one fifth–two thirds: ORIF	
Distal radius (distal third) and radioulnar dislocation	Galeazzi/ Piedmont	Supination/pronation (signs of instability: ulnar styloid fracture, widened distal radioulnar joint on posteroanterior view, dislocation on lateral view, ≥5-mm radial shortening)	ORIF of radius (volar), closed reduction with or without percutaneous pinning to radioulnar joint (in supination) if unstable	Angulation, distal subluxation, malunion, nonunion; displaced by gravity, pronator quadratus, brachioradialis

DCP, Dynamic compression plate; *ORIF,* open reduction and internal fixation.

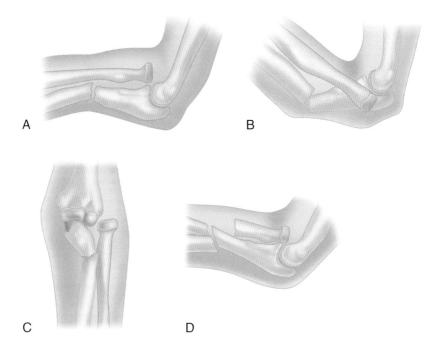

A

B

C

D

FIGURE 11-14 Monteggia fracture-dislocations. **A,** Type 1. **B,** Type 2. **C,** Type 3. **D,** Type 4. (From Crenshaw AH: Adult fractures and complex joint injuries of the elbow. In Stanley D, Kay NRM, editors: *Surgery of the elbow: practical and scientific aspects,* London, 1998, Arnold.)

- Interosseous membrane evaluation is important with Monteggia and Monteggia-equivalent injuries.
  - Physical examination—considered abnormal if greater than 3-mm instability is noted when the radius pulled proximally, indicating injury. If injury is greater than 6 mm, both the interosseous membrane and the triangular fibrocartilage complex are injured.
  - Confirm diagnosis with findings on MRI or ultrasonography.
  - Middle third is strongest and most important for stability.
- Treatment—all Monteggia fractures in adults should be treated with ORIF.
  - The radial head will normally reduce and be stable. If not, the most common cause is a nonanatomic reduction of the ulna.
  - If the ulna is anatomic and the radial head does not reduce, an open reduction with a separate approach is required to address the annular ligament.
- Complications
  - The complication rate is higher for Monteggia-equivalent and Bado type II injuries.
  - PIN injury
    - Usually resolves spontaneously and should be observed for 3 months
  - Redislocation/subluxation, synostosis, and loss of motion

- ■ **Both-bone forearm fractures**
- ■ Classification—displaced versus nondisplaced
- ■ Treatment
  - ORIF in adults
  - ORIF with **cancellous bone graft**
    - Significant segmental bone loss
    - Bone loss associated with open injury

- Routine use of bone graft for closed, comminuted fractures is no longer indicated.
- ■ Complications
  - Malunion (stiffness/deformity)
    - Restoration of the radial bow is directly related to functional outcome.
  - Nonunion
    - Typically due to technical error or use of IM fixation
    - Treat with ORIF and bone grafting.
  - Refracture after plate removal
    - Associated with premature plate removal at less than 12 to 18 months
    - After plate removal, a functional forearm brace should be worn for 6 weeks and activity protected for 3 months.
  - Synostosis
    - Associated with single-incision approach to ORIF
    - Treated with early excision, irradiation, and indomethacin
  - Posterior interosseous nerve injury
    - Henry (volar) approach to the middle and upper third of radial diaphysis
  - Vascular injury
- ■ **Ulna "nightstick" fractures**
- ■ Classification: stable (traditional definition is < 50% displacement) versus unstable (newer literature suggests that 25%-50% displacement or 10-15 degrees angulation is unstable)
- ■ Treatment
  - Distal two thirds, less than 50% displaced, and less than 10 degrees angulation—short arm cast or functional fracture brace with good interosseous mold
  - Proximal third, very distal shaft/head, over 50% displaced, or over 10 degrees angulation—ORIF

Table 11-14	Adult Wrist Fractures			
INJURY	**EPONYM**	**CLASSIFICATION**	**TREATMENT**	**COMPLICATIONS**
Distal radius fracture	Colles (dorsal displacement)	Frykman (I-VIII; even number = ulnar styloid fracture) I—extraarticular III—intraarticular radiocarpal joint fracture V—intraarticular radioulnar joint fracture VII—displaced intraarticular radiocarpal and radioulnar joint fractures	Distract, manipulate, splint 15 degrees palmar flexion and ulnar deviation, external fixation, and/or ORIF if comminuted/unstable; external fixation for severe comminution; ORIF for large fragments with a > 15-degree dorsal tilt, >1-2–mm articular displacement; bone graft comminuted fractures	Loss of reduction, nonunion, malunion, median neuropathy/carpal tunnel syndrome, weakness, tendon adhesion/rupture, instability, extensor pollicis longus rupture, DISI > 15 degrees (extension), ulnar side pain (shortening), CRPS, Volkmann ischemic contracture
	Smith (volar displacement)	Intraarticular vs. extraarticular	Distract, manipulate, splint in supination, flexion; CRPP vs. ORIF (volar approach)	Missed diagnosis, similar to Colles fracture
Dorsal rim of radius fracture	Dorsal Barton	Fernandez type II	Majority: ORIF with dorsal approach	Similar to Colles fracture
Radial styloid fracture	Chauffeur	Fernandez type II	Reduction, CRPP, cannulated screw or plate; immobilize in ulnar deviation	Similar to Colles fracture; rule out associated perilunate injury (ORIF)
Volar rim of radius fracture	Volar Barton	Fernandez type II	Majority: ORIF with volar buttress plate	Similar to Colles fracture
Distal radioulnar joint dissociation		Based on ulna displacement; fracture of base of ulnar styloid associated with TFCC tear	Dorsal—reduction, full supination, long-arm cast for 6 wk Volar—reduction (may require open reduction), long-arm cast for 6 wk in pronation	Osteochondral fracture, TFCC injury, ulnar nerve compression, instability, arthrosis, weak grip, decreased forearm rotation

CRPP, Closed reduction with percutaneous pinning; *CRPS,* complex regional pain syndrome; *DISI,* dorsal intercalated segment instability; *ORIF,* open reduction and internal fixation; *TFCC,* triangular fibrocartilage complex.

- **For nondisplaced fractures, there is no difference in outcome between surgical and nonsurgical treatment.**
- Complications: malunion/nonunion
- **Distal-third radius fracture with radioulnar dislocation (Galeazzi)**
- Diagnosis/classification: fracture of the radius (usually at junction of middle and distal thirds), with distal radioulnar joint (DRUJ) instability
  - DRUJ instability
    - DRUJ is unstable in 55% of patients when the radial fracture is less than 7.5 cm from the articular surface.
    - DRUJ is unstable in 6% of patients when the radial fracture is more than 7.5 cm away from the articular surface.
    - Signs of DRUJ instability include ulnar styloid fracture, widened DRUJ on posteroanterior view, dislocation on lateral view, and 5 mm or more of radial shortening.
- Treatment
  - Perform ORIF of the radius and then supinate the forearm and assess DRUJ.
    - Reduced and stable: protective splint and early motion
    - Reduced and unstable
      - Large ulnar styloid fragment: perform ORIF of styloid and immobilize in supination.
      - No fragment: **pin ulna to radius and immobilize in supination.**
    - Irreducible
      - Most commonly due to interposition of extensor carpi ulnaris tendon
      - Approach DRUJ via dorsal incision and remove block.

- Complications: malunion/nonunion and DRUJ subluxation

WRIST FRACTURES (TABLE 11-14)

- **Distal radius fractures**
- Classification
  - Frykman classification—types I to VIII (Figure 11-15)
    - Types II, IV, VI, and VIII—include the ulnar styloid
    - Type I—extraarticular
    - Type III—enters radiocarpal joint
    - Type V—enters radioulnar joint
    - Type VII—enters both joints
  - Melone classification (Figure 11-16)—describes radiocarpal joint as four fragments:
    - Radial styloid
    - Shaft
    - Volar medial
    - Dorsal medial
    - Types I to IV represent increasingly comminuted fractures of the aforementioned four anatomic regions and their parts.
    - Type V is an extremely comminuted unstable fracture without large identifiable facet fragments.
  - Fernandez classification (Figure 11-17)—based on the mechanism of injury and designed to guide treatment decision making
    - Type I—bending fractures
    - Type II—articular shear fractures
    - Type III—compression fractures
    - Type IV—fracture-dislocations (associated with ligamentous injury)
    - Type V—combined mechanisms

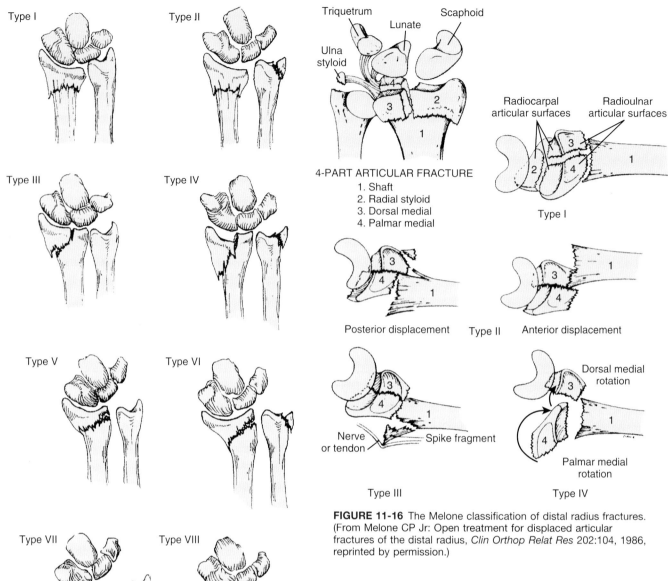

FIGURE 11-15 The Frykman classification of distal radius fractures. Note even numbers with ulnar styloid involvement. (From Kozin SH, Berlet AC: *Handbook of common orthopaedic fractures,* West Chester, PA, 1989, Medical Surveillance, pp 17, 19.)

4-PART ARTICULAR FRACTURE
1. Shaft
2. Radial styloid
3. Dorsal medial
4. Palmar medial

FIGURE 11-16 The Melone classification of distal radius fractures. (From Melone CP Jr: Open treatment for displaced articular fractures of the distal radius, *Clin Orthop Relat Res* 202:104, 1986, reprinted by permission.)

■ LaFontaine predictors of instability—patients with three or more factors have high chance of loss of reduction. Among these variables, radial shortening is the most predictive of instability, followed by dorsal comminution.
  • Dorsal angulation greater than 20°
  • Dorsal comminution greater than 50%, palmar comminution, intraarticular comminution
  • Initial displacement greater than 1 cm
  • Initial radial shortening greater than 5 mm
  • Associated ulnar fracture
  • Severe osteoporosis

■ Treatment—based on Fernandez classification
  • Type I—usually an extraarticular metaphyseal fracture. Comminution determines stability. The volarly displaced radial fracture is much more unstable. Use conservative treatment with reduction and casting if stable and CRPP versus internal/external fixation if unstable. **American Academy of Orthopaedic Surgeons Clinical Practice Guidelines gives a moderate strength of recommendation for surgical fixation of distal radius fractures.**
  • Type II—shearing injury of the joint surface (volar or dorsal lip or radial styloid). This type is usually unstable, and carpal subluxation frequently occurs. Treatment is with ORIF.
  • Type III—articular compression (die-punch) injuries follow patterns described by Melone.
    • Conservative treatment if nondisplaced
    • ORIF with disimpaction of the articular surface if displaced. Arthroscopy may be adjunct.
  • Type IV—rare and follows high-energy trauma
    • These are avulsion fractures with radiocarpal fracture dislocations.

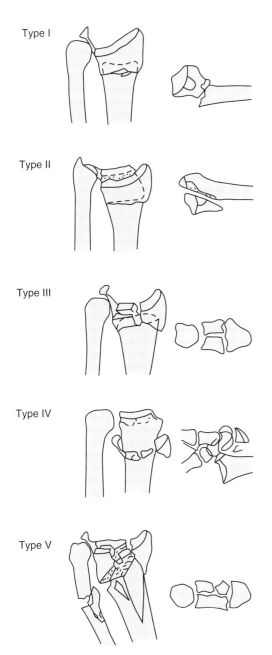

Type I

Type II

Type III

Type IV

Type V

FIGURE 11-17 The Fernandez classification of distal radius fractures (fracture types in adults based on the mechanism of injury). (From Tornetta P III, Baumgaertner M: *Orthopaedic knowledge update: trauma 3,* Rosemont, Ill, 2005, American Academy of Orthopaedic Surgeons, p 206.)

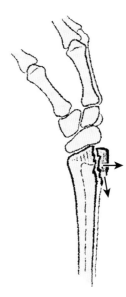

FIGURE 11-18 The Barton fracture (dorsal). (From Connolly JF, editor: *DePalma's the management of fractures and dislocations: an atlas,* ed 3, Philadelphia, 1981, WB Saunders, p 1032, reprinted by permission.)

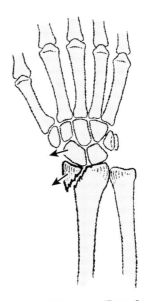

FIGURE 11-19 Radial styloid fractures. (From Connolly JF, editor: *DePalma's the management of fractures and dislocations: an atlas,* ed 3, Philadelphia, 1981, WB Saunders, p 1033, reprinted by permission.)

- Surgical repair of the avulsed styloid usually restores stability. Treat with closed or (more frequently) open reduction, pin or screw fixation, or tension wiring.
- Type V—combination fractures of types I to IV after high-energy trauma. These are very severe and unstable fractures. There are always associated injuries. Treatment is open, with combined methods.
■ Outcomes—restoration of anatomic alignment best predictor of a good outcome
- Loss of radial length and volar tilt is the most important; radial inclination is less important.
- Articular step-offs of more than 1 to 2 mm also predict poor outcome.
■ Complications—loss of reduction, malunion/nonunion, median nerve neuropathy, weakness, tendon adhesion,

instability, extensor pollicis longus rupture, dorsal intercalated segment instability (DISI), Volkmann ischemic contracture, and complex regional pain syndrome. Some studies have shown that vitamin C can reduce the likelihood of complex regional pain syndrome following distal radius fracture.

■ **Other variants and eponyms**
▤ Dorsal rim radius fractures—dorsal Barton (Figure 11-18)
- Classification—Fernandez type II
- Treatment—ORIF with dorsal approach in the vast majority
- Complications—same as for distal radius fracture
▤ Radial styloid fractures—chauffeur fracture (Figure 11-19)
- Diagnosis/classification—frequently high-energy trauma in young adults. Fernandez type II is associated with perilunate injuries.

- Treatment—CRPP or ORIF with screws; immobilize in ulnar deviation.
- Complications—same as for distal radius fracture
▪ Volar rim radius fractures—volar Barton fracture (Figure 11-20)
- Classification—Fernandez type II
- Treatment—usually with ORIF by means of the volar approach; closed reduction (rarely)
- Complications—same as for distal radius fracture
▪ DRUJ injuries
- Diagnosis/classification—fracture of the base of the ulnar styloid, associated with triangular fibrocartilage complex tear
- Treatment—closed or open reduction to achieve anatomic ulnar styloid reduction; immobilize in supination
- Complications—osteochondral fracture, ulnar nerve compression, instability, arthrosis, weak grip, and decreased forearm rotation

CARPAL INJURIES

See Chapter 7, "Hand, Upper Extremity, and Microvascular Surgery."

HAND INJURIES

See Chapter 7, "Hand, Upper Extremity, and Microvascular Surgery."

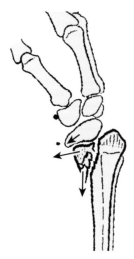

FIGURE 11-20 The Barton fracture (volar). (From Connolly JF, editor: *DePalma's the management of fractures and dislocations: an atlas,* ed 3, Philadelphia, 1981, WB Saunders, p 1028, reprinted by permission.)

SECTION 3 LOWER EXTREMITY AND PELVIS

 PELVIC AND ACETABULAR INJURIES

■ **Pelvic ring injuries (Table 11-15)**
▪ Diagnosis
- Mechanism of injury
- Often high energy
- Associated injuries common (chest, head, other orthopaedic)
- Nonpelvic sources of bleeding must be ruled out.
- Mortality usually related to nonpelvic injuries
- Radiographs
- Anteroposterior pelvis
- Inlet—evaluate anteroposterior displacement of sacroiliac joint and internal/external rotational deformity.
- Outlet—evaluate vertical displacement of sacroiliac joint and flexion of hemipelvis.
- CT—particularly useful to evaluate posterior pelvic injury patterns
▪ Classification
- Young-Burgess (Figure 11-21)—based on injury mechanism. Theorized to predict mortality, transfusion requirements, and associated nonorthopaedic injuries. Recent studies question its predictive value. One large series found it useful for predicting transfusion requirements but did not predict mortality or associated nonorthopaedic injuries well.
- Lateral compression (LC)—all have anterior transverse pubic ramus fracture.
- LC I—sacral compression fracture
- LC II—posterior iliac wing fracture
- LC III—contralateral anteroposterior compression injury ("windswept pelvis")
- Thought to be due to a rollover mechanism
- Anteroposterior compression (APC)—all have symphyseal diastasis.
- APC I—symphyseal diastasis less than 2.5 cm
- Stretching of anterior sacroiliac ligaments
- APC II—symphyseal diastasis greater than 2.5 cm with widening of sacroiliac joint anteriorly
- Rupture of sacrotuberous, sacrospinous, and anterior sacroiliac ligaments
- APC III—symphyseal diastasis greater than 2.5 cm with complete disruption of sacroiliac joint, both anteriorly and posteriorly. Highest transfusion requirements.
- Rupture of sacrotuberous, sacrospinous, and anterior and posterior sacroiliac ligaments
- Complete separation of hemipelvis from pelvic ring
- Vertical shear (VS)
- Usually due to a fall. Vertical displacement of hemipelvis commonly with complete disruption of the SI joint.
- Combined mechanism
- Stable types are lateral compression type I and anteroposterior compression type I

Table 11-15	Adult Pelvic Fractures			
INJURY	**EPONYM**	**CLASSIFICATION**	**TREATMENT**	**COMPLICATIONS**
Pelvic fracture		Young and Burgess	Emergent management (advanced trauma life support, resuscitation, embolization of bleeding arteries if necessary, binder/ external fixation/traction/ pelvic C-clamp based on injury pattern)	Posterior skin slough, life-threatening hemorrhage, gastrointestinal injury, genitourinary injury (bladder, urethra, impotency), neurologic injury, nonunion, posttraumatic degenerative joint disease, pain, deep venous thrombosis, pulmonary embolism, loss of reduction, sepsis, thrombophlebitis, malunion (leg-length discrepancy, sitting problems), vascular injuries (including aortic rupture), SI pain; APC type III highest rate of associated injury
Lateral compression		I (most common)—transverse rami fracture and sacral compression fracture	Protected weight bearing, pain control	
		II—rami fracture and posterior iliac wing fracture	Protected weight bearing or delayed ORIF	
		III—symphysis or rami and anterior and posterior SI ligament torn	Based on contralateral injury (ORIF of unstable injuries)	
Anteroposterior compression		I—symphysis (<2.5 cm) or rami (vertical) and anterior SI ligament stretched	Bed rest, early mobilization, pain control	
		II—symphysis or rami and anterior SI ligament torn	Acute external fixation/anterior ORIF if concurrent laparotomy	
		III—symphysis or rami and anterior and posterior SI ligament torn	Acute external fixation/anterior ORIF if concurrent laparotomy; posterior SI ORIF	
	Malgaigne	Vertical shear—anterior and posterior vertical displacement	Acute external fixation/anterior ORIF if concurrent laparotomy; posterior SI ORIF (SI screws, anterior SI plate, posterior transiliac sacral bars, spinal-pelvic fixation)	
		Combined mechanical—combination of other injuries	Based on injuries; ORIF if posterior SI displaced	
Sacral fracture	Denis—fracture location relative to foramen	Stable, nondisplaced	Nonoperative (weight bearing as tolerated if fracture incomplete, toe-touch weight bearing for complete fracture)	Neurologic (highest with zone II fractures), chronic low-back pain, malunion
		Unstable, displaced (>1 cm)	Percutaneous SI screws, posterior ORIF, transiliac sacral bars, open foraminal decompression for nerve root injury with zone II fractures	

APC, Anteroposterior compression; *ORIF,* open reduction and internal fixation; *SI,* sacroiliac.

- APC II, APC III, LC III, and VS may have stretching and tearing of veins and arteries causing hemorrhagic shock
- Associated injuries
  - APC pattern has associated urethral and bladder injuries. Incidence of spleen, liver, bowel, and pelvic vascular injury increases from APC-I to APC-III categories.
  - LC-I and LC-II pattern has associated brain, lung, and abdominal injuries.
  - LC-III pattern usually due to a crush injury to pelvis, sparing other organs from injury
  - Vertical shear pattern has similar injury pattern and mortality to APC-II and APC-III injuries.
- Combined mechanism pattern has organ injury pattern similar to lower-grade APC and LC patterns
- Cause of death in LC pattern is primarily due to brain injury, whereas in APC, pattern is primarily due to shock, sepsis, and ARDS.
- Tile—based on fracture stability
  - Stable (posterior arch intact)
    - Avulsion fractures
    - Iliac wing fractures
    - Transverse sacral fractures
  - Partially stable—rotationally unstable and vertically stable

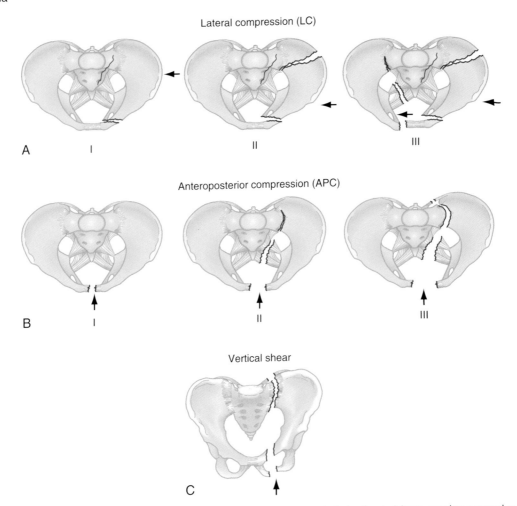

Lateral compression (LC)

A — I — II — III

Anteroposterior compression (APC)

B — I — II — III

Vertical shear

C

FIGURE 11-21 Young-Burgess classification. **A,** Lateral compression. Type I: a posteriorly directed force causing a sacral crushing injury and horizontal pubic ramus fractures ipsilaterally. Type II: a more anteriorly directed force causing horizontal pubic ramus fractures with an anterior sacral crushing injury and either disruption of the posterior sacroiliac joints or fractures through the iliac wing. Type III: an anteriorly directed force that is continued, causing external rotation of the contralateral side; the sacroiliac joint is opened posteriorly and the sacrotuberous and spinous ligaments are disrupted. **B,** Anteroposterior compression. Type I: symphysis disrupted but with intact posterior ligamentous structures. Type II: continuation of a type I fracture with disruption of the sacrospinous and potentially the sacrotuberous ligaments and an anterior sacroiliac joint opening. Type III: continuation force disrupts the sacroiliac ligaments. **C,** Vertical shear: vertical fractures in the rami and disruption of all posterior ligaments. This injury is equivalent to an anteroposterior type III or a completely unstable and rotationally unstable fracture. Arrow indicates the direction of force. (Redrawn from Young JWR, Burgess AR: *Radiologic management of pelvic ring fractures,* Baltimore, 1987, Urban & Schwarzenberg.)

- External rotation
  - Anterior pelvic disruption alone
  - Anterior sacroiliac ligaments too
  - Anterior and posterior sacroiliac ligaments
- Lateral compression
  - Ipsilateral
  - Contralateral (bucket handle)
  - Bilateral
- Unstable (complete disruption of posterior arch)
  - Unilateral
  - Bilateral but one side B type and one side C type
  - Bilateral C type
- Treatment
  - General principles
    - Emergent treatment: control hemorrhage and provisionally stabilize pelvic ring
    - Important to establish and follow a treatment protocol to avoid variation in treatment decision making (Figure 11-22)

- 85% of bleeding due to venous injury, only 15% arterial source
- Volume resuscitation and early blood transfusion
- Pelvic binder or wrapped sheet. External rotational deformity may also be reduced by taping feet together.
- Angiographic embolization
- Pelvic packing, initially popularized in Europe, provides tamponade of venous bleeding.
- External fixation
  - Place before emergent laparotomy
- Skeletal traction—for vertically unstable patterns
- Pelvic C clamp (rarely used)
- Nonoperative treatment
  - Indicated for stable fracture patterns
  - Weight bearing as tolerated for isolated anterior injuries
  - Protected weight bearing for ipsilateral anterior and posterior ring injuries

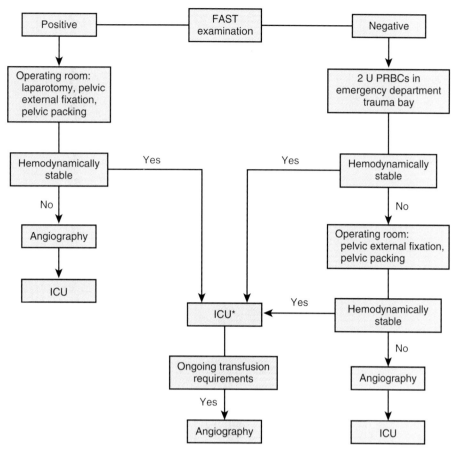

FIGURE 11-22 Algorithm for the treatment of patients with high-energy pelvic fracture who present with hemodynamic instability at Denver Health Medical Center. *Patients in whom a laparotomy was not done usually have an abdominal computed tomography scan en route to the intensive care unit (ICU). *FAST,* Focused abdominal sonography for trauma; *PRBCs,* packed red blood cells.

- Operative treatment
  - Indications
    - Symphysis diastasis greater than 2.5 cm. Degree of actual diastasis may not be apparent in patients who are placed in a pelvic binder prior to initial AP pelvic x-ray. May require intraoperative stress view examination.
    - Anterior and posterior sacroiliac ligament disruption
    - Vertical instability of posterior hemipelvis
    - Sacral fracture with displacement greater than 1 cm
  - Anterior injuries
    - ORIF with plate fixation
    - External fixation via pins through anterior-inferior iliac spine (biomechanically stronger than iliac wing but less well tolerated clinically) or iliac wing
      - The lateral femoral cutaneous nerve is most at risk.
  - Posterior injuries
    - Percutaneous iliosacral screw fixation
      - Vertical sacral fractures are at higher risk for loss of fixation.
    - Anterior plate fixation across the sacroiliac joint
    - Posterior transiliac sacral bars or sacral plating
    - Spinal-pelvic fixation considered for bilateral sacral fractures

- Vertically unstable patterns with anterior and posterior dislocations
  - Anterior ring internal fixation and percutaneous sacroiliac screw has been shown to be most stable fixation construct
  - Spinal-pelvic fixation may also be considered.
- Complications
  - Severe life-threatening hemorrhage
    - **Highest risk with APC II, APC III, and LC III patterns**
  - Neurologic injury
  - Urogenital injury/dysfunction
    - Urethral stricture most common in men
    - Dyspareunia and need for cesarean section childbirth common in women
  - Malunion
  - Nonunion
  - DVT and/or pulmonary embolus
    - DVT is the most common complication if thromboprophylaxis is not used.
  - Infection—open fracture and associated contaminated laparotomy
  - Death
    - Risk factors for death identified during initial treatment:
      - Blood transfusion requirement in first 24 hours

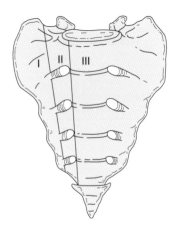

FIGURE 11-23 The Denis classification of sacral fractures. (From Browner BD et al, editors: *Skeletal trauma,* Philadelphia, 1992, WB Saunders, p 820.)

- Unstable fracture type (APC II, APC III, LC II, LC III, vertical shear, combined mechanism)
- Open fracture
- **Chronic instability following pelvic fracture can be best assessed with single leg stance views (Flamingo views)**

■ **Sacral fractures**

▨ Diagnosis
  - Mechanism of injury—high energy
  - Radiographs—AP pelvis, inlet, outlet, and lateral views
  - CT (usually required)
▨ Classification—Denis classification (Figure 11-23) based on fracture location relative to foramen (zones I, II, and III)
▨ Treatment
  - Nonoperative treatment
    - Indicated for stable and minimally displaced fractures
    - Weight bearing as tolerated for incomplete fractures in which the ilium is contiguous with the intact sacrum (e.g., anterior impaction fractures from lateral compression mechanism or isolated sacral alar fractures)
    - Touch-toe weight bearing for complete fractures
  - Operative treatment
    - Indicated for displaced fractures (>1 cm)
    - Percutaneous iliosacral screws
      - Appropriate fluoroscopic visualization of anatomic landmarks is mandatory before surgery.
      - The pelvic outlet radiograph allows optimal visualization of the S1 neural foramina to avoid injury.
      - The lateral sacral view identifies the sacral alar slope and minimizes risk to the L5 nerve root.
      - High incidence of sacral dysmorphism (20%-44%). Sacralization of L5 or lumbarization of S1. Risk of anterior screw penetration causing neurologic injury is much higher with anterosuperior sacral concavity. (Figure 11-24)
      - Radiographic signs of sacral dysmorphism best seen on outlet view: prominent mammillary processes, laterally downsloping sacral ala, residual vestigial disc space between S1 and S2, top of iliac wing at level of L5/S1 instead of at L4/5, noncircular S1 anterior neural tunnel

      - Radiographic signs of sacral dysmorphism best seen on axial CT scan: peaked or prow-shaped sacral promontory, tongue-in-groove sacroiliac articulation, oblique and narrow S1 sacral ala, wider S2 alar channel
    - Posterior plating
    - Transiliac sacral bars
    - Open foraminal decompression considered for neurologic injury associated with zone II fracture
▨ Complications
  - Neurologic injury
    - Highest incidence with displaced zone II fractures
    - L5 nerve root usually involved with zone II fractures
    - Cauda equina syndrome can be associated with zone III injuries.
  - Chronic low back pain
  - Malunion

■ **Acetabular fractures (Figure 11-25 and Table 11-16)**

▨ Diagnosis
  - Mechanism of injury
    - Pattern of injury dependent on position of hip and direction of impact
    - Flexed hip with axial load (dashboard injury mechanism) most common
  - Plain radiographs
    - AP pelvis—six cardinal lines (Figure 11-26)
    - **Obturator oblique—profiles anterior column and posterior wall. Best view to ensure that screw placed in anterior column does not penetrate into hip joint (Figure 11-27).**
    - **Iliac oblique—profiles posterior column and anterior wall (Figure 11-28)**
  - CT
    - Thin-cut (1-2 mm) axial
    - Three-dimensional reconstruction with femur subtracted
▨ Classification—Letournel classification (Figure 11-29) based on involvement of acetabular columns and walls
  - Simple types
    - Posterior wall (PW)
      - Most common simple type
    - Posterior column (PC)
    - Anterior wall (AW)
    - Anterior column (AC)
    - Transverse
      - Involves both the anterior and posterior columns
  - Associated types
    - Posterior column/posterior wall (PC/PW)
    - Transverse/posterior wall (TPW)
    - T-type
      - Transverse with vertical limbs through ischium
    - Anterior column/posterior hemitransverse (ACPHT)
      - Least common type
    - Associated both column (ABC)
      - Most common associated type
      - Dissociation of acetabular dome from intact ilium
        - "Spur sign" seen on obturator oblique view represents the posterior ilium that is undisplaced (Figure 11-30).
▨ Radiographs
  - A systematic evaluation can be used to classify most acetabular fractures using plain radiographs (see Figure 11-25):
    - Examine the iliopectineal and ilioischial lines.

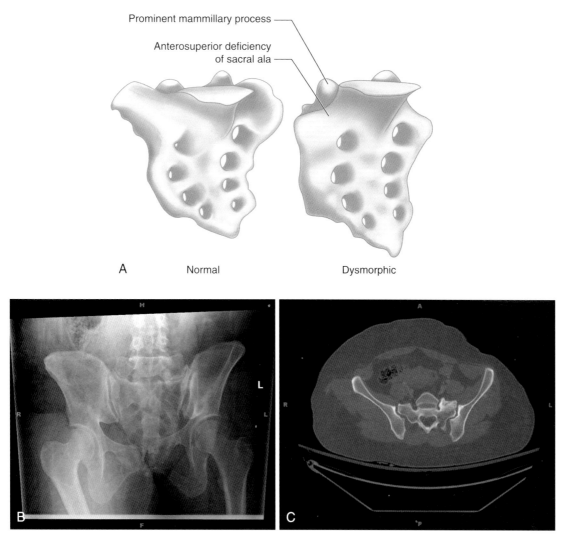

FIGURE 11-24 **A,** Schematic representation of the normal *(left)* and dysmorphic *(right)* sacrum. Characteristics of sacral dysmorphism include the presence of prominent mammillary processes and anterosuperior deficiency of the sacral ala. **B,** Outlet view showing classic features of sacral dysmorphism *(right)*. Iliac crest is at the same level as the upper sacral border, prominent mammillary processes, down sloping sacral ala and vestigial disc remnant. **C,** CT scan showing irregular tongue and groove contour of the sacroiliac joint.

- If both lines are intact:
  - Posterior wall fracture
- If only one line disrupted:
  - Iliopectineal line
    - Anterior wall fracture
    - Anterior column fracture
  - Ilioischial line
    - Posterior column fracture
    - Posterior column and posterior wall fracture
- If both lines disrupted:
  - Look at the obturator ring and determine if it is intact.
    - Obturator ring intact
      - Transverse fracture (Figure 11-31)
      - Transverse/posterior wall
    - Obturator ring disrupted
      - Look at iliac wing.
      - Iliac wing intact
        - T-type (Figure 11-32)
      - Iliac wing disrupted
        - Anterior column–posterior hemitransverse
        - Associated both column fracture

- CT
  - Typically used to evaluate posterior injuries, articular fragments, **marginal impaction,** and congruency of the hip joint
  - Axial CT may be useful to aid in fracture classification.
    - Vertical fracture line
      - Transverse or T-shaped fracture
      - If the wall can clearly be visualized, then anterior or posterior wall fracture
    - Horizontal fracture line
      - Column fracture
  - Sequential axial CT cuts that demonstrate no intact support between the acetabular articular surface and axial skeleton through the sacroiliac joint are associated both-column fractures
- Treatment
  - General principles
    - Restore articular congruity and hip stability.
    - Avoid injury to blood supply to femoral head.
    - DVT screening and prophylaxis

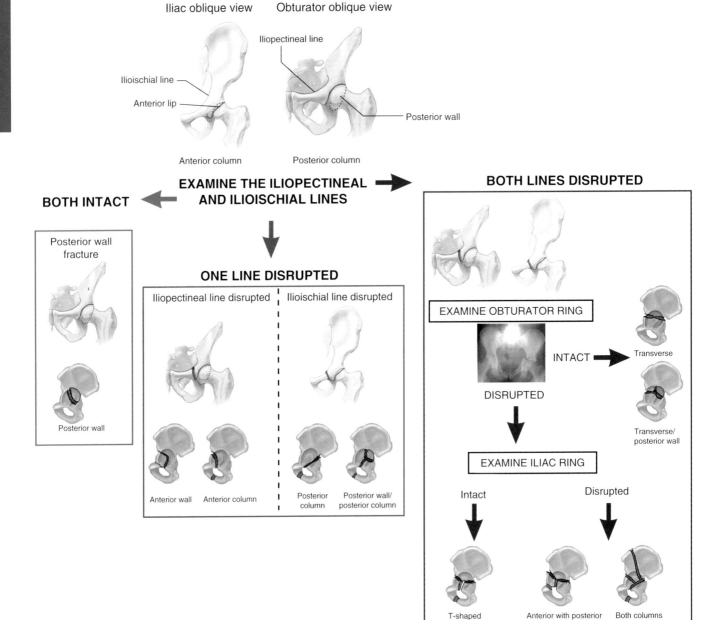

FIGURE 11-25 Acetabulum. Systematic evaluation for determining acetabular fracture type using plane radiographs.

- During surgery, extend hip and flex knee to minimize tension on sciatic nerve
- Patients are generally touch-down weight bearing postoperatively. Getting up from chair using the affected leg produces the greatest risk of fixation failure by creating the highest acetabular contact pressures.
- Nonoperative treatment
  - Indications
    - Nondisplaced or minimally displaced fracture (<1-mm step and <2-mm gap)
    - Roof arc angle greater than 45 degrees on AP, iliac oblique, and obturator oblique—CT correlate is a fracture greater than 10 mm from the dome apex.
    - Posterior wall fracture without instability (<20%-30% of posterior wall—exact number controversial)

- Operative dynamic stress examination may be considered to assess stability of posterior wall fracture.
- Fracture of both columns, with secondary congruence
- Severe comminution in the elderly in whom total hip replacement is planned after fracture healing
- Protected weight bearing for approximately 6 weeks
- For unstable injuries that cannot be operated on—femoral traction for 2 to 3 weeks, followed by toe-touch weight bearing for 3 to 4 weeks
- Operative treatment
  - Early surgery (<5 days from injury) is associated with improved fracture reduction compared to late surgery (10-14 days)
  - Indications

Table 11-16 | Adult Acetabular Fractures

CLASSIFICATION	TREATMENT	COMPLICATIONS

Letournel—based on involvement of acetabular columns and wall
Simple types:
  Anterior wall (AW)
  Anterior column (AC)
  Posterior wall (PW)—most common simple type
  Posterior column (PC)
  Transverse—involves both AC and PC
Associated types:
  PC/PW
  Transverse/PW—AC/posterior hemitransverse (ACPHT)—least common type
  T-type—transverse with vertical limb through ischium
  Associated both column (ABC)—dissociation of acetabular dome from axial skeleton. No part of articular surface remains attached to intact posterior ilium. "Spur sign" seen on obturator oblique view (most common associated type).
	Nonoperative: <1-mm step-off and < 2-mm gap; roof arc angle > 45 degrees on anteroposterior, inlet, and outlet views—computed tomographic correlate is fracture > 10 mm from dome apex; PW fractures without instability (<20% of PW); associated fractures of both columns (BCs) with secondary congruence; severe comminution in elderly in whom total hip arthroplasty is planned after fracture healing
	Relative contraindications to surgery: morbid obesity, physiologically elderly/nonambulatory, contaminated wound, delay to operation > 4 wk, presence of deep venous thrombosis with contraindication for filter
	Operative: displaced fracture, incongruous or unstable joint, intraarticular bone fragments, irreducible fracture-dislocation
	Surgical approaches:
	Kocher-Langenbeck (posterior approach) indicated for PW, PC, transverse, transverse/PW (when PW requires fixation), PC/PW, T-type
	Ilioinguinal (anterior approach) indicated for AW, AC, ACPHT, BCs
	Extensile approaches considered for fractures > 3 wk old and complex associated fractures
	Combined anterior and posterior approaches
	Extended iliofemoral
	Triradiate
	Posterior with trochanteric osteotomy
		Nerve injury (sciatic 16%-33%, femoral, superior gluteal), vascular injury (inferior gluteal artery), heterotopic ossification (3%-69%—consider radiation therapy or indomethacin), avascular necrosis (with posterior injury), chondrolysis, posttraumatic degenerative joint disease, soft tissue degloving (Morel-Lavallée lesion), osteonecrosis (damage to medial femoral circumflex artery), malreduction (delay to surgery), bleeding (shorter time to surgery)

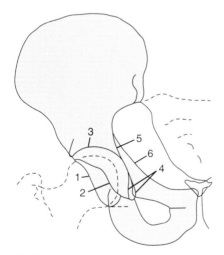

FIGURE 11-26 Six cardinal radiographic lines of the acetabulum. *1,* Posterior wall. *2,* Anterior wall. *3,* Roof. *4,* Teardrop. *5,* Ilioischial line. *6,* Iliopectineal line. (From Tornetta P III, Baumgaertner M: *Orthopaedic knowledge update: trauma 3,* Rosemont, Ill, 2005, American Academy of Orthopaedic Surgeons, p 264.)

- Relative contraindications to surgery
  - Morbid obesity
  - Physiologically elderly and nonambulatory
  - Presence of DVT, with contraindication to inferior vena cava filter
  - Contaminated wound compromising surgical approach
  - Delay to operation more than 3 weeks
- Surgical approaches
  - Kocher-Langenbeck
    - Posterior approach
    - **Indicated for PW, PC, transverse, transverse/PW (when PW requires fixation), PC/PW, and some T-type**
  - Ilioinguinal
    - Anterior approach procedure
    - Indicated for AW, AC, ACPHT, associated both column, and some T types (if limited posterior wall involved)
    - Can be divided into three "windows": lateral (iliac), middle (vascular), and medial (Stoppa)
    - **Ilioinguinal nerve travels with round ligament or spermatic cord through superficial inguinal ring**
    - **Injury to obturator nerve will cause hypesthesia of inner thigh.**
    - Injury to lateral femoral cutaneous nerve will cause hypesthesia of lateral thigh.
      - The modified Stoppa exposes the internal pelvis and **provides the best access to the quadrilateral surface.**

- Displacement with a greater than 1-mm step or greater than 2-mm gap associated with the roof is an angle less than 45 degrees on any view or documented instability with stress examination.
- Posterior wall fracture of greater than 20% to 30% or hip instability
- Intraarticular bone fragments
- Irreducible fracture-dislocation

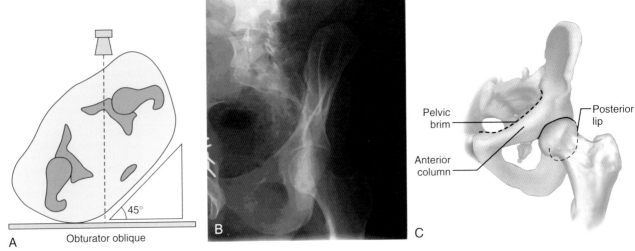

FIGURE 11-27 A, Obturator oblique view of pelvis obtained with the patient tilted 45 degrees, with the unaffected hip down and adjacent to the x-ray cassette. The x-ray beam was centered over the affected hip. **B,** Obturator oblique radiograph profiles the anterior column and the posterior wall of the acetabulum. **C,** Obturator oblique–related landmarks. (**A** and **B** from Tornetta P III, Baumgaertner M: *Orthopaedic knowledge update: trauma 3,* Rosemont, Ill, 2005, American Academy of Orthopaedic Surgeons, p 263; **C** from Schemitsch E: *Operative techniques: orthopaedic trauma surgery,* Philadelphia, 2010, Saunders.)

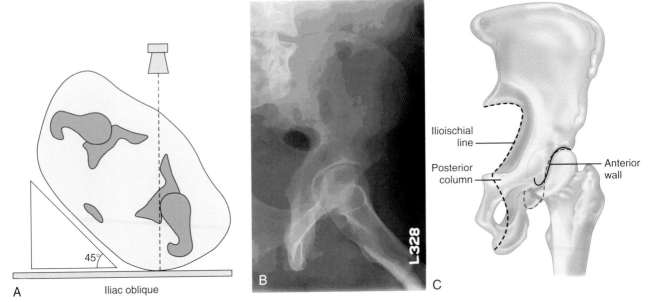

FIGURE 11-28 A, Iliac oblique view of pelvis obtained with the patient tilted 45 degrees, with the affected hip down and adjacent to the x-ray cassette. The x-ray beam was centered over the affected hip. **B,** Iliac oblique radiograph profiles the posterior column and the anterior wall of the acetabulum. **C,** Iliac oblique–related landmarks. (**A** and **B** from Tornetta P III, Baumgaertner M: *Orthopaedic knowledge update: trauma 3,* Rosemont, Ill, 2005, American Academy of Orthopaedic Surgeons, p 263; **C** from Schemitsch E: *Operative techniques: orthopaedic trauma surgery,* Philadelphia, 2010, Saunders.)

- **Corona mortis**: common (10%-30%) **vascular communication between external iliac and the obturator artery** typically seen about 5 cm medially from pubic symphysis. Needs to be ligated to prevent retraction of inadvertently injured vessel.
  - Extensile approaches considered for fractures more than 3 weeks old, complex associated fractures, and need for posterior column reduction
    - Combined anterior and posterior approaches

- Extended iliofemoral approach
- Triradiate
- Posterior with trochanteric osteotomy
- Treatment with ORIF and acute total hip arthroplasty
  - Relative indications:
    - Age older than 60 with presence of superomedial dome impaction on radiograph ("gull sign")
    - Associated displaced femoral neck fracture
    - Significant preexisting arthrosis

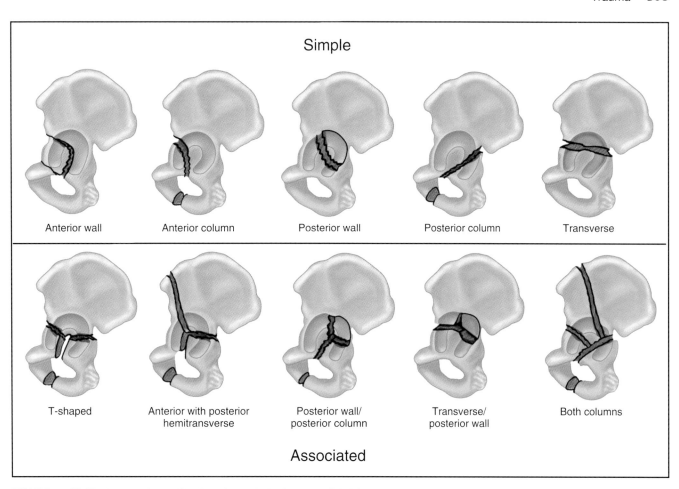

FIGURE 11-29 The Letournel classification of acetabular fractures. (Modified with permission from Letournel E, Judet R, editors: *Fractures of the acetabulum,* ed 2, Berlin, 1993, Springer-Verlag.)

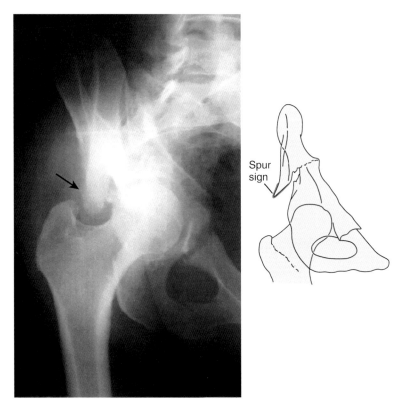

FIGURE 11-30 Spur sign. Obturator oblique radiograph and drawing of a both-column fracture. Note the medial translation of the dome of the acetabulum and the femoral head. The spur sign represents the intact portion of the iliac wing that remains in its anatomic position.

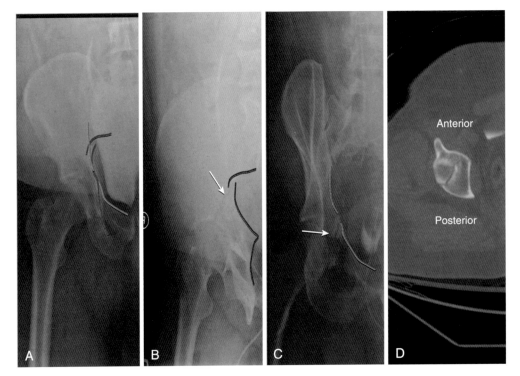

FIGURE 11-31 Imaging of a right acetabulum transverse fracture. In **A,** anteroposterior view showing disruption of both ilioischial *(red)* and iliopectineal *(blue)* lines. No rami fractures are seen (unlikely a T type). In **B,** iliac oblique view of the right hemipelvis revealing a fracture line *(white arrow)* breaking through the line demarcating the posterior column *(red)*. In **C,** obturator oblique view of the right hemipelvis revealing a fracture line *(white arrow)* breaking through the anterior column *(blue line)*. In **D,** axial CT cut of the transverse fracture extending from anterior to posterior.

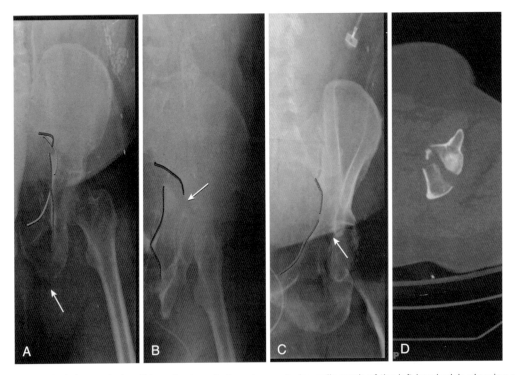

FIGURE 11-32 Imaging of a left acetabulum T-type fracture. In **A,** anteroposterior radiograph of the left hemipelvis showing a disruption of both iliopectineal *(blue)* and ilioischial *(red)* lines. Note the white arrow pointing at the fracture line extending down to the pubic rami (vertical stem of the T-type fracture). In **B,** iliac oblique radiograph of the left hemipelvis showing the fracture line breaching the posterior column *(red)*. In **C,** obturator oblique radiograph of the left hemipelvis showing the fracture extending through the anterior column. In **D,** axial CT cut of the T-type fracture extending from anterior to posterior (transverse stem) with a breach in the quadrilateral plate extending distally (vertical stem).

■ Complications
- Soft tissue degloving (Morel-Lavallée lesion) associated with higher infection rates
- DVT
  - Preoperative screening and inferior vena cava filter when DVT present. Postoperative screening and anticoagulation if DVT is present.
- Pulmonary embolism—treatment similar to that for DVT
- Heterotopic ossification
  - **Highest in extended iliofemoral approach.** Higher in extended approaches (20%-50%) than Kocher-Langenbeck (8%-25%), than anterior approach (2%-10%).
  - Prophylaxis with indomethacin (debatable efficacy) or external-beam radiation therapy of 600 cGy within 48 hours of surgery
- Neurologic injury
  - Sciatic nerve injury associated with posterior dislocations, especially peroneal division (<50% with full recovery)
  - Intraoperative monitoring is not associated with reduced iatrogenic nerve injury.
  - Hip extension and knee flexion reduce tension on sciatic nerve.
  - Iatrogenic injury to lateral femoral cutaneous nerve with anterior approach
- Osteonecrosis—the highest incidence with posterior fractures, especially fracture-dislocations; iatrogenic damage to medial femoral circumflex artery
- Posttraumatic DJD
  - Highest in patterns with posterior wall involvement
  - Quality of reduction is most important predictor.
- Malreduction
  - Associated with greater delay to surgery
- Bleeding—associated with shorter time to surgery
- Functional deficit—especially abductor weakness (posterior more than anterior approach)

FEMORAL AND HIP INJURIES (TABLES 11-17 AND 11-18)

■ **Hip dislocations**

▥ Diagnosis
- Mechanism of injury—axial load; position of hip determines direction of dislocation
  - Usually high-energy mechanism; very high rate of associated injuries either systemic or musculoskeletal; 93% rate of MRI abnormalities of ipsilateral knee
- Plain radiographs—AP and lateral views of the hip; AP pelvis and Judet views after reduction to evaluate associated acetabular fractures

- CT—performed after reduction to evaluate associated acetabular and/or femoral head fracture and loose bodies in joint

▥ Classification—based on direction of dislocation and presence or absence of associated acetabular or femoral head fracture
- Posterior dislocation—most common; associated with posterior wall acetabular fracture and anterior femoral head fracture—leg flexed, adducted, and internally rotated at hip
  - Ipsilateral associated knee injury; 30% rate of meniscal tear
- Anterior dislocation—uncommon; leg extended, abducted, and externally rotated at hip

▥ Treatment
- Emergent closed reduction
- Emergent open reduction if irreducible after closed reduction
  - AVN rate 2% to 10% if reduced within 6 hours and over 50% if reduction delayed more than 12 hours
  - Almost all cases of AVN appear within 2 years of injury.
- Evaluate stability after reduction.
- Traction and/or hip abduction pillow for unstable injuries pending definitive management of associated injuries (e.g., acetabular fracture)
- Postreduction radiographs (AP pelvis and Judet views) and CT to rule out associated acetabular fracture, femoral head fracture, and intraarticular loose bodies
- Weight bearing as tolerated (if hip is stable and without associated injuries)

▥ Complications
- Osteonecrosis (up to 15%)
- Posttraumatic arthritis; less common when associated with PW acetabular fracture
- Sciatic nerve injury (up to 20%); peroneal nerve division usually most affected
- Recurrent dislocation (rare)

■ **Femoral head fractures**

▥ Diagnosis
- Plain radiographs—AP and lateral views of hip
- CT—to evaluate location and size of fragment and rule out associated acetabular fracture

▥ Classification—Pipkin classification (Figure 11-33) based on location of fracture relative to fovea and presence or absence of associated fractures of the acetabulum or femoral neck
- Type I—fracture below fovea
- Type II—fracture above fovea
- Type III—associated femoral neck fracture
- Type IV—associated acetabular fracture

Table 11-17	Adult Hip Dislocations		
INJURY	**CLASSIFICATION**	**TREATMENT**	**COMPLICATIONS**
Hip dislocation	Direction: posterior (most common), anterior, obturator; associated fractures (acetabular, femoral head)	Emergent closed reduction (open if irreducible); computed tomography/plain films (Judet views) after reduction; traction/abduction pillow (depends on stability); weight bearing as tolerated if hip stable	Associated with increased-energy trauma and often associated with other injuries; femoral artery/nerve injuries (anterior dislocation), sciatic nerve injury (up to 20%; peroneal division most common), osteonecrosis (up to 15%), posttraumatic arthritis, recurrent dislocation (rare), posttraumatic degenerative joint disease (especially with retained fragments); instability (with > 30%-40% fracture of posterior wall); unrecognized femoral neck fracture

Table 11-18	Adult Hip Fractures		
INJURY	**CLASSIFICATION**	**TREATMENT**	**COMPLICATIONS**
Femoral head fracture	Pipkin—based on location of fracture relative to fovea and associated fractures of acetabulum or femoral neck	Restore articular congruity (ORIF when > 1-mm step-off), restore hip stability, remove loose bodies, treat associated fractures, avoid injury to femoral head blood supply	Osteonecrosis (up to 15%), posttraumatic arthritis, sciatic nerve injury (up to 20%), recurrent dislocation (rare); Pipkin III highest rate of avascular necrosis
	Type I—fracture below fovea	Nonoperative if small fragment, congruent joint, protected weight bearing; ORIF with anterior approach (headless countersunk screws)	
	Type II—fracture above fovea	Nonoperative if stable nondisplaced fragment, protected weight bearing; ORIF with anterior approach (headless countersunk screws)	
	Type III—associated femoral neck fracture	ORIF of femoral neck and head; arthroplasty if older patient	
	Type IV—associated acetabular fracture	ORIF of acetabulum and head via posterior approach; arthroplasty if older patient	
Femoral neck fracture	Garden (low energy in elderly) I—incomplete/valgus impaction (stable) II—complete, nondisplaced (stable) III—complete, partially displaced (unstable) IV—complete, totally displaced (unstable)	Based on orientation of trabecular lines and displacement Medical optimization; CRPP with 3 screws or sliding compression hip screw with derotation screw; prosthesis for elderly (>70-yr old physiologically), sick, pathologic fracture, Parkinson, rheumatoid arthritis, phenytoin (Dilantin) therapy with displaced fractures (Garden III or IV); results of unipolar vs. bipolar prosthesis similar; consider total hip arthroplasty for more active patients, acetabular degenerative joint disease (higher dislocation rate than hemiarthroplasty)	Osteonecrosis (10%-40%; injury to medial femoral circumflex), nonunion (10%-30% of displaced fractures), infection, malunion (accept < 15 degrees valgus and 10 degrees anteroposterior displacement); infection, pulmonary embolism, mortality (≈30% at 1 year; increases with advancing age, medical problems, males); cardiopulmonary decompensation with cemented stems
	Pauwels (high energy in the young)	Based on orientation of fracture line; increased vertical orientation associated with less stability; ORIF with sliding hip screw (fixed-angle device) for vertically oriented fracture lines	
Intertrochanteric fracture	Number of fracture fragments, ability to resist compressive loads when fixed	Nonoperative treatment with nondisplaced fractures in compliant patients, those with high operative risk	Excessive collapse (limb shortening, medialization of shaft, sliding hip screw ≫ IM device), prominent hardware; nail cutout (TAD > 25 mm); loss of fixation (increased with superolateral screws); joint penetration (screw ideally placed center-center and deep); mortality, infection
	Two-part: stable with little risk of collapse Three-part: intermediate stability Four-part and comminuted: least stable	ORIF with sliding compression hip screw and side plate most reliable; lag screw in center-center position (TAD < 25 mm); IM nail for unstable, reverse oblique, subtrochanteric fractures; calcar-replacing arthroplasty for patients with severe osteopenia, comminution	
Greater trochanteric fracture	Amount of displacement	ORIF if > 1 cm displacement in young patient	
Lesser trochanteric fracture	Amount of displacement	ORIF if > 2 cm displacement in young athlete	Consider pathologic fracture
Subtrochanteric fracture	Russell-Taylor—based on involvement of lesser trochanter and piriformis fossa	Restore limb length, alignment, rotation; indirect reduction (open or percutaneous if necessary); avoid piriformis entry when fossa involved; fixed-angle device (95-degree blade plate) for proximal comminution	Apex anterior and varus most common deformity; nonunion (minimized with IM nail), infection (increased with soft tissue dissection)
	IA—fracture below lesser trochanter	IM nail, standard proximal interlock	
	IB—fracture involves lesser trochanter; greater trochanter intact	IM nail, reconstructed interlock	
	IIA—greater trochanter involved, lesser trochanter intact	IM nail, standard proximal interlock	
	IIB—greater and lesser trochanters involved	ORIF with fixed-angle device (95-degree blade plate) vs. IM nail, reconstructed interlock	

CRPP, Closed reduction with percutaneous pinning; *IM,* intramedullary; *ORIF,* open reduction and internal fixation; *TAD,* tip-to-apex distance.

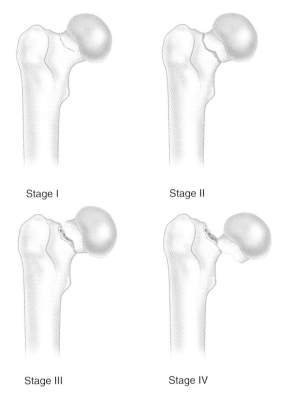

Stage I   Stage II

Stage III   Stage IV

FIGURE 11-33 Pipkin classification system of posterior hip dislocations associated with femoral head fractures. (From Browner BD, et al, editors: *Skeletal trauma,* ed 4, Philadelphia, 2008, Elsevier.)

- Treatment
  - General principles
    - Restore articular congruity of weight-bearing portion of head and hip stability.
    - Remove associated loose bodies.
    - Treat associated acetabular fracture if unstable.
    - Avoid injury to structures involved in blood supply to femoral head.
  - Nonoperative treatment
    - Indications
      - Pipkin type I—small fragment and congruent joint or nondisplaced larger fragment
      - Pipkin type II—nondisplaced; frequent (weekly) radiographs for 3 to 4 weeks to rule out secondary displacement
    - Protected weight bearing for 4 to 6 weeks
  - Operative treatment
    - Indications
      - Greater than 1-mm step-off (except small Pipkin type I)
      - Associated loose bodies in joint
      - Associated neck or acetabular fracture requiring surgical management
    - Fixation with headless countersunk lag screws
      - Anterior approach via Smith-Petersen approach for Pipkin types I and II without associated operative posterior wall fracture
      - Posterior approach for Pipkin type IV
    - Hip arthroplasty for older patient
- Complications
  - Same as those for hip dislocation

- AVN rate highest for Pipkin type III injuries. Rate of AVN is related to degree of displacement of femoral neck fracture.

■ **Femoral neck fractures**
- Diagnosis
  - Mechanism of injury
    - Low energy (fall from standing height) in elderly—associated with osteoporosis
    - High energy in young patients—associated with vertical fracture orientation and femoral shaft fractures
  - Nondisplaced fractures
    - Cross-table lateral view should be ordered because frog-leg lateral view could cause fracture displacement
  - MRI or bone scan to rule out occult fracture—MRI more sensitive if less than 24 hours from injury
- Classification
  - Garden classification (Figure 11-34) based on orientation of trabecular lines and displacement
    - Garden types I and II considered stable
    - Garden types III and IV considered unstable
  - Pauwels classification (Figure 11-35) based on orientation of fracture line
    - Increased vertical orientation associated with more shear force and reduced inherent stability
    - Nonunion and AVN associated with vertical patterns (Pauwels type III)
- Treatment
  - General principles
    - Rapid preoperative medical optimization
      - Mortality reduced if surgery within 48 hours
    - Stable fixation and early mobilization
  - Nonoperative treatment
    - Indications
      - Nondisplaced fractures in patients able to comply with weight-bearing restrictions
      - Displaced fractures in patients with extremely limited functional demands and/or those with high risk for surgery
        - Toe-touch weight bearing for 6 to 8 weeks
  - Operative treatment
    - Indications
      - Displaced fractures
      - Most nondisplaced fractures
    - Internal fixation
      - Indicated for Garden types I, II, and III fractures in young patients, occult fractures, and displaced fractures in young patients
      - Three parallel screws for Garden types I and II and occult fractures
        - V pattern of screw fixation
          - Since neck is devoid of substantial cancellous bone, fracture will settle until screw abuts intact cortical bone. Screws are ideally positioned so that shaft of screw abuts femoral neck fracture inferiorly and posteriorly to resist displacement (Figure 11-36).
      - Avoid start point distal to lesser trochanter (associated with increased risk of peri-implant subtrochanteric fracture)

- **Varus malreduction is correlated with failure of fixation following cannulated screw fixation of femoral neck fractures.**
  - Sliding hip screw (fixed-angle device) plus derotation screw indicated for basicervical fractures and vertically oriented fractures

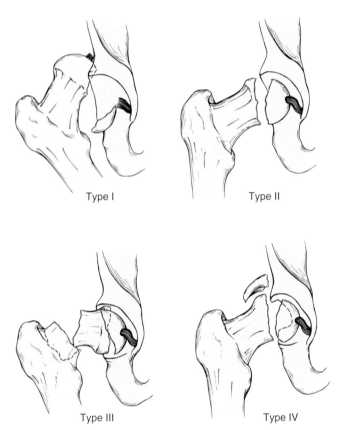

FIGURE 11-34 The Garden classification of femoral neck fractures. Grade I is an incomplete impacted fracture in valgus malalignment (generally stable). Grade II is a nondisplaced fracture. Grade III is an incompletely displaced fracture in varus malalignment. Grade IV is a completely displaced fracture with no engagement of the two fragments. The compression trabeculae in the femoral head line up with the trabeculae on the acetabular side. Displacement is generally more evident on the lateral view in grade IV. For prognostic purposes, these groupings can be lumped into nondisplaced/impacted (grades I and II) and displaced (grades III and IV) because the risk of nonunion and aseptic necrosis is similar within these grouped stages. (From Browner BD et al, editors: *Skeletal trauma,* ed 4, Philadelphia, 2008, Elsevier.)

- Anatomic reduction associated with the best results for displaced fractures in young patients
  - Open reduction often required
  - Anatomic reduction more critical than reduced time to fixation
- Decompression of intracapsular hematoma thought to reduce risk of AVN (not proven and controversial)
- Internal fixation associated with decreased perioperative morbidity (vs. hemiarthroplasty)
- Failure rate for internal fixation up to 30% requiring secondary procedure (typically arthroplasty)
- Hemiarthroplasty
  - Indicated for low-demand elderly patients with displaced fractures
  - Lower risk of dislocation than in total hip arthroplasty, especially in patients unable to comply with dislocation precautions (e.g., dementia, Parkinson disease)
  - Cemented femoral component better than uncemented component in patients with "stove pipe"–type canals (but higher cardiopulmonary complications if preexisting disease)
  - Functional results of unipolar and bipolar prostheses are similar.
- Total hip arthroplasty
  - Indicated for "active" elderly patients with displaced fractures
  - Preferred to hemiarthroplasty for patients with preexisting hip arthropathy (osteoarthritis and rheumatoid arthritis) and **has been shown to provide the best hip function after displaced femoral neck fracture**
  - Better functional results than those associated with hemiarthroplasty in active patients
  - Higher dislocation rate than hemiarthroplasty
- Complications
  - Osteonecrosis—10% to 40%; associated with injury to femoral head blood supply (terminal branch of the medial femoral circumflex artery)
    - Higher risk with greater initial displacement
    - Higher risk with poor or deficient reduction
    - Decompression of intracapsular hematoma may reduce risk (controversial).
    - Reduced time to reduction may reduce risk (controversial).

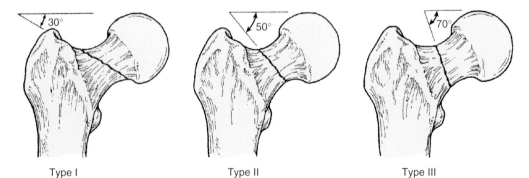

FIGURE 11-35 The Pauwels classification of femoral neck fractures. With progression from type I to type III, there are increasing shear forces placed across the fracture site. (From Evarts CM, editor: *Surgery of the musculoskeletal system,* ed 2, New York, 1990, Churchill Livingstone, p 2556.)

- Nonunion—occurs in 10% to 30% of displaced fractures
  - Higher risk with malreduction (particularly varus)
  - Treatment options include conversion to hip arthroplasty (worse results than those associated with primary arthroplasty) and valgus osteotomy.
- Infection
- Decreased functional status
  - Preinjury cognitive function and mobility predict postoperative functional outcome.
- Mortality—1-year mortality in elderly patients approximately 30%
- **Treatment of femoral fractures are one of the most common causes of malpractice suits against orthopaedic surgeons**.

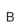 ■ **Intertrochanteric fractures**
- Diagnosis
  - Mechanism of injury: fall from standing height
  - Risk factors: osteoporosis, prior hip fracture, risk of falls
  - More common than femoral neck fracture in patients with preexisting hip arthritis

- Classification—based on the number of fracture fragments and ability to resist compression loads once they are reduced and fixed.
  - Two-part fractures—usually stable, with little risk of excessive collapse
  - Three-part fractures—intermediate stability
    - Size and location of lesser trochanteric fragment determine stability.
    - Large posterior medial fragments are less stable.
  - Four-part and severely comminuted fractures are the least stable. They have the highest risk for excessive shortening, varus collapse, and nonunion.
- Treatment
  - General principles
    - Stable fixation to allow early weight bearing
    - Minimize potential for implant failure
    - **Modifiable comorbidities should be corrected and surgery performed within first 48 hours**
  - Nonoperative treatment
    - Indications
      - Nondisplaced fractures in patients able to comply with non–weight-bearing restrictions
      - Displaced fractures in nonambulatory individuals or those with prohibitive operative risk

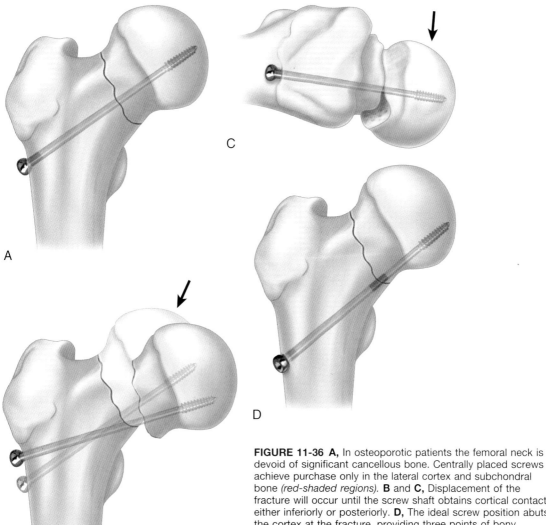

FIGURE 11-36 A, In osteoporotic patients the femoral neck is devoid of significant cancellous bone. Centrally placed screws achieve purchase only in the lateral cortex and subchondral bone *(red-shaded regions).* **B** and **C,** Displacement of the fracture will occur until the screw shaft obtains cortical contact either inferiorly or posteriorly. **D,** The ideal screw position abuts the cortex at the fracture, providing three points of bony support (lateral cortex, cortex adjacent to fracture, and subchondral bone of femoral head) to decrease the risk for loss of reduction and nonunion.

- Management with toe-touch weight bearing for 6 to 8 weeks
- Operative treatment
  - Indications
    - Displaced fractures
    - Most nondisplaced fractures
  - Internal fixation indicated for the vast majority of intertrochanteric fractures
    - Sliding hip screw device
      - Indicated for most intertrochanteric fractures except reverse oblique fractures, subtrochanteric fractures, and fractures without an intact lateral femoral cortex
      - High union rate
      - Associated with moderate amount of collapse, resulting limb shortening, and medialization when used for unstable fractures; more collapse than that seen with IM implants.
      - Lower peri-implant fracture rate than that seen with IM implants
      - Lag screw placed in center—center position with **tip-apex distance of less than 25 mm associated with lowest screw failure rate** (Figure 11-37)
      - Two-hole side plate sufficient for stable fractures
    - IM nail
      - Valid option for most intertrochanteric fractures, but best option for reverse oblique fractures, subtrochanteric fractures, and fractures without an intact lateral femoral cortex
      - Reduced collapse relative to sliding hip screw plate devices due to IM buttress effect of nail
      - Short nails indicated for standard obliquity fractures, with distal interlocking optional
      - Long nails indicated for standard obliquity, reverse obliquity, and subtrochanteric fractures
        - Risk of distal anterior perforation due to mismatch of anterior bow between femur and nail
      - Higher peri-implant fracture rate than that associated with sliding hip screw plate devices
      - Multiple screws into head fragment may provide improved rotational control (advantage controversial).
      - Single lag screw design should aim for center—center in head with **less than 25 mm tip-apex distance to minimize risk of screw cutout**
    - A 95-degree fixed-angle plate device or locking proximal femoral plate indicated for reverse obliquity, comminuted fracture, and nonunion repair
- Complications
  - Excessive collapse—stable fixation to allow early weight bearing
    - Results in limb shortening and medialization of shaft
    - Reduced abductor moment arm may cause functional deficit.
    - Associated with displacement of lesser trochanter
    - More collapse associated with sliding hip screw device than with IM implant
    - May result in painful, prominent hardware
  - Implant failure/cutout—associated with tip-apex distance (see Figure 11-37) greater than 25 mm
  - Peri-implant fracture

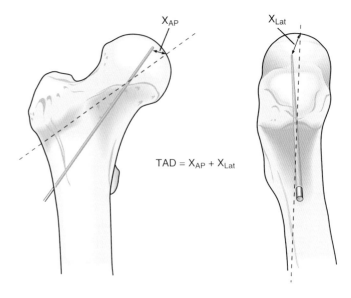

FIGURE 11-37 Tip-apex distance (TAD) should be less than 25 mm. (Redrawn from *Orthopaedic knowledge update: trauma 2,* Rosemont, Ill, 2000, American Academy of Orthopaedic Surgeons, p 127.)

$$TAD = X_{AP} + X_{Lat}$$

  - More common with nails than plates
  - Low risk with current nail designs
    - Smaller distal interlocking screws further from tip of nail than earlier designs
    - Reduced trochanteric bend compared with earlier designs
- Infection
- Mortality (often due to medical comorbidities)
  - American Surgical Association classification predicts mortality.

- **Subtrochanteric fractures**
- Diagnosis
  - Mechanism of injury—higher energy than intertrochanteric fractures
  - Plain radiographs
    - AP and lateral views of hip
    - AP and lateral views of femur
- Classification—Russell-Taylor classification (Figure 11-38) based on involvement of lesser trochanter and piriformis fossa
  - Type IA—fracture below lesser trochanter
  - Type IB—fracture involves lesser trochanter; greater trochanter intact
  - Type IIA—greater trochanter involved; lesser trochanter intact
  - Type IIB—greater and lesser trochanter involved
- Treatment
  - General principles
    - Restore limb length alignment and rotation.
    - Indirect reduction techniques obviate the need for bone grafting in acute fractures.
    - Nonoperative treatment rarely indicated
    - Operative treatment: implant must withstand high medial compressive loads and high lateral tensile loads.
      - Indications: most subtrochanteric fractures
      - IM fixation
        - Indirect reduction preserves biologic environment.

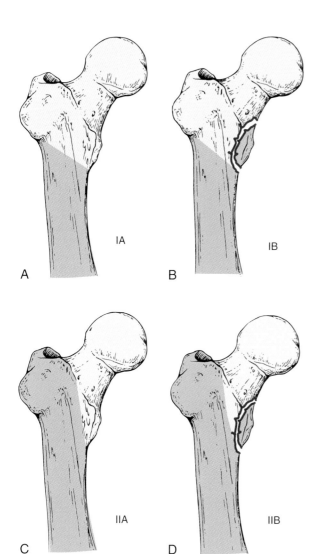

FIGURE 11-38 Russell-Taylor classification of subtrochanteric fractures. Fracture lines within red zones determine the type. In type I fractures, the piriformis fossa remains intact. Involvement of the piriformis fossa intramedullary nail entry site is the hallmark of type II fractures. Subtype A fractures do not involve the lesser trochanter, but in subtype B the lesser trochanter is a separate fragment. **A,** Type IA subtrochanteric fracture, suitable for first-generation locking nail. **B,** Type IB subtrochanteric fracture, which requires a cephalomedullary nail. **C,** Type IIA subtrochanteric fracture. The piriformis entry site is involved, but the lesser trochanter is intact. **D,** Type IIB subtrochanteric fracture. The nail entry site is involved, and lesser trochanteric comminution increases instability. (Modified from Tencer AF et al: *Orthop Biomech Lab Report #002,* Memphis, Tenn, 1985, Richards Medical Co.)

- Standard proximal interlocking for fractures with intact lesser trochanter
- Reconstruction interlocking for fractures with involvement of lesser trochanter
- Piriformis entry nail contraindicated for fractures involving piriformis fossa
  - Apex anterior and varus angulation are the most common deformities.
- The psoas and abductors lead to flexion, abduction, and external rotation of the proximal fragment.
  - Open or percutaneous reduction indicated when closed reduction inadequate (frequent); union rates same as with closed reduction

- Lateral positioning allows easier alignment of the distal segment to the flexed proximal segment.
- Fixed-angle plate fixation/proximal femoral locking plates
  - Indicated for fractures with proximal comminution and nonunion
  - 95-degree devices
  - Devices of 135 degrees contraindicated
  - Must avoid soft tissue stripping
  - Acute bone grafting usually not required when biological plating techniques are used
- Complications
  - Nonunion—minimized with IM nailing and biologic plating
  - Malalignment—varus and apex anterior angulation with IM nailing. Consider adjunctive reduction aids and percutaneous reduction.
  - Infection—associated with increased soft tissue dissection

■ **Femoral shaft fractures (Table 11-19)**
- Diagnosis
  - Mechanism of injury: often associated with high-energy mechanisms
  - Associated fractures and other injuries are common.
  - Associated neck fractures are uncommon (<10%) but when present, they are often missed (up to 50%). **Any patient who complains of hip pain during the early postoperative period following treatment of a femoral shaft fracture should have dedicated hip x-rays.**
  - Plain radiographs
    - AP and lateral views of femur
    - AP and cross-table lateral hip to rule out femoral neck fracture
  - CT scan to rule out occult femoral neck fracture
    - If the scan is obtained for abdominal or pelvic evaluation, it should be reviewed.
    - Consider dedicated thin-cut CT.
- Classification—Winquist-Hansen classification (Figure 11-39) based on degree of comminution and amount of cortical continuity
  - Type 0—no comminution
  - Type I—comminution less than 25%
  - Type II—comminution 25% to 50%
  - Type III—comminution greater than 50%
  - Type IV—comminution 100%
- Treatment
  - General principles
    - Restore limb length, alignment, and rotation.
    - Early stabilization reduces systemic complications associated with multiply injured patients.
  - Nonoperative treatment (rarely indicated)
    - Long leg cast or brace for nondisplaced distal shaft fracture
    - Pillow splint for nonambulatory individuals
  - Operative treatment—indicated for most fractures
    - IM nail
      - Indicated for most femoral shaft fractures
      - High union rates (>95%)
      - More hip problems with antegrade than retrograde insertion (pain/weakness).
      - **Quadriceps and abductors are weakest after antegrade femoral nailing.**

Table 11-19	Adult Femoral Shaft Fractures			
INJURY	**EPONYM/ OTHER NAME**	**CLASSIFICATION**	**TREATMENT**	**COMPLICATIONS**
Femoral fracture (2.0 cm below lesser trochanter to 8 cm from knee joint)		Winquist—based on degree of comminution and amount of cortical continuity I—transverse, comminution < 25% of circumference (e.g., butterfly fragment) II—comminution 25%-50% of circumference III—>50% comminution (unstable) IV—extensive (100%) comminution, no cortical contact, unstable V—segmental bone loss (unstable)	Most often high-energy mechanism; early stabilization as patient status permits; most fractures are treated by closed IM nail; statically locked, reamed nail for most fractures; antegrade (piriformis or trochanter) or retrograde; obesity a relative indication for trochanteric entry nail; multitrauma patients temporized with external fixation (damage control), converted to IM nail later; plate fixation for neck/shaft fractures, periprosthetic treatment (lower union, higher infection, longer time to weight bearing)	Infection (<5% closed fractures), nonunion (<5% closed fractures; treat with exchange nail vs. ORIF/ICBG), delayed union (exchange nail vs. dynamization), malalignment (malrotation, limb length discrepancy), hip pain/weakness (antegrade nail), knee pain (retrograde nail), pudendal nerve injury (excessive traction through post), missed knee ligament injury, knee stiffness (especially with distal external fixation), refracture, failure of fixation, deep venous thrombosis, pulmonary embolism, ARDS
Femoral neck and shaft fractures		Garden or Pauwels/ Winquist (2.5%-5.0% of femoral shaft fractures, but ≈ 30% are missed)	Neck takes priority; 135-degree fixed-angle device vs. parallel screws for neck, retrograde nail vs. plate for shaft; reconstruction nail for nondisplaced neck or intertrochanteric and shaft fractures	Infection, delayed union, nonunion, loss of fixation, avascular necrosis
Femoral and tibial shaft fractures	"Floating knee"		Retrograde nail for femur, antegrade nail for tibia	Multiple other injuries, fat emboli syndrome, ARDS

ARDS, Acute respiratory distress syndrome; *ICBG,* iliac crest bone graft; *IM,* intramedullary; *ORIF,* open reduction and internal fixation.

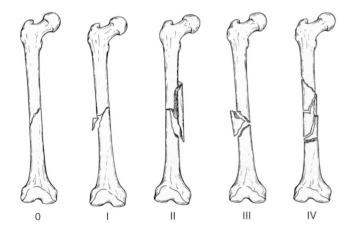

| 0 | I | II | III | IV |

FIGURE 11-39 Winquist-Hansen classification of femoral shaft comminution. *0,* Non-comminuted; *I,* single small wedge ("butterfly") fragment; *II,* wedge fragment, greater than 50% shaft cortical contact; *III,* wedge fragment, less than 50% shaft cortical contact; *IV,* segmental comminution, no shaft cortex contact between proximal and distal main fragments. (From Browner BD et al, editors: *Skeletal trauma,* ed 4, Philadelphia, 2008, Elsevier.)

- **More knee problems retrograde than antegrade insertion** (pain and chondral injury to patella if nail left proud)
- Piriformis and trochanteric starting points indicated when they are used with appropriately designed nails
  - Relative indications for retrograde femoral nail: morbid obesity, bilateral femoral shaft fractures (can be done without need to reposition patient), pregnancy (reduced abdominal radiation), ipsilateral tibial shaft fracture that will be treated with an IM nail, displaced ipsilateral femoral neck fracture that will be fixed with ORIF, ipsilateral acetabular fracture (to avoid contaminating acetabular surgical approach), multiply injured patients
  - Piriformis entry contraindicated when fracture extends to piriformis fossa
  - Anterior starting point in piriformis fossa associated with increased hoop stress and risk of iatrogenic comminution
  - Anterior trochanteric starting point with minimal hoop stress
  - Trochanteric starting point risks medial comminution of shaft due to off-axis starting point and varus if straight (no trochanteric bend) nail used
- Static interlocking for most fractures
- Reamed nailing for most fractures
  - Higher union rates than unreamed nails
  - Unreamed nails associated with decreased fat embolization; clinical relevance unclear
  - Appropriate reaming technique includes sharp reamers, slow advancement, less heat generation, and less embolization.
  - Minimum cortical reaming preferred
  - Nail diameter 1 to 2 mm smaller than largest reamer
- Multiply injured patients may benefit from delayed nailing with immediate provisional external fixation (damage control principles).

- Benefits include reduced blood loss, reduced hypothermia, and reduced inflammatory mediator release.
- External fixation
  - Indicated for provisional fixation
    - Application of damage control principles
    - Severe contamination requiring repeated access to medullary canal
    - Vascular injury
  - Safely converted to IM nail in absence of pin tract infection up to at least 3 weeks with equal union and infection rates
- Plate fixation
  - Indicated for periprosthetic fractures
  - Indicated for neck component of neck-shaft fractures
  - Reduced union rate, higher infection and implant failure rates, and longer time to weight bearing than with use of IM nail
- Complications
  - Infection—less than 5% of closed fractures
  - Nonunion—less than 5% of closed fractures
    - Exchange nailing less successful than repair with plate and screws and bone grafting
  - Delayed union—less than 5% of closed fractures
    - Dynamization less successful than exchange nailing
  - Malalignment
    - Proximal fracture more often malaligned with retrograde than antegrade nailing
    - Distal fractures more often malaligned with antegrade than retrograde nailing
    - **Malunion (rotation and length) is the most common complication following IM nailing of highly comminuted femoral shaft fractures.**
    - Malrotation difficult to diagnose, especially with comminuted fractures
      - Compare with contralateral limb before leaving operating room
      - Supine nailing has a higher incidence of internal rotation.
      - Lateral nailing has a higher incidence of external rotation.
      - Fracture table use has a higher incidence of internal rotation compared with manual traction.
  - Length discrepancy is associated with comminuted fractures.
  - Hip pain/weakness is associated with antegrade nailing.
  - Knee pain is associated with retrograde nailing.
  - Patellar chondral injury is associated with retrograde nailing, with nail left protruding into the knee joint.
  - Pudendal nerve injury is associated with excessive traction.
  - HO is associated with antegrade nailing (rarely clinically relevant).
  - Osteonecrosis in adolescents with open physes treated with a piriformis-starting IM nail
  - Significant shortening (i.e., 4 cm) results in medial mechanical axis deviation.
- Special circumstances
  - Obese patients
    - Higher complication rates with piriformis nailing
    - Relative indication for retrograde nailing

- Ipsilateral femoral neck and shaft fractures
  - Uncommon (<10%) but when present, missed in up to 50% of cases
  - **Neck fracture** management has the highest priority and **should be fixed first, generally followed by retrograde femoral IM nail or plate fixation for treatment of shaft fracture.**
    - Neck fracture often nondisplaced, vertical, and basicervical
    - Use of 135-degree sliding hip screw or parallel screws preferred for femoral neck
    - Reconstruction nail can be used for nondisplaced neck fractures or associated intertrochanteric and shaft fractures
      - Use of a cephalomedullary IM nail for fixation of displaced ipsilateral femoral neck and shaft fractures is associated with increased risk of femoral neck malreduction and AVN
- Multiply injured patient—consider damage control principles.
  - Provisional external fixator with conversion to IM nail when stable (within 3 weeks)
  - May be more applicable with associated lung/chest injury
- Periprosthetic fracture (See Chapter 5, Adult Reconstruction.)

■ **Supracondylar and intracondylar fractures**
- Diagnosis
  - Mechanism of injury—high energy in young patients and low energy in older patients
  - CT
    - If intracondylar extension
    - Coronal fracture (**Hoffa fracture**) incidence—40%
      - Lateral femoral condyle fracture incidence—80%
      - Plain radiographs frequently miss this injury.
- Classification—OTA classification (Figure 11-40) based on degree of comminution and articular involvement
  - 33-A—extraarticular
  - 33-B—simple articular (unicondylar)
  - 33-C—complex articular
- Treatment
  - General principles
    - Restore articular congruity.
    - Rigid stabilization of articular fracture
    - Indirect reduction of metaphyseal component to preserve vascularity to fracture fragments
    - Stable (not necessarily rigid) fixation of articular block to shaft
    - Early knee ROM
  - Nonoperative treatment—indicated for nondisplaced fractures
    - Brace or knee immobilized
    - Full-time bracing for 6 to 8 weeks
    - Closed-chain ROM at 3 to 4 weeks
  - Operative treatment—indicated for most displaced fractures
    - Plate fixation—indicated for most fractures
      - Fixed-angle plates required when metaphyseal comminution exists
        - Traditional 95-degree devices limited by number and location of distal fixation and are contraindicated in cases of associated Hoffa fractures

- **Locked plates** offer multiple fixed-angle points of fixation in distal fragment in multiple planes and **offer the advantage of use in cases with associated coronal (Hoffa) fractures**
  - Non–fixed-angle plates prone to varus collapse, especially in metaphyseal comminution
- High union rates (>80%) with indirect reduction technique without bone graft
- Lateral approach—indirect reduction of metaphyseal fracture and arthrotomy with direct reduction of articular component
  - Sagittal intraarticular split most common
  - Condyles are malrotated in sagittal plane with respect to each other.

- Coronal (Hoffa) fractures require interfragmentary lag screws.
- Laterally applied condylar plate spans fracture (locked plate preferred).
- Retrograde IM nail
  - Indicated for extraarticular fractures and simple intraarticular fractures
  - Reduced stability compared with plate fixation for osteoporotic fractures, especially those with wide metaphyseal flares
    - Blocking screws can help provide reduction and improved stability.
    - Fixed-angle distal interlocking screws may provide improved stability.

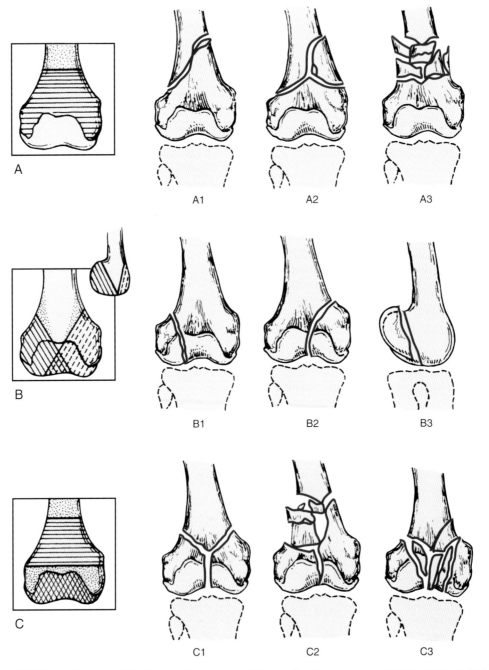

FIGURE 11-40 The AO/OTA classification of distal femoral fractures. In this classification system, which has been applied to all anatomic areas, the **A** category represents extraarticular fractures, **B** category represents partial articular fractures in which a part of the articular surface remains attached to the shaft, and the **C** category represents complete articular fractures. Subcategory numbers 1 to 3 in general represent increasing comminution. (From Browner BD et al, editors: *Skeletal trauma,* ed 4, Philadelphia, 2008, Elsevier.)

- Long nails that cross the femoral isthmus are preferred to short "supracondylar" nails.
- Arthroplasty
  - Indicated when associated with preexisting joint arthropathy and selected cases when stable internal fixation not achievable
  - Usually requires distal femoral replacement prosthesis
  - Reduced longevity compared with internal fixation
  - Allows immediate weight bearing
- Complications
  - Nonunion—associated with soft tissue stripping in metaphyseal region
  - Malalignment
    - Valgus malreduction most common (plate fixation) in coronal plane; hyperextension malreduction most common in sagittal plane
    - Malalignment more common with IM nails
  - Loss of fixation
    - Varus collapse most common
      - Plate fixation associated with toggle of distal non–fixed-angle screws used for comminuted metaphyseal fractures
      - IM nail fixation

- Proximal (diaphyseal) screw failure associated with short plates and nonlocked diaphyseal fixation. Plate fixation is associated with toggle of distal non–fixed-angle screws used for comminuted metaphyseal fractures.
- Infection—occurs in diabetic patients, especially those with active foot ulcers
- Knee pain/stiffness
- Painful hardware—avoid prominent medial screws.

KNEE INJURIES (TABLE 11-20)

■ Dislocation

- Diagnosis/classification
  - Direction (Kennedy)—anterior (30%-40%), posterior (30%-40%), medial, lateral, and rotatory (posterolateral the most common) (Figure 11-41)
  - Schenck anatomic classification of knee dislocation (KD)
    - KD I—dislocation with either anterior cruciate ligament (ACL) or posterior cruciate ligament (PCL) still intact (variable collateral involvement)
    - KD II—torn ACL/PCL

Table 11-20	Adult Knee Fractures and Dislocations			
INJURY	**EPONYM**	**CLASSIFICATION**	**TREATMENT**	**COMPLICATIONS**
Supracondylar fracture	"Hoffa" fracture (33-B3)	AO/OTA—degree of comminution and articular involvement 33-A—extraarticular 33-B—partially articular (unicondylar) 33-C—intraarticular	Restore articular congruity, rigid stabilization of articular fracture, preserve vascularity, stable fixation of joint to shaft, early ROM Nonoperative: brace or knee immobilizer, non–weight bearing for 6-8 wk, closed-chain ROM at 3-4 wk Plate fixation: most fractures; fixed-angle plate for metaphyseal comminution (nonfixed: varus collapse) Retrograde IM nail: extraarticular or simple intraarticular fractures, long nail preferred Arthroplasty when fixation not achievable, arthropathy present	Nonunion (soft tissue stripping of metaphyseal region), malalignment (valgus malreduction most common, nails ≫ plates), loss of fixation (varus collapse), infection, knee stiffness, DJD, unstable fixation, DVT, fracture fragments from missed coronal plane ("Hoffa fracture"), prominent hardware
Patella fracture		Nondisplaced, transverse, proximal or distal (30%) pole, comminuted, vertical (nonoperative)	Nonoperative: nondisplaced (<2 mm) with intact extensor mechanism; hinged knee brace in extension, progress in flexion after 2-3 wk ORIF (tension band wiring, screws) if patient cannot actively extend knee (extensor mechanism rupture) or there is >2-mm separation or incongruent articular surface (>2-mm step-off); excise fragments that are extremely comminuted; avoid patellectomy	Symptomatic hardware, loss of reduction, nonunion (<5%), infection, arthrofibrosis/ stiffness, quadriceps weakness, infection, DJD, extensor lag
Patella dislocation		Acute, recurrent, subluxation, habitual, usually lateral	Immobilize, controlled motion for 6 wk; arthroscopy for displaced or osteochondral fracture; recurrent: lateral release, medial plication (repair/ reconstruct MPFL); bony transplant if abnormal Q angle. Avoid surgery in those with habitual dislocation.	Redislocation
Knee dislocation		Anterior (30%-40%), posterior (30%-40%), lateral, medial, rotatory (anteromedial, anterolateral, posteromedial, posterolateral)	May present spontaneously reduced— easily missed; reduce dislocations emergently; open reduction if needed (posterolateral rotation); arteriogram based on physical examination findings (absent/asymmetric pulses); repair vascular injuries (5%-15%); ligament repair (within 2-3 wk) or reconstruction, allograft vs. autograft, early motion	Vascular injury (5%-15%, highest with KD-IV; ankle-brachial index > 0.9 associated with intact artery); neurologic injury (tibial/peroneal nerve), stiffness/arthrofibrosis (most common complication), ligamentous laxity

Continued

Table 11-20	Adult Knee Fractures and Dislocations—cont'd			
INJURY	**EPONYM**	**CLASSIFICATION**	**TREATMENT**	**COMPLICATIONS**
		Schenck anatomic classification: KD I—dislocation with anterior cruciate ligament (ACL) or posterior cruciate ligament (PCL) intact KD II—torn ACL/PCL KD III—torn ACL/PCL and either posterolateral corner (PLC) or posteromedial corner (PMC) KD IV—torn ACL/PCL/PLC/PMC KD V—fracture-dislocation		
Quadriceps rupture		Generally older than 40 and metabolic disorders (chronic renal failure, rheumatoid arthritis, steroid use), M ≫ F	Incomplete rupture: nonoperative management	Strength deficit; stiffness, inability to resume preinjury athletic/recreational activity; bilateral ruptures (identify underlying medical problem, repair both); DVT; chronic ruptures (allograft reconstruction, quadriceps tendon lengthening)
			Complete: repair through osseous drill holes or suture anchors; repair acutely: >2 wk or ≤ 5-cm retraction	
Patella tendon rupture		Younger than 40, overload of extensor mechanism; increased risk with metabolic disorders (rheumatoid arthritis, diabetes mellitus, infection)	Direct repair with nonabsorbable suture and locking (Krackow) stitch through drill holes; can protect repair with cerclage	Missed diagnosis (high-riding patella seen on radiographs), stiffness, extensor weakness

DJD, Degenerative joint disease; *DVT,* deep venous thrombosis; *IM,* intramedullary; *MPFL,* medial patellofemoral ligament; *ORIF,* open reduction and internal fixation; *ROM,* range of motion.

- KD III—most common
  - Torn ACL/PCL and either posterolateral corner (PLC-KD IIIL) or posteromedial corner (PMC-KD IIIM)
- KD IV—torn ACL/PCL/PLC/PMC
- KD V—fracture-dislocation
- More than 50% present reduced (easily missed diagnosis)
- Vascular injury—5% to 15% in recent studies
  - Selective arteriography with use of a physical examination (including ABI) rather than an immediate arteriogram is now the standard of care.
  - Most common finding in patients with vascular injury is a diminished or absent pedal pulse.
- Significant soft tissue injuries
- Treatment
  - Emergent reduction if patient did not present with fracture reduced
  - Revascularize within 6 hours if there is significant arterial injury.
  - Care for soft tissue injuries (open-knee dislocations).
  - Ligament repair or reconstruction
    - Reconstruction with allograft becoming the most common
    - Acute reconstruction may be better than chronic reconstruction.
  - Early motion rehabilitation
  - Possible role for hinged external fixator

- Complications
  - Vascular injury—highest with KD IV; ABI of greater than 0.9 associated with an intact artery
  - Neurologic injury—peroneal nerve injury common (≈25%), but up to 50% recover at least partially; may benefit from neurolysis.
  - Stiffness/arthrofibrosis—most common complication (38%)
  - Ligamentous laxity also very common (37%)
- **Patella fractures**
- Diagnosis/classification
  - Descriptive—transverse, vertical (rarely requires surgical treatment), comminuted, proximal or distal (30%) pole, and nondisplaced
  - Inability to extend knee or do a straight-leg raise demonstrates an incompetent extensor mechanism.
  - Displaced fracture is 3 mm fragment separation or 2 mm step-off.
- Treatment: preserve patella whenever possible (maintains lever arm for quadriceps function).
  - Nonoperative treatment: nondisplaced with intact extensor mechanism, hinged knee brace in extension, and progress in flexion after 2 to 3 weeks
  - Tension band wiring: simple fracture patterns, most common technique; can be done with K wires or cannulated screws (biomechanically stronger); may use wire or braided nonabsorbable suture (less hardware irritation)

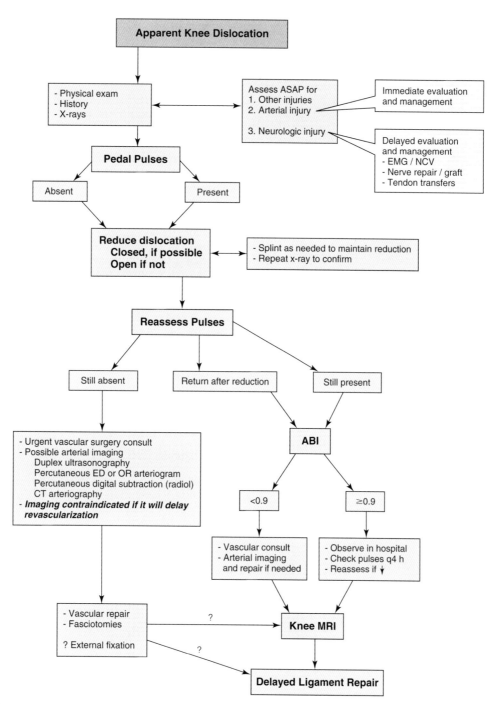

FIGURE 11-41 Treatment algorithm for dislocation of the knee. *ABI*, Ankle-brachial index; *ASAP*, as soon as possible; *CT*, computed tomography; *ED*, emergency department; *EMG/NCV*, electromyography/nerve conduction velocity; *MRI*, magnetic resonance imaging; *OR*, operating room. (From Browner BD et al, editors: *Skeletal trauma*, ed 4, Philadelphia, 2008, Elsevier.)

- Cerclage and tension band wiring: minimally displaced stellate fractures with significant comminution
- Partial patellectomy: useful with extraarticular distal pole fractures and also used with severely comminuted fractures; preserve the largest pieces and reattach patella ligament (Figure 11-42).
- **ORIF, when possible, is associated with better outcomes than partial patellectomy in comminuted and displaced fracture of the inferior pole of the patella.**
- ▦ Complications: **symptomatic hardware (very common)**, loss of reduction (22%), nonunion (<5%), infection, arthrofibrosis/stiffness

- ▪ **Patella dislocations**
- ▦ Diagnosis: frequently involves young adults or adolescents, usually laterally, and involves injury to the medial patellofemoral ligament
- ▦ Treatment: reduce and immobilize with controlled motion for 6 weeks.
- ▦ Complications: redislocation
- ▪ **Patella ligament rupture**
- ▦ Diagnosis/classification: occurs in patients younger than 40 with overload of extensor mechanism during athletic activity
  - Increased risk with metabolic disorders, rheumatologic disease, renal failure, corticosteroid injection, patellar

tendinitis, and infection. Diagnosis is frequently missed.

- Treatment: direct primary repair with a nonabsorbable suture and locking (Krackow) stitch through patellar drill holes; can supplement with semitendinosus graft and/or cerclage wire/suture to protect repair
- Complications: stiffness and extensor weakness

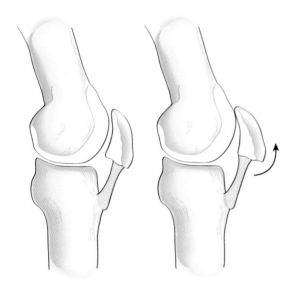

FIGURE 11-42 Anterior reattachment of the patellar ligament, which is recommended to prevent tilting of the patella superiorly. (Redrawn with permission from Marder RA et al: Effects of partial patellectomy and reattachment of the patellar tendon on patellofemoral contact areas and pressures, *J Bone Joint Surg Am* 75:35-45, 1993.)

■ **Quadriceps tendon rupture**

- Diagnosis: patients may be younger than 40, but this condition most commonly occurs in older patients with medical problems.
  - Association with renal failure, diabetes, rheumatoid arthritis, hyperparathyroidism, connective tissue disorders, steroid use, and intraarticular injections in 20% to 33%
  - Males are affected more often (up to 8 : 1); nondominant limb affected two times more often than dominant limb
- Treatment
  - Incomplete rupture: nonoperative management; warn of risk for future rupture.
  - Acute unilateral rupture: repair through osseous drill holes or suture anchors; repair acutely. Ruptures more than 2 weeks old may be retracted 5 cm.
  - Bilateral ruptures: identify underlying medical problem; otherwise, treat same as a unilateral rupture. Non–weight bearing and DVT prophylaxis are required.
  - Chronic tendon ruptures—less successful than acute ones; may require Codivilla procedure (V-Y lengthening) or quadriceps tendon lengthening
- Complications: strength deficit (33%-50% of patients), stiffness, inability to resume prior level of athletic/recreational activity (50%)

TIBIAL INJURIES (TABLE 11-21)

■ **Plateau fracture**

- Diagnosis/classification
  - Schatzker classification (Figure 11-43)
    - Type I—split
    - Type II—split depression

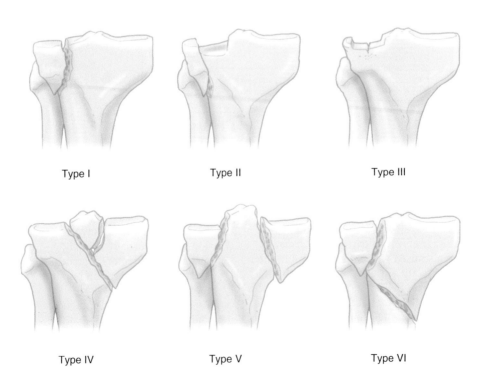

Type I   Type II   Type III

Type IV   Type V   Type VI

FIGURE 11-43 Schatzker classification of tibial plateau fractures. (Adapted from Lubowitz J et al: Part I: arthroscopic management of tibial plateau fractures, *Arthroscopy* 20:1063–1070, 2004.)

Table 11-21		Adult Tibia Fractures and Dislocations		
INJURY	**EPONYM/ OTHER NAME**	**CLASSIFICATION**	**TREATMENT**	**COMPLICATIONS**
Tibial plateau fracture		Schatzker classification I—split II—split depression III—pure depression IV—medial plateau split V—bicondylar with intact metaphysis VI—bicondylar with metaphyseal/ diaphyseal dissociation AO/OTA classification 41-A—extraarticular fracture 41-B—partial articular fracture (Schatzker I–IV) 41-C—complete articular/ bicondylar (Schatzker V and VI)	Magnetic resonance imaging can change treatment or classification in most cases (soft tissue injury); medial collateral ligament > ACL; lateral > bicondylar > medial (think dislocation with medial); spanning external fixation for high-energy injuries (soft tissue stabilization) Nonoperative: stable knees (<10 degrees varus/valgus in full extension, < 3 mm articular step-off); cast brace, early ROM, delayed weight bearing for 4-6 wk ORIF if articular step-off > 3 mm, condylar widening > 5 mm, knee unstable, medial and bicondylar; plate fixation (locked vs. nonlocked, single vs. dual [posteromedial] incision) vs. external fixation (bicondylar or severe soft tissue injury, wires > 15 mm from joint)	DJD, infection (surgical approach most important factor), malunion (varus collapse with nonoperative treatment or conventional plates/bicondylar fracture), ligament instability, peroneal nerve injury, compartment syndrome, stiffness, loss of reduction, avascular necrosis
Tibial spine fracture		I—anterior tilt II—complete anterior tilt III—no contact A—no rotation B—rotated	I/II/IIIA closed reduction, long-leg cast for 6 wk if knee can be brought into full extension; IIIB and all irreducible types require open reduction	Block to motion (arthroscopic loose-body removal), ACL laxity
Tibial tubercle fracture			ORIF with screw or staple	Loss of fixation, quadriceps weakness
Subchondral tibial fracture		Stable	Cast immobilization	Arterial injury, decreased ROM
		Displaced	ORIF with buttress plate	
Tibial stress fracture		Upper third (recruits)	Modify activity for 6-10 wk	Progression to complete fracture
Tibial shaft fracture		Gustilo and Anderson— open fracture grade Grade I—no periosteal stripping, <1-cm wound Grade II—no periosteal stripping, >1-cm wound Grade IIIA—periosteal stripping, no flap required Grade IIIB—periosteal stripping, flap required Grade IIIC—periosteal stripping, flap required, vascular injury requiring repair	Most respond to closed reduction, LLC, wedge as needed, PTB at 6-8 wk; IM nail for transverse oblique fracture of mid–one third or segmental and also for vascular injury, bilateral injury, pathologic fractures, severe ligamentous injuries to knee (statically locked IM nail); open fractures: unreamed nail up to and including some IIIB injuries, early flap coverage, delayed bone grafting. Consider early amputation in grade IIIC injuries, posterior tibial nerve injury, warm ischemia > 6 hr, and severe ipsilateral foot injury (unreconstructible limb).	Delayed union (>20 wk; increased with greater initial displacement and middle-third fractures; treatment includes fibulectomy and posterolateral bone graft), nonunion (posterolateral bone graft or reamed IM nail), infection (flap/graft or amputation), malunion (varus/ valgus, shortening [accept < 5 degrees varus/valgus, < 10 degrees anteroposterior angulation]), vascular injuries (upper fourth of anterior tibial artery), compartment syndrome, peroneal nerve injury, CRPS
Tibial plafond fracture	Pilon	Ruedi and Allgöwer I—minimally displaced II—incongruous III—comminuted	Long-leg cast and non–weight bearing ORIF if displaced and ankle involved; consider minimally invasive small-pin external fixation techniques	DJD (may require late fusion), infection, varus/valgus angulation, skin slough
Fibular shaft fracture		Middle to lower third (athletes)	Cast only if needed for pain relief	Missed syndesmotic injury
Proximal fibula fracture			Open if unstable	Injury to biceps, peroneal nerve
Proximal tibia-fibula dislocation		Anterior (most common), posterior, superior	Reduce (90 degrees flexion), ORIF fails with recurrence	
Chondral/ osteochondral fracture		Endogenous vs. exogenous	Arthroscopic evaluation of locked, acute condylar defects; remove small fragments (pin large fragments)	DJD

ACL, Anterior cruciate ligament; *CRPS,* complex regional pain syndrome; *DJD,* degenerative joint disease; *IM,* intramedullary; *ORIF,* open reduction and internal fixation; *PTB,* patella tendon–bearing cast; *ROM,* range of motion.

- Type III—pure depression (rare)
- Type IV—medial tibial (**highest risk of associated vascular injury**)
- Type V—bicondylar with intact metaphysis
- Type VI—bicondylar with metaphyseal/diaphyseal dissociation
  - AO/OTA classification
    - 41-A—extraarticular fracture
    - 41-B—partial articular fracture (Schatzker I-IV)
    - 41-C—complete articular/bicondylar (Schatzker V and VI)
  - MRI changes treatment or classification in most cases.
    - Soft tissue injury is demonstrated (50%-90% incidence).
    - MCL and ACL injuries in 30% to 50%
    - Meniscus tears in over 50% of cases
      - Lateral tears more common medial tears
        - Type II—lateral meniscal pathology
        - Type IV—medial meniscal pathology
      - Peripheral tears most common type
  - Order of frequency—lateral greater than bicondylar greater than medial (**think *knee dislocation* with medial plateau fractures**)
  - Elderly osteoporotic patients are less likely to suffer associated ligamentous injury, since their bone fails prior to the ligament.
  - The lateral plateau is more convex-shaped and situated more proximal than the medial plateau, which is more concave-shaped.
- Treatment
  - Nonoperative treatment indicated in stable knees (<10 degrees coronal plane instability with the knee in full extension) with less than 3 mm articular step-off. Cast brace, early ROM, and delayed weight bearing for at least 4 to 6 weeks.
  - Operative treatment indicated with articular step-off greater than 3 mm, condylar widening greater than 5 mm, instability of the knee, and all medial and bicondylar plateau fractures. The goal of treatment is restoration of normal alignment. **Maintenance of mechanical axis correlates most with a satisfactory clinical outcome.** Development of arthritis does not correlate with articular step-off.
    - ORIF
      - Plate fixation with early motion
      - Percutaneous locked plating for poor-quality bone in bicondylar fractures; no stripping
      - **Posteromedial coronal fragment** may not be captured via a lateral plate. Use a separate posteromedial incision and **posteromedial plate.**
      - Use of bone void fillers
        - Calcium phosphate cement has highest compressive strength
        - Lower rate of subsidence compared with autogenous iliac bone graft
        - Best treatment to prevent articular reduction loss in a split depression tibial plateau fracture is a lateral plate rafting screws and calcium phosphate cement
    - External fixation—ring fixation useful for bicondylar fractures with severe soft tissue injuries. Keep small wires at least 15 mm from the joint to avoid septic joint.

- Spanning external fixators—used temporarily with selected high-energy injuries to allow for a reduction in soft tissue swelling before definitive fixation
- Complications: degenerative joint disease (DJD), infection (surgical approach the most important factor), malunion (varus collapse with nonoperative or conventional plates in severe bicondylar fractures), ligament instability (left untreated, has an adverse impact on outcome), peroneal nerve injury
  - Compartment syndrome—increased risk with more proximal fractures. Anterior and lateral compartments are at highest risk.

■ **Shaft fractures**

■ Diagnosis
- Mechanism of injury
  - Low energy
    - Spiral oblique fracture
    - Tibia and fibula at different levels
    - Closed fracture with minor soft tissue trauma
    - **There is a high association of posterior malleolus fractures with spiral distal tibia fractures.**
  - High energy
    - Comminuted fracture
    - Tibia and fibula at same level
    - Transverse fracture pattern
    - Diastasis between tibia and fibula
    - Segmental fracture
    - Open fracture or closed with significant soft tissue trauma
- Most common long bone fracture
- Often associated with soft tissue injuries
  - Soft tissue management critical to outcome
  - Open fractures may require repeated incision and drainage.
    - Number of instances of débridement, type of irrigation, and pressure of irrigant controversial
    - Sharp débridement of nonviable soft tissue and bone the most important aspect of incision and drainage
    - **Severity of muscle injury has the highest impact on need for amputation.**

■ Classification
- OTA classification (Figure 11-44)—based on comminution
  - 42-A—simple (two parts)
  - 42-B—butterfly comminution
  - 42-C—comminuted, no direct contact between proximal and distal fragments
- High incidence of open fracture or associated severe soft tissue injury with closed fractures (See Table 11-5.)

■ Treatment
- General principles
  - Degree of shortening and translation seen on injury radiographs can be expected to be present at union with nonoperative management.
  - Angular and rotational alignment well controlled with cast
  - **Shortening is most difficult to control in oblique and comminuted fractures involving both tibia and fibula.**
  - Timely and thorough soft tissue management critical to outcome

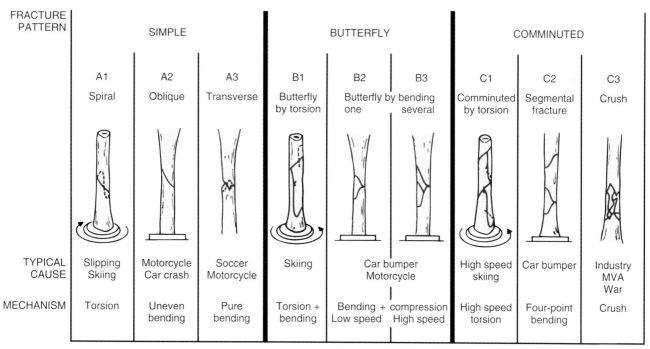

FIGURE 11-44 Johner and Wruhs classification system for tibial shaft fractures. Note that neither displacement nor soft tissue wound severity is considered in this system. Nine alphanumeric groups (A to C, 1 to 3) are illustrated in this figure. Each group can be separated into three subgroups, each of which may have three qualifications. The subgroups are the same for each of the A and B groups: 1 = fibula intact, 2 = fibula fracture at a different level, and 3 = fibula fracture at the same level. The qualifications are also the same for all the A and B groups: (1) = proximal, (2) = middle, and (3) = distal. The subgroups within group C1 are .1, two intermediate fragments; .2, three intermediate fragments; and .3, more than three intermediate fragments. The C1 qualifications are (1) pure diaphyseal, (2) proximal metadiaphyseal, and (3) distal metadiaphyseal. The C2 subgroups are .1, single intermediate segmental fragment; .2, intermediate segmental and wedge fragments; and .3, two intermediate segmental fragments. For C2.1, the qualifications are (1) pure diaphyseal, (2) proximal metadiaphyseal, (3) distal metadiaphyseal, (4) oblique lines, and (5) transverse and oblique lines. For C2.2 the qualifications are (1) pure diaphyseal, (2) proximal metadiaphyseal, (3) distal metadiaphyseal, (4) distal wedge, and (5) three wedges, proximal and distal. For C2.3, the qualifications are (1) pure diaphyseal, (2) proximal metadiaphyseal, and (3) distal metadiaphyseal. For group C3 the subgroups are .1, two or three intermediate fragments; .2, limited shattering (<4 cm); and .3, extensive shattering (>4 cm). Qualifications for C3.1 are (1) two intermediate fragments and (2) three intermediate fragments. For C3.2 and C3.3, qualifications are (1) pure diaphyseal, (2) proximal metadiaphyseal, and (3) distal metadiaphyseal. *MVA,* Motor vehicle accident. (Redrawn from Johner R, Wruhs O: *Clin Orthop* 178:7–25, 1983. In Browner N et al, editors: *Skeletal trauma,* ed 3, Philadelphia, 2002, Elsevier.)

- Restore limb length, alignment, and rotation.
- Stable fixation
- Early ROM of knee and ankle
- **Prompt administration (within 3 hours of injury) of antibiotics for open fractures is the most important factor in minimizing the risk of infection.**
- **BMP-2** is approved for use in open tibia fractures treated with IM fixation and has been shown to lead to **fewer reoperations in acute open tibia fractures.**
- BMP-7 is approved for treatment of tibial nonunion in cases where autogenous bone graft is not feasible.
- Nonoperative treatment
  - Indications
    - Low-energy fractures
    - Shortening less than 1 to 2 cm
    - Cortical apposition greater than 50%
    - Angulation maintained with cast
      - Varus—valgus less than 5 degrees
      - Flexion—extension less than 10 degrees
  - Long leg cast
    - Can control varus/valgus, flexion/extension, and rotation
    - Shortening and cortical apposition seen on injury radiograph are equivalent to shortening at union.

- Convert to functional brace at 4 to 6 weeks.
- Non–weight bearing for 4 to 6 weeks
- Operative treatment
  - Indications
    - Open fractures
    - Criteria for nonoperative management not met or failed nonoperative management
    - Soft tissue injury not amenable to cast
    - Ipsilateral femoral fracture
    - Polytrauma
    - Morbid obesity
  - IM nailing
    - Reduced time of immobilization compared with cast management
    - Earlier weight bearing than that achieved with cast
    - Union rate greater than 80% for closed injuries
    - Reamed nailing associated with higher union rates than those achieved with nonreamed nailing
      - Reamed nailing safe for open fractures
      - Severity of soft tissue injury more prognostic than reaming status
    - Static interlocking indicated for stable and unstable fractures
    - Dynamic interlocking indicated only for stable fracture (Winquist I or II)
    - Gaps at fracture site associated with nonunion

- **Proximal-third tibial fractures associated with valgus and apex anterior angulation**
- Avoidance of malreduction of proximal-third fractures achieved by the following:
  - Ensuring a laterally based starting point and anterior insertion angle; entry site should be in line with medial border of lateral tibial eminence
  - **Blocking screws placed in the metaphyseal segment at the concave side of the deformity narrow the available intramedullary space** and direct the nail toward a more centralized position (Figure 11-45).
  - **To prevent an apex anterior deformity, a blocking screw can be placed posterior to the nail in the proximal fracture.**
  - Provisional unicortical plates
  - Semiextended position for nailing
- External fixation
  - Temporary during application of damage control principles
  - Temporary or definitive for highly contaminated fractures
    - Definitive fixation with external fixation for type III open tibia fractures have significantly longer time to union and poorer functional outcomes compared with IM nailing.
  - Higher incidence of malalignment than IM nails
  - Circular frames indicated for very proximal and distal shaft fractures and when these fractures are associated with severe soft tissue injury
  - Can be safely converted to IM nail within 7 to 21 days (newer studies show longer than 7-day delay acceptable, but exact safe timing unknown)

- Plate fixation
  - For extreme proximal and distal shaft fractures
  - Higher infection risk than that for IM nailing in open fractures
  - Use of a **long 13-hole percutaneous plate,** such as a Less Invasive Stabilization System (LISS) plate, **places the superficial peroneal nerve at risk during percutaneous screw insertion for holes 11, 12, and 13.** A larger incision with blunt dissection should be used for insertion of screws in this region.
- Complications
  - Nonunion
    - Rule out infection.
    - Dynamization if axially stable
    - **Reamed-exchange nailing is preferred treatment for mid-diaphyseal tibial nonunions.**
    - Bone graft for bone defects
  - Malunion
    - Most common with proximal-third fractures
      - Valgus and apex anterior
    - May increase long-term risk of arthrosis, particularly in the ankle
      - More common with varus deformity
      - Rotational malalignment is common with distal-third fractures.
  - Delayed union
    - Risk factors for reoperation to achieve bony union within first postinjury year:
      - Transverse fracture pattern
      - Open fracture
      - Cortical contact less than 50%

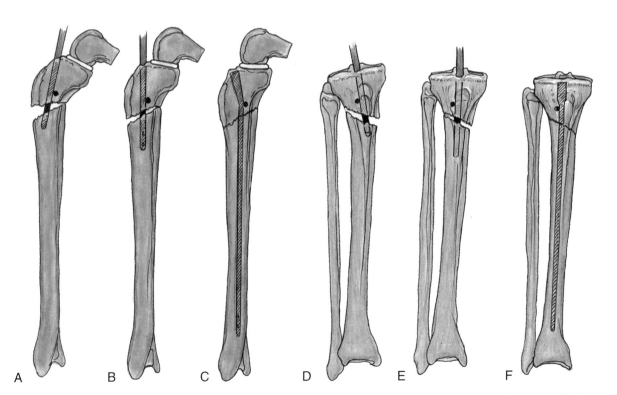

FIGURE 11-45 Shaft fractures. Blocking screws placed posteriorly and laterally to the central axes of the proximal fragment **(A-F).** (Reprinted with permission from Hiesterman TG et al: Intramedullary nailing of extra-articular proximal tibia fractures, *J Am Acad Orthop Surg* 19:690–700, 2011. © 2011 American Academy of Orthopaedic Surgeons.)

- Infection
  - Risk increases with increased severity of soft tissue injury and time to soft tissue coverage
  - Use of vacuum-assisted closure for wound does not alter risk of infection.
- Compartment syndrome
  - Diagnosed by compartment pressure within 30 mm Hg of diastolic blood pressure (ΔP)
  - Emergent fasciotomy indicated
  - Can occur even with open fractures

- Anterior knee pain—occurs in more than 30% of IM nailing cases; resolves with removal of nail in 50% of cases
- Ipsilateral femoral shaft and tibial shaft fractures ("floating knee")—treated by retrograde femoral nailing and antegrade tibial nailing
- **Tibial plafond fractures (pilon fractures) (see Chapter 6, Disorders of the Foot and Ankle.)**
- **Ankle and foot fractures (see Chapter 6, Disorders of the Foot and Ankle)**

SECTION 4 PEDIATRIC TRAUMA

INTRODUCTION

- **Several features of fractures and dislocations in children are not found in adults (see Tables 11-22 through 11-32 and Figures 11-46 through 11-64.)**
- Children's bones are more ductile than adults' bones, and bowing is thus unique to children.
- The terms *greenstick* and *torus* imply a partial fracture with some part of the bone intact.
- The periosteum in children is much thicker and often remains intact on the concave (compression) side, allowing for less displacement and better reduction of fractures.
- Children's fractures heal more quickly and with less immobilization than adults' fractures. Contractures are also less likely.
- Because bones are actively growing in pediatric fractures, malunion and growth plate injuries are important concerns. Remodeling is more thorough; thus, displacement and angulation that would not be acceptable in an adult are often acceptable in children.
- The exception to this rule is an intraarticular fracture, in which the same axioms apply. However, the presence of nearby physeal structures can affect fixation options.

CHILD ABUSE

- **Introduction**
- One must always be alert for the "battered child."
- All states now require physicians to report suspected child abuse. If child abuse is not diagnosed and reported there is a 30% to 50% chance of repeat abuse and a 5% to 10% chance of death from subsequent abuse.
- Suspicion should be raised when fractures are seen in children younger than age 5 years (90% of fractures due to abuse occur in children < 5), with multiple healing bruises, skin marks, burns, unreasonable histories, and signs of neglect, among other indications.
- Abuse accounts for 50% of fractures in children younger than age 1 year and 30% of fractures in children younger than age 3.
- The most common cause of femur fractures in nonambulatory children is abuse.
- Osteogenesis imperfecta is often in the differential diagnosis in a child with multiple fractures.
- **Fracture location**
- The most common locations of fractures in children of abuse are the humerus, tibia, and femur, in that order.
  - Spiral humerus fractures and distal humeral physeal separations are highly suggestive of child abuse.

- Spiral femur fractures in nonambulatory children are also highly suspicious.
- If suspicion is high, skeletal surveys are appropriate in children with delayed development and in some metaphyseal and spiral fractures.
- Corner fractures (at junction of metaphysis and physis) and posterior rib fractures are described as pathognomonic for abuse (Figure 11-46).
- However, diaphyseal fractures are more common in abuse cases (four times as likely as metaphyseal fractures).
- Skeletal surveys are not as helpful in children older than 5 years. Instead, a bone scan may be done as an alternative or adjunctive study.
- Nonorthopaedic injuries found in abuse include skin injuries, head injuries, burns, and blunt abdominal visceral injuries.
- **Treatment**
- In addition to normal fracture care, early involvement of social workers and pediatricians is essential to evaluate for possibility of child abuse and initiate necessary protective actions.

PHYSEAL FRACTURES

- **Introduction**
- Fracture of the physis, or growth plate, is more likely than injury to attached ligaments; thus, assume that there is a fracture of the physis until evidence proves otherwise (young children rarely get sprains).
- **Characteristics**
- Although physeal fractures are classically thought to be through the zone of provisional calcification (within the zone of hypertrophy) of the growth plate, the fracture can be through many different layers.
- Blood supply of epiphysis is tenuous, and injuries can disrupt small physeal vessels supplying the growth center. This can lead to many complications associated with these injuries (e.g., limb-length discrepancies, malunion, bony bars).
- Most common physeal injuries occur in distal radius, followed by distal tibia
- **Classification**
- The Salter-Harris (SH) classification modified by Rang is the gold standard for physeal injuries (Figure 11-47; Table 11-22).
  - It can be recalled using the mnemonic **SALTR**
    - I—**S**lipped—separation physis
    - II—**A**bove—metaphysis and physis

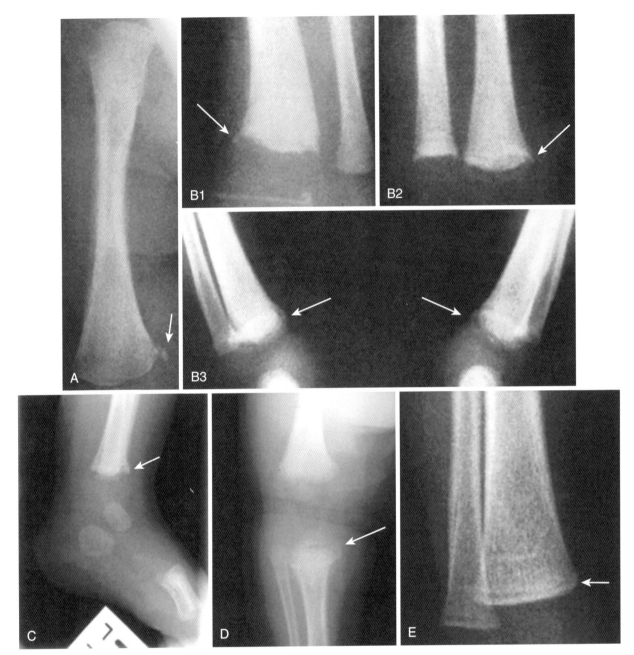

FIGURE 11-46 Metaphyseal fractures. Radiographs of the right femur **(A)** and both ankles **(B)** of a 2-month-old abused infant demonstrating metaphyseal corner fractures of the distal femur and both distal tibia *(arrows)*. Angled tangential view reveals the "bucket handle" appearance of the fracture. **C,** Radiograph of the left ankle of an infant demonstrates a metaphyseal corner fracture of the distal tibia *(arrow)*. **D,** Angled tangential view of the right lower limb of an abused infant demonstrates the "bucket handle" appearance *(arrow)*. **E,** Radiograph of the right ankle of a 6-week-old abused neonate with subtle metaphyseal fractures evident as a metaphyseal lucent line *(arrow)*. (From Adam A, Dixon A, editors: *Grainger & Allison's diagnostic radiology,* ed 5, Edinburgh, UK, 2007, Elsevier.)

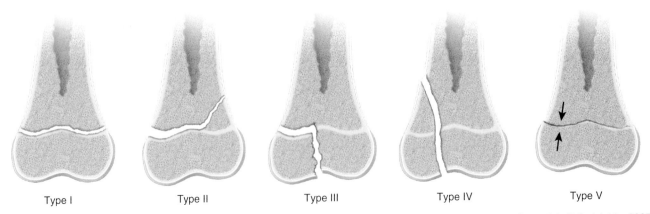

Type I Type II Type III Type IV Type V

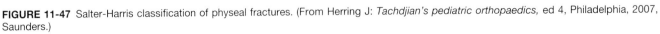

FIGURE 11-47 Salter-Harris classification of physeal fractures. (From Herring J: *Tachdjian's pediatric orthopaedics,* ed 4, Philadelphia, 2007, Saunders.)

Table 11-22	Salter-Harris Classification of Physeal Injuries	
TYPE	**DESCRIPTION**	**PROGNOSIS**
I	Transverse fractures through physis	Excellent
II	Fractures through physis, with metaphyseal fragment	Excellent
III	Fractures through physis and epiphysis	Good but with potential for intraarticular deformity; may require ORIF
IV	Fractures through epiphysis, physis, and metaphysis	Good but unstable; fragment requires ORIF
V	Crush injury to physis	Poor, with growth arrest
VI	Injury to perichondrial ring	Good; may cause angular deformities

ORIF, Open reduction and internal fixation.

- III—Lower—epiphysis and physis
- IV—Through—metaphysis, physis, epiphysis
- V—Ruined—crushed physis
  - SH type I fracture is through the zone of hypertrophic cells of the physis.

■ **Treatment and results**
▦ Gentle reduction should be attempted initially for SH I and II fractures, sometimes using conscious sedation protocols. With reduction and immobilization, these fractures will do well without a significant amount of growth arrest (except in the distal femur).
▦ SH III and IV fractures are intraarticular by definition and usually require ORIF. Follow-up radiographs are required for all physeal injuries.
▦ Remodeling is also common in pediatric fractures (up to 20 degrees). This depends on the location and age of the patient.
▦ Harris-Park growth arrest lines (transverse radiodense lines) may be the only evidence of a physeal injury on follow-up radiographs.

■ **Partial growth arrest**
▦ Physeal bars or bridges result from growth plate injuries that arrest a part of the physis and leave the uninjured physis to grow normally. This results in angular growth and deformity.
▦ Physeal bridge resection with interposition of a fat graft or artificial material is reserved for patients with over 2 cm of growth remaining and less than 50% physeal involvement.
▦ Treatment of smaller peripheral bars in young patients have the highest success rate.
▦ MRI and CT can help define the location and amount of physeal closure.
▦ Arrest involving more than 50% of the physis should be treated with ipsilateral completion of the arrest and contralateral epiphysiodesis or ipsilateral limb lengthening.

PEDIATRIC POLYTRAUMA

■ **Introduction**
▦ Trauma is the most common cause of death in children older than age 1 year.
- Death and long-term morbidity are most closely associated with the severity of traumatic brain injury.
▦ Most common causes of polytrauma are fall from height and motor vehicle collision

■ **Treatment**
▦ Children may remain hemodynamically stable for some time despite significant blood loss. Intraosseous infusion may be needed owing to difficulty in quickly obtaining IV access. Crystalloid fluid bolus 20 mL/kg. If hemodynamic stability recurs or persists despite 2 or 3

boluses, should begin blood transfusion (10 mL/kg). Estimate of pediatric blood volume is 75 to 80 mL/kg.
▦ Cervical spine immobilization for children younger than age 6 years requires use of a backboard with occipital cutout because of the large head size of children.
- Adult backboard use can result in neck flexion.
▦ Timing of orthopaedic management
- Early operative fixation (within 2-3 days) decreases intensive care unit and overall hospital stay.

SHOULDER AND ARM INJURIES (TABLE 11-23)

■ **Clavicle fractures**
▦ Principles and presentation
- Most frequent fracture in children
- 90% of obstetric fractures; often associated with brachial plexus palsies
- Birth injury mechanism—direct pressure from symphysis pubis
- Older children mechanism—fall on an outstretched hand; direct trauma to clavicle or acromion
▦ Diagnosis and radiographs
- Ultrasound for obstetric fractures
- Cephalic tilt views (cephalic tilt of 35-40 degrees)
- Apical oblique view (ipsilateral side rotated 45 degrees and cephalic tilt of 20 degrees toward beam)
- CT axial imaging for medial clavicle fractures and physeal separation evaluations
▦ Classification—Allman
- Middle third (80%)
- Lateral third (10%-15%)
  - Distal to coracoclavicular ligaments
- Medial third (5%-10%)
▦ Treatment
- Newborn: nonoperative treatment
- Adolescents: nonoperative treatment (standard of care)
- Sternoclavicular physeal fracture-dislocations
  - Anterior: closed reduction, often unstable but can remodel
  - Posterior: reduction with CT surgery backup after CT scan to evaluate for mediastinal impingement
- Operative treatment controversial for middle-third clavicle fractures
  - Absolute indications: open fractures, neurovascular compromise
  - Relative indications: nonunion, malunion, displacement greater than 2.0 cm
  - Pin fixation should be avoided.
  - Plate fixation or intramedullary nailing acceptable operative options

Table 11-23	Pediatric Shoulder Trauma		
INJURY	**CLASSIFICATION**	**TREATMENT**	**COMPLICATIONS**
Humeral shaft fracture	Neonate	Small splint or splint to side	Compartment syndrome, radial nerve palsy, rotational palsy
	< age 3 yr	Collar and cuff OK	
	age 3-12	Sarmiento brace	
	> age 12	Sarmiento brace	
Proximal humeral physis fracture	SH (I most common in < age 5 yr)	Sling if minimally displaced, gentle manipulation for displaced fractures, CRPP vs. ORIF for < 50% apposition, >45 degrees angulation	
Proximal humeral metaphysis fracture (common)	Based on location	Sling	
Midshaft clavicle fracture	≤ age 2	Supportive sling if symptomatic	Rare: malunion or nonunion, neurovascular compromise
	> age 2	Figure-eight brace vs. sling	
Medial clavicle fracture	Usually SH I or II physeal separations	Sling for 1 wk	
Lateral clavicle fracture	I—nondisplaced; intact AC and CC ligaments	Sling vs. figure-eight brace Type II may need ORIF	
	IIA—clavicle displaced superiorly; fracture medial to CC ligament		
	IIB—clavicle displaced superiorly; conoid ligaments tear		
AC joint injury	Same as adult	Same as adult	Watch for coracoid fracture
SC joint injury	Anterior and posterior	Same as adult	
Clavicle dislocation (rare)	Anterior and posterior	ORIF with repair of periosteal tube	
Scapula fracture	Anterior and posterior	Same as adult	
Glenohumeral dislocation	Anterior and posterior	Initial immobilization followed by rehabilitation; reconstruction for recurrent instability	Recent research shows > 60% chance of redislocation when patient is < age 21

AC, Acromioclavicular; *CC,* coracoclavicular; *ORIF,* open reduction and internal fixation; *CRPP,* closed reduction with percutaneous pinning; *SC,* sternoclavicular; *SH,* Salter-Harris.

- Complications
  - Nonunion (1%-3%)—rare in children; beware of congenital pseudarthrosis
  - Malunion—rare in younger populations; rates increase as age increases.
  - Neurovascular compromise
  - Pneumothorax
- **Proximal humerus fractures**
- Principles and presentation
  - In 80% to 90% humeral growth occurs at proximal physis; increased remodeling potential (Figure 11-48)
  - Less than 5% of pediatric fractures
  - Three ossification centers (humeral head, greater and lesser tuberosities) coalesce at ages 6 to 7.
  - Proximal fragments rotated into abduction and external rotation by rotator cuff muscles
  - Distal fragments pulled into adduction and shortened by the pectoralis major and deltoid
    - Accordingly, gravity can be a useful reduction aid.
  - Blocks to closed reduction can include long head of biceps tendon, joint capsule, and periosteum
- Diagnosis and radiographs
  - AP, scapular Y, and axillary views
- Classification
  - SH classification commonly applied to these fractures
  - SH I fractures most common in children younger than age 5
  - SH II fractures most common in children older than age 12
  - Metaphyseal fractures common in children between ages 5 and 12
  - "Little Leaguer shoulder" represents an SH I fracture.

- Treatment
  - Nonoperative treatment with temporary immobilization is usual treatment owing to remodeling potential (see Figure 11-48)
  - Operative indications
    - Absolute: open fractures, neurovascular injuries, intraarticular extension
    - Relative: young children (<12 years); 70 degrees and 100% displacement acceptable
    - Age older than 12 years, controversial, 30 to 40 degrees, and 50% displacement
- Complications
  - Malunion—varus deformity well tolerated owing to shoulder motion
- **Diaphyseal humerus fractures**
- Principles and presentation
  - Uncommon in children
  - Radial nerve palsy can accompany middle- or distal-third fractures; usually neurapraxia and transient
- Diagnosis and radiographs
  - AP and lateral radiographs of humerus
  - Always evaluate elbow and shoulder appropriately.
- Treatment
  - Nonoperative treatment with sling or clam-shell type splint immobilization
  - Operative indications: open fractures, vascular compromise after reduction
- Complications
  - Radial nerve palsy—usually transient; exploration rarely indicated

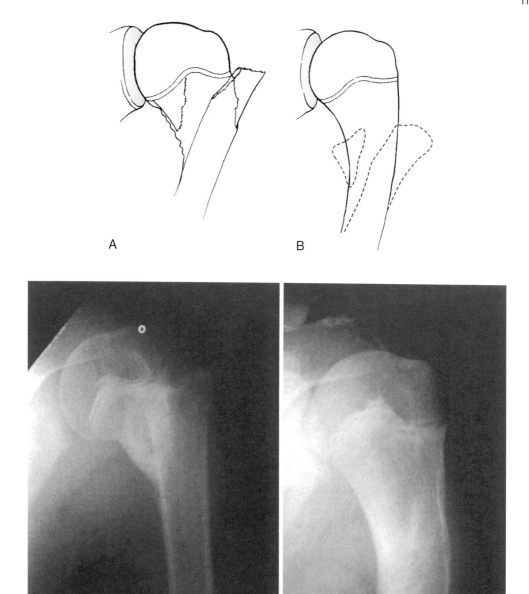

FIGURE 11-48 The remodeling potential of the proximal end of the humerus is great because of the amount of growth (80% of the entire humerus) coming from the proximal physis, as well as the universal motion of the shoulder joint. **A** and **C**, Early remodeling. **B** and **D**, Late remodeling. (From Herring J: *Tachdjian's pediatric orthopaedics,* ed 4, Philadelphia, 2007, Saunders.)

ELBOW INJURIES (TABLE 11-24)

■ Principles of elbow fractures

■ Skeletal anatomy (Figure 11-49)
  • Secondary ossification centers in order of ossification can be recalled using the mnemonic **CRITOE**, and age at ossification can be roughly estimated based on odd numbers 1, 3, 5, 7, 9, 11:
    • **C**apitellum
    • **R**adial head
    • **I**nternal (medial) epicondyle
    • **T**rochlea
    • **O**lecranon
    • **E**xternal (lateral) epicondyle
  • Radial head, trochlea, and olecranon may appear as multiple ossification sites.

■ Radiographic anatomy
  • A five-part systematic approach is key to avoiding missing injury (Figure 11-50):
    • Proximal radius should align with capitellum in all views.
    • Long axis of ulna should align and be slightly medial to humerus on AP radiograph.
    • Anterior humeral line should bisect capitellum on true lateral radiograph.
    • Humeral-capitellar (Baumann) angle should be in valgus and fall between 9 and 26 degrees.
    • Soft tissue shadows may demonstrate an anatomic anterior fat pad.
  • Abnormalities in radiographic anatomy (Box 11-1)

Table 11-24 Pediatric Elbow Trauma

INJURY	EPONYM/OTHER NAME	CLASSIFICATION	TREATMENT	COMPLICATIONS
Supracondylar fracture (6-8 yr old) (see Figure 11-52)		I—extension (98%), nondisplaced	Immobilize 3 wk. Minimally displaced (<2 mm), splint	Nerve injury (AIN and radial), vascular injury (1%), decreased ROM; if pulse present but then lost, explore; if no pulse present but pink hand, watch; if no pulse present and cold, explore HO, cubitus varus (5%-10%), ipsilateral fractures Nerve injury (ulnar), malunion (decreased extension)
		II—displaced (posterior cortex intact)	Reduce; cast vs. CRPP (must re-create Baumann angle) (see Figure 11-52)	
		III—displaced (posterior periosteal hinge intact)	Reduce; CRPP vs. open pinning	
		IV—displaced (posterior periosteal hinge disrupted)	Reduce; CRPP vs. open pinning	
		Flexion (distal fragment anterior)	Reduce; CRPP vs. ORIF	
Lateral condyle fracture (6 yr old) (see Figure 11-53)		Milch I—SH IV Milch II—SH II into trochlea	Minimally displaced (<2 mm), splint; displaced, ORIF with pins or cannulated screws	Overgrowth/spur "fish tail" deformity, nonunion, cubitus valgus, AVN, ulnar nerve palsy
Medial condyle fracture (age 9-14 yr)		Nondisplaced—<10 mm displacement		Cubitus varus, AVN
Displaced—>10 mm displacement			Minimally displaced, splint Displaced, ORIF	
Entire distal humeral physis fracture (age < 7 yr)		A—infant (SH I) B—age 7 mo-3 yr (SH I) C—age 3-7 yr (SH II)	Closed reduction, long-arm cast; displaced, CRPP	Child abuse, common late diagnosis, cubitus varus
Medial epicondylar apophysis fracture (age 11 yr) (see Figure 11-54)	Little Leaguer elbow	I—acute injuries		Highly associated with elbow dislocation (50%), valgus instability, loss of extension
		A—nondisplaced	Immobilize 1 wk	
		B—minimally displaced	Immobilize 1 wk	
		C—significantly displaced (may be dislocated)	ORIF for valgus instability; otherwise, early ROM	
		D—entrapment of fragment in joint	Manipulative extraction, ORIF (especially with ulnar nerve entrapment)	
		E—fracture through epicondylar apophysis	Immobilization vs. ORIF	
		II—chronic tension stress injury	Change in throwing activities	
T condylar fracture		Based on fracture	ORIF with cannulated screws	Decreased ROM
Radial head and neck fractures (age < 4 yr)		A—SH I or II physeal fracture B—SH IV fracture C—transmetaphyseal fracture D and E—with elbow dislocation	Immobilize if < 60 degrees in pronation/supination; ORIF if markedly displaced or > 60 degrees primarily	Decreased ROM, radial head overgrowth, neck notching, AVN, synostosis, nonunion
Proximal olecranon physis fracture (rare)		I—physeal-metaphyseal border (younger children) II—physis with large metaphyseal fragment (older children)		
Olecranon metaphysis fracture		A—flexion	If undisplaced (<3 mm), immobilize 3 wk; ORIF if defect	Rare: delay/nonunion
		B—extension	Reduction in extension Immobilize in hyperflexion	
		C—shear	ORIF if periosteal tear	
Elbow dislocation (age 11-20 yr)		Based on direction of dislocation	Reduction and cast for < 2 wk	Watch for associated fractures and nerve injuries (ulnar > median), HO, recurrent dislocation
Radial head subluxation (age 15 mo-3 yr)	Nursemaid's elbow		Stretching of annular ligaments Reduce (supination/flexion)	

AIN, Anterior interosseous nerve; *AVN,* avascular necrosis; *CRPP,* closed reduction with percutaneous pinning; *HO,* heterotopic ossification; *ORIF,* open reduction and internal fixation; *ROM,* range of motion; *SH,* Salter-Harris.

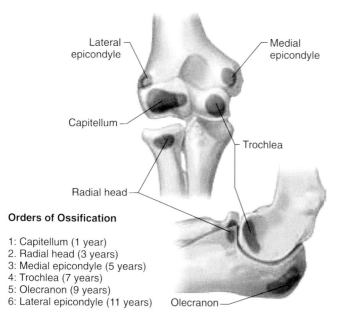

Lateral epicondyle

Medial epicondyle

Capitellum

Trochlea

Radial head

Orders of Ossification

1: Capitellum (1 year)
2. Radial head (3 years)
3. Medial epicondyle (5 years)
4. Trochlea (7 years)
5. Olecranon (9 years)
6. Lateral epicondyle (11 years)

Olecranon

FIGURE 11-49 Ossification centers of the elbow in order of appearance and approximate age of ossification.

Box 11-1	Abnormalities in Pediatric Radiographic Anatomy

RADIOGRAPHIC ABNORMALITY	LIKELY INJURY
Radius does not point to capitellum	Lateral condyle fracture Radial neck fracture Monteggia fracture or equivalent Elbow dislocation
Long axis of ulna not in line or not slightly medial to long axis of humerus	Radial head and capitellum correctly aligned → transphyseal injury or displaced supracondylar Radius not pointing to capitellum → elbow dislocation
Anterior humeral line does not bisect capitellum	First, ensure true lateral radiograph Center of capitellum posterior → extension-type supracondylar fracture Center of capitellum anterior → flexion-type supracondylar fracture
Baumann angle abnormal	Inadequate reduction of supracondylar fracture
Posterior fat pad present	76% rate of occult fracture when no other radiographic abnormality identified

- Complications
  - Fishtail deformity of distal humerus may result from malunion, osteonecrosis, growth arrest, or some combination of these factors. Uncommon but challenging complication to treat that may be seen following both supracondylar and lateral condylar fractures. Results in loss of motion with proximal forearm migration, ulnotrochlear incongruity, and radial head dislocation.
- **Distal humerus fractures**
- Distal humeral physeal separation (Figure 11-51)
  - Principles and presentation
    - Usually occur in pediatric patients younger than age 6 to 7 years

- **Consider evaluation for child abuse** in young patients with questionable presentation.
  - Young patients may present with pseudoparalysis.
  - Often confused for elbow dislocations (which are rare in young children)
- Diagnosis and radiographs
  - Radiographs demonstrate intact relationship between radius and capitellum. Radius and ulna lose normal relationship with distal end of humerus.
  - Ultrasound or MRI evaluation may be necessary for young children.
  - Arthrography can be used to evaluate for intraarticular extension.
- Treatment
  - Closed reduction and percutaneous pinning
  - Avoid closed reduction if diagnosis is made late to avoid iatrogenic injury to the physis.
- Complications
  - Misdiagnosis is most common, and these injuries can be mistaken for elbow dislocations or soft tissue injuries.
    - Physeal separations are typically medial, whereas elbow dislocations are typically lateral.
- Supracondylar humerus fractures
  - Principles and presentation
    - 50% to 60% of fractures
    - 95% to 98% extension type; typically occur from a fall on outstretched hand with elbow in extension or hyperextension
    - 2% to 5% flexion type; typically occur from a fall onto the flexed elbow
    - Peak incidence in children between ages 5 and 8
    - 1% associated with vascular injuries
    - Anterior interosseous nerve (AIN) injury most common for extension-type fractures; usually neurapraxia
    - Ulnar nerve injury usually iatrogenic from medial pinning and also the most common nerve injury from flexion type
    - Posteromedial angulation associated with radial nerve injury (the second most common neuropraxia after AIN palsy)
    - Posterolateral angulation associated with brachial artery and median nerve injury
    - Immediate surgery indicated in presence of vascular compromise (pale, cool hand)
    - Most injuries can be splinted in a nonflexed position and treated the following day with no adverse impact on outcome.
  - Diagnosis and radiographs
    - AP and lateral radiographs essential
      - AP view should be examined for Baumann angle; may need to compare with contralateral arm
      - Lateral radiograph should be examined to see if the anterior humeral line intersects the middle third of the capitellar ossification center.
      - Anterior and posterior fat pad signs should be examined.
        - Anterior fat pad displacement has low specificity and can be normal.
        - Posterior fat pad displacement is always pathologic and can indicate a nondisplaced fracture.
  - Classification and treatment—Gartland classification (Figure 11-52)

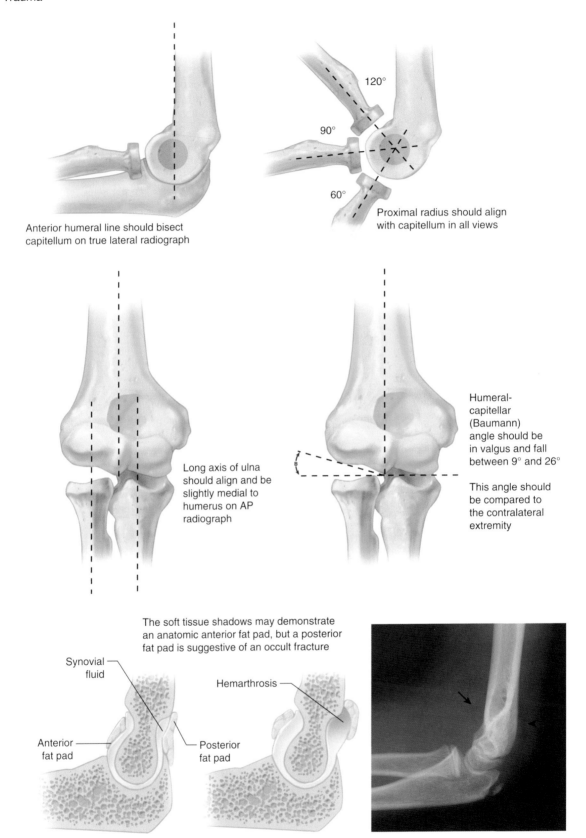

Anterior humeral line should bisect capitellum on true lateral radiograph

120°

90°

60°

Proximal radius should align with capitellum in all views

Long axis of ulna should align and be slightly medial to humerus on AP radiograph

Humeral-capitellar (Baumann) angle should be in valgus and fall between 9° and 26°

This angle should be compared to the contralateral extremity

The soft tissue shadows may demonstrate an anatomic anterior fat pad, but a posterior fat pad is suggestive of an occult fracture

Synovial fluid

Hemarthrosis

Anterior fat pad

Posterior fat pad

FIGURE 11-50 Radiographic anatomy of the pediatric elbow.

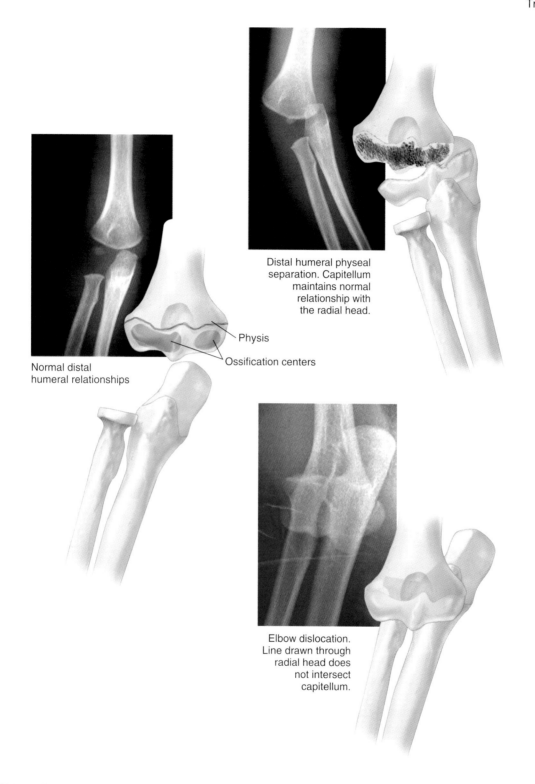

Normal distal
humeral relationships

Physis

Ossification centers

Distal humeral physeal
separation. Capitellum
maintains normal
relationship with
the radial head.

Elbow dislocation.
Line drawn through
radial head does
not intersect
capitellum.

FIGURE 11-51 Injuries about the distal end of the humerus comparing distal humeral physeal separations and elbow dislocations.

- Type I—nondisplaced
  - Treated closed in a long-arm cast for 2 to 3 weeks
- Type II—displaced with intact posterior cortex
  - Closed treatment for type II fractures is appropriate if all of the following criteria are met:
    - No significant swelling
    - Anterior humeral line intersects the capitellum
    - No medial distal humeral cortical impaction
  - Otherwise, closed reduction and percutaneous pinning is appropriate for type II fractures with

postoperative long-arm immobilization at 90 degrees of flexion.
- Type III—completely displaced; can be displaced posteromedially or posterolaterally
  - Treated with closed reduction and percutaneous pinning
  - ORIF rarely needed
    - Rotationally unstable fractures, open fractures, or those associated with neurovascular injuries
    - Anterior approach preferred

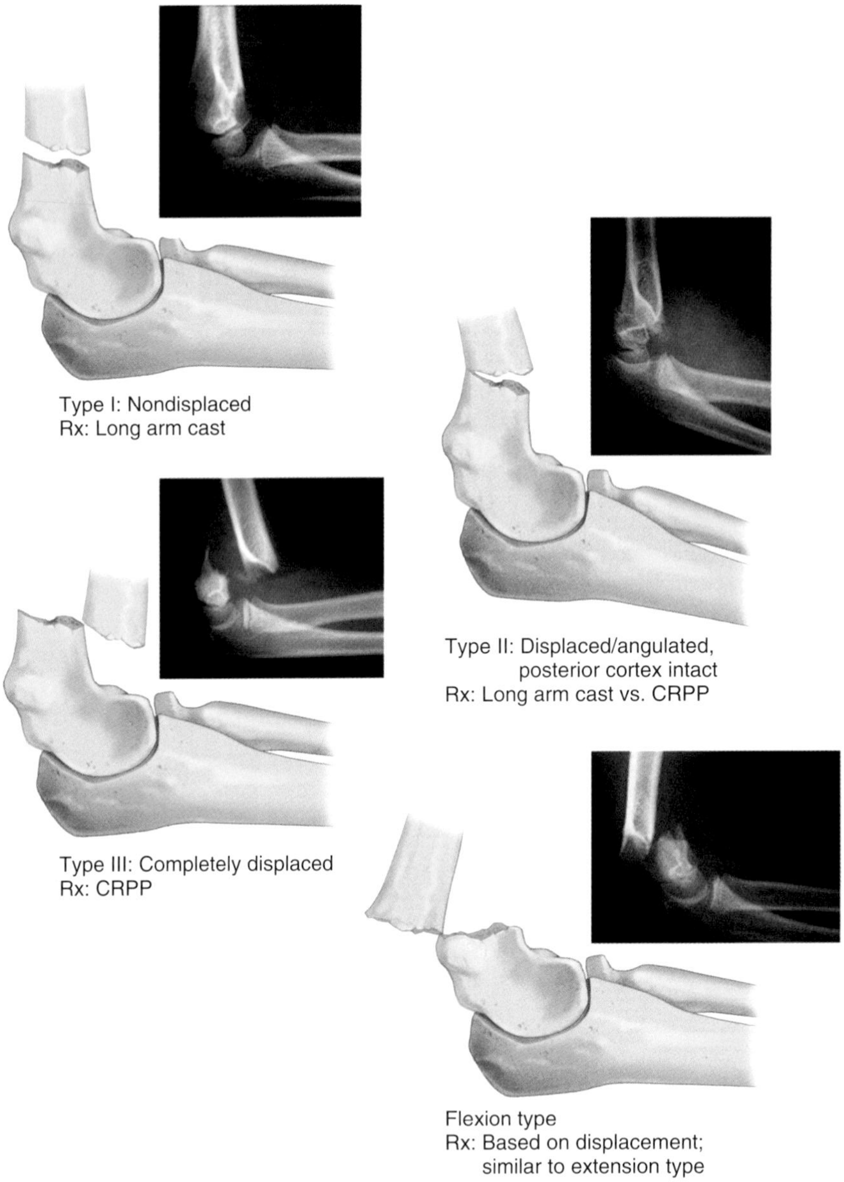

Type I: Nondisplaced
Rx: Long arm cast

Type II: Displaced/angulated,
posterior cortex intact
Rx: Long arm cast vs. CRPP

Type III: Completely displaced
Rx: CRPP

Flexion type
Rx: Based on displacement;
similar to extension type

FIGURE 11-52 Supracondylar fractures. *CRPP,* Closed reduction with percutaneous pinning; *Rx,* treatment.

- Crossed pin and lateral-entry pin configurations often used
  - Crossed pin considered more stable biomechanically
  - Medial pin can risk iatrogenic ulnar nerve (3%-8%).
  - Lateral-entry pin configuration has shown similar clinical results as crossed pin fixation when there is appropriate pin spread and engagement of both humeral columns. **Use a divergent wire technique with wires placed laterally to minimize complications and maximize the likelihood of successful outcomes.**
- Flexion type
  - Similar management to extension type based on degree of displacement
  - Minimally displaced treated with immobilization in extension
  - Displaced treated with closed reduction and percutaneous pinning

- Supracondylar fracture with associated vascular injury
  - Well-perfused hand, absent pulse ("pink, pulseless hand") (controversial)
    - Urgent closed reduction and percutaneous pinning
    - Pulse returns in majority of cases. If not, observe as an inpatient and splint extremity.
    - If hand becomes poorly perfused, obtain vascular consultation and consider intervention.
  - Poorly perfused hand, absent pulse
    - Urgent closed reduction and percutaneous pinning. Arteriography generally not warranted; location of injury is generally known.
    - If perfusion restored, observe as an inpatient.
    - If hand remains poorly perfused, obtain vascular consultation.

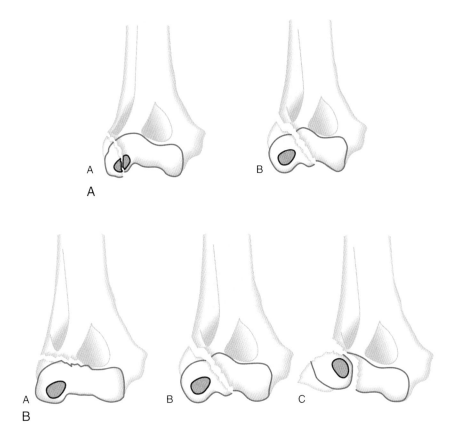

FIGURE 11-53 A, Lateral condyle drawing—Milch classification. *(A)* Milch type I fracture. The fracture line is through the ossific center of the capitellum; *(B)* Milch type II fracture. The fracture line is lateral to the ossific center of the capitellum. **B,** Lateral condyle drawing—Jakob classification. *(A)* Type I fracture. The fracture line does not enter the articular surface, permitting it to remain stable. *(B)* Type II fracture. Fracture extends into the articular surface but is minimally displaced. *(C)* Type III fracture. Fracture extends into the articular surface and is highly displaced. (From Miller MD et al, editors: *DeLee & Drez's orthopaedic sports medicine,* ed 3, Philadelphia, 2009, Saunders.)

- Complications
  - Iatrogenic ulnar nerve injury with medial pin use (3%-8%)
  - Compartment syndrome
    - Volkmann ischemic contracture is the most serious complication; beware of antecubital swelling and pressure from splint/cast.
  - Angular deformity
    - Cubitus varus is typically the result of malunion, not growth arrest. It results in a gunstock deformity associated with poor cosmesis but does not generally affect function.
    - Cubitus valgus is the result of malunion and can lead to tardy ulnar nerve palsy.
    - Recurvatum is poorly tolerated.
  - Stiffness
    - Rare if cast removal is done appropriately
- Lateral condyle fractures
  - Principles and presentation
    - 17% of distal humeral fractures
    - Peak incidence around 6 years old
    - Loss of motion can be severe owing to intraarticular extension if the diagnosis is missed.
    - Increased incidence of growth disturbance
  - Diagnosis and radiographs
    - AP, lateral, and oblique radiographs (**especially internal oblique, which is most likely to accurately show maximum degree of displacement**)

- Arthrogram can help distinguish transphyseal fractures from lateral condyle fractures.
- Classification—Milch (historical; does not dictate treatment) (Figure 11-53)
  - Milch I—SH type IV fracture; fracture courses through ossific center of capitellum; less common
  - Milch II—SH type II fracture; fracture courses medial to ossific center of capitellum; more common
- Classification—Jakob (more clinically useful)
  - Type I—less than 2 mm displacement; intact intraarticular cartilage hinge
    - Can be treated with long-arm immobilization but can displace; needs to be followed closely
  - Type II—2 to 4 mm displacement
    - Generally treated with closed reduction and percutaneous pinning
  - Type III—greater than 4 mm displacement
    - Closed reduction and percutaneous pinning if intraarticular reduction confirmed on arthrogram
    - Open reduction can be necessary to ensure intraarticular reduction
      - Must preserve posterior blood supply
- Complications
  - Lateral overgrowth or prominence (spurring) occurs in up to 50% of cases
    - Correlated with greater initial fracture displacement. May be diminished with accurate lateral periosteal alignment. Does not affect function.

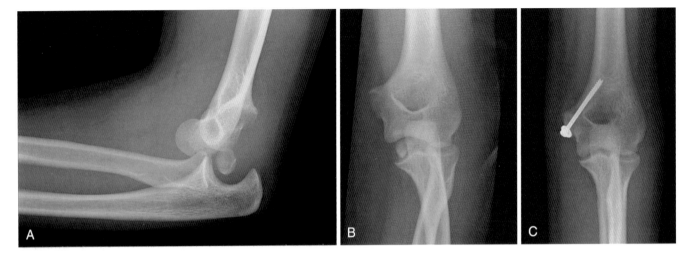

FIGURE 11-54 Medial epicondyle fracture following elbow dislocation. **A,** Lateral view with intraarticular medial epicondyle fragment. **B,** Anteroposterior view after reduction with incarcerated fragment. **C,** Internal fixation with a single cannulated 3.5-mm screw and washer. (From Miller MD et al, editors: *DeLee & Drez's orthopaedic sports medicine,* ed 3, Philadelphia, 2009, Saunders.)

- High incidence of delayed union or nonunion
  - Fracture fragment bathed in synovial fluid; relatively tenuous blood supply and primarily cartilage
- Stiffness
  - Because of longer immobilization often needed and intraarticular extension
- Angular deformity
  - Cubitus valgus more common; due to lateral growth arrest
  - Tardy ulnar nerve palsy may result.
- Osteonecrosis of lateral condyle
  - Iatrogenic—avoid dissection posterior to fragment to reduce risk of blood supply damage
- Medial condyle fractures
  - Principles and presentation
    - Rare injury, less than 1% of elbow fractures
    - 8 to 12 years old
    - Can be mistaken for more common medial epicondylar fractures
  - Diagnosis and radiographs
    - AP, lateral, oblique views
    - In young children, arthrogram may help show intraarticular component.
  - Classification—Milch (same as lateral condyle)
    - Type I—through apex of trochlea (SH type II); very rare
    - Type II—through groove between capitellum and trochlea (SH type IV)
  - Treatment
    - Similar treatment protocol as lateral condyle fractures
  - Complications
    - Missed diagnosis; usually confused for a medial epicondylar fracture
- Medial epicondyle fractures
  - Principles and presentation
    - Traction injury resulting in an avulsion of the apophysis by the medial collateral ligament and flexor mass
    - Last ossification center to fuse with metaphysis
    - **Associated with elbow dislocation approximately 50% of the time (most common fracture associated with an elbow dislocation in children)**

- Valgus force with contraction of flexor-supinator mass (same mechanism as in elbow dislocation)
- Can be incarcerated after reduction in 15% to 18% of cases (Figure 11-54)
- Little Leaguer elbow is an overuse injury akin to SH 1 injury of the medial epicondyle physis.
- Ulnar nerve symptoms can accompany injury secondary to stretch during trauma or swelling.
- Diagnosis and radiographs
  - AP, lateral, oblique views
  - If apophysis is missing from an AP view, carefully evaluate lateral and oblique views for possible incarceration.
- Classification
  - Based on the amount of displacement whether it is incarcerated in the joint
- Treatment
  - Most can be treated nonoperatively with excellent functional results.
  - The amount of displacement that would necessitate surgical reduction and fixation in young athletic patients is controversial.
  - More than 5 mm was a traditional amount of acceptable displacement; however, has been shown to be difficult to assess the true displacement on standard radiographs.
  - Incarceration of the fragment is an indication for surgical treatment.
- Complications
  - Missed incarceration
  - Ulnar nerve symptoms (10%-16%)
  - Nonunion—reported to occur in up to 60% of cases, but good functional outcomes reported even with radiographic nonunion
  - Loss of extension—20%

■ **Radial head and neck fractures**
▪ Principles and presentation
  - 5% of pediatric elbow fractures
  - 90% are physeal or metaphyseal; rarely involve the head
  - Often valgus injuries
  - Associated with elbow dislocations and medial epicondyle fractures

- Diagnosis and radiographs
  - AP, lateral, oblique views
  - Radiocapitellar view (Greenspan)—oblique lateral directed 40 degrees proximally
- Classification—Wilkins
  - Type A—SH I or II physeal fractures
  - Type B—SH III or IV intraarticular fractures (rare)
  - Type C—metaphyseal fractures
- Treatment
  - Multiple closed reduction maneuvers
    - Patterson maneuver
    - Israeli technique
  - Indications for surgery
    - Less than 20 to 30 degrees of angulation and no translation acceptable; treated in long-arm immobilization
    - More than 30 degrees angulation, translation greater than 3 to 4 mm, and more than 45 degrees of rotation are indications for surgical intervention.
    - Surgical treatment using percutaneous wire correction or retrograde insertion of a wire with rotation of the wire accounting for reduction (Metaizeau)
    - Open reduction occasionally needed through a lateral approach
  - Complications
    - Decreased ROM: usually loss of pronation and supination
    - Radial head overgrowth (20%-40%)
    - Physeal arrest—can lead to cubitus valgus deformity
    - AVN of the radial head—70% of AVN cases associated with open reduction
    - Neurologic injury—posterior interosseous nerve most commonly injured
    - Radioulnar synostosis—associated with open reduction

Radial head subluxation

- Principles and presentation
  - Also known as "nursemaid's elbow"
  - Mechanism is usually traction on an extended elbow in children younger than age 5; peak age is 2 to 3 years.
  - Arm usually held in slight flexion and pronation
  - Annular ligament subluxates over the radial head.
- Diagnosis and radiographs
  - Usually normal and usually not necessary if clinical picture is appropriate
- Treatment
  - Closed reduction achieved by placing thumb over radial head as elbow is progressively supinated and flexed
  - Immobilization is generally not needed.
- Complications
  - Recurrence can be common in young patients but uncommon after age 5 as the distal attachment of the annular ligament strengthens.

Monteggia fractures

- Principles and presentation
  - Proximal ulna fracture associated with a radial head dislocation
  - Radial head dislocation in children without an obvious fracture can often be secondary to plastic deformation of the ulna.
  - Peak incidence between ages 4 and 10 years

- Diagnosis and radiographs
  - All forearm fractures should be accompanied by elbow radiographs to evaluate for radial head dislocation; all radial head dislocations should be accompanied by forearm radiographs.
- Classification—Bado (see Figure 11-14)
  - Anterior radial head dislocation and apex anterior proximal ulna fracture
  - Posterior radial head dislocation and apex posterior proximal ulna fracture
  - Lateral radial head dislocation and apex lateral proximal ulna fracture
  - Radial head fracture-dislocation and proximal ulna fracture
- Treatment
  - Nonoperative treatment usually unsuccessful in adults
  - If ulnar length restored either by closed reduction or intramedullary fixation, radial head reduction can be successfully maintained
  - Chronic Monteggia fractures may require ulnar osteotomy and annular ligament reconstruction.
- Complications
  - Neurovascular—posterior interosseous nerve neurapraxia (10%)

FOREARM FRACTURES (TABLE 11-25)

Diaphyseal ulna and radius fractures

- Principles and presentation
  - Forearm fractures make up 45% of all pediatric fractures; male predominance.
  - 80% occur after age 5 years
  - Mechanism is usually a fall on an outstretched hand.
    - Pronation can lead to a flexion injury with dorsal angulation.
    - Supination can lead to an extension injury with volar angulation.
- Diagnosis and radiographs
  - AP and lateral views of the forearm
  - Radiographic evaluation of the elbow and wrist also important
- Classification
  - Can be described as incomplete (greenstick fractures) or complete fractures
  - Otherwise can be described by direction of apex angulation and amount of displacement
- Treatment
  - Nonoperative treatment with closed reduction and long-arm immobilization is usually successful in children.
  - In general, apex dorsal angulation should be accompanied by immobilization in supination.
  - In general, apex volar angulation should be accompanied by immobilization in pronation.
  - Location of the fracture and associated deforming forces may dictate the proper arm rotation of immobilization:
    - Proximal-third fractures in supination
    - Middle-third fractures in neutral
    - Distal-third fractures in pronation
  - Indications for surgery include open fractures, neurovascular compromise, compartment syndrome,

Table 11-25	Pediatric Radial and Ulnar Shaft Trauma			
INJURY	**EPONYM/ OTHER NAME**	**CLASSIFICATION**	**TREATMENT**	**COMPLICATIONS**
Radius and ulna fractures	"Both-bone"	Greenstick, compression, complete	Correct rotation, with pronation/ supination and < 10 degrees angulation: long-arm cast 3-4 wk if < age 10 yr; bayonet apposition OK if growth remains	Refracture, limb ischemia, malunion (especially in < age 10 yr with inadequate reduction), nerve injury, synostosis
Plastic deformation		Based on bones involved (ulna > radius)	Reduction with pressure as a fulcrum, the most deformed bone first; must reduce > 20 degrees in age 4 yr, less in older children	Persistence of deformity
Ulna fracture and radial head dislocation (see Figure 11-14)	Monteggia	Type I—ulna angulation and radial head anterior (extension)	Reduce (traction flexion); long-arm cast, 100 degrees flexion in supination	Late diagnosis (reconstruct annular ligament), decreased ROM Missed wrist injury, nonunion, persistent radial head dislocation, periarticular ossification
		Type II—ulna angulation and radial head posterior (flexion)	Reduce (traction extension); long-arm cast in some extension	
		Type III—ulna anterior angulation, radial head lateral (adduction)	Reduce (extension); long-arm cast, 90 degrees flexion in supination	
		Type IV—ulna and proximal-third radius fracture (both anterior angulation)	Reduce (supinate); may require ORIF	
Radial head dislocation (anterior)	Monteggia equivalent		Supination and pressure on radial head; long-arm cast, 100 degrees flexion in supination	Synostosis, PIN injury, loss of reduction
Ulna and radial neck fractures	Check for Monteggia equivalent		Reduce (traction, pressure on radial head, varus stress); long-arm cast, 90 degrees flexion	
Ulna and proximal radius fractures	Check for Monteggia equivalent		Reduce (traction supination); long-arm cast, 90 degrees in supination	
Radius fracture and distal radioulnar dislocation	Galeazzi		Reduce (traction supination if ulna dorsal, pronation if ulna volar); ORIF if > age 12 yr or reduction fails	Malunion, nerve injury (AIN), radioulnar subluxation, loss of radial bow

AIN, Anterior interosseous nerve; *ORIF*, open reduction and internal fixation; *PIN*, posterior interosseous nerve; *ROM*, range of motion.

over 15 to 20 degrees of angulation in patients younger than age 10 years, over 10 degrees of angulation in patients older than 10, bayonet apposition in patients older than 10, and greater than 30 degrees of malrotation.
- Fixation can be with plate/screws or intramedullary rods. For ulnar shaft fractures the IM rod is inserted into the olecranon and advanced distally. For radial shaft fractures the IM rod is inserted into the dorsal aspect of the distal radius through a small longitudinal incision placed over the fourth extensor compartment and advanced proximally.
- Complications
  - Compartment syndrome
    - Caution with multiple false pass attempts of the IM rod across the fracture site
    - Low threshold to open the fracture site if having difficulty in passing the IM rod across the fracture site
  - Malunion
    - Contributing factors include quality of initial reduction, quality of initial reduction in relation to initial displacement, and delay in diagnosis.
    - Mild loss of supination and/or pronation
  - Refracture
    - 5% to 12%

■ Distal ulna and radius fractures
▨ Principles and presentation
- Very common in pediatric patients
- Important to evaluate forearm and elbow for associated injuries
▨ Diagnosis and radiographs
- AP and lateral views of the wrist
- Radiographic evaluation of the forearm and elbow is also often necessary.
▨ Classification
- Generally classified by the SH classification of physeal injuries
- Metaphyseal fractures can be buckle or incomplete fractures or complete fractures.
▨ Treatment
- Generally treated with closed reduction and immobilization
- Acceptable sagittal angulation is up to 30 degrees in patients with more than 5 years of growth remaining, with 5 degrees less accepted for each year less than 5 years of growth remaining.
- Acceptable coronal angulation is up to 10 to 15 degrees in patients with greater than 5 years of growth remaining.
- Surgical indications to pin these fractures include failure to maintain adequate closed reduction with

Table 11-26 Pediatric Hand and Wrist Trauma

INJURY	EPONYM/OTHER NAME	CLASSIFICATION	TREATMENT	COMPLICATIONS
Phalanx fracture (watch for mallet equivalent)		Based on phalanx and SH classification	Closed reduction for most; ORIF if condylar, SH III/IV > 25 degrees if < 10 yr old, >10 degrees if > 10 yr old; dynamic traction for pilon equivalents	Residual deformities, tendon imbalance, nail deformities
MC fracture		Based on location	Reduce; ORIF if irreducible	Avascular necrosis of metacarpal head
Thumb MC fracture	Type D = Bennett equivalent	Type A—metaphyseal Type B—SH II (medial) Type C—SH II (lateral) Type D—SH III	Closed reduction except for type D, which requires ORIF	
Interphalangeal dislocation			Closed reduction and splint; ORIF if unable to obtain or maintain a congruous reduction	
MCP dislocation			Attempt closed reduction; ORIF if irreducible	
CMC dislocation			Reduce with finger traps; CRPP with Kirschner wire to carpus and adjacent MC	
Distal radius fracture		SH fractures I-V	CRPP types III and IV	Deformity, loss of reduction, infection with open fracture, Volkmann contracture, growth arrest, malunion, refracture, TFCC tears, carpal tunnel syndrome
Torus	Tension side intact	Short-arm cast for 3 wk		
Greenstick	Tension side with plastic deformation	Reduce if angulation > 10 degrees		
Complete	Both cortices disrupted	Reduce and place in long-arm cast		

CMC, Carpometacarpal; *CRPP,* closed reduction with percutaneous pinning; *MC,* metacarpal; *MCP,* metacarpophalangeal joint; *ORIF,* open reduction and internal fixation; *SH,* Salter-Harris; *TFCC,* triangular fibrocartilage complex.

casting alone, ipsilateral distal humerus fracture requiring operative intervention, and soft tissue concerns that would not allow for casting.

- Complications
  - Similar to those of diaphyseal forearm fractures
  - Distal ulnar physeal fractures are uncommon but have a 50% rate of physeal arrest, compared to 4% for distal radius physeal fractures.
  - Loss of reduction can occur with a poorly molded cast. Loss of reduction is associated with a cast index (sagittal width/coronal width) above 0.84

PEDIATRIC SCAPHOID FRACTURE (TABLE 11-26)

- **Scaphoid (navicular) bone: most lateral of proximal row of carpal bones**
- Principles and presentation
  - Usually due to a fall on an outstretched hand
  - Presents with snuffbox tenderness
  - Usually avulsion injuries of the distal pole
- Diagnosis and radiographs
  - If suspected but not apparent on plain x-ray, CT scan should be obtained
- Treatment
  - Thumb spica cast for 4 to 8 weeks
  - Displaced midwaist fractures can result in AVN or nonunion and should be managed operatively.

LOWER EXTREMITY

- **Pelvis fractures (Table 11-27)**
- Principles and presentation
  - Less common in pediatric patients but associated (>50%) with multiple injuries and visceral injuries in the polytrauma patient
  - Avulsion fractures can be seen in adolescence, especially in athletes.
  - Ischial avulsions result from the pull of the hamstring or adductors (Figure 11-55).
  - Anterior superior iliac spine avulsions result from the pull of the sartorius.
  - Anterior inferior iliac spine avulsions result from the pull of the rectus femoris.
  - Iliac crest avulsions result from the pull of the abdominal muscles and tensor fascia lata.
  - Lesser trochanter avulsions result from the pull of the iliopsoas.
- Diagnosis and radiographs
  - AP, Judet views (acetabulum), inlet/outlet views (pelvic ring)
  - CT often necessary because 50% of all pelvic fractures may be missed on a plain AP pelvis view
- Classification
  - Tile
    - Type A—stable
    - Type B—rotationally unstable but vertically stable
    - Type C—rotationally and vertically unstable

Table 11-27	Pediatric Pelvic Fracture*			
CLASSIFICATION (KEY AND CORNWELL)	**EPONYM**	**TREATMENT**		**COMPLICATIONS**
I—RING INTACT				
Avulsions (ASIS, AIIS, IT)		BR flexed hip for 2 wk; guarded WB for 4 wk		Loss of reduction, delayed union
Pubis/ischium	Duverney	BR 3-7 days; limited WB for 4 wk		DJD, malunion, organ injury
Iliac wing		BR with leg abducted; progress to full WB		Sacral nerve injury
Sacrum/coccyx		BR 3-6 wk, conservative management if < 1 cm displaced, otherwise ORIF		
II—SINGLE BREAK IN RING				
Ipsilateral rami		BR 2-4 wk; non-WB		
Symphysis pubis		BR with sling or spica; ORIF if undergoing laparotomy or widely displaced		
SI joint (rare)		BR with progressive WB		
III—DOUBLE BREAK IN RING	Straddle			
Bilateral pubic rami	Malgaigne	BR with flexed hip 2-4 wk		Often unstable, with associated injuries
Anterior and posterior ring with migration		Skeletal traction; external fixator for 3-6 wk		
IV—ACETABULAR FRACTURES				
Small fragment with dislocation		BR followed by progressive ambulation		
Linear: nondisplaced		Treat associated pelvic fracture		
Linear: hip unstable		Skeletal traction; ORIF if incongruous		
Central		Lateral traction for reduction; ORIF if severe		HO, especially if severe

AIIS, Anterior inferior iliac spine; *ASIS,* anterior superior iliac spine; *BR,* bed rest; *DJD,* degenerative joint disease; *HO,* heterotopic ossification; *IT,* ischial tuberosity; *ORIF,* open reduction and internal fixation; *SI,* sacroiliac; *WB,* weight bearing.
*In general, less than adults because of remodeling.

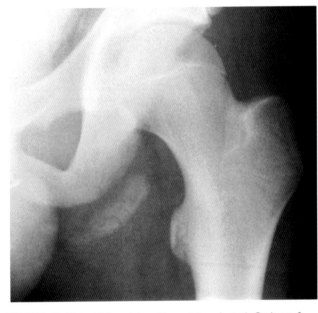

FIGURE 11-55 Ischial avulsion. (From Adam A et al: *Grainger & Allison's diagnostic radiology,* ed 5, Philadelphia, 2008, Churchill Livingstone.)

- Treatment
  - Pelvic ring fractures in the polytrauma patient who is hemodynamically unstable may necessitate placement of external fixation.
  - Vertically unstable and intraarticular displacement of acetabular fractures in pediatric patients are surgical indications.
  - Nonoperative treatment is usually indicated for avulsion fractures with gradual return to athletics.
  - Operative treatment of avulsion fractures may be necessary if these progress to symptomatic nonunions.
- Complications
  - Premature closure of the triradiate cartilage
  - Leg-length discrepancies

- Neurovascular injuries
- Heterotopic ossification

■ Hip dislocations (Table 11-28)
- Principles and presentation
  - More common than hip fractures in pediatric patients
  - New research may suggest an association with femoral acetabular impingement in athletes sustaining these injuries without high-energy trauma.
- Diagnosis and radiographs
  - AP pelvis and cross-table lateral views
  - CT scan or MRI may be necessary post reduction to confirm the adequacy of the reduction and rule out incarcerated fragments.
- Classification
  - Generally described based on the direction of dislocation (anterior vs. posterior)
  - Posterior dislocations are 10 times more common than anterior dislocations.
- Treatment
  - Gentle closed reduction with sedation as soon as possible to reduce risk of AVN
  - Caution with causing a physeal fracture of the proximal femur with too much force (usually from inadequate sedation)
  - Open reduction is indicated for failed closed reduction, nonconcentric reduction, or dislocation with associated femoral head, neck, or acetabular fracture.
- Complications
  - AVN—8% to 10%
    - Decreased incidence in patients younger than age 5 years
    - Increased incidence a delay in reduction

■ Femoral neck fractures (see Table 11-28)
- Principles and presentation
  - Rare in pediatric patients
  - Usually the result of severe high-energy trauma (75%-80%)

Table 11-28 | Pediatric Hip Trauma

INJURY	CLASSIFICATION	TREATMENT	COMPLICATIONS
Hip fracture (see Figure 11-56)	Delbet		
	IA—transepiphyseal with dislocation	Closed reduction or ORIF with pin	AVN close to 100%
	IB—transepiphyseal without dislocation	CRPP with spica	AVN in up to 60%
	II—transcervical	CRPP with spica	Coxa vara (25%): treat with subtrochanteric valgus osteotomy
	IIIA—cervical trochanteric (displaced)	CRPP with spica	Nonunion (6%)
	IIIB—cervical trochanteric (nondisplaced)	Spica cast in abduction	Growth arrest
	IV—intertrochanteric	Spica cast; ORIF if unstable	May cross physis if it creates greater fracture stability
Femoral neck stress fracture	Devas		Displacement causes more problems; varus deformities
	Superior transverse	CRPP (otherwise is displaced) NWB	
	Inferior (compressive)		
Traumatic dislocation	Posterior or anterior	Closed reduction; open if joint incongruous	AVN (10%), recurrent dislocation, HO, DJD

AVN, Avascular necrosis; *CRPP*, closed reduction with percutaneous pinning; *DJD*, degenerative joint disease; *HO*, heterotopic ossification; *NWB*, non–weight bearing; *ORIF*, open reduction and internal fixation.

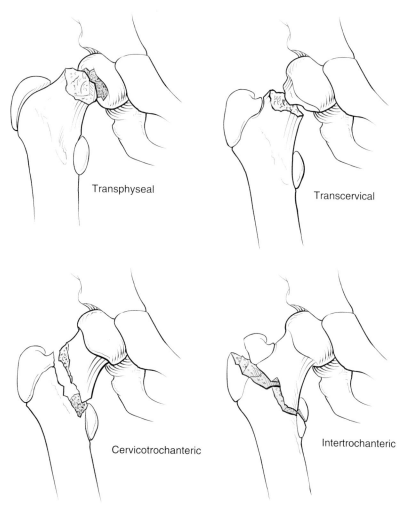

FIGURE 11-56 Delbet classification of children's hip fractures. (From Herring J: *Tachdjian's pediatric orthopaedics,* ed 4, Philadelphia, 2007, Saunders.)

■ Diagnosis and radiographs
- AP pelvis and cross-table lateral views
- CT and MRI can help in the cases of nondisplaced fractures or stress fractures.

■ Classification—Delbet (Figure 11-56)
- Type I—transphyseal fractures
  - Very high risk of AVN (approaches 100%)
- Type II—transcervical fractures
  - Moderate risk of AVN (50%)
- Type III—basicervical or cervicothoracic fractures
  - Low risk of AVN (20%-30%)
- Type IV—intertrochanteric fractures
  - Very low risk of AVN (10%-15%)

Table 11-29	Pediatric Femoral Shaft Trauma		
INJURY	**CLASSIFICATION**	**TREATMENT**	**COMPLICATIONS**
Femur fracture (including subtrochanteric fractures)	age ≤ 6 yr	Spica cast; may need short period of traction if shortened > 2 cm and followed by spica casting	LLD: Angular deformity (avoid > 10 degrees frontal and > 10 degrees sagittal malalignment)
	age 6-13 yr	Current trend to use flexible titanium nails, with possible additional immobilization, but may also use external fixation (higher refracture rate), plate (need to remove, causes large scar formation), or traction (rare)	Rotational deformity (>10 degrees); expect 0.9 cm overgrowth in children < age 10
	≥ age 14 yr	IM nail (trochanteric entry)	AVN reported with IM nails in children with growth remaining

AVN, Avascular necrosis; *IM*, intramedullary; *LLD*, leg-length discrepancy.

- Treatment
  - Types I to III represent a surgical emergency and should be treated with ORIF; smooth pins should be used for younger patients and threaded pins in adolescent patients.
  - Postoperative spica casting may be necessary in some cases especially younger children and more severe injuries
- Complications
  - AVN
  - Coxa vara
  - Nonunion
  - Physeal arrest
- **Diaphyseal femur fractures (Table 11-29)**
- Principles and presentation
  - Bimodal age distribution in pediatric patients, with peaks between ages 2 and 4 years and later in adolescence
  - Consider child abuse in pediatric patients not yet walking.
- Diagnosis and radiographs
  - AP and lateral views of the femur
  - Ipsilateral knee and hip views should be obtained to rule out associated injuries.
- Treatment
  - Based on fracture pattern and patient age
  - Infants younger than age 6 months can be treated in Pavlik harness.
  - Patients younger than age 5 to 6 years can be treated with early spica casting or traction with delayed spica casting especially if minimal (<2 cm) shortening.
  - Patients between ages 5 and 11 can be treated with several approaches:
    - Flexible intramedullary nailing is appropriate for more stable simple fracture patterns without significant shortening and is associated with poorer results in children older than 11 years and in heavier obese children.
    - Submuscular plate fixation is appropriate for more unstable fracture patterns, especially with shortening and comminution.
    - External fixation is appropriate for the polytrauma patient, open fractures, or those with soft tissue management concerns and is usually placed laterally to avoid the quadriceps.
  - Patients older than age 11 and those approaching skeletal maturity can be usually treated with antegrade intramedullary nailing.
    - Trochanteric or lateral entry nailing required

- Must avoid piriformis entry nailing because this risks the vascularity to the femoral head
- External fixation is always an option in emergency setting in which the patient may be hemodynamically unstable, multiply injured, or has open fractures.
- Complications
  - Malunion—rotational deformities do not remodel and need to be controlled at the time of reduction and fixation. Greater sagittal angulation is acceptable secondary to better remodeling capability than varus/valgus angulation.
  - Leg-length discrepancy
    - Overgrowth
      - Overgrowth of 0.7 to 2.0 cm is common in younger children (<10 years old). It is most common during the 2 years after injury.
    - Shortening
      - **Up to 2.0 cm of shortening is acceptable in young children with the potential for overgrowth. Thus older children and those with more than 2.0 cm of shortening need to have either traction applied to restore length or appropriate ORIF to address shortening.**
- **Distal femur fractures (Table 11-30)**
- Principles and presentation
  - Most distal femoral physeal fractures occur in adolescence (two thirds).
  - Often the result of direct trauma with some degree of rotation or angulation
    - Physis often fails on the tension side, whereas metaphysis often fails on the compression side, resulting in the Thurston-Holland fragment (in SH type II physeal fractures) (Figure 11-57).
  - Must be considered in adolescent patients possibly misdiagnosed with collateral ligament injuries
- Diagnosis and radiographs (Figure 11-58)
  - AP, lateral, oblique views of the knee
  - Stress views may help delineate subtle physeal injuries.
  - CT or MRI may be necessary to evaluate for intraarticular extension
  - Angiograph is occasionally necessary to evaluate for a vascular injury, especially those physeal fractures with wide displacement and posterior spiked fragments with a clinical presentation that warrants evaluation.
- Classification (see Figure 11-44)
  - SH physeal fracture classification is often used to describe these injuries.
- Treatment

Table 11-30	**Pediatric Knee Trauma**			
INJURY	**EPONYM/ OTHER NAME**	**CLASSIFICATION**	**TREATMENT**	**COMPLICATIONS**
Distal femoral epiphysis fracture (see Figures 11-57 and 11-58)	"Wagon wheel"	SH I-IV (II most common)	Closed reduction: LLC; CRPP in SH III or IV; open if soft tissue interposition or displaced III and IV	Popliteal artery or peroneal nerve injury, recurrent displacement; growth plate injuries because of undulating physis
Proximal tibial epiphysis fracture		SH I-IV (II most common)	Nondisplaced: long-leg cast in 30 degrees of flexion Displaced: CRPP	Popliteal artery injury, growth plate injury
Floating knee		Letts		Infection, nonunion, malunion, injuries
		A—both fractures diaphyseal	ORIF in one, closed reduction in the other	
		B—one fracture diaphyseal and one metaphyseal	ORIF of diaphyseal and closed reduction of metaphyseal	
		C—one fracture diaphyseal and one epiphyseal	CRPP of epiphyseal and ORIF of diaphyseal	
		D—one fracture open and one closed	Débride/external fixation, open and closed reductions of closed fracture	
		E—both fractures open	Débride/external fixation of both	
Tibial tubercle avulsion fracture (age 14-16 yr in jumping sport) (see Figure 11-61)		Ogden		
		1—small distal piece fractured	If minimally displaced with extension, then cast; otherwise, ORIF	Genu recurvatum, decreased ROM, laxity
		2—fracture at junction of primary and secondary ossification centers		
		3—fracture through one epiphysis (SH III)		
Tibial spine fracture (most common hemarthrosis in preadolescent) (see Figure 11-60)		Meyers and McKeever		
		I—incomplete/ nondisplaced	Attempt closed reduction in extension for all; if it remains displaced, then may use arthroscope and ACL guide to fix with suture	Meniscal entrapment
		II—hinged (posterior rim intact)		
		III—completely displaced		
Patella fracture		Nondisplaced	Aspiration and cast vs. brace in 5 degrees of flexion	Patella alta, extensor lag, infection
		Displaced (>2 mm)	ORIF with tension band	
Sleeve fracture (see Figure 11-59)		Avulsion of the distal pole and articular cartilage	ORIF with tension band	
Femorotibial dislocation		Same as in adults	Same as in adults: arteriogram	Popliteal artery injury
Patella dislocation		Same as in adults	Closed-reduction cast for 3 wk; consider fixing MPFL; open if fragment	Predisposition: Down syndrome, arthrogryposis

ACL, Anterior cruciate ligament; *CRPP,* closed reduction with percutaneous pinning; *LLC,* long-leg cast; *MPFL,* medial patellofemoral ligament; *ORIF,* open reduction and internal fixation; *ROM,* range of motion; *SH,* Salter-Harris.

- Nonoperative treatment with cast immobilization appropriate for nondisplaced fractures
- Operative treatment indicated for open fractures, intraarticular fractures, or displacement through the physis
- Smooth wires can be placed across the physis temporarily to hold the physeal reduction.
- Fixation across the Thurston-Holland fragment to the rest of the metaphysis may help the reduction but generally cannot hold the reduction of the physis alone.

- Complications
  - Growth arrest—very common (30%-50%); patients and families should be counseled about this at the time of initial evaluation; can also result in limb-length discrepancies and angular deformities, depending on the amount of physis arrested and age of the patient.
  - Vascular injury (<2%)—especially with hyperextension injuries that have a posterior spike
  - Peroneal nerve palsy (3%)—especially with varus injuries

- Knee instability (possibly up to 40%)—some degree of stretch of the cruciate ligaments is thought to occur during these injuries. Whether this stretch and instability causes functional deficits is unclear.
- **Hardware irritation is a common cause of pain in healed fractures.**

■ **Patella (see Table 11-30)**

▨ Principles and presentation
- Presents similar to adult patellar fractures
- Be aware of bipartite patella (5%)
- Can be missed secondary to difficult to visualize radiographically cartilaginous avulsion injury—"**patellar sleeve**" fracture
  - Must look for patella alta and defect (Figure 11-59)

▨ Diagnosis and radiographs
- AP, lateral, and sunrise views

▨ Treatment
- Similar to adult patellar fractures
- Indications for **surgical reduction and internal fixation** include extensor lag, **inability to do a straight-leg raise**, and intraarticular displacement.
- Tension band constructs are often used if bone stock is sufficient.
- Soft tissue repair techniques with careful attention to repair of the retinacular structures if repair of the cartilaginous sleeve fracture is needed

▨ Complications
- Loss of ROM; fixation technique should allow for early motion.

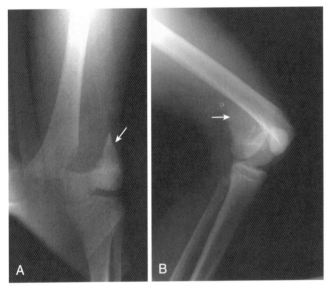

FIGURE 11-57 Anteroposterior **(A)** and lateral **(B)** images of a typical Salter-Harris type II fracture of the distal femur in a 15-year-old boy who sustained a valgus force to the knee while playing football. Note the significant displacement in the lateral Thurston-Holland fragment *(arrow)*. (From Herring J: *Tachdjian's pediatric orthopaedics,* ed 4, Philadelphia, 2007, Saunders.)

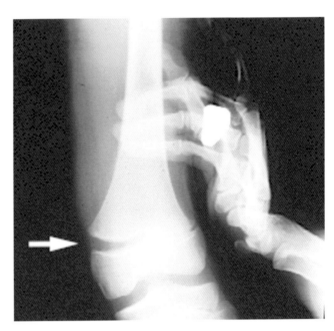

FIGURE 11-58 Stress radiograph of a physeal injury of the distal femur. An anteroposterior radiograph with valgus stress applied reveals unstable physeal disruption. (From Townsend C et al: *Sabiston textbook of surgery,* ed 18, Philadelphia, 2007, Elsevier.)

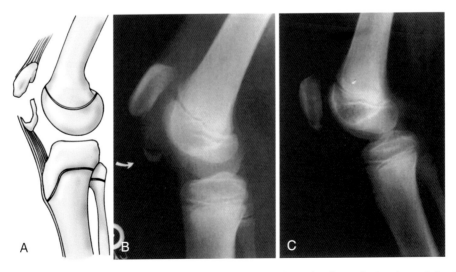

FIGURE 11-59 **A,** Schematic representation of a sleeve fracture of the patella. **B,** Lateral radiograph showing patella alta (note that the large articular cartilage segment attached to the bony distal fragment is not visualized). **C,** Lateral radiograph following operative repair. (From Scott WM, editor: *Insall & Scott surgery of the knee,* ed 4, Philadelphia, 2005, Elsevier.)

■ Proximal tibia (see Table 11-30)

▨ Tibial spine fractures
- Principles and presentation
  - Similar to ACL ruptures in terms of mechanism of injury; often while landing with a rotational component; hyperextension and valgus forces predominant
  - Present with hemarthrosis
  - Often have an unstable Lachman or pivot shift test
  - SH type III fracture
  - Occurs most commonly in children ages 8 to 14
  - 40% rate of associated injuries, including meniscal tears, collateral ligament injury, capsular injury and osteochondral fractures
- Diagnosis and radiographs
  - AP and lateral views
  - An AP view taken perpendicular to the tibial plateau accounting for the 5 to 10 degrees of posterior tibial slope can help visualize the often small osseous fragment.
- Classification—Meyers and McKeever (Figure 11-60)
  - Type I—nondisplaced spine fragment
  - Type II—anterior angulation and displacement of the spine fragment hinging on the posterior cortex
  - Type III—completely displaced fragment

- Treatment
  - Type I and type II fractures that reduce with extension can be treated nonoperatively with initial immobilization in extension; ROM can be progressed once bony union is achieved, usually at 4 to 6 weeks.
  - Type II fractures that do not reduce and type III fractures are treated with operative fixation (both open and arthroscopic techniques can be used).
    - Often anterior horn of either meniscus can be found trapped in fracture site
      - Lateral meniscus was thought to be found most commonly trapped, but Kocher et al. found the medial meniscus to be trapped more commonly.
    - Fixation can be achieved with screw fixation if the fragment is big enough; otherwise, suture fixation is suggested
- Complications
  - Knee stiffness and loss of extension—very common; loss of extension found in up to 60%
  - Late anterior instability—up to 60%; possibly secondary to ligamentous stretch; unclear whether clinically significant
  - Malunion can lead to impingement (similar to a Cyclops lesion after ACL reconstruction)

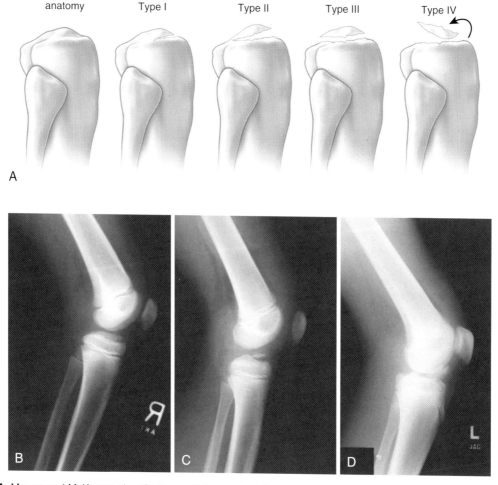

FIGURE 11-60 **A,** Meyers and McKeever classification of tibial spine injuries in children. **B,** Lateral radiograph demonstrating a nondisplaced type I tibial spine injury. **C,** Lateral radiograph demonstrating a type II tibial spine injury. **D,** Lateral radiograph demonstrating a type III tibial spine injury. (From Herring J: *Tachdjian's pediatric orthopaedics*, ed 4, Philadelphia, 2007, Saunders.)

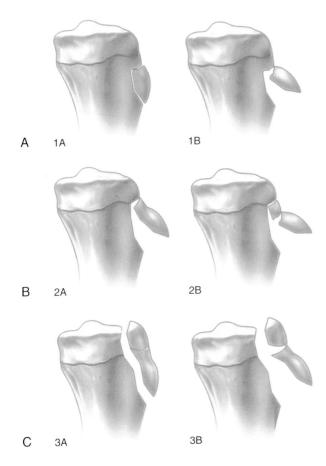

A 1A 1B

B 2A 2B

C 3A 3B

FIGURE 11-61 Ogden modification of the Watson-Jones classification of tibial tubercle fractures. **A,** Type 1A, fracture distal to the junction of proximal tibia and tubercle ossification centers with minimal displacement. Type 1B, fragment is displaced. **B,** Type 2A, fracture at the junction of the proximal tibia and tubercle ossification centers with minimal displacement. Type 2B, fragment is comminuted and the distal fragment is displaced. **C,** Type 3A, fracture extends into the joint. Type 3B, fracture extends into the joint with fragment comminution. (From Herring J: *Tachdjian's pediatric orthopaedics,* ed 4, Philadelphia, 2007, Saunders.)

- Tibial tuberosity fractures
  - Principles and presentation
    - Most common between ages 14 and 16 years; often occurs in athletes
    - Tibial tubercle and tibial plateau physis closes from posterior to anterior and from medial to lateral.
    - Predisposing factors include patella baja, tight hamstrings, and history of Osgood-Schlatter disease.
  - Diagnosis and radiographs
    - AP and lateral views
    - Patellar alta often observed on the lateral view
  - Classification—Ogden modification of Watson-Jones (Figure 11-61)
    - Type I—small fragment displaced proximally
    - Type II—secondary ossification completely displaced proximally
    - Type III—fracture extends intraarticularly
    - A+B versions of each type denote increasing comminution and displacement.
  - Treatment
    - Nondisplaced fractures can be treated with long-leg immobilization in a manner similar to tibial spine fractures.

- Displaced fractures should be treated with ORIF.
  - Screws can be used in most of these patients because they are approaching skeletal maturity.
  - Intraarticular reduction must be confirmed for type III fractures (arthroscopically or through an arthrotomy).
- Complications
  - Compartment syndrome—anterior tibial recurrent artery can be tethered and torn as it enters anterior compartment from the trifurcation posteriorly; increased risk of swelling.
  - Growth arrest—most patients are approaching skeletal maturity; however, young patients may suffer from a recurvatum deformity if a growth arrest occurs.
- Proximal tibial physeal fractures
  - Principles and presentation
    - More uncommon but often unstable
    - Vascular injury is the most serious sequela, given the popliteal artery is tethered behind the knee.
  - Diagnosis and radiographs
    - AP and lateral views of the knee
    - Like the distal femur, stress views may help delineate a subtle injury, but care must be taken to not stretch the neurovascular structures.
    - CT or MRI can help delineate an intraarticular extension or displacement.
  - Classification
    - SH classification of physeal fractures often used
  - Treatment
    - Nondisplaced fractures can be treated with immobilization but need to be followed closely because these injuries can be unstable.
    - Displaced fractures can be treated with reduction, and smooth pin fixation that crosses the physis can be used when necessary.
    - Intraarticular fractures (SH types III and IV) should be visualized by arthroscopy or arthrotomy to confirm reduction.
  - Complications
    - Neurovascular injury—popliteal injury possible during initial trauma; peroneal nerve susceptible to stretch injuries from varus displacement
    - Growth arrest—can result in leg-length discrepancies; partial arrests or bars can be associated with angular deformities.
- Proximal tibia metaphyseal fractures
  - Principles and presentation
    - Common in 3- to 6-year-old children
    - Heal rapidly but often present with late genu valgum (Cozen phenomenon) (Figure 11-62)
      - Unknown cause but resolve spontaneously over time
  - Diagnosis and radiographs
    - Standard AP, lateral views of the knee ± tibia
  - Treatment
    - Closed reduction and long-leg cast immobilization
  - Complications
    - Cozen phenomenon; resolves spontaneously
- **Tibial shaft (Table 11-31)**
- Principles and presentation
  - Common; accounts for 15% of all pediatric fractures
  - Average age: 8 years

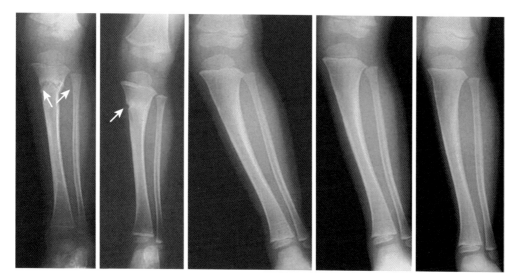

FIGURE 11-62 Posttraumatic tibial valgus with subsequent resolution. (Reprinted with permission from Macnicol MF: Paediatric knee problems, *Orthop Trauma* 24:369–380, 2010.)

Table 11-31	Pediatric Tibial Shaft Trauma			
INJURY	**EPONYM/ OTHER NAME**	**CLASSIFICATION**	**TREATMENT**	**COMPLICATIONS**
Tibia-fibula fracture	Greenstick	Incomplete	Long-leg cast in slight flexion for 6-8 wk unless > 10 degrees AP or > 5 degrees varus/valgus; then must do manipulation	Angular deformity (valgus)
		Complete	Closed reduction and cast	LLD (may see overgrowth if < age 10), malrotation, vascular injury
Tibial spiral fracture		Spiral fracture in children < age 6 yr	Long-leg cast for 3-4 wk	
Bike spoke injury		Soft tissue disruption	Admit and observe	Compartment syndrome; need for soft tissue coverage
Proximal tibial metaphysis fracture (see Figure 11-62)	Cozen	Greenstick in age 3-6 yr (complete in older children)	Long-leg cast in varus for 6 wk	Genu valgum, arterial injury, physeal injury

AP, Anteroposterior; *LLD,* leg length discrepancy.

- 30% associated with a fibular fracture
- Most commonly secondary to pedestrian versus motor vehicle accidents (50%)
- "Toddler's fracture" is a nondisplaced oblique or spiral tibial shaft fracture with intact fibula.
  - Typically occurs in child younger than age 6 who sustained a twisting injury
  - Occasionally mistaken for infection, because radiographs are often normal
- Diagnosis and radiographs
  - AP and lateral views of tibia and fibula
  - Radiographic evaluation of the ipsilateral ankle and knee usually required
- Treatment
  - Closed reduction and casting can be used for nondisplaced fractures and adequately reduced fractures.
    - Toddler's fractures should be placed into a long-leg cast for 2 weeks, and repeat radiographs obtained to demonstrate presence of callus, thus confirming diagnosis.
  - Indications for surgery include open fractures, neurovascular compromise, more than 5 degrees

valgus angulation, more than 5 degrees posterior angulation, and more than 5 to 10 degrees varus or anterior angulation.
  - Operative fixation techniques include percutaneous pinning (younger patients), screw and plate fixation, external fixation (especially in open fractures), and intramedullary nail fixation (either flexible nails or rigid nails in older patients).
- Complications
  - Compartment syndrome
  - Leg-length discrepancy
  - Angular deformity
  - Unrecognized physeal injury proximally or distally
- **Distal tibia/ankle fractures (Table 11-32)**
- Principles and presentation
  - 25% to 38% of all physeal injuries
  - Second most common physeal injury (distal radius is most common)
  - Physeal injuries in the distal tibia and fibula are typically seen between ages 8 and 15 years.
  - Mechanism of injury is similar to that for adult ankle fractures; occasional direct trauma, usually rotation around a fixed foot and ankle

Table 11-32 Pediatric Ankle and Foot Trauma

INJURY	EPONYM/OTHER NAME	CLASSIFICATION	TREATMENT	COMPLICATIONS
Ankle fracture		SH and Dias-Tachdjian (see Figure 11-47)	If SH I or II injury, treat with short-leg walking cast; if SH III or IV injury, treat with CRPP vs. ORIF	Angular deformity, bony bridge (poor prognosis with distal tibia), LLD, DJD, rotational deformity, AVN
	Juvenile Tillaux (see Figure 11-63)	SH III of lateral tibial physis (because distal-medial tibial physis is closed in this age group)	May use long-leg cast if < 2 mm displacement; if greater, treat with ORIF and visualization of joint line	
	Wagstaff	SH III of distal fibular physis	Closed reduction and cast; ORIF if necessary	
	Triplane (see Figure 11-64)	Complex SH IV, with components in all three planes	ORIF if > 2 mm articular step-off (fixation achieved parallel to physis in metaphysis and epiphysis)	Must use CT to delineate fracture
Talus fracture		Same as in adults	Closed reduction and cast unless > 5 mm or 5 degrees of displacement	AVN
Calcaneus fracture	Essex-Lopresti	Same as in adults	Same as in adults	
Tarsometatarsal fracture		Fracture of base of second metatarsal and cuboid fracture	Closed reduction vs. CRPP if unstable	
Base of the fifth metatarsal fracture	Jones/pseudo-Jones	Same as in adults	Same as in adults	Nonunion

AVN, Avascular necrosis; *CRPP,* closed reduction/percutaneous pinning; *CT,* computed tomography; *DJD,* degenerative joint disease; *LLC,* long-leg cast; *LLD,* leg-length discrepancy; *ORIF,* open reduction and internal fixation; *SH,* Salter-Harris.

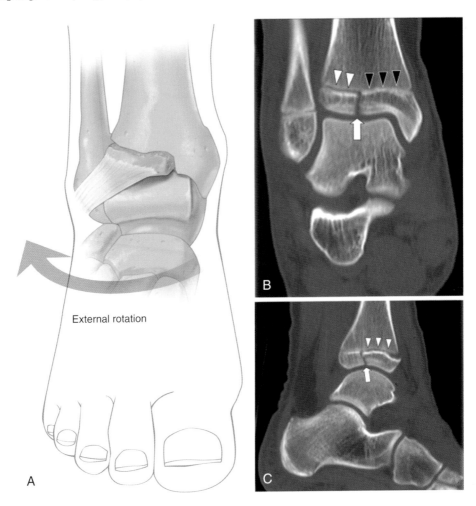

FIGURE 11-63 A, Tillaux fracture. **B,** Coronal computed tomography (CT) scan shows the Salter-Harris type III fracture with a longitudinal component through the epiphysis *(arrow)* and a transverse component through the unfused lateral physis *(white arrowheads).* The fused medial physis is indicated by the black arrowheads. **C,** Sagittal CT scan shows the Salter-Harris type III fracture with a longitudinal component through the epiphysis *(arrow)* and a transverse component through the unfused physis *(arrowheads).*

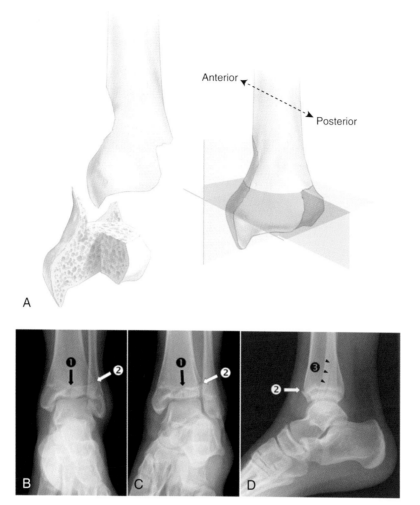

FIGURE 11-64 Triplane fractures are usually Salter-Harris type IV fractures. **A,** Schematic depiction showing the orientation of the three fracture planes. Anteroposterior **(B)** and mortise **(C)** radiographs. When minimally displaced, the fracture margins can be difficult to see on radiographs. The *black arrow* points to the epiphysis fracture, running vertically in the sagittal plane (plane 1). The *white arrow* points to the physis fracture, running horizontally in the axial plane (plane 2). **D,** Lateral non–weight-bearing radiograph. The *arrow* points to the physis fracture, running horizontally in the axial plane. The *arrowheads* point to the metaphysis fracture, running obliquely vertically in the coronal plane (plane 3).

- The distal tibial physis closes in a predictable pattern from central to medial, and the anterolateral portion closes last; this gives rise to unique "transitional" type physeal fractures.
- **Tillaux fractures are SH type III fractures of the distal tibia** (Figure 11-63).
  - External rotation force fractures off the anterolateral portion of the distal tibia.
  - Usually in patients between 12 and 14 years old
  - **Evaluate with CT scan**
- Triplane fractures are usually SH type IV fracture of the distal tibia that occurs in three planes (Figure 11-64):
  - Sagittal plane fracture occurs through the epiphysis (seen on AP or mortise view).
  - Axial plane fracture occurs through the physis.
  - Coronal plane fracture occurs through the metaphysis (seen on lateral view).
  - Thurston-Holland metaphyseal fragment is generally posterolateral.
  - Occurs most commonly in children ages 12 to 15 who have partial distal tibial physis closure

- Distal tibial physis closure begins centrally, then medially, then laterally
- Similar mechanism of external rotation through a partial closed physis
- Diagnosis and radiographs
  - AP, mortise, and lateral views of the ankle
  - Proximal tibial views occasionally needed to rule out a Maisonneuve-type high fibular fracture
  - CT scan may be needed to examine the displacement of intraarticular extension of triplane or Tillaux-type fractures.
- Classification
  - SH physeal fracture classification is generally used to describe these injuries.
  - Triplane can be described by the number of fracture fragments (two, three, or four parts) and their location.
- Treatment
  - Nondisplaced fractures of the distal tibial and fibular physes can often be treated with immobilization and no weight bearing.
  - Less than 2 mm of intraarticular displacement is generally considered the appropriate amount that can

be tolerated; more displacement should be treated with ORIF or closed reduction and percutaneous pin or screw fixation.

- ■ Complications
  - Growth arrest
    - Partial arrests can result in angular deformity; distal fibular arrests will result in a valgus deformity; medial tibial physeal arrests are associated with varus deformities.
    - Complete arrests can result in leg-length discrepancies; contralateral epiphysiodesis can address these issues if prompt diagnosis and remaining skeletal growth allows.
  - Posttraumatic arthrosis
    - Unrecognized intraarticular displacement or inadequate reduction can result in premature arthritic changes.

ACKNOWLEDGMENTS

The editors would like to express our gratitude to David A. Volgas, William M. Ricci, Daniel J. Sucato, Todd A. Milbrandt, and Matthew R. Craig for their contributions to this chapter in the fifth edition; to David B. Weiss, Matthew D. Milewski, Stephen R. Thompson, and James P. Stannard for their contributions to this chapter in the sixth edition; and to Matthew R. Schmitz for his contribution to this chapter in the seventh edition. We would also like to thank MS for his review of the Pediatric Trauma section.

SELECTED BIBLIOGRAPHY

The selected bibliography for this chapter can be found on https://expertconsult.inkling.com.

TESTABLE CONCEPTS

SECTION 1 CARE OF THE MULTIPLY INJURED PATIENT

I. Principles of Trauma Care

- Failure to respond to a 2-L crystalloid bolus in a trauma patient should be considered to have an estimated blood loss greater than 30% of blood volume and require early blood product transfusion.
- Massive transfusion should be a 1:1:1 ratio of packed red blood cells, fresh frozen plasma, and platelets.
- The end points of adequate resuscitation are not clear. Hemodynamic parameter use is inadequate. Base deficit, as measured by lactate level, is a proxy for amount of anaerobic metabolism by the body.
  - Lactate levels and base deficit are used to guide the adequacy of resuscitation.
- Hemorrhagic shock presents as increased heart rate and systemic vascular resistance. Central venous pressure and pulmonary capillary wedge pressure are low.
- Neurogenic shock presents as a low heart rate, low blood pressure, and failure to respond to crystalloids. Treatment is with dobutamine and dopamine.
- Damage control orthopaedics should be employed in severely injured patients with elevated lactate levels. Acute stabilization is achieved primarily via external fixation.
- Pregnant patients should be placed into the left lateral decubitus position to alleviate potential vena cava compression by the uterus.

II. Care of Injuries to Specific Tissues

- Compartment syndrome is a clinical diagnosis with pain out of proportion to the injury and pain with passive stretch.
  - Intracompartmental pressure measurement is abnormal if pressure is within 30 mm of the diastolic pressure (ΔP) or greater than 30 mm of the absolute pressure (criteria are debated).
  - Anesthesia may lower the diastolic blood pressure and give abnormally low ΔP values.
- Motor recovery potential after repair is poorest for the peroneal nerve. The best results are seen in the radial, musculocutaneous, and femoral nerves.
- Traumatic arthrotomies may be detected via a saline load test or reverse arthrocentesis. The knee may require more than 150 mL for correct diagnosis. However, small puncture wounds may be missed.

- Open segmental fractures and farm injuries are automatically Gustilo type III.
  - Types I and II → first-generation cephalosporin
  - Type III → cephalosporin and aminoglycoside
  - Farm → cephalosporin, aminoglycoside, and penicillin
- Osteoporotic fractures
  - World Health Organization Fracture Risk Assessment Tool (FRAX) calculates the 10-year risk of hip fracture.
  - Low-energy stress fractures associated with bisphosphonate use in patients treated for osteoporosis; fracture characterized by cortical thickening, mostly transverse pattern, minimal comminution
  - Fracture of the proximal humerus consistently predicts patient's risk for a subsequent low-energy hip fracture.

III. Biomechanics of Fracture Healing

- Stability determines strain. Strain determines the type of healing. Fractures with less than 2% of strain result in primary bone healing, whereas strain between 2% and 10% results in secondary bone healing.
  - Examples of absolute stability include lag screws, compression plating, and rigid locked plating (in nonbridging mode).

IV. Biomechanics of Open Reduction and Internal Fixation (ORIF)

- Compression plating screw insertional order is neutral position, then compression on opposite side of fracture, then lag screw (if placing through plate).
  - May need pre-bend to eliminate gapping opposite plate
  - Tight contact of plate to bone when initially applied causes decreased periosteal blood flow and temporary osteopenia.
- Bridge plating spans an area of comminution with fixation above and below the fracture. It allows some elastic deformation.
- Submuscular plating advantages include retained medullary and periosteal bone perfusion.
- Locking plates are most useful in unstable short-segment metaphyseal fractures and osteoporotic bone.
  - Other indications: periprosthetic fractures, proximal humerus fractures, intraarticular distal femur and proximal tibia fractures, and humeral shaft nonunions in the elderly
  - Multiaxial locking screws increase options for fixation in working around periprosthetic fractures but do not offer strength or pullout advantages.

TESTABLE CONCEPTS

- Locking plates with unicortical locked screws are weaker in torsion compared with bicortical screws.
- Locked plating screws typically fail simultaneously rather than sequentially.
- IM nail stiffness depends on material, size, and wall thickness.
- Increased diameter results in increased stiffness at a ratio of radius to the power of 3 in bending and to the power of 4 in torsion.
- The working length is the portion of the nail that is unsupported by bone when loaded.
- Increased working length produces increased interfragmentary motion and may delay union.

SECTION 2 UPPER EXTREMITY

I. Shoulder Injuries

- Sternoclavicular dislocation is most commonly anterior. The majority will remain unstable, but these are typically asymptomatic.
    - The medial clavicular epiphysis is the last to close at a mean age of 25 years. In patients younger than this, sternoclavicular dislocation is often a Salter-Harris (SH) type I or II fracture.
- Clavicle fractures are most commonly middle third. Open clavicle fractures are associated with high rates of pulmonary and closed-head injuries.
    - Treatment is controversial. Most middle-third fractures are treated nonoperatively in a sling. There is no difference between sling and figure-eight bandage in outcomes.
    - Risk of nonunion after midshaft fractures is higher in females, elderly, and fractures that are displaced, shortened more than 2 cm, or comminuted.
    - Operative treatment is recommended for displaced and shortened clavicle fractures, owing to higher rates of nonunion and decreased shoulder strength and endurance.
- Scapula fractures are associated with pulmonary contusion, pneumothorax, clavicle fracture (i.e., floating shoulder), rib fracture, head injury, brachial plexus injury, upper extremity vascular injury, pelvic or acetabular fracture, and spine fracture. These fractures are generally treated nonoperatively.
- Glenoid neck fractures are almost always treated nonoperatively.
    - Operative treatment is indicated when the glenoid neck and humeral head are translocated anterior to the proximal fragment or are medially displaced. Preferred surgical approach is posterior between infraspinatus and teres minor.
- Scapulothoracic dislocation should be suspected when there is a neurologic and/or vascular deficit. Lateral displacement of the scapula more than 1 cm on a chest radiograph is also suggestive. Functional outcome is based on the severity of the associated neurologic injury.
- Proximal humerus fracture treatment can be divided based on the Neer classification. Two-part fractures treated nonoperatively should have immediate physical therapy to facilitate faster recovery.
    - Three- and four-part fractures may be treated with ORIF for young patients and hemiarthroplasty for elderly. During hemiarthroplasty, attention must be paid to humeral height, humeral version, and tuberosity reconstruction. The insertion of pectoralis major is a reliable landmark for determining height.
    - Avascular necrosis (AVN) can be predicted by the Hertel criteria: disruption of the medial periosteal hinge, medial metadiaphyseal extension less than 8 mm, and increasing fracture complexity.

- Locking plate constructs are associated with significant rates of screw cutout.
- Nonunion of the greater tuberosity after arthroplasty results in a loss of active shoulder elevation.
- Shoulder dislocation must be evaluated with an axillary radiograph. The most common associated injury at arthroscopy is an anteroinferior labral tear. There is a high incidence of rotator cuff injury in patients older than age 45 years after a shoulder dislocation.
    - Inferior dislocation (luxation erecta) commonly presents with the arm abducted between 110 and 160 degrees.
    - Fixed posterior dislocation—physical examination shows a lack of external rotation.

II. Humeral Injuries

- Humeral shaft fractures may be treated nonoperatively if there is less than 20 degrees of anterior angulation, less than 30 degrees of valgus/varus angulation, or less than 3 cm of shortening.
- Indications for fixation include those fractures outside nonoperative parameters, open fracture, floating elbow, polytrauma, pathologic fracture, and associated brachial plexus injury.
    - ORIF (with plate/screws) has higher union rates and decreased secondary operations. Weight bearing to tolerance is safe after plate fixation.
    - Intramedullary nails may be used for segmental or pathologic fractures. Complications include a higher rate of reoperation and shoulder pain. Distal locking options vary by nail design. Lateral to medial screws put radial nerve at risk, whereas anterior to posterior screws put musculocutaneous nerve at risk. Mini open incisions are recommended for interlocking screws.
- Radial nerve palsy occurs in 5% to 10% of cases.
    - *When to observe:*
        - The vast majority (up to 92%) resolve with observation for 3 to 4 months.
        - Brachioradialis followed by extensor carpi radialis longus are the first to return, whereas the extensor pollicis longus and extensor indicis proprius are last to return.
    - *When to explore:*
        - Open fracture: there is a higher likelihood of transection; perform ORIF of fracture at time of exploration.
    - *Controversial whether to observe or explore:*
        - Secondary nerve palsy (i.e., after fracture manipulation)
        - Spiral or oblique fracture of distal third (Holstein-Lewis fracture)
- Humeral shaft nonunion should be treated with compression plate and bone grafting if atrophic. Locking plates may be used in elderly patients.
- Distal humerus fractures involving both columns should be treated with ORIF using a posterior approach with two plates applied to either column.
    - Total elbow arthroplasty is a treatment option in severely comminuted fractures in patients older than age 65 years, particularly if they have rheumatoid arthritis.
    - The most frequent complication is stiffness, which is treated with static-progressive splinting.
    - No benefit from ulnar nerve transposition during ORIF
    - Elbow muscle strength typically decreases 25%.
- Coronal shear fractures should be treated with ORIF via a lateral approach.

III. Elbow Injuries

- Olecranon fractures treated with a tension band construct should have the wire loop dorsal to the midaxis of the ulna, thus transforming tensile forces at the fracture site into compressive forces at the articular surface.
  - Kirschner wires should be buried in the anterior cortex of the ulna for increased stability. Protrusion through the anterior cortex, however, is associated with reduced forearm rotation.
  - Plate fixation is the preferred technique for oblique fractures that extend distal to the coronoid process; this is more stable than tension band wiring.
  - Excision with triceps advancement is reserved for nonreconstructible proximal olecranon fractures in elderly low-demand patients.
- Radial head fractures that are nondisplaced may be treated in a splint for no more than 7 days, followed by early motion.
  - Comminuted fractures less than three places may be treated with ORIF. Otherwise, treat with metallic radial head replacement.
  - Safe zone for ORIF of a head fracture is a 110-degree arc between the radial styloid and the Lister tubercle.
  - Posterior interosseous nerve is at risk; arm must be pronated to avoid injury.
- Simple elbow dislocations may be treated with brief immobilization.
- "Terrible triad" of the elbow is a complex dislocation with lateral collateral ligament injury, radial head fracture, and coronoid fracture. The lateral collateral ligament injury is most commonly a ligamentous avulsion from the origin on the distal humerus. This injury is always unstable and requires treatment.
  - Perform coronoid ORIF, radial head ORIF or replacement, lateral collateral ligament repair (typically to distal humerus), and possible medial collateral ligament repair, depending on stability.

IV. Forearm Fractures

- Monteggia fractures are ulnar fractures with associated radial head dislocation.
  - Treat with ORIF. The radial head will normally reduce and be stable.
  - Nonanatomic reduction of the ulna followed by interposition of the annular ligament are the most common causes for failure of radial head reduction.
  - Posterior radial head dislocation (Bado type II) or radial head fractures (Monteggia equivalent) are associated with higher complications. Posterior interosseous nerve injury is most frequent, typically resolves spontaneously, and should be observed for 3 months.
- Both-bone forearm fractures are almost universally treated with ORIF.
  - Restoration of the radial bow is directly related to functional outcome.
  - Refracture risk is elevated with removal of hardware in less than 12 to 18 months.
  - Synostosis is associated with single incision approach to ORIF and treated with early excision, irradiation, and indomethacin.
- Galeazzi fractures are radius fractures with distal radioulnar joint instability.
  - ORIF of the radius should be performed, followed by intraoperative assessment of the distal radioulnar joint.
  - Irreducible distal radioulnar joint is most commonly due to interposition of the extensor carpi ulnaris tendon. Recommended approach is dorsal to remove the block.

SECTION 3 LOWER EXTREMITY AND PELVIS

I. Pelvic and Acetabular Injuries

Pelvic Fractures

- Pelvic ring injuries are commonly classified using the Young-Burgess system.
  - APC I → stretching of anterior sacroiliac ligaments
  - APC II → rupture of the anterior sacroiliac sacrotuberous and sacrospinous ligaments
  - APC III → rupture of sacrotuberous, sacrospinous, and anterior and posterior sacroiliac ligaments
- Emergent treatment of a hemodynamically unstable patient with a pelvic ring injury:
  - Volume resuscitation
  - Pelvic binder
  - Angiographic embolization
  - External fixation—place before emergent laparotomy
  - Skeletal traction—for vertically unstable patterns
  - Pelvic C clamp (rarely used)
- Nonoperative treatment is indicated for stable fracture patterns
  - Weight bearing as tolerated for isolated anterior injuries
- Anterior injuries are generally treated with plate fixation. External fixation with pins in the AIIS region is stronger than iliac wing pins but not stronger than internal fixation. The lateral femoral cutaneous nerve is most at risk "during ex fix pin placement."
- Posterior injuries with a vertically oriented sacral fracture are at higher risk for loss of fixation.
- Vertically unstable patterns with anterior and posterior dislocations can be treated with anterior ring internal fixation and percutaneous sacroiliac screw fixation. This is the most stable fixation construct.
- The risk of severe life-threatening hemorrhage is highest in anteroposterior compression types II and III and lateral compression type III patterns and vertical shear.
- Urogenital injury is common.
  - Men: urethral stricture
  - Women: dyspareunia and need for cesarean section childbirth
- The most common complication of pelvic ring injury is deep venous thrombosis if thromboprophylaxis is not employed.
- Risk factors for death during initial treatment:
  - Blood transfusion requirement in first 24 hours
  - Unstable fracture type (anteroposterior compression types II and III, lateral compression types II and III, vertical shear, combined mechanism)
- Percutaneous sacroiliac screw insertion requires appropriate fluoroscopic visualization of anatomic landmarks. Use the pelvic outlet radiograph to visualize the S1 neural foramina. The lateral sacral view identifies the sacral alar slope and minimizes risk to the L5 nerve root.

Acetabular Fractures

- The obturator oblique view profiles the anterior column and posterior wall. The iliac oblique view profiles the posterior column and anterior wall.
- The Letournel classification divides acetabular fractures into five simple and five associated types.
- The associated both-column fracture represents a dissociation of the acetabular dome from the intact ilium. A "spur sign" is seen on the obturator oblique view and represents the intact portion of the iliac wing.
- Cardinal radiographic features of fracture types:
  - Posterior wall—iliopectineal and ilioischial lines intact
  - Posterior column or posterior column/posterior wall—ilioischial line disrupted
  - Anterior wall or anterior column—iliopectineal line disrupted

- Transverse or transverse/posterior wall—iliopectineal, ilioischial lines disrupted, obturator ring intact
- Both column or anterior column posterior hemi-transverse—"T-type" iliopectineal, ilioischial, iliac wing and obturator foramen disrupted
- General guidelines for surgical approach based on fracture type:
  - Kocher-Langenbeck (posterior): posterior wall, posterior column, transverse, transverse/posterior wall (when posterior wall requires fixation), posterior column/posterior wall, and some T types
  - Ilioinguinal (anterior): anterior wall, anterior column, anterior column posterior hemitransverse, associated both column, and some T types (if limited posterior wall involved). The ilioinguinal nerve travels with the round ligament or spermatic cord through the superficial inguinal ring.
  - Extensile approaches: fractures more than 3 weeks old, complex associated fractures, and need for posterior column reduction
- Treatment with ORIF and acute total hip arthroplasty relative indications are age older than 60 years with presence of superomedial dome impaction on radiograph ("gull sign"), associated displaced femoral neck fracture, or significant preexisting arthrosis.
- Risk of neurologic injury can be reduced with hip extension and knee flexion.
- Quality of reduction is the most important predictor of posttraumatic osteoarthritis. Malreduction is associated with a greater delay to surgery.

II. Femoral and Hip Injuries

Hip Dislocations

- Hip dislocations require emergent closed reductions in an attempt to ameliorate the risk of osteonecrosis.
  - Posterior wall and anterior femoral head fractures are common associated injuries. There is a 30% rate of labral tear.

Femoral Head Fractures

- Treatment principles include restoration of articular congruity of the weight-bearing portion of the femoral head and to remove associated loose bodies.
- Smith-Petersen approach for ORIF recommended for Pipkin types I and II. Type IV fractures are typically fixed via a posterior approach.

Femoral Neck Fractures

- High-energy femoral neck fractures are typically vertical and associated femoral neck fractures.
- AP radiographs should be obtained with the legs in internal rotation to compensate for femoral anteversion.
- Treatment of femoral neck fractures is controversial and includes cannulated screws, sliding hip screws, hemiarthroplasty, and total hip arthroplasty.
  - Cannulated screw fixation start points should be above the lesser trochanter to decrease risk of peri-implant subtrochanteric fracture.
  - Hemiarthroplasty is associated with a lower risk of dislocation than in total hip arthroplasty, especially in patients unable to comply with dislocation precautions (e.g., dementia, Parkinson disease)
  - In "active" elderly patients, better functional results are seen with total hip arthroplasty.
- Osteonecrosis risk is increased with greater initial displacement and poor reduction.
- Nonunion risk is higher with varus malreduction. Treatment options include conversion to hip arthroplasty (worse results than those associated with primary arthroplasty) and valgus osteotomy.

- Preinjury cognitive function and mobility predict postoperative functional outcome.

Intertrochanteric Hip Fractures

- Size and location of the lesser trochanteric fragment determine stability.
- A sliding hip screw device is indicated for most fractures.
  - *Exceptions:* reverse obliquity fractures, subtrochanteric fractures, and fractures without an intact lateral femoral wall
  - These fractures are associated with a moderate amount of collapse, resulting limb shortening, and medialization when used for unstable fractures. Collapse is more than that seen with intramedullary implants.
- Long intramedullary nails are indicated for standard and reverse obliquity and subtrochanteric fractures.
  - Mismatch of anterior bow between femur and nail risks distal anterior perforation.
- Implant failure/cutout is associated with a tip-apex distance greater than 25 mm.
- Peri-implant fracture is more common with nails compared with plates.
- American Surgical Association classification predicts mortality in patients with intertrochanteric hip fractures.

Subtrochanteric Fractures

- Apex anterior and varus angulation are the most common deformities. The psoas and abductors lead to flexion, abduction, and external rotation of the proximal fragment.
- Lateral positioning allows easier alignment of the distal segment to the flexed proximal segment.

Femoral Shaft Fractures

- Piriformis and trochanteric starting points are indicated when they are used with appropriately designed nails.
  - Piriformis entry is contraindicated when fracture extends to piriformis fossa and in children with open physes (osteonecrosis).
  - Anterior starting point in piriformis fossa is associated with increased hoop stress and risk of iatrogenic comminution.
  - Anterior trochanteric starting point is associated with minimal hoop stress.
- Trochanteric starting point risks medial comminution of shaft owing to off-axis starting point and varus if straight (no trochanteric bend) nail used.
- Static interlocking for most fractures
- Reamed nailing for most fractures
  - Higher union rates than unreamed nails
- Multitrauma patients may benefit from delayed nailing with immediate provisional external fixation (damage control principles). Benefits include reduced blood loss, reduced hypothermia, and reduced inflammatory mediator release.
  - External fixation can be safely converted to intramedullary nailing in absence of pin tract infection for up to at least 3 weeks with equal union and infection rates.
- Nonunion treatment is more successful with plate/screw/bone graft constructs compared with exchanged nailing. Dynamization is less successful than exchange nailing for treating delayed union.
- Malalignment is difficult to diagnose, but comparison must be made to the contralateral limb before leaving the operating room. Use of a fracture table is associated with increased risk of malalignment.
- Ipsilateral femoral neck and shaft fractures are uncommon (<10%), but when present they are missed in up to 50% of cases.
  - Neck component is typically vertical in orientation. It has the highest priority.

- Preferred technique is to use parallel screws or sliding hip screw for the neck, followed by retrograde nail or plate fixation for the shaft.

Supracondylar Femur Fractures

- Intracondylar extension warrants CT evaluation for a coronal fracture (Hoffa fracture).
  - 40% incidence, with 80% affecting lateral femoral condyle
- Plate fixation is indicated for most fractures. Non–fixed-angle plates are prone to varus collapse, especially in metaphyseal comminution. Avoid prominent medial screws.

III. Knee Injuries

- Vascular injury is present in 5% to 15% of knee dislocations. Selective arteriography with the use of a physical examination (including ankle-brachial index < 0.9) rather than an immediate arteriogram is now the standard of care.
- Patella fractures may be treated nonoperatively or with tension band wiring, cerclage, and tension band wiring and partial patellectomy.
  - Partial patellectomy is useful for extraarticular distal pole fractures. Preserve the patella wherever possible, however.
  - ORIF, when possible, is associated with better outcomes than partial patellectomy in comminuted and displaced fracture of the inferior pole of the patella.

IV. Tibial Injuries

Tibial Plateau Fractures

- Meniscus tears occur in more than 50% of tibial plateau fractures. Lateral is more common than medial: Schatzker II—lateral; Schatzker IV—medial. Peripheral tears are the most common type.
- Medial fractures are uncommon. Think *knee dislocation* with spontaneous reduction.
- The goal of treatment is restoration of normal alignment. Posttraumatic arthrosis development does *not* correlate with articular step-off.
- Spanning external fixators are used temporarily with selected high-energy injuries to allow for a reduction in soft tissue swelling before definitive fixation.
- Use percutaneous locked plating for poor-quality bone in bicondylar fractures. Avoid stripping.
- Posteromedial fragments may not be captured via a lateral pate. Use a separate posteromedial incision if second plate is needed.
- Use of bone void fillers
  - Calcium phosphate cement has highest compressive strength.
  - Lower rate of subsidence compared with autogenous iliac bone graft

Tibial Shaft Fractures

- Indications for nonoperative management:
  - Shortening less than 1 to 2 cm
  - Cortical apposition greater than 50%
  - Varus-valgus less than 5 degrees
  - Flexion-extension less than 10 degrees
  - Shortening is the most difficult deformity to correct. Shortening and cortical apposition seen on injury radiograph are equivalent to shortening at union.
- Operative management in intramedullary nailing is associated with reduced time of immobilization compared with cast management and earlier weight bearing than that achieved with a cast.
- Avoidance of malreduction of proximal-third fractures associated with valgus and apex anterior angulation is achieved by:
  - Ensuring a laterally based starting point and anterior insertion angle
  - Blocking screws placed posteriorly and laterally to the central axes of the proximal fragment

- Definitive fixation with external fixation for type III open tibia fractures have significantly longer time to union and poorer functional outcomes compared with intramedullary nailing.
- Plate fixation for extreme proximal and distal shaft fractures is associated with a higher infection risk than that for intramedullary nailing in opening fractures.
  - Use of a 13-hole percutaneous plate, such as a Less Invasive Stabilization System (LISS) plate, places the superficial peroneal nerve at risk during percutaneous screw insertion for holes 11, 12, and 13. A larger incision with blunt dissection should be used for insertion of screws in this region.
- Nonunion should be treated with reamed-exchange nailing after infection has been ruled out.
- Malunion is most common with proximal-third fractures, resulting in valgus and apex anterior angulation.
  - This may increase long-term risk of arthrosis, particularly in the ankle (more common with varus deformity).
  - Rotational malalignment is common with distal-third fractures.
- Risk factors for reoperation to achieve bony union within the first year:
  - Transverse fracture pattern, open fracture, cortical contact less than 50%
- Infection risk increases with severity of soft tissue injury and time to soft tissue coverage. Use of wound vacuum-assisted closure does not alter the risk of infection.
- Anterior knee pain occurs in more than 30% of intramedullary nail cases and resolves with removal of the nail in 50% of cases.

SECTION 4   PEDIATRIC TRAUMA

I. Introduction

- Suspected child abuse must be reported. Suspicion should be raised in children younger than 3 years who have inconsistent or developmentally incorrect histories.
- Skin injuries are most common (bruising), followed by fractures and head injuries.
  - Skeletal surveys are most helpful in children younger than age 5. If older than age 5, consider bone scan as alternative or adjunct.
  - The most common locations of fractures, in order of frequency, are the humerus, tibia, and femur.
  - Spiral femur fractures in nonambulatory children, as well as distal humeral physeal separations, are highly suggestive of abuse.
  - Corner fractures at the junction of the metaphysis and physis are said to be pathognomonic for abuse. They are four times less common than diaphyseal fractures, however.
- SH type I fractures involve the zone of hypertrophy in the physis.
- Polytrauma outcomes are most closely linked with the severity of traumatic brain injury.

Upper Extremity Fractures

- Clavicle fractures represent 90% of obstetric fractures, frequently associated with brachial plexus palsies and almost universally treated nonoperatively.
- Proximal humerus fractures have increased remodeling potential because 80% to 90% of humeral growth occurs at the proximal physis.
  - In children younger than age 12 years, 70-degree angulation and 100% displacement may be accepted.
  - The distal fragment is shortened and adducted by the deltoid and pectoralis major. Gravity can be a useful reduction aid.
- All pediatric elbow fractures should have a systematic evaluation of radiographic anatomy (see Figure 11-48).
- Distal humeral physeal separations occur in the young child and raise suspicion of child abuse. This injury is often confused with an elbow dislocation.

TESTABLE CONCEPTS

- Radiographs demonstrate an intact relationship between the radius and capitellum with loss of relationship between the radius/ulna and distal humerus.
- Treatment is with closed reduction and percutaneous pinning (CRPP).
- Supracondylar humerus fractures are 98% extension type and 2% flexion type.
  - Most common nerve injury:
    - Extension-type—anterior interosseous nerve
    - Flexion-type—ulnar nerve
  - Gartland classification guides treatment
    - I—nondisplaced—long-arm cast
    - II—displaced with intact posterior cortex—long-arm cast if no swelling, anterior humeral line intersects capitellum, and no medial distal humeral cortical impaction; otherwise, CRPP
    - III—displaced—CRPP; crossed pins more stable biomechanically
  - Vascular abnormalities should be first treated with reduction, not angiography.
  - Complications of treatment include iatrogenic ulnar nerve injury and cubitus varus from malunion/malreduction.
- Lateral condyle fractures are historically classified using the Milch system, with a type I representing a SH type IV fracture and a type II representing a SH type II fracture. The Jakob classification, however, is more clinically useful.
  - Amount of displacement guides treatment
    - Less than 2 mm—cast and closely observe
    - 2 to 4 mm—CRPP
    - More than 4 mm—CRPP if arthrogram shows perfect reduction; otherwise, ORIF to ensure articular reduction
  - During ORIF, the blood supply arises posteriorly and should be protected.
  - This is one of the rare pediatric fractures that may proceed to nonunion.
- Medial epicondyle fractures that occur in adolescents represent an apophyseal avulsion injury of the flexor mass and medial collateral ligament.
  - A 50% association occurs with elbow dislocation (most common fracture associated with an elbow dislocation in children), which can result in an incarcerated fragment in 15% of cases.
    - Close attention must be given to identifying the apophysis on the AP view. If it is missing, look for an incarcerated fragment on a lateral or oblique view.
  - Most injuries are treated nonoperatively, but this is controversial.
  - Treatment of an incarcerated fragment is ORIF.
  - Never excise a medial epicondyle fracture.
- Radial neck fractures can be managed nonoperatively according to the "rule of 3s."
  - Less than 30-degree angulation, less than 3-mm translation, and less than one third of radial head involvement
  - There are multiple techniques for closed reduction.
- Radial head subluxation ("nursemaid's elbow") occurs when the annular ligament subluxates over the radial head. Closed reduction is achieved by supination and flexion with a thumb placed over the radial head.
- Monteggia fractures can be classified as in adults. Plastic deformations and incomplete injuries may be treated with closed reduction and casting.
  - The key feature in treatment is based on ulnar length restoration. This will generally result in radial head reduction.
  - Diaphyseal "both bone" forearm fractures are generally treated nonoperatively with closed reduction and long-arm casting.

- Apex dorsal angulation—supination
- Apex volar angulation—pronation
- Distal radius fractures can be treated nonoperatively in the majority of cases.
  - Acceptable sagittal angulation is up to 30 degrees in patients with greater than 5 years of growth remaining, with 5 degrees less accepted for each year less than 5 years of growth remaining.

VII. Lower Extremity
- Avulsion fractures of the pelvis are relatively common in the pediatric population and generally treated nonoperatively.
- Femoral neck fractures resulting in AVN can be predicted using the Delbet classification, with type I transphyseal fractures approaching 100% risk.
  - Transphyseal, transcervical, and basicervical fractures represent a surgical emergency.
- Diaphyseal femur fracture management is based on fracture pattern and age of the patient.
  - Birth to 6 months—Pavlik
  - 6 months to 6 years—spica casting
  - 6 to 11 years—flexible nails for stable fractures and submuscular plating for unstable and external fixation for polytrauma
  - Older than 11 years—trochanteric-starting intramedullary nail
- Distal femur physeal fractures should be suspected in adolescent patients with "knee sprains" and can be diagnosed with stress views.
  - Nonoperative treatment is reserved for nondisplaced fractures.
  - Displaced fractures are treated with CRPP and casting versus ORIF.
  - Growth arrest occurs in approximately 50% of cases, resulting in either limb-length discrepancy (1 cm/yr) or angular deformity.
  - Up to 40% of patients sustain injury to the cruciate ligaments.
- Patellar sleeve fractures should be suspected when radiographs demonstrate patella alta. Indications for surgery include extensor lag, inability to straight-leg raise, and intraarticular displacement. A tension band construct can be used if bone-stock permits it.
- Tibial spine fractures are similar to anterior cruciate ligament ruptures in terms of mechanism.
  - Meyers and McKeever classification guides treatment:
    - I—nondisplaced—casting
    - II—anterior hinge—reduction in extension and casting
    - III—displaced—operative fixation
  - Both stiffness (arthrofibrosis) and late anterior instability are common complications occurring in up to 60% of cases. It is unclear whether late anterior instability is clinically significant.
- Tibial tuberosity fractures can be treated nonoperatively for nondisplaced fractures. The anterior tibial recurrent artery may be injured and increases the risk for compartment syndrome.
- Proximal tibial metaphyseal fractures may be termed *Cozen fractures* based on the phenomenon he described. These minimally displaced fractures present as late genu valgum that spontaneously resolves.
- Toddler's fracture is a nondisplaced oblique or spiral tibial shaft fracture with intact fibula. It may not be apparent on radiographs and can be confused with tibial osteomyelitis. Treatment is with a long-leg cast and repeat radiographs in 2 weeks looking for evidence of callus to confirm the diagnosis.
- Tillaux fractures are SH type III fractures due to external rotational force; evaluate with CT scan.
- Triplane fracture is an SH type IV fracture due to external rotational force through a partially closed physis. It appears as SH type III on AP radiographs and type II on lateral radiographs. CT may be particularly helpful.
  - Less than 2 mm displacement may be treated nonoperatively.

CHAPTER 12

PRINCIPLES OF PRACTICE

Marc McCord DeHart

CONTENTS

SECTION 1 PRINCIPLES OF PRACTICE

INTRODUCTION (Figure 12-1)

- ■ **Profession, ethics, and laws**
- ■ The orthopaedic profession represents an occupation where our work is based upon mastery of a complex body of knowledge and skills. This demands demonstrating an adequate understanding of the science we use and the routine practice of the art of medicine used for the service of others.
- ■ Codes of ethics are the governing rules our community of professionals have agreed upon as standards of conduct that define the essentials of honorable behavior for orthopaedic surgeons.
  - Four major principles in medical ethics can be easily defined, but their application can be complex:
    - **Nonmaleficence:** a basic obligation not to inflict harm on their patients, either intentionally or carelessly, summed up first by Hippocrates: "Do no harm"
    - **Beneficence:** obligation to intervene to benefit the well-being of an individual
    - **Autonomy**: personal rule of the self, free from both controlling interferences by others and from personal limitations that prevent meaningful choice
    - **Justice**: distributive justice (allocation of limited healthcare resources)
      - Rights-based justice (patient rights)
      - Legal justice (upholding the law)
- ■ Laws are the external regulations and rules that are created and enforced through government to guide behavior.
- ■ Morals are personally held beliefs concerning what behavior is acceptable and frequently directs an individual orthopaedic surgeon's actions.
- ■ **Conflicts and focus of ethics:**
- ■ Although the aspiration of our profession has changed very little over the centuries, our understanding of the science behind our practice, the laws that govern our activities, and the business realities that face us every day constantly change. With this change comes conflict.
- ■ When conflicts of interest arise among medical care, business goals, and legal considerations, ethical resolutions focus on the best interest of our patients.
- ■ The **physician-patient relationship is the central focus of all ethical concerns**.
- ■ **Documents have been developed by the American Academy of Orthopaedic Surgeons (AAOS) with the help of other organizations to outline ethical principles of medicine and orthopaedic surgery:**
  - ■ *Medical Professionalism in the New Millennium: A Physician Charter* (2002)
  - ■ *Principles of Medical Ethics and Professionalism in Orthopaedic Surgery* (2002)
  - ■ *Code of Ethics and Professionalism for Orthopaedic Surgeons* (2011)
  - ■ *Guide to Professionalism and Ethics in the Practice of Orthopaedic Surgery* (2013)
  - ■ AAOS Standards of Professionalism

MEDICAL PROFESSIONALISM IN THE NEW MILLENNIUM: A PHYSICIAN CHARTER (2002)

(Available at: http://www.abimfoundation.org/en/Professionalism/Physician-Charter.)

- ■ **The AAOS adopted the charter crafted by physicians throughout the industrialized world who were concerned about changes in healthcare delivery systems that threaten professional values.**
- ■ Three fundamental principles of professionalism define the basis of the contract between the field of medicine and society:
  - Primacy of patient welfare: serve the patient's interest
    - Altruism—selflessness—builds trust, which is key to patient-physician relationship

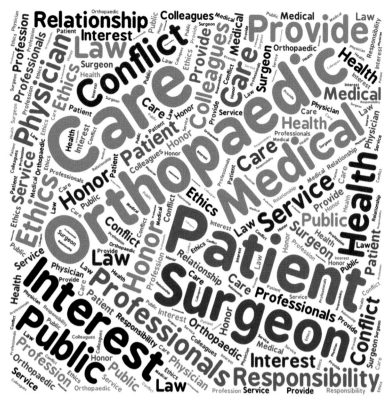

FIGURE 12-1 Word cloud created from AAOS *Principles of Medical Ethics and Professionalism in Orthopaedic Surgery.* (Available at: http://www.aaos.org/about/papers/ethics/prin.asp. Accessed October, 26, 2015.)

- Autonomy: respect a patient's informed choices
  - Honest information on treatment's benefits and risks needed for choice
- Social justice: promote fair distribution of healthcare resources
- **The charter also defines a set of 10 professional "commitments" that apply to physicians:**
- Professional competence: individual commitment to lifelong learning
  - Profession must strive to ensure all members are competent
- Honesty with patients: good information must be provided before and after treatment.
  - Reporting mistakes:
    - Enhances patient and societal trust
    - Encourages prevention and improvement
- Patient confidentiality: privacy reinforces trust and encourages patient disclosure.
  - May need to be broken when the patient endangers others
- Appropriate relations: patients must never be exploited for sexual or financial advantage.
- Improving the quality of care: professionals and their organizations must
  - Maintain clinical competence, reduce errors, create mechanisms to improve care
- Improving access to care:
  - Healthcare systems objective: to provide a uniform and adequate standard of care
  - Eliminate barriers based on laws, education, finances, geography, and social issues
- Just distribution of finite resources: promote wise and cost-effective use of limited resources

- Scientific knowledge: promote research, create new knowledge, and use it appropriately
- Managing conflicts of interest: must recognize and disclose to patients and public
  - Private gain from drug, equipment, and insurance companies
  - When reporting results of clinical trials or guidelines
- Professional responsibilities:
  - Work collaboratively to maximize patient care.
  - Be respectful of one another.
  - Participate in self-regulating and self-disciplining others.
  - Define educational and standard-setting process.
  - Engage in self-assessment and accepting scrutiny.

ASPIRATIONAL DOCUMENTS

- **All can be found at: http://www.aaos.org/about/papers/ethics.asp**
- *Principles of Medical Ethics and Professionalism in Orthopaedic Surgery* (2002)
- *Code of Ethics and Professionalism for Orthopaedic Surgeons* (2011)
- *Guide to Professionalism and Ethics in the Practice of Orthopaedic Surgery* (2013)
- **Take legal requirements into account but may call for a standard of behavior that is often higher than the law**
- **Define the "essentials of honorable behavior," briefly summarized:**
- Physician-patient relationship is the "central focus of all ethical concerns."
  - Relationship based on trust, confidentiality, and honesty
    - Must present facts in understandable terms

- Also has a contractual basis:
  - Patient and physician free to enter/discontinue relationship
  - Within third-party constraints
  - No discontinuation without adequate notice
  - Obligation to care only for those conditions where competent
  - Obligation to assist in transfer to appropriate care
  - No illegal discrimination
- Conduct of the orthopaedic surgeon must have the following goals:
  - Emphasize the patient's best interests
  - Provide "competent and compassionate care"
  - Obey the law and maintain professional dignity and discipline
- Conflicts of interest are common
  - Must be resolved in the best interest of the patient
  - Most common conflicts: medical facility ownership
    - If not obvious must disclose
      - Relationships with industry
    - All payments should be disclosed to patients
- Other sections of the code address additional important issues:
  - Maintaining competence
  - Relationships with orthopaedic surgeons, nurses, and allied health professionals
  - Relationship to the public
  - General principles of care
  - Research and academic responsibilities
  - Responsibility to society as a whole

STANDARDS OF PROFESSIONALISM

- ■ **Mandatory minimum levels of acceptable conduct for orthopaedic surgeons can be found at: http://www3.aaos.org/member/profcomp/sop.cfm**
- Different from prior aspirational documents
- **AAOS Standards of Professionalism are unique;** they represent the **minimal level of acceptable conduct** to remain a member of our academy.
- Nonadherence to these principles can result in loss of membership.
- Violations of these standards:
  - Are grounds for formal complaints to AAOS
  - Subject to review by the AAOS Professional Compliance Program
  - Actions are outlined by the AAOS Bylaws and include:
    - Censuring, suspension for a time, or expulsion from AAOS
    - May result in action outlined in **reporting:**
      - To the National Practitioner Data Bank
      - To state medical licensing boards
      - To American Board of Orthopaedic Surgery
- ■ **Providing musculoskeletal services to patients (2008):**
- Responsibility to the patient is paramount:
  - Provide equal treatment of patients regardless of race, color, ethnicity, gender, sexual orientation, religion, or national origin.
  - Provide needed and appropriate care or refer to a qualified alternative provider.
  - Present pertinent medical facts and obtain informed consent.
  - Advocate for the patient and provide the most appropriate care.

- Safeguard patient confidentiality and privacy.
- Maintain appropriate relations with patients.
- Respect a patient's request for additional opinions.
- Pursue lifelong scientific and medical learning.
- Only provide services and use techniques for which one is qualified by personal education, training, or experience.
- If impaired by substance abuse, seek professional care and limit or cease practice as directed.
- If impaired by mental or physical disability, seek professional care and limit or cease practice as directed.
- Disclose to the patient any conflict of interest, financial or otherwise, that may influence care.
- Do not enter into a relationship in which the surgeon pays for the right to care for patients with musculoskeletal disorders.
- Make a reasonable effort to ensure that the academic institution, hospital, or employer does not pay for the right to care for patients.
- Do not couple a marketing agreement or provision of services, supplies, equipment, or personnel with required patient referrals.

- ■ **Professional relationships (2005)**
- Responsibility to the patient is paramount:
  - Maintain fairness, respect, and confidentiality with colleagues and other professionals.
  - Act in a professional manner with colleagues and other professionals.
  - Work collaboratively to reduce medical errors, increase patient safety, and improve outcomes.
  - Facilitate and cooperate in transferring patient care.

- ■ **Orthopaedic expert witness testimony (2010)**
- Standards of professionalism:
  - Do not testify falsely.
  - Provide fair and impartial opinions.
  - Evaluate care by standards of time, place, and context as delivered.
  - Do not condemn standard care or condone substandard care.
  - Explain the basis for any opinion that varies from standard.
  - Seek and review all pertinent records.
  - Have knowledge and experience, and respond accurately to questions.
  - Have current valid unrestricted license to practice medicine.
  - Have current board certification in orthopaedic surgery (i.e., American Board of Orthopaedic Surgery).
  - Have an active practice or familiarity with current practices to warrant expert designation.
  - Accurately represent credentials, qualifications, experience, or background.
  - Fees should not be contingent on trial outcome.
  - Expect reasonable compensation that is based on expertise, time, and effort needed to address issue.

- ■ **Research and academic responsibilities (2006)**
- Standards of professionalism:
  - Responsibility to patient is paramount.
  - Informed consent is required.
  - Honor withdrawal requests.
  - Seek peer review and follow regulations.
  - Be truthful with patients and colleagues.
  - Report fraudulent or deceptive research.

- Claim credit only if substantial contributions were made.
- Give credit when presenting other's ideas, language, data, graphics, or scientific protocols.
- Expose fraud and deception.
- Make significant contributions when publishing manuscripts.
- Disclose existence of duplicate publications.
- Include and credit or acknowledge all substantial contributors.
- Acknowledge funding sources or consulting agreements.

■ **Advertising by orthopaedic surgeons (2007)**

▦ Advertising must not suggest any of the following:
- A diagnosis can be made without consultation.
- One treatment is appropriate for all patients.
- A treatment is without risk.

▦ Other imperatives:
- Do not use false or misleading statements.
- Use no misleading representation about ability to provide medical treatment.
- Use no false or misleading images or photographs.
- Use no misrepresentations that communicate a false degree of relief, safety, effectiveness, or benefits of treatment.
- Surgeons will be held responsible for any violations of their office or public relations firms retained.
- Surgeons will make efforts to ensure that advertisements by academic institutions, hospitals, and private practices are not false or misleading.
- Advertisements shall abide by state and federal laws and regulations related to professional credentials.
- Provide no false or misleading certification levels.
- Provide no false or misleading representation of procedure volume or academic appointments or associations.
- Provide no false or misleading statements regarding development or study of surgical procedures.

■ **Orthopaedist-industry conflicts of interest (2007)**

▦ Standards of professionalism:
- Surgeons shall regard their responsibility to the patient as paramount.
- Surgeons shall prescribe drugs, devices, and treatments on the basis of medical considerations, regardless of benefit from industry.
- Surgeons shall be subject to discipline by AAOS Professional Compliance Program if convicted of federal or state conflict-of-interest laws.
- Surgeons shall resolve conflicts of interest in the best interest of the patient, respecting the patient's autonomy.
- Surgeons shall notify the patient when withdrawing from a patient-physician relationship if a conflict cannot be resolved in the best interest of the patient.
- Surgeons shall decline subsidies or support from industry except: gifts of $100 or less, medical textbooks, or educational material for patients.
- Surgeons shall disclose any relationship with an industry to colleagues, institution, and other entities.
- Surgeons shall disclose to patients any financial arrangement, including royalties, stock options, and consulting arrangements with an industry.
- Surgeons shall refuse any direct financial inducement to use a particular implant, device, or drug.

- Surgeons shall enter into **consulting agreements** with industry only when agreements are made in advance in writing and have the following features:
  - They include **documentation of an actual need for the service.**
  - They include **proof that the service was provided.**
  - They include **evidence that physician pay for consulting is consistent with fair market value.**
  - They are **not based on the volume or value of business the physician generates.**
- Surgeons shall participate only in meetings conducted in clinical, educational, or conference settings conducive to effective exchange of information.
- Surgeons shall accept **no financial support to attend social functions with no educational element.**
- Surgeons shall accept **no financial support to attend continuing medical education (CME) events** except in the following situations:
  - As residents/fellows when selected by and paid by their training institution or CME sponsor
  - As faculty members of CME programs: allowed honoraria, travel/lodging/meal expenses from sponsor
- Surgeons shall accept only tuition, travel accommodations, and modest hospitality when attending industry-sponsored non-CME events.
- Surgeons shall accept no financial support for guests or other persons who have no professional interest in attending meetings.
- Surgeons shall disclose any financial relationship with regard to procedure or device when reporting clinical research and experience.
- Surgeons shall truthfully report research results with no bias from funding sources, regardless of positive or negative findings.

CHILD, ELDER, AND SPOUSAL ABUSE

■ **Child abuse**

▦ U.S. Child Abuse Prevention and Treatment Act of 1974 **requires orthopaedic surgeons to report all suspected cases of child abuse to local authorities.**

▦ Failure to report might result in state disciplinary actions.
- Child protective services and social workers should be alerted, and the events and home circumstances should be investigated.
- Legal immunity for reporting physicians when acting in good faith, even if the information is protected by the physician-patient privilege

■ **Elder abuse**

▦ Many states have legislation to protect physician liability from reporting.

▦ Risk factors: increasing age, functional disability, cognitive impairment, higher rates of child abuse within the regional population
- Gender is not a risk factor.

■ **Spousal abuse**

▦ One in four women experience domestic violence.

▦ Reporting of suspected spousal abuse is not required.
- Corresponding absence of legal protection for physicians

▦ May encourage a patient to seek self-protection

▦ A court order may be obtained to permit reporting.

- Risk factors for spousal abuse:
  - Pregnancy
  - Age of 19 to 29 years
  - Low socioeconomic status
  - African American race

SEXUAL MISCONDUCT

- **Description and identification**
- Even situations of consensual sexual relationships may create potential for sexual exploitation and loss of objectivity:
  - Professional supervisor-trainee relationship
  - Boss-employee relationship
  - Physician-patient relationship
- Sexual harassment in employment can cause claims under the Civil Rights Act.
  - Quid pro quo: harassment is directly linked to employment or advancement.
  - Hostile environment harassment:
  - Verbal or physical conduct (e.g., gestures, innuendo, humor, pictures) of a sexual nature
  - General gender-based hostility
- **"Reasonable woman" test is the adopted standard for offensive behavior.**
  - If a "reasonable woman" would have found the behavior objectionable, then harassment may have occurred
- Sexual misconduct with patients is a form of exploitation.
  - Unethical and may represent malpractice or even criminal acts of assault
  - Courts say a **patient is unable to give meaningful consent to sexual/romantic advances.**

THE IMPAIRED PHYSICIAN

- **"Impairment" can include chemical impairment, dependence, misconduct, or incompetence.**
- Resident, fellow, or attending physician who discovers impairment should report
- Can be reported to state and local agencies
- Must act in good faith with reasonable evidence
- If patient at risk for harm, assert authority to relieve impaired physician of patient's care
- Address the problem with the senior hospital staff as soon as possible.

RESEARCH

- **Research is considered "ethical" when:**
- Primary goal is to improve methods of detection or treatment of illness
- **Designed to produce useful, reproducible information**
- Is not redundant
- Is not primarily to further the interests of individuals or institutions, financially or professionally
- Results are reported honestly, accurately, and in a timely manner.
- **Both positive and negative results are reported.**
- **Sponsorship by industry not tied to results**
- **Human research subjects:**
- Voluntary only
- Informed consent before participating in any research protocol

- Medical care not contingent upon participation
- Allowed to withdraw from the study at any time
- Demonstrate understanding of the information
- Able to make a responsible decision
- **Animal use in research**
- Humane use of animals in research is justified.
- Use of animals is ethical when:
  - No suitable alternatives available
  - Number of animals used is minimized.
  - Standards of animal care are maintained.
  - Approved by local Animal Care and Use Committee
- **Responsibilities of the principal investigator:**
- All aspects of the research even when duties delegated to others
- Accurately representing the efforts of individuals/agencies involved
- Citing contributions from other researchers or publications
- **Responsibilities of coauthors:**
- Make a significant contribution: study design, data collection, project assistance.
- Sign an affidavit of manuscript review agreement before publication.
- Resident research should be conducted under the supervision of an attending surgeon.
- Attending surgeon must contribute to the work in actual fact or in a consultative capacity.

MEDICAL LIABILITY

- **Definitions**
- **Malpractice:** negligence by a healthcare provider that **results in injury** to a patient
- **Negligence:** failure to be as diligent and select care a reasonable/prudent person would exercise under the same or similar conditions
- **Medical negligence comprises four elements: duty, breach of duty, causation, and damages.**
- **Duty:** begins when surgeon offers and patient accepts offer of care
  - Duty to provide care that meets "standard of care"
    - Equal to the same care ordinarily executed by same medical specialty
    - Established by "expert testimony"
    - *Res ipsa loquitur* ("the thing speaks for itself"): do not need expert testimony
      - Wrong-site surgery, retained instrument/sponge
- **Breach of duty:** when action or inaction deviates from the standard of care
  - Act of **commission** (doing what should not have been done)
  - Act of **omission** (failing to do what should have been done)
- **Causation:** when breach was the direct cause of injuries
- **Damages:** financial loss awarded as compensation for injuries
  - Compensatory damages: dollars to restore plaintiff's loss from injury
  - Nominal damages: smaller sums paid for invasion of rights
  - Punitive damages: sums to penalize defendant for egregious conduct
- **Physician-patient communication: frequently cited as most common factor in initiation of malpractice lawsuits**

- Errors in treatment should be disclosed to the patient.
- The law requires proof of the allegation by a preponderance of the evidence.
- **Statute of limitations: time limit for plaintiff to file a malpractice suit**
- Often approximately 2 years (varies by state)
- For minors, generally 2 years from incident or until eighteenth birthday
- If error not disclosed, may extend the duration of statute
- **Liability status of residents and fellows**
- Residents and fellows are licensed physicians.
- Function as employees
- Responsible for their own actions
- Act as agent for their supervisors
- Supervisors are responsible for their trainees (vicarious liability).
- Residents/fellows held to same standard as board-certified surgeons
- Should function at the level of their training
- Should consult their supervisors to avoid the risk of acting independently
- Must disclose residency or fellow status to patients

- Failure to inform a patient may result in claims: fraud, deceit, misrepresentation, assault, battery, lack of informed consent
- **Medical record:**
- Tells the story of patient care and allows continuity between providers
- Is a **legal document and best defense in malpractice suit**
  - Should not be altered (may be amended)
  - **Errors should be "lined out"**
- Is a business document justifying appropriate reimbursement when allowed by contract
- Must be **maintained for 7 years after last treatment**
- Data in records belong to patient and are confidential
  - Patient must provide written authorization to release
  - May require patient to pay costs of copies
  - HIPAA Privacy Rule regulates use and disclosure of Protected Health Information

SELECTED BIBLIOGRAPHY

The selected bibliography for this chapter can be found on https://expertconsult.inkling.com.

TESTABLE CONCEPTS

- Four major principles in medical ethics:
  - Nonmaleficence: "Do no harm"
  - Beneficence: do good
  - Autonomy: personal rule of the self
  - Justice: equal treatment
- Conflicts of interest are common and must be resolved in the best interest of the patient.
- Most common conflicts: facility ownership and relationships with industry where physician should disclose payment to patients
- AAOS Standards of Professionalism represent the minimal level of acceptable conduct to remain a member of our academy.
  - Violations can be reported to: National Practitioner Data Bank, state medical licensing boards, and American Board of Orthopaedic Surgery.

- Child abuse laws require reporting all suspected cases of child abuse to local authorities.
- Medical negligence comprises four elements:
  - Duty—physician accepts care
  - Breach of duty—acts of omission or commission
  - Causation—breach was responsible for injury
  - Damages—financial payments paid by defendant to plaintiff
- Physician-patient communication the most common factor cited in malpractice cases
- Supervisors are responsible for their trainees (vicarious liability).
- Residents/fellows held to same standard as board-certified surgeons

CHAPTER 13

BIOSTATISTICS AND RESEARCH DESIGN

Joseph M. Hart

CONTENTS

SECTION 1 INTRODUCTION

Critical review of medical research is essential for orthopaedic surgeons in promoting evidence-based decision making and practice. Experiments are conducted in both the clinical and basic sciences, and decisions are often based on the results of these experiments and associated statistical analyses. It is the responsibility of physicians to be astute appraisers of the most current evidence that supports or refutes clinical decisions that affect patient care.

Research starts with developing a question that is important to a particular area of investigation or clinical practice. Questions often arise from anecdotal observations during clinical practice. Research is best accomplished in teams with complimentary skillsets among the selected investigators. As a research study is planned, the most appropriate research design is selected to match the primary research question. A study population is defined, and the most appropriate outcome measures and variables are selected. It is important that the research team collaborate so that their combined expertise can contribute to the study aims.

This chapter describes some important concepts to consider in designing a research study and analyzing and interpreting results.

SELECTING A RESEARCH STUDY DESIGN (Figure 13-1)

- Research starts with asking a clinically relevant question, determining an appropriate outcome measure (data), and deciding on the most rigorous and feasible design.
- Research designs are selected to test a specific theoretical hypothesis in a way that provides the highest level of evidence.

- Research designs should be rigorous and controlled to provide highest-quality outcomes.

EVIDENCE-BASED MEDICINE

- Aims to apply evidence from the highest-quality research studies to the practice of medicine
- Also known as *evidence-based practice*
- Greater influence on decision making is based on findings from the best-designed and most rigorous studies.
- The "levels of evidence" in medical research (see Figure 13-1): a hierarchy for various research applications and questions based on several factors affecting the quality of a research design.
- Diagnostic, prognostic, or therapeutic research designs with higher levels of evidence have a greater influence on clinical recommendations. There are many factors that may affect the quality of a research design (see later discussion of flaws in research designs):
  - Level I: high-quality clinical trials (randomized, controlled, blinded, etc.)
  - Level II: cohort studies or lesser-quality clinical trials
  - Level III: case-control studies
  - Level IV: case series studies
  - Level V: expert opinions

CLINICAL RESEARCH DESIGNS

- Clinical study design is an essential element of research to determine among a study team in advance of study initiation.

		TYPE OF STUDY			
	Level	**Therapeutic Studies** (Investigating the results of treatment)	**Prognostic Studies** (Investigating the outcome of disease)	**Diagnostic Studies** (Investigating a diagnostic test)	**Economic and Decision Analyses** (Developing an economic or decision model)

	Level I	1. Randomized controlled trial
		  a. Significant difference
		  b. No significant difference but narrow confidence intervals
		2. Systematic review[2] of level I randomized controlled trials (studies were homogeneous)
			1. Prospective study[1]
			2. Systematic review[2] of level I studies
				1. Testing of previously developed diagnostic criteria in series of consecutive patients (with universally applied reference "gold" standard)
				2. Systematic review[2] of level I studies
					1. Clinically sensible costs and alternatives; values obtained from many studies; multiway sensitivity analyses
					2. Systematic review[2] of level I studies

	Level II	1. Prospective cohort study[3] 2. Poor-quality randomized controlled trial (e.g., <80% follow-up) 3. Systematic review[2] of level II studies or nonhomogeneous level I studies	1. Retrospective study[4] 2. Study of untreated controls from a previous randomized controlled trial 3. Systematic review[2] of level II studies	1. Development of diagnostic criteria on basis of consecutive patients (with universally applied reference "gold" standard) 2. Systematic review[2] of level II studies	1. Clinically sensible costs and alternatives; values obtained from limited studies; multiway sensitivity analyses 2. Systematic review[2] of level II studies
	Level III	1. Case-control study[5] 2. Retrospective cohort study[4] 3. Systematic review[2] of level III studies	Case-control study[5]	1. Study of nonconsecutive patients (no consistently applied reference "gold" standard) 2. Systematic review[2] of level III studies	1. Limited alternatives and costs; poor estimates 2. Systematic review[2] of level III studies
	Level IV	Case series	Case series	1. Case-control study 2. Poor reference standard	No sensitivity analysis
	Level V	Expert opinion	Expert opinion	Expert opinion	Expert opinion

[1]All patients were enrolled at the same point in their disease course (inception cohort) with ≥80% follow-up of enrolled patients.
[2]A study of results from two or more previous studies.
[3]Patients were compared with a control group of patients treated at the same time and institution.
[4]The study was initiated after treatment was performed.
[5]Patients with a particular outcome ("cases" with, for example, a failed arthroplasty) were compared with those who did not have the outcome ("controls" with, for example, a total hip arthroplasty that did not fail).

Confidence that study conclusions and recommendations are valid →

FIGURE 13-1 Study design characteristics that are considered when various types of studies are assigned a "level of evidence." (Adapted from Wright JG et al: Introducing levels of evidence to the journal, *J Bone Joint Surg Am* 85:1–3, 2003.)

Designs can be observational or experimental and can be prospective, retrospective, or longitudinal.

- **Prospective studies are designed to start in the present and collect data forward in time. For example, an exposure or potential risk factor has occurred and patients are followed forward in time to determine the occurrence of an outcome of interest.**
- **Retrospective studies are designed to assess outcomes that have already occurred or data that have been collected in the past. Chart review of medical records is a typical application of retrospective research designs in orthopaedic research.**
- **Longitudinal studies involve repeated assessments over a long period of time. A longitudinal study can be performed on historical (retrospective) data.**
- **Observational research designs can be prospective, retrospective, or longitudinal. Common observational designs are as follows (Figure 13-2):**
- Case reports:
  - Descriptions of unique injures, disease occurrences, or outcomes in a single patient
  - No attempts at advanced data analysis are made.
  - Cause-effect relationships and generalizability are not made.
- Case series:
  - Outcomes are measured in patients with a similar disease/injury to determine outcomes retrospectively.
  - No attempts are made at estimating frequencies or distributions.
- Case-control studies:
  - **Outcomes measured in patients with similar disease/injury are compared to a control group** (see later discussion of flaws in research designs for more information about control groups).
  - Odds ratios (not relative risks) are appropriate measures of association from data collected in these study designs (see Concepts in Epidemiologic Research Studies)
- Cohort study:
  - **Groups of patients with a similar characteristic or exposure/risk factor are studied forward in time (prospective) or from existing data (retrospective).**
  - Cohort studies are appropriate for estimating incidence of disease/injury and relative risks.
- Cross-sectional study designs
  - **A specific patient population is studied at a given point in time.**
  - **All measurements are made at once with no follow-up period.**
  - Considered "snapshots" that are useful for describing the prevalence of a particular injury/disease of interest at a particular point in time
- **Experimental research designs**
- Clinical trials are designed to allocate treatments and track outcomes prospectively to test a specific hypothesis.
  - The gold standard and highest level of evidence clinical trial is the randomized controlled trial (RCT).
- Clinical trials with parallel design: treatments are allocated to different subjects/patients in random or nonrandom manner.
  - Example: patients are randomly assigned to receive one of the study interventions only. This allocation is

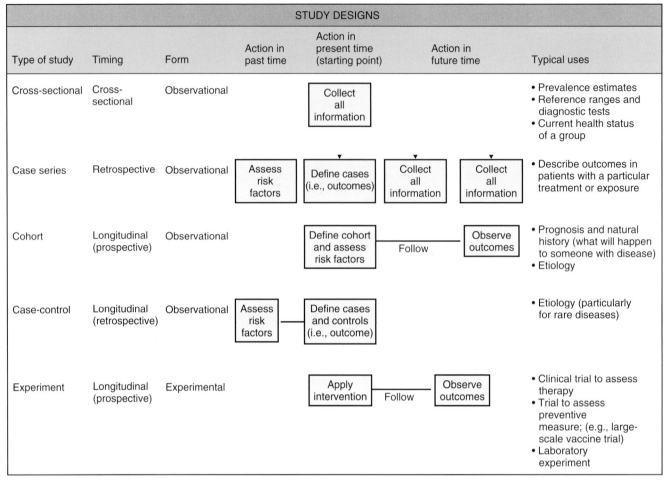

FIGURE 13-2 Characteristics and typical uses of various research designs common in orthopaedic research. (Modified from Petrie A, Sabin C: *Medical statistics at a glance,* Oxford, UK, 2000, Blackwell Science.)

typically randomized and blinded (see discussion of prior blinding and randomization).

■ Clinical trials with crossover designs: each subject receives two or more interventions in a predetermined or random order.

• Patients are followed prospectively for a period of time while receiving treatment A, then start receiving treatment B and are followed for an additional period of time. One of the "treatment conditions" can be a control condition.

■ Clinical studies can be designed to determine superiority of one treatment versus another or to determine whether one treatment is no worse than another (noninferiority) or just as effective (equivalency).

BEWARE OF THESE COMMON FLAWS IN RESEARCH DESIGNS

■ Confounding variables are factors extraneous to a research design that potentially influence the outcome. Conclusions regarding cause-effect relationships may be explained by confounding variables instead of the treatment/intervention being studied and must therefore be controlled for in the research design (via matching, randomization, etc.) or accounted for in statistical analyses (see ANCOVA later).

■ **Bias is unintentional systematic error that will threaten the internal validity of a study. Sources of bias include selection (sampling) bias, nonresponder (loss to follow-up) bias, observer/interviewer bias, recall bias, and so on.**

■ Protection against these threats can be achieved through randomization (i.e., random allocation of treatment[s]) to ensure bias and confounding factors are equally distributed among the study groups. Single blinding (examiner or patient) or double blinding (examiner and patient) is important for minimizing bias.

■ Control groups can help account for potential placebo effect of interventions.

■ Control groups may receive a standard-of-care intervention, no intervention, a placebo (i.e., inactive substance), or sham intervention.

■ Control data may have been collected in the past (historical controls) or may occur in sequence with other study intervention(s) (crossover design).

■ Control subjects are often matched based on specific characteristics (e.g., gender, age, etc.), which helps account for potential confounding sources that may influence the impact of research findings.

■ The strongest research design will use randomly allocated, blinded and concurrent, matched controls.

■ Descriptive and controlled laboratory studies are common in basic science research but may involve many of the common concepts of clinical research and apply similar statistical methods and design methods to protect against sources of bias and confounding.

■ Design limitations may challenge the internal or external validity of a research study. Internal validity describes the quality of a research design and how well the study is controlled and can be reproduced. External validity is the ability for generalization to a whole population of interest.

HOW MANY SUBJECTS ARE NEEDED TO COMPLETE A RESEARCH STUDY?

- Research studies should have enough subjects/samples to get valid results that can be generalized to a population while minimizing unnecessary work or risk to subjects.
- Sample size estimates are based on the desired statistical power (often termed *power analyses*).
- Statistical power is the probability of finding differences among groups when differences actually exist (i.e., avoiding type II error).
- We want to be able to find these differences with our statistical tests 80% of the time or more.
- Sample sizes are justified as the number of subjects needed to find a statistically significant difference or association (i.e., $P < 0.05$) while maintaining statistical power greater than 80%.
- Higher sample sizes and/or highly precise measurements (lower variability) are necessary to find small differences between study groups.
- Power analyses can be done before the study starts (a priori) or after the study has been completed (post hoc).
- Studies with low power have higher likelihood of missing statistical differences when they actually exist (i.e., type II error).

WHAT OUTCOMES SHOULD BE INCLUDED IN A RESEARCH STUDY?

- Selecting the most appropriate outcome for a study is an important decision made in advance by the research team.
- Primary outcome measures match the primary purpose of the study.
- Secondary and tertiary outcomes may also be included as additional (sometimes exploratory) measures that are important to achieving the goals of the study.
  - Typically, sample size estimates for a study are based off the primary outcome measure.
- Subjective data are opinions, judgments, or feelings (e.g., in clinical research, patient-reported outcomes are subjective). Objective data are measured by a valid or reliable instrument (see Validity and Reliability).
- Primer on sampling and data distributions
- Population: all individuals who share a specific characteristic of clinical or scientific interest.
  - **Parameters** describe the characteristics of a population.
- Random sampling affords all members of a specific population equal chance of being studied/enrolled in a clinical study.
- Sample populations are representative subsets of the whole population. Statistics describe the characteristics of a sample and are intended to be generalized to the whole population.
- Populations are delimited based on inclusion and exclusion criteria that are set before a study starts.
- Types of data collected from samples:
  - **Discrete data have an infinite number of possible values** (age, height, distance, percentages, time, etc.).

- **Categorical data have a limited/finite number of possible values or categories** (excellent/good/fair/poor, male/female, satisfied/unsatisfied, etc.).
  - Binary categorical data only have two options (yes/no, etc.).
  - Categorical data can be ordered (severity: mild, moderate, severe) or unordered (gender, race).
- Data can be plotted in frequency distributions (histograms) to summarize basic characteristics of the study sample (Figure 13-3).
- Continuous data are often converted into categorical or binary data through the use of cutoff points. Cutoff points can be arbitrary or evidence based.
  - Evidence-based establishment of cutoff points uses receiver operating characteristic (ROC) curves and identifying a point that maximizes sensitivity and/or specificity of a particular test.
  - Example: a numerical value can be established as a cutoff point for white blood cell count to identify whether or not an infection exists.
  - Arrays of continuous data can be separated into percentiles to identify upper/lower halves, thirds, quartiles, and so forth.

DESCRIBING YOUR DATA WITH SIMPLE STATISTICS

- Data distribution is a histogram describing the frequency of occurrence of each data value. Distributions can be described using descriptive statistics such as the following:
- **Mean** is calculated as the sum of all scores divided by the number of samples (n).
- **Median** is the value that separates a dataset into equal halves, where half of the values are higher and half are lower than the median.
- **Mode** is the most frequently occurring data point.
- **Range** is the difference between the highest value and the lowest value in a dataset.
- **Standard deviation (SD)** is a value that describes the dispersion or variability of the data.
  - SD is higher when data are more "spread out."
- The **confidence interval (CI)** quantifies the precision of the mean or other statistic, such as an odds ratio (OR) or relative risk (RR).
  - Datasets that are highly variable (large SDs) will have larger CIs and hence less accurate estimates of the characteristics of a population.
  - A 95% CI consists of a range of values within which we are 95% certain that the actual population parameter [mean/OR/RR] lies.
    - Example: mean = 40.5 [95% CI, 35.5-45.5] indicates that we are 95% confident that the population mean lies somewhere between 35.5 and 45.5.
- How to determine whether a data distribution is normal (see Figure 13-3)
  - Because many statistical tests rely on a normal data distribution, the following factors are important to consider when analyzing your research results:
    - Normally distributed data take a bell-shaped curve. The mean, median, and mode are the same value in a gaussian (normally distributed) distribution.
    - Skewed data distributions are asymmetric and may be due to outliers. Data distributions can be skewed to the left (negative skew) or skewed to the right (positive skew). This can be calculated as a numeric

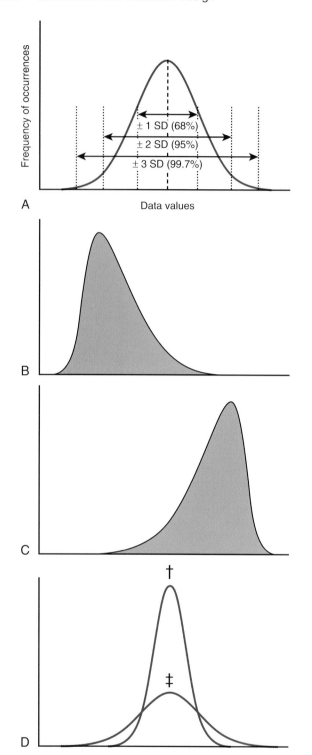

FIGURE 13-3 Data histograms. **A,** Dispersion of normally distributed data with regard to standard deviation. **B,** Data that are skewed to the right (positive skew). **C,** Data that are skewed to the left (negative skew). **D,** Data exhibiting excessively high (†) and low (‡) kurtosis.

value to determine the skewness of a data distribution
- **Kurtosis** is a measure of the relative concentration of data points within a distribution. If data values cluster closely, the dataset is more kurtotic. This can be calculated as a numeric value to determine the extent of kurtosis in a data distribution.

- **Outliers** are data point(s) that are considerably different than the rest of the data set. Outliers can cause data distributions to be skewed.

CONCEPTS IN EPIDEMIOLOGIC RESEARCH STUDIES

- **Epidemiology is the study of the distribution and determinants of disease. The following are common measures used in this type of research:**
- **Prevalence** is the proportion of existing injuries/disease cases conditions within a particular population.
- **Incidence** (absolute risk) is the proportion of new injuries/disease cases within a specified time interval (requires a follow up period).
- Can be reported with respect to the number of exposures.
  - Example: if 12 of 100 athletes on a sports team experience a sports injury over a 10-game season, the **incidence rate** would be 12 injures per 1000 athlete exposures.
- RR is a ratio between the incidence of an outcome between two cohorts. Typically a treated/exposed cohort (in the numerator of the ratio) is compared to an untreated (control) group/unexposed group (in the denominator of the ratio). Values can range from 0 to infinity and are interpreted as follows:
  - RR = 1.0: indicates the incidence of an outcome is equal between groups
  - RR > 1.0: indicates the incidence of an outcome is greater in the treated/exposed group (higher incidence value in the numerator)
  - RR < 1.0: indicates the incidence of an outcome is greater in the untreated/unexposed group (higher incidence value in the denominator)
- ORs are calculated as a ratio between the probabilities of an outcome in two cohorts.
  - ORs are well suited for binary data or studies where only prevalence can be calculated.
- Interpreting RR and OR
  - OR and RR values are interpreted similarly.
  - When comparing outcomes between two groups, an RR or OR value of 0.5 would indicate that treated/exposed patients have half the likelihood of experiencing a particular outcome compared to the untreated/control group.
  - A value of 2.5 would indicate 2.5 times greater likelihood for experiencing the outcome in a treated/exposed group compared to the untreated/control group.
  - An RR or OR whose CI crosses 1 is not considered to be "significant."

- **Clinical usefulness of diagnostic tests (Figure 13-4)**
- A 2 × 2 contingency table can be used to plot occurrences of a disease/outcome of interest in those who had a positive or negative diagnostic test.
  - True positives: the number of individuals who had a positive diagnostic test and actually DO have the disease/outcome of interest
  - True negatives: the number of individuals who had a negative diagnostic test and actually DO NOT have the disease/outcome of interest
  - False positives: the number of individuals who had a positive diagnostic test but DO NOT actually have the disease/outcome of interest

	Disease present (+)	Disease absent (−)	
Diagnostic test (+)	True positives	False positives	Positive predictive value = $\dfrac{\text{True positives}}{\text{Total patients with positive test result*}}$
Diagnostic test (−)	False negatives	True negatives	Negative predictive value = $\dfrac{\text{True negatives}}{\text{Total patients with negative test result}^{\dagger}}$
	Sensitivity = $\dfrac{\text{True positives}}{\text{Total patients with disease}^{\ddagger}}$	Specificity = $\dfrac{\text{True negatives}}{\text{Total patients without disease}^{\S}}$	

FIGURE 13-4 Calculations of specificity, sensitivity, and positive and negative predictive values are presented in relation to a 2 × 2 contingency table. Data from all patients (N) can be calculated by summing the four boxes in the contingency table. *Total patients with positive diagnostic test results = number of patients with true-positive results + number of those with false-negative results. †Total patients with negative diagnostic test results = number of patients with false-negative results + number of those with true-negative results. ‡Total patients with disease = number of patients with true-positive results + number of those with false-negative results. §Total patients without disease = number of patients with false-positive results + number of those with true-negative results.

- False negatives: the number of individuals who had a negative diagnostic test but actually DO have the disease/outcome of interest
- Analysis of diagnostic ability
  - Sensitivity:
    - **The likelihood of a positive test result in patients who actually have the disease/condition of interest (i.e., ability to detect true positives among those with a disease)**
    - Calculated as the proportion of patients with a disease/condition of interest who have a positive diagnostic test

$$\text{Sensitivity} = \frac{\text{True positives}}{\text{Total patients with disease}}$$

- Total patients with the disease of interest = true positive + false-negative test results
- **Sensitive tests are used for screening** because they have few false-negative results. They are unlikely to miss an affected individual.
- When the result of a highly sensitive (Sn) test is negative, the condition can be ruled OUT (mnemonic: SnOUT).
- Specificity:
  - **The likelihood of a negative test result in those patients who actually DO NOT have the disease/condition of interest (i.e., ability to detect true negatives among those without a disease)**
  - Calculated as the proportion of patients without a disease/condition of interest who have a negative test

$$\text{Specificity} = \frac{\text{True negatives}}{\text{Total patients without disease}}$$

- Total patients without the disease or condition of interest = true negatives + false positives

- **Specific tests are used for confirmation** because they are tests that have few false-positive results and are therefore unlikely to result in false treatment of a healthy individual.
- When the result of a highly specific (Sp) test is positive, the condition can be ruled IN (mnemonic: SpIN).
- **Positive predictive value:** the likelihood that patients with a positive test result actually DO have the disease/condition of interest
  - Calculated as the proportion of patients who have a positive test result and actually have the disease of interest (i.e., correctly diagnosed with a positive test)

$$\text{Positive predictive value} = \frac{\text{True positives}}{\text{Total patients who tested positive}}$$

- Total number of patients who tested positive = true positives + false positives.
- **Negative predictive value:** the likelihood that patients with a negative test result actually DO NOT have the disease/condition of interest
  - Calculated as the proportion of patients with a negative test result who do not have the disease of interest (i.e., correctly diagnosed with a negative test).

$$\text{Negative predictive value}$$
$$= \frac{\text{True negatives}}{\text{Total patients who tested negative}}$$

- Total number of patients who tested negative = true negatives + false negatives
- Likelihood ratio
  - Probability that a disease exists, given a test result; likelihood ratios consider both specificity and sensitivity of a given test.

- Likelihood ratios close to 1.0 provide little confidence regarding presence/absence of a disease.
- Positive likelihood ratios greater than 1.0 indicate higher probability of disease when diagnostic test is positive.
  - Calculated as the ratio between the true-positive rate (sensitivity) and the false-positive rate (1-specificity).

$$(+) \text{ Likelihood ratio} = \frac{\text{Sensitivity}}{(1 - \text{Specificity})}$$

- Negative likelihood ratios less than 1.0 indicate higher probability that the disease is absent given a negative test.
  - Calculated as the ratio between the false-negative rate (1-sensitivity) and the true-negative rate (specificity).

$$(-) \text{ Likelihood ratio} = \frac{(1 - \text{Sensitivity})}{\text{Specificity}}$$

- Receiver operating characteristic (ROC) curves are graphical representations of the overall clinical utility of a particular diagnostic test that can be used to compare accuracy of different tests in diagnosing a particular condition (Figure 13-5).
  - Tradeoffs between sensitivity and specificity must be considered when identifying the best diagnostic tests.
  - ROC curves plot the true-positive rate (sensitivity) and the false-positive rate (1-specificity) on a graph.
  - The area under the ROC curve ranges from 0.5 (useless test, no better than a random guess) to 1.0 (perfect diagnostic ability).

TESTING YOUR HYPOTHESES WITH STATISTICS

■ Statistical tests are prescribed to match the purpose and design of a particular research study. Statistical tests are used to answer research questions. Statistics are merely tools to describe data and make inferences. Interpretation of statistical findings is left to expert scientists and clinicians.

■ Statistical analyses will differ based on whether a researcher wants to compare groups to identify differences, establish relationships between groups, and so on (Table 13-1).

■ Inferential statistics are used to test specific hypotheses about associations and/or differences among groups of subject/sample data.

▥ The dependent variable is what is being measured as the outcome. There can be multiple dependent variables depending on how many outcome measures are desired.

▥ The independent variables include the conditions or groupings of the experiment that are systematically manipulated by the investigator.

- For example, a researcher is measuring pain and prescription medication use in patients receiving treatment A or B or C in patients with shoulder pain. The dependent variables are "pain" and "prescription medicine use." The independent variable is "treatment condition" with three levels: "A," "B," or "C"

▥ Inferential statistics can be generally divided into parametric tests and nonparametric tests. The goal of inferential statistics is to estimate parameters, therefore

Table 13-1	Decision-Making Guide for Common Parametric and Nonparametric Statistical Tests for the Desired Study Purpose		
DESIRED ANALYSIS	**PARAMETRIC STATISTICS[1]**	**NONPARAMETRIC STATISTICS[2]**
Comparison of Two Groups		
Paired	Dependent (paired) samples *t*-test	Wilcoxon signed rank test
Unpaired	Independent samples *t*-test[1]	Mann-Whitney *U* test
Comparison of Three or More Groups		
One outcome variable	Analysis of variance (ANOVA)	Kruskal-Wallis test
Repeated observations in same patient	Repeated measures ANOVA	Friedman test
Multiple dependent variables	Multivariate analysis of variance (MANOVA)	
Analysis including a covariate	Analysis of covariance (ANCOVA)	
Establishing Relationship/ Association	Pearson product moment correlation coefficient	Spearman rho correlation coefficient
Prediction		
From one predictor variable	Simple regression	Logistic regression
From more than one predictor variable	Multiple regression	
Comparisons of Categorical Data		
Two or more variables	Chi-square	Chi-square
Better for low sample size	Fisher exact test	Fisher exact test

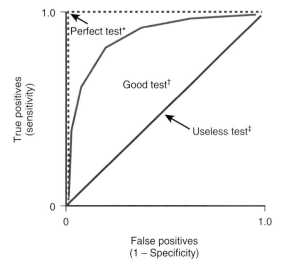

FIGURE 13-5 Graphic plot showing receiver operating characteristic (ROC) curves for perfect tests (*area under the curve value = 1.0), good tests (†area under the curve is less than 1.0 but greater than 0.5), and useless tests (‡area under curve = 0.5).

[1]Appropriate for normally distributed continuous data.
[2]Alternative tests appropriate for non–normally distributed data and/or small sample sizes.

default should be to parametric tests. Nonparametric alternatives are justified if the basic underlying assumptions for using parametric statistics are violated or if the sample sizes are very small.

- Parametric statistics are appropriate for continuous data and rely on the assumption that data are normally distributed.
  - Use the mean and SD when comparing groups or identifying associations.
  - The mean of a dataset is greatly influenced by outliers, so these tests may not be as robust for skewed datasets.
- Nonparametric statistics are appropriate for categorical and non–normally distributed data.
  - Use the median and ranks as more robust alternatives when data are non-normally distributed.

WHAT STATISTICAL TEST TO USE FOR DIFFERENT ANALYSES IN RESEARCH

- The decision on what statistical test to use is based on several factors inherent to research designs. Statistical analyses should always match the purpose of the study and the primary research question asked by the researchers (Figure 13-6).
- Some important distinctions are:
  - How many groups are being studied?
  - Are the measures being recorded in the same or different subjects (or samples)?

- Are the data continuous or categorical?
- Are the data normally distributed?
- When comparing two groups of data, the *t*-test is used; there are two variations:
  - Dependent (paired) samples *t*-test:
    - Appropriate for comparing continuous normally distributed data collected two times on the same subjects
    - Example: two time points measured in the same patient (e.g., before/after intervention)
    - Also appropriate for side-by-side comparison within the same subject or in matched pairs of subjects
    - The nonparametric equivalent is the Wilcoxon signed rank sum test.
  - Independent samples *t*-test
    - **Appropriate for comparing continuous normally distributed data from two separate groups**
    - Example: two groups of patients who received a different treatment
    - Nonparametric equivalent: Mann-Whitney *U* test
- **When comparing three or more groups, an analysis of variance (ANOVA) test is used.** This is also known as the *F*-test.
  - ANOVA is appropriate when comparing three or more groups of continuous normally distributed data.
    - Nonparametric equivalent: Kruskal-Wallis test
  - Repeated measures ANOVA is a variation of the ANOVA test that is appropriate for

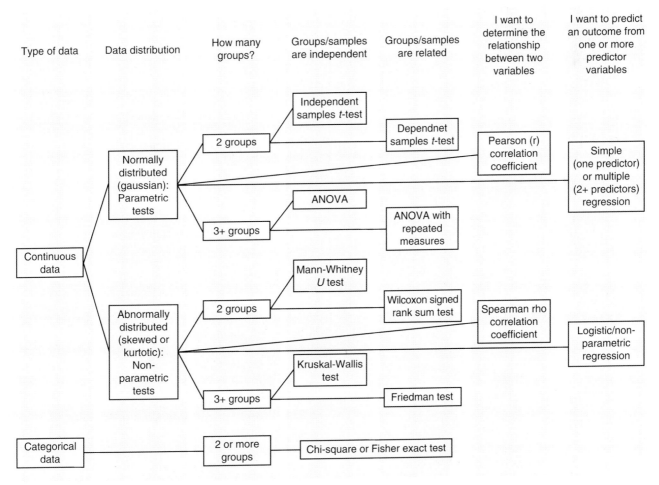

FIGURE 13-6 Flow chart to guide basic decision making for statistical tests.

sequential measurements recorded on the same subjects.
- For example, this test would be used to compare a dependent variable (outcome measure) recorded at three or more time points (baseline, 1 month post intervention, 2 months post intervention).
- Nonparametric alternative: Friedman test
- Multivariate ANOVA (MANOVA): variation of the ANOVA test that is used when multiple dependent variables are compared among three or more groups
- Analysis of covariance (ANCOVA) is an appropriate test when confounding factors must be accounted for in the statistical test.
- Post hoc testing is necessary after any ANOVA test to determine the exact location of differences among groups.
  - ANOVA tests describe whether or not a statistically significant difference exists somewhere among the study groups.
  - For example, when comparing three levels of the independent variable treatment condition (A, B, or C), post hoc testing will specifically compare A vs. B, B vs. C, and A vs. C to determine the exact location of group differences. Post hoc testing is only appropriate if the ANOVA test is statistically significant (see section below).
  - Common post hoc tests: Tukey HSD, Sidak, Dunnet, Scheffe, and others
- Factorial designs for multiple independent variables
  - Hypotheses regarding an interaction among three different treatment groups from pre/post intervention will have a 2 × 3 factorial design.
    - "2 × 3" indicates two independent variables—example, the first (time) has two levels (pre/post test) and the second (treatment condition) has three levels, treatments A, B, or C
- Correlation and regression
  - Correlation coefficients
    - Describe the strength of a relationship between two variables
    - Pearson product correlation coefficient (r) used for continuous normally distributed data
    - Spearman rho correlation coefficient (ρ) is the nonparametric equivalent.
    - Values range from −1.0 to 1.0; less than ±0.33 are "weak," between ±0.33 and 0.66 are "moderate," and higher than ±0.66 are "strong."
    - Positive correlation coefficients indicate direct relationships suggesting that patients who scored high on one scale also scored high on the other.
    - Negative correlation coefficients indicate inverse/indirect relationships suggesting that patients who score high on one scale will score low on the other.
  - Simple linear regression
    - Describes the ability of one independent (predictor) variable to predict a dependent variable (outcome) variable
    - The coefficient of determination (R^2) is the square of r (Pearson product correlation coefficient) and indicates the proportion of variance explained in one variable by another.
    - R^2 ranges from 0 to 1.0, where higher values indicate more variance explained.

- Multivariate linear regression describes the ability of several independent variables to predict a dependent variable.
- Logistic regression is used when the outcome is categorical and the predictor variables can be either categorical or non–normally distributed continuous data.
- Statistical tests for categorical data
  - Chi-square (χ^2) test
    - **Used for two or more groups of categorical data**
    - Example: to compare treatment A versus B when the outcome is either "satisfied or unsatisfied," the chi-square test can be used to identify relationships between "treatment condition" and "outcome category."
      - If the result of the test is statistically significant, frequencies of each outcome can be visually compared between the two treatment groups to describe which treatment is superior.
  - Fisher exact test
    - Similar to the chi-square test but better for small sample sizes or when the number of occurrences in one of the categories is low (e.g., if only one patient in treatment group A had an unsatisfactory outcome, this test is preferred)

VALIDITY AND RELIABILITY

- Can be assessed using statistical techniques similar to correlation coefficients
- The intraclass correlation coefficient evaluates agreement between two measures on the same scale.
- Accuracy/validity
- An instrument or test with the ability to accurately describe truth/reality is said to be valid.
- A validation study is designed to compare measures recorded from a gold-standard method with a new or experimental method. The data should be on the same measurement scale to determine agreement between the two instruments or techniques.
- Precision/reliability
- The ability to precisely describe a characteristic with repeated measurements can be tested statistically.
- The precision of an instrument or technique can be tested for interobserver (measures taken by different examiners on the same patient) or intraobserver (reliability of measures recorded by the same examiner at consecutive times) reliability. Measures should be on the same scale to determine agreement.
- The **intraclass correlation coefficient** (ICC) is a common statistical method for statistically testing the agreement between two sets of data. Values range from 0 to 1.0 (1.0 = perfect accuracy/precision).
- For binary or categorical data, a κ (kappa) statistic can be used to determine agreement. The κ statistic has the same scale (0 to 1.0) as the ICC.

INTERPRETATION OF STATISTICAL TEST RESULTS

- When interpreting the result of a statistical test, it is important to establish whether or not your findings (e.g., a difference or relationship) was due to chance. It is also extremely important to determine if your findings have clinical importance.
- Probability values (P values)

▨ Inferential test statistics (*t*-statistic, *F*-statistic, *r* coefficient, etc.) are accompanied by a probability (*P*) value. These values are on a 0% to 100% scale and indicate the probability that the differences/relationships among study data occurred by chance.

▨ **P values less than 0.05 mean there is less than 5% chance that the observed difference/relationship has occurred by chance alone and not the study intervention.**

▨ A test is identified as statistically significant if the *P* value is 0.05 or less (willing to commit type I error 5/100 times).
  • Note: decision regarding the threshold for defining statistical significance is arbitrary, but this amount of error (alpha or type I error [see later]) is generally accepted.

▨ Therefore, based on the *P* value, we either reject the null hypothesis, which stated that there were no differences or no association existed (i.e., *P* < 0.05), or fail to reject the null hypothesis (*P* > 0.05).

▨ Bonferroni correction to the *P* value:
  • Adjusted threshold for statistical significance when performing multiple *t*-tests for each of several dependent (outcome) variables (used to protect against type I error that may occur)
  • Calculated as 0.05/k where *k* is the number of comparisons being made
    • For example, when comparing two groups using a *t*-test for each of three outcome variables, the *t*-test is only statistically significant if the *P* value is less than or equal to 0.05/3 = 0.017

▪ **Statistical significance does not imply clinical importance. Therefore if a study result includes a statistically significant difference, it remains essential to determine whether that difference is clinically important.**

▪ **Minimal clinically important differences (MCID) is a method to describe the importance of an observed difference during a statistical test.**

▨ Describe the least change in a patient-oriented outcome measure that would be perceived as being beneficial to the patient or would necessitate treatment

▨ Many of the more commonly used patient-oriented outcome instruments have research-established MCID values—or a change in outcome that would change the course of a disease or its treatment.

▨ Expert and experienced clinicians should also consider whether observed differences are important enough to change practice.

▪ **Effect sizes (e.g., Cohen's d) are a standardized method of expressing the magnitude of differences between study groups or before/after treatment in the unit of the SD. (Effect size = 1 means that the mean difference equals the SD). The larger the value, the greater the effect (e.g., of treatment).**

▨ Calculated as the mean difference (e.g., between two treatment groups or from pre/post treatment) divided by the SD (typically SD pooled between groups or the SD of the reference/control group). Equation:

$$\text{Effect size} = \frac{Mean_{Group\,1} - Mean_{Group\,2}}{\text{Standard deviation}_{pooled}}$$

▨ Interpretation of effect sizes: greater than 0.8 are "strong," less than 0.2 are "small" (between these values can be interpreted as "medium")

▨ Effect sizes are similar to percentage differences, except the denominator is the SD. Therefore datasets that are highly variable may have lower effect sizes even if the mean difference is high.

▪ **Statistical error primer**

▨ Type I error (alpha [α] error)
  • Probability that a statistical test is WRONG when the null hypothesis is rejected (i.e., claiming that groups are different when they actually are not)
  • It is accepted that this may occur 5 times out of 100, so the probability value threshold for statistical significance is 0.05 or 5%.

▨ Type II error (beta [β] error)
  • Probability that a statistical test is WRONG when failing to reject the null hypothesis (i.e., claiming that two groups are NOT different when they actually are)
  • It is accepted that this may occur up to 20% of the time.

SELECTED BIBLIOGRAPHY

The selected bibliography for this chapter can be found on https://expertconsult.inkling.com.

TESTABLE CONCEPTS

I. Selecting a Research Study Design

- Research designs are selected to test a specific theoretical hypothesis in a way that provides the highest level of evidence. Research designs should be rigorous and controlled to provide highest-quality outcomes.

II. Evidence-Based Medicine

- Findings from the best-designed and most rigorous studies have the greatest influence on decision making. Such studies are of higher quality and are the most valid.
- Specific levels of evidence are assigned to published manuscripts; in level I, the highest level, results are the most valid and can best describe cause-effect relationships.
- In general, well-designed randomized and blinded clinical trials are graded as level I, prospective cohort studies as level II, case-control studies as level III, case series as level IV, and case reports or expert opinions as level V (see Figure 13-1).

III. Clinical Research Designs

- Observational studies can be prospective or retrospective. Common designs include case series (patients with a common injury or disease), case-control studies (similar to case series but with a defined control group, typically retrospective), cohort (defined groups of subjects to monitor over time), and cross-sectional (measurements taken on a single occasion with no retrospective or prospective review). Case reports are descriptions of a single unique observation of a patient.
- Clinical trials are experimental studies in which a research hypothesis is tested through a specific intervention.
- The gold standard of experimental research designs is the randomized, blinded, and controlled clinical trial. These design types require greater time and resources; however, findings from a well-designed randomized controlled trial are considered highly influential.

IV. Beware of These Common Flaws in Research Designs

- Bias is unintentional systematic error that threatens the internal validity of a study. Randomization, matching, blinding, and using control conditions are methods to protect against the numerous forms of bias.

V. How Many Subjects Are Needed to Complete a Research Study?

- Sample size estimates are used to determine the necessary number of subjects or observations needed for statistically significant results and are based on the desired statistical power (these estimates are often termed power analyses).
- Statistical power is the probability of finding differences among groups when differences actually exist (i.e., avoiding type II error). Higher sample sizes or highly precise measurements (lower variability) are needed to find small differences between study groups.

VI. What Outcomes Should Be Included in a Research Study?

- Data from research studies can be discrete (infinite possible values) or categorical (finite possible values); the latter type of data can be binary (only two options), ordered (e.g., a scale of intensity or severity), or unordered (e.g., race).

VII. Describing Your Data with Simple Statistics

- Descriptive statistics include mean, median, mode, and standard deviation (SD).

- Confidence intervals (CIs) provide a range of values around a point estimate (e.g., mean, relative risk [RR], odds ratio [OR]) that describe the level of confidence in the ability of the study data to accurately describe truth.

VIII. Concepts in Epidemiologic Research Studies

- Common epidemiologic measures of the distribution and determinants of disease include prevalence, incidence, OR, and RR.
- Prevalence is the proportion of existing injuries or disease cases within a particular population. Incidence is the proportion of new injuries or disease cases within a specified time interval.
- Incidence can be calculated from prospective or longitudinal study designs because a follow-up period is required. Prevalence is calculated from cross-sectional designs to describe injury distribution at a particular time point.
- ORs and RRs can be calculated from clinical studies that are designed to determine associations among risk factor exposure and patient outcomes.
- RR and OR describe the risk and odds of a particular outcome of interest between two groups: typically a group in which subjects are treated or exposed and a reference or control group. RR is calculated as the ratio between the incidence rates of an outcome in two cohorts.
- Reliability is the reproducibility of a test or measure; similarly, precision is the repeatability of the results. Validity is the ability of a measure, test, or instrument to represent truth and reality; similarly, accuracy describes the ability of a test to differentiate between correct and incorrect outcomes.
- Sensitivity is a ratio (true-positive test results divided by the number of patients with disease) that describes the proportion of patients who actually have a disease or condition and whose diagnostic test result is positive. Because highly sensitive tests (Sn) yield few false-negative results, a negative (N) result would confidently rule "OUT" the condition of interest (mnemonic: "SnNOUT").
- Specificity is a ratio (true-negative test results divided by the number of patients without disease) that describes the proportion of patients who do not have the disease or condition and whose diagnostic test result is negative. Because highly specific tests (Sp) yield few false-positives, a positive (P) test would confidently rule "IN" the condition of interest (SpPIN).
- Like specificity and sensitivity, likelihood ratios, positive predictive values, and negative predictive values are calculated from 2×2 contingency tables and can describe the accuracy of diagnostic tests.

IX. Testing Your Hypotheses with Statistics

- Statistical tests can be parametric (appropriate for normally distributed continuous data) or nonparametric (appropriate for skewed data, categorical data, or small sample sizes). Each parametric test has a nonparametric equivalent.

X. What Statistical Test to Use for Different Analyses in Research

- For comparing two groups of normally distributed data, the independent samples t-test is used (paired samples if the groups are matched or measures recorded in the same individual over time). For comparisons of three or more groups, the ANOVA is used for repeated measures, ANCOVA if there is a covariate, and MANOVA if there are many dependent variables. The Pearson product moment correlation coefficient is used for correlations.

TESTABLE CONCEPTS

- The chi-square test is used for comparing categorical data. When sample sizes are small, the Fisher exact test is used.
- For nonparametric tests, Mann-Whitney U test is for comparing two groups; the Wilcoxon test is for paired groups, the Friedman test is for comparisons of three or more groups, and the Spearman rho correlation coefficient is for correlations.

XI. Validity and Reliability

- An instrument or test with the ability to accurately describe truth/reality is said to be valid. Studies can be designed to test the validity of a particular instrument or test.
- Precision is the ability for the same testers (intraobserver reliability) or different testers (interobserver reliability) achieving similar measurement or diagnostic outcomes.
- Precision or accuracy can be tested statistically using intraclass correlation coefficients (continuous data) or κ statistics (binary data).

XII. Interpretation of Statistical Test Results

- Type I error (α error, false-positive error) is the probability that a statistical test result is wrong when the null hypothesis is rejected (i.e., concluding that groups are different when they actually are not). Researchers are willing to accept this error in 5% of tests.
- Type II error (β error, false-negative error) is the probability that a statistical test result is wrong when the test fails to reject the null hypothesis (i.e., concluding that two groups are not different when they actually are).
- P values lower than 0.05 mean that the probability that the observed difference or relationship has occurred by chance alone, not because of the study intervention, is less than 5%.
- Effect sizes are used to describe the magnitude of a treatment effect. They are calculated as the difference between treatment groups divided by the SD (typically pooled SD, or the SD of the reference or control group).

INDEX